Complications in Surgery and Their Management

Fourth Edition

JAMES D. HARDY, M.D.

Professor and Chairman
Department of Surgery
University of Mississippi
School of Medicine
Jackson, Mississippi

With contributions by 50 authorities

1981

W. B. SAUNDERS COMPANY   Philadelphia   London   Toronto   Sydney

W. B. Saunders Company: West Washington Square
Philadelphia, PA 19105

1 St. Anne's Road
Eastbourne, East Sussex BN21 3UN, England

1 Goldthorne Avenue
Toronto, Ontario M8Z 5T9, Canada

9 Waltham Street
Artarmon, N.S.W. 2064, Australia

Library of Congress Cataloging in Publication Data

Main entry under title:

Complications in surgery and their management.

Fourth ed. of: Management of surgical complications.

1. Surgery—Complications and sequelae.   I. Hardy, James
   D., 1918–   .   II. Management of surgical complica-
   tions. [DNLM: 1. Postoperative complications—Therapy.
   WO 184 C738]

RD98.C65 1981   617'. 01   80–54380

ISBN 0–7216–4509–7   AACR2

Listed here is the latest translated edition of this book together with
the language of the translation and the publisher.

Italian (*3rd Edition*)—Piccin Editore, Padova, Italy

Spanish (*3rd Edition*)—Nueva Editorial Interamericana S.A. de C.V.,
            Mexico City, Mexico

Complications in Surgery and Their Management   ISBN 0-7216-4509-7

Last digit is the print number: 9   8   7   6   5   4   3   2   1

TO
CURTIS P. ARTZ

CONTRIBUTORS

BENJAMIN L. AARON, M.D.

Associate Professor of Surgery and Director, Division of Thoracic Surgery, George Washington University School of Medicine and Health Sciences. Attending Surgeon (Thoracic), George Washington University Hospital, Washington, D.C.

Complications of Pulmonary Resection

PAUL C. ADKINS, M.D. (Deceased)

Former Professor and Chairman, Department of Surgery, George Washington University School of Medicine and Health Sciences. Former Attending Surgeon (Thoracic), George Washington University Hospital, Washington, D.C.

Complications of Pulmonary Resection

WILLIAM A. ALTEMEIER, M.D.

Christian R. Holmes Professor Emeritus of Surgery, University of Cincinnati College of Medicine. Attending Physician, Cincinnati General Hospital, Children's Hospital, Holmes Hospital, and Cincinnati Veterans Administration Hospital, Cincinnati, Ohio.

Complications of Appendectomy

JOSEPH D. ANSELY, M.D.

Assistant Professor of Surgery, Department of Surgery, Emory University School of Medicine. Chief of Vascular Surgery Service, Veterans Administration Hospital, Decatur, Georgia.

Complications of Portal-Systemic Shunt Surgery

OLIVER H. BEAHRS, M.D.

Professor of Surgery, Emeritus, Mayo Medical School, Rochester, Minnesota.

Complications of Surgery for Cancer of the Head and Neck

JOHN L. CAMERON, M.D.

Professor of Surgery, Johns Hopkins University. Consulting Surgeon, Loch Raven Veterans Administration Hospital. Consultant in Gastroenterology, Naval Hospital, Bethesda, Maryland. Consultant in Surgery, Walter Reed Army Hospital, Washington, D.C.

Complications Following Operations Upon the Biliary Tract and Their Management

WILLIAM R. CULBERTSON, M.D.

Professor of Surgery, University of Cincinnati College of Medicine. Attending Physician, Cincinnati General Hospital, Children's Hospital, Holmes Hospital, and Cincinnati Veterans Administration Hospital, Cincinnati, Ohio.

Complications of Appendectomy

JOHN HERSCHEL DAVIS, M.D.

Professor and Chairman, Department of Surgery, and Associate Dean for Clinical Affairs, University of Vermont College of Medicine. Executive Director, University Health Center, Inc., University of Vermont College of Medicine, Burlington, Vermont.

Miscellaneous Complications in the Preoperative and Postoperative Periods

ALAN R. DIMICK, M.D.

Associate Professor of Surgery, University of Alabama School of Medicine. Director, Burn Center, and Staff Surgeon, University of Alabama Hospitals, Birmingham, Alabama.

Complications of Burns and Burn Treatment

CHARLES ECKERT, M.D.

Professor of Surgery, Albany Medical College of Union University. Attending Surgeon, Albany Medical Center Hospital; Consultant, Veterans Administration Medical Center and St. Peter's Hospital, Albany, New York.

Complications of Adrenal Surgery

F. HENRY ELLIS, JR., M.D., Ph.D.

Clinical Professor of Surgery, Harvard Medical School. Chief, Division of Thoracic and Cardiovascular Surgery, Lahey Clinic Medical Center, Burlington, Massachusetts, and New England Deaconess Hospital, Boston, Massachusetts.

Complications of Esophageal and Diaphragmatic Surgery

C. THOMAS FITTS, M.D.

Professor of Surgery, Medical University of South Carolina College of Medicine. Attending Surgeon, Medical University Hospital; Consultant, Charleston Naval Hospital and Charleston Veterans Administration Hospital; Staff Physician, Charleston County Hospital, Charleston, South Carolina.

Miscellaneous Complications in the Preoperative and Postoperative Periods

ROBERT J. FLEMMA, M.D.

Clinical Professor of Surgery, The Medical College of Wisconsin, Milwaukee, Wisconsin.

Complications of Surgery of the Heart and Adjacent Great Vessels

JOHN E. FORESTNER, M.D.

Assistant Professor, Department of Anesthesiology, Emory University School of Medicine. Attending Anesthesiologist, Henrietta Egleston Hospital for Children, Scottish Rite Hospital for Crippled Children, and Grady Memorial Hospital, Atlanta, Georgia.

Complications of Anesthesia

ALAN E. FREELAND, M.D.

Associate Professor of Surgery (Orthopaedic), University of Mississippi School of Medicine. Attending Physician, University of Mississippi Medical Center, Jackson, Mississippi.

Complications of Common Fractures and Dislocations

DONALD E. FRY, M.D.

Assistant Professor and Director, Price Institute of Surgical Research, University of Louisville School of Medicine. Attending Physician, Veterans Administration Hospital, University Hospital, Norton-Children's Hospitals, Jewish Hospital, and Audubon Hospital, Louisville, Kentucky.

Infection and Fever in the Surgical Patient

FRANK GLENN, M.D.

Professor of Surgery Emeritus, Cornell University Medical College. Attending Surgeon, The New York Hospital, New York, New York.

Complications Following Operations upon the Biliary Tract and Their Management

LAZAR J. GREENFIELD, M.D.

Stuart McGuire Professor and Chairman, Department of Surgery, Virginia Commonwealth University, Medical College of Virginia, School of Medicine. Chief of Surgery, Medical College of Virginia Hospitals; Consultant, McGuire Veterans Administration Hospital, and Richmond Metropolitan Hospital, Richmond, Virginia.

Shock

JAMES D. HARDY, M.D.

Professor and Chairman, Department of Surgery, University of Mississippi School of Medicine. Surgeon-in-Chief, University Hospital, Jackson, Mississippi.

Complications of Thyroid and Parathyroid Surgery; Complications of Gastric Surgery

STEPHEN E. HEDBERG, M.D.

Clinical Assistant Professor of Surgery, Harvard Medical School. Associate Visiting Surgeon and Senior Endoscopist in Gastrointestinal Surgery, Massachusetts General Hospital, Boston, Massachusetts.

Complications in Surgery of the Colon and Rectum

THOMAS K. HUNT, M.D.

Professor of Surgery, University of California, San Francisco, School of Medicine. Attending Physician, University of California Hospital, San Francisco, California.

Wound Complications

OLGA JONASSON, M.D.

Professor of Surgery, University of Illinois College of Medicine. Chief of Surgery, Cook County Hospital; Attending Surgeon, University of Illinois Hospital, Chicago, Illinois.

Acute Renal Insufficiency Complicating Surgery and Trauma

GEORGE L. JORDAN, JR., M.D.

Distinguished Service Professor of Surgery, Baylor College of Medicine. Chief of Medical Staff, Harris County Hospital District; Attending Surgeon, The Methodist Hospital; Consultant in Surgery, Veterans Administration Hospital; Associate Attending Surgeon, St. Luke's Episcopal Hospital, Houston, Texas.

Complications of Pancreatic and Splenic Surgery

JAMES R. JUDE, M.D.

Clinical Professor of Surgery, University of Miami School of Medicine. Attending Surgeon, Jackson Memorial Hospital, Mercy Hospital, Northridge General Hospital, and Baptist Hospital, Miami, Florida.

Cardiac Arrest and Resuscitation

JOHN P. KAPP, M.D., Ph.D.

Associate Professor of Neurosurgery, University of Mississippi School of Medicine. Attending Physician, University of Mississippi Medical Center, and Veterans Administration Hospital, Jackson, Mississippi.

Complications Involving the Nervous System

JOHN S. KUKORA, M.D.

Assistant Professor of Surgery, University of Mississippi School of Medicine. Attending Surgeon, University of Mississippi Medical Center, and Veterans Administration Hospital, Jackson, Mississippi.

Complications of Thyroid and Parathyroid Surgery

GORDON R. LANG, M.D.

Associate Professor of Clinical Medicine, University of Illinois College of Medicine. Director, Dialysis Unit, and Associate Director, Section of Nephrology, St. Joseph Hospital; Attending Physician, Roosevelt Memorial Hospital; Assistant Attending Physician, University of Illinois Hospital, Chicago, Illinois.

Acute Renal Insufficiency Complicating Surgery and Trauma

HOWARD K. LEONARDI, M.D.

Staff Member, Overholt Thoracic Clinic; Staff Surgeon, New England Deaconess Hospital, Boston, Massachusetts.

Complications of Esophageal and Diaphragmatic Surgery

DERWARD LEPLEY, JR., M.D.

Professor and Chairman, Department of Thoracic and Cardiovascular Surgery, The Medical College of Wisconsin, Milwaukee, Wisconsin.

Complications of Surgery of the Heart and Adjacent Great Vessels

JOHN R. LURAIN, M.D.

Assistant Professor of Obstetrics and Gynecology, Northwestern University Medical School. Assistant Director, Division of Gynecologic Oncology, Prentice Women's Hospital and Maternity Center, Northwestern Memorial Hospital, Chicago, Illinois.

Complications of Gynecologic Surgery

ROBERT M. MILES, M.D.

Professor of Surgery, University of Tennessee College of Medicine. Chief, Surgical Service, Baptist Memorial Hospital; Consultant in Surgery, Veterans Administration Hospital, Memphis, Tennessee.

Complications of Surgery That Involve the Venous System

RICHARD C. MILLER, M.D.

Professor of Surgery and Chief of Pediatric Surgery, University of Mississippi Medical Center. Associate Dean for Clinical Affairs, School of Medicine and Medical Director, University Hospital, Jackson, Mississippi.

Complications of Gastrointestinal Surgery in Infancy

FRANCIS S. MORRISON, M.D.

Professor of Internal Medicine, University of Mississippi School of Medicine. Attending Physician, University Hospital; Consultant, Teaching Staff, Veterans Administration Hospital and Methodist Rehabilitation Center, Jackson, Mississippi.

Hemorrhagic Complications in Surgery

PETER V. MOULDER, M.D.

Professor of Surgery, Tulane University School of Medicine. Attending Physician, Tulane Medical Center and Charity Hospital of New Orleans, New Orleans, Louisiana; Consulting Physician, Veterans Administration Hospital, Alexandria, Louisiana.

Postoperative Pulmonary Complications

DONALD C. MULLEN, M.D.

Associate Clinical Professor of Surgery, The Medical College of Wisconsin, Milwaukee, Wisconsin.

Complications of Surgery of the Heart and Adjacent Great Vessels

MICHAEL NEWTON, M.D., M.B.B.Ch.

Professor of Obstetrics and Gynecology, and Head, Section of Graduate Education, Department of Obstetrics and Gynecology, Northwestern University Medical School. Director, Division of Gynecologic Oncology, Prentice Women's Hospital and Maternity Center, Northwestern Memorial Hospital, Chicago, Illinois.

Complications of Gynecologic Surgery

LLOYD M. NYHUS, M.D.

Professor and Head, Department of Surgery, University of Illinois College of Medicine. Surgeon-in-Chief, University of Illinois Hospital, Chicago, Illinois.

Complications of Hernial Repair

W. SPENCER PAYNE, M.D.

Professor of Surgery, Mayo Medical School. Consultant, Section of Thoracic, Cardiovascular and General Surgery, Mayo Clinic, Rochester, Minnesota.

Complications of Esophageal and Diaphragmatic Surgery

HIRAM C. POLK, JR., M.D.

Professor and Chairman, Department of Surgery, University of Louisville School of Medicine. Attending Physician, University Hospital, Veterans Administration Hospital, Norton-Children's Hospitals, Jewish Hospital, and St. Anthony Hospital, Louisville, Kentucky.

Infection and Fever in the Surgical Patient

CHARLES W. PUTNAM, M.D.

Associate Professor of Surgery, University of Arizona College of Medicine. Chief, Surgical Service, Veterans Administration Medical Center; Attending Surgeon, University of Arizona Health Services Center, Tucson, Arizona.

Complications of Transplantation

JOHN H. C. RANSON, M.A., B.M., B.Ch.

Professor of Surgery, New York University School of Medicine. Attending Surgeon, New York University Hospital, Bellevue Hospital, and Manhattan Veterans Administration Hospital, New York, New York.

Complications of Small Intestine Surgery

NORMAN M. RICH, M.D.

Professor and Chairman, Department of Surgery, Uniformed Services University of the Health Sciences. Senior Vascular Surgeon, Walter Reed Army Medical Center, Bethesda, Maryland.

Complications of Surgery of the Abdominal Aorta and of Aortic Branches

GUY F. ROBBINS, M.D.

Clinical Associate Professor of Surgery, Cornell University Medical College. Senior Attending Surgeon, Breast Service, Department of Surgery, Sloan-Kettering Institute for Cancer Research, New York, New York.

Complications Following the Surgical Treatment of Women with Potentially Curable Carcinoma of the Breast

WILLIAM SCHUMER, M.D.

Professor and Chairman, Department of Surgery, and Professor, Department of Biochemistry, University of Health Sciences/The Chicago Medical School. Chief, General Surgery Section, Veterans Administration Medical Center; Chief, University Service, Department of Surgery, Saint Mary of Nazareth Hospital Center, Chicago, Illinois.

Complications of Parenteral Fluid Therapy and Other States of Postoperative Fluid Disequilibrium

HARRY M. SHIZGAL, M.D.

Professor of Surgery, McGill University Faculty of Medicine. Associate Surgeon, Royal Victoria Hospital, Montreal, Quebec, Canada.

Nutritional Complications in the Surgical Patient

ROBERT B. SMITH, III, M.D.

Professor of Surgery, Emory University School of Medicine. Chief of Surgical Service, Veterans Administration Medical Center; Staff Surgeon, Emory University Hospital, Henrietta Egleston Hospital for Children, and Grady Memorial Hospital, Atlanta, Georgia.

Complications of Portal-Systemic Shunt Surgery

ROBERT R. SMITH, M.D.

Professor and Chairman, Department of Neurosurgery, University of Mississippi School of Medicine. Attending Physician, University of Mississippi Medical Center, and Mississippi Methodist Hospital and Rehabilitation Center, Jackson, Mississippi, and Mercy Regional Medical Center, Vicksburg, Mississippi; Consultant, Veterans Administration Hospital, Jackson, Mississippi.

Complications Involving the Nervous System

THOMAS E. STARZL, M.D., Ph.D.

Professor of Surgery, University of Pittsburgh School of Medicine, and Presbyterian University Hospital. Attending Physician, Veterans Administration Medical Center, Pittsburgh, Pennsylvania.

Complications of Transplantation

WATTS R. WEBB, M.D.

Professor and Chairman, Department of Surgery, Tulane University School of Medicine. Chief of Surgery, Tulane Medical Center. Consulting Physician, Touro Infirmary and Baptist Hospital, New Orleans, Louisiana; Lallie Kemp Charity Hospital, Independence, Louisiana; and Huey P. Long Memorial Hospital and Veterans Administration Hospital, Alexandria, Louisiana.

Postoperative Pulmonary Complications

CLAUDE E. WELCH, M.D.

Clinical Professor of Surgery, Harvard Medical School. Visiting Surgeon, Massachusetts General Hospital, Boston, Massachusetts.

Complications in Surgery of the Colon and Rectum

JOHN E. WOODS, M.D.

Professor and Head, Section of Plastic Surgery, Mayo Medical School. Consultant, Head and Neck and General Surgery, Department of Surgery, Mayo Clinic, Rochester, Minnesota.

Complications of Surgery for Cancer of the Head and Neck

PUBLISHER'S FOREWORD

James D. Hardy was born in Birmingham, Alabama, and received his undergraduate education at the University of Alabama. He came north in 1938 to medical school and received his medical degree at the University of Pennsylvania in 1942. He served a medical residency at the University of Pennsylvania Hospital from 1943 to 1944, became a resident in general surgery in 1946 after service in the United States Army, and was Chief Resident in General Surgery from 1948 to 1949 under Dr. I. S. Ravdin and a resident in Thoracic Surgery from 1949 to 1951 under Dr. Julian Johnson.

In 1954, after three years as Director of Surgical Research at the University of Tennessee, he accepted his present appointment as Professor and Chairman of the Department of Surgery and Director of Surgical Research at the University of Mississippi Medical Center.

His principal area of investigation has been the pathophysiology of surgical disease, and he has been one of the most significant of modern contributors to the elucidation of surgical physiology. He has also done pioneering work in the field of transplantation of organs and has had extensive experience in vascular surgery. He is a Past President of the American Surgical Association, the Society for Surgery of the Alimentary Tract, the Southern Surgical Association, and the Society of University Surgeons. He is currently President of the United States Chapter of the International Society of Surgery and President of the American College of Surgeons.

IN MEMORIAM

CURTIS PRICE ARTZ

1915–1977

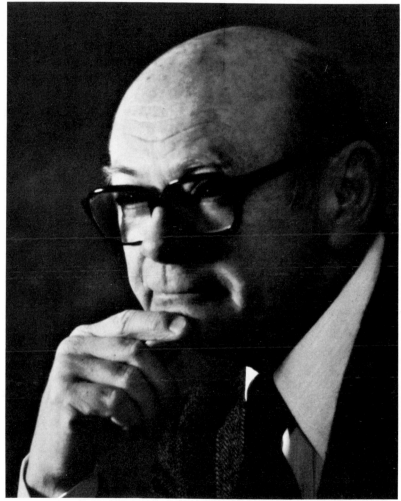

ELSON–ALEXANDRE

The previous three editions of "Complications" were joint editorial efforts of Dr. Artz and myself. We alternated the major responsibility, but each edition contained much from both of us. The development of this fourth edition has been an especially poignant one. Dr. Artz and I were closely associated from 1956 until his untimely death in 1977, first as colleagues on the faculty of the University of Mississippi Medical Center and later as Co-editors of this book and in many other endeavors.

Dr. Artz was a man of many talents. Known by all his colleagues for his energy and enthusiasm, he was an excellent surgeon with special expertise in burn management. He was greatly admired as a teacher, a reflection of his mastery of organization and his superbly articulated interest in his subject. He was a part of many enterprises, surgical societies, and other people's lives. He was an outstanding leader and loyal friend. He was Professor and Chairman of the Department of Surgery at the Medical University of South Carolina at the time of his death. It has been a great loss.

JAMES D. HARDY

PREFACE

Much has changed in clinical surgical practice since the third edition of "Complications" was published six years ago. A large number of new operations and procedures have been developed. Many remarkable, and in some cases even stunning, advances in diagnosis and in treatment have occurred. And, yes, new types of complications have accompanied the new investigative and therapeutic modalities. Thus, all of these considerations have rendered a new edition of this reference source imperative.

Accordingly, the entire material presented in the third edition has been searchingly examined, obsolete items deleted, others altered to accord with current knowledge, and new material added in every chapter. Too, a number of new authors have joined the volume, and each has brought on board a new and different insight and experience with respect to each specific complication or problem considered.

We are pleased with this volume. The editor extends his warmest appreciation to the authors for their authoritative contributions, to Mrs. Virginia W. Keith and Mrs. Sandra M. Day for their dedicated editorial assistance, to Mr. Carroll C. Cann, Medical Editor of the W. B. Saunders Company, and to the publishers themselves.

JAMES D. HARDY

CONTENTS

Chapter 12

NUTRITIONAL COMPLICATIONS IN THE SURGICAL

Harry M. Shizgal

Chapter 13

COMPLICATIONS OF SURGERY FOR CANCER OF THE

Oliver H. Beahrs and John E. Woods

Chapter 18
COMPLICATIONS OF SURGERY OF THE ABDOMINAL
AORTA AND OF AORTIC BRANCHES
Norman M. Rich

Chapter 19
COMPLICATIONS OF GASTRIC SURGERY (Distal Subtotal
Gastrectomy, Esophagogastrectomy and Total Gastrectomy,
Vagotomy, Pyloroplasty, and Gastrostomy)
James D. Hardy

Chapter 23
COMPLICATIONS OF PORTAL-SYSTEMIC SHUNT SURGERY 579
Robert B. Smith, III, and Joseph D. Ansley

Chapter 24
COMPLICATIONS OF APPENDECTOMY................................. 606
W. A. Altemeier and W. R. Culbertson

Chapter 34
COMPLICATIONS OF GYNECOLOGIC SURGERY 860
Michael Newton and John R. Lurain

1

INFECTION AND FEVER IN THE SURGICAL PATIENT

Hiram C. Polk, Jr. and
Donald E. Fry

Since the mid-nineteenth century, a host of independent observations and studies has broadened understanding of the infection process. Semmelweis noted that contagion that passed from the physician to the patient was responsible for the dreaded childbed fever and subsequent septic deaths of postpartum patients. Pasteur and Koch recognized bacteria as pathogens in human infection. Finally, Lister demonstrated the usefulness of antisepsis, which has paved the way for the evolution of asepsis and disclosed the need for even more sophisticated efforts to control infection, the most persistent of the surgeon's enemies.

While these contributions have made significant impact on the frequency and consequences of infection, particularly in the surgical patient, the millennium of infection-free operations has not been realized. As greater technological advances have allowed prolonged survival of critically ill patients, the immunocompromised host now has become the target of an entire new generation of difficult infection-related problems. Only with improved understanding of the complete infection process can prevention and treatment regimens best be applied in the surgical setting.

HOST-PATHOGEN RELATIONSHIPS

Sources of Infection

The origin of contamination that results in clinical infection directly influences subsequent prevention and treatment efforts.

Hiram C. Polk, Jr. was born in Mississippi and graduated from Millsaps College and Harvard Medical School. After taking his surgical training at Barnes Hospital in St. Louis, he joined the faculty of the University of Miami and six years later was named Professor and Chairman of the Department of Surgery of the University of Louisville. Dr. Polk has served in positions of major responsibility in many national surgical societies and is one of the genuine leaders in American surgery. He has published widely in a number of fields, but he is a recognized expert in surgical infections.

Donald Edmund Fry was born in Ohio and graduated from both college and medical school at Ohio State University. He served his residency training at the University of Louisville, where he is now Assistant Professor of Surgery. Dr. Fry is a member of a number of professional organizations and has a special interest in the management of infections in surgical patients.

Community-acquired infections are initiated before a patient's contact with the hospital environment. Such pathogens tend to be less difficult management problems, since they have not been exposed to the chronic selective pressures created by the antibiotic-laden atmosphere and concentration of critically ill patients in contemporary hospitals. Streptococcal cellulitis and pneumococcal pneumonia typify community-based infections.

On the other hand, the hospital-acquired pathogens have usually evolved through patterns of chemotherapeutic resistance that reflect generations of antibiotic exposure. Bacteria that in bygone days were not considered potentially pathogenic, e.g., Serratia species, have now emerged as clinically significant. Many non-bacterial pathogens such as *Candida albicans* and *Pneumocystis carinii* have also become recognized as nosocomial problems. Appreciation of community-based versus hospital-acquired pathogens allows the clinician to anticipate resistance patterns and special treatment in the postoperative patient.

Host-Pathogen Interaction

A specific series of events occurs incident to bacterial contamination of the host tissues. The inflammatory response is initiated with alterations of capillary permeability and resultant extravasation of protein-rich plasma fluids. As the first line of host defense, the neutrophil becomes marginated to the vascular endothelium at the site of the evolving inflammatory response. By diapedesis the neutrophil moves out of the intravascular compartment and into the interstitial space. Chemoattractants released during the initial phases of inflammation direct the neutrophil toward the offending bacterial contaminants. Opsonization of the potential pathogen occurs from adherence of non-specific proteins from the plasma that facilitate the process of phagocytosis, or engulfment, of the organism once the neutrophil has made contact. The role of natural or spontaneously occurring specific antibody in this process may be very important but is largely unknown and unstudied. The process is then completed by the process of intracellular killing, when potent lysosomal enzymes enter the phagosome and digestion

of the pathogen occurs. The neutrophil represents the initial defense mechanism with mononuclear phagocytic cells invading the inflamed area 24 to 48 hours after contamination. These processes are quite predictable in most tissues, with the notable exception of the lung, where resident alveolar macrophages are constantly present to deal with pulmonary contaminants. Recruitment of systemic cellular elements then occurs as a secondary event.

Predisposing Factors

Numerous local and systemic factors may compromise the ability of host defense mechanisms to deal with contamination (Table 1–1). While the mechanism whereby many of these factors exert their influence is poorly defined, adjuvant effects in maximizing the pathogenic potential of a given bacterial inoculum are well documented.

Most local factors that predispose to infection relate to adequacy of tissue blood supply. Because of regional blood flow differences, facial wounds are less prone to infection than are upper extremity wounds, which in turn are less vulnerable to infection than are lower extremity wounds, even when the quantity of contamination is comparable. The use of local vasoconstrictive agents, such as epinephrine with local anes-

TABLE 1–1   PREDISPOSING FACTORS
TO INFECTION

Preoperative Factors
    Hypovolemia
    Protein-calorie malnutrition
    Alcoholism
    Chronic corticosteroid use
    Remote infection
    Extended preoperative hospitalization
    Nicks/cuts from surgical preparation of operative
        site

Intraoperative Factors
    Disregard for asepsis
    Poor hemostasis/hematoma
    Excess electrocautery
    Foreign bodies
    Excessive dead space in wounds
    Drains through surgical incision

Postoperative Factors
    Prolonged Foley catheterization
    Prolonged endotracheal intubation
    Prolonged intravenous cannulation
    Poor oral hygiene
    Inadequate nutritional support

thesia, reduces wound blood supply and, a priori, enhances the likelihood of infection. Of course, the blood supply is extremely inadequate in devitalized tissue, where the dying tissue serves as an ideal pabulum for bacterial growth and also is removed from available circulating host-defense elements. Similarly, foreign bodies provide a protected environment for bacterial contaminants. Finally, dead space within wounds serves as a drainage basin for fibrinous debris and bacteria.

Hemoglobin is a potent adjuvant to local bacterial proliferation. Hematomas within experimental wounds clearly reduce the bacterial inoculum necessary to cause infection. The addition of lysed red cells with contamination into the peritoneal cavity in the experimental laboratory dramatically potentiates the virulence of bacteria. While considerable speculation surrounds the mechanism of the adjuvant effects of hemoglobin, the surgical implications of hemostasis are as evident in the laboratory as at the bedside.

Many systemic factors also predispose to vulnerability of the host from a microbial challenge. The very young infant and the aged patient appear to have frequent infections. Such a predisposition in neonates relates to inadequately developed host defense, while elderly patients often experience a progressive decline in immunocompetence.

Obesity increases the likelihood of infection, particularly in surgical and traumatic wounds, probably due to the relatively poor blood supply of large reservoirs of subcutaneous adipose tissue. Similarly, it appears that chronic or acute, severe malnutrition predisposes to infection.

Many systemic illnesses are identified with increased rates of infection. Patients with disseminated malignancy are at increased risk, at least in part owing to the cachectic influences of the primary neoplasm and immunosuppressive influences of systemic chemotherapy. Diabetes and hepatic cirrhosis each exert a systemic predisposition for infection. Furthermore, there is increasing clinical and experimental evidence that the patient with an active infection is at increased risk for developing a second remote septic focus.

Many aspects of multiple trauma appear to contribute to the increased frequency of infection. Hypovolemic shock and systemic hypoxemia are most notable in this regard. Experimental soft tissue trauma appears to exhaust available non-specific opsonic proteins. Major burns and some attendant topical therapies both seem to provoke specific host defense deficiencies.

Finally, selected medications and drugs contribute to increased frequency and severity of infection; chronic corticosteroid use has clearly been so recognized. Both acute and chronic alcohol ingestion also appear to have an immuno-inhibitory effect.

POSTOPERATIVE FEVER AND INFECTION

Infections that follow operative procedures are an all-too-common complication in surgical patients. The spectrum of postoperative infections varies dramatically from troublesome wound infections to intraperitoneal infections that represent the major threat to patient survival. Reduction in morbidity and mortality in patients with postoperative infection can be achieved only by a thorough understanding of prevention, early diagnosis, and definitive therapeutic intervention.

Clinical manifestations of postoperative infection generally result in either local or systemic signs and symptoms. Local signs of postoperative infection include the traditional cardinal signs of the infection: specifically, *calor, dolor, rubor,* and *tumor.* All of these signs of inflammation represent clinical evidence of the non-specific inflammatory response. In surgical patients, clinical evidence of the non-specific inflammatory response should serve as a significant indicator of an emerging infection.

Systemic manifestations of postoperative infection usually are consequences of the host febrile response. Chills, rigors, and elevated core body temperature all represent systemic manifestations of the febrile response. A specific series of pathophysiological events triggers the febrile response. Agents that provoke fever are referred to as either endogenous or exogenous pyrogens. In patients with postoperative fever, the exogenous pyrogens are usually bacterial organisms. These exogenous pyrogens are then phagocytosed by neutrophils, monocytes, and other phagocytic cells of the reticuloendothelial system. Phagocytosis of these exogenous pyrogens results in the release of endogenous pyrogen from the phagocytic cell into the systemic circulation. These endogenous pyrogens then affect the temperature control center in the hypothalamus, and this in turn triggers a series of physiological events that result in elevation of the core body temperature. Peripheral vasoconstriction takes place early in the evolution of fever and results in the chills and shivering that commonly occur as the patient's core temperature begins to rise. While vasoconstriction does reduce heat dissipation, the increased oxygen consumption consistently noted in the febrile patient suggests that intrinsic metabolic rates are accelerated and that actual heat production is increased. Thus, both local and systemic manifestations of postoperative infection are meaningful indicators in establishing a clinical diagnosis of infection and in monitoring the results of subsequent therapeutic interventions.

The diagnostic and therapeutic efforts in the patient with postoperative fever should be directed toward recognition and eradication of the primary source of exogenous pyrogens. Characteristics of the postoperative fever may be significant in definition of the primary cause. Fever that begins within 24 hours after operation usually suggests atelectasis. While wound infections and abdominal abscess are usually not identifiable until the fifth to tenth postoperative day, these patients usually have fever beginning very early in the postoperative course. Abscesses commonly have a recurrent, spiking pattern. Infections arising from environmental contamination during the postoperative period will commonly show an antecedent period of no fever prior to temperature elevation. Foley catheter and intravenous cannula–associated infections commonly fit this pattern.

A comprehensive physical examination is essential to the initial assessment of postoperative fever. Specific attention should be focused upon identifying signs of inflammation, such as unusual surgical wound tenderness. Rhonchi or rales on pulmonary examination in the early postoperative period may point to a pulmonary cause of fever.

The specifics of diagnosis and treatment are detailed below as each infectious cause of postoperative fever is discussed. The likely causes are detailed in Table 1–2. Again, specific treatment requires a diagnosis. Commonly, postoperative infections require mechanical treatment and not antibiotics (e.g., atelectasis, wound infection). The em-

TABLE 1–2   THE COMMON INFECTIOUS CAUSES OF FEVER IN THE POSTOPERATIVE PERIOD

Source of Fever	Predisposing Factors	Prevention	Diagnosis	Treatment
Pulmonary	Atelectasis; aspiration; endotracheal intubation; respirator-assisted ventilation.	Cough, deep breathing; early ambulation; nasogastric decompression of stomach; rapid weaning from respirator.	Radiographic; culture of purulent sputum.	Aggressive pulmonary toilet; specific antibiotics.
Surgical wound	See Table 1–1.	See Table 1–4.	Unusual wound tenderness; suppurative drainage; always culture the wound!	Remove all sutures; drain the wound; debride non-viable tissue; antibiotics only for invasive infection.
Intra-abdominal abscess	Acute gastrointestinal/ biliary perforation.	Earlier surgical intervention in peritonitis.	Radiographic; CT scanning; emerging organ failure; persistent sepsis in spite of antibiotic therapy.	Surgical drainage; adjunctive systemic antibiotics.
Urinary tract sepsis	Foley catheterization.	Asepsis in catheter management.	Pyuria on urinalysis; $> 10^5$ bacteria/ml. of urine.	Specific antibiotic therapy.
Intravenous catheter sepsis	Hyperalimentation; prolonged central or peripheral intravenous cannulation.	Asepsis in placement and management of intravenous cannulae.	Clinical defervescence with catheter removal; pus from vein.	Remove cannula; excision of septic peripheral vein.

TABLE 1–3 NON-INFECTIOUS CAUSES OF FEVER RELEVANT IN POSTOPERATIVE SURGICAL PATIENTS

Non-infectious Cause	Diagnosis*	Treatment
Drug fever	Eosinophilia; high index of suspicion.	Cessation of drug in question.
Malignant hyperthermia	Intraoperative/postoperative fever to 40–42° C.	Antipyretics; systemic hypothermia therapy (e.g., ice packs); fluid support.
Thyroid storm	Clinical and chemical evidence of hyperthyroidism.	Propylthiouracil; propranolol.
Hypothalamic trauma	Basilar skull fracture; labile hyper- and hypothermia.	Antipyretics; systemic hypothermic therapy; support care.
Malignancy	Tissue diagnosis; particularly lymphoma.	Primary treatment of malignancy.

*All diagnoses presume that thorough clinical evaluation has eliminated an infectious cause of fever.

pirical initiation of antibiotic therapy for postoperative fever is inappropriate except in the most unusual cases and should rarely be so employed. While non-infectious causes of postoperative fever are rare, they do occur and should be borne in mind (Table 1–3).

Wound Infection

Wound infections represent a potential threat to every surgical incision. However, all surgical incisions are not subject to the same risk factors and, accordingly, the probability of subsequent infection is different. Because of this highly variable frequency of postoperative infection, it has been necessary to define a classification system that provides a means for estimating the likelihood of infection in the postoperative period (Table 1–4).

Refined-clean wounds are surgical incisions that have an extraordinarily low probability of significant intraoperative contamination and resultant clinical infection. These surgical incisions do not intrude into anatomical locations that are normally colonized with bacteria. Likewise, these incisions are not in areas where the skin is heavily colonized, such as the perineum or groin. Infection rates in refined-clean wounds should be less than 1 per cent as exemplified by the elective craniotomy.

Simple clean wounds vary only from refined-clean wounds in the sense that these incisions may extend through cutaneous areas that are known to have substantial bacterial contamination. The inguinal hernia incision represents a clean surgical wound, since its anticipated infection rate is less than 2 per cent. Because of its proximity to the contaminated groin and perineal

TABLE 1–4 PRACTICAL CLASSIFICATION OF SURGICAL WOUNDS

Type of Wound	Source of Contamination	Frequency of Infection	Preventive Measures of Importance	Examples
Refined-clean	Extrinsic to patient	<1%	Asepsis? Ultraviolet light or laminar flow air system	Craniotomy incision
Clean	Extrinsic or resident cutaneous flora	1–2%	Asepsis	Inguinal herniorrhaphy
Clean-contaminated	Endogenous flora	10–30%	Preoperative systemic antibiotics	Elective colon resection
Dirty	Endogenous flora	>40%	Preoperative systemic antibiotics; delayed primary closure	Perforated diverticulitis

areas, infection rates will be slightly higher than in the refined-clean incision.

Clean-contaminated (or potentially contaminated) wounds are those surgical incisions where substantial bacterial contamination regularly occurs. However, these wounds do not include those where active infection or massive bacteriological contamination is present. An example of a clean-contaminated wound is the elective colon resection. Preoperative mechanical bowel preparation and other preventive measures prevent contamination from being massive, but major contamination is nevertheless inevitable. Infection rates in this class of surgical wounds are between 10 and 30 per cent in the absence of specific preventive measures to be subsequently discussed.

Finally, the contaminated or dirty wounds are those surgical incisions where active infection is encountered or massive bacterial contamination is present. Thus, the abdominal incision for draining an intraperitoneal abscess or the abdominal incision in the patient with a left colon gunshot wound both represent circumstances of massive bacterial contamination and a high probability of subsequent wound sepsis. Infection in such wounds tends to be the rule rather than the exception.

In general, infections arising in refined-clean and clean surgical incisions are consequences of contamination exogenous to the patient. Infections in clean-contaminated and contaminated incisions are consequences of contamination endogenous to the patient. Thus, because staphylococcal organisms primarily represent exogenous pathogens, the frequency of staphylococcal wound infections in refined-clean and clean procedures can serve as a useful infection surveillance tool to gauge the adequacy of overall sterile technique procedures in the operating room.

Numerous preventive measures are available to the surgeon to reduce the overall frequency of operative wound infection. First, careful preoperative preparation can reduce both the number of potential pathogenic bacteria and the number of systemic factors that might predispose to subsequent infectious complications. The site of the planned operative wound can be frequently scrubbed, preferably by the patient himself, prior to the procedure, with any number of

acceptable antiseptic detergents (povidone-iodine; chlorhexidine). Patients with active infections remote from the surgical wound should have these infections treated adequately before an elective operative procedure. The duration of a patient's preoperative hospitalization should be kept to an absolute minimum, since excessive preoperative hospitalization will result in increased refined-clean and clean operative wound infection rates. Thus, when it is a feasible alternative or in those cases where wound infection would be a particularly catastrophic event (total hip replacement, arterial prosthetic graft, heart valve replacement), discharge from the hospital with subsequent readmission may even be advisable.

Preoperative preparation may be required to reduce systemic risk factors that also might predispose to infection. Specifically, nutritional support by the most practical means available should achieve positive nitrogen balance and reduce potential contributions of protein-calorie malnutrition as a factor in subsequent infection complications. Furthermore, hypovolemia and anemia require preoperative correction to eliminate potential contributions that these variables may make to subsequent septic problems.

Meticulous attention to technical considerations during the conduct of the operative procedure is of particular significance in reducing subsequent wound infection rates. Because of the foreign body effects of braided suture material, ligatures within the wound should be used sparingly. Excessive use of electrocautery will also result in tissue injury and non-viable foci for bacterial proliferation and subsequent infection. Nevertheless, adequate hemostasis remains an important objective in the surgical wound, and considerable care should be exercised in achieving that goal. If excessive dead space in obese patients necessitates wound drainage, then only closed catheter drainage is considered an acceptable alternative. Penrose drains that exit through the surgical wound are simply not acceptable, although they are still widely used.

Two additional methods have gained limited popularity in attempts to control airborne contamination. Because of its bactericidal effects, ultraviolet irradiation in the operating room has been advocated. This cumbersome method requires special clothing and hoods to protect the operating personnel from the harmful effects of ultraviolet irradiation. Similarly, laminar flow air-handling devices have also achieved regional popularity, particularly during total hip replacement procedures. Since both of these techniques are directed at reducing contamination, it is proper that they be applied only in refined-clean operative wounds. Because of the usually low wound infection rates in refined-clean wounds, it is not surprising that only a few studies have documented the clinical efficacy of either of these modalities.

Prophylaxis of surgical wound infection by the use of antibiotics has achieved considerable levels of popularity, despite the fact that these antibiotics are often inappropriately employed for prevention. Early studies attempting to define the effectiveness of antibiotics in preventing surgical wound infection were generally inadequate studies. In most of these attempts the types of surgical wounds in control and experimental groups were not regulated; the temporal relationships of contamination and antibiotic administration were inconsistent; and data and conclusions were often generated from retrospective analysis.

Experimental studies by Miles and associates clearly defined the requirements for the prevention of cutaneous infections by employing systemic antibiotic prophylaxis. These studies demonstrated that systemic antibiotics administered prior to dermal contamination completely prevented subsequent infection. Furthermore, antibiotics administered 1 to 4 hours after dermal contamination were significantly less beneficial than those administered prior to contamination. Finally, these studies illustrated that antibiotics administered 4 hours or more after contamination had no effect whatsoever.

Subsequent prospective randomized clinical trials have verified these experimental observations as being clinically practical. These studies have demonstrated that the immediate preoperative administration of a systemic antibiotic was effective in reducing surgical wound infection rates. Furthermore, studies by Stone and associates have shown that administration of the antibiotic beginning 8 to 12 hours preoperatively is of no more value than beginning the drug within 1 hour of the operative procedure. Also, initiation of the antibiotic following the operative procedure had no effect upon wound infection rates. Finally, Stone demonstrated that prolonged postoperative administration of systemic antibiotic prophylaxis is no better than the immediate perioperative administration of antibiotics alone.

From these numerous clinical and experimental studies, the following principles of systemic prophylactic antibiotic administration for the prevention of surgical wound infections can be formulated:

1. Antibiotics must be administered prior to initiation of the surgical wound but need to be continued only through the period of operative contamination. Preventive antibiotics do not need to be administered days in advance nor days following the operative procedure. The priority of systemic prophylaxis is to have an active antibiotic within the incision at operation, not before nor subsequent to the contamination.

2. Systemic prophylactic antibiotics should be used only in those cases in which there is a high frequency of wound infection, e.g., elective colon surgery, or in which the risk of a subsequent infection is particularly catastrophic, e.g., total hip or arterial prosthetic graft placement.

3. The systemic prophylactic antibiotic chosen should have minimum toxicity. Previous studies by Caldwell and Cluff have shown a 5 per cent complication rate associated with antibiotic administration in hospitalized patients. Low toxicity antibiotics should only be chosen for prevention purposes.

4. Only antibiotics that have a proven record of effectiveness and prevention should be employed. By virtue of many studies that have documented the effectiveness of cephaloridine in the prevention of surgical wound infection, this information has been extrapolated by some to mean that all cephalosporin antibiotics are equally effective in the prevention of surgical wound infections. Prospective randomized trials have clearly demonstrated that cephalothin is not an effective prophylactic antibiotic. Subsequent pharmacokinetic studies have documented the poor tissue concentrations of cephalothin in the prophylactic setting.

Therapeutic equivalency for antibiotic prophylaxis cannot be interpreted from in vitro culture and sensitivity data but can be established only by comparative trials.

The oral antibiotic bowel preparation represents an alternative method for the prevention of surgical wound infections in patients undergoing elective colon surgery; its goal is to reduce the number of bacteria available to contaminate the wound. This technique employs orally administered, poorly absorbed antibiotics to reduce potential contaminating aerobic and anaerobic enteric bacteria. Prospective clinical trials with neomycin-tetracycline, neomycin-erythromycin, and neomycin-metronidazole have all shown protection from wound infection in patients having these regimens. Whether systemic antibiotic prophylaxis or the oral antibiotic bowel preparation is preferable or whether the two methods together will provide additional benefit remains an issue that is not resolved by currently available clinical data. Preliminary data indicate that the two methods are not additive.

Despite all efforts at prevention, surgical wound infections continue to occur in the postoperative period. Overt clinical evidence of wound infection is not usually evident until the fifth to eighth postoperative day. Prior to that time, the cardinal signs of inflammation about the surgical wound may be seen and fever often antedates the subsequent discharge of pus from the incision and confirmation of the diagnosis.

Surgical principles in the management of infection apply to the handling of wound infection. All cutaneous sutures are removed and the wound is opened to allow complete surgical drainage of purulent material which is carefully cultured. Bold surgeons may attempt to remove only a portion of the cutaneous sutures, but this limited approach may lead to disaster. The smoldering, inadequately drained wound infection may progress to a necrotizing fasciitis, and for this reason all suture material should be removed from the infected incision. Surgical debridement of fibrinous material adherent to the subcutaneous tissue is advisable, and the wound is then loosely packed with coarse mesh gauze. There is no uniformity of opinion as to the types of antiseptic solutions that might be employed with the coarse mesh gauze. Indeed, some surgeons prefer simple saline, wet-to-dry dressings. Regardless of the potion applied to the wound, frequent changes of dressings, using sterile surgical technique and meticulous mechanical debridement, where indicated, are the hallmarks of managing these wound infections. Occasionally, infected wounds may resolve quickly and delayed primary closure may be attempted, although this is not without the risk of recurrent suppuration. In general, secondary closure is the preferable option. Systemic antibiotic therapy for simple wound infections is indicated only when there is evidence of cellulitis into adjacent tissues or when there is evidence of necrotizing infection. When evidence of invasive infection is present at the time of drainage, an immediate Gram stain of purulent material may guide in antibiotic selection until culture data are available. Since predicting which wounds will ultimately require supplemental systemic antibiotic therapy is difficult, every surgical wound must be cultured!

Intra-Abdominal Infection

Peritonitis represents the majority of infections occurring within the abdominal cavity, and it usually occurs secondary to bacterial contamination arising from biliary or enteric sources. Perforating injuries or spontaneous gastrointestinal perforations are the most common causes of this contamination and peritonitis. Primary peritonitis owing to peritoneal contamination from hematogenous or lymphatic sources is more a medical curiosity than a common problem. The surgeon is specifically concerned with the problems of secondary peritonitis in which contamination arises from a specific mechanical defect in a visceral structure.

Following contamination, bacteria are disseminated throughout the entire peritoneal cavity. Dissemination occurs as a function of the normal flow patterns of peritoneal fluid. For this reason, peritonitis is considered a diffuse process involving the entire peritoneal cavity.

Three possible outcomes can be observed in the natural history of the patient with peritonitis. First, the bacterial contamination may be quantitatively small or the patient's host defense may be so effective as to result in complete resolution of the acute process. This is occasionally seen in younger patients with perforated peptic ulcers. Second, the contamination may be quantitatively very large or the patient's host defense may be inadequate, with resultant death occurring in the acute phase of the infection. Third, a relative stalemate may evolve between the bacterial contaminant and host defense, resulting in loculation and abdominal abscess formation. Survival depends on the ultimate management of these collections.

Early clinical diagnosis of acute peritonitis in patients is essential. Most patients relate an acute physiological event that initiated symptoms of abdominal pain. The physical examination characteristically demonstrates diffuse tenderness and involuntary muscle guarding or even abdominal wall rigidity. Laboratory and x-ray studies may demonstrate leukocytosis or free intraperitoneal air but, by and large, a careful clinical examination is the keystone of the diagnosis.

Abdominal exploration is the treatment of choice for the patient with acute peritonitis. Volume resuscitation is expeditiously pursued with establishment of a satisfactory urinary output representing the clinical endpoint of this biological titration. Antibiotics appropriate for the anticipated enteric bacterial pathogens are initiated preoperatively. While considerable numbers of discussions have centered on which antibiotic or combination of antibiotics is appropriate in these circumstances, very early administration of these drugs is uniformly agreed upon.

At laparotomy, the mechanical defect responsible for the peritoneal contamination is either repaired, resected, or exteriorized as deemed appropriate. Pus and non-viable tissue are removed. Because of the generalized character of acute peritonitis within the intra-abdominal cavity, the use of drains is discouraged.

The postoperative care of the patient with acute peritonitis requires continued volume support, nasogastric decompression, and continuation of systemic antibiotic therapy for 5 to 7 days postoperatively. The role of intraperitoneal antibiotic administration remains incompletely defined. A favorable clinical response is usually indicated by the lysis of fever and the gradual return of gastrointestinal function. The persistence of clinical sepsis after the seventh postoperative day should serve as a clinical indicator of abdominal abscess and not as an indication for extended systemic antibiotic therapy.

Among diagnostic dilemmas in surgery, no problem is greater than abdominal abscess. The physical examination is frequently compromised in the patient with a recent laparotomy incision. The abscess mass itself is rarely palpable, except when it is in the pelvis. Chest and abdominal roentgenograms may demonstrate a pleural effusion, an elevated hemidiaphragm, or extraluminal air, but generally they are not helpful in many patients. Abdominal ultrasound and various scanning techniques have been useful only in the hands of a selected few individuals. Computerized tomography may facilitate diagnosis. The emergence of organ failure in the postoperative period recently has served as a useful clinical indicator of continued intra-abdominal infection that requires surgical management. Occasionally, persistent sepsis in the high-risk patient may be the only objective evidence of abdominal abscess.

Surgical management continues to be the only effective treatment for abdominal abscess. Only by complete evacuation of the intra-abdominal purulence can clinical resolution of the intra-abdominal infection be achieved. The operative methods for drainage of abdominal abscess continue to be controversial. A limited abdominal exploration may be justified in the patient whose abscess is well localized by preoperative evaluation and who is also tolerating the clinical infection with relatively little difficulty. This limited approach prevents complications of inadvertent enterotomy and fistulization. However, the patient without preoperative localization of the abscess cavity or the patient who is not tolerating the systemic manifestations of sepsis should have a complete exploratory operation on the abdomen. This approach avoids missed multiple abscesses or inadequately drained established abscesses in those patients who desperately need complete and thorough surgical drainage.

As opposed to the patients with acute peritonitis, those with localized abscess cavities should have drains used. Generally, active sump drainage is preferred over passive drainage, and dependent drainage is considered more desirable than non-dependent drainage.

Patients having abdominal abscesses drained are usually also receiving antibiotic therapy; if not, antibiotics should be initiated preoperatively. Broad spectrum antibiotics usually are chosen to combat the polymicrobial character of intra-abdominal infections. Gram stains of abdominal pus invariably show a multitude of different organisms, and cultures usually show numerous gram-negative aerobic rods and a variable number of enteric anaerobic organisms, including *Bacteroides fragilis*. While specific antimicrobial coverage continues to be a controversial issue, we feel that only the aerobic enteric rods ordinarily require specific antibiotic therapy in conjunction with surgical drainage.

Pulmonary Infections

Pneumonitis

Pulmonary infections are common in surgical patients, particularly in the postoperative period. These infections may assume any one of three separate but similar clinical patterns. First, pulmonary infections may arise as a consequence of postoperative atelectasis. Atelectasis represents the collapse of alveoli and small airways owing to inadequate tidal volumes, thus entrapping bacteria and setting the stage for invasive infection. When atelectasis is not adequately treated, invasive pulmonary infection results. Second, endotracheal intubation and ventilation assistance are commonly employed in patients undergoing major operative procedures. While the ventilator has been essential in providing respiratory support, it has also served as a reservoir of potential bacterial pathogens. The combination of the direct access provided by the endotracheal tube, the critically ill and potentially immunosuppressed patient, and the presence of a ventilator as a source of pathogen, all too frequently leads to respirator-associated pulmonary infections. Third, aspiration pneumonitis may also

occur in those patients who have an altered sensorium secondary to head injury, drugs, hypovolemia, or sepsis from another site.

Based on these three classifications of pneumonia, it is evident that all can be prevented. Aggressive measures in the prevention and treatment of atelectasis are early ambulation, coughing and deep breathing postoperatively, chest physiotherapy for more difficult cases, and even nasotracheal suctioning for refractory atelectasis; these measures will reduce postoperative pneumonia complications. Patients on ventilators require meticulous placement technique to avoid introduction of bacteria into the patient's airway and scrupulous, periodic cleansing of ventilator equipment. Obviously, rapid weaning from the respirator will also reduce the period of time the patient is at risk for contamination via this route. Finally, gastric decompression with the nasogastric tube should be considered part of the airway management of any patient with an altered sensorium.

The diagnosis of pneumonitis is primarily made radiographically. Infiltrates are characteristically present. Culture and bacterial sensitivity of purulent sputum will provide guidelines for antibiotic therapy. Bronchoscopy may be both diagnostic and therapeutic, particularly in the patient with suspected aspiration. There is some evidence that sequential quantitative sputum cultures may provide an earlier diagnosis.

As noted above, antibiotic therapy should be specifically tailored to culture and sensitivity data. Unfortunately, most postoperative pulmonary infections are due to increasingly resistant gram-negative organisms and usually require very broad spectrum antibiotic therapy. Antibiotic therapy should be discontinued as soon as clinical resolution is evident. Finally, systemic antibiotic prophylaxis is not useful in the prevention of pneumonitis and will only hasten the emergence of resistant bacterial strains.

Empyema

Suppurative infections of the pleural space are most commonly identified following pneumonitis or blunt and penetrating injuries of the chest wall. These injuries result in either hemothorax or hydrothorax and, if improperly treated or if secondary contamination intervenes, then the setting for empyema is complete. Empyemas following tuberculosis are now relatively uncommon. The most effective means of preventing empyema is rapid and effective evacuation of the pleural space in patients sustaining chest wall injury. Patients who have had a chest tube placed to treat hemothorax but who have retained a clot within the pleural space require an additional chest tube to achieve evacuation. Depending on the patient's overall condition, a retained clotted hemothorax that is refractory to chest tube drainage should be considered an indication for immediate removal by thoracotomy.

Diagnosis of empyemas is usually made from two-dimensional chest roentgenograms. With this approach, needle aspiration of the suspicious area will allow confirmation of the diagnosis and afford materials for both Gram stain and culture. After diagnostic confirmation by needle aspiration, closed chest drainage can be achieved by placement of a chest tube. More difficult drainage problems may require resection of a rib. Finally, the pleuropulmonary peel adjacent to the visceral pleura of the lung may restrict normal pulmonary function, and accordingly, decortication may be required to preserve ultimate pulmonary function.

Antibiotic therapy for empyemas is purely adjunctive to the primary drainage procedure. Because the source of bacterial contamination responsible for the empyema may be either exogenous or endogenous, the primary pathogen has a high degree of variability and makes utilization of the Gram stain essential in making initial antibiotic choices. Culture and sensitivity data will allow further refinement of antibiotic choices when they are available.

Urinary Tract Infection

Urinary tract infections are the most common nosocomial infection in postoperative surgical patients. These infections are associated most commonly with Foley catheterization but may also occur in patients with urinary outflow obstruction, e.g., prostatic hypertrophy, anorectal operations, and spinal anesthetics.

Post-catheterization infections occur because bacteria gain direct access to the urinary bladder. This contamination may occur either at the time of catheter placement or during its subsequent management. Contamination introduced at the time of catheter placement usually is a consequence of casual technique. The indwelling catheter then becomes a source of contamination because of violations of the closed catheter drainage system that permits contaminants direct access to the urinary bladder.

Unlike the community-acquired urinary tract infection, the signs and symptoms of post-catheterization urosepsis are often non-specific. Symptoms such as dysuria or even hematuria in the patient post-catheterization are quite common and may be consequences of catheter irritation and not necessarily from infection. In general, fever is the most common clinical manifestation of post–Foley catheterization urinary tract infections. Pyuria identified in the urinalysis then justifies a urine culture. A culture with greater than 100,000 bacteria per ml. of urine requires treatment.

These post-catheterization infections are, for the most part, preventable. Attention to meticulous sterile technique in the placement of catheters will minimize contamination of the patient. It is essential that the closed catheter drainage system be maintained throughout the entire time that the patient has an indwelling catheter in place. The catheter should be appropriately anchored so that to-and-fro movement of the catheter within the urethra prevents retrograde translocation of catheter contaminants. Finally, removal of the Foley catheter as soon as it has served its purpose is equally effective in reducing the incidence of these infections.

Antibiotic treatment should be based upon culture and sensitivity data. The organisms responsible for post-catheterization urinary tract infections tend to reflect the hospital environment and accordingly Pseudomonas, Klebsiella, and other hospital pathogens represent the primary microbes. Antibiotic treatment should be discontinued after clinical resolution of the infectious process. Recurrence of a urinary tract infection following catheterization and appropriate antibiotic treatment may warrant investigations into possible urinary outlet obstruction, which may be secondary to either intrinsic patient disease (prostatic hypertrophy) or iatrogenic urinary tract injury from the catheterization process.

Septic Thrombophlebitis

Thrombophlebitis at the intravenous infusion site is a relatively common event in patients receiving prolonged intravenous fluids or locally noxious drugs. Occasionally, bacterial contamination may be superimposed upon these primary chemical processes, resulting in a suppurative infection within the vessel lumen. Unlike chemical thrombophlebitis, however, septic thrombophlebitis requires more treatment than simple removal of the intravenous catheter.

The diagnosis of septic thrombophlebitis can be quite difficult. The infusion site commonly looks identical to those in patients with a simple chemical phlebitis in that there is mild inflammation and tissue reaction. Actually, the infusion site may look totally innocuous, without any evidence of the cardinal signs of inflammation. However, the patient may have positive blood cultures with high spiking fever as a consequence of the bacterial shower originating from the septic vein.

The diagnosis can be confirmed only by local exploration of old infusion sites and looking for pus within the veins. Commonly, gross examination will confirm the diagnosis in an unequivocal fashion. Periodically, examination of the clotted vein may be equivocal, and culture of the luminal contents or even histological examination for bacteria may be required to confirm the diagnosis. In the patient with positive blood cultures but a seemingly occult primary focus of infection, exploration of multiple intravenous infusion sites may be necessary, regardless of their apparently innocuous appearance, to rule out septic thrombophlebitis as the cause.

The prevention of septic thrombophlebitis requires a renewed commitment to asep-

tic technique in the placement of intravenous catheters. Likewise, prolonged maintenance of infusion sites is likely to create the local chemical reaction that will allow secondary bacterial contamination to initiate a septic process. Thus, the routine changing of intravenous sites, e.g., every 48 hours, may also reduce the frequency of septic thrombophlebitis. The role of topical antimicrobial therapy at the site remains unclear. Because lower extremity infusion sites have been identified as having an unusually high incidence of this complication, lower extremity cutdowns and intravenous sites should be used only when other sites are impractical.

The treatment of septic thrombophlebitis is surgical. The entire length of infected vein must be excised. Partial excision will result only in continuation of the systemic bacterial shower. Antibiotic therapy is employed only as an adjunctive measure and may not be of particular value in the overall results of treating this complication. The pathogens commonly identified in septic thrombophlebitis represent the gram-negative rods prevalent in the hospital environment.

Central Venous Catheter Sepsis

The subclavian and internal jugular vein catheters are being used with increased frequency for monitoring central venous pressure, for the administration of parenteral hyperalimentation solutions, and for fluid administration in those patients with limited extremity infusion sites. These catheters, while serving a very real purpose, have at the same time provided a direct access route for potential bacterial pathogens into the central venous circulation.

The diagnosis of central venous catheter sepsis can be most difficult. Patients who require these catheters commonly have additional potential or documented sources of infection. Replacement of these catheters can be a technically exasperating procedure, and therefore the physician on empirical evidence alone usually will not remove one of these catheters because of a septic episode.

Indeed, the diagnosis of central venous catheter sepsis is usually based upon the clinical results of catheter removal. If removing the catheter results in resolution of the fever, catheter sepsis is generally concluded to have been the cause. Cultures of the catheter are usually significant only if they are negative. A negative culture means that catheter sepsis was not likely. However, a positive catheter culture may have been positive because of contamination upon removal, contamination from remote foci, or because the catheter was truly infected.

Again, the pathogens responsible for catheter sepsis are characteristic of the hospital environment. Fungal pathogens, specifically *Candida albicans,* are quite common in patients with central venous catheters who are receiving parenteral hyperalimentation. A blood culture positive for a fungal organism in a patient with a central venous catheter is an absolute indication for removal of that catheter.

Prevention of central venous catheter sepsis requires careful technique in catheter placement, day-to-day attention to the care and dressing of the catheter entrance site, and early removal of the catheter when clinical circumstances make this a feasible alternative. Patients receiving hyperalimentation solutions should never have these catheters used for blood sampling or for the administration of medications.

The treatment for central venous catheter sepsis is catheter withdrawal. Antibiotics are commonly used as adjunctive treatments to removal of the catheter. Antifungal chemotherapy should not be continued in those patients whose fungal sepsis clearly defervesces with removal of the catheter.

Postoperative Parotitis

Postoperative suppurative parotitis is an uncommon but particularly troublesome infectious complication. Normal saliva from healthy patients has intrinsic bacteriostatic activity. This property makes spontaneous salivary gland infection very unusual in the absence of salivary duct obstruction, except in the elderly and/or debilitated patient. Parotitis in the immunoincompetent, chronically ill patient is associated with poor oral hygiene, dehydration, and anticholinergic drug administration that reduces salivary flow.

The diagnosis is usually evident by palpatory examination of the swollen, tender parotid gland. Sialography may be required to rule out ductal obstruction. *Staphylococcus aureus* has been the most common pathogen in the past, although the opportunistic gram-negative rods, e.g., Pseudomonas, have become more prevalent in those patients who have received long-term systemic antibiotic therapy.

Prevention of parotitis requires attention to those factors that predispose the patient to these infections; adequate oral hygiene, avoidance of dehydration, and attention to anticholinergic drug use are important. Long-term, indwelling nasogastric tubes are also predisposing factors and gastrostomy placement should be considered in patients requiring sustained gastric intubation.

Treatment requires systemic antibiotic therapy initially. The Gram stain of suppuration expressed from the intraoral opening of Stensen's duct will provide appropriate guidelines for early antibiotic administration. Culture and sensitivity data will allow confirmation of the Gram stain and a more specific antibiotic choice. Staphylococcal infections are best treated with systemic nafcillin. This agent is preferred to alternative choices, e.g., methicillin or oxacillin, because it has less renal toxicity in high-dose treatment ranges. It also has a broader gram-positive spectrum than alternative choices, which may be very significant before specific culture data are available. The aminoglycosides are commonly required for gram-negative parotitis. Palpable fluctuants require surgical drainage; failure of clinical response of the affected gland to systemic antibiotic therapy may also warrant surgical intervention.

Foreign Body Infections

Numerous permanently implanted foreign materials are currently used in day-to-day surgical practice. Postoperative infections associated with placement of prosthetic heart valves, placement of total hip prosthesis, and synthetic arterial replacement materials are formidable problems. In general, management of surgical foreign body infections demands that the prosthetic device in question be removed. The magnitude of these problems cannot be covered in detail, and the reader is referred to more comprehensive discussions.

SPECIAL PROBLEMS IN SURGICAL INFECTION

Burn Wound Sepsis

After there is thermal injury to the skin, devitalized tissue forms a densely adherent eschar. This eschar is rapidly colonized by bacteria and, because of its avascular character, bacterial proliferation proceeds rapidly. If unchecked, the bacterial proliferation within the eschar will result in invasion of these organisms into adjacent viable tissue and result in invasive infection in the burn wound. This invasive infection has the effect of increasing the depth of tissue loss as well as posing a formidable risk to the patient's life.

The prevention of burn wound sepsis requires appropriate application of both surgical principles and topical chemotherapy. Early and continued debridement of non-viable tissue as it separates from the wound is essential in all phases of the burn patient's care. All mechanical efforts are directed toward achieving the earliest closure of the burn wounds.

Three different compounds have been employed as topical treatments in preventing bacterial proliferation within the eschar. Aqueous silver nitrate (0.5 per cent) is a proven topical treatment but does have the adverse metabolic complications of electrolyte dilution, namely hyponatremia. Furthermore, it does not penetrate the eschar to an appreciable depth. Mafenide acetate is an effective topical agent that has excellent eschar penetration properties. However, its carbonic anhydrase inhibition activity results in a systemic metabolic acidosis and prolonged hyperpnea. Finally, silver sulfadiazine is a third proven topical treatment that is largely free of metabolic complications but is associated with a leukopenia syndrome. While these topical compounds have been effective in the prophylaxis and treatment of burn wound sepsis, administration of systemic antibiotics to prevent burn wound colonization and infection is not recommended. Systemic prophylaxis does not prevent invasive burn wound infection but does tend to select out more resistant bacterial species as the subsequent pathogen.

Invasive burn wound sepsis usually is characterized by fever and colonization of the eschar with greater than 10^5 organisms per gram of tissue. Antibiotic therapy should be directed toward the culture-proven pathogen in the wound. In anticipation of burn wound sepsis as a potential complication, the surgeon should periodically perform a biopsy on the eschar so that constant information is available as to probable causative pathogens if burn wound sepsis emerges. Periodic examination of the wounds with the Wood's lamp may identify critical levels of Pseudomonas contamination. Systemic antibiotic therapy for the treatment of invasive infection should be discontinued as soon as there is favorable clinical response. Prolonged use of systemic antibiotics will hasten the emergence of Candida overgrowth, as well as further selective pressures to facilitate the emergence of resistant bacterial strains.

Clostridial Infections

Clostridial infections are among the oldest recognized anaerobic infections. Clostridial myositis, cellulitis, and tetanus are major concerns for the surgeon. Clostridial myositis, or gas gangrene, represents a rapidly progressive, necrotizing infection involving the skeletal muscle. These infections arise secondary to traumatic injury that is accompanied by contamination with *Clostridium perfringens*. This bacterial species elaborates an exotoxin that results in necrosis of adjacent viable muscle. This muscle necrosis creates the anaerobic environment necessary for survival of these obligate anaerobes.

The diagnosis of clostridial myositis is made by noting severe swelling and pain at the injury site that is accompanied by a brown, watery discharge. Crepitation is commonly heard upon deep palpation, and roentgenographic studies will document subfascial air. Adequate local debridement of the primary injury site is the best prevention for clostridial myositis. Similarly, the treatment of clostridial myositis requires aggressive and extensive debridement of those muscle groups involved with the infectious process and high-dose antibiotic therapy, with penicillin as the drug of choice. Since clostridial exotoxin plays a crucial role in the pathophysiology of this infectious process, the administration of gas gangrene antitoxin should be initiated as soon as the diagnosis is established.

Clostridial cellulitis may occur synchronously with clostridial myositis but is a separate disease process that may occur exclusive of myositis. Clostridial cellulitis commonly follows a superficial traumatic injury. The diagnosis is usually easier to make than that of clostridial myositis, since the crepitation in the soft tissue is readily audible because of its more superficial location. Similarly, as in myositis, clostridial cellulitis requires large doses of penicillin and aggressive local debridement of non-viable skin and subcutaneous tissue.

Tetanus, more commonly known as lockjaw, is a consequence of traumatic wound contamination with the organism *Clostridium tetani*. Like other clostridial pathogens, the tetanus organism elaborates a potent exotoxin that has characteristic neurotoxicity. The treatment of established tetanus requires extensive supportive care, antiseizure medications, and prolonged respiratory support. Tetanus immune globulin is employed as soon as the diagnosis is made, while systemic antibiotic therapy is of relatively little value.

Ideally, tetanus is completely preventable. All children should have active immunization with three doses of tetanus toxoid (0.5 ml.) over a six-month period. An additional dose of tetanus toxoid should be administered every 10 years thereafter. Booster doses may be administered for high-risk trauma wounds occurring more than 5 years after the last tetanus toxoid dose. Patients presenting with traumatic injury who have not had immunization against tetanus are candidates for immediate treatment with tetanus immune globulin in addition to the initial doses of tetanus toxoid.

Synergistic Infections

Traditional concepts of infections in man, as detailed by Robert Koch, ascribe one pathogen only for each infectious process. However, polymicrobial infections with synergistic relationships existing among the component bacteria have been recognized. Meleney first described a synergistic necrotizing infection of the abdominal wall due to anaerobic streptococcal and aerobic staphylococcal pathogens. Intra-abdominal infections, in fact, are characteristically synergistic polymicrobial infections involving the organism *Bacteroides fragilis* in symbiosis with the aerobic, but facultative, gram-negative enteric bacteria.

While many details of the synergistic relationship of the aerobic and anaerobic organisms remain unknown, some aspects of this relationship have been defined. The facultative aerobic organism appears to consume available oxygen within the environment and thus maintains a low oxidation-reduction potential necessary for obligate anaerobic bacteria to survive. In return, the anaerobic organism may elaborate certain growth factors that potentiate multiplication of the aerobic portion of the relationship, or it may secrete enzymes, such as beta-lactamase, superoxide dismutase, or heparinase, that facilitate the invasive properties of the facultative symbiont.

The treatment of synergistic, polymicrobial infections requires aggressive local surgical debridement to disrupt the anaerobic environment that is so crucial for maintenance of the synergistic relationship. These principles apply whether pertaining to a necrotizing wound infection or an abscess within the peritoneal cavity. Antibiotic therapy for synergistic infections remains a controversial subject with most authors advocating antibiotic treatment directed against both halves of the synergistic pair. Others feel that antibiotic treatment need only address the aerobic component of these infections. Regardless of antibiotic philosophy, the important components of the treatment of synergistic infections are thorough surgical debridement and drainage.

Systemic Candidiasis

As additional broad spectrum antibiotics have become available, systemic fungal infections have become a greater cause for concern. Systemic candidiasis occurs in two clinical settings: (1) the contaminated catheter as noted above, or (2) systemic dissemination of fungi secondary to Candida overgrowth in the gastrointestinal tract. The subsequent discussion will deal only with the latter phenomenon.

Systemic candidiasis occurs as a consequence of Candida overgrowth in the gastrointestinal tract. This overgrowth is a consequence of broad spectrum antibiotic therapy that disrupts the normal bacterial predominance of the microflora in the gastrointestinal tract. The predominance of Candida organisms results in persorption or direct transmucosal movement of these organisms into the portal circulation. In the chronically ill patient, portal candidemia is not cleared by the hepatic reticuloendothelial system, and accordingly, the organisms gain access to the systemic circulation.

Establishment of a diagnosis of systemic candidiasis is difficult. Because peripheral filtration of *Candida* organisms ordinarily occurs with a high degree of efficiency, traditional venous blood cultures have a low frequency of being positive. Thus, arterial rather than venous blood cultures should be performed. Systemic candidiasis is suggested in those patients with chronic illness who have been on long-term systemic antibiotic therapy and who have otherwise unexplained persistent sepsis. The presence of Candida in the urine in patients with unexplained sepsis is an absolute indication for arterial blood cultures. Prevention of systemic candidiasis requires correction of the predisposing clinical factors. While direct immunostimulation is currently not feasible, systemic nutritional support by the most practical means available is important. Systemic antibiotic therapy should be limited in both its duration and spectrum of activity when practical. Oral Nystatin may suppress Candida overgrowth within the gastrointestinal tract but cannot regularly be used to replace more discreet usage of systemic antibiotic therapy.

The treatment of systemic candidiasis requires discontinuation of systemic antibiotic therapy. All indwelling central venous catheters should be removed to eliminate this possibility of Candida dissemination. Systemic antifungal chemotherapy usually consists of either amphotericin B or 5-fluorocytosine.

Pneumocystis Carinii Pneumonitis

One of the most notable, newly recognized, non-bacterial pathogens is the parasite *Pneumocystis carinii*. This pathogen characteristically affects the compromised host. The cancer patient receiving high doses of systemic antineoplastic chemotherapy and the deliberately immunosuppressed transplantation patient represent the prototype population that is affected by this pathogen.

These pulmonary infections begin as bilateral, central hilar infiltrates of the lung. They rapidly progress to severe diffuse parenchymal involvement. Rapid deterioration of pulmonary function, with respirator-dependence necessary to maintain oxygenation, is the general rule.

The diagnosis of Pneumocystis requires an open lung biopsy and methenamine silver staining of the tissue. This pathogen cannot be identified by conventional staining techniques of expectorated sputum, nor can the organism be cultured. The treatment of Pneumocystis pulmonary infections is with the drug combination of trimethoprim and sulfamethoxazole.

ANTIMICROBIAL CHEMOTHERAPY

Numerous antibiotics are available for treatment of surgical patients. All have pharmacokinetic, microbiological, and toxicity differences that pose formidable problems when attempting to select the most appropriate drug for a particular infection. Establishment of specific selection criteria can be useful in making an optimal choice to provide maximum patient benefit.

First, the pathogen should be sensitive to the antibiotic. Thus, culture and sensitivity data should be obtained on all surgical infections. When the acute character of the infection necessitates antibiotic therapy prior to the availability of sensitivity data, then drug therapy should be directed against the anticipated pathogens. The Gram stain can assist in this selection process. Therapy can then be tailored more specifically when sensitivity data are available.

Second, since clinical isolates are usually sensitive to several antibiotics, the drug with the narrowest possible spectrum should be chosen. For example, staphylococcal pathogens are usually sensitive to both nafcillin and cephalothin. However, cephalothin has a modest spectrum of gram-negative coverage that nafcillin does not have. Thus, nafcillin becomes the preferable choice for these staphylococcal infections. The choice of antibiotics with the narrowest antimicrobial spectrum will minimize selection pressure responsible for the evolution of bacterial resistance.

Finally, the toxicity and route of excretion should be carefully considered. Less toxic drugs should be selected when comparable sensitivities exist. Since all antibiotics are metabolized or excreted via the liver or the kidney, the integrity of hepatic or renal function is important in the selection proc-

ess and in establishment of a proper dose schedule.

The general choices of antibiotics for specific pathogens are listed in Table 1–5. These choices commonly reflect personal preference as well as objective bases for their selection. Emerging patterns of bacterial resistance require sensitivity documentation of all cultured pathogens.

FUTURE PROSPECTS IN INFECTION

The last four decades have seemingly brought about major improvements in the prevention and treatment of infection in surgical patients. Effective use of preventive antibiotics can reduce infection rates. Systemic antibiotics and generally improved

TABLE 1–5 ANTIBIOTIC CHOICES* FOR INFECTIONS CAUSED BY COMMONLY IDENTIFIED SURGICAL PATHOGENS

Pathogen	Site of Infection	Antibiotic Choice
Aerobic gram-positive		
Streptococcus		
Group A	Soft tissue cellulitis	Penicillin G
Group D	Intra-abdominal and wound infection	High-dose Penicillin G
Staphylococcus	Surgical wounds; soft tissue cellulitis; occasional pneumonitis	Nafcillin
Pneumococcus	Pulmonary	Penicillin G
Aerobic gram-negative		
Escherichia coli	All sites	Cephalosporin
Klebsiella-Enterobacter	All sites	Cephalosporin
Proteus		
Indole-negative	All sites	Ampicillin
Indole-positive	All sites	Aminoglycoside
Salmonella	Enteritis	Chloramphenicol
Hemophilus influenzae	Upper respiratory tract infections	Ampicillin
Pseudomonas	Pneumonitis; urinary tract	Tobramycin
Serratia	Pneumonitis; urinary tract	Tobramycin
Anaerobic gram-positive		
Clostridia species	Myonecrosis; cellulitis	High-dose Penicillin G
Anaerobic gram-negative		
Bacteroides species	Wounds; intra-abdominal	Clindamycin/ Chloramphenicol
Fungi		
Candida species	Catheter sepsis; primary candidiasis	Amphotericin B
Protozoan		
Pneumocystis carinii	Pulmonary	Trimethaprim/ Sulfamethoxazole

*Selections are the authors' preferences and must be confirmed by specific sensitivity data. The use of antibiotics in surgical patients presupposes that adequate mechanical treatment of the primary focus of infection has been completed or is being contemplated.

supportive care of critically ill patients have improved results in patients who have severe life-threatening infections. However, the same technology that has had such a significant impact upon the critically ill patients has, at the same time, paradoxically created the severely immunocompromised host and an environment teeming with resistant hordes of exotic bacterial, viral, and even protozoan pathogens. Careful examination of the microbiological changes over the antibiotic era of the past 40 years leads to the conclusion that the short generation time of microorganisms virtually guarantees that any new antimicrobial chemotherapy will have only a transient period of effectiveness prior to the emergence of microbial resistance.

Future prospects for improved prevention and treatment of surgical infection hinge upon two pivotal issues. (1) Better definition of the mechanisms involved in the compromised host is needed. Also, methods of modulation of the immune response may hold promise for enhancement of the patient's defense against contamination that is inevitable from ubiquitous, potential pathogens. The ability to stimulate non-specific host defense is particularly attractive, since this should minimize the capability of microbial invaders to create a resistant niche in the protection that has characterized antibiotics or specific bacterial vaccines. (2) Advances in the metabolic support of critically ill patients should reduce the disruptive impact of infections upon host homeostasis. The recognition of multiple organ failure as the final expression of infection underscores the need for more comprehensive understanding of these host-pathogen metabolic relationships and the resultant pathophysiologic derangements that are fatal events in severely infected patients.

Until additional weapons are added to the surgical arsenal in the battle against microbial invaders, the stringent application of currently known standards of care must continue. The importance of attention to technique in all phases of patient care must always be remembered. Careful application of known methods of prevention is equally essential. While antibiotics have been useful in treatment, the surgeon should not abandon time-honored principles of drainage and debridement that were successfully used to manage numerous infection problems before the advent of antimicrobial chemotherapy. Only by a continued commitment to these established principles can the surgeon and the patient expect the least impact of invasive infection on surgical care.

Bibliography

1. Burke, B. A., and Good, R. A.: *Pneumocystis carinii* infection. Medicine *52*:23, 1973.
2. Caldwell, J. R., and Cluff, L. E.: Adverse reaction to antimicrobial agents. J.A.M.A. *230*:77, 1974.
3. Clarke, J. S., Condon, R. E., Bartlett, J. G., et al.: Preoperative oral antibiotics reduce septic complications of colon operations: Result of prospective randomized, double-blind clinical study. Ann. Surg. *186*:251, 1977.
4. Cruse, P. J. E., and Foord, R.: A five-year prospective study of 23,649 surgical wounds. Arch. Surg. *107*:206, 1973.
5. Dinarello, C. A., and Wolff, S. M.: Pathogenesis of fever in man. N. Engl. J. Med. *298*:607, 1978.
6. Feller, I., Flora, J. D., Jr., and Bawol, R.: Baseline results of therapy for burned patients. J.A.M.A. *236*:1943, 1976.
7. Fry, D. E., Garrison, R. N., Heitsch, R., et al.: Determinants of death in patients with intra-abdominal abscess. Surgery *88*:517, 1980.
8. Fry, D. E., Garrison, R. N., and Polk, H. C., Jr.: Clinical implications in bacteroides bacteremia. Surg. Gynecol. Obstet. *149*:189, 1979.
9. Fry, D. E., Pearlstein, L., Fulton, R. L., and Polk, H. C., Jr.: Multiple system organ failure: The role of uncontrolled infection. Arch. Surg. *115*:136, 1980.
10. Hart, D., Postlewait, R. W., Brown, I. W., et al.: Postoperative wound infection: A further report on ultraviolet irradiation with comments on the recent (1964) national council cooperative study report. Ann. Surg. *167*:728, 1968.
11. Kunin, C. M., and McCormack, R. C.: Prevention of catheter-induced urinary tract infections by sterile closed drainage. N. Engl. J. Med. *274*:1155, 1966.
12. Meleney, F. L.: Bacterial synergism in disease processes with a confirmation of the synergistic bacterial etiology of a certain type of progressive gangrene of the abdominal wall. Ann. Surg. *94*:961, 1931.
13. Miles, A. A., Miles, E. M., and Burke, J.: The value and duration of defense reactions of the skin to primary lodgment of bacteria. Br. J. Exp. Pathol. *38*:79, 1957.
14. Polk, H. C., Jr.: Quantitative tracheal cultures in surgical patients requiring mechanical ventilatory assistance. Surgery *78*:485, 1975.

15. Polk, H. C., Jr., Fry, D. E., and Flint, L. M.: Dissemination and causes of infection. Surg. Clin. North Am. *56*:817, 1976.

16. Polk, H. C., Jr., and Lopez-Mayor, J. R.: Postoperative wound infection: A prospective study of determinant factors and prevention. Surgery *66*:97, 1969.

17. Polk, H. C., Jr., Trachtenberg, L., and Finn, M. P.: Human incisional antibiotic activity: The basis for prophylaxis in selected operations. J.A.M.A. *244*:1353, 1980.

18. Postoperative wound infections: The influence of ultraviolet irradiation of the operating room and of various other factors. National Academy of Sciences, National Research Council, Division of Medical Sciences, Ad Hoc Committee on Trauma. Ann. Surg. (Suppl. 2):1, 1964.

19. Pruitt, B. A., McManus, W. F., Kim, S. H., and Treat, R. C.: Diagnosis and treatment of cannula-related intravenous sepsis in burn patients. Ann. Surg. *191*:546, 1980.

20. Ryan, J. A., Abel, R. M., Abbott, W. M., et al.: Catheter complications in total parenteral nutrition. N. Engl. J. Med. *290*:757, 1974.

21. Spratt, J. S.: The etiology and therapy of acute pyogenic parotitis. Surg. Gynecol. Obstet. *112*:391, 1961.

22. Stone, H. H., Haney, B. B., Kolb, L. D., et al.: Prophylactic and preventive antibiotic therapy: Time, duration, and economics. Ann. Surg. *189*:691, 1979.

23. Stone, H. H., Hooper, C. A., Kolb, L. D., et al.: Antibiotic prophylaxis in gastric, biliary, and colonic surgery. Ann. Surg. *184*:443, 1976.

24. Stone, H. H., Kolb, L. D., Currie, C. A., et al.: Candida sepsis: Pathogenesis and principles of treatment. Ann. Surg. *179*:697, 1974.

25. Stone, H. H., Kolb, L. D., and Geheber, C. E.: Incidence and significance of intraperitoneal anaerobic bacteria. Ann. Surg. *181*:705, 1975.

26. Washington, J. A., Dearing, W. H., Judd, E. S., et al.: Effect of preoperative antibiotic regimen on development of infection after intestinal surgery: Prospective, randomized, double-blind study. Ann. Surg. *180*:567, 1974.

27. Wright, R. L., and Burke, J. F.: Effect of ultraviolet radiation on postoperative neurosurgical repair. J. Neurosurg. *31*:533, 1969.

2

WOUND COMPLICATIONS

Thomas K. Hunt

All surgeons are faced with the problem of wound complications. The incidence depends on the type of operation, the patient's disease and condition, and the technical proficiency and judgment of the surgeon. Most large surgical services have an infection rate of about 2 to 4 per cent in clean wounds. Other complications such as dehiscence, hernia, and hematoma raise the complication rate in clean wounds to about 5 per cent. In contaminated cases and in trauma surgery, the complication rate is higher. In emergency operations upon unprepared bowel or infected urinary tract, the rate of wound complications in reported series are as high as 50 to 60 per cent. However, these figures for all categories are higher than they need be, as several investigators have noted.[2, 3, 4, 6, 9, 10, 27]

If surgeons had perfect foresight, serious wound complications would be rare, since techniques for their prevention are available. Part of the surgeon's trade is the fine art of assessing the risk of wound complications and taking the appropriate steps to prevent or treat them.

THE BASIC NATURE OF WOUNDS

The science of wound healing is too complex to be fully summarized here. The reader is referred to several comprehensive volumes that have recently been published.[7, 9, 10, 20, 22, 24] Certain aspects of repair processes will be explained because they are particularly important and are frequently the points on which the success or failure of repair depend.

During the first 3 days after injury, damaged vascular structures thrombose; plasma and lymph exude into the wounded tissue. Inflammatory cells appear and perform their poorly understood functions. Polymorphs and lymphocytes seem unnecessary for primary, uncomplicated healing.[10, 24, 26] They are, however, necessary for normal resistance to infection; and they may perform lytic functions in secondary repair.

Monocytes, which accumulate slowly in the first 2 days, probably receive signals that injury has occurred by sensing the changes in tissue complement and by sensing chemotactic factors released in fibrin polymerization and lysis. These cells then ingest foreign material and tissue debris. In this process, they appear to become "activated" to release a protein substance(s) that causes local cells to divide into fibroblasts and incites lateral growth of local venular endothelial cells, thus establishing both fibroplasia and angiogenesis. Platelet interaction with thrombin causes release of platelet factor which has the same capacities.[9, 10, 11, 24]

Thomas K. Hunt, born in Chicago, was elected to Phi Beta Kappa at Harvard College and to Alpha Omega Alpha at Harvard Medical School. After interning on the Harvard Service of the Boston City Hospital, he entered the United States Army, thereafter joining Dr. J. Engelbert Dunphy at the University of Oregon Medical School. His widely acknowledged studies of wound healing led to his being named Director of the Surgical Wound Healing Laboratory, University of California at San Francisco, in 1965. Serving in this capacity and as Professor of Surgery, Dr. Hunt is an outstanding clinical surgeon, one of the world's leading authorities in the field of wound healing and related problems.

About 2 days after injury, a few fibroblasts appear, and by the fifth or sixth day, many fibroblasts are rapidly synthesizing collagen. This state continues until the end of the second or third week. During this time, the tensile strength of the closed wound increases rapidly. In the open wound, granulation tissue is formed. Nevertheless, by the end of the second or even third week, skin fascia and tendons have gained only a small fraction of their ultimate strength. During this "proliferative phase," the healing ridge, an induration that characteristically extends about 0.5 cm. on each side of the wound, should appear.[21] Its absence after 7 or 8 days may be the first sign of inadequate healing and impending wound disruption.

After about the third week, or after an open wound becomes closed, the hyperplastic wound tissue begins to resorb and the wound begins to resemble normal connective tissue histologically. Collagen synthesis slows but does not stop. The wound collagen, which up to this time has been almost amorphous, becomes more fibrous, and these fibers intertwine with the normal collagen fibers at the edge of the wound. Although the wound seems static, rapid collagen turnover and gain in tensile strength continue for at least 6 months. The final result is a scar that is relatively strong but inelastic and brittle.

Secondary healing follows essentially the same sequence. However, the emphasis is shifted toward contraction of surrounding skin, epithelization, and the synthesis of new tissue to fill the defect. Nutritional requirements for secondary healing are far greater than for primary repair. If the wound is on the body surface, it is exposed to drying, to injury, and to bacterial contamination. Far more tissue synthesis and epithelization are required. All these processes increase the nutritional and circulatory requirements. Secondary healing, therefore, is more precarious than primary and may not even be possible in an ischemic extremity in which primary healing might occur. In particular, primary healing may occur, albeit slowly, in steroid-treated patients, whereas secondary healing frequently fails.[10, 22, 24]

FIBROPLASIA AND COLLAGEN SYNTHESIS. The fibroblast is the dominant cell in healing tissue and the source of collagen and mucopolysaccharide. Each chain (alpha chain) of the collagen triple helix is synthesized on the ribosomal network of the fibroblast. This step requires an energy source, amino acids and carbohydrate. As the amino-acid chain is assembled, or shortly thereafter, some of the proline and lysine molecules in it are hydroxylated by an essential step that requires iron, ascorbic acid, molecular oxygen, and alphaketoglutarate.[7] If this step is not completed, it is difficult for collagen to be excreted from the cell. After the chain is complete, it is cross-linked (probably by hydrogen bonding) with the two other similar chains and the collagen molecule is formed. The molecule is transported in the Golgi apparatus to the extracellular space.

Before the collagen molecule (monomer) can be polymerized into fibrils, however, a terminal peptide chain on each end of the molecule, the procollagen peptide, is cleaved away. These peptides are essential to the synthesis of collagen and contain sulfated amino acids, which are not present in the finished collagen molecule. This may explain in part the requirement for large amounts of sulfated amino acids for wound healing. On the other hand, mucopolysaccharides, which play an as-yet-unclear role in wound healing, also contain large amounts of sulfate.

The submicroscopic soluble collagen molecules polymerize along their long axes with an overlap of approximately 25 per cent to form the characteristic strong insoluble fibers. Intermolecular cross-binding occurs mainly (but not totally) through covalent linkages between adjacent lysine molecules.[7]

TISSUE LYSIS. Collagen lysis occurs concomitantly with collagen deposition. Wound collagen "turns over" rapidly. The collagen molecule is degraded by a combination of collagenase and proteases. These enzymes are contained in epidermal cells, fibroblasts, and several types of white cells. Partly by successive depositions and removals, the wound collagen, first deposited in disorganized, often gelatinous masses, is slowly remodeled into mechanically more useful patterns. This explains why, in the later phases of healing, wound strength gains while total collagen content diminishes. This is also why apparently healed wounds can break down, as in scurvy, when collagen synthesis is impaired but lysis continues unabated.

NEOVASCULARIZATION. Connective tissue repair is dependent upon neovascularization for nutrition and removal of metabolites. Connective tissue can grow only approximately 100 μ beyond the advancing capillary. In primary wounds, cut vessels on each side of the wound reunite, and some circulation is reconstituted across the wound as early as 3 or 4 days after suture. In dead-space wounds the granulation tissue grows together by advancement and fusion of capillary beds.

The process of angiogenesis is essential to meet the metabolic needs of reparative tissues. Somehow, the host vasculature joins that of a skin graft to establish the early nutrition. Some new circulation generates later. The new vessels are extremely fragile. Immobilization, obviously, is essential to successful skin grafting as well as to successful repair of "mechanically active" tissues such as bone, cartilage, and tendon.

EPITHELIZATION. Epithelium repairs by proliferation and migration of cells. Within 2 days after wounding, increased mitoses are seen in the basal layer of squamous epithelium near the wound, and the new cells migrate across the wound, skipping over established basal cells.[25] As the cells migrate they find a plane with a suitable environment. If the superficial tissue is dry or necrotic, the epithelium grows under it and cleaves it from the viable tissue. If there is no surface necrosis, the epithelium migrates across the surface.[25]

Mitoses are seen only at the edge of the wound, and the new cells migrate across. The reparative cells apparently prepare for the hypoxic conditions of repair by acquiring enzymes suitable for glycolysis. In the process of repair, they derive a greater amount of energy from glycolysis than do normal cells.[15] Nevertheless, they retain the ability to use oxygen when it is available, and epithelization is slightly faster in the presence of added oxygen.[10, 25]

CONTRACTION. Contraction is the process by which open wounds in soft tissue spontaneously close by inward migration of normal tissue.[10] It should not be confused with "contracture," which refers to loss of motion from shrinkage of existing scar tissue. The force of contraction, and possibly some of the force that leads to contracture, is apparently supplied by "myofibroblasts" with microscopic features of both smooth muscle and fibroblast. Strips of contracting wound shorten in response to smooth-muscle stimulators. Contraction proceeds more rapidly when the wound is exposed to smooth-muscle stimulators and is slowed by smooth-muscle relaxants. It is almost stopped by anti-inflammatory steroids.[11] Contraction, obviously, is most effective in the loose skin of the neck and abdomen.

HEALING AS A RESULTANT OF OPPOSING FORCES. Healing can be regarded as a battle between tissue synthesis and lysis (Fig. 2–1). Collagen lysis is a part of the general catabolic process that follows injury and starvation, and collagen is a prime source of amino acids for the reserve pool. When lysis is exaggerated, it leaves the wound unusually weak unless collagen synthesis is correspondingly increased. Cortisol released by stress causes some lysis of collagen. Exogenous cortisol causes fragile skin and osteoporotic bone (Cushing's syndrome).

Infection and inflammation decrease the collagen content of tissue far more than does simple scalpel injury. Excessive inflammation and infection are probably the most potent causes of excessive lysis and failure of tissue surfaces to unite.[9, 10, 12]

Collagen synthesis, on the other hand, is also easily hindered. Starvation sufficient to

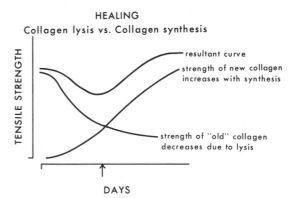

HEALING
Collagen lysis vs. Collagen synthesis

resultant curve
strength of new collagen increases with synthesis
strength of "old" collagen decreases due to lysis

TENSILE STRENGTH

DAYS

Figure 2–1 Interaction of collagen synthesis and lysis. Pathological healing is likely to result if the synthesis curve is delayed (moved to the right) or if lysis is exaggerated and its curve is moved downward. (From Hunt, T. K.: Wound healing. *In* Paparella, M. M., and Shumrick, D. A.: (Eds.): Otolaryngology. Vol. I. Philadelphia, W. B. Saunders Company, 1973.)

cause a weight loss of 15 per cent or more in some experimental animals has been reported to delay collagen synthesis. Feeding methionine or cysteine restores almost to normal healing retarded by protein depletion (at least in animals). Lysine deficiency also impairs healing in animals. Appropriate experiments in man have not been performed.

Ascorbic acid deficiency, or scurvy, severely impairs collagen synthesis in man. It is now relatively rare but still occurs in the alcohol or drug addict, the fad dieter, and the severely injured patient. Zinc deficiency also seems to delay collagen synthesis.

Anti-inflammatory steroids given in the first few days after injury inhibit inflammation, inactivate macrophages, and thereby delay all subsequent events, including fibroplasia and epithelization. Steroids also increase susceptibility to infection. Therapeutic steroids given at any time during the course of secondary healing will impair contraction, granulation, and epithelization. Fortunately, vitamin A, given either locally or systemically, will stimulate steroid-inhibited inflammation.[11] Thereafter, fibroplasia and epithelization are stimulated. Since patients who are taking steroids have an increased risk of suture-line failure, this effect of vitamin A is clinically useful. Vitamin A does not seem to restore contraction, however.[11] Dose relationships are unknown. Oral doses of 25,000 units of vitamin A are probably adequate, except possibly in severely injured patients. Locally applied vitamin A in commercially available creams seems adequate for use on steroid retarded open wounds. It is usually applied several times daily.

Severe trauma, even at a distance from the wound, impairs nutritional blood flow and fibroplasia. Restoration of blood volume improves healing but does not make it normal after trauma.[3, 28]

As noted previously, molecular oxygen is required for collagen synthesis. Wounding diminishes blood and oxygen supply, whereas inflammation and fibroplasia increase the need for oxygen. Wounds normally are hypoxic.[14, 15] Anything that deprives the wound of oxygen slows collagen synthesis and probably increases susceptibility to infection. Any factor that increases arterial Po_2 within safe limits increases collagen synthesis and reduces susceptibility to infection.[10, 13, 14, 15, 16]

Hypovolemia causes vasoconstriction, which impairs healing. In hypovolemia, increased arterial Po_2 cannot restore wound oxygen tension to normal. Normovolemic anemia, however, does not interfere with oxygen transport to the wound or with healing until the anemia is very severe.[8] Hematocrit values in the range of 20 to 30 per cent do not significantly influence wound healing and do not change wound Po_2 unless the anemia is secondary to hypovolemia. Perhaps the only exceptions to this rule occur in patients whose cardiac reserve cannot compensate for the anemia and the increased blood flow requirements. Because injury damages vascularity and thus increases diffusion resistance, wound oxygen supply is governed by arterial Po_2 (not hemoglobin content) under normal circumstances of blood flow to the wound.[10]

Many drugs interfere with collagen synthesis. Some of these that are used frequently in medical practice are actinomycin D, nitrogen mustards, cyclophosphamide, 5-fluorouracil, methotrexate, chloramphenicol, and dicumarol. In very large doses, penicillamine interferes with cross-linking of collagen.[10]

Radiation injury interferes with fibroblast function just as it interferes with tumor-cell function. However, healing is not impaired in the 6 weeks after the completion of well managed radiotherapy. More than 6 weeks after therapy, one sees radiation changes of progressive fibrosis of vessels and diminution of vascular supply. The notoriously poor healing in areas of irradiation injury is analogous to the poor healing seen in scleroderma. The risk of poor healing is proportional to the visible radiation damage.[10]

The healing area absolutely requires an adequate blood flow. Wounds closed under tension and narrow-base flaps heal poorly. Shock, hypotension, and intravascular thrombosis all can actually *prevent* healing.

Diabetics tend to heal poorly. Well-controlled diabetics, however, rarely have healing problems except in ischemic, neuropathic tissue. According to animal experiments, diabetic "control" is especially important during the first few days (the inflammatory phase) of repair.[6]

LACK OF HEALING.   Wounds mature according to a sequence which should be familiar to every surgeon. He should be ready to note and admit that wound healing is falling behind schedule. Then, using a detailed knowledge of wound healing, he must review all possible causes. Contrary to the "law of parsimony", impaired wound healing is as often due to multiple causes as it is to one cause. Exogenous steroids are probably the most common cause of delayed repair seen in practice, and the use of vitamin A is indicated, as already noted. Present data indicate (but do not yet prove) that vitamin A does not reduce the immunosuppressive action of cortisone, and it probably can be used safely to stimulate steroid-retarded wound healing even in the presence of a transplanted organ.

Malnutrition is probably the second most common cause of delayed repair. One can test individually for serum zinc, vitamin C, and albumin. On the other hand, the nutrients that are usually lacking are inexpensive and have few side effects, even when given in great quantities.

The presence of sepsis, either in the wound or elsewhere, will slow repair. The mechanism is not known, and it may be that nutritional supplementation will return the retarded, uninfected wound to normal healing despite distant sepsis. At present, surgical correction of fistulas and drainage of sepsis are essential to normal repair.

Poor healing may require temporary withdrawal of cytotoxic drugs in order to achieve closure so that the future use of these drugs can be uncomplicated. It is folly to continue such drugs as 5-fluorouracil in the immediate postoperative period if the integrity of a precarious colon or esophageal anastomosis is at stake. The surgeon must often choose whether he wants good repair or drug effect. Fortunately, a brief respite from drugs is usually sufficient to stimulate or allow adequate repair.

Supplemental oxygen will insure greater take of skin grafts and may make the difference between adequate healing and none at all in cases in which healing has been retarded by inadequate local blood flow caused by diabetes, scleroderma, or radiation injury. In any case, the maintenance of normal blood volume is essential to insure adequate oxygenation via the vascular route.

WOUND DEHISCENCE

Wound dehiscence is a major complication that is particularly significant in the abdomen and joints. Dehiscence of an abdominal wound is associated with a mortality rate of approximately 20 per cent. It occurs about once in every 200 surgical procedures, but the rate varies widely depending on the surgeon, the patient, and the type of operation. In an abdominal wound, total dehiscence may lead to evisceration; and partial, deep dehiscence may lead to ventral hernia. Dehiscence of the synovial membrane may greatly prolong morbidity, particularly after operations on the knee and shoulder. Dehiscence of chest wounds is rare except after median sternotomy. Impending separation of an abdominal wound is often preceded by serosanguineous drainage; and that of a lateral thoracotomy wound, by parodoxical motion.

Dehiscence essentially represents failure to heal. Infection is present in approximately half. Hypoproteinemia, advanced age, and hypertension may contribute to dehiscence.[19] Other mechanisms are probable but are still clinically unproven. Dehiscence usually occurs between the fifth and eighth day after operation. This is as one would expect from exaggerated wound collagen lysis when synthetic mechanisms are not adequate to replace the lysed collagen. Almost all cases of dehiscence occur in patients in whom a healing ridge has not developed by the fifth to eighth day (see Fig. 2–1).[21]

In most cases of dehiscence, reexploration reveals that the sutures have torn through the tissue rather than being dissolved or untied. Tying sutures too tightly strangulates wound circulation and is probably the most common technical error leading to dehiscence. Studies have shown that a few surgeons will have many wounds with dehiscence, and others will have extremely few. Surgical technique is important.[5, 10]

Other technical errors include using a light suture closure in a heavy, muscular patient who will cough forcefully postoperatively; using a light closure in patients who are severely ill and can be expected not to heal; failure to combat severe abdominal distention; and using too many sutures. Preventing dehiscence requires assessment of "wound risk" so that these errors can be

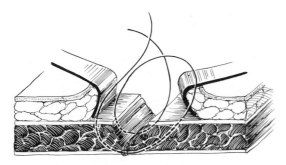

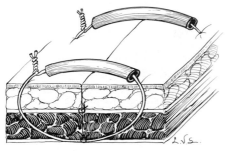

Figure 2–2 Wire sutures placed correctly with "bolster" to prevent wound dehiscence.

loosened or tightened as necessary later. The skin should be protected with "bolsters" or one of the frames available commercially. Sutures should be placed about 2.5 cm. apart and 2.5 cm. back from the wound (Fig. 2–2). This closure is painful and also carries a slight risk of injury to deeper structures and consequent fistula formation. These sutures also require daily dressing, cleansing, and adjustment of the wires. In sternotomies, plastic sutures can be used safely since it is not necessary to include the skin, and sutures rarely cut through.

The most secure closure for general abdominal use is buried No. 28 wire or equally heavy monofilament plastic in the fascia, with well over 1 cm. of fascia taken in each bite and the sutures spaced about as far apart as they are wide.[18] The "Tom Jones" suture (Fig. 2–3) or far-far, near-near suture is used by many, but others prefer widely spaced, large simple sutures alternating with enough smaller, looser sutures to achieve accurate approximation of the edges of the wound. I use this closure for major abdominal wounds in all but the most healthy and the most ill patients; and with it, dehiscence is extremely rare.

In general, wounds in the upper abdomen are less secure than those in the lower.

avoided. The most "dehiscence-proof" closure is done with heavy No. 22 to 24 wire through all layers except peritoneum, which is closed separately if possible. Wire should be used because it can be twisted tightly and

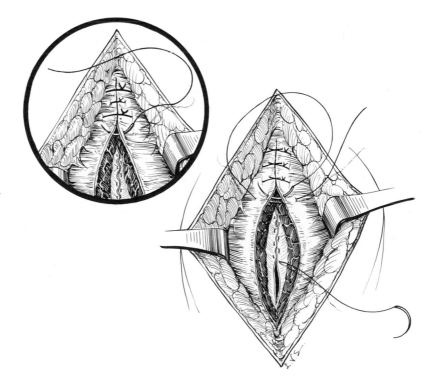

Figure 2–3 Tom Jones suture.

The widely heralded safety factor of the transverse incision is small, if real at all, under modern conditions.

When dehiscence occurs, the surgeon has two choices: to do nothing except provide external support, pack the wound to prevent evisceration, and accept the hernia that inevitably follows; or to reanesthetize the patient, take out the *entire* closure, and substitute a retention suture closure with large wires. The individual layers are usually too friable to be closed anatomically. If infection is present, the skin should be left open. The usefulness of adjustable wire closure cannot be stressed too strongly. Tied plastic through-and-through sutures are either strangulating or too loose. They lead to fistula formation in too many patients. Dehisced wounds are usually edematous. The edema will eventually subside and the sutures will need to be tightened. If healing still has not occurred, a loose, nonadjustable suture merely limits the distance of separation of the wound edges. The suture "bowstrings" across the gap and will "saw" through viscera and cause fistulas.

When dehiscence occurs, a defect of healing must be suspected and corrected, unless the problem is obviously mechanical.

WOUND PAIN

Wound pain is the most common complaint of surgical patients. When retention sutures are used, wound pain may be localized to one or more particular spots. The pain will usually diminish in time. Hypesthesia, due to nerve damage, is the next most common complaint. The patient will become accustomed to the hypesthesia, and sensation will improve somewhat. After several months, patients rarely are concerned about hypesthesia. If a painful area persists, it may be due to a small stitch abscess, an encysted retention suture, a neuroma, or a hernia.

Painful sutures can be removed under local anesthesia. Neuromas usually cause discrete tender spots that when irritated cause radiating pain. They can be removed easily under local anesthesia.

SERUM COLLECTION

Serum collections are most frequent in wounds that have a large potential dead space, such as mastectomy wounds or wounds in obese patients. The fluid, though similar to plasma, is characterized by deficiency of oxygen, alpha globulin, and gamma globulin, and excess of hydrogen ion and carbon dioxide. This fluid possesses some natural resistance to infection, and the levels of antibiotics in it can be equated with serum antibiotic levels if necessary.[1, 2, 10] The danger of infection following aseptic aspiration of serum collections is not great, but the collection usually recurs. If a serum collection is large, placement of a dependent stab wound and a small drain together with a pressure dressing on the wound is easier and better than aspiration. When the dead space has been obliterated by drainage, susceptibility to infection is greatly diminished.

HEMORRHAGE

Wound hemorrhage occurs most frequently in patients with hypertension or coagulation defects associated with trauma and massive transfusion. Most wound hematomas result from surgically controllable bleeding. The diffuse oozing from the wound that accompanies coagulation defects usually is associated with bleeding into a body cavity as well and is rarely accompanied by hematoma formation. The treatment for an expanding hematoma is to reopen the wound under sterile conditions and locate and ligate the bleeding vessel. Procrastination leads to continued bleeding, hard and painful hematomas, and possible wound infection.

DRAINS

Wound drainage is one of the most unnecessarily used procedures in surgery. Drainage of an established abscess or to allow egress of an undesirable substance (such as pus, bile, or extravasated blood) when it is expected to come from a specific spot at which a drain can be placed is necessary and prudent; but drainage in generalized peritonitis, for example, is not. I rarely insert drains for possible blood collections. Routine drainage of splenectomy wounds has proved to be harmful rather than helpful. Drains provide a channel for bacteria to enter as well as for other substances to leave; because of the danger of infection, drainage through primary surgical wounds is rarely indicated. A stab wound can be used more easily and safely for drainage.

Drains must be soft. Hard plastic sump drains cause fistulas by eroding into surrounding bowel or even blood vessels. Soft sump drains can be purchased or improvised. One dependent drain, however, is worth a dozen nondependent sump drains.

Drainage of duodenal and colon suture lines is controversial. In no case should a drain lie in contact with a crucial suture line, but drains probably should be brought near traumatic wounds in the duodenum. I generally prefer not to drain colon suture lines; if drainage is thought to be necessary, colostomy probably should be done. A presacral drain near difficult low anterior anastomosis may prevent pelvic sepsis, however.

SUTURE SINUSES

Sinus tracts form when multifilament nonabsorbable sutures become infected and the infection works its way to the surface. Formation of a sinus tract in or near the wound weeks or more after surgery usually has a foreign body at its source. Gentle exploration with an ordinary crochet hook frequently removes the suture. If a suture cannot be found, waiting a few weeks for spontaneous ejection may be wise. However, no patient should have to tolerate a draining sinus for many weeks or months. If the sinus persists, it is best to open the entire affected portion of the wound and remove all local suture material under local anesthesia and good lighting conditions. Occasionally, the incautiously used probe opens the bowel or joint space.

INFECTION

Wound infections generally appear from the fifth to tenth postoperative day although they may appear as early as 1 day or as late as many years after operation. Most occur in subcutaneous tissue. The first sign usually is fever, and unexplained fever requires inspection of the wound. Wound pain may also reappear. The wound rarely appears severely inflamed, but local edema made obvious by tight skin sutures is often prominent.

Firm or fluctuant areas, crepitus, or tenderness can be detected with minimal pain and contamination if surgical soap is poured on the wound and used as a lubricant, and palpation is done gently with the gloved hand. The rare infection deep to the fascia may be difficult to find. If there is doubt about its existence and a decision must be made, the surgeon can carefully open the wound in the suspected area. If no pus is found, the wound can be closed again with tapes.

Before antibiotics were introduced, streptococcal and staphylococcal infections were common. When antibiotics became available many surgeons felt that their prophylactic use would end wound infections. When the unforeseen problem of resistant strains emerged, staphylococcal infections again became prominent. Operating room and dressing discipline coupled with reduced use of antibiotics controlled the staphylococcus epidemic. Now, most infections are due to endogenous bacteria, many of them gram-negative and anaerobes. When an individual hospital or ward has an outbreak of infections, the source must be found and eliminated.

No means have yet been devised to eliminate bacteria completely from the wound. With extraordinary precautions, such as operating through ports in sterilized plastic chambers, external contamination can be excluded, but even then the patient himself contributes bacteria within the wound. All wounds are contaminated. Nevertheless, prevention of infection is still the most important aspect of care of the patient.

There are three main steps in preventing infection: (1) gentle, clean surgery; (2) reduction of contamination; and (3) support of the patient's defenses.[1, 2, 3, 4, 5, 13]

The surgeon who traumatizes tissue, leaves foreign bodies or hematomas, uses mass ligatures, or exposes the wound to drying or pressure from retractors is inviting infection. This cannot be emphasized too strongly. Repair of a hernia on a kitchen table by a good, gentle surgeon would probably be safer than rough treatment by an indecisive surgeon in a modern operating room.

Preparation of the skin tends to become part of an operative ritual whose performance is reassuring but not necessarily effective. There are countless skin preparations, but none has proved more effective than soap and water followed by a 1 per cent aqueous iodine solution. The risk of iodine "burn" is small with *aqueous* iodine.

Many means of reducing air contamination have been devised, but except in extreme cases, no one has convincingly related "fallout" contamination with wound infection rates. Operating theater ventilation must be effective and clean, but expensive air-flow systems add little or no benefit.

Plastic protectors inserted into the wound and over its surface are effective in preventing wound contamination.[23] Contaminated wounds can be washed gently with Ringer's lactate solution in order to remove dead tissue and surface bacteria. In some cases irrigation with antibiotic solutions is probably effective.

Closure techniques also influence infection rates. Subcutaneous sutures are foreign bodies in the most infection-prone part of the wound. They should be used sparingly, and principally when large dead spaces are sure to result if they are omitted. Using skin tapes instead of skin sutures lowers infection rates in contaminated wounds (Fig. 2–4). Bleeding from the wound sometimes obviates the use of tapes. If so, the wound can be sutured and the sutures replaced with tapes on the second day. This method retains most of the advantages of skin tapes.[5]

Severely contaminated wounds in which infection is likely are best left open and closed secondarily.[27] In civilian practice this usually means that the deep layers are closed while skin and subcutaneous tissue are left open and covered with sterile (and occlusive) dressings. The wound is inspected on the fifth day, and closed (preferably with skin tapes) if *no* sign of infection is seen. A clean granulating open wound is superior to a wound infection. Scarring from secondary healing is usually less than anticipated. This method prevents abscess formation and increased "wound morbidity" in a large percentage of patients.

Most sutured or taped wounds can safely be left without dressings, but wounds are susceptible to surface contamination for the first 24 to 48 hours (less if tapes are used instead of sutures). If contamination is likely, protective dressings should be used.

The patient has many defenses against infection which the surgeon can support. Sufficient blood volume, adequate arterial

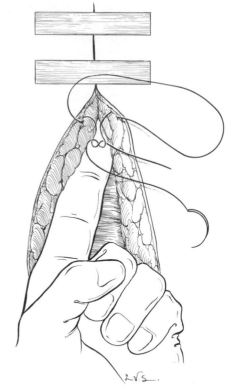

Figure 2–4   Use of skin tapes to lessen the risk of infection in a contaminated wound.

oxygenation, and good nutrition all help to prevent infection.[10]

The use of antibiotics as a means of *preventing* surgical wound infection is still somewhat controversial. There is an inevitable and deplorable tendency to use them "just to be sure," especially for operations in which foreign substances are implanted. Good studies show that antibiotics are of little value in preventing infections after basically clean surgery. Whenever antibiotics are used unnecessarily, an unwarranted risk is taken not only in that patient but in future patients as well.

Severely contaminated wounds are a different matter. Careful selection of antibiotics that have a reasonable chance of being effective against the contaminating organisms and administration early enough so that their concentration in the blood is adequate *by the time of wounding* can lower but will not eliminate a contaminated high risk of infection after surgery.[1, 2, 10] Penicillin should be given for obviously contaminated traumatic wounds containing contused tissue, as tetanus prophylaxis. Most surgeons use antibiotics as part of standard operative therapy for penetrating wounds of the abdomen.[2] If an old wound that was once infected is to be reopened, the patient should be given antibiotics that are specifically effective against the organism that caused the old infection. Many studies demonstrate that most of the effect to be obtained from prophylactic antibiotics is achieved a few hours after operation. The only way to prevent disastrous ecological changes in hospital flora is to start antibiotics immediately prior to operation and discontinue them by the next day or within the day that intravascular tubes are removed from patients in whom vital foreign bodies have been implanted.

Wound infections are treated by opening the wound and allowing it to drain. Antibiotics are usually not necessary unless the infection is invasive. Bacterial culture is necessary: (1) to help locate the source of infection and prevent its spread to other patients; (2) as a preview of the bacteriologic aspects in case other infections develop deep to the wound; (3) for selection of prophylactic antibiotics should the wound have to be entered again; and (4) if the infection should become invasive if the host resistance falls.

ANAEROBIC INFECTIONS. Infections of surgical and traumatic wounds with anaerobic organisms are now being reported more frequently, probably because of improvements in microbiologic technique. *Bacteroides fragilis* and microaerophilic streptococcus infections are now commonly seen. The low oxidation-reduction potential present in wounded tissue makes it vulnerable to these organisms, and when degenerating muscle and foreign body are added, the stage is set for advancing anaerobic infection.

Invasive anaerobic gangrene is a disastrous complication that requires spectacular efforts in management. A threefold approach employing débridement, hyperbaric oxygen, and antibiotics must be taken. The first step is to gain surgical control of the disease by débriding all dead tissue. Large amounts of tissue, even full-thickness abdominal wall (in which temporary placement of plastic mesh will prevent evisceration), may need to be removed. The differentiation between live and dead and between infected and noninfected tissue may be difficult to make. Therefore, the wound should be inspected within the next 24 hours and redébrided if necessary.

In the case of clostridial gangrene, hyperbaric oxygen treatment, if available, can save tissue and even life. However, in many patients with spreading anaerobic infections delivery of oxygen to the peripheral tissues is decreased. For this reason, measures should be taken to support blood volume and the oxygen transport mechanisms.

Antibiotics should be used vigorously. A gram-stained smear of infected tissue should be examined immediately. If streptococci or clostridia are found, massive doses of penicillin should be given. Gram-negative rods and the fetid odor of Bacteroides call for other specific therapy. Mixed infections of streptococcus and various types of gram-negative organisms are frequently responsible for "synergistic bacterial gangrene." In this case the choice of antibiotic is more difficult and must be determined by culture, preferably with direct sensitivity studies.

In the repair of the huge tissue defects that may result, homografts or pigskin xenografts are helpful in preparing the tissue for final closure. If used as temporary dressings, they do not inhibit wound contraction but do decrease bacterial counts in the wound. In most cases, after an abdominal wall of granulation and fibrous tissue is formed, infected plastic mesh can be removed, if necessary, and the hernia repaired at a later date.

HYPERTROPHIC SCARS, CONTRACTED SCARS, AND KELOIDS

The major prophylaxis against hypertrophic scar is proper placement of incisions. Incisions that cross isotonic lines, particularly in highly movable areas, often result in hypertrophic scars; in accidental wounds so placed, hypertrophy may be prevented by immobilization. In other cases, as soon as hypertrophy is obvious, injection of anti-inflammatory corticosteroids can reverse the process, but too much corticoid can cause an atrophic scar.

Keloids develop in surgical, traumatic and

injection wounds, particularly in members of the dark-skinned races (including Orientals), although Caucasians are occasionally affected. Keloids are by far most commonly seen in the area between the ears and the mid-chest. They too can be treated by injecting steroids during the formative phases, but once a large keloid is established, steroids are relatively ineffective. Resection and primary closure, followed by steroid injection as soon as primary healing is achieved, can reduce the mass of the keloid. Irradiation therapy is said to be effective, but must be given immediately after operation. The cause of keloids is unknown, but both the collagen synthesis and collagen lysis in the keloid are increased. Current theories implicate autoimmune mechanisms.[16]

The best means of predicting and preventing keloid formation is to find out whether the patient has had previous keloids. If so, careful closure, with use of skin tapes or subcuticular closure, and early corticoid injection are useful.

Contracted scars are prevented or treated in much the same way as hypertrophic wounds. In relatively young scars, pressure dressings will reduce the mass, and traction will restore the length of the scar and motion of the contracted joint.[17] Once the scar is adequately lengthened, splinting for several months (perhaps accompanied by steroid injections) will usually prevent further contracture.[17]

REOPERATION THROUGH EXISTING WOUNDS

When a recently sutured wound is reopened, or when dehiscence due solely to mechanical causes occurs, the wound can be reclosed and will heal to tensile integrity almost as rapidly as if it had never been reopened. That is, a wound resutured on the eighth day after the original wound, becomes 3 days later an "11-day wound," not a "3-day wound." This is because the wound has already undergone the inflammatory phase and some of the early fibroplasia, and no further time is lost in remustering these forces.[10] Early reoperation should be done through the original wound if it is surgically appropriate. It

makes no sense to excise the wound and close it in fresh tissue unless infected foreign body or scarred skin that would be difficult to close has been removed.

In reentering war wounds and wounds that were known to have been contaminated by soil or foreign body, penicillin prophylaxis is warranted because of the risk of tetanus and gas gangrene following reexploration. The risk of reinfection decreases with time, and many believe that no prophylaxis is required if a year has elapsed since the original procedure. I have seen reinfection occur years after operation, however, and I believe that specific prophylactic antibiotics are warranted for any reentry through previously infected tissue.

HERNIA

Hernia formation is a common complication of abdominal and flank wounds; its incidence after primary healing is about 1 per cent. The incidence after wound infection rises to about 10 per cent, and after dehiscence and reclosure the chance of hernia formation is about 30 per cent. A hernia will form in any tissue defect the surgeon leaves behind. Defects can be due to a loose suture or to one that is too tight and has "cut through" the tissue that surrounds it. Frequently, there is not just a single hernia but a complex of several small hernias. Recent studies indicate that closure of peritoneum subtracts little from the incidence of incisional hernia.

Repair of incisional hernias can be difficult. Patients who are grossly overweight rarely undergo successful repair. Loss of 30 per cent of weight increases reparability dramatically. Except under unusual circumstances, the repair should not be done until the old wound has stopped remodeling — that is, at least 6 months, or even better, a year after wounding. Too early repair dooms the patient to recurrence.

In repairing ventral hernias, the entire wound should be examined from the peritoneal side for satellite hernias. Successful repair cannot be accomplished if tissue is under tension, and relaxing incisions in the anterior rectus may be useful. Most experienced surgeons prefer to join unscarred tissue over hernia defects rather than to suture the hard scarred hernial ring. I try to suture the ring as a deep layer, then develop an edge of unscarred anterior fascia and close it as a second layer. Occasionally, insertion of a prosthetic mesh is necessary; at present, polypropylene mesh is the material of choice. When this is used, monofilament plastic sutures should be used as well. It is important to close a tissue layer beneath the plastic mesh. Otherwise, satellite hernias around the mesh and between the sutures are liable to develop. Since infection is so prominent a feature of hernia formation, old infections of the wound to be repaired should be treated.

In a few patients, hernias will form because of connective tissue abnormalities such as Ehlers-Danlos syndrome and probably other as-yet-uncharacterized disorders. Usually, such patients have had several unsuccessful repairs. In treating these patients, the surgeon must then give careful consideration to whether the hernia can be surgically repaired, because such hernias usually become larger with each unsuccessful repair. When repair is attempted, closure should be reinforced and all one knows about fostering repair should be used. Nevertheless, when one is faced with an incisional hernia that has resisted several repairs, one should not assume that he can solve the problem simply because he is "better" than all the past surgeons. There may be a patient factor to account for the problem.

Bibliography

1. Alexander, J. W., Sykes, N. S., Mitchell, M. M., and Fisher, M. W.: Concentration of selected intravenously administered antibiotics in experimental surgical wounds. J. Trauma 13:423, 1973.
2. Altemeier, W. A., Burke, J. F., Pruitt, B. A., and Sandusky, W. R.: Manual on Control of Infection in Surgical Patients. American College of Surgeons. Philadelphia, J. B. Lippincott Company, 1976.
   This book, in my mind, is required reading for all surgeons. Several references in this chapter refer to separate parts of the book.
3. Conolly, W. B., Hunt, T. K., Sonne, M., and Dunphy, J. E.: Influence of distant trauma on local wound infection. Surg., Gynecol. Obstet. 128:713, 1969.
4. Cruse, P. J. E., and Foord, R.: A five-year prospective study of 23,649 surgical wounds. Arch. Surg. 107:206, 1973.
5. Edlich, R. F., Rodeheaver, G., Thacker, J. G., and

6. Goodson, W. H., III, and Hunt, T. K.: Wound healing and the diabetic patient. Surg., Gynecol. Obstet. 149:600, 1979.
7. Grant, M. E., and Prockop, D. J.: The biosynthesis of collagen. N. Engl. J. Med. 286:194, 1972.
   Part 1 of a two part exhaustive review.
8. Heughan, C., Grislis, G., and Hunt, T. K.: The effect of anemia on wound healing. Ann. Surg. 179:163, 1974.
9. Hunt, T. K. (Ed.): Wound Healing and Wound Infection. New York, Appleton-Century-Crofts, 1980.
   A recent research compendium with many chapters useful to the practicing surgeon and student of wound healing.
10. Hunt, T. K., and Dunphy, J. E. (Eds.): Fundamentals of Wound Management. New York, Appleton-Century-Crofts, 1979.
    A book devoted to summarizing the basic science of wound healing for practical use. References to this book refer to chapters by T. K. Hunt (healing), J. F. Burke (infection), J. E. Meakins (infection), S. Levenson (nutrition), and R. Edlich (surgical techniques).
11. Hunt, T. K., Ehrlich, H. P., Garcia, J. A., and Dunphy, J. E.: Effect of vitamin A on reversing the inhibitory effect of cortisone on healing of open wounds in animals and man. Ann. Surg. 170:633, 1969.
12. Hunt, T. K., and Hawley, P. R.: Surgical judgment and colonic anastomoses. Dis. Colon Rectum. 12:167, 1969.
13. Hunt, T. K., Linsey, M., Grislis, G., Sonne, M., and Jawetz, E.: The effect of differing ambient oxygen tensions on wound infections. Ann. Surg. 181:35, 1975.
14. Hunt, T. K., and Pai, M. P.: The effect of varying ambient oxygen tensions on wound metabolism and collagen synthesis. Surg. Gynecol. Obstet. 135:561, 1972.
15. Im, M. J. C., and Hoopes, J. E.: Energy metabolism in healing skin wounds. J. Surg. Res. 10:459, 1970.
16. Ketchum, L. D., Cohen, I. K., and Masters, F. W.: Hypertrophic scar and keloids: A collective review. Plast. Reconstr. Surg. 53:140, 1974.
17. Larson, D. L., Abston, S., Evans, E. B., Dobrovsky, M., and Linares, H. A.: Techniques for decreasing scar formation and contractures in the burned patient. J. Trauma 11:807, 1971.
18. McCallum, G. T., and Link, R. F.: The effect of closure techniques on abdominal disruption. Surg. Gynecol. Obstet. 119:75, 1964.
19. May, J., Chalmers, J. P., Lowenthal, J., and Rountree, P. M.: Factors in the patient contribution to surgical sepsis. Surg. Gynecol. Obstet. 122:28, 1966.
20. Montandon, D., D'Andisan, T., and Gabbiani, G.: The mechanism of wound contraction and epithelization. Clin. Plast. Surg. 4:325, July, 1977.
    This volume also contains a number of other authoritative reviews on assorted topics in wound healing.

Edgerton, M. T.: Technical factors in wound management. In Hunt, T. K., and Dunphy, J. E. (Eds.): Fundamentals of Wound Management. New York, Appleton-Century-Crofts, 1979, pp. 364–454.

21. Pareira, M. D., and Serkes, K. D.: Prediction of wound disruption by use of the healing ridge. Surg. Gynecol Obstet. *115*:72, 1962.

22. Peacock, E. E., and Van Winkle, W., Jr.: Wound Repair. 2nd Ed. Philadelphia, W.B. Saunders Company, 1970.
    A highly authoritative book with emphasis on skin and tendon repair and collagen biology in wounds.

23. Raahave, D.: Aseptic barriers of plastic to prevent bacterial contamination of operation wounds. Acta Chir. Scand. *140*:603, 1974.

24. Ross, R.: Inflammation, cell proliferation and connective tissue formation in wound repair. *In* Hunt, T. K. (Ed.): Wound Healing and Wound Infection. New York, Appleton-Century-Crofts, 1980.

25. Rovee, D. T., Kurowsky, C. A., Labun, J., and Downes, A. M.: Effect of local wound environment on epidermal healing. *In* Maibach, H. I., and Rovee, D. T. (Ed.): Epidermal Wound Healing. Chicago, Year Book Medical Publishers, Inc., 1972, p. 159.
    The most inclusive and authoritative single reference on epithelization.

26. Stein, J. M., and Levenson, S. M.: Effect of the inflammatory reaction on subsequent wound healing. Surg. Forum *17*:484, 1966.

27. Verrier, E. D., Bossart, J., and Heer, F. W.: Reduction of infection rates in abdominal incisions by delayed wound closure techniques. Am. J. Surg. *138*:22, 1979.

28. Zederfeldt, B. H., and Hunt, T. K.: The effects of trauma on respiratory gases in healing wounds. Cur. Top. Surg. Res. *1*:297, 1969.

3

SHOCK

Lazar J. Greenfield

HISTORICAL PERSPECTIVE

The current emphasis on adequate fluid volume replacement in shock therapy can be traced to a classic study in experimental shock reported by Alfred Blalock in 1930.[7] Prior to that time, the relationship between trauma and shock was based on a theory favoring toxic action of a histaminelike substance, with production of generalized vasodilatation. Dr. Blalock showed that sufficient blood and plasma were sequestered in a traumatized extremity to explain the resulting shock on the basis of hypovolemia. These observations were extended to clinical practice, and the administration of blood and plasma expanders markedly improved the results of resuscitation of the wounded in World War II. During this same period the first efforts to obtain hemodynamic data from patients in shock were made by Cournand and his associates,[14] who introduced the concept of therapy based on objective measurements made at the bedside of the patient.

As knowledge increased and financial support became available, special shock study units were established in medical centers across the country where more sophisticated clinical investigation could be performed. Data from these studies over the past 15 years have provided new insight into the full spectrum of clinical shock states and required revision of most time-honored concepts of shock based on hypotension and reduced cardiac output alone. We must acknowledge now that some forms of septic shock are associated with normal or increased cardiac output, and a more appropriate definition of shock must recognize the more fundamental cellular problem. Accordingly, we may define shock as a generalized imbalance between the metabolic needs of vital organs and available blood flow, leading to inadequate cellular function.

DIAGNOSIS OF SHOCK

CRITERIA. The clinical picture of a patient in shock will vary with antecedent circumstances, but characteristically it is associated with signs of poor perfusion, i.e., weakness, paleness, hypotension, and a systolic blood pressure less than 80 mm. Hg. Generally a reduction in blood volume of 30 to 40 per cent is required to produce these effects. The adrenergic response to these events results in sweating, hyperventilation, tachycardia, and peripheral vasoconstric-

Lazar John Greenfield, born in Houston, attended Rice University and was elected to Alpha Omega Alpha at Baylor University College of Medicine. He interned and served his residency at the Johns Hopkins Hospital, with an interim 2 years at the National Heart Institute. In 1966 he joined the surgical staff of the University of Oklahoma as Assistant Professor and became full Professor of Surgery in 1971. In 1968 he became a John and Mary R. Markle Scholar and has received numerous important national appointments and memberships. In 1974 he was appointed Stuart McGuire Professor and Chairman, Department of Surgery at the Medical College of Virginia, Virginia Commonwealth University. Dr. Greenfield has long had a special interest in the circulation, and his research and writings in the field of experimental and clinical shock have been extensive.

TABLE 3–1 CLASSIFICATION OF SHOCK

   I. Hypovolemic
    A. External loss, e.g., blood, plasma, water
    B. Sequestration – distributive abnormality
       1. Intravascular
         a. Arteriolar resistance loss, e.g., spinal shock
         b. Capacitance pooling, venous system, e.g., endotoxin
       2. Extravascular
         a. Exudative, e.g., peritonitis
         b. Traumatic, e.g., hematoma
  II. Cardiogenic
    A. Intrinsic power
       1. Focal, e.g., infarct or aneurysm
       2. Generalized, e.g., drug effect or ischemia
    B. Extrinsic factors
       1. Obstructive, e.g., pulmonary embolus
       2. Compressive, e.g., cardiac tamponade
 III. Peripheral vascular
    A. Neural factors, e.g., neurogenic shock (fainting)
    B. Humoral factors, e.g., anaphylactic shock, histamine shock

tion producing cool extremities. There is initial anxiety with minimal alteration in level of consciousness, followed by apathy, and finally stupor. The only complaint may be intense thirst, even in the presence of severe wounds. Rectal temperature is usually reduced.

Further objective confirmation of the diagnosis is obtained from signs of poor organ function, specifically, oliguria, with urine output of less than 25 ml. per hour, and a progressive metabolic acidosis. Measurement of cardiac output will usually show reduction below 2.5 liters per minute per square meter, but this value alone is insufficient for diagnosis, since patients with chronic heart failure can tolerate similar depression without the progressive deterioration characteristic of the patient in shock.

CLASSIFICATION OF SHOCK. Each of the many efforts at classification of shock was designed to encompass existing knowledge of physiological mechanisms and was subsequently rendered obsolete by discovery of new mechanisms and areas of overlap. Much of current research in shock is directed toward sorting out mechanisms to establish cause and effect. However, the deterioration of a particular organ system rarely occurs at a discrete point in time, and multisystem derangements are more characteristic of progressive stages of shock.

The classification proposed (Table 3–1) recognizes individual and combined derangements of the factors responsible for cardiovascular integrity: circulating volume, peripheral vascular resistance, and adequacy of the pump. This also suggests a mechanistic basis for therapy. It must be recognized, however, that shock may be a useful defense, for example, by temporarily reducing activity and intravascular pressure so that further blood loss is prevented and blood clotting can occur.

PATHOPHYSIOLOGY AND COMPENSATORY MECHANISMS

HYPOVOLEMIC SHOCK

Arterial Pressure and Cardiac Output Changes

In the dog, rapid bleeding to a mean systemic arterial pressure of 50 mm. Hg is followed by a tendency for spontaneous recovery of arterial pressure toward control values over a period of 20 to 30 minutes. However, if the animal is bled continuously into an elevated reservoir so that the height of the reservoir determines the pressure, the compensatory mechanisms that would restore pressure result instead in further blood being added to the reservoir slowly over a 2-hour period.

After the maximal shed volume is attained, blood will begin to return to the animal as mean arterial pressure falls below the established level. Most experimental studies of this type show that once 40 to 50 per cent of the shed volume has returned to the animal, rapid infusion of the remainder results in only temporary improvement in arterial pressure. The subsequent course is usually progressive deterioration to death. At some point in this deterioration even massive transfusions of whole blood are ineffective and the condition fulfills the criteria for irreversible hemorrhagic shock.

In man, the blood volume of 5 to 6 liters represents 7 to 8 per cent of body weight and is distributed mostly in the venous system and heart (70 per cent). Acute blood loss up to 30 per cent can be tolerated because of compensatory mechanisms described below, but when more than 40 per cent of the blood volume is lost, cerebral and cardiac function fail.

Similar effects can be observed experimentally without external blood loss following the administration of a lethal dose of endotoxin. It has been well demonstrated in primates that this response of reduction in cardiac output and arterial pressure is secondary to decreased venous return to the heart as venous pooling occurs in the splanchnic bed.[41]

These observations in animals provide us with useful information but cannot be freely translated to the care of patients. The mesenteric pooling and intestinal bleeding characteristic of terminal shock in dogs are not usually found in patients and presumably are due to decreased mucin and mucosal metabolism and trypsin activation in the dog.[8]

It has been demonstrated in man that larger volumes of fluids than the amount lost are required in late shock to maintain blood pressure and cardiac output. This may be due to decreased arteriolar or capacitance-bed vasoconstriction, opening of arteriovenous shunts, sequestration of fluids in injured areas, blood sludging, or alterations in capillary or cell membrane permeability.[56] Furthermore, the nature of the hypovolemic insult in man is usually

sudden rather than protracted and bears little similarity to the elevated reservoir preparation. Thus, experimental efforts to simulate clinical situations are hampered by differing species responses and anesthesia in animals so that the need continues for better models of clinical problems and more investigations in patients at the bedside.

Compensatory Reflexes

BARORECEPTOR REFLEXES. The carotid sinuses and aortic arch contain baroreceptors sensitive to reduction in mean arterial pressure and pulse pressure. The initial responses to hemorrhage are an increase in sympathetic tone and a reduction in vagal tone. These responses result in tachycardia, a positive inotropic effect on cardiac muscle, arteriolar vasoconstriction, and enhancement of venomotor tone. Contraction of the spleen in the dog results in autotransfusion of blood but is not significant in man, whose blood reservoirs are principally the hepatic, cutaneous, and pulmonary vascular beds.

The increase in total peripheral resistance by arteriolar vasoconstriction is primarily at the expense of the cutaneous, skeletal muscle, renal, and splanchnic beds. However, splanchnic blood flow may remain in the control range in certain subhuman primate species. The coronary and cerebral circulation are spared this constrictor response and consequently enjoy an increased percentage of the reduced cardiac output. If the vasoconstriction is prolonged, however, ischemic damage can result, particularly in the kidney.

CHEMORECEPTOR REFLEXES. Reductions in mean systemic arterial pressure below 60 mm. Hg do not elicit the baroreceptor response but may result in sufficient stagnant hypoxia to stimulate the chemoreceptors. This results in enhanced peripheral vasoconstriction and more hyperventilation, which may improve venous return.

CEREBRAL ISCHEMIA. Compensatory adjustments to hypotension in the circulatory and respiratory systems preferentially maintain circulation and metabolism in the brain and heart. With progressive reduction in systemic arterial pressure to mean levels below 40 mm. Hg, however, a generalized sympathetic discharge occurs in response to inadequate cerebral perfusion. This response is of much greater magnitude than that resulting from the baroreceptors but may not persist as increased vagal tone results from progressive cerebral ischemia.

TRANSCAPILLARY REFILL. As a result of there being greater precapillary arteriolar vasoconstriction than postcapillary venoconstriction, capillary hydrostatic pressure falls to levels favoring intravascular movement of interstitial fluid by the Starling relationship. Reasonably large quantities of fluid are available approximating 0.25 ml. per minute per kilogram body weight or roughly 1.0 liter of fluid per hour in addition to protein stores available in the liver and transported largely through lymph channels. As the depleted blood volume is replaced, there is a gradual fall in hematocrit. The speed at which hemodilution occurs in man is generally slower than in the dog.[28] Conservation of external secretions is also noted, increasing the subjective sensation of thirst.[45]

RENAL RESPONSES. Increased conservation of fluid and electrolytes results from a decreased glomerular filtration rate as arterial pressure falls and there is subsequent reduction in water and electrolyte excretion. The decrease in renal blood flow results in the secretion of renin from the juxtaglomerular apparatus. This enzyme converts angiotensinogen to angiotensin, which acts as a vasopressor and promotes the release of aldosterone from the adrenal cortex. Aldosterone in turn acts on renal tubules to promote sodium and water resorption.

In addition, vasopressin is secreted by the posterior pituitary gland in response to hemorrhage and to both baroreceptor and left atrial low-pressure reflexes. Vasopressin as the antidiuretic hormone is responsible for further conservation of water, and its effect is enhanced in shock by a reduced rate of inactivation.[76]

ADRENAL RESPONSE. The adrenal medulla responds to the sympathetic discharge and hypotension by release of the catecholamines epinephrine and norepinephrine in a 5:1 ratio, respectively. These agents enhance the alpha and beta effects of the sympathetic response, promoting vasoconstriction and positive inotropism.

The other hormonal agents released during shock, renin and vasopressin, also serve to increase vasoconstriction, as already mentioned.

Decompensatory Mechanisms

When a reactive mechanism tends to exaggerate the effects of the original insult it is termed positive feedback and may institute a vicious cycle of progressive deterioration. The preponderant influences of negative feedback mechanisms as opposed to positive feedback factors will favor survival if no extraneous therapeutic factors are brought into play.

CARDIAC FAILURE. Although most investigators agree that the heart eventually fails in shock, there is considerable disagreement on the role of cardiac failure in earlier stages. Clinical experience with cardiopulmonary bypass suggests that even diseased hearts have remarkable reserve, demonstrating good functional return after prolonged periods of low perfusion pressure and even ischemic arrest. It is not too surprising, then, that a significant influence of a "myocardial depressant factor" or MDF,[49] acting to impair cardiac performance early in shock, has not been supported by the work of other investigators.[33, 79]

Progressive deterioration of ventricular function is ordinarily observed after 4 hours of hypotension[15] and results in further decline in arterial pressure and lack of response to fluid volume resuscitation. This may be due in part to depletion of myocardial norepinephrine.[27] The reduction in tissue perfusion increases the release of acid metabolites, which decrease peripheral resistance and blood pressure further, thereby further impairing tissue perfusion.

CEREBRAL ISCHEMIA. The compensatory hyperventilation in shock resulting in the lowering of Pa_{CO_2} may have a deleterious effect on cerebral perfusion since reduced carbon dioxide tension causes cerebral vasoconstriction. As mentioned previously, the initial sympathetic response to inadequate cerebral blood flow may be followed by a loss of sympathetic tone as cardiac and vasomotor centers become depressed and vagal effects become dominant. The combination of reduced peripheral resistance and bradycardia then leads to further deterioration of cerebral compensatory mechanisms.

ABNORMAL HEMATOLOGIC FACTORS. The initial response to hemorrhage under the influence of catecholamines, reduced pH, and increased circulating thromboplastin usually involves a period of hypercoagulability that may even result in intravascular thrombosis. This phase is followed by decreased coagulability and fibrinolysis that may lead to bleeding phenomena as seen typically in the intestine of the dog. Disseminated intravascular coagulation has been observed in certain clinical conditions and, if recognized by falling fibrinogen levels and the presence of fibrin split products, requires treatment by heparin administration. More commonly, large-volume transfusions utilize blood that is deficient in clotting factors, and the bleeding disorder that results can be treated best by the administration of fresh platelets, fresh frozen plasma, and fresh whole blood. The viscosity of blood is also dependent on blood flow and rises sharply as flow conditions are reduced, or if excessive hemoconcentration occurs. This effect is particularly deleterious in the microcirculation, where the rate of flow is normally low.

METABOLIC ACIDOSIS. The combination of reduced renal blood flow limiting hydrogen ion excretion and generalized tissue underperfusion leading to lacticacidemia results in a profound metabolic acidosis in shock. Ventilatory compensation by hyperventilation to eliminate carbon dioxide usually is inadequate, and the reduced arterial pH diminishes the vascular response to circulating catecholamines and eventually depresses the myocardium.

IMMUNOLOGIC DEPRESSION. The reticuloendothelial system bears the responsibility for detoxification and antibacterial defense, principally clearing portal blood flow in the liver. Depression of this system results from prolonged hypotension in the intestine secondary to release of a depressor substance.[50] The deficit in circulating opsonic α_2SB glycoprotein has been corrected in a preliminary study by infusion of cryoprecipitate.[65a] The mucosal barrier in the intestine similarly is less effective, permitting greater ingress of bacteria and toxins. Experimentally, sterilization of the intestine adds a significant measure of protection against the mortality from hemorrhagic shock preparations.

ARTERIAL AND VENOUS CLOSURE MECHANISMS. Transmural hydrostatic pressures are opposed by elastic and muscular components of the vessel wall, and when the distending pressure falls below a critical level ("critical closing pressure"), the vessel may close completely, with interruption of all blood flow. This can produce ischemic capillary damage, so that restoration of perfusion may be associated with edema formation and impaired tissue function. There are also important species differences in regional vascular responses since the dog, unlike man, has a strong hepatic vein sphincter mechanism that may be responsible for the predominance of splanchnic congestion in that animal.

CARDIOGENIC SHOCK

Definition

Primary cardiogenic shock is usually secondary to myocardial infarction with a concomitant loss of contractile force over a significant area of left ventricle or rhythm disturbance with inadequate cardiac output. Secondary cardiogenic shock, as indicated earlier, is defined by inadequate output despite filling pressures and is usually a result of prolonged coronary underperfusion. The mortality rate of the development of shock in patients with myocardial infarction approximates 60 per cent.[23]

Pathophysiology

The combination of pain, anxiety, and low cardiac output results in a massive sympathoadrenal response that produces sweating, tachycardia, and intense vasoconstriction. In some patients a relative hypovolemia may be observed, favoring a response to cautious fluid administration. Since there is primary concern with left ventricular function in these patients, there is a particular need for pulmonary arterial catheter monitoring, especially during fluid administration. When inotropic agents and diuretics fail to correct cardiac failure, systemic arteriolar dilator drugs can augment pump performance and reduce myocardial oxygen requirements by reducing afterload, thereby increasing ventricular emptying and stroke volume.

Between a quarter and one-half of patients in cardiogenic shock have an arrhythmia, usually ventricular premature contractions. Since this occurrence may precede development of ventricular fibrillation, these patients require constant electrocardiographic monitoring; this is one reason why the coronary care unit evolved. In some patients, bradycardia, requiring administration of isoproterenol or atropine, or permanent heart block, necessitating placement of a permanent pacemaker lead, may develop.

Inotropic Agents

By definition, a positive inotropic agent increases myocardial contractility but may not have a chronotropic effect.

CATECHOLAMINES. The rate of secretion of the catecholamines epinephrine and norepinephrine from the adrenal medulla is determined by activity of the sympathetic nervous system. The system obviously would be stimulated maximally in a patient in shock with hypotension.

The effect of the catecholamines on the oxygen consumption of the heart is mediated through their actions increasing both developed wall tension and myocardial contractility.[17] Each of these effects in the failing heart would be expected to increase oxygen consumption, but if initial ventricular volume is large with greater wall tension, improved cardiac performance may reduce volume and wall tension and decrease oxygen consumption. This would tend to offset the increase that results from enhanced contractility. The adverse effect of raising wall tension on myocardial energy needs signals a note of caution against the excessive elevation of afterload by vasoconstrictor agents to maintain an elevated aortic blood pressure. Similarly, a critically low blood pressure in a patient with cardiogenic shock will reduce coronary blood flow further, possibly leading to further ischemia and necrosis (positive feedback mechanism).

The clinical use of inotropic agents in cardiogenic shock must be based on consideration of these antecedent factors. With a major concern for adequate coronary perfusion, the use of isoproterenol would seem less justifiable, since its effects on myocardial energy requirements by increasing contractility would not be offset by increased systemic pressures necessary to improve coronary perfusion. Observations in patients support these conclusions, with increased myocardial lactate production observed after isoproterenol as opposed to

norepinephrine.[58] It would be more logical to use dopamine regulated to maintain systemic blood pressures 20 to 30 mm. Hg less than the estimated control values, since this agent causes less tachycardia and less increase in myocardial oxygen consumption. The use of combined inotropic-vasodilator therapy with preload control has proven to be very effective in managing postoperative cardiac failure.[54a]

DIGITALIS. The administration of digitalis in cardiogenic shock is controversial and generally reserved for those patients with clear-cut evidence of congestive heart failure or cardiomegaly. In this situation, the rapidly metabolized glycosides would be preferred, with hemodynamic response used as a guide to dosage in an effort to avoid toxicity in a heart that is usually regarded as hypersensitive to digitalis. Other inotropic agents such as glucagon have been used clinically with variable results, and further discussion of the uses of these drugs will be found in the section on vasoactive agents.

REFRACTORY CARDIOGENIC SHOCK. Persistence of low cardiac output without a rhythm disturbance or hypovolemia is associated with a prohibitive mortality rate. Deterioration after a temporary response to inotropic agents is similarly lethal and has prompted a more aggressive approach to provide mechanical circulatory support. The development of effective counterpulsation devices, particularly the intra-aortic balloon pump, has provided a means for diastolic augmentation of coronary blood flow while reducing left ventricular work. This support alone can salvage a number of patients. If low cardiac output persists or further deterioration occurs after 24 hours of counterpulsation, the patient is a candidate for coronary arteriography in the hope of identifying a lesion favorable for arterial bypass. Under circumstances favorable for operation, 30 to 40 per cent of these patients can be saved whose survival would be extremely unlikely without operation.[63]

SEPTIC SHOCK

Incidence

There is considerable evidence that the incidence of bacteremia and septic shock is increasing in most hospitals as more patients survive major trauma, have their resistance altered, and are subjected to an increasing variety of intracorporeal procedures often involving implantation of prostheses and long-term infusion and ventilation. The routine administration of antibiotics post-operatively has been incriminated in the rising incidence of gram-negative infections, but a more frequent factor is the contamination of intravenous catheters.[70] Since iatrogenic factors are common, the most appropriate therapy would be preventive: meticulous aseptic technique and no reliance on antibiotic prophylaxis.

Experimental Models

CANINE. The classic studies of the effects of purified *Escherichia coli* endotoxin on dogs elicited a pattern characterized by portal hypertension, rapid decreases in venous return, and early decrease in systemic arterial pressure. Decreased renal blood flow and urine output and a rising hematocrit with decline in arterial pH also were observed. Following the infusion of live *E. coli* organisms, however, there was only a gradual decline in venous return not associated with elevated portal vein pressure.[42] Similarly, there was a gradual decrease in total peripheral resistance and mean systemic arterial pressure. The renal response to live organisms was often exactly opposite of that to endotoxin — vasodilatation, hypoxemia, and polyuria. In the lung, the effects were similar — microembolic aggregates of leukocytes and early systemic hypoxia.[38]

PRIMATE. Responses more similar to human septic shock have been observed in monkeys to which either endotoxin or live *E. coli* organisms were administered. There was early onset of hypotension, decreased peripheral resistance and cardiac output, and both hyperventilation and hypoxia of greater magnitude after administration of endotoxin. A later increase in peripheral resistance was related to elevation of plasma catecholamine levels. The pulmonary lesion seen ultrastructurally was similar to that in the dog, with leukocyte plugging of pulmonary capillaries and endothelial cellular damage.

OTHER EXPERIMENTAL ANIMALS. The effects of endotoxin and live organisms have been studied in a variety of other species, often for selective effects observed more commonly in a particular animal model. Both rats[44] and rabbits[4] have been observed to develop disseminated intravascular coagulation and have been used for study of the therapeutic effects of heparin; the results have been variable. Similar observations of intravascular coagulation have been noted in swine after administration of endotoxin.[9]

Clinical Patterns

HYPERDYNAMIC STATE. The application of hemodynamic investigative techniques to critically ill patients at the bedside sheds considerable light on the status of the circulation in early septic shock. Instead of the anticipated low cardiac output with systemic hypotension, nearly all patients studied have been found to have normal or elevated cardiac output with reduced peripheral vascular resistance.[59] This is the clinical picture of "warm shock" with peripheral vasodilatation. This finding tends to be misleading since decreased oxygen uptake and utilization also were observed.[19] In addition, there is a decreased level of 2,3-diphosphoglycerate in the red blood cells associated with a shift to the left of the oxyhemoglobin dissociation curve, making oxygen less available to the tissues and more adherent to hemoglobin.[55] Some of these patients may show a normal arteriovenous oxygen difference suggesting an appropriate response to increased tissue oxygen utilization. This early adaptation may be associated with no alteration in venous Po_2 or pH.

Efforts to differentiate patterns of response to gram-negative from those to gram-positive organisms have been controversial,[75] and it does not appear that there are predictable syndromes for different infections. However, a marked hyperlipidemia has been observed in patients with gram-negative bacillary infections but not in those with severe infections with gram-positive cocci.[24] In one series of gram-negative bacteremias, coagulation abnormalities or thrombocytopenia were found in 64 per cent of patients.[47a] Evidence of disseminated intravascular coagulation (DIC) was found in 10 per cent of them and produced spontaneous subcutaneous or visceral bleeding in 3 per cent.

Systemic arterial hypoxemia is often found but usually is not related to hypoventilation since arterial P_{CO_2} tensions also are reduced. In spite of hypoxia, there is a narrowed arteriovenous oxygen difference reflecting reduced oxygen consumption and leading to a progressive metabolic acidosis with accumulations of lactate and pyruvate.[12] A positive correlation between the level of arterial blood lactate and oxygen uptake has been found.[20] The same investigators also observed an increase in capillary blood flow proportional to increased cardiac output in the dog with sepsis, suggesting that a primary cellular defect is responsible for the reduced oxygen uptake rather than arteriovenous shunting of blood. In this situation the increase in cardiac output may represent a compensatory effort to maintain oxygen uptake at the highest possible level.

HYPODYNAMIC STATE. In contrast to the "warm shock" associated with the hyperdynamic pattern of septic shock, in hypodynamic shock the extremities are cool, as a result of vasoconstriction, and cardiac output is reduced. This pattern is associated with hypovolemia and is seen most commonly in the surgical patient with sepsis complicated by extensive "third-space" losses (Fig. 3–1); for example, the patient with peritonitis, extensive burns, or intestinal obstruction complicated by sepsis would be more likely to show a lower blood volume and cardiac index with an increased peripheral vascular resistance.

Measurement of the filling pressures of the right or left heart by central venous or pulmonary arterial catheters, respectively, will provide the confirmation of this diagnosis and indicate a need for infusion of colloid or crystalloid based on the clinical situation. The hypodynamic picture has also been noted frequently in the presence of extensive gram-negative bacillary pneumonia[83] and may be related to an increase in pulmonary vascular resistance or sequestration of protein-containing fluid in the lung exaggerated by the presence of hypoxia. A similar picture may also be seen in patients with preexisting heart disease in whom sepsis develops.

After sufficient fluid volume to restore ventricular filling pressures to normal is administered, the cardiac output usually will increase to normal or elevated levels. However, it is unusual for the peripheral vascu-

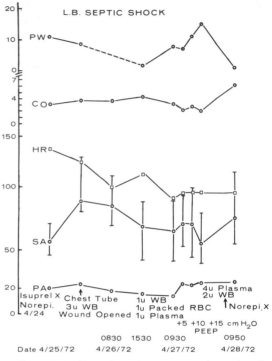

Figure 3–1 Hemodynamic responses of a patient in septic shock with a wound abscess who had required norepinephrine and isoproterenol to maintain blood pressure. After drainage of the abscess and transfusion of whole blood (WB) there was transient improvement in systemic pressure (SA) and heart rate (HR), but pulmonary wedge pressures (PW) and cardiac output (CO) remained low. An additional 4500 ml. of colloid was required to increase CO and SA so that administration of the vasopressors could be discontinued.

lar resistance to be reduced to normal levels; in this situation with persisting vasoconstriction, some investigators have advocated the use of alpha-adrenergic blocking agents to improve tissue blood flow. With the use of these agents, however, it must be recognized that additional fluid volume will be required to maintain satisfactory perfusion pressures when vasodilation occurs.

The hyperdynamic state may progress to the hypodynamic condition as the length of time the patient is in shock becomes extended. Under these circumstances the response to volume loading and drugs is poor, and the prognosis is grave.

DECOMPENSATION GROUP. Siegel and his associates[68] have defined a third group of patients characterized by severe clinical sepsis and unresponsiveness to therapy. These patients show signs of myocardial failure with elevated ventricular filling pressures, lowered systemic arterial pressures, and variably normal cardiac output. The arteriovenous oxygen difference is widened, and there is marked lowering of venous pH with elevated venous Pco_2. Accordingly, the tissues seem to be unable to satisfy their metabolic requirements, and the 12-hour survival time is only 38 per cent. In this group, as in all other patients with septic complications, survival was possible only if adequate surgical drainage of the septic focus could be accomplished. With adequate drainage it was possible to document shifting of a patient from this preterminal category to one of the other groups. This favorable change is less likely to occur once signs of cardiac failure are prominent, however, since this usually is a late result of shock leading to multisystem organ failure.

CELLULAR FUNCTION IN SHOCK

Energy Metabolism

Since the final result of inadequate perfusion is cellular dysfunction, it is important to recognize the limitations of cellular adaptation. The essential substrates such as glucose, fatty acids, amino acids, and glycerol are transported through the cell membrane by an energy-dependent transfer system. A lack of oxygen can prevent their transport and utilization since anaerobic glycolysis is less effective than the aerobic citric acid cycle. Participation of the substrates in the glycolytic cycle or through gluconeogenesis for fatty acids and amino acids is essential for energy production.

Studies of primate tissue homogenates following hemorrhagic shock showed a metabolic block in the reaction pyruvate to acetyl coenzyme A and citrate.[65] It has also been documented that lack of oxygen results in utilization of the anaerobic glycolytic cycle only. The pyruvate that could not be transformed to citrate or oxaloacetate in the tricarboxylic cycle was converted to lactate, which provided a good index of anaerobic metabolism.

Specific mitochondrial function studies on cardiac and skeletal muscle and liver in humans and animals have shown that endotoxin depresses mitochondrial respiration both in vivo and in vitro. Eventually there is uncoupling of oxidation and respiration, signifying that the energy produced by oxidation of substrates is not taken up by the phosphate acceptors in a high-energy bond. Similar dysfunction in ion transport and respiratory activity after endotoxin has been reported by Mela and her associates,[54] who also described alteration of the mitochondrial membrane. The utilization of oxygen without production of ATP may explain the clinical picture of an energy deficit despite high oxygen consumption.

Protein Metabolism

The response to hemorrhagic shock in the rat includes an increase in protein metabolism, and as the hypoxic liver fails to metabolize amino acids, the blood amino nitrogen increases.[21] The tendency for these amino acids to enter the glycolytic and oxidative cycles to help produce adenosine triphosphate (ATP) is enhanced by the glucocorticoid hormones, which are released as a result of stress. Corticoids also stimulate production of the liver enzyme tryptophane pyrrolase, usually decreased in endotoxin shock,[6] and the resulting production of nicotinic acid, which participates in the respiratory enzyme system, is one of the justifications used for the administration of exogenous steroids.

The energy deficit in both endotoxic and hemorrhagic shock and subsequent irreversibility have also been correlated with the loss of the purine bases adenine and guanine, which are needed for high-energy phosphate synthesis.[16]

Fat Metabolism

The catabolism of triglycerides to free fatty acids and glycerol is accelerated by catecholamines and glucocorticoids and provides an important source of energy during stress. However, the by-products of metabolic degradation of fatty acids include large quantities of ketone and acetone bodies, which the liver may not be able to oxidize during shock. Similarly, metabolism of ketones for energy by peripheral tissues, which can occur under normal circumstances, is reduced by hypoxemia, and increased metabolic acidosis results.

Electrolyte Metabolism

The loss of cellular energy interferes with the function of the cell membrane pump and allows loss of intracellular potassium to the extracellular space. The existing metabolic acidosis contributes further to the hyperkalemia and may interfere with cardiac function. A corresponding decrease in serum sodium concentration is usually observed, and occasionally a decrease in serum calcium is also seen.

The loss of intracellular potassium may interfere with protein synthesis at the level of amino acid incorporation into the polypeptide chain. In the lymphocyte, this effect can alter immunoprotein synthesis and may further impair toxin defense mechanisms in the shock patient. The role of potassium in neutralizing phosphate esters may also be adversely affected, with further interference with ATP production.

Intracellular edema also results from loss of function of the sodium-potassium pump, depression of resting transmembrane potential, and depletion of extracellular fluid.[45a] This may explain some of the concealed or "third-space" losses characteristic of patients with trauma or shock.

Lysosomal Enzymes

The intracellular organelle described by de Duve et al.[18] as a lysosome contains inactive acid hydrolases. If the liproprotein membrane becomes permeable or is disrupted, the enzymes are activated and have been demonstrated to hydrolyze ribonucleic acid, phosphate esters, and mitochondrial membranes, with resultant disruption of oxidative phosphorylation. Lysosomal rupture has been described in shock by a number of investigators and has been associated with increased circulating levels of acid phosphatase, β-glucuronidase, and proteinase. Efforts to correlate these findings with the irreversible stage of shock are controversial and are not supported by ultrastructural microscopic findings.[43] Protection of the lysosomal membrane against pH changes after steroid administration has been demonstrated[46] and is frequently cited to justify this treatment, although a primary role of the lysosomes remains to be proven.

TREATMENT OF SHOCK

APPROACH TO THE PATIENT

A systematic approach to the management of shock regardless of etiology has been utilized by Weil;[78] it is based on a sequence of therapeutic maneuvers that also provide valuable diagnostic information.

Ventilation

The most frequent single cause of death in a shock unit is failure of respiratory gas exchange.[57] Adequacy of ventilation is particularly critical in the immediate postoperative or post-traumatic period, and insufficiency should be suspected if there is weak, shallow, or labored breathing with inadequate air movement on auscultation of the chest.

ARTERIAL BLOOD GASES. The key to rapid assessment of adequacy of ventilation is prompt determination of the partial pressures of oxygen and carbon dioxide in arterial blood (Pa_{O_2} and Pa_{CO_2}) and arterial pH. Elevation of Pa_{CO_2} above 46 mm. Hg with arterial pH less than 7.30 is diagnostic of respiratory acidosis. The Pa_{CO_2} may or may not have fallen to abnormal levels (less than 70 mm. Hg for a patient breathing room air).

RESPIRATOR THERAPY. Abnormal blood gas findings obligate the physician to provide mechanical ventilatory assistance by means of a pressure-cycled or volume-cycled respirator, and respiratory therapy should be applied early in the course rather than after severe hypercarbia has developed. When signs of shock are present, patients require greater minute ventilation and levels of inspired oxygen, and often show reduced pulmonary compliance. These requirements can be satisfied best by use of a volume-cycled respirator with naso-tracheal intubation for controlled ventilation. If control of ventilation is required for periods longer than several days, tracheostomy should be considered in order to avoid the complications of laryngeal damage, necrosis of alar cartilage, and sinusitis. During the period of nasotracheal intubation, tube changes may be required if there are thick secretions that obstruct the lumen of the tube.

The respirator used should be adjusted to provide adequate ventilation, usually in the range of 8 to 12 ml. per kilogram body weight, for tidal volume. One should measure actual expired volume rather than relying on indicator settings, which are usually inaccurate. Respiratory rate should be adjusted to avoid respiratory alkalosis, with $Paco_2$ below levels of 30 mm. Hg, which interferes with cerebral perfusion and oxyhemoglobin dissociation. Maintenance of more normal levels of $Paco_2$ in the range of 35 mm. Hg can be facilitated by the addition of lengths of tubing to increase external dead space or more commonly by slower rates of intermittent mandatory ventilation. Pao_2 can usually be maintained at 80 to 100 mm. Hg when FIo_2 (ratio of inspired oxygen concentration) is 0.4. If FIo_2 is raised to 0.6 without improvement in Pao_2, then end-expiratory pressure should be employed. The Pao_2 level should not be maintained above 150 to 200 mm. Hg because of the risk of oxygen toxicity.

Peak inflation pressures, which are normally less than 20 cm. H_2O, may reach levels of 30 to 50 cm. H_2O in patients with pulmonary consolidation or interstitial pulmonary edema. The specific problems posed by the "wet-lung syndrome" will be discussed in a later section.

Excessive peak inflation pressure can be deleterious to the lung and interfere with pulmonary blood flow[32] and venous return. A valuable clinical sign of such excessive phasic inflation pressure is the presence of a paradoxical pulse that diminishes in volume during maximal inflation. Such a finding should be corrected by reducing tidal volume of the respirator until the pulse volume is more constant throughout the ventilatory cycle. The insertion of a Swan-Ganz catheter flow directed into the pulmonary artery allows measurement of pulmonary capillary wedge pressure to insure adequate filling pressure of the left ventricle. Catheters that have thermistor beads attached allow sequential direct measurement of cardiac output by the thermodilution technique. Another hazard of high inflation pressures with or without the addition of positive end-expiratory pressure is pneumothorax. Immediate treatment by insertion of a chest tube in the second intercostal space or needle decompression can be life-saving.

Perfusion

PRIORITY. Restoration of circulatory volume should be the primary consideration after adequacy of ventilation is assured. No other treatment is more efficient in bringing about rapid improvement in circulatory status than fluid replacement, and the most common clinical error is to underestimate the need for it (Fig. 3–2). The choice of

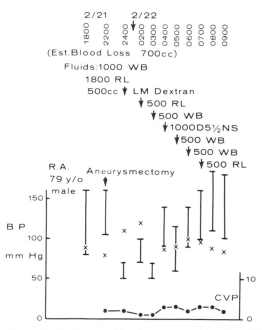

Figure 3–2 Systemic blood pressure and heart rate (X) in a 79-year-old man who underwent emergency aneurysmectomy with an estimated blood loss of 700 ml. Immediately after operation, he had hypotension and tachycardia with a low central venous pressure (CVP) that improved only after transfusion of an additional 1500 ml. of whole blood and 2000 ml. of lactated Ringer's solution (RL).

fluids for replacement must be based on the antecedent pathologic condition, but in most postoperative and post-traumatic situations blood and saline will be most effective in restoring adequate intravascular volume. The need for continued blood transfusions in the immediate postoperative period must be weighed against the value of early reoperation to control bleeding. Usually the latter should be resorted to before the blood bank is exhausted and the patient has lost coagulability.

FLUID MANAGEMENT. In the resuscitation of patients who have not been recently operated upon, the use of crystalloid solutions has been proven effective for volume repletion providing rapid restoration of cardiac output and oxygen consumption.[2] Occasionally, exsanguinating hemorrhage may require the administration of type O, Rh-negative blood of low antibody titer for survival. Since time is a critical factor in shock, the use of blood substitutes often is necessary until blood is cross-matched, and a variety of agents are available. The basis for use of saline solutions in volumes exceeding measured blood losses is the demonstrated extracellular fluid deficit ascribed by Shires[67] to redistribution and sequestration in traumatized tissues. In accordance with this principle, Ringer's lactate as a balanced electrolyte solution is usually administered in volumes proportional to four times the red cell mass plus the volume of plasma lost, on the basis of the work of Grayson.[29] Preference for Ringer's lactate solution is based on its buffering capacity in an acidotic patient, which is an advantage over isotonic saline at a low pH. The concern about administration of lactate in the face of lactic-acidemia has not proven to be justified when blood flow and cardiac output are improved by the infusion.[3] Of more concern are the sequelae of significant hemodilution with reduction in hematocrit, oxygen transport, and plasma proteins. There is experimental evidence that significant hemodilution is poorly tolerated[74] and can contribute to the development of pulmonary interstitial edema.[77] Also, some impairment in host defense owing to the absence of plasma opsonics may result from use of packed red blood cells as opposed to whole blood.[13a] However, most clinical situations requiring volume resuscitation can be dealt with effectively by administration of Ringer's lactate solution and either packed red blood cells or whole blood without adverse effects. Autotransfusion devices also can be used under emergency circumstances of major blood loss provided that the additional anticoagulation required can be controlled and that significant bacterial contamination has not occurred.

Dextran preparations can be helpful in initial resuscitation and tend to remain in the intravascular compartment, but administration of more than 1500 ml. may produce problems with coagulation or blood cross-matching, and allergic responses may occur. Although some investigators report improved microcirculation with use of low-molecular-weight dextran,[26] most of the changes can be explained by hemodilution,[61] and survival in experimental shock is not improved.[31] Other colloid agents have been studied, including hydroxyethyl starch, which showed initial promise[1] but did not prove to have significant advantages over dextran.

Vasoactive and Inotropic Drugs in Shock

PATHOPHYSIOLOGY. Efforts to incriminate excessive vasoconstriction in the deterioration of organ function are based on the time factor of reduced tissue perfusion. Recognizing the role of vasoconstriction as a compensatory mechanism alone minimizes treatment errors and use of drugs that exaggerate or attempt to remove this response. There remains no substitute for adequate fluid replacement in shock.

DRUGS IN USE. *Methoxamine* is a selective alpha-adrenergic stimulator inducing vasoconstriction without an inotropic effect. Although an elevation of systemic pressure might be observed after its administration in shock, the effects on tissue perfusion would be deleterious.

Metaraminol is a strong vasoconstrictor with a positive inotropic effect. Some of its effects are mediated through norepinephrine although it has less renal vasopressor effect.

Epinephrine increases myocardial contractility as a beta-adrenergic stimulator without alpha-adrenergic effects except at higher dosage levels. A chronotropic effect is observed with increase in stroke volume producing increased cardiac output in normovolemic situations.

Dopamine is an intermediate in the synthesis of epinephrine and norepinephrine with an effect on the heart similar to that of epinephrine. It has less chronotropic effect, however, and less tendency to produce arrhythmias. Peripherally it causes muscular and splanchnic vasoconstriction at higher doses although some renal-sparing effect has been observed in humans.

Dobutamine is a synthetic catecholamine that acts directly to increase myocardial contractility without inducing marked tachycardia or greatly changing peripheral arterial resistance. It acts directly on β_1-adrenergic receptors in the myocardium, but unlike dopamine it does not stimulate the heart indirectly by releasing norepinephrine from nerve endings.[70a]

Norepinephrine is the sympathetic system chemical mediator with both alpha- and beta-adrenergic activity. It increases peripheral vascular resistance and has both inotropic and chronotropic effects on the heart. It may be used in conjunction with an alpha-adrenergic blocking agent to minimize the vasoconstrictor effect and selectively increase cardiac output.

Isoproterenol is a beta-adrenergic stimulator that has both inotropic and chronotropic effects. Some degree of vasodilatation occurs peripherally, with reduction of peripheral resistance. The tendency for the drug to reduce the refractory period of heart muscle seems to facilitate development of arrhythmias.

Mephentermine is an adrenergic drug with both inotropic and chronotropic effects. In the periphery it increases venous tone and may increase arteriolar resistance slightly. Most of its cardiac effects are mediated through norepinephrine.

Angiotensin is a synthetic polypeptide with greater pressor effect than norepinephrine and longer duration of action. It apparently has no effect on the heart.

Phenoxybenzamine is an alpha-adrenergic blocking agent that acts as a potent vasodilator to decrease total peripheral resistance. It also increases capacitance further by dilatation of veins and should not be administered to hypovolemic patients. Its use in resuscitated shock patients to improve tissue perfusion and increase cardiac output has not been associated with improved survival rates.[80]

Phentolamine and *chlorpromazine* both have milder alpha-adrenergic blocking effects and chlorpromazine has additional sedating effects.

Steroid administration in shock has been based on a combination of effects, usually with unpredictable hemodynamic results despite massive doses. At best, reports tend to show some vasodilatation in patients with vasoconstriction and some vasoconstriction in those with vasodilatation.[80] One double-blind randomized study of administration of dexamethasone or methylprednisolone to patients in septic shock showed a significant reduction in mortality rate in the steroid treated groups with no difference in results between the two agents.[64a]

Beta-adrenergic blocking agents have been advocated for treatment of refractory shock on the basis of reducing the beta-stimulated vasodilatation in pulmonary and splanchnic areas. Both experimental and clinical studies of the use of *propranolol* have been conducted, and favorable results have been reported in patients with the refractory hyperdynamic syndrome of septic shock.[5] Use of the drug may result in significant cardiodepression, however.

Glucagon has been used in critically ill patients for its positive inotropic effect, but it also can be demonstrated to increase peripheral vasoconstriction.[69] Beneficial results in patients in the hyperdynamic state were also reported.

Cardiac Performance

EVALUATION BY CENTRAL VENOUS PRESSURE MEASUREMENT. Adequacy of cardiac output becomes a point of concern if signs of improvement in blood pressure and perfusion do not result from fluid administration. In order to discriminate between pump failure and inadequate volume replacement, challenges of a fixed volume of fluid, usually 200 cc., are used to assess the functional response to this fluid load delivered over a 10 to 15 minute period.

The easiest means of assessing the cardiac response to the fluid load is by measurement of ventricular filling pressure as re-

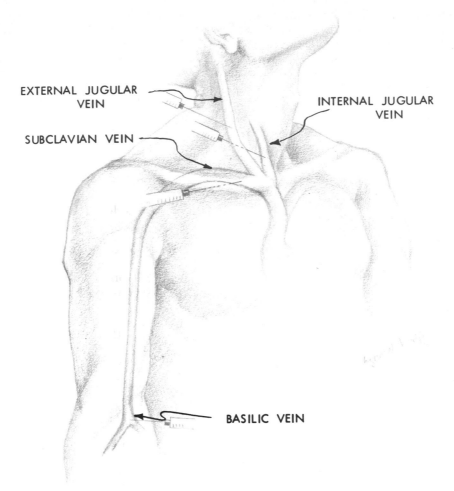

EXTERNAL JUGULAR
VEIN

INTERNAL JUGULAR
VEIN

SUBCLAVIAN VEIN

BASILIC VEIN

Figure 3–3 Routes of access for the measurement of central venous pressure (CVP). Catheters can be directed percutaneously into the superior vena cava from any of the veins shown.

flected for the right heart by the central venous pressure (CVP). CVP has been used in regulation of fluid therapy despite considerable evidence of limitations of its reliability. By definition, central venous pressure can be measured only by a catheter whose tip is within the thorax, and placement is usually accomplished via an arm vein or the external jugular or by percutaneous infraclavicular or supraclavicular puncture of the subclavian vein (Fig. 3–3).

The normal range of CVP is from 2 to 10 cm. H_2O, and its clinical usefulness for the patient in shock is limited to encouraging further fluid administration when the readings remain low (0 to 5 cm. H_2O). As volume is restored, the CVP tends to rise, but there is no absolute end point. The response of the CVP to the trial fluid load of 200 cc.

saline, as mentioned previously, should be less than an increase of 2 cm. above the control level. If it exceeds this response, then further fluid administration may produce congestive failure, and attention must be directed to improving cardiac performance by digitalis or other inotropic agents. There is good experimental evidence that the CVP may not reflect circulatory overload[72] and that there is poor correlation between CVP levels and fluid requirements for resuscitation in patients.[82]

PULMONARY ARTERIAL PRESSURE MEASUREMENT. Of more value clinically is direct measurement of the pulmonary arterial pressure in critically ill patients as a guide to fluid therapy. This has been facilitated by the use of a flow-directed cardiac catheter as described originally by Lategola and Rahn,[48] and popularized by Swan, Ganz, et al.[73] After passage of the catheter into the superior vena cava by venous cutdown in the arm, the balloon is inflated and the catheter permitted to follow the flow into the pulmonary artery. Catheter position can be confirmed by portable chest x-ray, although the sequence of typical right ventricular and pulmonary arterial tracings is usually adequate for clinical use. Electrocardiographic monitoring can also be used to determine passage of the catheter through the right ventricle in catheters equipped with a lead at the tip, and it is possible to measure cardiac output by thermodilution with a thermistor-tipped catheter in the pulmonary artery. Passage of the open-tipped catheter farther out in the pulmonary artery results in wedging of it peripherally into an arteriole that reflects mean left atrial pressure through the pulmonary capillary bed. This position can be confirmed by aspiration of fully oxygenated blood from the catheter.

Monitoring of the pulmonary wedge pressure (PWP) or pulmonary arterial end-diastolic pressure (PAEDP) has been shown to provide a more accurate reflection of the filling pressure of the left ventricle and to be more sensitive to fluid overloading than the CVP. Even in patients in shock, the PWP is a reliable indicator of left ventricular end-diastolic pressure, showing abnormal elevation when it is greater than 15 mm. Hg and normal to low filling pressure when it is less than 10 mm. Hg.[64] In addition, the pulmonary arterial catheter permits sampling of true mixed venous blood that indirectly reflects circulatory status by the level of oxygen tension. Mixed venous Po_2 of less than 30 mm. Hg is associated with inadequate cardiac output and a poor prognosis.

Differential Diagnosis

Most of the initial efforts in resuscitation of the patient in shock provide at the same time diagnostic information in terms of response to treatment or lack thereof. It is necessary, however, to exclude other significant complications that may be overlooked.

PNEUMOTHORAX. In any patient supported by positive-pressure ventilation, and particularly in those patients requiring high inflation pressures, tension pneumothorax is a constant threat and must always be excluded in the patient whose condition is deteriorating. A similar concern is necessary for those patients who have been resuscitated by closed-chest massage, which frequently results in rib fractures and potential pulmonary disruption from overinflation or compression injury. Similarly, placement of CVP catheters by infraclavicular puncture and occasionally from supraclavicular approaches can produce pleural and pulmonary injuries directly, and misplacement of the catheter can lead to extravascular fluid administration.

Tube thoracostomy is the preferred method of management and must be utilized in patients with pneumothorax who require positive-pressure ventilation. The chest catheter should be introduced through the second intercostal space anteriorly and angled toward the apex of the thorax.

MYOCARDIAL INFARCTION. The occurrence of shock carries potential risk of coronary thrombosis in patients with pre-existing coronary arteriosclerotic disease and may of course be the primary cause of it. A complete electrocardiographic examination is necessary to exclude this complication, and it is usually advisable to maintain oscilloscopic monitoring of cardiac rate and rhythm using lead II connections. Availability of an electrocardiographic tracing provides a valuable reference for comparison in patients with changing patterns, but usually only non-specific ST and T wave changes are seen during shock and resuscitation. The electrocardiogram is not a reliable guide to adequacy of cardiac output.

PULMONARY EMBOLISM. In many patients with serious underlying diseases and periods of hypotension, venous thrombosis develops that is asymptomatic and not evident on routine examination. Detachment of these thrombi can result in the full spectrum of embolic disease from silent microemboli to acute massive thromboembolism and sudden death. The hypotensive hypoxic patient with an elevated CVP and hypocarbia should be presumed to have a massive pulmonary embolism until the diagnosis is excluded by lung scan or pulmonary arteriogram or both.

PULMONARY ASPIRATION. There is increasing evidence that aspiration of gastric contents occurs more frequently than is suspected, particularly in anesthetized patients. As the primary cause of shock, however, it is less common and usually recognized by the presence of particulate matter in the pharynx and increased airway resistance. As a complication of shock it is a constant threat in patients who are not adequately decompressed by nasogastric suction and in whom gastric dilatation develops secondarily to low splanchnic perfusion pressure.

OBSTRUCTIVE UROPATHY. In the older patient, urinary retention with infection can cause septic shock. This problem is usually recognized early by the chief complaint and should not develop as a complication in shock, since bladder catheter drainage is established early to monitor hourly urine output.

Monitoring the Patient (Fig. 3–4)

As indicated in previous sections, the following information should be available in all shock patients (Tables 3–2 and 3–3):

ARTERIAL PRESSURE. Direct measurement by insertion of a radial artery catheter is the optimal method of monitoring systemic pressure by connection to a pressure transducer and oscillographic or direct-writing recorder. This catheter also provides access for arterial blood samples for pH and blood gas determinations without repeated arterial punctures.

Arterial pressures obtained by cuff and sphygmomanometer are inaccurate in most

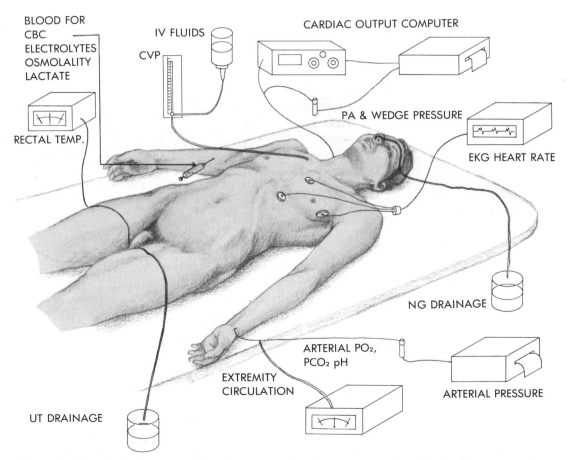

Figure 3–4 Comprehensive approach to the patient in shock permitting rapid assessment of response to therapy. Although some of the hemodynamic determinations are not commonly available, they should be added whenever possible to permit evaluation of drug and fluid responses.

TABLE 3–2 GUIDELINES FOR NORMAL HEMODYNAMIC MEASUREMENTS IN PATIENTS

Determination	Normal Adult Range
Central venous pressure	5–10 cm. H_2O
Pulmonary arterial pressure	25–30/8–10 mm. Hg
Pulmonary wedge pressure	8–10 mm. Hg
Systemic arterial pressure	120/80 mm. Hg
Cardiac index	3.0–4.5 l./min./M^2
Heart rate	70–80/min.
Hematocrit	37–45%

shock patients with vasoconstriction and small pulse volume. Improved accuracy is possible with Doppler techniques, but these indirect methods do not permit sampling of arterial blood or precise evaluation of beat-to-beat pressure which is useful during resuscitation in cardiac arrest by closed-chest massage.

CENTRAL VENOUS PRESSURE. Insertion of a catheter into the superior vena cava is possible by a variety of routes (see Fig. 3–3). There is relatively less risk from the percutaneous insertion via brachial or external jugular veins, although the direct insertion via the subclavian and internal jugular veins has become more fashionable. The small but significant risk of the latter approaches should dictate appropriate caution in their use, since air embolism, arterial hemorrhage, pneumothorax, sepsis, catheter shearing, and intrapleural placement all can be lethal complications in shock patients. Position of the catheter should be checked by portable chest x-ray. Meticulous technique must be used to avoid contamination of the catheter; this should include application of topical antibiotics and removal and culture of the tip at the earliest sign of infection.

INTAKE AND OUTPUT. The hourly measurement of urine output is essential to document response to resuscitation in the shock patient and can be recorded accurately from an indwelling bladder catheter. Similarly, nasogastric and other external losses must be recorded and replaced with appropriate volumes of fluids and electrolytes. Weighing the patient daily can be a useful adjunct to fluid management but is often hampered by numerous connecting tubes and other hardware.

ELECTROCARDIOGRAPH. The application of limb leads has for the most part been replaced by positioning of three leads in a triangle on the thorax to provide oscillographic display of rate and rhythm. This should not, however, be considered a substitute for the full 12-lead electrocardiogram, which should be the basis for comparison to evaluate myocardial damage and changes in rhythm.

RESPIRATOR. Frequent and careful assessment of respiratory function is essential to prevent malfunction or suboptimal per-

TABLE 3–3 GUIDELINES FOR NORMAL RESPIRATORY FUNCTION MEASUREMENTS IN PATIENTS

Determination	Normal Adult Range
Arterial Po_2 (on room air)	80–100 mm. Hg
Arterial Pco_2	37–45 mm. Hg
Arterial pH	7.35–7.45
Venous Po_2	35–50 mm. Hg
Venous Pco_2	42–51 mm. Hg
Venous pH	7.30–7.40
Alveolar-arterial oxygen difference ($A-aDo_2$)	
Room air	5–10 mm. Hg
100% O_2	10–60 mm. Hg
Dead space–tidal volume ratio (V_D/V_T)	0.3–0.35
Vital capacity	3–4.8 l.
Respiratory rate	12–15/min.
Compliance	10–30 ml./cm. H_2O

formance. Monitoring of expired air for tidal volume and peak inflation pressure is helpful as a guide to effective ventilation and early alterations in pulmonary compliance (see Table 3–3).

HEMODYNAMIC MEASUREMENTS. As outlined previously, the placement of a pulmonary arterial catheter provides more accurate and useful information than the CVP. Similarly, the direct measurement of cardiac output by indicator or thermodilution techniques will be of increasing value in evaluating response to treatment (see Table 3–2).

DATA FLOW SHEET. The organization of large volumes of data is essential for continuous evaluation of response to therapy and to avoid overlooking early signs of organ dysfunction. Most flow sheets list the parameters to be followed on the ordinate and the chronologic intervals, usually days, on the abscissa. In addition to the standard listings of serum electrolytes, arterial pH and blood gases, hemogram values, and urine output, it is helpful to add data on body weight, respirator settings, plasma and urine osmolalities, coagulation studies, drugs in use, and culture reports.

Review and evaluation of these data should be mentioned in progress notes, and a plan for management should be included that will avoid uncoordinated orders being written by a variety of physicians. In this regard it is essential that a responsible physician be designated to coordinate suggestions made by a variety of consultants to avoid the confusion of multidisciplinary therapy.

OTHER ADJUNCTS

Temperature. Measurements of temperature gradients between the periphery and body core have been found useful by Weil, who also advocated comparing peripheral and central hematocrits.[78] These values provide further data on the degree of vasoconstriction and retarded peripheral blood flow.

Blood Volume. Blood volume determinations are of limited usefulness in patients in shock owing to the wide range of normality and prolonged equilibration times.[82] Using radioiodinated serum albumin is likely to increase the error because of losses of albumin from increased capillary permeability, particularly in patients with sepsis. Somewhat more accurate results can be obtained from the use of chromium-51–tagged red

blood cells, which are less likely to disappear from the intravascular space.

Oxygen Consumption. Following hemorrhagic or cardiogenic shock there may be little alteration in oxygen consumption until the terminal stage is reached. At this point cellular metabolism has probably been altered irreversibly and accordingly low values suggest a poor prognosis. Initial low values may be seen in about one-fourth of patients in septic shock and would imply a similarly poor prognosis.

The shift from aerobic to anaerobic metabolism usually results in the production of excess lactate and a metabolic acidosis. However, in some patients with reduced oxygen consumption, anaerobic metabolism also may be impaired[62] and less alteration may be observed in levels of lactate and standard bicarbonate. This failure to develop a base deficit can be misleading and conceal the extent of cellular metabolic failure.

Breakdown Products. Various vasoactive substances have been demonstrated in shock patients, including serotonin, catecholamines, histamine, and polypeptides such as bradykinin. The role of these agents in the pathophysiology of clinical shock remains controversial, but further studies of these substances and other lysosomal enzymes may prove useful in elucidating the stages of shock.

Level of Consciousness. Adequacy of organ perfusion and blood gases often may be detected earliest by changes in the patient's alertness, orientation, and sensorium. The most reliable observations in this regard are often made by members of the patient's family or nurses who have been caring for him. Routine evaluation of the sensorium should be made at regular intervals.

SPECIFIC ORGAN FAILURE

Pulmonary Insufficiency

PATHOGENESIS OF "SHOCK LUNG." Recognition of a syndrome of progressive pulmonary insufficiency following resuscitation from shock or trauma achieved prominence as a result of experiences with military casualties in Southeast Asia, where, as in other major wars, specific organ management problems were brought to light. In the Vietnam conflict the survival of massively injured casualties proved the effectiveness of rapid transport and fluid resuscitation but introduced new complications. The clinical picture was one of onset 24 to 48 hours after successful hemodynamic resuscitation of signs of respiratory failure that was often progressive and refractory to treatment, was characterized by relentlessly advancing opacification of the chest radiograph, and terminated in hypoxic death. The characteristic congested and hemorrhagic appearance of the lungs at autopsy gave rise to the term "wet-lung syndrome." Histologically there were signs of congestive atelectasis, intra-alveolar hyaline membranes, and interstitial pulmonary edema.[52] The relationship of these findings to experimental fat embolism,[30] intravascular coagulation,[36] pulmonary hypoperfusion,[10, 39] oxygen toxicity,[11] altered capillary permeability,[37] overinfusion of crystalloids,[77] secondary infection,[51] aspiration of gastric contents,[35] pulmonary contusion,[60] transfusion microemboli,[13] and blood-borne vasospastic factors[22] has been studied extensively, but it has not been possible to incriminate any single factor as the major determinant. Even the most common insult of massive crystalloid fluid resuscitation was difficult to incriminate since hemodilution edema was shown to be less damaging to pulmonary function than hydrostatic edema in the isolated lung preparation.[34] Most commonly, if fluid overload has not occurred during resuscitation, progressive pulmonary insufficiency can be attributed to unrecognized sepsis, aspiration, or direct lung injury.

The earlier pulmonary lesion that has been observed in patients in septic shock presumably results from rapid development of microembolic aggregates of leukocytes.[38] Physiological studies in patients confirm the presence of interstitial pulmonary edema from a non-cardiac cause.[58] Normal serum albumin levels in these patients excluded the possibility of lowered oncotic pressure as an etiologic factor under the Starling relationship of capillary fluid exchange. Experimental studies show a direct effect of bacteria on pulmonary capillary permeability that is not altered favorably by the administration of albumin.[18a]

PROPHYLAXIS AND THERAPY. Recognition of the probability of increased capillary permeability and of the necessity to preserve plasma oncotic pressure provides the rationale for prophylaxis by avoidance of infusion of excessive crystalloid fluids and filtration of blood to prevent microemboli. In this situation the CVP can be misleading, since overloading can occur without unusual elevation or signs of right heart failure. Here the pulmonary arterial catheter is a better guide in avoiding diastolic or wedge pressures greater than 12 mm. Hg.

It is usually possible to predict which patients with trauma or septic shock are most likely candidates for pulmonary insufficiency. In this group early positive-pressure ventilation provides support of gas exchange and limitation of edema formation as outlined earlier. If Pa_{O_2} remains below 65 mm. Hg in spite of increase of FI_{O_2} to 0.6, then it is advisable to add positive end-expiratory pressure in 5 cm. increments to the level necessary to produce a significant rise in Pa_{O_2}. In addition, administration of diuretic agents may be useful, along with restriction of salt and of water intake to 1500 ml. a day. Progressive deterioration is common, however, with signs of increasing pulmonary arteriovenous shunting indicated by increasing alveolar-arterial oxygen difference (A-aD_{O_2}, Table 3–3). Alveolar oxygen tension (Pa_{O_2}) can be estimated after ventilation with 100 per cent oxygen for 15 minutes by the equation: $Pa_{O_2} = PI_{O_2} - Pa_{CO_2}$, where PI_{O_2} = inspired oxygen tension = barometric pressure − water vapor pressure (47 mm. Hg), and Pa_{CO_2} = alveolar carbon dioxide tension, which can be assumed to equal arterial carbon dioxide tension. This equation assumes a respiratory exchange ratio of 1.0, whereas the usual ratio is less than 1.0.

In the face of relentless progression of pulmonary insufficiency, or if the initial attempts to treat a full-blown lesion are unsuccessful, some efforts have been made to provide extracorporeal oxygenation by venovenous or venoarterial partial bypass support. If technical problems related to hemorrhage, infection, and hemolysis can be solved, it should be possible to provide continuous extracorporeal circulatory and respiratory support to permit resolution and healing of the pulmonary lesion. This is probably more likely to prove of benefit in the long run than pulmonary transplantation.

Renal Function in Shock

RENAL FAILURE. Whether acute renal failure develops as a result of prolonged hypovolemic hypotension is a matter of debate. In most instances of clinical renal failure, there is associated abdominal injury, preexisting renal disease, dehydration, salt losses, or pigment excretion. When the normal kidney is subjected to a period of ischemia it should retain the capability for restoration of function if adequate volume and perfusing pressure are restored.

Oliguria can be defined in the critically ill patient as a urine volume less than 30 cc. per hour; it demands immediate attention and efforts to improve urine flow.

FUNCTIONAL EVALUATION

Glomerular Filtration Rate. As an index of the glomerular filtration rate (GFR), a simple determination of the levels of creatinine in both plasma and urine permits rapid assessment by the formula for clearance:

$$GFR = \frac{Vol. \times Concentration\ in\ urine}{Plasma\ creatinine}$$

Proximal Tubular Function. The function of the proximal tubules is concerned with sodium recovery and measurement of the urinary sodium permits assessment of tubular work. In the patient resuscitated from shock but with persistent oliguria, the presence of urinary sodium greater than 60 mEq. per liter is an indication that tubular function is adequate. Higher levels of urinary sodium, approaching the concentration in plasma, reflect tubular damage.

Distal Tubular Function. Measurement of the ratio of urine to plasma osmolality can provide information regarding water resorption by the distal tubules. Preservation of the ability to concentrate urine to levels greater than 400 milliosmoles suggests active tubular function and probably favorable response to hydration and diuretics. However, the restoration of perfusion pressure to the kidney may not restore the medullary osmotic gradient, and so renal handling of solutes and water may remain abnormal.[47]

TREATMENT. Restoration of circulating volume and perfusion pressure to the kidneys should result in prompt increase in urine output if the period of ischemia has not been prolonged.

If oliguria persists in the face of adequate renal perfusion, the use of a loop diuretic such as furosemide can be advocated. Repetitive administration of the diuretic with or without an osmotic agent such as mannitol should be attempted before the diagnosis of renal failure is made. Total lack of response confirms the diagnosis of acute renal failure, however, and requires restriction of fluid intake and management as outlined in Chapter 6.

FUTURE DIRECTIONS IN SHOCK

The trend of investigation in shock over many years has been toward the cell and the microcirculation. The demonstration of a vascular endothelial lesion[25] and early cellular membrane transport defects[17] suggests more widespread injury than would be suspected from evidence of specific organ failure. Similarly, there is evidence that circulatory derangements in shock are enhanced by microaggregation of platelets.

There is great interest in oxygen utilization at the cellular level and its relationship to oxyhemoglobin dissociation, oxygen delivery, and arteriovenous shunting. Further studies of the role of uncoupling of oxidative phosphorylation should be of value in understanding the biochemical changes in shock. It is to be hoped that this information will permit new therapeutic approaches such as substrate manipulation.

Other factors that influence response to shock can be shown to be significant in specific experimental preparations, but years of investigation have not clarified the roles in man of lysosomal enzymes, toxic factors, prostaglandins, disseminated intravascular coagulation, vasoactive amines, immunological reactions, and hypoinsulinism.

Probably the most certain feature of shock is that it will remain a fertile field of investigation for many years to come.

Bibliography

1. Ballinger, W. F., II, Murray, G. F., and Morse, E. E.: Preliminary report on the use of hydroxyethyl starch solution in man. J. Surg. Res., 6:180, 1966.

2. Baue, A. E., Tragus, E. T., and Parkins, W. M.: A comparison of isotonic and hypertonic solutions and blood on blood flow and oxygen consumption in the initial treatment of hemorrhagic shock. J. Trauma 7:743, 1967.

3. Baue, A. E., Tragus, E. T., and Wolfson, S. K., Jr., et al.: Hemodynamic and metabolic effects of Ringer's lactate solution in hemorrhagic shock. Ann. Surg. 166:29, 1967.

3a. Beiting, C. V., Kozak, K. J., Dreffer, R. L., Stinnett, J. D., and Alexander, V. W.: Whole blood vs. packed red cells for resuscitation of hemorrhagic shock: An examination of host defense parameters in dogs. Surgery 84:194, 1978.

4. Beller, F. K., Graeff, H., and Gorstein, T.: Disseminated intravascular coagulation during the continuous infusion of endotoxin in rabbits. Morphologic and physiologic studies. Am. J. Obstet. Gynecol. 103:544, 1969.

5. Berk, J. L., Hagen, J. F., Maly, G., and Koo, R.: The treatment of shock with beta adrenergic blockade. Arch. Surg. 104:46, 1972.

6. Berry, L. J., and Smythe, D. S.: Effects of bacterial endotoxins on metabolism. VII. Enzyme induction and cortisone protection. J. Exper. Med. 120:721, 1964.

7. Blalock, A.: Experimental shock: The cause of low blood pressure produced by muscle injury. Arch. Surg. 20:959, 1930.

8. Bounous, G., McArdle, A. H., Hodges, D. M., Hampson, L. D., and Gurd, F. N.: Biosynthesis of intestinal mucin in shock: Relationship to tryptic hemorrhagic enteritis and permeability to curare. Ann. Surg. 164:13, 1966.

9. Brown, P., Coalson, J., Elkins, R. C., and Greenfield, L. J.: Unpublished data.

10. Chernick, V., Hodson, W. A., and Greenfield, L. J.: The effect of chronic pulmonary artery ligation on pulmonary mechanics and surfactant. J. Appl. Physiol. 21:1315, 1966.

11. Coalson, J. J., Beller, J. E., and Greenfield, L. J.: Effects of 100 per cent oxygen ventilation on pulmonary ultrastructure and mechanics. J. Pathol. 104:267, 1971.

12. Cohn, J. D., Greenspan, M., Goldstein, C. R., Gudwin, A. L., Siegel, J. H., and DelGuercio, L. R. M.: Arteriovenous shunting in high cardiac output shock syndromes. Surg. Gynecol. Obstet. 127:282, 1968.

13. Connell, R. S., and Swank, R. L.: Pulmonary fine structure after hemorrhagic shock and transfusion of aging blood. Symposia 6th European Conference on Microcirculation, Aalborg 1970. Basel, S. Karger, 1971, pp. 49–58.

14. Cournand, A., Riley, R. L., Bradley, S. E., Breed, E. D., Noble, R. P., Louson, H. D., Gregerson, M. I., and Richards, D. W.: Studies of the circulation in clinical shock. Surgery 13:964, 1943.

15. Crowell, J. W., and Guyton, A. C.: Further evidence favoring a cardiac mechanism in irreversible hemorrhagic shock. Am. J. Physiol. 203:248, 1962.

16. Crowell, J. W., Jones, C. E., and Smith, E. E.: Effect of allopurinol on hemorrhagic shock. Am. J. Physiol. 216:744, 1969.

17. Cunningham, J. N., Jr., Shires, G. T., and Wagner, Y.: Cellular transport defects in hemorrhagic shock. Surgery 70:215, 1971.

18. de Duve, C., Pressman, B. C., Gianetto, R., Watiaux, R., and Appleman, F.: Tissue fractionation studies: Intracellular distribution patterns of enzymes in rat-liver tissue. Biochem. J. 60:604, 1955.

18a. Demling, R. H., Will, J. A., and Perea, A.: Effect of albumin infusion on pulmonary microvascular and protein transport. J. Surg. Res. 27:321, 1979.

19. Duff, J. H., Groves, A. C., McLean, A. P., et al.: Defective oxygen consumption in septic shock. Surg. Gynecol. Obstet. 128:1051, 1969.

20. Duff, J. H., Wright, C. J., McLean, A. P. H., and MacLean, L. D.: Oxygen consumption in septic shock. In Forscher, B. K., Lillehei, R. C., and Stubbs, S. S. (Eds.): Shock in Low and High-Flow States. Amsterdam, Excerpta Medica, 1972, pp. 235–239.

21. Engel, F. L., Winton, M. G., and Long, C. N. H.: Biochemical studies on shock: Metabolism of amino acids and carbohydrates during hemorrhagic shock in the rat. J. Exp. Med. 77:397, 1943.

22. Farrington, G. H., Saravis, C. A., Cossette, G. R., et al.: Blood-borne factors in the pulmonary response to sepsis (acute experimental peritonitis). Surgery 68:136, 1970.

23. Friedberg, C. K.: Cardiogenic shock in acute myocardial infarction. Circulation 23:325, 1961.

24. Gallin, J. I., Kaye, D., and O'Leary, W. M.: Serum lipids in infection. N. Engl. J. Med. 281:1081, 1969.

25. Gaynor, E., Bouvier, C. A., and Spaet, T. H.: Vascular lesions: Possible pathogenetic basis of the generalized Shwartzman reaction. Science 170:986, 1970.

26. Gelin, L. E., and Ingelman, B.: Rheomacrodex — A new dextran solution for rheological treatment of impaired capillary flow. Acta Chir. Scand. 122:294, 1961.

27. Glaviano, V. V., and Coleman, B.: Myocardial depletion of norepinephrine in hemorrhagic hypotension. Proc. Soc. Exp. Biol. Med. 107:761, 1961.

28. Grant, R. T., and Reeve, E. B.: Observations on the General Effects of Injury in Man with Special Reference to Wound Shock. (Med. Res. Council Special Report Series, No. 227). London, H. M. Stationery Office, 1951.

29. Grayson, T. L., White, J. E., and Moyer, C. A.: Oxygen consumptions: Concentrations of inorganic ions in urine, serum, and duodenal fluid,

hematocrits, urinary excretions, pulse rates and blood pressure during duodenal depletions of sodium salts in normal and alcoholic man. Ann. Surg. 158:840, 1963.

30. Greenfield, L. J., Barkett, V. M., and Coalson, J. J.: The role of surfactant in the pulmonary response to trauma. J. Trauma 8:735, 1968.

31. Greenfield, L. J., and Blalock, A.: Effect of low molecular weight dextran on survival following hemorrhagic shock. Surgery 55:684, 1964.

32. Greenfield, L. J., Ebert, P. A., and Benson, D. W.: Effect of positive pressure ventilation on surface tension properties of lung extracts. Anesthesiology 25:312, 1964.

33. Greenfield, L. J., McCurdy, J. R., Hinshaw, L. B., and Elkins, R. C.: Preservation of myocardial function during cross-circulation in terminal endotoxin shock. Surgery 72:111, 1972.

34. Greenfield, L. J., Reif, M. E., Coalson, J. J., McCurdy, J. R., and Elkins, R. C.: Comparative effects of interstitial pulmonary edema produced by venous hypertension or hemodilution in perfused lungs. Surgery, 71:857, 1972.

35. Greenfield, L. J., Singleton, R. T., McCaffree, D., R., and Coalson, J. J.: Pulmonary effects of experimental graded aspiration of hydrochloric acid. Ann. Surg. 170:74, 1969.

36. Hardaway, R. M.: Syndromes of Disseminated Intravascular Coagulation; with Special Reference to Shock and Hemorrhage. Springfield, Ill., Charles C Thomas, 1966.

37. Harrison, L. H., Beller, J. E., Hinshaw, L. B., Coalson, J. J., and Greenfield, L. J.: Effects of endotoxin on pulmonary capillary permeability, ultrastructure and surfactant. Surg. Gynecol. Obstet. 129:723, 1969.

38. Harrison, L. H., Hinshaw, L. B., Coalson, J. J., and Greenfield, L. J.: Effects of E. coli septic shock on pulmonary hemodynamics and capillary permeability. J. Thorac. Cardiovasc. Surg. 61:795, 1971.

39. Henry, J. N., McArdle, A. H., Scott, H. J., et al.: A study of the acute and chronic respiratory pathophysiology of hemorrhagic shock. J. Thorac. Cardiovasc. Surg. 54:666, 1967.

40. Hinshaw, L. B., Greenfield, L. J., Owen, S. E., Archer, L. T., and Guenter, C. A.: Cardiac response to circulating factors in endotoxin shock. Am. J. Physiol. 222:1047, 1972.

41. Hinshaw, L. B., Shanbour, L. L., Greenfield, L. J., and Coalson, J. J.: Mechanism of decreased venous return in subhuman primate administered endotoxin. Arch. Surg. 100:600, 1970.

42. Hinshaw, L. B., Solomon, L. A., Holmes, D. D., and Greenfield, L. J.: Comparison of canine responses to E. coli organisms and endotoxin. Surg. Gynecol. Obstet. 127:981, 1968.

43. Holden, W. D., DePalma, R. G., Drucker, W. R., and McKalen, A.: Ultrastructural changes in hemorrhagic shock. Electron microscopic study of liver, kidney, and striated muscle cells in rats. Ann. Surg. 162:517, 1965.

44. Horwitz, D. L., Ballantine, T. V. N., Coran, A. G., and Herman, C. M.: Heparin treatment of live E. coli bacteremia in rats. J. Surg. Res. 13:120, 1972.

45. Howard, J. M.: Gastric and salivary secretion following injury: Systemic response to injury. Ann. Surg. 141:342, 1955.

45a. Illner, H., and Shires, G. T.: The effect of hemorrhagic shock on potassium transport in skeletal muscle. Surg. Gynecol. Obstet. 150:17, 1980.

46. Janoff, A., Weissmann, G., Zweifach, B. W., and Thomas, L.: Pathogenesis of experimental shock. IV. Studies on lysosomes in normal and tolerant animals subjected to lethal trauma and endotoxemia. J. Exp. Med. 116:451, 1962.

47. Kramer, K.: Renal failure in shock. In Bock, K. D. (Ed.): Shock: Pathogenesis and Therapy: An International Symposium. Berlin, Springer-Verlag, 1962, pp. 134–144.

47a. Koeger, B. E., Craven, D. E., and McCabe, W. R.: Gram-negative bacteremia. IV. Re-evaluation of clinical features and treatment in 62 patients. Am. J. Med. 68:344, 1980.

48. Lategola, M., and Rahn, J.: A self-guiding catheter for cardiac and pulmonary arterial catheterization and occlusion. Proc. Soc. Exp. Biol. Med. 84:667, 1953.

49. Lefer, A. M., Cowgill, R., Marshall, F. F., et al.: Characterization of a myocardial depressant factor present in hemorrhagic shock. Am. J. Physiol. 213:492, 1967.

50. Levy, M. N., and Blattberg, B.: Blood factors in shock. In Hershey, S. G. (Ed.): Shock. Boston, Little, Brown and Company, 1964, pp. 65–67.

51. Lewin, I., Weil, M. H., Shubin, J., et al.: Pulmonary failure associated with clinical shock states. J. Trauma 11:22, 1971.

52. Martin, A. J., Jr., Soloway, H. B., and Simmons, R. L.: Pathologic anatomy of the lungs following shock and trauma. J. Trauma 8:687, 1968.

53. McLean, A. P., Duff, J. H., and MacLean, L. D.: Lung lesions associated with septic shock. J. Trauma 8:891, 1968.

54. Mela, L., Miller, L. D., Diaco, J. F., and Sugerman, H. J.: Effect of E. coli endotoxin on mitochondrial energy-linked functions. Surgery 68:541, 1970.

54a. Miller, D. C., Stinson, E. B., Oyer, P. E., Derby, G. C., Reitz, B. A., and Shumway, N. E.: Postoperative enhancement of left ventricular performance by combined inotropic vasodilator therapy with preload control. Surgery 88:108, 1980.

55. Miller, L. D., Oski, F. A., Diaco, J. F., et al.: The affinity of hemoglobin for oxygen: Its control and in vivo significance. Surgery 68:187, 1970.

56. Moore, F. D.: Metabolic Care of the Surgical Patient. Philadelphia, W. B. Saunders Company, 1959.

57. Moore, F. D., Lyons, J. H., Jr., Pierce, E. C., Jr., Morgan, A. P., Jr., Drinker, P. A., MacArthur, J. A., and Dammin, G. J.: Post-Traumatic Pulmonary Insufficiency: Pathophysiology of Respiratory Failure and Principles of Respiratory Care after Surgical Operations, Trauma, Hemorrhage, Burns and Shock. Philadelphia, W. B. Saunders Company, 1969.

58. Mueller, H., Ayres, S. M., and Grace, W. J.: Principal defects which account for shock following acute myocardial infarction in man. Implications for treatment. Crit. Care Med. 1:27, 1973.

59. Neely, W. A., Berry, D. W., Rushton, F. W., and

Hardy, J. D.: Septic shock: Clinical physiological, and pathological survey of 244 patients. Ann. Surg. *173*:657, 1971.

60. Nichols, R. T., Pearch, H. J., and Greenfield, L. J.: Effects of experimental pulmonary contusion on respiratory exchange and lung mechanics. Arch. Surg. *96*:723, 1968.

61. Replogle, R. L., Kundler, H., and Gross, R. E.: Studies on the hemodynamic importance of blood viscosity. J. Thorac. Cardiovasc. Surg. *50*:658, 1965.

62. Rush, B. F., Jr., Rosenberg, J. E., and Spencer, F. C.: Changes in oxygen consumption in shock: Correlation with other known parameters. J. Surg. Res. *5*:252, 1965.

63. Sanders, C. A., Buckley, M. J., Leinbach, R. C., Mundth, E. D., and Austen, W. G.: Mechanical circulatory assistance. Current status and experience with combining circulatory assistance. Emergency coronary angiography, and acute myocardial revascularization. Circulation *45*:1292, 1972.

64. Schienman, M., Evans, G. T., Weiss, A., and Rapaport, E.: Relationship between pulmonary artery end-diastolic pressure and left ventricular filling pressure in patients in shock. Circulation *47*:317, 1973.

64a. Schumer, W.: Steroids in the treatment of clinical septic shock. Ann. Surg. *184*:333, 1976.

65. Schumer, W.: Localization of the energy pathway block in shock. Surgery, *64*:55, 1968.

65a. Scovill, W. A., Saba, T. M., Blumenstock, F. A., Bernard, H., and Powers, S. R. Jr.: Opsonic α_2 surface binding glycoprotein therapy during sepsis. Ann. Surg. *188*:521, 1978.

66. Selkurt, E. E.: Role of ADH in the loss of renal concentrating ability in primate hemorrhagic shock. Proc. Soc. Exp. Biol. Med. *142*:1310, 1973.

67. Shires, T., and Carrico, C. J.: Current status of the shock problem. Curr. Probl. Surg. *3*:67, 1966.

68. Siegel, J. H., Goldwyn, R. M., and Friedman, H. P.: Pattern and process in the evolution of human septic shock. Surgery *70*:232, 1971.

69. Siegel, J. H., Levine, M. J., McConn, R., and DelGuercio, L. R. M.: The effect of glucagon infusion on cardiovascular function in the critically ill. Surg. Gynecol. Obstet. *131*:505, 1970.

70. Smits, H., and Freedman, L. R.: Prolonged venous catheterization as a cause of sepsis. N. Engl. J. Med. *276*:1229, 1967.

70a. Sonnenblick, E. H., Frishman, W. H., and LeJeritel, J. H.: Dobutamine: A new synthetic cardioactive sympathetic amine. N. Engl. J. Med. *300*:17, 1979.

71. Sonnenblick, E. H., and Skelton, C. L.: Myocardial energetics: Basic principles and clinical implications. N. Engl. J. Med. *285*:668, 1971.

72. Spencer, F. C., Yu, S. C., and Rossi, N. P.: Intracardiac pressure changes with overtransfusion of normal dogs. Ann. Surg. *162*;74, 1965.

73. Swan, H. J., Ganz, W., Forrester, J., et al.: Catheterization of the heart in man with use of a flow-directed balloon-tipped catheter. N. Engl. J. Med. *283*:447, 1970.

74. Takaori, M., and Safar, P.: Treatment of massive hemorrhage with colloid and crystalloid solutions. Studies in dogs. J.A.M.A. *199*:297, 1967.

75. Udhoji, V. N., and Weil, M. H.: Hemodynamic and metabolic studies on shock associated with bacteremia: Observation on 16 patients. Ann. Intern. Med. *62*:966, 1965.

76. Usami, S., and Chieu, S.: Role of hepatic blood flow in regulating plasma concentration of antidiuretic hormone after hemorrhage. Proc. Soc. Exp. Biol. Med. *113*:606, 1963.

77. Weedn, R. J., Cook, J. H., McElreath, R. L., and Greenfield, L. J.: Wet-lung syndrome after crystalloid and colloid volume repletion. Curr. Top. Surg. Res. *2*:335, 1970.

78. Weil, M. H., and Shubin, H.: The "VIP" approach to the bedside management of shock. J.A.M.A. *207*:337, 1969.

79. Wilson, J. M., Gay, W. A., Jr., and Ebert, P. A.: The effects of oligemic hypotension of myocardial function. Surgery *73*:657, 1973.

80. Wilson, R. F., Ali, M., Anand, V., McCarthy, B., Pitt, J., Hayes, D., Percivel, A., and LeBlanc, L. P.: Effects of vasoactive agents in clinical septic shock. *In* Forscher, B. K. (Ed.): Shock in Low and High-Flow States. Amsterdam, Excerpta Medica, 1972, pp. 269–281.

81. Wilson, R. F., Khambhla, A., and Mammen, E. F.: Coagulation changes in shock. Circulation *36* (Suppl. II):273, 1967.

82. Wilson, R. F., Sarver, E., and Birks, R.: Central venous pressure and blood volume determinations in clinical shock. Surg. Gynecol. Obstet. *132*:631, 1971.

83. Wilson, R. F., Sarver, E. J., and LeBlanc, P. L.: Factors affecting hemodynamics in clinical shock with sepsis. Ann. Surg. *174*:939, 1971.

4

HEMORRHAGIC COMPLICATIONS IN SURGERY

Francis S. Morrison

In order to discuss a rational approach to diagnosis and management of bleeding problems it will first be necessary to review the normal hemostatic mechanism. A sound background in enzyme chemistry is almost a prerequisite for thorough understanding of the complexities of the clotting system. The system is composed of a myriad of interdependent and interacting catalysts, as well as inhibitors, all in a state of dynamic equilibrium. Clearly, any test of the system must be viewed as a vignette of only one frame of a motion picture sequence.

Fortunately, however, understanding of concept rather than detail will permit management of the overwhelming majority of these problems. A rather superficial understanding of the hemostatic mechanism will suffice if it is correct. Such understanding will permit a logical analysis of what may be going on, how it can be conveniently established, and what can be done about it.

THE HEMOSTATIC MECHANISM

PRIMARY HEMOSTASIS. The first major concept of importance is the separation of primary hemostasis from coagulation. The formation of a primary hemostatic plug is not a function of the coagulation system, but the result of the interaction between platelet and vessel. A severed or injured vessel exposes collagen to circulating platelets. The platelets adhere to collagen, and this induces changes in the platelet itself that result in release of several intrinsic substances. One of the released substances is adenosine diphosphate (ADP), which causes platelets to cohere and thus form an aggregate or platelet plug. The release of vasoactive amines assists in retracting the open vessel around this platelet plug. Bleeding ceases, and primary hemostasis is complete (Fig. 4–1).

Without an adequate number of normally functioning platelets, there can be no platelet plug and no hemostasis. It is only after the formation of this platelet plug that the coagulation mechanism results in the deposition of fibrin and the formation of the definitive hemostatic plug.

Clinically, abnormalities in primary hemostasis result in bruising and petechiae. Occasionally "mucous-membrane" bleeding such as nosebleeds or gastrointestinal bleed-

Francis S. Morrison was born in Chicago. He was graduated with honors from Mississippi State University and received his medical degree from the University of Mississippi Medical School. After his internship and medical residency at the Hospital of the University of Pennsylvania, he became a Trainee in Hematology under Dr. W. Dameshek at the Tufts-New England Medical Center in Boston. He also attended the Massachusetts Institute of Technology in 1962–63 and in 1965–66 was Visiting Investigator at the Experimental Hematology Research Unit, St. Mary's Hospital Medical School in London. In 1969 he joined the faculty of the University of Mississippi Medical School as Assistant Professor of Medicine, Director of the Division of Hematology and the Transfusion Service of the University Hospital. He now holds the rank of Professor and is an outstanding teacher and clinician in the fields of hematology, blood coagulation and transfusion problems.

THE HEMOSTATIC MECHANISM

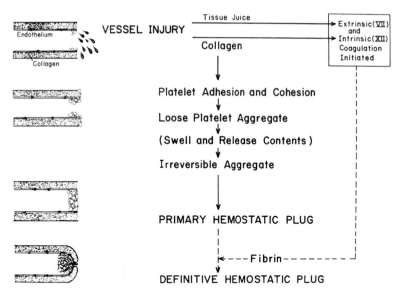

Figure 4–1 Primary hemostasis. Figure 4–2 shows in more detail how coagulation completes the process.

ing occurs. Bleeding is immediate with trauma or surgery and, if not too severe, will respond to direct pressure.

THE DEFINITIVE HEMOSTATIC PLUG. Primary hemostasis, namely, the formation of the platelet plug, is closely accompanied by the stepwise activation of a "cascade" of circulating clotting factors. These are counterbalanced by numerous specific inhibitors, as well as physiologic degradation. There is still not complete agreement on all aspects of the coagulation sequence, but a pragmatic approach will not require such agreement.

While primary hemostasis is taking place, both the extrinsic and the intrinsic coagulation systems are activated. The result of both is the activation of factor X, which, in the presence of platelet lipid and factor V, converts prothrombin to thrombin. Thrombin converts fibrinogen to a loose fibrin clot interwoven through the platelet plug. Factor XIII then acts to effect a firm fibrin clot and platelets once again function by inducing retraction of the clot into the definitive hemostatic plug (Fig. 4–2).

The clinical manifestations of deficiencies in the clotting mechanism are quite variable and will be mentioned when specific deficiencies are discussed. In general, however, purpura or petechial eruptions are not seen. Traumatic bleeding into joints resulting in

arthropathy is common. Also characteristic is rebleeding after immediate hemostasis has occurred. With severance of large vessels massive bleeding may result.

COAGULATION

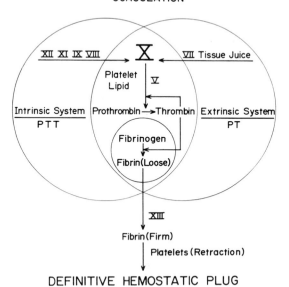

DEFINITIVE HEMOSTATIC PLUG

Figure 4–2 The intrinsic and extrinsic systems have in common the steps from activated factor X through the formation of a fibrin clot. The partial thromboplastin time (PTT) is influenced by those factors enclosed in the circle on the left. The prothrombin time (PT) is influenced by those factors enclosed in the circle on the right. The thrombin time reflects the influence of only the substances enclosed in the small circle.

TABLE 4–1   COAGULATION FACTORS

Numeral	Common Names
I	Fibrinogen
II	Prothrombin
III	Tissue thromboplastin
IV	Calcium
V	Proaccelerin, labile factor, accelerator (AC) globulin
VII	Proconvertin, stable factor
VIII	Antihemophilic factor (AHF), antihemophilic globulin (AHG)
IX	Christmas factor, plasma thromboplastin component (PTC)
X	Stuart-Prower factor
XI	Plasma thromboplastin antecedent (PTA)
XII	Hageman factor, surface contact factor
XIII	Fibrin-stabilizing factor
PF3	Platelet factor 3, platelet phospholipid
PF4	Platelet antiheparin activity

NORMAL FORCES COUNTERACTING THE HEMOSTATIC MECHANISM. Once the clotting mechanism has been initiated, the process accelerates rapidly. It is obviously very important that the fibrin plug be localized to the injured site and the remainder of the blood continue to circulate. Numerous counteracting factors exist to maintain the delicate balance. Probably the flow rate is of prime importance. Activated factors that are not in a terminal vessel and involved in a dead-end pocket, forming fibrin, will be rapidly diluted and carried away. These activated factors are degraded by the reticuloendothelial system, primarily in the liver.

The formation of fibrin is also normally associated with the release of factors that activate the fibrinolytic mechanism. These activators derive from endothelium and lysosomes, as well as other sources. They act on an inert precursor, plasminogen, to form plasmin which then can degrade and lyse fibrin. This event, of course, tends to limit fibrin extension through the body. Plasmin also degrades factor V, factor VIII, and fibrinogen, as well as other proteins, but has no effect on platelets.

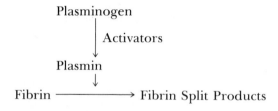

This reaction is controlled physiologically by inactivators and may be blocked by the administration of epsilon-aminocaproic acid (EACA).

LABORATORY SCREENING FOR HEMOSTATIC DEFECTS

It should be mentioned at the outset that there is no laboratory substitute for a carefully obtained history. Patients with congenital defects of hemostasis usually have had some clinical manifestation very early in life. Excessive bleeding at circumcision or with dental extractions frequently is the first indication of an abnormality. Menorrhagia, easy bruisability, nosebleeds, gastrointestinal bleeding, or hematoma may be the initial clinical presentation. Repeated hemarthroses may result in arthropathy before the underlying problem has been recognized. Family history is also important since the pattern of inheritance may help to identify a congenital defect. Von Willebrand's disease is considered an autosomal dominant disorder, although the clinical spectrum suggests variable penetrance. Hemophilias A and B are both sex-linked recessive defects. All the other genetic defects of coagulation have autosomal recessive inheritance patterns.

Numerous laboratory tests have been devised in order to define precisely the abnormalities of hemostasis and also, it would occasionally seem, in order to confuse the clinician. The laboratory evaluation of hemostasis either as a preoperative study or in the diagnosis of a bleeding patient must be rapid and relatively simple and should distinguish among all the more common causes of bleeding. The more sophisticated, and hence less available and less easily interpreted, techniques should be relegated to coagulationists. A group of six simple, readily available tests will sufficiently identify the problems so as to permit rational management in most situations.

1. *The bleeding time (BT)* is the test of primary hemostasis. This test has been difficult to interpret in the past because of difficulty in standardization and a wide range of normal, both between individuals and between sequential determinations in the same individual. In 1969 a standardized technique for the bleeding time was described that purported to obviate these two difficulties and in fact our experience and that of others corroborates the early work. The standardized bleeding time has become a most useful screening test for evaluation of platelet function. This test will be abnormal when there is a quantitative or qualitative defect in platelets. It is not prolonged in the hemophilias or other coagulation defects. Some vascular problems may also produce an abnormal result but these are rarely a problem.

2. *The platelet count* obviously will be necessary to differentiate between numerical and functional deficiencies of the platelets. In general, a platelet count of 100,000 per cubic millimeter or more is necessary for a normal BT. However, in conditions resulting in rapid platelet turnover and hence predominance of young platelets, lower counts can still produce a normal BT.

3. *Examination of the peripheral blood smear* will permit confirmation of the platelet count as well as evaluation of platelet morphology. Bizarre shape, giant platelets, and the absence of any clumping all suggest the possibility of functional aberration. Furthermore, the blood film examination may reveal abnormalities of red cell morphology suggestive of disseminated intravascular coagulation. Fragmented, torn, or helmet-shaped cells are typical of microangiopathic disease and, therefore, provide a helpful clue to this particular bleeding disorder.

4. *The partial thromboplastin time (PTT)* is a convenient screen for abnormalities of the intrinsic system of coagulation exclusive of any contribution from platelets. It is a simple test and is quite sensitive. An abnormal PTT, if the prothrombin time is normal, suggests a congenital disorder such as one of the hemophilias. Heparin therapy is also probably best monitored with this test. Some laboratories use the prothrombin consumption test in place of the PTT, but the PC is affected by platelet abnormalities and is also less sensitive and, therefore, less useful as a screening test.

5. *The prothrombin time (PT)* is sensitive to deficiencies of the extrinsic system down through the formation of fibrin. Adequate levels of factors VII, X, V, prothrombin, and fibrinogen are necessary for a normal PT.

6. *The thrombin time (TT)* detects severely deficient fibrinogen or the presence of anticoagulants, including fibrin split products. Therefore, it is prolonged by both primary and secondary fibrinolysis.

Other Tests. Although not necessary as part

TABLE 4–2 PATTERNS OF SCREENING TEST RESULTS IN COMMON BLEEDING DISORDERS

Disorder	BT	Platelets	PTT	PT	TT
Thrombocytopenia	↑	↓	N	N	N
Thrombocytopathy	↑	N	N	N	N
Von Willebrand's disease	↑	N	N ↑	N	N
Hemophilia	N	N	↑	N	N
Chronic liver disease	N	N	↑	↑	N ↑
Acute liver necrosis	↑	N ↓	↑	↑	↑
Acute DIC	↑	↓	↑	↑	↑
Vitamin K deficiency	N	N	↑	↑	N
Coumarin drugs	N	N	↑	↑	N
Heparin	N	N	↑	↑	↑

Arrows indicate increase (prolonged) or decrease
N = normal
N ↑ = occasionally increased

of routine screening, certain other laboratory tests can be helpful in specific situations. A clot-solubility test will detect deficiency of factor XIII. An assay of clottable protein or an immunologic method to detect a significantly reduced fibrinogen level is frequently useful. A test for fibrinolytic activity usually merely reflects an active compensatory defense mechanism and not primary fibrinolysis and therefore can be misleading. The thromboplastin generation test (TGT) can be used to specifically identify deficient coagulation factors but is by no means a screening test. Assays for specific factors should be available when needed. Clot retraction and platelet aggregation and adhesiveness are useful in precisely defining platelet functional abnormalities. Means for detection of fibrin split products, such as

ethanol gelation, protamine precipitation, or staphylococcal clumping, are alternatives to the thrombin time and occasionally provide additional information. The whole-blood clotting time is only of historic interest, and its usage reflects primarily the habit of the user.

When used in conjunction with a careful history, the recommended battery of six screening tests almost invariably will demonstrate and define fairly well any significant bleeding disorder. Occasionally, they will point the direction to more specific assays of deficient factors. Specific treatment then will correct the defect in hemostasis and permit even elective surgery. These same tests performed in the presence of unexpected bleeding can direct the clinician to appropriate treatment.

DISORDERS OF HEMOSTASIS

Those disorders of hemostasis that antedate the surgical procedure and that occasionally necessitate special preparation of the patient will be considered first, and then the disorders that commonly become manifest during surgery or in the postoperative period will be discussed.

PREEXISTING HEMOSTATIC DEFECTS

THROMBOCYTOPENIA. This is probably the most common disorder of hemostasis. The normal platelet count is 150,000 to 400,000 per cubic millimeter. Less than this number is defined as thrombocytopenia. However, unless the count is less than 100,000, there is neither prolongation in bleeding time nor hazard encountered in surgery unless there is another abnormality compounding the problem. Thrombocytopenia, like any deficiency of a system in equilibrium, is either caused by decreased production or the result of increased destruction, or utilization, beyond the capacity for compensation.

In those conditions associated with decreased production of platelets, such as myelophthisis, leukemia, or hypoplasia of the marrow, infusion of sufficient platelets to obtain a platelet count of approximately

100,000 per cubic millimeter will permit any required surgery. This objective usually requires infusion of eight to ten units of properly prepared platelet concentrates in an adult and about half this number in a child. Transfused platelets should have a half-life of 4 to 5 days in the circulation.

In idiopathic (immunologic) thrombocytopenic purpura (ITP), platelets are destroyed by an autoantibody. In the acute form, splenectomy is not indicated and corticosteroids will effect a prompt increment in platelet count. In the chronic form, on the other hand, splenectomy is usually performed at some time in the course of the disease. Despite the fact that transfused platelets may be cleared from the circulation in minutes, some clinicians choose to transfuse multiple units of platelet concentrate immediately before surgery. As soon as the splenic vessels are ligated, a marked improvement in hemostasis can almost invariably be observed.

In the presence of splenomegaly, thrombocytopenia is common and is largely due to pooling of platelets in the spleen. Much larger numbers of transfused platelets are usually necessary to effect the desired increment, but the survival time of those platelets that circulate is usually quite normal.

Thrombocytopenia is an expected finding in disseminated intravascular coagulation (DIC) and may be either severe or mild. It is the result of consumption of platelets, along with other clotting factors, and this fact has suggested the appellation "consumption coagulopathy" for this clinical syndrome. Specific treatment of DIC with heparin and removing the cause when possible is more urgent than platelet replacement and the latter is, in fact, usually not necessary. This condition will be discussed later in more detail.

THROMBOCYTOPATHY. Used in a general sense, this term indicates a functional defect in platelets. This is actually a group of disorders requiring sophisticated tests for precise definition. As a group, thrombocytopathies are characterized by a prolonged bleeding time associated with an adequate number of platelets. There has been extensive investigation into the adhesive and cohesive as well as other properties of platelets. As we understand more, we can better define specific platelet functional defects. For our present purposes we are concerned only with the overall contribution of platelets to primary hemostasis so that a deficiency of this function can be identified and specific treatment instituted. Abnormalities may be inherited or may be the result of acquired disease. Treatment in any case consists of transfusion of normal platelets.

Glanzmann's disease (thrombasthenia) is a commonly mentioned but rare inherited disorder characterized by lack of normal clumping of platelets on the blood smear and a prolonged bleeding time. These platelets also effect poor clot retraction and fail to aggregate in response to adenosine diphosphate.

The very high platelet counts occasionally seen in myeloproliferative diseases such as polycythemia myeloid metaplasia, or chronic granulocytic leukemia are not uncommonly associated with bleeding. These platelets have been demonstrated to be functionally abnormal. Liver disease and renal failure also frequently result in functionally abnormal platelets. Platelet transfusion should probably be reserved, in these conditions, for treatment when bleeding occurs.

An interesting inherited disorder associated with defective platelet function is von Willebrand's disease. This disorder is characterized by a prolonged bleeding time, a mild to moderate decrease in factor VIII in the plasma, and an inordinate and prolonged beneficial response to transfused plasma. Platelet adhesiveness has also been found to be abnormal. This is a mendelian dominant condition with variable penetrance and is probably one of the more common hereditary bleeding disorders. The management of these patients is much easier than that of those with hemophilia and consists of transfusion of plasma, approximately 10 ml. per kilogram a day, beginning 2 days before surgery. The abnormal bleeding time will usually be corrected only transiently after each transfusion, but adequate hemostasis will still be attained. Cryoprecipitates, which will be discussed later, are useful since they contain the needed factors.

VASCULAR PURPURA. For completeness, the vascular purpuras should be mentioned. This group of disorders includes a list of hereditary abnormalities of connective tissue which result in failure of the small vessel to maintain its integrity. Pseudoxanthoma elasticum, Ehlers-Danlos syndrome, purpura simplex and osteogenesis imperfecta are a few of these disorders. Bruising is common. Bleeding may or may not be a problem. The bleeding time may be abnormal but all other tests are normal. Only local and supportive measures are possible.

DEFICIENCIES OF THE INTRINSIC CLOTTING SYSTEM

The term hemophilia, in a broad sense, applies to any inherited deficiency of the first stage of the intrinsic system of coagulation. It is characterized, therefore, by an abnormal PTT but normal results in the other five tests. "Classic hemophilia" applies to deficiency of factor VIII (hemophilia A). Factor IX deficiency (hemophilia B) is less common. Both are sex-linked recessive genetic disorders. The history, therefore, reveals bleeding in some of the male members of a lineage. Females in this lineage may be carriers of the trait but this is usually difficult to demonstrate even by assay of the factor since the range of normal is wide.

Classic hemophilia in the female requires a match between a male hemophiliac and a female carrier of the trait. This is clearly an unusual event. Only about two-thirds of hemophiliacs will have a positive family history at all. Some of the remainder are the direct result of mutation. The clinical severity of the disease is usually similar in all affected members of a given family. It is, therefore, unusual for a severe case of hemophilia to occur in a lineage characterized by mild disease.

The bleeding time is normal in hemophilia but recurrent late bleeding is the rule. With the severance of large vessels, hemostasis is impossible without replacement of the missing factor. The deficient factor must be identified and assayed and replacement must be accomplished prior to surgery. Adequate factor levels must be maintained for 1 to 2 weeks after operation.

In hemophilia A, hemostasis requires a factor VIII level of 30 to 40 per cent of normal. This usually requires, in the adult, the administration of the amount of factor VIII in six to eight units of blood. Since the biologic half-life of factor VIII is less than 12 hours, half the initial dose must be given at 12-hour intervals. Clearly, this fluid volume is difficult to attain when blood or plasma is used, and therefore concentrates are needed. Factor VIII replacement is made more difficult because of the lability of the factor in storage. It must be stored in the frozen or lyophilized state. Such replacement therapy is extremely expensive; it is usually wise, therefore, to schedule several elective surgical procedures at one time. The almost universal availability of cryoprecipitates may ultimately make replacement less expensive as well as reducing waste of this blood product.

Occasionally, in the hemophiliac, antibodies to the transfused protein factor develop, and very large quantities become necessary to effect the desired circulating level. These situations are more difficult to manage but the principle is the same. Enough of the deficient factor must be given to attain a level of 30 to 40 per cent of the normal. Quantitative assay is necessary in order to determine precisely how much is required. High doses of corticosteroids may be given simultaneously in an effort to help overcome the inhibition of factor VIII activity.

The commercially available concentrates are prepared from pooled plasma and are lyophilized. These preparations carry a higher risk of transmission of hepatitis than nonpooled preparations but are more convenient and more precisely standardized for use. Cryoprecipitate is obtained as a by-product of modern standard blood component therapy and constitutes the cold-precipitable proteins, primarily fibrinogen and factor VIII, present in a standard unit of blood. Because the amount of factor VIII in cryoprecipitates is more variable and because there is some loss of it in preparation, replacement with cryoprecipitates requires more units than replacement with lyophilized concentrate. The advantages of cryoprecipitates lie in ready availability in any modern blood bank and the obvious economy of utilizing an otherwise wasted natural resource. Furthermore, the incidence of hepatitis after use of nonpooled plasma products is always less than after use of pooled preparations.

Deficiency of factor IX (hemophilia B) is usually easier to manage for several reasons. The turnover time of factor IX in the plasma is longer than that of factor VIII, and therefore less frequent administration is possible. Factor IX is also more stable on storage and thus less difficult to provide. Furthermore, a blood level lower than the required levels of factor VIII is quite compatible with normal hemostasis.

The initial clearance curve of factor IX in the plasma is much steeper than that of factor VIII, because of a larger distribution space, but the over-all biologic half-life is twice that of factor VIII. Because of this, a large loading dose, equivalent to 60 ml. of plasma per kilogram of body weight, should be given before surgery. This can be given slowly over a 24-hour period. One-fourth this amount given every 24 hours after the loading dose will usually provide an adequate plasma level in the patient. The actual level should, of course, be assayed routinely in order to be certain that an acceptable level of about 25 per cent of normal is obtained. Antibodies to administered factor IX have been found, but this occurrence is very rare. Concentrates of factor IX are commercially available; these concentrates are also rich in factors VII, X, and II.

The danger of hepatitis from these plasma products is always a consideration and some have recommended prophylactic administration of immune gamma globulin while the defect is being corrected. This question is not settled as yet, and until sufficient data are available no recommendation can be made. However, single donor plasma should be used when possible.

Factor XI deficiency is much rarer and usually is not associated with a history of inordinate overt bleeding or joint problems. However, serious bleeding can occur in these patients during and after surgery. The screening tests are normal except for the prolonged PTT as in the hemophilias. The factor XI activity should be assayed for confirmation after the more common deficiencies of factor VIII or IX are excluded. No concentrate of factor XI is available, and so treatment is accomplished with plasma collected in plastic bags to avoid activation of factor XI by activated factor XII.

Factor XII deficiency has no clinical significance. Even with the challenge of major surgery, hemostasis presents no problem. This factor is called "contact" factor and in its absence the PTT is markedly prolonged. Factor XII deficiency must, therefore, be differentiated from the other causes of isolated prolongation of the PTT that do require treatment.

DEFICIENCIES OF THE EXTRINSIC CLOTTING SYSTEM

As previously mentioned the prothrombin time (PT) reflects the function of the entire extrinsic system. As can be seen in the coagulation diagram (Fig. 4–2), only factor VII is involved solely in the extrinsic system.

Deficiency of factor VII is characterized by a prolonged PT but normal results in all the other tests. Not all patients with severe deficiency of this factor will experience abnormal bleeding at surgery. When bleeding does occur, it is not massive. The effective replacement level approximates 5 per cent of normal, and this is easily attained by transfusion when necessary. The factor is stable under standard storage conditions and therefore fresh plasma is not required.

Factor V deficiency is very similar to factor VII deficiency except that the PTT is usually abnormal and the patients tend to have more serious bleeding with surgery. Replacement requires *fresh* frozen plasma, 10 ml. per kilogram a day preoperatively and for a week after surgery.

Hereditary deficiency of factor X or prothrombin is extremely rare. The PT and the PTT are prolonged but the remaining screening tests are normal. Assay is necessary to identify the deficiency. There are no reports of surgery other than dental extraction in patients with these deficiency states, and very little is known about patient response. Stored plasma will replace these factors.

Fibrinogen deficiency is most commonly acquired as a result of defibrination in disseminated intravascular coagulation (DIC) but occasionally is inherited. Patients with hereditary afibrinogenemia have almost no fibrinogen in their plasma. They may go long periods of time without problems unless operated upon or otherwise injured. They cannot form a clot, and so the thrombin time obviously is abnormal, as are any tests relying on clot formation as an end point. Qualitative abnormalities of fibrinogen also have been described.

Fibrinogen is present in cryoprecipitates and should be transfused to a level of about 200 mg. per 100 ml. before surgery. About one-fifth of the loading dose should be given daily for a week after surgery. Both deficiency of fibrinogen and qualitatively abnormal fibrinogen have been associated with wound dehiscence.

Factor XIII deficiency has also been associated with poor wound healing. Characteristically hemostasis is normal until the day after surgery and then rebleeding occurs. Diagnosis can be made by observing dissolution of a clot in urea. Usually the diagnosis is not made because transfusion — for blood loss — corrects the deficiency for weeks.

Vitamin K-Dependent Group. Much more common than the inherited deficiencies of individual factors in the extrinsic system is the combined deficiency of VII, IX, X, and II, which is the result of vitamin K deficiency, liver disease, or coumarin drugs. In fact, in severe liver disease only factor VIII is *not* affected, but it is convenient to include the coagulation defects associated with liver disease in the discussion of factors of the vitamin K-dependent group. With adequate supply of this fat-soluble vitamin, the liver synthesizes factors VII, IX, X, and II. Deficiency of the vitamin may result from dietary inadequacy, prolonged intravenous feeding, steatorrhea, obstructive biliary disease, or alteration of intestinal flora by antibiotics. The simplest way to distinguish liver disease from vitamin K deficiency as a cause for a prolonged prothrombin time is to administer parenteral vitamin K_1. If the prothrombin time is not almost completely corrected within 24 hours, deficiency of the vitamin is not the problem. If liver disease is the problem, the factors can be replaced conveniently by transfusion of plasma. Necessary surgery can then be accomplished. The salutary effect will last only a few days, however, unless the liver recovers and is able to synthesize the necessary proteins.

CIRCULATING ANTICOAGULANTS. In addition to the previously mentioned antibodies to factor VIII elicited in hemophiliacs, similar antibodies can occur spontaneously, especially in patients with autoimmune disease. The screening tests suggest hemophilia but normal plasma will not correct the defect. The abnormal test results with test plasma and normal plasma are made worse by incubating the two together prior to testing. Antibodies to factor V, as well as to factor XIII, have also been reported. Some of these anticoagulants pose serious clinical problems and may not respond to any therapeutic maneuver. Sometimes they disappear either spontaneously or concomitantly with corticosteroid or immunosuppressive treatment. Exchange transfusion may be of temporary benefit. Elective surgery should be postponed in these patients and emergency surgery undertaken with the knowledge that it may not be possible to stop the bleeding.

DISSEMINATED INTRAVASCULAR COAGULATION (DIC). This syndrome has enjoyed immense popularity in recent years. A plethora of papers have appeared ascribing the initiation of this process to almost every imaginable disease, drug, or organism.

The most obvious clinical setting is, of course, the long-recognized hypofibrinogenemia associated with obstetric catastrophes. The recommended treatment until not long ago was replacement of fibrinogen. Evacuation of the uterus was also recommended, and this latter maneuver probably accounted for the survival of many of these patients.

If a thromboplastic substance, such as amniotic fluid, gains access to the circulation, diffuse coagulation may be expected. The fibrinolytic mechanism is also activated in an attempt to keep the circulation open by lysing fibrin. The effect of this sequence is: (1) clotting factors are consumed (primarily factors VIII and V, fibrinogen, and platelets and, to a lesser extent, factors II, VII, IX, X, and XIII); (2) fibrin split products are formed and interfere with fibrin polymerization, thus acting as anticoagulant and prolonging the thrombin time; and (3) the fibrin plugs in the microvasculature induce morphologic changes in the red cell. Torn, sheared red cells, resembling helmets and fragments, characterize what has been called the microangiopathic blood picture.

Bleeding may be minimal to massive but the process may be lethal even without bleeding if, for example, fibrin deposition results in renal cortical necrosis. It would seem that transfusion of fibrinogen would merely feed a fire and hasten tragedy. Possibly the evacuation of the uterus in obstetric catastrophes — that is, removal of the cause — permitted the clotting system to regain an equilibrium compatible with survival. Septic abortion is particularly hazardous since gram-negative organisms may themselves initiate the process.

Other common clinical settings include hemolytic transfusion reactions, any severe infection, massive tissue trauma, malignancy, and even shock and burns.

Especially in those cases in which the inciting agent cannot be removed immediately, the process must be interrupted by the use of heparin. It is extremely dangerous to give fibrinogen or even whole blood without first stopping the process. The antifibrinolytic agent epsilon-aminocaproic acid (EACA) may, in fact, block the only physiologic defense of the kidneys the patient has. Heparin is necessary, and therein lies the problem. A certain degree of reluctance on the part of the physician to give a potent anticoagulant to a hemorrhaging patient is understandable. In fact, if the diagnosis is incorrect the result could well be worsening of an already desperate situation.

The first requirement for diagnosis is awareness of the possibility. The screening tests are ordered, and the blood smear is examined. The red cell morphology is observed, and severe thrombocytopenia usually will also be obvious on the smear. Thrombocytopenia may be moderate or severe but must be present. The PTT, PT, and TT all are prolonged. If the fibrinogen level is determined it is found to be less than 150 mg. per 100 ml. Some rapid test for fibrin split products should also be available. Various tests, such as protamine precipitation, ethanol gelation, and the TT, reflect fibrin split products and in borderline cases this may be useful. Severe hepatic necrosis can produce most of these findings, but factor VIII assay will not be low and this fact may occasionally be useful.

Minimal criteria for diagnosis, in the absence of liver disease, would be: (1) platelet count under 150,000 per cubic millimeter; (2) fibrinogen under 150 mg. per 100 ml.; (3) prothrombin time greater than 15 sec. (control 12); and (4) microangiopathic blood smear. If only two of these are present some demonstration of fibrin split products is mandatory.

A dose of 100 USP units of heparin per kilogram body weight should be given intravenously every 4 hours. This probably should be continued for 24 hours after the causative factor has been removed. Replacement of the consumed clotting factors by transfusing platelets, fresh frozen plasma, and/or cryoprecipitate after heparin is begun will cause no problem but may not be necessary.

OPERATIVE AND POSTOPERATIVE BLEEDING

When the history and physical examination give no reason to anticipate a bleeding disorder and the preoperative screening tests are all normal, the possible causes for unexpected bleeding are reduced considerably. The incidence of this event has been reported from various sources to be between 0.05 and 4.0 per cent. A definite plan is necessary to facilitate management. Such a plan must entail three elements: informed deliberate judgment; a few well-chosen tests; and knowledge of appropriate treatment.

The causes of bleeding in this particular clinical situation are listed in approximate order of frequency.

1. Surgical or mechanical fault.
2. Thrombocytopenia, especially with extracorporeal circulation or after use of more than five units of stored blood.
3. Disseminated intravascular coagulation (DIC) associated with hemolytic transfusion or other causes.
4. Unsuspected mild coagulation defect.
5. Post-transfusion purpura (rare).

Far and away the most common cause of operative or postoperative bleeding in a patient with a negative history and physical examination, as well as normal screening tests, is failure to tie bleeding vessels. Almost all experienced surgeons would agree with this. For whatever reason, possibly because of pressure of retraction or torsion of tissue during the operation, even though a field appears dry at closure, rebleeding occurs afterward. The extent of bleeding frequently suggests the cause. Bleeding confined to the pleural cavity or pericardium, with dry venipuncture sites, strongly suggests a local problem. Postoperative internal bleeding that requires constant replacement is likely to be surgical in origin if a bleeding problem was not evident with the first incision. Despite the fact that a mechanical fault is most likely the problem, other causes must be excluded in order to justify exploration.

Thrombocytopenia commonly occurs while the operation is still in progress. The usual setting is as follows: Excessive bleeding, usually mechanical, is treated with numerous transfusions of stored blood which is essentially free of viable platelets; more bleeding occurs and more platelet-free blood is given. Platelet concentrates should be used routinely after five units of blood are required. A quick look at a stained blood smear or a platelet count will of course identify this problem.

DIC during or after surgery is most frequently the result of an incompatible blood transfusion. Whatever the cause, a generalized oozing may indicate the development of this complication. Because anesthesia may prevent one of the early signs of transfusion incompatibility, namely, the shaking chill, one must be alert to other signs. A fall in blood pressure may also go unappreciated since the blood may have been given because of a falling pressure. It is imperative that a blood transfusion be discontinued when generalized oozing occurs. The blood type and other information on the label should, of course, be checked; but several other things should be observed immediately. Prompt recovery of blood pressure and cessation of oozing would suggest that the blood had been responsible. Cessation of oozing without return of blood pressure is less informative since hypotension may itself reduce bleeding. Agglutinated red cells may be observed on the scalpel blade if looked for. If hemolysis is occurring, a centrifuged specimen of blood will reveal hemoglobin in the plasma on inspection. While the blood bank is preparing more blood and cross-matching the discontinued blood again, salt solutions should be used to maintain circulatory volume and to assure adequate hydration. An osmotic diuretic such as mannitol should be administered since it has been established that this can provide some protection from severe renal tubular necrosis. The DIC that frequently attends this clinical setting is transient and usually requires no treatment once the causative agent has been removed.

DIC may occur as the result of endotoxins in transfused blood or thromboplastins released during surgery. The most common operative procedures that have been associated with DIC are surgery of the lung, pancreas, prostate, and aortic aneurysms. The onset may be in the postoperative period when oozing at venipuncture sites is noted. Management is precisely as outlined earlier.

Unsuspected mild deficiencies of clotting factors are unusual problems after careful screening, but when they occur the diagnosis and management seldom pose new problems. For example, very mild classic hemophilia may escape detection and cause serious bleeding. Attempts to keep up with blood loss by transfusion of stored blood further reduces the level of factor VIII; thus a repeat PTT at this time would be more likely to suggest the problem and treatment can be given as outlined previously. Most of the clotting deficiencies, of course, are being treated quite satisfactorily simply by the expedient of blood replacement since low levels of the factors involved are sufficient and stored blood contains all but platelets and factors VIII and V.

Post-transfusion purpura (PTP) is a rare condition, but when it occurs it presents a very alarming clinical picture and therefore warrants mention. The setting is typically a patient recovering uneventfully from an uncomplicated surgical procedure wherein a transfusion was administered. One week after the surgery severe purpura and bleeding occur. Platelet count reveals severe thrombocytopenia. Usually the patient is a middle-aged woman who has previously been pregnant. Transfusion of platelets or blood after onset of the condition may be associated with a severe reaction, and there is no increment in platelet count. A very high titer antibody to 98 per cent of donor platelets can be demonstrated (anti Pl^{A1}). Since the patient's own platelets do not carry this antigen it is likely that another, or cross-reacting, antibody also exists. The titer of the responsible antibody is probably too low to be measured in vitro but sufficient to cause the thrombocytopenia. The self-limited course ranges from 2 to 6 weeks unless exchange transfusion is accomplished. The risk of severe thrombocytopenia in this age group is such that these patients should probably undergo plasma exchange as soon as the diagnosis is made. It is very important to recognize that platelet transfusion is contraindicated, since the transfused platelets will not circulate; and furthermore, transfusion can result in a severe, even life-threatening, reaction.

MISCELLANEOUS REPORTS

It has been known for some time that patients being treated with coumarin anticoagulants, well-controlled in the therapeutic range of the prothrombin time, can withstand major surgery without excessive bleeding. Although a slight reduction in dosage may be prudent, the use of vitamin K is probably not indicated since rebound phenomena are possible. Furthermore, if bleeding is encountered, transfusion of stored blood will immediately replace the deficient factors far more expeditiously than vitamin K administration.

As a means of reducing thrombosis and emboli in high-risk patients it has been suggested that low doses of heparin (5000 units given subcutaneously 2 hours *before* surgery and every 12 hours throughout the postoperative period) may be very useful. No increase in bleeding was observed in patients thus treated as compared to a control group of similar but unheparinized patients. This dosage has no detectable effect on the laboratory screening tests but apparently is effective in reducing thrombosis and thromboembolism. A corollary of these studies would justify the inference that heparinized patients requiring surgery could be maintained on heparin at this reduced dosage level. This would avoid the possibility of rebound after abrupt termination of heparin therapy. The peak dosage attained by this treatment is approximately one-tenth that of the more conventional dose schedules. Intramuscular heparin, especially in the hip, should always be avoided since local bleeding can go completely unrecognized and dissection into the retroperitoneal space may occur.

Epsilon-aminocaproic acid (EACA) is probably the drug most overused, and most improperly used, in bleeding patients. The only indication for this drug is the existence of primary fibrinolysis. This is an exceedingly unusual event and must be documented as being primary since use of the drug in secondary fibrinolysis, before heparin, can cause much harm. In addition to generalized fibrin deposition and renal cortical necrosis produced when EACA has been used in treatment of DIC, the drug has been associated with blockage of the ureters in hemophiliacs, and with glomerular capillary thrombosis and subendocardial hemorrhage. In prostatic surgery, local fibrinolysis is common because of the presence of urokinase in the urine and local plasmin activation. EACA is concentrated by the kidney, and so a low dosage, 1 gm. every 3 hours, has been found useful. It should be remembered, however, that hematuria after prostatic surgery is commonly the result of DIC. Therefore, the routine use of EACA, without appropriate studies to rule out DIC, would seem to be inordinately hazardous.

Aspirin significantly prolongs the bleeding time by altering platelet function, but this does not as a rule cause a significant surgical problem. The presence of aspirin can, however, exaggerate problems in the presence of other defects in hemostasis. Not uncommonly, blood from donors who have taken aspirin contains functionally abnormal platelets.

A useless procedure occasionally utilized in the operating room is the application of hot packs to a bleeding area. In the first place the heat dilates vessels and increases bleeding. If the packs are hot enough (I have seen them too hot to hold), actual tissue damage and denaturation of coagulation enzymes might occur. In contrast, cold, in the form of a Popsicle in the mouth, for example, may be a useful maneuver in stopping oral bleeding.

The administration of calcium after transfusion of large volumes of citrated blood has also been recommended, but the concentration of calcium needed for normal coagulation is such that this is never necessary. Mobilization from the body's considerable stores will more than adequately compensate for the infused citrate. Hypocalcemia, even to the extent of clinical tetany, has had no demonstrable effect on hemostasis. In fact, there is probably no basis for the fear of "citrate intoxication," even as far as electrocardiographic changes are concerned.

Vitamin C is useful in scurvy but has no demonstrated beneficial effect on the hemostatic mechanism otherwise. Vitamins P and E have been suggested as treatment for bleeding. It is interesting that the latter has also been recommended for prevention of thromboses. These agents, like rutin, antihistamines, bioflavonoids, lipotropic agents, adrenochromes, dried platelets, extracts of various hormones, and other nostrums, do not replace a missing factor nor do they tie a bleeding vessel. Adequate specific replacement therapy and careful ligation are what is necessary in the prevention and management of hemorrhagic complications in surgery.

Bibliography

1. Allen, J. G.: The case for the single transfusion. N. Engl. J. Med. *287*:984, 1972.
2. Barkhan, P.: Haematological consequences of major surgery. Br. J. Haematol. *17*:221, 1969.
3. Basu, D., Gallus, A., Hirsh, J., and Cade, J.: A prospective study of the value of monitoring heparin treatment with the activated partial thromboplastin time. N. Engl. J. Med. *287*:324, 1972.
4. Becker, G. A., and Aster, R. H.: Platelet transfusion therapy. Med. Clin. North Am. *56*:81, 1972.
5. Biggs, R. (Ed.): Human Blood Coagulation and Its Disorders. Philadelphia, F. A. Davis Company, 1972.
6. Colman, R. W., Robboy, S. J., and Minna J. D.: Disseminated intravascular coagulation (DIC): An approach. Am. J. Med. *52*:679, 1972.

7. Colman, R. W., and Rodriguez-Erdmann, F.: Terminology of intravascular coagulation. N. Engl. J. Med. *282*:99, 1970.

8. Crosby, W. H.: The problem of oozing during surgery. Anesthesiology *20*:685, 1959.

9. Crosby, W. H., and Howard, J. M.: The hematologic response to wounding and to resuscitation accomplished by large transfusions of stored blood. A study of battle casualties in Korea. Blood *9*:439, 1954.

10. Deykin, D.: Thrombogenesis. N. Engl. J. Med., *276*:622, 1967.

11. Deykin, D.: Regulation of heparin therapy. N. Engl. J. Med. *287*:355, 1972.

12. Deykin, D.: The clinical challenge of disseminated intravascular coagulation. N. Engl. J. Med. *283*:636, 1970.

13. Diamond, L. K., and Porter, F. S.: The inadequacies of routine bleeding and clotting times. N. Engl. J. Med. *259*:1025, 1958.

14. Hardaway, R. M., McKay, D. G., Wahle, G. H., and Hall, R. M.: Pathologic study of intravascular coagulation following incompatible blood transfusion in dogs. I. Intravenous injection of incompatible blood. II. Intra-aortic injection of incompatible blood. Am. J. Surg. *91*:24, 32, 1956.

15. Harker, L. A., and Slichter, S. J.: The bleeding time as a screening test for evaluation of platelet function. N. Engl. J. Med. *287*:155, 1972.

16. Jackson, D. P., Sorensen, D. K., Cronkite, E. P., Bond, V. P., and Fliedner, T. M.: Effectiveness of transfusions of fresh and lyophilized platelets in controlling bleeding due to thrombocytopenia. J. Clin. Invest. *38*:1689, 1959.

17. Kakkar, V. V., Spindler, J., Flute, P. T., Corrigan, T., Fossard, D. P., Crellin, R. Q., Wessler, S., and Yin, E. T.: Efficacy of low doses of heparin in prevention of deep-vein thrombosis after major surgery. Lancet *2*:101, 1972.

18. Karpatkin, S., and Weiss, H. J.: Deficiency of glutathione peroxidase associated with high levels of reduced glutathione in Glanzmann's thrombasthenia. N. Engl. J. Med. *287*:1062, 1972.

19. Kasper, C. K., and Rapaport, S. I.: Bleeding times and platelet aggregation after analgesics in hemophilia. Ann. Intern. Med. *77*:189, 1972.

20. Kim, B. K., and Baldini, M.: Reversal reaction and viability of frozen human platelets. (Abstract) Cryobiology *9*:29, 1972.

21. Levine, P. H.: Emergency search for a bleeding diathesis. Arch. Int. Med. *130*:445, 1972.

22. Mielke, C. H., Jr., Kaneshiro, M. M., Maher, I. A., Weiner, J. M., and Rapaport, S. I.: The standardized normal Ivy bleeding time and its prolongation by aspirin. Blood *34*:204, 1969.

23. Morrison, F. S.: Platelet transfusion. Vox Sang. *11*:656, 1966.

24. Morrison, F. S.: Preservation of blood platelets. Cryobiology *5*:29, 1968.

25. Morrison, F. S., and Mollison, P. L.: Posttransfusion purpura. N. Engl. J. Med. *275*:243, 1966.

26. Morrison, F. S., and Wurzel, H. A.: Retroperitoneal hemorrhage during heparin therapy. Am. J. Cardiol. *13*:329, 1964.

27. Morrison, F. S. (Ed.): Hemostasis for Blood Bankers. Washington, D.C., American Association of Blood Banks, 1977.

28. Morrison, F. S. (Ed.): Hemophilia. Washington, D.C., American Association of Blood Banks, 1978.

29. Müllertz, S., and Storm, O.: Anticoagulant therapy with dicumarol maintained during major surgery. Circulation *10*:213, 1954.

30. Nicolaides, A. N., Desai, S., Douglas, J. N., Fourides, G., Dupont, P. A., Lewis, J. D., Dodsworth, H., Luck, R. J., and Jamieson, C. W.: Small doses of subcutaneous sodium heparin in preventing deep venous thrombosis after major surgery. Lancet *2*:890, 1972.

31. O'Brien, J. R., Jamieson, S., Etherington, M., and Klaber, M. R.: Platelet function in venous thrombosis and low-dosage heparin. Lancet *2*:1302, 1972.

32. Penick, G. D., Averett, H. E., Jr., Peters, R. M., and Brinkhous, K. M.: The hemorrhagic syndrome complicating extracorporeal shunting of blood: An experimental study of its pathogenesis. Thromb. Diath. Haemorrh. *2*:218, 1958.

33. Petrucci, J. V.: Red cell (packed cell) transfusions: An appeal to reason. Md. State Med. J. *20*:61, 1971.

34. Ratnoff, O. D.: Epsilon aminocaproic acid — A dangerous weapon. N. Engl. J. Med. *280*:1124, 1969.

35. Rock, R. C., Bove, J. R., and Nemerson, Y.: Heparin treatment of intravascular coagulation accompanying hemolytic transfusion reactions. Transfusion *9*:57, 1969.

36. Rosenfield, R. E., Berkman, E. M., and Camp, F. R., Jr.: Transfusion reactions. *In* Conn, H. F. (Ed.): Current Therapy 1971. Philadelphia, W. B. Saunders Company, 1971.

37. Rustad, H., and Myhre, E.: Surgery during anticoagulant treatment. Acta Med. Scand. *173*:115, 1963.

38. Salzman, E. W., and Britten, A.: Hemorrhage and Thrombosis. Boston, Little, Brown and Company, 1965.

39. Schorr, J. B., and Marx, G. F.: New trends in intraoperative blood replacement. Anesth. Analg. *49*:646, 1970.

40. Simone, J. V.: Disseminated intravascular coagulation. Adv. Intern. Med. *15*:339, 1969.

41. Spaet, T.: Clinical implications of acquired blood coagulation abnormalities. Blood *23*:839, 1964.

42. Sutor, A. H., Bowie, E. J. W., and Owen, C. A., Jr.: Effect of aspirin, sodium salicylate, and acetaminophen on bleeding. Mayo Clin. Proc. *46*:178, 1971.

43. Ulin, A. W., Gollub, S., and Ehlich, E. W.: Unexplained bleeding in the surgical patient (hemorrhage associated with massive transfusion). Physiologic studies and clinical applications. Surg. Clin. North Am. *40*:1569, 1960.

44. Van Crevald, S.: Hemorrhagic diathesis in congenital heart disease — Influence of operation under hypothermia and of whole blood transfusions. Ann. Paediat. *190*:342, 1958.

45. Williams, W. J., Beutler, E., Ersler, A. L., and Rundles, R. W.: Hematology. 2nd ed. New York, McGraw-Hill Book Company, 1977.

5

COMPLICATIONS OF PARENTERAL FLUID THERAPY AND OTHER STATES OF POSTOPERATIVE FLUID DISEQUILIBRIUM

William Schumer*

The technological advances of the past 20 years have changed the characteristics and complications of fluid therapy administration. Heretofore, high fluid pyrogenicity coupled with inadequate methodology for the evaluation of specific fluid therapeutic requirements forced the physician to use the subcutaneous route (clysis). This technique, however, was not free of such complications as extravasation, sloughing, and indefinite absorption patterns, frequently resulting in profound metabolic derangements. Therefore, the development of minimally pyrogenous prepackaged intravenous solutions and new methodology for

determining specific metabolic and electrolytic fluid therapy requirements made the intravenous technique the desirable route of fluid administration. But these advances have not entirely eliminated complications of enteral and parenteral therapy as they will be discussed in this chapter.

COMPLICATIONS OF METHODS OF ADMINISTRATION

Needle

The use of metallic needles has declined in recent years because of the difficulty in maintaining them in place intravascularly. Common complications are perforation, hematoma, pain, and injury to the vessel, all of which promote clotting and subsequent venous obstruction. Thus, when Meyer in-

*We wish to acknowledge the late Dr. John A. Moncrief's contribution to this chapter. Portions of the chapter he authored in earlier editions of Management of Surgical Complications have been included in the present text.

William Schumer was born in Chicago and graduated from the Chicago Medical School, where he also earned a Master's Degree in Biochemistry. He took his internship and residency training at the Mount Sinai Hospital Medical Center of Chicago and subsequently joined the faculty as an Assistant Professor. In 1967 he became Associate Professor and later Professor at the University of Illinois College of Medicine. In 1975, he was appointed Professor and Chairman of the Department of Surgery at the University of Health Sciences, the Chicago Medical School. Dr. Schumer has long been interested in the physiology and management of shock, and his contributions in this and related fields have been the subject of many important publications.

troduced polyethylene catheters for simple long-term venous system cannulation, the "metallic needle age" was practically over, the only remnant being the use of small bore pediatric scalp or butterfly needles which, although easily dislodged, are almost free of complications.

Plastic Catheters

The polyethylene catheter, introduced by Meyer in 1945, was an improvement over the rigid metallic needle in that it lessened the injury to the venous intima. However, there were serious problems associated with its use. First, it was inserted through a large bore needle, and, since polyethylene does not have "memory," once the catheter was bent it remained thus. If the insertion was unsuccessful, the physician unaware of the "memory" problem pulled out the bent catheter and sheared off its tip on the sharp bevel of the needle, and this tip had to be surgically removed (Fig. 5–1). Also, the polyethylene catheter was thrombogenic.

The polyvinyl catheter does not have "memory" but is too rigid, so tissue reactions develop; however, there are fewer problems with retained catheter segments. More recently, there has been increasing use of Teflon and Silastic catheters. Teflon is more rigid than either polyvinyl or polyethylene, thus allowing the external insertion of a

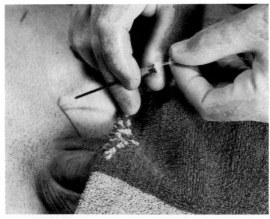

Figure 5–1. Technique of inserting femoral catheter to demonstrate the ease with which the catheter can be sheared off if withdrawn through the needle. Femoral catheter techniques have for the most part been supplanted by the subclavian catheter but the method of shearing the plastic catheter is the same in both locations.

Teflon catheter into the vein by placing it over the needle, which diminishes the possibility of shearing the catheter when it is withdrawn. This technique cannot be used with polyethylene and polyvinyl, since they pleat accordion-like around the needle at insertion. Teflon is not thrombogenic and causes minimal tissue reaction. The extreme pliability of Silastic catheters prevents perforation and — almost completely — thrombosis. It is inserted through a large bore needle or by venous cutdown, and because of minimal tissue reaction it may remain in place indefinitely. Silastic catheters are now being utilized in prolonged total parenteral nutrition.

Technical Error

Hematoma

A local hematoma of varying severity may result from laceration or perforation of the vein wall during insertion of a long-beveled needle or a rigid polyethylene or polyvinyl catheter. The appearance of either edema, hematoma, and/or skin discoloration at the insertion site is easily recognized when cannulating superficial veins, but difficult when cannulating the large veins of the chest, lower limbs, and abdomen. Treatment consists of discontinuation of intravenous fluids, elevation of the extremities, and warm compresses to the affected area. Slow reabsorption of the hematoma usually follows.

Perforation or Laceration of Vessel

Laceration of the large veins of either the chest, abdomen, or lower limbs may be diagnosed by observing the clinical symptoms produced by impingement of the contiguous structure, secondary to either the hematoma or the contents of the parenteral solution. Perforation of the chest vein is a severe complication that can be recognized by the clinical signs of chest pain radiating to the neck and/or distention of the neck veins. A diagnosis of extravasation or major perforation should be considered when a patient develops dyspnea, chest pain, cyanosis, and/or shock following placement of a catheter into a subclavian or large vein. The injury may be localized by roentgenogram examination and thoracentesis. The treatment may vary from thoracentesis for small blood loss to closed thoracotomy tube insertion, or exploratory thoracotomy for massive hematoma. A large mediastinal hematoma may produce superior vena caval obstruction necessitating either cervical exploration, median sternotomy, or anterior thoracotomy to evacuate the hematoma and accomplish hemostasis (Fig. 5–2).

Abdominal venous perforation and/or laceration is more difficult to diagnose because of the resiliency and expanse of the posterior peritoneal space. There may be vague abdominal complaints and because of the dissecting nature of the hematoma, ecchymoses of the lateral abdominal wall and umbilicus similar to those of hemorrhagic pancreatitis may be present (Grey Turner sign). Ordinarily when the catheter is removed the bleeding subsides, resulting in a hematoma tamponade. If after adequate blood volume restitution hypovolemic shock persists, then an exploratory laparotomy should be performed to accomplish hemostasis and evacuation of the hematoma.

MYOCARDIAL PERFORATION. This complication occurs when the tip of the long central venous pressure or pulmonary artery pressure catheter injures the heart, causing either atrial and ventricular irritability or irritation of the tricuspid valve, the latter leading to thrombosis. The most common injuries are gradual myocardial perforation producing either a blood tamponade, a perfusate tamponade or an acute perforation secondary to introduction of a pulmonary artery pressure catheter. Less common is coronary sinus obstruction resulting in venous outflow disruption and pericardial effusion and tamponade. Recognition of these complications involves a roentgenographic examination immediately after inserting the catheter. Treatment consists of removal of the catheter from the heart; this treatment is usually sufficient because the perforation seals itself. Rarely is pericardial aspiration or myocardial suturing necessary (Fig. 5–3).

PNEUMOTHORAX. This complication may occur when the subclavian route is utilized for the introduction of intravenous catheters. Both the supraclavicular and intraclavicular routes have been implicated in this complication, since the apical pleura lies only 5 mm. from the posterior wall of the subclavian vein after it passes over the first rib.

The symptoms are those typical of any pneumothorax, their severity depending upon the magnitude of the pneumothorax and the presence or absence of any tension

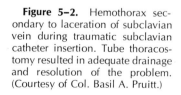

Figure 5–2. Hemothorax secondary to laceration of subclavian vein during traumatic subclavian catheter insertion. Tube thoracostomy resulted in adequate drainage and resolution of the problem. (Courtesy of Col. Basil A. Pruitt.)

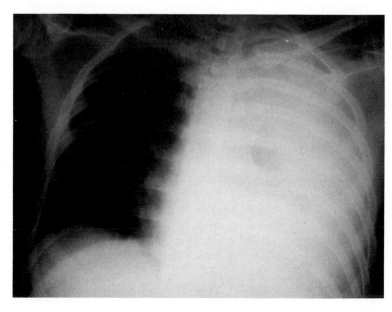

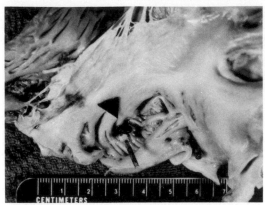

Figure 5–3. Perforation of the wall of the right atrium by a plastic cannula. This complication of subclavian catheter insertion resulted in a fatal pericardial tamponade with Ringer's lactate solution. (Courtesy of Col. Basil A. Pruitt.)

component. Ordinarily, the patient complains of shortness of breath and chest pain, and upon auscultation, diminished breath sounds can be detected; occasionally, there may be a moderate shift of the mediastinum.

Therapy is directed to reexpansion of the lung — thoracentesis for minimal pneumothorax; tube thoracostomy for recurrent, significant, or tension pneumothorax; and tracheostomy when marked subcutaneous emphysema and respiratory embarrassment are present. Ordinarily, the pneumothorax results from the laceration of the apical pleura by the needle used to insert the subclavian catheter.

Pneumothorax is such a common complication after insertion of the subclavian catheter that a chest film should be routinely obtained to detect the presence of even subclinical evidence of pneumothorax.

THORACIC DUCT INJURY. This injury may occur during subclavian vein cannulation when either the supraclavicular or external jugular vein route is used, and it also may occur during internal jugular vein cannulation. Minimal swelling and hydrothorax of the left side of the neck usually signal the diagnosis. Aspiration of the chest reveals cloudy to creamy yellow fluid in the pleural space; its lymphocytic nature is confirmed by the high triglyceride content and the almost complete dominance of lymphocytes among the white cell population in the field.

Therapy consists of removal of the jugular catheter and conservative management of the laceration with bed rest, low-fat diet, and repeated aspiration of the chest. If after 2 to 4 days the amount of chyle accumulation is not diminishing, surgical intervention under local anesthesia should be accomplished. Ordinarily the duct can be readily identified, and both the proximal and distal stumps should be ligated. Postoperatively, there is rapid resolution of the pleural effusion, and the chest tube can then be removed.

Extravasation Injuries

Extravasation necrosis is signified by localized pain usually attributable to vasospasm but disproportionately intense relative to any evidence of soft tissue fluid accumulation. Discoloration of the skin overlying the area is followed by varying degrees of sensory loss and subsequent moderate intradermal edema. The area becomes indurated during the next 24 to 48 hours, and following the resolution of the intradermal edema the involved area becomes depressed below the surrounding skin with the sharply demarcated margins clearly delineating the impending necrosis. Further discoloration rapidly progresses until finally there is blackening of the skin (Fig. 5–4). In Upton and associates' 1979 review of extravasation injuries, the following mechanisms of extravasation necrosis were described:

1. Osmotically active substances such as urea, calcium, potassium, and diatrizoate, when injected as a bolus into the interstitial subcutaneous space may cause intracellular uptake of the osmotically active cations (calcium and potassium), producing cellular swelling and death. Urea may produce cell death by intracellular dehydration.

2. Ischemic necrosis may be caused when extravasated vasopressors and cationic solutions such as dopamine, epinephrine, and norepinephrine produce vasoconstriction and ischemia with consequent accumulation of large intracellular concentrations of lactic acid that induce lysosomal enzyme release. Cations such as calcium and potassium cause ischemic necrosis by prolonged depolarization and contraction of the pre- and post-capillary sphincters, and finally, gangrene of the affected area occurs.

3. Direct cellular toxicity may be caused by extravasated agents such as adriamycin, a DNA replication inhibitor, and methotrexate, a folate antagonist that interrupts purine biosynthesis. The extent of cellular death and tissue necrosis is dependent on the dosage and concentration of the cytotoxic drug administered. Diazepam, tetracycline, and pentothal are painful when extravasated and exert their necrosing effect by localized intimal damage and subsequent small vessel thrombosis.

4. Mechanical compression capillary perfusion occurs when intravenous fluids are administered with a mechanical infusion pump. Increased extracellular hydrostatic pressure causes increased interstitial pressure and venous compression, ultimately compromising arterial blood flow.

5. Bacterial colonization secondary to any of the above extravasation processes is an additive factor to the extent and depth of tissue loss.

The following guidelines for the preven-

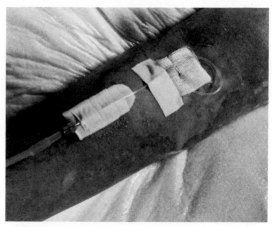

Figure 5–5. Technique of splinting the polyethylene tubing at the point at which it joins the adaptor or needle to prevent puncture or severance at this point. The catheter lying free between the skin entry point and the adaptor may be readily severed during dressing change if extreme care is not used. (Courtesy of Col. Basil A. Pruitt.)

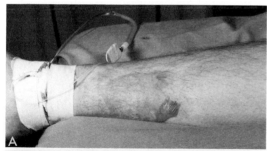

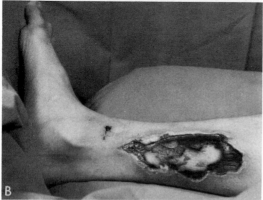

Figure 5–4. *A,* Early appearance of impending ischemic slough secondary to infiltration of solution containing 40 mEq. per liter of potassium chloride. *B,* Appearance of wound following stabilization of the ischemic necrosis and prior to surgical débridement. Skin grafting of defect was necessary. (Courtesy of Col. Basil A. Pruitt.)

tion of extravasation during intravenous fluid therapy administration are recommended:

1. Use large central veins. Lower limbs should be avoided, particularly in the elderly with preexisting vascular disease.

2. Multiple perforations or repeated use of the same vein should be avoided, especially when administering the above drugs.

3. Use soft plastic catheters and avoid metal needles.

4. Avoid infusing under any pressure; monitor all perfusion pump infusions.

5. Avoid infusing high-risk drugs directly over tendons, nerves, and blood vessels, especially those of the dorsum of the hand and wrist.

6. Avoid camouflaging the intravenous administration site with dressings and armboards so that monitoring may be facilitated (Fig. 5–5).

The specific treatment for extravasation injuries of intravenous fluid administration is listed in Table 5–1.

Septic and Aseptic Complications

Sepsis

It has been stated that "for all intents and purposes the patient receiving intravenous

TABLE 5–1 TREATMENT OF MAJOR INTRAVENOUS EXTRAVASATION INJURIES

Causative Agents	Treatment
Osmotically Active Solutions and Cations 30% urea, hypertonic glucose, calcium gluconate, calcium chloride, diatrizoate, bicarbonate, potassium chloride	Clysis within 60 minutes with 0.9% N sodium chloride and hyaluronidase in dosages of 150 units per liter at 10× volume of the causative agent; corticosteroids may be indicated; antibiotics*
Vasopressors Dopamine, aramine, epinephrine, norepinephrine	Early administration of phentolamine and piperoxan hydrochloride; local infiltration with phentolamine; antibiotics*
Cytotoxic Agents Adriamycin, methotrexate, sodium salt	Observation; antibiotics*; grafting
Mechanical Obstruction	Discontinuance of the pump infusion; local hyaluronidase; antibiotics*

*Recommended antibiotics are cephalosporins or ampicillins, followed by culture and sensitivity tests to determine further antibiotic therapy.

Note: If necrosis occurs, resect non-viable tissue and either close primarily or allow to heal by secondary intention, and then graft.

therapy has a hollow conduit directly connecting his bloodstream with the possible contamination of the outside world and its abundant microflora." The skin, the most important host defense, has been compromised, thus enhancing the chances for a septic episode. Sepsis owing to intravenous therapy may be caused by (1) contaminated additive fluids or drugs, and/or (2) conduits such as intravenous delivery sets, catheters, plastic containers, central venous pressure sets, filters, and connectors.

FLUID, DRUG, AND CONDUIT CONTAMINATION. Contamination of intravenous solutions (additives or drugs) continues to be reported. In 1970, liners in the threaded caps of parenteral solution bottles were found to contain *Enterobacter cloacae* and *E. agglomerans*. This contamination caused an outbreak of septicemia and septic shock of epidemic proportions — by April, 1971, 378 patients were involved — that was terminated by discontinuing the use of and by nationwide total recall of the manufacturer's infusion products. Three subsequent outbreaks of infection traced to intrinsically contaminated intravenous fluid were reported between April, 1971, and January, 1972, in England and the United States, emphasizing that no specific design should automatically be assumed to be safe.

In our hospital we routinely use the "light test" as a method of determining whether the solutions are usable; solutions that are cloudy or contain precipitates or particulates are discarded. Intravenous fluids may contain cultures of *Klebsiella pneumoniae*, *Enterobacter aerogenes*, *Serratia marcescens*, *Pseudomonas aeruginosa*, *Citrobacter freundii*, and *Pseudomonas cepacia*. The technique for reducing the incidence of fluid contamination is to change routinely, every 24 hours, the complete administration sets — bottles, bags, and complete delivery apparatus. In-line bacterial filters have also been advocated; however, their effectiveness has not been tested with controlled studies. Contamination of intravenous solutions may also occur during the preparation of parenteral nutrition. These fluids should be prepared in a central pharmacy area by a trained pharmacist and not on the ward by a nurse. Airborne contamination of these solutions can be eliminated by using the aseptic technique of wearing gloves, mask, and gown, and preparing the solutions under a laminar flow hood. Another advantage the central pharmacy offers is the reduction of drug incompatibility and medication errors.

CATHETER-RELATED SEPSIS. This is an ever-present risk in parenteral feeding, especially in total parenteral nutrition (TPN). The rates of positive catheter cultures have been reported to range from 3.8 to 5.7 per cent; rates of associated septicemia ranged from zero to as high as 8 per cent. Particularly high rates of positive cultures and sepsis were associated with surgical cutdowns and percutaneously placed

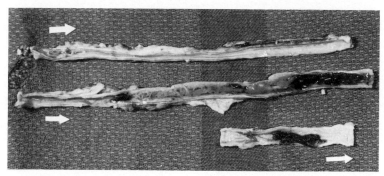

Figure 5–6.   An excised segment of vein involved in a process of septic phlebitis secondary to a long-standing cutdown utilizing a plastic cannula. The darkened areas indicate the areas of septic phlebitis. Note that there are skip areas and that the septic thrombus resides at a considerable distance from the cutdown site which is near the location of the top arrow. (From O'Neill, J. A., et al.: Suppurative thrombophlebitis — A lethal complication of intravenous therapy. J. Trauma, 8:256, 1968, © The Williams & Wilkins Company, Baltimore.)

subclavian catheters. The highest rates found were in association with neonatal umbilical catheters. The incidence of catheter-related septicemia ranged from 2 to 5 per cent with plastic catheters left in longer than 48 hours. Therefore, this observation formed the basis for the principle of removing intravenous catheters, whenever possible, within 48 to 72 hours of insertion. This may be a difficult principle to apply, especially in those very ill patients with poor veins; thus, their catheters should be inserted under strict surgical asepsis — sterile gloves, drapes, and mask, and in a treatment room away from hospital traffic. The insertion site should be scrubbed and cleansed and chemically disinfected with iodine. Once the catheter is inserted and firmly anchored, the site should be aseptically cleansed daily with iodine, and the veins should be palpated to determine the presence of tenderness, thrombosis, or inflammation.

SEPTIC PHLEBITIS. Despite the observance of careful aseptic principles and techniques, catheter sepsis may develop into septic phlebitis, one of the leading causes of septic shock and, ultimately, death. The vein becomes a site of purulence, discharging massive numbers of microorganisms into the bloodstream. *Staphylococcus aureus,* Enterobacter, and Serratia have been frequently implicated. In one series central venous suppuration was found in 18 per cent of autopsies of burn patients; suppuration in this location was almost uniformly lethal. In non-burn patients suppurative phlebitis may occur in cannulations of the lower limbs. Diagnosis of this condition is based on signs of septicemia: fever, chills, and toxicity, and if septic shock is present, a decreasing blood pressure. Expressing pus from the catheter or vein after removal of the catheter is the best way of diagnosing venous suppuration (Figs. 5–6 and 5–7).

Septic phlebitis treatment, which is similar to that of septicemia, is as follows:

1. Incision, drainage, and resection of the septic vein.

2. Antibiotics — immediately treat with amphotericin for fungal infection; second or third generation cephalosporins for bacterial infection. Culture and sensitivity tests determine further antibiotic therapy.

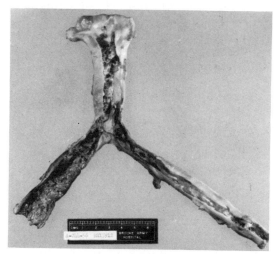

Figure 5–7.   Septic thrombus involving the inferior vena cava and both iliac vessels secondary to prolonged use of an indwelling femoral catheter.

3. Treat septic shock with intravenous fluids and corticosteroids.

4. Large vein ligation and heparin administration for emboli.

Today, greater emphasis is placed upon the appearance of Candida infection at catheter sites, particularly with the demonstration that the amino acid–glucose mixtures utilized in hyperalimentation are an excellent culture medium for Candida. The incidence of infection is difficult to ascertain with any great accuracy but apparently depends on the technique used in the aseptic insertion of the plastic cannula. The frequency appears to rise most sharply after the cannulas have been in place for more than 4 days, and although the local application of antibiotics to the cutdown site shows some evidence of inhibiting bacterial infection, such a benefit has not been definitely established. With the rising incidence of Candida sepsis (particularly with the hyperalimentation techniques), it has recently been recommended that amphotericin be used prophylactically 2 to 3 times weekly. The procedure is to instill 0.6 mg. of a 1.0 mg./ml. solution of amphotericin into the intravenous line, flush it through, and reintroduce the same amount and flush it through for 5 to 10 minutes. This technique has decreased the incidence of Candida sepsis in the catheter system.

Aseptic Phlebitis

Aseptic inflammation of the cannulated vein associated with thrombosis is a common sequela of intravenous therapy. The contributory factors are as follows:

1. Anatomic location — lower limbs have a relatively slow blood flow, and when the muscle pump is impaired during intravenous administration, venous flow retardation occurs followed by thrombosis.

2. Prolonged duration of catheter insertion.

3. Catheter tip irritation.

4. Large bore size catheters.

5. Infusate type — certain infusates and drugs are irritating: Hypertonic glucose, methicillin, cephalosporins, barbiturates, cytotoxic agents, and potassium chloride.

6. As described previously, catheter types and characteristics may bear on the incidence of phlebogenicity.

7. Acidity or alkalinity of the infusate has been recently shown to cause phlebitis.

The prophylactic treatment of infusion phlebitis is as follows:

1. Change catheters every 24 to 48 hours, whenever possible.

2. Use small bore catheters, whenever possible.

3. Buffering and inline filters, especially those measuring 0.45 μ, have been effective.

4. Use large veins (superior vena cava) to infuse irritating solutions.

5. Avoid infusing in the lower limbs.

Active treatment consists of removal of the catheter, application of warm compresses to the affected area, and elevation of the limb.

Embolism

Air Embolism

Air embolism can occur at any time when there is a leak in the system, either as the result of a hole in the plastic catheter or while the catheter is being inserted through the percutaneous needle utilized for its introduction into the venous channel. To obviate such an occurrence during insertion of the cannula, it is customary to have the patient perform a Valsalva maneuver at the time the stylet is removed from the needle and the plastic cannula is inserted.

The diagnosis of air embolism is made on the basis of obvious evidence of an impediment to the function of the right side of the heart, including dyspnea. Distention of neck veins can be detected clinically, and measurement of venous pressure indicates a sharp rise, cyanosis develops rapidly, blood pressure falls, the pulse becomes weak and rapid, and signs of cerebral ischemia may supervene. Auscultation of the chest reveals a "churning" sound over the precordium. Treatment is directed at attempting to allow the air in the right side of the heart to escape by placing the patient in the left lateral decubitus position with the head down. If this is not sufficient to cause resolution of symptoms promptly, a thoracotomy with removal of the air by needle aspiration should be accomplished. While preparations are made for the thoracotomy, an attempt to aspirate the air through a cardiac catheter should be attempted. Minor- to moderate-sized air emboli may produce only transient symptoms and not require heroic measures.

Catheter Embolism

This complication of intravenous plastic catheters was reported with distressing frequency in earlier years, but an awareness of the etiology has resulted in a marked diminution of the frequency in recent years. As noted previously, in percutaneous insertion a portion of the catheter may be sheared off by the sharp bevel of the needle through which it is being introduced. This cutting of the catheter occurs when the operator withdraws the plastic catheter even for a short distance before the needle through which it is being inserted is withdrawn. Cases have also been reported in which the indwelling plastic catheter has for some reason broken within the lumen of the vein, setting free a fragment into the vascular system, or occasionally the plastic catheter has slipped from its connection to the external adaptor and entered the vascular lumen.

Another cause of catheter embolus is the severance of the catheter at the time of the dressing change. In one collected review of the literature the length of the catheter found within the vascular compartment varied from 3.5 cm. to 72 cm. Catheter segments have been reported in the pulmonary artery, jugular vein, inferior vena cava, subclavian vein, arm veins, leg veins, and pudendal vein, and even as a paradoxical embolus to the right renal artery (Fig. 5–8). In addition, catheter segments have been demonstrated within the chambers of the right side of the heart. Such occurrences can be minimized by careful attention to the management of the catheter and the catheter site, as well as by the utilization of radiopaque catheters and the careful measurement of the length of the catheter before insertion and after removal. Discovery of the presence of a free fragment of catheter has ordinarily been made within minutes or days of the occurrence, and in most instances, even in those in which the catheter fragment could not be retrieved, no known harmful effects have been demonstrated. In some instances,

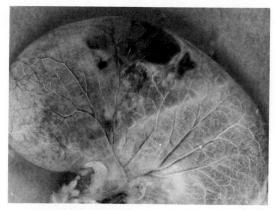

Figure 5–8. Renal infarct secondary to plastic catheter embolus to renal artery through a patent foramen ovale. (Courtesy of Col. Basil A. Pruitt.)

however, thrombosis or sepsis or both have been a serious consequence.

If a catheter fragment becomes loose in a superficial vein and can be demonstrated to lie within a superficial venous channel, prompt surgical removal is the proper treatment. The application of a tourniquet to the extremity at a point proximal to the location of the catheter fragment will aid in preventing its dislodgement during the surgical manipulation.

Non-operative retrieval of these catheter segments from cardiac chambers has been accomplished by means of a wire snare introduced through a cardiac catheter. The snare is utilized to trap the catheter fragment; then the snare and the cardiac catheter are withdrawn along with the entrapped catheter fragment. Such a technique may be used in retrieval of catheter segments from the main vascular channels. In every case in which location of the catheter is possible, either by consequence of its radiopaque nature or by means of venography or arteriography, an attempt should be made to remove it even if operative intervention is necessary.

Thrombosis and Embolism

Treatment of thrombosis and embolization occurring secondary to catheter insertion is described in Chapter 9 of this book and is similar to that of idiopathic thrombosis: removal of the catheter and heparinization. If embolization continues, insert a vena

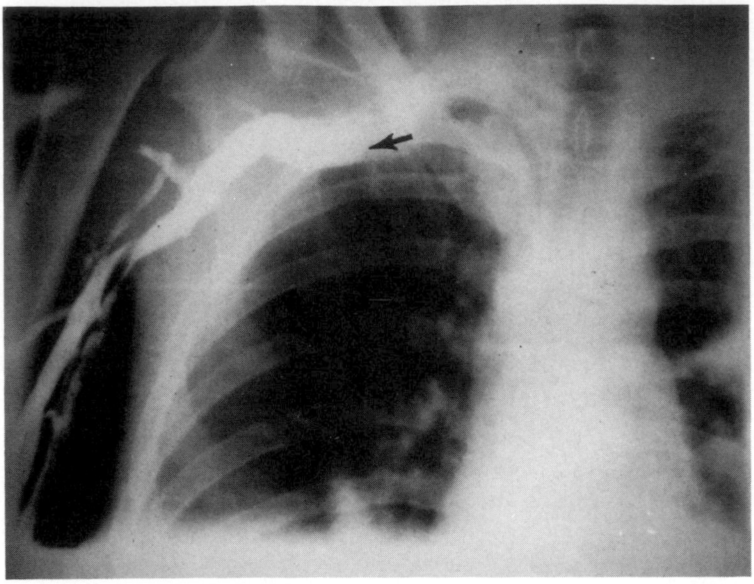

Figure 5–9. Thrombosis of right subclavian vein demonstrated by venogram obtained 2 weeks after the onset of right arm swelling. Arrow points to margin of the thrombus which was at the point of the insertion of right subclavian catheter. (From Warden, G. D., et al.: Central venous thrombosis: A hazard of medical progress. J. Trauma, *13*:620, 1973. © The Williams & Wilkins Co., Baltimore.)

caval umbrella or clip, or ligate the inferior vena cava (Fig. 5–9).

METABOLIC COMPLICATIONS OF TOTAL PARENTERAL NUTRITION

Metabolic problems primarily associated with the use of parenteral hyperalimentation are shown in Table 5–2. These are divided into metabolic complications of glucose, protein, fat, vitamins, and trace elements.

Glucose Metabolism

Hyperglycemia

With the usual techniques of intravenous hyperalimentation (IVH), careful monitoring of the blood sugar and urine sugar is necessary. Ideally, the blood sugar should be maintained below 200 mg./dl. and the urine sugar in the range of 1+ to 2+ values. Anything above these levels is considered hyperglycemia and results from the too-rapid infusion of the hypertonic glucose-amino acid mixture, so that the ability of the body to metabolize the sugar is exceeded, and the excess is spilled into the urine as glycosuria. The body initially responds by a slow increase of insulin production to meet the requirements of this extra sugar load. For this reason, alimentation is begun with small quantities of hypertonic solutions, approximately 1000 cc. per day, with gradual increases as the patient's clinical tolerance of additional sugar load, measured by blood and urine sugar levels, is demonstrated.

Hyperglycemia can also occur if there is an uneven administration of the hyperalimentation mixture as in alternating rapid and slow infusions during the day. It is imperative that a constant infusion of glucose be maintained throughout the 24-hour period of administration. Monitoring of urine and blood sugar every 3 to 4 hours is necessary until the patient is well adjusted; once glucose equilibrium has occurred, monitoring can be discontinued.

The most significant danger of hyperglycemia is the development of hyperosmotic, hyperglycemic, non-ketotic coma. Coma is the result of the osmotic diuresis forced by the glycosuria secondary to the hyperglycemia. Onset is usually slow and inapparent and may be overlooked until one is well aware of the possibility of its occurrence. In a recent study Kaminski reported that hyperglycemia and glucosuria must be avoided during TPN by supplying exogenous insulin when endogenous insulin fails to meet the demands of a hypercaloric infusion. Patients with a positive family or per-

TABLE 5-2 METABOLIC PROBLEMS ASSOCIATED WITH PARENTERAL HYPERALIMENTATION*

Problems	Possible Etiologies
I. Glucose metabolism	
A. Hyperglycemia, glycosuria, osmotic diuresis, hyperosmolar nonketotic dehydration and coma	Excessive total dose or rate of infusion of glucose; inadequate endogenous insulin
B. Ketoacidosis in diabetes mellitus	Inadequate erdogenous insulin response; inadequate exogenous insulin therapy
C. Post-infusion hypoglycemia	Persistence of endogenous insulin production secondary to prolonged stimulation of islet cells by high carbohydrate infusion
D. Hyperlactacidemia	Excessive glycolytic cycle fluxing due to increased glucose substrate
II. Amino acid metabolism	
A. Hyperchloremic metabolic acidosis	Excessive chloride and monohydrochloride content of crystalline amino acid solutions
B. Serum amino acid imbalances	Unphysiologic amino acid profile of the nutrient solution
C. Hyperammonemia	Excessive ammonia in protein hydrolysate solutions; arginine, ornithine, aspartic acid and/or glutamic acid deficiency in amino acid solutions; primary hepatic disorder
D. Prerenal azotemia	Excessive protein hydrolysate or amino acid infusion
III. Calcium and phosphorous metabolism	
A. Hypophosphatemia	Inadequate phosphorus administration, redistribution of serum phosphorus into cells and/or bone
1. Decreased erythrocyte 2,3-diphosphoglycerate	
2. Increased affinity of hemoglobin for oxygen	
3. Aberrations of erythrocyte intermediary metabolites	
B. Hypocalcemia	Inadequate calcium administration; reciprocal response to phosphorus repletion without simultaneous calcium infusion
C. Hypercalcemia	Excessive calcium administration with or without high doses of albumin
D. Vitamin D deficiency; Hypervitaminosis D	Inadequate or excessive vitamin D administration
IV. Essential fatty acid metabolism	
A. Serum deficiencies of phospholipid linoleic and/or arachidonic acids; serum elevations of $\Delta 5, 8, 11$-eicosatrienoic acid	Inadequate essential fatty acid administration; inadequate vitamin E administration
V. Miscellaneous	
A. Hypokalemia	Inadequate potassium intake relative to increased requirements for protein anabolism
B. Hyperkalemia	Excessive potassium administration especially in metabolic acidosis
C. Hypomagnesemia	Inadequate magnesium administration relative to increased requirements for protein anabolism
D. Anemia	Iron deficiency; folic acid deficiency; vitamin B_{12} deficiency; copper deficiency
E. Bleeding	Vitamin K deficiency
F. Hypervitaminosis A	Excessive Vitamin A administration
G. Elevations in SGOT, SGPT and serum alkaline phosphatase	Enzyme induction secondary to accelerated glucose metabolism, possible hepatotoxicity secondary to amino acid imbalance; excessive glycogen and/or fat deposition in the liver

*From Dudrick, S. J., MacFadyen, B. V., Jr., Van Buren, C. T., Ruberg, R. L., and Maynard, A. T.: Parenteral hyperalimentation: Metabolic problems and solutions. Ann. Surg. 176:239, 1972.

sonal diabetic history belong to a high-risk group. Osmotic diuresis, secondary to untreated hyperglycemia, produces a water deficit in excess of a sodium deficit. The lack of ketosis in hyperosmotic, hyperglycemic, non-ketotic diabetes (HHND) is probably due initially to endogenous insulin levels that are adequate for preventing lipolysis but inadequate for preventing hyperglycemia and glucosuria. Later, the hyperglycemia itself is anti-ketogenic. Stress stimulates glyconeogenesis-glycogenolysis produced by the effect of catechol, glucagon, and cortisol. Total parenteral nutrition during these metabolic events can compound the naturally occurring hyperglycemia of stress. During brief periods of surgical stress, a reduction in the concentration of infused glucose and potassium will prevent hyperglycemia and hyperkalemia. If TPN at hypercaloric concentrations is to be continued during prolonged non-surgical stress, the hyperglycemic effects of the stress hormones may be forcibly reversed by administration of exogenous insulin. If HHND inadvertently develops, TPN should be stopped and replacement of the water and sodium deficit should precede insulin administration.

The course of HHND is characterized by progressive lethargy, mental confusion, coma, and death. This again emphasizes the necessity to maintain an even rate of infusion and a constant check on the blood sugar and the urine sugar. The fact that the patient is well-adjusted at one time during the course of his intravenous hyperalimentation does not obviate the possibility of hyperglycemia and coma occurring as a consequence of the development of the additional stress or sepsis. One cannot emphasize too strongly the necessity for close monitoring of these patients.

Hypoglycemia

Since the normal response to the infusion of the hyperglycemic mixture is a gradual increase in insulin production, sudden changes in the rate of infusion of the hypertonic glucose mixture can produce hypoglycemia. Any abrupt change in the concentration of glucose in the presence of the increased outpouring of insulin from the pancreas can result in a marked decrease in serum glucose. This decrease may occur if the infusion is terminated abruptly or the rate is slowed. This problem must also be kept in mind when hyperalimentation therapy is being terminated in a patient whose condition has improved. Any termination of intravenous hyperalimentation must be done gradually. If hyperalimentation is to be discontinued during surgery, infusion of a mixture of a 5 per cent glucose in water or 5 per cent glucose in saline should be substituted. Concomitantly, monitoring of urine sugar level should be performed, and if there is any change, an immediate blood sugar determination should be obtained.

Hyperlactacidemia

This is another complication of glucose metabolism that produces metabolic acidosis. Woods reported that when using a combination of amino acids and sorbitol a hyperlactacidemia developed. However, this also has been reported with the use of glucose and amino acids. The resultant lactic acid increase produces lactic acidosis. Cessation of the infusion of high concentrations of glucose and amino acids decreases hyperlactacidemia.

Protein Metabolism

The use of large volumes of 3 to 7 per cent amino acid solutions has been implicated in the production of acidosis and elevated blood ammonia levels (in patients with hepatocellular disease), encephalopathy (in cirrhotic patients receiving aromatic amino acids or phenylalanine), cholestasis (manifested by increased serum bilirubin), and increases in leucine aminopeptidase or alkaline phosphatase (after crystalline amino acid infusion). In both adult and pediatric patients there may be serum amino acid changes characterized by decreased levels of isoleucine and increased levels of aspartic acid, glutamic acid, serine, proline, glycine, alanine, threonine, and lysine.

Some patients develop histidine deficiency, manifested by a skin rash. Prerenal azotemia will occur when low-dextrose-to-nitrogen-ratio solutions are administered. Usually the BUN will not be excessively high but may cause some osmotic diuresis. Prerenal azotemia will occur in dehydrated patients. Patients who are dehydrated should not receive parenteral feeding until adequate hydration has been established.

Patients with renal failure are unable to excrete endogenously produced urea. Moreover, fluid restriction is necessary because of the inability to excrete water. For that reason dextrose concentrations higher than those usually employed in TPN (dextrose:nitrogen ratio — 900:1) are advantageous because such solutions minimize urea formation by depressing gluconeogenesis, provide maximal calories with minimal fluid, and minimize hyperkalemia.

In patients with hepatic insufficiency, administration of greater than 40 gm. of protein may cause hepatic encephalopathy. New solutions with high levels of branched-chain amino acids may treat or prevent this potential complication and allow these patients to receive the benefits of parenteral feeding.

Lipid Metabolism

Disorders of lipid metabolism also occur in patients fed therapeutic nutrition regimens. If enterally fed, the patient with inability to absorb long-chain fatty acids will benefit by special formulas containing fat sources in the form of medium-chain triglycerides that are absorbed directly into the portal system without requiring pancreatic enzymes. In most patients, however, fat contained in the various Defined Formula Diets will suffice to meet fat requirements of 2 to 4 per cent of daily calories. During intravenous nutrition using dextrose and amino acids as the primary food source, essential fatty acid deficiency will occur within 3 days of initiation of treatment. For that reason, on alternate days patients should receive intravenous fat. New commercial preparations of fat may allow increased concentrations to be administered. Fatty acid deficiency is characterized by a flaky, erythematous dermatitis primarily of the legs, chest, and face. Rubbing safflower oil on the skin or administering safflower oil or fat orally to patients who can absorb minimal amounts of lipids provides a satisfactory and less expensive alternative to intravenous fat. It is possible that administration of fat may produce hyperlipidemia and exacerbation of pancreatitis. Therefore, patients receiving intravenous fat should have triglyceride levels monitored, and these levels should be within normal values 3 hours after the infusion.

Electrolyte Metabolism

Electrolyte values are normal in patients with malnutrition who maintain a relatively steady state among the various components of body cell mass. However, when refeeding is initiated, a deficiency of micronutrients required for tissue anabolism such as potassium, phosphate, zinc, chromium, manganese, and other micro- and macronutrients will frequently be uncovered. A patient receiving dextrose–amino acid infusion requires a ratio of potassium to glucose of 40 to 100 mEq./1000 Kcal. Hypophosphatemia of a profound nature will develop if the patient is previously severely malnourished. The deficiency is compounded by an intracellular shift of inorganic phosphate with low serum values, which results in low red cell organic phosphates, primarily diphosphoglycerate and adenosine triphosphate. Clinical manifestations of this syndrome are hyperventilation, high cardiac output, and hemolytic anemia (phosphate < 1.0 mg./dl.). Severely malnourished patients should have electrolyte determinations every 6 to 8 hours until a steady state is reached. In addition, calcium and magnesium are required to prevent tetany.

Trace Elements

Malnourished patients and particularly those with gastrointestinal losses will develop zinc deficiency. As zinc is required for wound healing, immunity, and growth, it should be administered concomitantly with TPN. Zinc deficiency is clinically diagnosed by a characteristic skin lesion (acrodermatitis enteropathica), low serum zinc values, and hair loss.

Copper deficiency frequently occurs during TPN. Copper is essential for cytochrome

C oxidase, ceruloplasmin, and other oxidases. Copper deficiency is characterized by leukopenia with lymphocytosis.

Chromium deficiency is relatively rare and may occur during prolonged TPN — 6 months or longer. As chromium is essential for normal glucose metabolism, deficiency is characterized by a diabetic blood sugar pattern and peripheral neuropathy.

Vitamin Metabolism

The exact vitamin concentration required to prevent deficiency is at present unclear, but commercial preparations are usually adequate. Vitamin B-12, folate, and vitamin K need to be added to the fat- and the water-soluble vitamins.

POSTOPERATIVE FLUID DISEQUILIBRIUM

Hyposmotic State

Postoperative fluid administration can produce both a hyposmotic and a hyperosmotic state. Moore showed that the hyposmotic state is more common and difficult to treat. Metabolically, the organism responds to surgery or injury by producing a dilutional state resulting from the release of antidiuretic factors and aldosterone. These hormones induce water retention that is compounded by tissue destruction and an abnormal retention of sodium-free water. This dilutional state may be present preoperatively in patients who, because of their prolonged disease stress, have developed expanded extracellular and plasma volumes. If this dilution is unrecognized, they are taken to surgery with this excess water, and further dilution occurs when postoperative volume losses are replaced. Hypervolemia may occur, and in very young or elderly patients this may lead to cardiac function embarrassment or failure.

Diagnosis of hyposmotic or dilutional states is based on a high index of suspicion when treating cachectic patients or those with prolonged illness and on laboratory findings of increased plasma volume and decreased total protein and hematocrit measurements. The treatment consists of red cell blood volume replacement and the judicious administration of diuretics to reduce excess plasma volume as well as restriction of fluid intake.

Hyperosmotic State

Contrariwise, there are postoperative or traumatic states during which fluid losses predominate over solute losses, producing a hyperosmotic state. The non-ketotic hyperosmotic state is caused by severe osmotic diuresis secondary to the diarrhea produced by enteral hyperosmotic feedings. Other causes of osmotic diuresis are infusion of hypertonic glucose, of large amounts of mannitol, of such diuretics as furosemide, diuril, and hydrodiuril, as well as losses of fluid due to heat prostration. Burns and, rarely, postoperative dehydration also produce hyperosmotic states.

Diagnosis of the hyperosmotic state is based on laboratory findings of increased levels of serum osmolality and sodium, hematocrit, and protein, and of decreased plasma volume. Treatment is simple, consisting of administration of 5 per cent glucose and water.

Gastric Outlet Obstruction

In certain pathologic conditions such as gastric outlet obstruction, duodenal or jejunal fistula, pancreatic fistula, enterocolitis, ulcerative colitis, and small and large bowel obstruction, fluid disequilibrium is associated with absolute losses of cations and anions that may or may not alter acid-base balance. Once the diagnosis is established, these losses can be forecast and either prevented or treated. Depending on the site of loss or obstruction, the common denominator of these pathologic conditions is the subtraction of water or electrolyte (Table 5–3).

Ordinarily, the fluid loss pattern for gastric outlet obstruction consists of losses in chloride, hydrogen ion, potassium, sodium, and water, all leading to hypochloremia, hypokalemia, and alkalemia with dehydration. The degree of the alkalemia depends on both the patient's age and the amount of acid being produced by the parietal cell mass. Elderly patients have decreased hydrogen ion excretion that consequently in-

TABLE 5–3 VOLUME AND ELECTROLYTIC COMPOSITION OF GASTROINTESTINAL SECRETION

Fluid	Average Volume (ml./24 h.)	Electrolytic Concentration (mEq./L.)				
		Na$^+$	K$^+$	Cl$^-$	HCO$_3^-$	H$^+$
Plasma		135–145	· 3.6–5.5	95–105	24.6–28.8	0.30–0.40
Gastric Juice	2500	31–90	4.3–12.0	52–124	0	90.0
Bile Juice	700–1000	134–156	3.9–63.0	83–110	38.0	
Pancreatic Juice	1000–1500	113–153	2.6–7.4	54–95	110.0	
Succus Entericus (Jejunum)	3000–5000	72–120	3.5–6.8	69–127	30.0	
Succus Entericus (Ileum)	3000–5000	112–142	4.5–14.0	93–122	30.0	
Cecal Stool	3000	48–116	11.1–28.3	35–70	15.0	
Feces	100	10	10	15	15.0	

creases the isoelectrolytic water loss. Patients with hypersecretion may lose as much as 60 to 80 mEq./L. of hydrogen ion. Hypokalemia is caused by the kidney's retention of sodium and bicarbonate at the expense of potassium excretion (aldosterone effect). The treatment for hypokalemic hypochloremic alkalosis consists of the judicious administration of 0.9 N NaCl with 40 mEq. KCl with careful monitoring of serum potassium, pH, and volume. Profound alkalemia is treated with NH$_4$Cl or 0.1 N HCl with careful monitoring to prevent ammonia intoxication and acidosis, respectively. Parenteral nutrition to replace energy deficit may be indicated.

Duodenal or Jejunal Fistula

Most commonly, fluid disequilibrium is secondary to complication of the surgical treatment of duodenal or gastric ulcer. The duodenal stump or gastrojejunal fistula produced during a Billroth I or II procedure may subsequently blow out or leak (suture disruption), leading to the formation of a fistula at the site of the stump or gastrojejunal anastomosis. The duodenal contents include bile, pancreatic juice, and duodenal succus entericus, all of which can produce a fluid loss of 3000 to 4000 cc. per day. Each liter of this fluid also contains 150 mEq. of bicarbonate; therefore, as much as 500 mEq./L. per day can be lost, leading to a subtraction metabolic acidosis and marked dehydration if not adequately replaced. The treatment for this condition is replacement of basic fluid needs arising from insensible and respiratory losses, as well as administration of the fistula output equivalent — Ringer's solution plus 44 mEq. NaHCO$_3$.

Obstruction

Acid-base and water alterations in small bowel obstruction and regional enteritis are dependent on the obstruction site. High jejunal obstruction produces the same subtraction acidosis as that shown by jejunal fistula, except that in this instance, the loss is due to vomiting or aggressive intestinal tube suction. A low obstruction produces similar losses, except that acid-base imbalances are uncommon because there is an isotonic and isoelectrolytic loss. The main problem is that water loss and dehydration may ensue and produce circulatory collapse. The treatment consists of water loss replacement with Ringer's solution. Large colon obstruction produces a similar water loss, but with much less cation and anion losses; thus treatment with Ringer's solution is also indicated.

Enteritis and Colitis

Patients with enteritis or colitis present a different problem because of their diarrheic losses. The diarrheic stool of Crohn's disease and of ulcerative colitis contains undigested food, proteins, and high potassium concentrations. Therefore, besides dehydration there can be a hypokalemic and protein catabolic state. This condition is treated by administering anti-diarrheic agents and anabolic parenteral fluids containing adequate concentrations of potassium chloride.

Bibliography

1. Abernathy, C., and Dickinson, T.: Massive air emboli from intravenous infusion pump: Etiology and prevention. Am. J. Surg. *137*:274, 1979.
2. Arnold, R., Elliot, E., and Holmes, B.: The importance of frequent examination of infusion sites in preventing postinfusion phlebitis. Surg. Gynecol. Obstet. *145*:19, 1977.
3. Ayalon, A., Anner, H., Berlatzky, Y., and Schiller, M.: Complications of the infusion pump. Lancet *2*:891, 1978.
4. Aynsley-Green, A., Baum, J., Alberti, K., and Woods, H.: Hyperlactataemia during intravenous feeding in childhood. Arch. Dis. Child. *49*:647, 1974.
5. Batstone, G., Alberti, K., and Dewar, A.: Reversible lactic acidosis associated with repeated intravenous infusions of sorbitol and ethanol. Postgrad. Med. J. *53*:567, 1977.
6. Belani, K.: Hydrothorax and central venous catheters. J. Pediatr. *95*:813, 1979.
7. Bogen, J.: Local complications in 167 patients with indwelling venous catheters. Surg. Gynecol. Obstet. *110*:112, 1960.
8. Boltax, R., Dineen, J., and Scarpa, F.: Gangrene resulting from infiltrated dopamine solution. N. Engl. J. Med. *296*:823, 1977.
9. Bowers, D., Jr., and Lynch, J.: Adriamycin extravasation. Plast. Reconstr. Surg. *61*:86, 1978.
10. Buxton, A., Highsmith, A., Garner, J., West, M., Stamm, W., Dixon, R., and McGowan, J.: Contamination of intravenous infusion fluid: Effects of changing administration sets. Ann. Intern. Med. *90*:764, 1979.
11. Collin, J., and Collin, C.: Infusion thrombophlebitis. Lancet *2*:458, 1975.
12. Connon, J.: Diarrhea possibly caused by total parenteral nutrition. N. Engl. J. Med. *301*:273, 1979.
13. DeLuca, P., Rapp, R., Bivins, B., McKean, H., and Griffen, W.: Filtration and infusion phlebitis: A double-blind prospective clinical study. Am. J. Hosp. Pharm. *32*:1001, 1975.
14. Duma, R.: Thomas Latta, What Have We Done? The hazards of intravenous therapy. N. Engl. J. Med. *294*:1178, 1976.
15. Ebels, T., and van der Heide, J.: Dopamine-induced ischaemia. Lancet *2*:762, 1977.
16. Finberg, L.: The relationship of intravenous infusions and intracranial hemorrhage — A commentary. J. Pediatr. *91*:777, 1977.
17. Fleming, C., Smith, L., and Hodges, R.: Essential fatty acid deficiency in adults receiving total parenteral nutrition. Am. J. Clin. Nutr. *29*:976, 1976.
18. Frazer, I., Eke, N., and Laing, M.: Is infusion phlebitis preventable? Br. Med. J. *2*:232, 1977.
19. Freeman, J., and Litton, A.: Preponderance of gram-positive infections during parenteral alimentation. Surg. Gynecol. Obstet. *139*:905, 1974.
20. Fukui, S., Takada, Y., and Hayasaka, J.: Hyperalimentation and its problems in the cases of long term nutrition. Acta Chir. Scand. *466*:88, 1976.
21. Garnica, A.: The hepatotoxicity of parenteral protein hydrolysate-containing solutions. Ann. Clin. Lab. Sci. *6*:446, 1976.
22. Gaze, N. R.: Tissue necrosis caused by commonly used intravenous infusions. Lancet *2*:417, 1978.
23. Guillou, P., Morgan, D., and Hill, G. (Goligher, J. C.): Hypophosphataemia: A complication of 'innocuous' dextrose-saline. Br. J. Surg. *63*:667, 1976.
24. Heller, R., Kirchner, S., O'Neill, J. A., Jr., Hough, A., Howard, L., Kramer, S., and Green, H.: Skeletal changes of copper deficiency in infants receiving prolonged total parenteral nutrition. J. Pediatr. *92*:947, 1978.
25. Hessov, I., Allen, J., Arendt, K., and Gravholt, L.: Infusion thrombophlebitis in a surgical department. Acta Chir. Scand. *143*:151, 1977.
26. Hessov, I., Bojsen-Moller, M., and Melsen, F.: Do fat emulsions protect against infusion thrombophlebitis? Intensive Care Med. *4*:155, 1978.
27. Indar, R.: Dangers of indwelling polyethylene cannulae in deep veins. Lancet *1*:284, 1959.
28. Jarret, F., Maki, D., and Chan, C-K.: Management of septic thrombosis of the inferior vena cava caused by candida. Arch. Surg. *113*:637, 1978.
29. Jeejeebhoy, K., Chu, R., Marliss, E., Greenberg, G., and Bruce-Robertson, A.: Chromium deficiency, glucose intolerance, and neuropathy reversed by chromium supplementation, in a patient receiving long-term total parenteral nutrition. Am. J. Clin. Nutr. *30*:531, 1977.
30. Kaminski, M., Jr.: Hyperosmolar hyperglycemic non-ketotic dehydration. Etiology, pathophysiology and prevention during total parenteral alimentation. *In* Manni, C., et al. (Eds.): Total Parenteral Alimentation. Amsterdam, Excerpta Medica, 1976.
31. Kaminski, M., Jr., and Harris, D.: Prolonged uncomplicated intravascular catheterization. Am. J. I.V. Ther. p. 19, June, 1976.
32. Kay, R., Tasman-Jones, C., Pybus, J., Whiting, R., and Black, H.: A syndrome of acute zinc deficiency during total parenteral alimentation in man. Ann. Surg. *183*:331, 1976.
33. Kirkpatrick, J., Mullin, T., and Dahn, M.: Alterations in the glucose-mediated regulation of growth hormone associated with sepsis. Surg. Forum *30*:52, 1979.
34. Kirkpatrick, J., and Gobeille, R.: Selective hyperalimentation: A new look at an old problem. J. Trauma *17*:725, 1977.
35. Kramer, J., and Goodwin, J.: Wernicke's encephalopathy: Complication of intravenous hyperalimentation. J.A.M.A. *238*:2176, 1977.
36. Lowe, R., Moss, G., Jilek, J., and Levine, H.: Crystalloid vs. colloid in the etiology of pulmonary failure after trauma: A randomized trial in man. Surgery *81*:676, 1977.
37. Maki, D.: Preventing infection in intravenous therapy. Anesth. Analg. *56*:141, 1977.
38. Maki, D., Rhame, F., Mackel, D., and Bennett, J.: Nationwide epidemic of septicemia caused by

contaminated intravenous products. I. Epidemiologic and clinical features. Am. J. Med. *60*:471, 1976.

39. Maki, D., and Martin, W.: Nationwide epidemic of septicemia caused by contaminated infusion products. IV. Growth of microbial pathogens in fluids for intravenous infusion. J. Infect. Dis. *131*:267, 1975.

40. McCarthy, D., May, R., Maher, M., and Brennan, M.: Trace metal and essential fatty acid deficiency during total parenteral nutrition. Am. J. Dig. Dis. *23*:1009, 1978.

41. Miller, R., and Grogan, J. B.: Efficacy of inline bacterial filters in reducing contamination of intravenous nutritional solutions. Am. J. Surg. *130*:585, 1975.

42. Moncrief, J. A.: Complication of parenteral fluid therapy. *In* Artz, C. P., and Hardy, J. D. (Eds.): Management of Surgical Complications. 3rd Ed. Philadelphia, W. B. Saunders Company, 1975.

43. Moncrief, J.: Femoral catheters. Ann. Surg. *147*:166, 1958.

44. Mukherjee, G., and Guharay, B.: Digital gangrene and skin necrosis following extravasation of infusion fluid. J. Indian Med. Assoc. *68*:77, 1977.

45. Mullen, J., Oleaga, J., and Ring, E.: Catheter migration during home hyperalimentation. J.A.M.A. *238*:1946, 1977.

46. Papile, L., Burstein, J., Burstein, R., Koffler, H., and Koops, B.: Relationship of intravenous sodium bicarbonate infusions and cerebral intraventricular hemorrhage. J. Pediatr. *93*:834, 1978.

47. Peters, R., and Hogan, J.: Fluid overload and post-traumatic respiratory distress syndrome. J. Trauma *18*:83, 1978.

48. Reinhardt, G., Gelbart, S., and Greenlee, H.: Catheter infection factors affecting total parenteral nutrition. Am. Surg. *44*:401, 1978.

49. Roberts, J.: Cutaneous and subcutaneous complications of calcium infusions. JACEP *6*:31, 1977.

50. Rodrigues, R., and Wolff, W.: Fungal septicemia in surgical patients. Ann. Surg. *180*:741, 1974.

51. Ryan, J. A., Jr.: Complications of total parenteral nutrition. *In* Fischer, J. E. (Ed.): Total Parenteral Nutrition. Boston, Little, Brown and Company, 1976.

52. Schumer, W.: High caloric solutions in traumatized patients. *In* Fox, C. L., Jr., and Nahas, G. G. (Eds.): Body Fluid Replacement in the Surgical Patient: A Symposium. New York, Grune and Stratton, 1970.

53. Schumer, W.: Adverse effects of xylitol in parenteral alimentation. Metabolism *20*:345, 1971.

54. Wretlind, A., and Schumer, W.: Carbohydrates and fats colloquium. *In* White, P. L., and Nagy, M. E. (Eds.): Total Parenteral Nutrition. Acton, Mass., Publishing Sciences Group, Inc., 1974.

55. Shah, P., Zafar, M., and Patel, A.: Folate deficiency during intravenous hyperalimentation. J. Med. *8*:383, 1977.

56. Smitherman, M., Ballantine, T., and Grosfeld, J.: Catheter complications with total parenteral nutrition in the first year of life. J. Indiana State Med. Assoc. *71*:478, 1978.

57. Spriggs, D., and Brantley, R.: Thoracic and abdominal extravasation: A complication of hyperalimentation in infants. Am. J. Roentgenol. *128*:419, 1977.

58. Stein, L., Beraud, J-J., Morissette, M., Da Luz, P., Weil, M., and Shubin, H.: Pulmonary edema during volume infusion. Circulation *52*:483, 1975.

59. Thong, M., and Tay, L.: Septicaemia from prolonged intravenous infusions. Arch. Dis. Child. *50*:886, 1975.

60. Touloukian, R.: Isosmolar coma during parenteral alimentation with protein hydrolystate in excess of 4 gm/kg/day. J. Pediatr. *86*:270, 1975.

61. Tovey, S.: Hazard of air embolism with multiple infusion apparatus. Br. Med. J. *4*:462, 1975.

62. Upton, J., Mulliken, J., and Murray, J.: Major intravenous extravasation injuries. Am. J. Surg. *137*:497, 1979.

63. Wardrop, C., Heatley, R., Tennant, G., and Hughes, L.: Acute folate deficiency in surgical patients on aminoacid/ethanol intravenous nutrition. Lancet *2*:640, 1975.

64. Watkins, J., and Clarke, R. S. J.: Report of a symposium: Adverse responses to intravenous agents. Br. J. Anaesth. *50*:1159, 1978.

65. Weiss, Y., and Nissan, S.: A method for reducing the incidence of infusion phlebitis. Surg. Gynecol. Obstet. *141*:73, 1975.

66. Woods, H.: The metabolic complications of intravenous nutrition. Int. J. Vitam. Nutr. Res. *15*:54, 1976.

67. Woodhouse, C.: Movelat in the prophylaxis of infusion thrombophlebitis. Br. Med. J. *1*:454, 1979.

68. Wyatt, H.: First aid when contaminated infusion fluid is suspected. Scand. J. Infect. Dis. *10*:95, 1978.

69. Yosowitz, P., Ekland, D., Shaw, R., and Parsons, R.: Peripheral intravenous infiltration necrosis. Ann. Surg. *182*:553, 1975.

6

ACUTE RENAL INSUFFICIENCY COMPLICATING SURGERY AND TRAUMA

Gordon R. Lang
and Olga Jonasson

Through complex processes of excretion or conservation of solutes filtered from the plasma, the kidneys maintain a nearly constant internal environment. In an adult the production of a normal urine flow rate of 1 ml. per minute requires a blood flow of approximately 1 liter per minute, or 20 per cent of the cardiac output. While the combined weight of the kidneys in an adult is only 300 grams, 10 per cent of basal oxygen consumption takes place in the kidneys. The high metabolic requirements for blood flow and oxygen render the kidney very susceptible to damage from decreases in blood volume or cardiac output. In addition, the kidneys receive a large exposure to circulating toxins secondary to the high renal blood flow, and filtered toxins will likely become concentrated during excretion through the kidneys, directly exposing tubular epithelial cells to high levels of the toxic agent (Table 6–1).

It is not surprising, then, that failure of renal function can and does occur in a variety of circumstances. The causes of acute renal failure are classified into three

Gordon R. Lang received his B.A. degree in history from Duke University and his doctorate from the University of Buffalo School of Medicine. He served his medical residency at the University of Illinois Hospitals and at present is Associate Professor of Clinical Medicine at the Abraham Lincoln School of Medicine, University of Illinois. He is Director of the Dialysis Unit at Saint Joseph Hospital.

Olga Jonasson is a graduate of the University of Illinois College of Medicine. Her graduate training in General Surgery was done at the University of Illinois under the direction of Warren H. Cole. She has done research fellowships in immunology at the Walter Reed Army Institute of Research under Elmer Becker and at the Massachusetts General Hospital under Henry Winn. Dr. Jonasson is a national leader in surgery and serves in numerous important national capacities. She has been a member of the faculty of the University of Illinois since 1967 and is presently Professor of Surgery and Chief of Surgery at Cook County Hospital.

TABLE 6–1 COMMON NEPHROTOXIC AGENTS

Antibiotics	Sulfonamides, aminoglycosides (gentamicin, kanamycin, tobramycin), cephalosporins, methacillin, amphotericin, vancomycin, bacitracin, polymyxin
Analgesics	Phenacetin
Anesthetics	Methoxyfluorane (Penthrane)
X-ray Contrast Agents	Iodinated contrast media (acetrizoate, iopanoic acid, iothalamate, diatrizoate)
Toxins	Ethylene glycol (antifreeze), organic solvents, methyl alcohol, heavy metals, pesticides

broad categories: *prerenal* azotemia (renal underperfusion), *postrenal* azotemia (obstructive uropathy), and acute *renal* parenchymal failure (ARF) (Table 6–2).

PRERENAL AZOTEMIA

Within limits, renal blood flow remains fairly constant despite fluctuations in systemic blood pressure, blood volume, or systemic peripheral resistance. The capacity for autoregulation of renal blood flow is mediated through the renal afferent arterioles which respond to pressure gradients and vasoactive substances such as angiotensin II, prostaglandins, and catecholamines with modifications of renal vascular resistance. When perfusion pressures decrease below the limits of physiologic autoregulation, intense vasoconstriction of preglomer-

TABLE 6–2 ETIOLOGY OF ACUTE RENAL FAILURE

I. Prerenal azotemia
  a. Decreased effective arterial volume
    1. Hypotension
    2. Hypovolemia
      a. hemorrhage
      b. third space losses
      c. burns
  b. Hepatorenal syndrome
II. Postrenal azotemia
  a. Obstruction of upper tracts from tumor, stone, surgical error, etc.
  b. Lower urinary tract obstruction from prostatic enlargement, cervical cancer, bladder tumor, neurogenic bladder dysfunction, etc.
III. Renal
  a. Ischemia
  b. Toxins

ular (afferent) arterioles occurs, and renal blood flow falls abruptly. The glomerular filtration rate slows as glomerular perfusion is lowered, reducing the volume of filtrate in the tubules. Composition of the filtrate is further altered by the action of aldosterone (conserving sodium by promotion of sodium reabsorption) and antidiuretic hormone (conserving water by promotion of water reabsorption); secretion of both of these hormones is increased in response to hypovolemia. Therefore, blood volume is ultimately conserved by production of a low filtrate volume from which sodium and water are actively reabsorbed, resulting in a urine of small volume (oliguria) with high specific gravity and low sodium concentration. Tubular fluid flow rate is slow and more urea is reabsorbed in the tubules, decreasing the ratio of urine to blood urea from a normal 30:1 to 15–20:1 and resulting in increased plasma urea concentration (azotemia).

Decreased effective arterial volume with poor renal perfusion is the key to the development of prerenal azotemia. Autoregulation of renal blood flow and conservation of salt and water are normal responses to this event. Prerenal azotemia becomes irreversible only when renal blood flow is reduced so severely that oxygen and substrate delivery to the kidney is inadequate to keep the renal tubular cells alive. Until cell death occurs, all of the compensatory physiologic changes of prerenal azotemia can be reversed through improvement in renal perfusion.

Recognition of the factors that lead to renal hypoperfusion is an important step in the prevention of prerenal azotemia. Two of the most important factors are *hypotension* and *hypovolemia*.

Hemorrhage and hypotension from cardiogenic shock are obvious causes of prerenal azotemia. Much less obvious are "third space" (neither intracellular nor intravascular) fluid sequestrations associated with soft tissue trauma, sepsis, peritonitis, bowel obstruction, burns, diarrhea, and pancreatitis.

Systemic arterial blood pressure may not accurately reflect effective circulating blood volume if catecholamine-mediated increase in systemic vascular resistance has occurred. Measurement of central venous pressure or left atrial pressure (pulmonary capillary wedge pressure — PCWP) is necessary to identify the marked contraction of blood volume in many instances of third space loss. It is not uncommon for liters of plasma volume to become sequestered in obstructed bowel loops or into an inflamed retroperitoneum. Prompt recognition of a severely contracted plasma volume is necessary if the progression from prerenal reversible azotemia to irreversible acute renal failure is to be prevented. Hypovolemia or a clinical suspicion of third space losses should be confirmed by hemodynamic monitoring (central venous pressure measurement, insertion of a Swan-Ganz pulmonary artery catheter, and measurement of the pulmonary capillary wedge pressure and cardiac output) and promptly treated with intravenous crystalloid infusions (Ringer's lactate or 0.9 N saline).

The diagnosis of prerenal azotemia is made by documentation of oliguria, azotemia, a concentrated urine with a sodium content of less than 20 mEq./l., and a urine:plasma urea ratio of approximately 10:1. The urine potassium will be high, reflecting the high aldosterone levels. Patients with preexisting chronic renal disease, especially interstitial nephritis or pyelonephritis, may lack the capacity to conserve sodium efficiently in response to hypovolemia or a decreased cardiac output. Such patients are at greatly increased risk for developing irreversible renal failure and must be monitored closely in order to correct plasma volume deficits accurately, even if the diagnosis of prerenal azotemia is in doubt.

Patients with severe liver disease may develop the so-called hepatorenal syndrome, characterized by hepatic failure and severe renal underperfusion. This form of prerenal azotemia may be impossible to reverse, since successful treatment depends upon restoration of liver function.

POSTRENAL AZOTEMIA

Complete anuria rarely occurs in the absence of bilateral ureteral or lower urinary tract obstruction. Therefore, obstruction should be strongly considered in an anuric patient and ruled out with appropriate diagnostic tests. Obstruction of the upper tract of one kidney will not cause obvious impairment of renal function, since the remaining kidney, if normal, will promptly adapt with increase in renal blood flow and glomerular filtration rate. However, *chronic* obstructive lower tract pathology will result in anatomic and functional abnormalities. Increased back-pressure will reduce glomerular filtration rate and increase urea reabsorption. Prolonged obstruction to urine flow then causes renal vasoconstriction, possibly mediated by renal prostaglandins,[60] and renal blood flow decreases. Ischemic damage to the nephrons will be added to the damage from obstruction, and cortical atrophy will eventually occur.

Chronic obstruction alters the expected capabilities of the kidney in salt and water excretion, so that sodium may be lost and the urine becomes isosmolar. Polyuria or oliguria may be seen. Because of these confusing findings obstructive uropathy should be considered in all patients with renal failure and ruled out by appropriate tests. Diagnostic ultrasound is especially useful and is a readily available non-invasive test that will demonstrate dilation of renal pelvis, ureter, or bladder and give a good estimate of renal cortical thickness. A high-dose infusion intravenous urogram may be useful to rule out obstructive uropathy if ultrasound is unavailable; it is relatively safe in a well-hydrated patient.

A renal scan with radioiodinated Hippuran will also demonstrate outflow obstruction, although late in the disease when renal blood flow and glomerular filtration are reduced the findings may be obscured. Cystoscopy and unilateral retrograde pyelography may be necessary if obstruction remains a possibility. Prompt recognition of obstruction as the cause of acute renal failure is important, since relief of the obstruction, especially if accomplished early (within 7 days), may restore normal renal function.

ACUTE RENAL PARENCHYMAL FAILURE — ARF

Acute renal failure (ARF) is due to poor renal perfusion with ischemia of the renal parenchyma and cell death. The precipitat-

TABLE 6–3 PATHOGENESIS OF ACUTE RENAL FAILURE

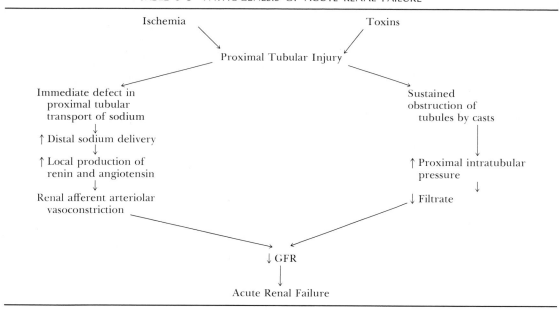

ing cause of ARF is renal vasoconstriction, usually triggered by a reduction in cardiac output. Reduction of renal blood flow is especially severe in the outer cortex where cell damage is often the greatest. The consequences of preglomerular arteriolar vasoconstriction are that glomerular filtration rate falls abruptly and intratubular fluid pressures drop; and that the peritubular capillary blood flow falls and ischemic necrosis of patchy areas of tubular epithelium occurs. Morphologic studies have shown that the brush border of the proximal tubular epithelial cells is especially sensitive to the effects of ischemia.[28] In experimental models of ARF, it can be demonstrated that these microvilli and other debris drop into the tubular lumen and cause tubular obstruction, which further decreases glomerular filtration rates as back-pressure in the nephron rises.[4, 18, 53] It can also be demonstrated experimentally that substances within the lumen of damaged tubules leak back into the interstitium, further decreasing urine flow. Free hemoglobin from a mismatched blood transfusion reaction, myoglobin from crush injuries, or plasma protein in a patient with multiple myeloma will also obstruct tubular lumina but only when glomerular filtration rates have fallen owing to a decrease in renal blood flow. Vasoconstriction in response to inadequate

renal perfusion is the common denominator of ARF (Table 6–3).

In contrast to prerenal azotemia, ARF may be irreversible, or it may take days to weeks to reverse. The urine contains casts and tubular cells, has a specific gravity of 1.010 and osmolarity equal to that of plasma, and has a high sodium content owing to failure of the damaged tubular epithelium to reabsorb salt. Urea is inadequately filtered and much of what appears in the glomerular filtrate leaks back and is taken up by the peritubular capillaries, so that urine urea concentration is low and the urine:plasma urea ratio is reduced to less than 10:1.

The pathophysiology of ARF is still not clearly understood. The many studies performed have supported various theories. However, the methods used have varied, making it difficult to relate these experimental results to the human with ARF. The mechanisms proposed as important in the development and maintenance of ARF are intrarenal tubular obstruction;[39] back-diffusion of solutes across necrotic tubular epithelium;[9, 42] shunting of blood flow from outer cortex to juxtamedullary nephrons;[56] and primary diminution in glomerular filtration rate (GFR) mediated through local renin-angiotensin produced by the juxtaglomerular apparatus (JGA).[29, 30]

Many investigators have postulated that intrarenal obstruction, possibly associated with back diffusion, is the main pathophysiologic factor in ARF.[3, 20, 25] Rats with ARF caused by clamping of the renal artery have been examined with micropuncture studies of the nephron by Arendshorst et al.[5] These studies have shown obstruction of tubular lumina with proteinaceous material, especially in medullary portions, and a marked increase in proximal intratubular pressure. These investigators concluded that early in the course of ARF tubular obstruction played the most important role.

Tanner and Steinhausen found an increase in proximal intratubular pressure (PIP) in micropuncture studies of rats that had had 1 hour of renal ischemia.[54] The GFR was depressed, owing to the increased PIP, which has also been observed with ureteral obstruction.[2] Microinjection with high pressure into the tubules will result in a decrease in PIP, supposedly related to flushing out of the obstruction, although back-leak secondary to leaking tubules could be responsible for this observation.

In the maintenance of ARF there is a cessation of filtration secondary to preglomerular vasoconstriction, resulting in a drop in proximal intratubular pressure. If volume expansion is used to increase renal blood flow and GFR, the PIP will then increase, indicating that tubular obstruction has not been relieved. In the recovery phase there is progressive repair of tubular epithelium with return of PIP to normal.[4, 23]

Other evidence that supports the primary role of tubular obstruction in the initiation of ARF includes the observation that dye markers in the proximal tubules fail to pass into the distal tubules,[54] that GFR can be increased to 70 per cent of normal by micropipette collection of filtrate proximal to the obstruction,[52] and that polyuria is present if some tubules remain patent.[22]

Obstruction could be caused by any of three factors: (1) intraluminal casts;[39, 45, 54] (2) compression of tubules owing to an increase in interstitial pressure;[31] or (3) swelling of tubule cells.[12] Morphologic studies in patients with ARF by Bohle et al.[10] do not support the theory of tubular obstruction by casts. The degree of renal failure could not be correlated with presence or absence of casts, and in many cases of ARF casts cannot be demonstrated. Acute tubular necrosis (ATN) certainly occurs after exposure to nephrotoxins. However, the minimal and patchy areas of tubular necrosis usually seen in patients even with severe ARF speak against acute tubular necrosis as the most important aspect of ARF in man.

Renal blood flow (RBF) remains reduced throughout the period of ARF in man. Total RBF may be only one-fourth to one-half of normal. Renal angiography demonstrates severe narrowing of cortical blood vessels, and other methods of demonstrating renal blood flow confirm these findings.[32, 46] While the initiating event of ARF after exposure to toxins may be different, the end result is the same, that is, severe sustained preglomerular vasoconstriction, even in the face of normalization of blood volume and cardiac output.[33] This may be accompanied by a decrease in efferent arteriolar vasomotor tone, which further diminishes effective filtration pressure.

The vasomotor abnormalities of afferent arteriolar vasoconstriction that occur in ARF have been studied by many workers.[11, 32, 33, 41, 46, 47, 58] Much data exist to support the hypothesis that local production of renin-angiotensin by the JGA is responsible for preglomerular vasoconstriction.[24, 29, 36, 37] Renin release appears to be secondary to sodium loss from the tubules. Sodium delivery to the macula densa, a specialized area of distal convoluted tubular epithelium lying adjacent to the JGA, is increased because of tubular damage and decreased ability to reabsorb sodium. The increased sodium concentration sensed by the macula densa sends a signal to the JGA that results in release of renin and local production of angiotensin with constriction of afferent arterioles. Thus, GFR is reduced in an attempt to avoid excessive loss of sodium and resultant loss of plasma volume.[49, 55]

Angiotensin-converting enzyme inhibitors, which should block the conversion of angiotensin I (produced from substrate by the enzymatic action of renin) to the active form angiotensin II, do not alter the vasoconstriction or the course of ARF.[6, 34, 50] Likewise, saralasin, a competitive inhibitor of angiotensin, is ineffective in reversing ARF.[7] As shown by Baranowski et al.,[8] the converting enzyme in the kidney may have properties different from those of the converting enzyme in the lung, which may explain the lack of effect of plasma-converting enzyme inhibitors in ARF. On the other hand, propranolol has protected animals from ARF in certain experiments, presumably by blocking renin release.[13, 17, 26] Plasma renin levels are consistently elevated in ARF and return to normal as recovery occurs.[16, 35, 40, 44, 57, 59] However, vasodilators directly infused into the renal artery fail to change the course of ARF even while increasing RBF. Undoubtedly, the cause of persistent failure to open up is complex and most likely involves several processes: vasoconstriction, tubular obstruction, and back-leak.

PRACTICAL CONSIDERATIONS IN DIAGNOSIS AND MANAGEMENT OF ACUTE AZOTEMIA AND OLIGURIA

Acute renal failure can often be prevented. It is possible to interrupt the continuum from prerenal azotemia to ARF by prompt restoration of adequate renal perfusion, but the longer the duration of prerenal azotemia, the greater the likelihood that ARF will develop. Recognition of plasma volume contraction, the most common cause of inadequate renal perfusion in the surgical patient, is paramount. Volume status of the patient can be evaluated by clinical and laboratory parameters. Clinical evaluation will determine skin and tissue turgor, systemic blood pressure (and the presence or absence of orthostatic change in blood pressure), tachycardia, ascites, sepsis, and possible sources of third space fluid sequestration such as soft tissue trauma, peritonitis, or bowel obstruction. However, it must be stressed that with clinical examination alone it may be difficult to determine the *effective* arterial volume of a patient accurately; for example, a patient with ascites may have a markedly decreased effective arterial volume, while total body sodium and water are elevated. It is often necessary to use hemodynamic measurements of central venous pressure and left atrial pressure (PCWP) as objective parameters in plasma volume assessment (Table 6–4).

In patients with azotemia, the laboratory also becomes a useful tool (Table 6–5). Effective arterial volume is reflected by the fractional excretion of sodium. In reversible conditions associated with plasma volume

TABLE 6–4 EVALUATION OF ACUTE AZOTEMIA OR OLIGURIA IN THE SURGICAL PATIENT

I. Clinical Assessment
  a. Hypotension, dehydration, causes for third space losses, sepsis, liver failure
  b. Cardiogenic shock, decreased cardiac output
II. Central venous pressure measurement, establishment of IV lines
III. Blood chemistry determinations
  a. Electrolytes, especially potassium
  b. Calcium, phosphorus
  c. Urea, creatinine
IV. Hematologic values
  a. Platelet count
  b. Hematocrit
V. Determination of urine output
  a. Anuria
    1. Physical examination: pelvic, rectal, abdominal
    2. Catheterization of urinary bladder
    3. Ultrasound examination of kidneys, bladder
    4. Renal scan
    5. Cytoscopy and unilateral retrograde pyelogram
  b. Oliguria
    1. Specific gravity and osmolarity
    2. Microscopic examination
    3. Sodium, creatinine, and urea concentrations

contraction (prerenal azotemia), the kidney will avidly retain sodium; upon development of ARF, the kidney will then lose sodium. The excreted fraction of filtered sodium, FE_{Na}, is determined from the following formulae:[21]

$$FE_{Na} = \frac{Na\ excreted}{Na\ filtered} \times 100$$

or

$$FE_{Na} = \frac{U_{Na} \times V}{P_{Na} \times GFR} \times 100$$

or

$$FE_{Na} = \frac{U_{Na} \times V}{P_{Na} \times C_{Cr}} \times 100$$

or

$$FE_{Na} = \frac{U_{Na} \times V}{P_{Na} \times \dfrac{U_{Cr} \times U_v}{P_{Cr}}} \times 100$$

or

$$FE_{Na} = \frac{U_{Na} \times P_{Cr}}{P_{Na} \times U_{Cr}} \times 100$$

or

$$FE_{Na} = \frac{U}{P} Na \left/ \frac{U}{P} Cr \times 100 \right.$$

TABLE 6–5   FLOW SHEET FOR ACUTE AZOTEMIA OR OLIGURIA

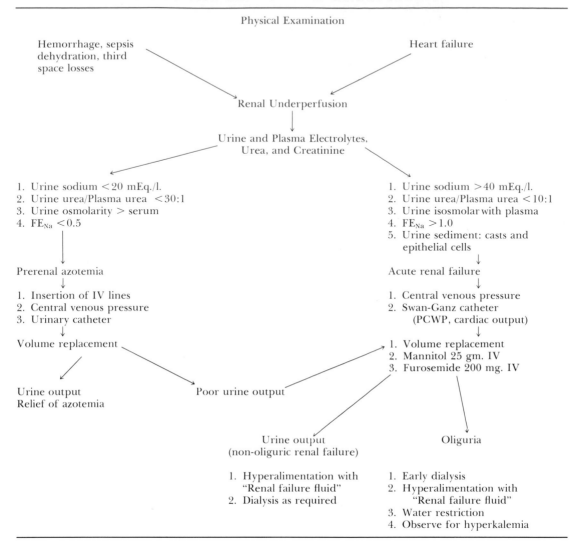

The FE_{Na} is less than 0.5 in patients with decreased effective arterial volume (prerenal azotemia), in contrast to patients with acute oliguric renal failure, acute non-oliguric renal failure, acute obstructive uropathy, and acute glomerulonephritis. In all of these other conditions, the FE_{Na} exceeds 1.0,[38] although this concept has recently been challenged.[43]

A simple estimate of the FE_{Na} can be obtained by measurement of the urine sodium concentration. Values less than 20 mEq./l. are usually associated with plasma volume contraction (prerenal). Values greater than 40 mEq./l. are usually associated with acute renal failure.[38]

Treatment of oliguria in the patient without obstructive uropathy is the vigorous replacement of plasma volume with crystalloids, preferably normal saline or Ringer's solution. Hemodynamic monitoring of the PCWP by a Swan-Ganz catheter should be employed in any elderly or severely oliguric patient, so that precise volume replacement can be achieved without cardiac overloading.

Should volume replacement not result in adequate urine output, mannitol 25 gm. I.V. push and furosemide 200 mg. I.V. push (over 20 minutes, to avoid ototoxicity) are given. If the patient has an adequate plasma volume, this therapeutic trial usually results in a resumption of urinary flow. If urine flow does not occur, the diagnosis of ARF must be made and the patient treated by fluid restriction and dialysis when indicated.

The normal adult must excrete approximately 500 ml. of maximally concentrated urine per day in order to remove the waste products of metabolism. If this cannot be achieved, fluid intake must be restricted to replacement of insensible and calculated water losses plus urine output, minus the water of oxidation produced by the breakdown of endogenous fats and proteins. Insensible losses through the skin and respiration total approximately 900 ml. in an afebrile, stable patient but increase with fever or severe catabolic conditions such as trauma, major surgery, or burns. Fluid is also lost via nasogastric suction or drains and must be measured and added to the estimated insensible losses. Water produced by oxidation of endogenous fats and proteins equals approximately 400 ml./day. Therefore, in a stable, afebrile patient who is not losing fluid through drains or intestinal suction, the amount of fluid to be replaced is approximately 500 ml. per day plus urine output. Sodium is retained during oliguria and does not need to be replaced. Hyponatremia in ARF is almost always due to overhydration and is treated by water restriction and dialysis.

Development of ARF in the postsurgical or post-trauma period is especially serious because of tissue destruction and the increased rate of catabolism that these patients exhibit. The development of uremia is accelerated as body protein is catabolized and electrolyte imbalances occur. Principal among these is hyperkalemia, caused by breakdown of cells and shifting of potassium from the intracellular to the extracellular pool. Hyperkalemia is exaggerated after the increased tissue damage of trauma or major surgery. Ketoacidosis also occurs as fats are catabolized for energy sources.

The mortality of ARF in the postsurgical or post-trauma patient is 50 to 60 per cent.[51] Most of this mortality is due to fluid and electrolyte imbalance or to sepsis occurring in the catabolic and uremic patient with markedly diminished resistance to infection.

An important advance in management of these postsurgical catabolic patients in ARF has been described by Abel and Fischer,[1] and by Dudrick and associates.[19] Their work has been based on the observations of Rose and Dekker in normal volunteers[48] that essential amino acids could be directly incorporated into body protein if adequate calories were provided and no other source of exogenous protein were present. An intravenous solution has been made available, which provides the essential L-amino acids in crystalline form. Adding glucose to provide 800 non-protein calories per gram of nitrogen, the intravenous preparation of "renal failure fluid" can be given to patients with ARF via a central venous line. Quite remarkable results are achieved. The carbohydrate and amino acids are utilized, decreasing the consumption of fat and lean muscle mass for gluconeogenesis. Endogenous urea is recycled into protein, thus decreasing the blood urea concentration and reducing the level of uremia. Tissue breakdown is inhibited; therefore, potassium release, hyperkalemia, and ketoacidosis are reduced. Hyperphosphatemia and attendant hypocalcemia are also minimized. By providing adequate substrate and energy, the necessary protein synthesis for renal tubular regeneration can take place and the duration of ARF may be shortened, thus reducing the occurrence of late complications of ARF due to impaired host resistance. A prospective double-blind study was conducted by Abel and associates;[1] postsurgical patients with ARF treated with "renal failure fluid" had a 75 per cent survival, compared with a 44 per cent survival of similar patients treated with hypertonic glucose only. The benefits were most marked in patients with severe ARF requiring dialysis. The treated patients also had significantly earlier improvement in renal function. We strongly recommend that ARF patients be treated early in the course of their disease with intravenous or enteral feedings of glucose and essential amino acids and "renal failure fluid", now readily available commercially (Nephramine).

Serum potassium, calcium, blood urea nitrogen, and creatinine should be measured daily during ARF. Hyperkalemia can be life-threatening; if the serum potassium is found to be above 6.5 mEq./l., the patient should be treated as an emergency, and given an I.V. bolus of 44 mEq. of sodium bicarbonate, 50 gm. of hypertonic glucose, and 10 units of regular insulin. This treatment will drive potassium into cells and temporarily relieve hyperkalemia. If the serum potassium is above 7.5 mEq./l. or if electrocardiogram changes of peaking of the T waves, widening of the QRS complex, and prolonged Q-T interval occur, calcium salts should be given to antagonize the effect of potassium on the myocardium, as 10 per cent calcium chloride, 5 to 10 ml. I.V. over 2 to 5 minutes while observing the ECG. Long-term control of hyperkalemia may be necessary especially in the post-trauma patient with tissue injury. Sodium polystyrene sulfonate (Kayexalate), a sodium ion-exchange resin, may be given as a retention enema (40 gm. in 200 ml. of 25 per cent sorbitol every 6 hours). More often, dialysis is instituted.

We have found that many complications of uremia can be avoided by early and frequent hemodialysis, and we initiate dialy-

TABLE 6–6   INTERVAL EXTENSION METHOD OF DRUG THERAPY IN RENAL FAILURE*

| | | GFR ml./min. | | |
		>50	10–50	<10
		(Hours between usual calculated doses)		
Aminoglycosides				
1. *All* of the aminoglycoside antibiotics are excreted by the kidney and are nephrotoxic and ototoxic.	Amikacin	12–18	24–36	36–48
	Gentamicin	8–12	12–24	24–48
	Kanamycin	24	24–72	72–96
2. Dose reduction is mandatory in renal failure.	Tobramycin	8–12	12–24	24–48
3. Gentamicin is one of the most common causes of ARF in elderly surgical patients.				
4. Blood levels are best guide to therapy.				
Cephalosporins				
1. Excretion of cephalosporins is mainly by the kidney.	Cefaclor	8	12–24	24–48
	Cefadroxil	8	12–24	24–48
2. Dose reduction is necessary in renal failure	Cefamandole	6	6–9	9
	Cefazolin	8	12	24–48
3. Nephrotoxicity is markedly increased when given in combination with aminoglycosides, or in patients with volume depletion.	Cefoxitin	8	8–12	24
	Cephalothin	6	6	8–12
	Cephalexin	6	6	6–12
	Cephapirin	6	6	12
	Cephadine	8	12–24	24–48
Penicillins				
1. Excretion of most penicillins is by the kidney.	Amoxicillin	6	6–12	12–16
	Ampicillin	6	6–12	12–16
2. Seizures and coagulopathy are major toxic manifestations.	Carbenicillin	8–12	12–24	24–48
	Cloxacillin	No change	No change	No change
3. High loads of sodium or potassium may be given inadvertently.	Dicloxacillin	No change	No change	No change
	Methicillin	4	4	8–12
	Nafcillin	No change	No change	No change
	Oxacillin	No change	No change	No change
	Penicillin	8	8–12	12–18
	Ticarcillin	8–12	12–24	24–48
Tetracyclines				
1. Tetracyclines are anti-anabolic in action and increase catabolism, causing elevation of BUN and potentiating acidosis.	Doxycycline	12	2–18	18–24
	Minocycline	12	18–24	24–36
	Vancomycin	24–72	72–240	240
	Naladixic Acid	No change	No change	AVOID
	Nitrofurantoin	No change	AVOID	AVOID
Cardiac glycosides				
1. Toxicity of the cardiac glycosides is enhanced by dialysis (removal of potassium).	Digoxin	24	30–40	40–48
	Digitoxin	24	24	30–36
2. Serum levels are best guide to therapy.				

*Adapted from Bennett, W. M., et al.: Drug therapy in renal failure: Dosing guidelines for adults. Ann. Intern. Med. *93*:62, 1980.

sis in the surgical patient when the blood urea nitrogen reaches 90 mg./dl. Most patients with acute renal failure, especially postoperatively or following trauma, need frequent dialysis. Water can be removed by ultrafiltration, permitting additional fluid intake or correcting volume overload, and electrolyte abnormalities can be readily corrected. In the presence of massive tissue injury, hyperkalemia may still be a problem, and Kayexalate enemas should be given between dialysis treatments if the potassium reaches 5.5 to 6.0 mEq. per liter. Patients who are hypercatabolic (BUN rise greater than 30 mg./dl. in 24 hours) will need daily dialysis.

Hypertension in the patient with ARF is usually due to overhydration and is best treated by removing excessive salt and water through dialysis. Life-threatening hypertension can be temporarily controlled with diazoxide, 300 mg. I.V. push or with a constant infusion of sodium nitroprusside, 100 gm./l. of 5 per cent dextrose in water.

Drugs that are excreted by the kidney must be given in reduced doses or at protracted intervals. A loading dose of the normal calculated amount is given, and daily total doses thereafter must be reduced or given less often. A rough guide to the use of certain commonly used drugs is provided in Table 6–6. However, measurements of blood levels of the drugs are necessary to assure that proper peak and trough levels are achieved.

SURGERY IN THE PATIENT WITH IMPAIRED RENAL FUNCTION

Surgery in the patient with impaired renal function has become a common occurrence. Such patients are at high risk for the development of ARF in the postoperative period. With the use of appropriate preventive measures, worsening of renal function or the development of acute renal failure can be avoided. Adequate hydration at all times is essential; patients with renal insufficiency should always be given intravenous fluids when placed N.P.O. or when given bowel purgatives in preparation for tests or surgery.

Recent experimental studies[15, 27] have identified a role for mannitol and furosemide in preventing ARF. Volume expansion with mannitol was effective in preventing a decrease in renal blood flow. The rise in the proximal intratubular pressure as glomerular filtration increases after mannitol has been given may also protect against the development of tubular obstruction. Volume expansion with isotonic saline alone was not as effective as mannitol, although oliguria was prevented. Furosemide exerts its effect by increasing renal blood flow through increased renal prostaglandin production, and by interruption of the tubuloglomerular feedback mechanism. The effector in the tubuloglomerular feedback mechanism (increased sodium delivery to the macula densa) is afferent arteriolar vasoconstriction which, when interrupted by furosemide, permits afferent arteriolar vasodilation. Another effect of furosemide is to increase salt and water excretion outside the control of prostaglandin or tubuloglomerular feedback, and this increase in solute excretion exerts a protective effect.[27]

The clinical approach to the preoperative patient with preexisting renal insufficiency or to the patient who is about to undergo a procedure that carries a high risk for development of ARF (such as complicated open heart surgery with long perfusion times or resection of abdominal aortic aneurysm) is to properly hydrate the patient with 0.9 N saline or Ringer's solution. One half hour before induction of anesthesia, mannitol 25 gm. and furosemide 200 mg. are given I.V. over 20 minutes. An indwelling urinary catheter must be placed, and urine output is continuously monitored and replaced with 0.9 N saline or Ringer's solution.

This same procedure should be used in a high-risk patient prior to radiographic studies requiring an intravenous iodinated contrast medium (intravenous urogram, angiogram, or computerized axial tomography). The older diabetic patient is especially prone to develop ARF following intravenous contrast studies and should be pretreated on a routine basis.

Bibliography

1. Abel, R. M., Beck, C. H., Jr., Abbott, W. M., Ryan, J. A., Jr., Barnett, G. O., and Fischer, J. E.: Improved survival from acute renal failure after

treatment with intravenous essential L-amino acids and glucose: Results of a prospective, double-blind study. N. Engl. J. Med. *288*:695, 1973.

2. Andreucci, V. E., Herrera-Acosta, J., Rector, F. D. J., and Seldin, D. W.: Effective glomerular filtration pressure and single nephron filtration rate during hydropenia, elevated ureteral pressure, and acute volume expansion with isotonic saline. J. Clin. Invest. *50*:2230, 1971.

3. Arendshorst, W. J., Finn, W. F., and Gottschalk, C. W.: Pathogenesis of acute renal insufficiency after temporary renal ischemia in the rat. (Abstract) Proc. Am. Soc. Nephrol., Washington, D.C., 1973.

4. Arendshorst, W. J., Finn, W. F., and Gottschalk, C. W.: Pathogenesis of acute renal failure following temporary ischemia in the rat. Circ. Res. *37*:558, 1975.

5. Arendshorst, W. J., Finn, W. F., and Gottschalk, C. W. (with the technical assistance of Lucas, H. K.): Micropuncture study of acute renal failure following temporary renal ischemia in the rat. Kidney Int. *10*:100, 1976.

6. Baranowski, R. L., Dach, J., Kurtzman, N. A., and Gutierrez, L.: The effect of angiotensin II on glycerol induced acute renal failure. Kidney Int. *6*:20a, 1974.

7. Baranowski, R. L., O'Connor, G. J., McCreary, J. T., and Kurtzman, N. A.: The effect of 1-sarcosine, 8-leucyl angiotensin II on the pressor effect of infused angiotensin II. Arch. Intern. Pharm. Ther. *217*:322, 1975.

8. Baranowski, R. L., Westenfelder, C., and Kurtzman, N. A.: Renal angiotensin I converting enzyme differs from that of lung and is not inhibited by captopril (SQ14225) or the nonapeptide SQ 2881. Clin. Res. *27*:494a, 1979.

9. Bibec, T. U. L., Mylle, M., Baines, A. D., Gottschalk, C. W., Oliver, J. R., and MacDowell, M. C.: A study by micropuncture and microdissection of acute renal damage in rats. Am. J. Med. *44*:664, 1968.

10. Bohle, A., Jahnecke, J., Meyer, D., and Schubert, G. E.: Morphology of acute renal failure: Comparative data from biopsy and autopsy. Kidney Int. *10*:9, 1976.

11. Brun, C., Crone, C., Davidsen, H. G., Fabricius, J., Hansen, A. T., Lassen, N. A., and Munck, O.: Renal blood flow in anuric human subject determined by use of radioactive krypton 85. Proc. Soc. Exp. Biol. Med. *89*:687, 1955.

12. Burwell, R. G.: Changes in the proximal tubule of the rabbit kidney after temporary complete renal ischemia. J. Pathol. Bacteriol. *70*:387, 1955.

13. Chevalier, R. L., and Finn, W. F.: Effects of propranolol on post-ischemic acute renal failure. Nephron *25*:77, 1980.

14. Cronin, R. E., de Torrente, A., Miller, P. D., Bulger, R. E., Burke, T. J., and Schrier, R. W.: Pathogenic mechanisms in early norepinephrine-induced acute renal failure: Functional and histological correlates of protection. Kidney Int. *14*:115, 1978.

15. de Torrente, A., Miller, P. D., Cronin, R. E., Paulsen, P. E., Erickson, A. L., and Schrier, R. W.: Effects of furosemide and acetylcholine in norepinephrine-induced acute renal failure. Am. J. Physiol. *235*:131, 1978.

16. DiBona, G. F., and Swain, L. L.: The renin-angiotensin system in acute renal failure in the rat. Lab. Invest. *25*:528, 1971.

17. Dollery, C. J., Paterson, J. W., and Conolly, M. E.: Clinical pharmacology of beta-receptor blocking drugs. Clin. Pharmacol. Ther. *10*:765, 1969.

18. Donohoe, J. D., Venkatachalan, M. A., Bernard, D. B., and Levinsky, N. G.: Tubular leakage and obstruction after renal ischemia: Structural-functional correlations. Kidney Int. *13*:208, 1978.

19. Dudrick, S. J., Steiger, E., and Long, J. M.: Renal failure in surgical patients: Treatment with intravenous essential amino acids and hypertonic glucose. Surgery *68*:180, 1970.

20. Eisenbach, G. M., and Steinhausen, M.: Micropuncture studies after temporary ischemia in the rat. Pflugers Arch. Ges. Physiol. *343*:11, 1973.

21. Espinel, C. H.: The FE_{Na} test: Use in the differential diagnosis of acute renal failure. J.A.M.A. *236*:579, 1976.

22. Finn, W. F.: Anesthetic-induced variation in the renal response to ischemia. Kidney Int. *14*:724, 1978.

23. Finn, W. F.: Post-ischemic acute renal failure. Initiation, maintenance, and recovery. Invest. Urol. *17*:427, 1980.

24. Flamenbaum, W.: Pathophysiology of acute renal failure. Arch. Intern. Med. *131*:911, 1973.

25. Frega, S. N., Di Bona, D. R., Guertler, B., and Leaf, A.: Ischemic renal injury. Kidney Int. *10*:17, 1976.

26. Gavendo, S., Kapuler, S., Serban, I., Iaina, A., and Eliahou, H.: Beta-adrenergic receptors in rat kidneys. (Abstract) Kidney Int. *15*:581, 1979.

27. Gerber, J. G., and Nies, A. S.: Furosemide-induced vasodilatation: Importance of the state of hydration and filtration. Kidney Int. *18*:454, 1980.

28. Glaumann, G., Glaumann, H., and Trump, B. F.: Studies of cellular recovery from ischemia. III. Ultrastructural studies of the recovery of recta of the proximal tubular (P_3) segment of the rat kidney from temporary ischemia. Virchows Arch. Cell Pathol. *25*:281, 1977.

29. Goormaghtigh, N.: Vascular and circulatory changes in renal cortex in the anuric crush-syndrome. Proc. Soc. Exp. Biol. Med. *59*:303, 1945.

30. Goormaghtigh, N.: The renal arteriolar changes in the anuric crush-syndrome. Am. J. Pathol. *23*:513, 1947.

31. Gottschalk, C. W., and Mylle, M.: Micropuncture of the rat kidney during osmotic diuresis. Am. J. Physiol. *189*:323, 1957.

32. Hollenberg, N. K., Epstein, M., Rosen, S., et al.: Acute oliguric renal failure in man: Evidence for preferential renal cortical ischemia. Medicine *47*:455, 1968.

33. Hollenberg, N. K., Adams, D. F., Oken, D. E., et al.: Acute renal failure due to nephrotoxins: Renal hemodynamic and angiographic studies in man. N. Engl. J. Med. *282*:1329, 1970.

34. Ishikawa, I., and Hollenberg, N. K.: Pharmacologic interruption of the renin-angiotensin system in myohemoglobinuric acute renal failure. Kidney Int. *10*:183, 1976.

35. Kokot, F., and Kuska, J.: Plasma renin activity in acute renal insufficiency. Nephron 6:125, 1969.

36. MacGregor, J., Briggs, J. D., Brown, J. J., Chinn, R. H., Gauras, H., Lever, A. F., MacAdam, R. F., Medina, A., Morton, J. J., Oliver, N. W. J., Paton, A., Powell-Jackson, J. D., Robertson, J. J. S., and Waite, M. A.: Renin and renal function in modern diuretic therapy in the treatment of cardiovascular and renal disease. Excerpta Med. 71–83, 1973.

37. Matthews, P. G., Morgan, T. O., and Johnston, C. I.: The renin-angiotensin system in acute renal failure in rats. Clin. Sci. Mol. Med. 47:79, 1974.

38. Miller, T. R., Anderson, R. J., Linas, S. L., Henrich, W. L., Berns, A. S., Gabow, P. A., and Schrier, R. W.: Urinary diagnostic indices in acute renal failure: A prospective study. Ann. Intern. Med. 89:47, 1978.

39. Minnani, S.: Nierenveränderungen nach Verschuttung. Arch. Pathol. Angr. 245:247, 1923.

40. Ochoa, E., Finkielman, S., and Agrest, A.: Angiotensin blood levels during the evolution of acute renal failure. Clin. Sci. 38:225, 1970.

41. Oken, D. E.,: Nosologic considerations in the nomenclature of acute renal failure. Nephron 8:505, 1971.

42. Oliver, J., MacDowell, M., and Tracey, A.: The pathogenesis of acute renal failure associated with traumatic and toxic injury: Renal ischemia, nephrotoxic damage, and ischemuric episode. J. Clin. Invest. 30:1305, 1951.

43. Pru, C., and Kiellstrand, C.: The clinical usefulness of the FE$_{Na}$ test. (Abstract) Clin. Dial. Transplant. Forum 10:49, 1980.

44. Raugh, W., Oster, P., Dietz, R., and Gross, F.: Angiotensin II in acute renal failure of the rat. Acta Endocrinol. 73 (S 177):193, 1973.

45. Reimer, K. A., Ganote, C. E., and Jennings, R. B.: Alterations in renal cortex following ischemic injury. III. Ultrastructure of proximal tubules after ischemia or autolysis. Lab. Invest. 26:347, 1972.

46. Reubi, F. C., Vorburger, C., and Tuckman, J.: Renal distribution volumes of indocyanine green ($_{51}$Cr) EDTA and $_{24}$Na in man during acute renal failure. J. Clin. Invest. 52:223, 1973.

47. Reubi, F. C., and Vorburger, C.: Renal hemodynamics in acute renal failure after shock in man. Kidney Int. 10:137, 1976.

48. Rose, W. C., and Dekker, E. E.: Urea as a source of nitrogen for the biosynthesis of amino acids. J. Biol. Chem. 223:107, 1956.

49. Schnermann, J.: Regulation of single nephron filtration rate by feedback: Facts and theories. Clin. Nephrol. 3:75, 1975.

50. Semple, P. F., Brown, J. J., Lever, A. F., MacGregor, J., Morton, J. J., Powell-Jackson, J. D., and Robertson, J. I. S.: Renin, angiotensin II and III in acute renal failure: Note on the measurement of angiotensin II and III in rat blood. Kidney Int. 10:169, 1976.

51. Stott, R. B., Cameron, J. S., Ogg, C. S., and Bewick, M.: Why the persistently high mortality in acute renal failure? Lancet 2:75, 1972.

52. Tanner, G. A., Sloan, K. L., and Sophasan, S.: Effects of renal artery occlusion on kidney function in the rat. Kidney Int. 4:377, 1973.

53. Tanner, G. A., and Sophasan, S.: Kidney pressures after temporary renal artery occlusion in the rat. Am. J. Physiol. 230:1173, 1976.

54. Tanner, G. A., and Steinhausen, M.: Tubular obstruction in ischemia-induced acute renal failure in the rat. Kidney Int. 10:65, 1976.

55. Thurau, K., Vogt, C., and Dahlheim, H.: Renin activity in the juxtaglomerular apparatus of the rat kidney during post-ischemic acute renal failure. Kidney Int. 10:177, 1976.

56. Trueta, J., Barclay, A. E., Daniel, P. M., Franklin, K. G., and Prichard, M. M. L.: Studies of the Renal Circulation. Springfield, Ill., Charles C Thomas, 1947.

57. Vogt, C., Stowe, N., Dahlheim, H., Wobert, W., and Thurau, R.: Mechanisms determining GFR after renal ischemia. Pflugers Arch. Gest. Physiol. 343:R42, 1973.

58. Walker, J. G., Silva, H., Lawson, T. R., Ryder, J. A., and Shaldon, S.: Renal blood flow in acute renal failure measured by renal arterial infusion of indocyanine green. Proc. Soc. Exp. Biol. Med. 112:932, 1963.

59. Weber, P. C., Held, E., Uhlich, E., and Eigler, J.: Reaction constants of renin in juxtaglomerular apparatus and plasma renin activity after renal ischemia and hemorrhage. Kidney Int. 7:331, 1975.

60. Wilson, D. R.: Pathophysiology of obstructive nephropathy. Kidney Int. 18:281, 1980.

GENERAL REFERENCES

61. Bennett, W. M., Muther, R. S., Parker, R. A., et al.: Drug therapy in renal failure: Dosing guidelines for adults. Ann. Intern. Med. 93:62, 1980.

62. Finn, W. F.: Acute renal failure. In Early, L. E., and Gottschalk, C. W. (Eds.): Strauss and Welt's Diseases of the Kidney. 3rd Ed. Boston, Little, Brown and Company, 1979.

63. Guyton, A. C.: Textbook of Medical Physiology. 5th Ed. Philadelphia, W. B. Saunders Company, 1976.

64. Levinsky, N. G.: Pathophysiology of acute renal failure. N. Engl. J. Med. 296:1453, 1970.

7

POSTOPERATIVE PULMONARY COMPLICATIONS

Including Complications of Bronchoscopy

Watts R. Webb
and Peter V. Moulder

In spite of many advances in the care of the surgical patient, pulmonary problems continue to constitute the most frequent postoperative complications, particularly after surgery of the thorax or abdomen. They are less frequent, but nevertheless common, after other types of surgery. Although innumerable factors play a role, the basic problem is one of maintenance of a clear tracheobronchial airway, since atelectasis, pneumonia, lung abscess, and postoperative pulmonary edema are usually secondary to partial or complete obstruction by retained or aspirated secretions.

ATELECTASIS AND PNEUMONIA

Atelectasis and pneumonia are the most common of all postoperative complications. The Mayo Clinic report[38] on surgery of the stomach and duodenum for 1950 noted that 25 per cent of the hospital deaths were due to pneumonia. Moersch[24] found atelectasis in 10 per cent of operations on the thorax or upper part of the abdomen and in 4 per cent of operations on the lower portion. Similarly, Stringer[35] found that 26 of 55 patients showed abnormal x-ray signs after gastrectomy, and of these, 13 had signs of

Watts Rankin Webb is a Mississippian who was educated at Johns Hopkins. As Chief of Surgery at Mississippi State Sanatorium he gained national recognition in the surgical treatment of tuberculosis. For several years he was an outstanding professor in the Department of Surgery at the University of Mississippi and later he was Professor of Surgery and Chairman of Cardiovascular Surgery at the University of Texas Southwestern Medical School. Later, he was Professor and Chairman of the Department of Surgery of the Upstate Medical Center, State University of New York. At present, he is Professor and Chairman of the Department of Surgery of Tulane University School of Medicine. His accomplishments as a medical educator and investigator have been a great tribute to his former teachers, Dr. Evarts A. Graham and Dr. Thomas Burford.

Peter Vincent Moulder, a native of Jackson, Michigan, graduated from the University of Notre Dame and received his M.D. degree from the University of Chicago. There he received general and thoracic surgical training with Dr. Lester Dragstedt and Dr. W. E. Adams. He served as Professor of Surgery at the University of Chicago and later at the University of Pennsylvania, and the University of Florida before joining the staff of Tulane University. He has made many outstanding contributions, particularly in surgical physiology of the heart and lungs.

partial or massive atelectasis. In a review of 300 consecutive patients seen in 1944, Clendon and Pygott[10] found 38 per cent of the abdominal group — but only 2.7 per cent of the non-abdominal group — to show evidence of respiratory complications, while Thoren[37] found pulmonary changes in 41.9 per cent of a carefully studied group of patients subjected to gallbladder surgery. Clendon and Pygott[10] extensively reviewed several series to point out the greater number of pulmonary complications of upper abdominal surgery versus lower abdominal surgery, and also the increasing incidence of pulmonary complications in recent years as older patients and more complicated procedures are involved. Kurzweg[19] summarizes the incidence of postop-

erative complications as averaging 2.5 to 3 per cent of all operations, 10 to 20 per cent in abdominal surgery, and 20 to 30 per cent in upper abdominal surgery. Many of these obviously go unsuspected unless specifically sought by careful clinical and x-ray studies.

ETIOLOGY. At some risk of oversimplification it can be stated categorically that the ultimate pathway of production of postoperative atelectasis and pneumonia is obstruction of the tracheobronchial airway. Palmer and Sellick[28] list 31 possible etiologic factors in postoperative atelectasis that essentially fall into the following major groups: (1) changes in bronchial secretion; (2) defective expulsion mechanism; and (3) reduction of bronchial caliber. These in-

PATHOGENESIS OF PULMONARY SUPPURATION AND ATELECTASIS

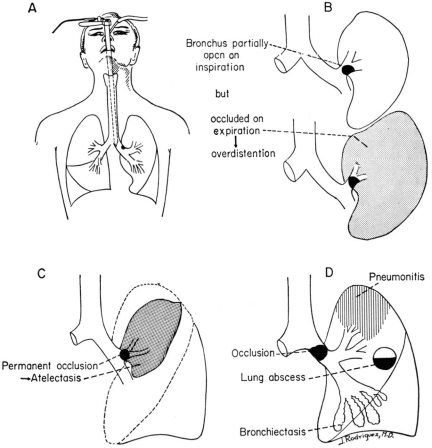

Figure 7–1 Diagram showing role of bronchial obstruction as an etiologic factor in pulmonary suppuration and insufficiency. (From Hardy, J. D.: Pathophysiology in Surgery. Baltimore, Williams & Wilkins Company, 1958.)

clude the many factors that tend to increase the incidence of obstruction, e.g., narcotics, which may suppress the cough reflex, prolonged postoperative immobilization, splinting from pain or constricting bandages, dehydration, pulmonary congestion, aspiration of foreign material, and weakness of the respiratory muscles. Swank and Smedal,[36] in an illuminating study, found pulmonary complications in 65 per cent of a group of young soldiers following stuporous states induced by deep Sodium Amytal narcosis.

Pneumonitis routinely follows persistent atelectasis. One of the important factors was demonstrated by Shields,[34] who found experimentally that intravenously injected organisms are selectively localized in any segment of lung, however small, in which there is bronchial obstruction or interrupted or impaired ventilation.

PREDISPOSING FACTORS. There is an increased complication rate in those who smoke or who suffer from bronchitis, and this is not affected by discontinuance of smoking 4 days or less before the operation.[30] A simple preoperative cough test (Green[15]) will frequently detect the susceptible patients, since a "self-propagating" paroxysm of coughing or the sound of a "wet" cough is the most significant sign of preoperative bronchitis or the presence of potentially obstructing material. Preoperative bronchitis was detected in 46 per cent of the men and 21 per cent of the women in their surgical population, the usual etiologic factor being 20 or more cigarettes per day. Asthma, obesity, emphysema, and thoracic kyphoscoliosis likewise are usually associated with an abnormal cough test and predispose to postoperative difficulties.

One must regard as susceptible to postoperative respiratory complications any patient who is subjected to an appreciable period of respiratory depression or interference with the ability to cough vigorously. These are proportionate to (1) the depth and duration of the anesthesia; (2) the length of depression of ventilation whether by a Trendelenburg, lateral, or prone position, by the use of heavy preoperative or postoperative sedation, or by postoperative stupor or coma; and (3) the reduction of ventilatory power by emphysema, asthma,

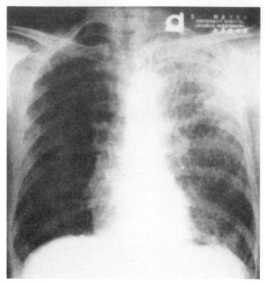

Figure 7–2 Aspiration pneumonitis in a 61-year-old man with abdominal carcinomatosis.

obesity, large abdominal hernia, or flabby musculature.

Other perpetuating factors include pain that prevents coughing and ambulation, nasogastric tubes that stimulate secretions in the nasopharynx that may be aspirated, and intravenous administration of fluids over prolonged periods which immobilize the patient.

The surgeon must weigh the depression of respiratory function caused by narcotic analgesics against their value as pain relievers. In general, narcotic analgesics are administered in doses insufficient for effective pain relief because of fear of respiratory interference. (This is true of morphine in particular.) Since the use of narcotic analgesics and nerve blocks cannot be done by simple orders (e.g., every four hours or q.i.d.), the surgeon must devise a system in which the interaction between the patient and the nurse and others responsible for the patient's care produces an optimal situation. The following guidelines have proven useful. In the very early postoperative period an analgesic is administered intravenously in small hourly doses. Relief of pain and absence of respiratory depression can be assessed rapidly. Once the appropriate dose of analgesic is found, then an appropriate regimen of q. 1 to 2 hours can be ordered, and for the first 24 to 48 hours the intravenous route is used. Longer intervals not only allow pain to return but also lead to a need for larger doses to control the pain. Morphine sulfate, which is particularly useful in thoracic surgical procedures and other extremely painful situations, is especially suited to this format. The use of nerve blockade can be complementary.

Interest has increased in the use of *intra*operative nerve block, especially with long-acting agents. However, extensive use in the 1940's and the 1950's led to a few cases in which spinal cord damage and paralysis resulted, and, therefore, this method was discontinued. Postoperative nerve blocks performed through the chest wall are much safer, as the site of the injection is well away from the spinal canal projections. It is important to block a number of intercostal nerves above and below the site of the surgical incision or trauma. Flooding with a ¼ per cent solution of lidocaine and epinephrine will help area pain.

The effects of the site of the operative procedure have been beautifully explored by Anscombe,[2] who followed serially for several days the vital capacity, maximum expiratory rate, and maximum inspiratory rate after various operations. All measurements were greatly reduced by upper abdominal procedures, the vital capacity often dropping to 40 per cent of preoperative control. The reduction was not necessarily related to the severity of the procedures, for an abdominoperineal resection of the rectum produced only moderate and transient changes. On the other hand, abdominal rigidity such as that following simple closure of a perforated peptic ulcer reduced pulmonary mechanical power the greatest of all, even though there was rather rapid recovery. These findings parallel those of Beecher,[4] Churchill,[9] and Powers,[31] who demonstrated significant postoperative changes in vital capacity and found that these are directly proportional to the incidence of pulmonary complications. This decrease in vital capacity is not readily perceived clinically, since tidal and minute volumes may be sufficient for adequate oxygenation in spite of inactivity of a significant portion of the bellows mechanism. It is, however, the bellows effect that maintains

the "bronchial toilet" to prevent the pulmonary complications.

DIAGNOSIS. Incipient atelectasis may be detected by the presence of moist rales usually localized posteriorly or toward the bases, or by diminished breath sounds with bronchial breathing over a localized segment of the lung. The sudden onset of fever and rapid pulse, as classically described, though common in massive atelectasis, is usually a late sign. Shift of the trachea, mediastinum, and heart to the involved side results from massive atelectasis, but not from the more common segmental atelectases. An inspiratory lag of the involved side likewise is present in late or extensive atelectasis, or in the presence of an associated pneumonia with pleurisy. A roentgenogram of the chest will usually confirm the diagnosis, but again, the earliest sign of an incipient atelectasis is bronchial breathing, which offers a means of detection with the stethoscope long before other physical signs or the x-ray film become diagnostic.

PROPHYLACTIC MEASURES. Prophylaxis should be started in elective surgery at least 2 weeks preoperatively, with the cessation of smoking and with parenteral and aerosol antibiotics as indicated, to clear the residual bronchitis. Weight should be reduced, bronchospasm relaxed, and the general condition improved as far as possible. A preoperative regimen of respiratory exercises emphasizing deep abdominal diaphragmatic breathing and productive coughing is most rewarding. Patients should be immobilized for only as short a time as is consistent with their disease process. Additional caution should be taken with the extremes of age — infancy, because of the small size of the bronchi so readily susceptible to obstruction, and the older age group, because of muscular weakness and frequent respiratory infections.

A unique set of patients needs consideration in this context — namely, those who have been at complete bed rest, nearly immobile, during medical or recuperative therapy; for example, a patient with a severe myocardial infarction. Prior to anesthesia and surgery there must be vigorous ventilation of the respiratory system to clear stagnant, inspissated secretions ("plugs"), or disaster can ensue. Superior segments of

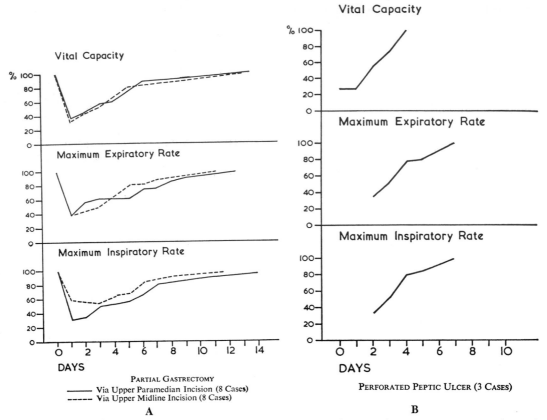

Figure 7–3 Sequential studies of vital capacity, maximum expiratory velocity, and maximum inspiratory velocity after upper abdominal surgery. Note the extreme depression from peritonitis following simple closure of perforated peptic ulcers (*B*), which is more pronounced than that caused by the more extensive surgical procedure of gastrectomy (*A*). One hundred per cent represents the norm for the individual patient. Postoperative airway obstructive phenomena correlate with depression of the bellows effect demonstrated here, even though respiratory volumes or oxygenation may be adequate. (Figures A and B reproduced by kind permission from Pulmonary Complications of Abdominal Surgery (1957) by A. R. Anscombe, M. S., F. R. C. S. London: Lloyd-Luke [Medical Books]).

lower lobes are particularly vulnerable sites for accumulation of such material, and there is usually an associated atelectasis.

TREATMENT.   There has been a traditional utilization of the "stir-up" regimen, which depends upon adequate doses of narcotics to allay pain and good nursing care for the stimulation of ventilation, frequent coughing, and changes in position.

Mucolytic agents given either by nebulization or by direct instillation into the trachea through a percutaneously inserted plastic catheter have proven invaluable in liquefying tracheobronchial secretions for complete evacuation.[40] These aid in the early clearing of bronchitis, or the more complete evacuation of purulent material in any pulmonary septic process. Because of their use, patients can be brought to the operating room much clearer of secretions and thus at less risk of respiratory complications. Also, during operation mucolytic agents such as acetylcysteine (Mucomyst) are injected frequently through the endotracheal tube to aid in the liquefaction and complete evacuation of any mucoid or purulent secretions which otherwise might obstruct the tracheobronchial airway or spill into the dependent portions of the lung.

The next steps are endotracheal suctioning with a soft catheter and, whenever necessary, bronchoscopy. Following a dictum, such as "perform a temporary tracheostomy if one or two repetitions of bronchoscopy fail," can lead to using this modality too soon. Rapid implementation of other methods and verification of their effectiveness should be accomplished so that the problem does not proceed to extensive pneumonitis. Despite the fact that tracheostomy is not commonly needed now as compared to previous times, it must not be ignored, since it remains a useful modality. Antibiotics of proven or at least presumptive effectiveness should be utilized in the presence of known bronchitis or during operative procedures on the lung, since these are always associated with traumatic edema which predisposes to pneumonia. Our preference in elective cases is penicillin alone, or a semi-synthetic, penicillinase-resistant penicillin alone, which is effective against the gram-positive cocci and mouth organisms that are the most common cause of postoperative pneumonias. This does not predispose to the development of fungus infections or superinfections with organisms resistant to the broad-spectrum antibiotics.

DeTakats[13] demonstrated that blunt injury to the chest and intraperitoneal manipulation, especially traction on the mesentery, increase bronchial secretions and induce widespread bronchoconstriction, which can be relieved by bilateral vagotomy or by administration of large doses of atropine. We have seen postoperative and post-traumatic bronchorrheas lead to massive atelectasis and even suffocation and cardiac arrest — all of which could have been prevented by atropine and endotracheal suctioning.

Many authors[26, 32] have utilized intermittent positive-pressure breathing (IPPB), to inflate the lungs and nebulize aerosols to reduce the incidence of postoperative complications. Mucus and other secretions are not washed further down the respiratory tract by the IPPB-aerosol therapy, but are expelled, since the peak instantaneous expiratory flow velocity is greater than the peak instantaneous inspiratory flow velocity. The net result is to work secretions outward in an expectorantlike action.

IPPB is effective as a vehicle for nebulization but much less effective for pulmonary re-expansion. Any patient with shallow breathing will have progressive diminution of his functional residual capacity (FRC), which is that volume of air remaining in the lung after quiet exhalation. Air is absorbed from the dependent lung, which has relatively less ventilation than the upper part of the lung. This results in progressive microatelectasis. Positive end-expiratory pressure (PEEP) is used to maintain the FRC at normal or above. PEEP is more effective in maintaining full alveolar expansion than blow bottles or IPPB.

LUNG ABSCESS

ETIOLOGY. A lung abscess is initiated most frequently by aspiration of foreign material. Classically, the principal offending operations have been teeth extractions and tonsillectomies, for the aspirate contains

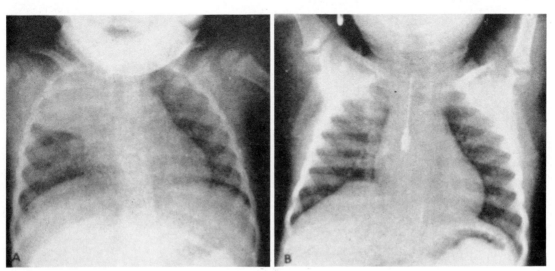

Figure 7–4 *A*, Roentgenogram showing postoperative right upper lobe pneumonia in a 14-month-old child. *B*, Film made 2 days later after hourly injections of acetylcysteine through a percutaneous indwelling intratracheal catheter. The needle is in the external end of the catheter several inches from the site of insertion.

blood and purulent matter with the mouth organisms which produce an acute putrid abscess. Posture must be incriminated here, since, contrary to the usual experience, over 33,000 tonsillectomies were performed at the Johns Hopkins Hospital without a single resultant lung abscess, because of the adoption of the Trendelenburg position during and immediately after tonsillectomies.

Aspiration of gastric contents is likewise an ever-present possibility. Culver, Makel, and Beecher[12] demonstrated by preoperative oral administration of dyes that 76 per cent of their patients regurgitated. Aspirated material could be identified in the trachea in nearly all of these. In a similar study of nearly 1000 patients by Berson and Adriani,[5] regurgitated material was identified in the pharynx in 25 per cent and in the trachea in 14 per cent. Aspiration into the trachea could be totally prevented by a cuffed endotracheal tube.[7]

Remember also that repeated aspiration occurs — after one episode the preventive measures must still be implemented. Central nervous system depression and a number of specific neurological disorders predispose to this state, and continuous prevention and control must be instituted.

PROPHYLAXIS. Prevention requires emptying the stomach preoperatively by fasting, by aspiration, or by induced vomiting. When this is impractical or impossible, as in precipitate operations or intestinal obstruction, use of the Trendelenburg position and initial insertion of a cuffed orotracheal airway under topical anesthesia will prevent dangerous aspiration of gastric contents. Recognized or suspected aspiration should be treated with immediate endotracheal suctioning and/or bronchoscopy. Even though the acid pepsin may cause a severe bronchitis and pneumonitis, if the larger elements are removed and heavy antibiotic and steroid coverage is administered, an abscess can usually be prevented.

The frequency of transbronchial aspiration from a lung abscess or tuberculous cavity to produce suffocation, daughter abscesses, or generalized spread of tuberculous disease emphasizes the need for care in the operative handling of these patients. A double-lumen endotracheal catheter or endobronchial intubation by a single-lumen catheter can localize the secretions or bleeding to a single lung. Certainly the use of the prone or supine position is preferable to the usual lateral thoracotomy position, since the

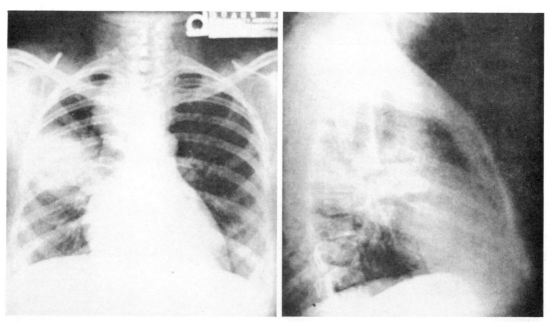

Figure 7–5   Posteroanterior (A) and right lateral (B) roentgenograms showing a lung abscess in the lateral (axillary) division of the anterior segment of the right upper lobe. This is a frequent site of gravitational aspiration, usually causing a putrid abscess abutting on the pleural surface, which makes drainage, if required, simple and safe.

diseased segment can be placed dependent to retain secretions until the entering bronchus can be ligated.

TREATMENT. Treatment consists primarily of continuous postural drainage, the use of bronchodilators and mucolytic agents, large doses of effective antibiotics, both parenteral and aerosol, and repeated bronchoscopies as needed. Those unresponsive will require drainage[16] or resection for ultimate cure, though fortunately most postoperative abscesses that are treated early and vigorously will clear with an adequate medical regimen.

In these situations as well as in the de novo lung abscess, longer treatment periods have led to success primarily because of the potency and diverse number of available antibiotics. *However*, do not forget the danger of lethal hemorrhage associated with abscesses; in particular, the thick-walled abscess with obstructed bronchus (rounded cavity with air-fluid level) already demonstrating bleeding potential with hemoptysis. These abscesses must be treated promptly with appropriate pulmonary resection.

RESPIRATORY INSUFFICIENCY

ETIOLOGY. Inadequate respiratory exchange can be precipitated in the postoperative period by most of the same factors that tend to produce atelectasis; since it is frequently due to bronchospasm, those patients with asthma, chronic bronchitis, or emphysema are particularly susceptible. Cardiac failure, pulmonary congestion, oversedation with various drugs and anesthetic agents, fractured ribs, splinting of the thoracic or abdominal wall, and laryngotracheobronchial edema all further predispose to pulmonary insufficiency. Likewise, resection of pulmonary tissue[16] or collapse of the lung by thoracoplasty, pneumothorax, or hemothorax will reduce the pulmonary reserve.[2] Initially, inadequate alveolar ventilation may be manifested by few clinical signs except restlessness and anxiety, though later air hunger, labored respirations, carphology, circumoral grayish pallor, cyanosis, and hypoxemic metabolic acidosis may become apparent.

TREATMENT. As always, prevention is preferable by protecting as far as possible the integrity of the chest wall, assuring complete expansion of the lung, and maintenance of a patent airway. Extreme gentleness should be observed in manipulation within the larynx or trachea, whether by the anesthesiologist's endotracheal tube or the suctioning endotracheal catheter. Bronchospasm should be vigorously treated with the various bronchodilators, including isoproterenol, aminophylline, epinephrine, or the adrenocortical steroids.

Ventilation can likewise be assisted materially by positive-pressure breathing used continuously, or preferably with intermittent mandatory ventilation (IMV). Respiratory support increases ventilation while reducing the cost of the work of breathing, which is most important in many postoperative and post-traumatic states. The energy required for respiration may rise from the normal 1 to 2 per cent to 50 per cent of the total cardiac work. Inadequate alveolar ventilation leads to hypoxemia with cellular anaerobic metabolism, increasing organic anaerobic acid metabolites, and a falling pH, thus producing metabolic as well as respiratory acidosis. Ventilatory support improves both peripheral and myocardial oxygenation, and this latter improves cardiac function, cardiac output, and peripheral perfusion.

The guiding principle is to achieve adequate alveolar ventilation which will maintain the arterial P_{CO_2} around 40 mm. Hg and the oxygen saturation at 80 mm. Hg or more without reducing cardiac output by excessive pressures. Positive-pressure ventilation tends to raise the intrathoracic mean pressure to reduce cardiac filling, but this is overcome by lengthening expiratory time to at least twice the inspiratory phase.

In patients with pulmonary edema or physiologic shunting (alveoli that are perfused but not ventilated) the addition of 5 to 15 mm. Hg positive end-expiratory pressure (PEEP) may be of great value. In most acute situations the shunting is proportional to the decrease in the functional residual capacity (FRC). The FRC tends to be low in disease states and trauma, particularly with loss of surfactant. The FRC is increased by PEEP and reverses the process of microatelectasis in poorly ventilated areas. While it tends to reduce cardiac output, this effect can be minimized by maintaining an optimal blood volume and by the use of spontaneous respiration with IMV.

No external monitor works as well as the normal respiratory center. The use of spontaneous respiration with IMV with or without PEEP allows the patient to resume breathing on his own at the earliest possible moment. The IMV delivers a large volume of air at positive pressure only as frequently as needed to maintain a normal blood Pco_2. This also acts as a deep sigh to maintain inflation. Both PEEP and the rate of assisted ventilations are reduced as rapidly as the patient can return to normal self-respiration. Although ventilation can be crudely estimated from observation of chest wall motion, measurement of the total volume is preferable either by a volume-regulated machine or a meter to record expired air. Periodic determinations of the pH, Pco_2, and Po_2 constitute the best method of assaying the adequacy of alveolar exchange. The rate of diffusion of carbon dioxide is so great that it is never elevated because of alveolar membrane thickening. A Pco_2 above 40 indicates underventilation, and below 40, overventilation, whether primary or compensatory. If the patient has a metabolic acidosis in the face of adequate ventilation, tissue oxygen supply is inadequate, and a higher percentage of oxygen should be administered in the same ventilatory volume. Obviously if there is a problem of oxygen transport due to low hemoglobin or cardiovascular insufficiency, attention should be directed toward these.

Tight-fitting masks or nasotracheal or orotracheal tubes are adequate for short-term support, but should be replaced by tracheostomy if very long-term assisted ventilation is required. Tracheostomies are of value by reducing the dead space, bypassing the partial obstruction of the larynx, and facilitating control of tracheobronchial secretions, and at times are all that is needed to achieve adequate air exchange. The tracheostomy tube cuff should be long and of large diameter to distribute the pressure on the tracheal mucosa to prevent necrosis. The lowest possible inflation pressure that will prevent leakage is used. Whenever the cuff is deflated, the trachea should be suctioned to aspirate any secretions that have collected above the cuff. It is possible for the cuff to slip and partially occlude the airway or to become deflated and cause inadequate ventilation. The incidence of ulceration and perforation of the trachea has been drastically reduced since the introduction of the softer, more malleable, plastic tracheostomy tubes and cuffs.

Crusting of secretions is a serious and often lethal complication that can be reduced by adequate humidification with warm mist. Normally, inspired air is fully humidified and warmed to body temperature before exhalation, and this process is dehydrating to the lungs. Since fully humidified air at room temperature contains only half the moisture it can hold at body temperature, the air must be warmed as well as saturated. Frequent instillation of a mucolytic agent such as acetylcysteine will further aid by liquefying mucoid or purulent encrustations. Frequent aspiration with a soft, small-caliber, non-traumatic catheter remains extremely important. In fact, with the use of warm mist and acetylcysteine, plugging of the tracheal cannula is no longer seen. Use of the inner cannula of the tracheostomy tube is not necessary, and this greatly increases the airway lumen, which is of extreme value particularly in infants.

THE ACUTE RESPIRATORY DISTRESS SYNDROME*

In recent years rapid evacuation, improved resuscitation, and accurate monitoring of severely traumatized patients have led to the recognition of a serious and often fatal pulmonary condition that theretofore either went undiagnosed or was concealed by the death of the patient.[39] This pulmonary complication has been called "shock lung" or, more comprehensively, acute respiratory distress syndrome.[3]

It has been estimated that between one-third and one-half of those patients dying in intensive care units throughout this country die from such pulmonary derangements. Radiologically this syndrome may resemble acute pulmonary edema, fat embolism, irradiation damage, bacterial or fungal pneumonitis, or blast injury, while clinically it is

---

*Tables 1 and 2 are derived from Webb, W. R., Wax, S. D., and Murakami, T.: The shock lung: Pathogenesis and treatment. J. Mississippi Med. Assoc., *13*:77, 1972.

characterized by progressive acute pulmonary insufficiency.

The clinical course is characterized by progressive dyspnea, tachypnea, restriction of thoracic motion, hypotension, and resistant cyanosis with decreasing arterial oxygen tensions.

In the various clinical situations many factors play a role, such as overinfusion of crystalloids or colloids, overtransfusion, oxygen toxicity, inadequate ventilation, fat emboli, blood and fibrin clots,[23, 33] aspiration, changes in surfactant,[45] neurogenic factors, and circulating vasoactive substances. Multiple transfusions deliver a large volume of clot since present commercial blood filters have a pore size of 170μ. Thus any clot less than this size is delivered intravenously, and each unit of blood contains 1 to 5 ml. of small platelet, leukocytic, and red cell thrombi. The lung acts as a screen for such thrombi and also for vasoactive peptides, since it is the only organ in the body that is perfused by all circulating blood. Also it is unique in being the first capillary bed for oxygen and for absorbed foods and other substances from the liver.

Sepsis is often the cause of respiratory failure and almost always is a later complicating factor in pulmonary problems initiated by other causes.[6] The lung itself may be the primary site of an infection, or it may be colonized by bacteria carried by the blood from protracted sepsis of a remote site.

Physiologically there can be only a limited scope of response — manifested by either mechanical changes or changes in diffusion (gas exchange). During shock there is a fall in pulmonary arterial and right and left atrial pressures. However, pressures in the small pulmonary veins remain elevated, leading to higher back pressure in the capillaries and capillary congestion.[18, 25] This is further increased by excessive infusions or transfusions.

The work of breathing and the energy cost of expanding the lung increase appreciably.[29] Failure to stimulate deep breathing leads to multiple areas of micro-atelectasis, loss of surfactant, decreasing lung compliance, and a falling arterial Po_2.[17, 20] In addition, inactivity of the patient permits progressive congestion of the dependent lung. This increases airway resistance and decreases lung compliance, both of which increase the work of breathing. Retained secretions result in bronchial obstruction and bronchoconstriction, again increasing airway resistance. The oxygen cost of breathing may be more than doubled following abdominal surgery alone.

TREATMENT. The rationale of therapy in any patient developing pulmonary complications includes: (1) prevention of alveolar collapse; (2) maintaining ventilation; (3) preventing and treating infection; and (4) treating the underlying pathology to improve perfusion and minimize subsequent cellular injury (Table 7-1).

The most important principle is that of accuracy of therapy, such as replacement of adequate blood when blood has been lost and administration of electrolyte solutions or colloids as indicated. In addition, the accuracy of administration of oxygen in the inspired atmosphere and control of blood gases must be assured.

Adequate humidity and mucolytic agents are important in all situations, but particularly when an endotracheal or tracheostomy tube is being used. Adequate moisture can be added to the inspired air only by heating the mist to body temperature or by use of ultrasonic nebulizers.

In situations where excessive fluids have been administered or there is inflammatory edema of the lung — as in fat embolism — the newer loop diuretics such as furosemide and ethacrynic acid are particularly effective in aiding the removal of the edema fluid by excretion of the excess.

In most patients, Pa_{O_2} of 70 to 80 mm. Hg is adequate. Any concentration of oxygen in the inspired air above 40 per cent, if continued for longer than a few minutes, will begin to have toxic effects on pulmonary epithelium and endothelium. Obviously in some instances it is imperative to utilize high concentrations of oxygen, but this should be reduced as rapidly as possible (Table 7-2).

An expiratory retard with a positive end-

TABLE 7-1 INDICATIONS FOR RESPIRATORY SUPPORT

	Oxygen Therapy Chest Physiotherapy	Intubation Ventilation
Respiration rate	25–35/min.	>35
Vital capacity	30–15 ml./kg.	<15
Po_2	70 (40 per cent O_2)	<70
Pco_2	45–60	>60

TABLE 7–2 RESPIRATORY THERAPY

Humidity and Mucolytic Agents
Oxygen-Enriched Atmosphere
Postural Changes
Fluid Restriction and Diuretics
Corticosteroids
Intubation-Tracheostomy
Slow Deep Respirations
Positive End-Expiratory Pressure (PEEP) and
 Intermittent Mandatory Ventilation (IMV)
Antibiotics (on indication)

expiratory pressure (PEEP) of 5 to 15 cm. H_2O is very effective in preventing the progressive micro-atelectasis that causes arteriovenous shunting in the lung. While this may slightly decrease the blood flow to the thorax and through the lungs in patients with hypovolemia, this effect can easily be overcome by restoring blood volume to normal. In addition, each patient should have a deep forceful inspiration (sigh) several times an hour and a change in posture at least hourly to prevent the deleterious effects of static hypotension.

Our studies, using motion picture films of direct microscopic observations of the lung and its capillary congestion during shock, have demonstrated the beneficial effects of massive doses of corticosteroids (prednisone 30 mg./kg.) in preventing sludging of the blood and alveolar congestion. There is minimal danger of this increasing infection since the steroid is administered only during the first day of therapy.

MONITORING. Monitoring should include a daily weight check, chest x-ray, an accurate record of intake and output, hematocrit, plasma electrolytes, blood gases, pH, and vital capacity with an estimate of the effective compliance. The last can easily be gauged by the pressure required for the respirator to deliver the selected volume of inspiratory gas. Additional measures that may be useful at times include estimates of the alveolar-arterial oxygen gradient and the ratio of dead space to tidal volume (computed from nomograms from the arterial P_{CO_2} and the end-expiratory P_{CO_2}).

PULMONARY EDEMA

Pulmonary edema during or immediately after operations occurs rather infrequently, but sporadic reports testify to its occurrence as a definite problem.[21] Although the etiology may be cardiac failure, especially after a myocardial infarction or a cardiac operation, in many cases there is an underlying basis of hypoxia. Once again, regardless of etiology, whether cardiac, hypoxic, or toxic, one common factor — partial or complete obstruction by edema fluid — develops, so that these patients die by drowning. Ordinarily edema fluid is removed by coughing or lymphatic absorption. The latter, however, is rarely effective in these instances, since lymph flow is slowed and the high protein content of the edema fluid prevents rapid capillary reabsorption.

As a result of the ensuing bronchial obstruction, a variable degree of hypoxia develops, leading to pulmonary arterial hypertension and capillary dilatation, with resultant congestion, stasis, mucosal edema, and further transudation of edema fluid, with increasing obstruction and greater hypoxia.

TREATMENT. Treatment consists in the insertion of a cuffed endotracheal tube either orally or through a tracheostomy, with administration of oxygen under intermittent inspiratory positive pressure or increased expiratory resistance.[43] Aspiration is performed through the endotracheal tube as frequently as may be necessary, even once per minute, to remove the accumulating endobronchial edema fluid. In addition, all the adjunctive measures are used, including intravenous administration of digitalis or aminophylline, restriction of fluids, administration of diuretics, rotating tourniquets on the extremities, and actual phlebotomies. Luisada[21] advocates ethyl alcohol vapor to lower surface tension and prevent froth formation in the small bronchioles and alveoli, and thus avert progressive hypoxia and edema. Should shock be superimposed, as is prone to happen, the problem becomes much more complex, for many of the measures beneficial for one, such as positive pressure and reduced blood volume, may be instrumental in precipitating or aggravating shock. In this situation partial cardiopulmonary bypass with a membrane oxygenator may give the required temporary support — even for a period of days.

These episodes are often acute, and an early favorable response can be anticipated, particularly when the heart is normal or any preexisting valvular disease has been corrected at operation.

PLEURAL EFFUSIONS AND EMPYEMA

Pleural effusions are rarely seen in the postoperative period other than after intrathoracic surgery, except after pneumonia, pulmonary emboli, or subphrenic abscesses. Because of the tremendous resistance of the pleura, empyemas are rare, regardless of any massive single contamination that may have occurred, if complete reexpansion of the lung is obtained immediately. Repeated contamination, dead space, air pockets, and undrained fluid accumulations, however, are conducive to infection. Even in chronic infections such as tuberculosis, proper management will prevent empyemas unless a bronchopleural fistula is present. On the other hand, resections for fungal infections such as histoplasmosis and coccidioidomycosis,[11] which are more virulent and freely cross tissue planes and for which there are no very effective antibiotic drugs, are often followed by pleural complications, both early and late.

TREATMENT. Treatment consists in the use of appropriate antibiotics and removal of the pleural effusion, which may be accomplished by thoracenteses or, if recurrent, by the introduction of a large intercostal catheter attached to water-seal drainage. Decortication and open drainage have a decreasing place but are still necessary when conservative measures fail.[41]

MEDIASTINAL EMPHYSEMA

Air may enter the mediastinum (1) after trauma involving the trachea or esophagus, (2) spontaneously from rupture of pulmonary alveoli, or (3) during operative procedures in the neck in which the pretracheal fascia has been opened. Forbes and his co-workers[14] demonstrated that after opening of the pretracheal fascia, as in a tracheotomy or thyroidectomy, air may be sucked into the mediastinum to produce mediastinal emphysema, and then rupture through the mediastinal pleura to produce a tension pneumothorax. This process is augmented by the labored respiration usually seen in those cases requiring an emergency tracheotomy. Bowden and Schweizer[8] reported 18

cases of pneumothorax and two of mediastinal emphysema after operations on the head and neck, which developed presumably by this same mechanism of aspiration of air into the mediastinum along the fascial planes. Experimental observations[44] have demonstrated that the hemodynamic effects are not due to pressure within the mediastinum, which in experimental animals and man could not be maintained even as high as 5 mm. Hg, since the air promptly escapes into the pleura, subcutaneous tissues, or retroperitoneal spaces. All symptoms produced appear to be due to the associated pneumothorax. This type of mediastinal emphysema, of course, is completely different from the malignant interstitial emphysema of the lungs which is accompanied by mediastinal emphysema, as studied extensively by the Macklins.[22] In this condition the air dissects from the alveoli along vascular sheaths and compresses the pulmonary capillaries and may, in addition, cause "airlock" of the alveoli, impairing ventilation.

In the usual postoperative or post-traumatic pneumomediastinum, proper *treatment* consists first in decompressing the accompanying tension pneumothorax. Cervical mediastinotomy may be of value in the occasional case of mediastinal emphysema, but it appears to be of value more in preventing further accumulations of air in the thorax than in decompressing the mediastinum. If a cervical mediastinotomy is performed for mediastinal emphysema, the pretracheal fascia which forms the anterior sheath of the visceral space in the neck must be opened to decompress the mediastinum. The usual accompanying subcutaneous emphysema is of no physiologic import.

COMPLICATIONS OF SPECIFIC THORACIC PROCEDURES

Tube Thoracostomy

Thoracostomy tubes are inserted routinely after thoracic surgery, and frequently after traumatic wounds, for removal of air or blood or for drainage of effusions or empyemas. Ordinarily the thoracostomy is innocuous, but various minor difficulties may arise. The most troublesome is bleeding from intercostal arteries or veins damaged at the time of introduction of the tube.

If, under local anesthesia, a stab wound is made through the skin, through the subcutaneous tissues, and through the muscular fascia, but no further, and the tube is inserted just above the inferior rib, this complication will be rare. Similarly, after incision of the skin, the tube may be safely inserted with a blunt instrument such as a curved Kelly clamp. Should bleeding occur, pressure from the tube may be hemostatic, although at times the incision must be extended sufficiently to expose and ligate the vessel. This can be performed under local anesthesia, even though it necessitates an open pneumothorax for a short time.

The most common complication of tube thoracostomy is that it is ineffective. A state of nearly complete or complete expansion of the lung with a minimum of residual fluid in the pleural space must be attained and documented. Repositioning of a tube, additional tubes, enzymatic or instrumental breakdown of debris, positive-pressure ventilation, pneumoperitoneum, and chest physiotherapy must be used as needed.

Laceration of the lung is fairly common if a trocar is used to introduce a thoracostomy tube for a minimal pneumothorax or hemothorax. A safe rule is to insert a catheter only if there is room for a needle to be inserted safely. Only under the most emergent circumstances of tension supported by classic physical signs should a trocar be inserted without a diagnostic chest roentgenogram having been obtained. We have seen numerous pulmonary lacerations result when catheters have been inserted into well-expanded lungs.

Inadvertent placement of the catheter subdiaphragmatically is not uncommon, particularly in disease states in which the diaphragm is elevated. Penetration of the liver is the most common accident and may lead to profuse bleeding, bile peritonitis, or a subdiaphragmatic abscess. The spleen, stomach, and colon have also been damaged on occasion, the latter two especially when a diaphragmatic hernia is not recognized. The pleural space should be identified first by thoracentesis or the gloved finger and the trocar passed in a cranial direction to avoid the upward doming of the diaphragm.

PAIN.   Pain from the pressure of a thoracostomy tube against the adjacent intercos-

tal nerve is a frequent occurrence — in fact, almost routine. Nearly all thoracostomy patients have a genuine sense of relief after removal of the thoracostomy tubes. Occasionally a traumatic intercostal neuritis persists for some weeks or months. This often responds to a single intercostal block with a local anesthetic, and almost always to repeated intercostal blocks, preferably performed paravertebrally.

If too stiff a tube is used and inserted too far, it may prevent complete reexpansion of the lung. Likewise, tubes may be extruded unless sealed in place by being taped to the bandage and also tied in by a suture through the skin and subcutaneous tissue, which then circumscribes the tube. Sutures or safety pins should not be inserted through the tube, since they allow leakage of air back into the pleural space. A leaking tube or connector may suggest persistent air leakage from the lung and simulate a bronchopleural fistula. If a tube is maintained in place for several days, air will usually leak through the loosened tube tract. When this occurs, it is best to replace the tube through a new site.

SUBCUTANEOUS EMPHYSEMA. In the presence of continued leakage of air from the lung, the pleural opening afforded by the thoracostomy tube allows a ready route for the development of subcutaneous emphysema. This is particularly true if the tube becomes plugged or partially extruded, or if the tube is unable to evacuate the air as fast as it is accumulating within the chest. Subcutaneous emphysema, though mildly uncomfortable and distressing in appearance, causes no particular physiologic derangement.

INFECTION. Osteomyelitis of the accompanying rib or a local cellulitis or abscess is rarely seen, unless the tubes have to be maintained in position for an extended time. Local infection will usually respond to removal of the tube and local drainage. A definite osteomyelitis will require rib resection. Tubes left in place after their function has been served predispose to development of an empyema and should be removed the instant they are no longer functional.

Water-seal bottles, particularly the glass adapters or rods, are apt to be broken, allowing aspiration of air and development of a tension pneumothorax. Less frequently the water bottles may be raised above the level of the patient's chest to siphon the contained fluid into the pleural cavity. Both accidents are easily remedied by reestablishment of the water seal and suction.

Thoracentesis

Thoracentesis is one of the most frequently utilized and safest of diagnostic and therapeutic procedures. Nevertheless various complications do supervene, the most common of which is a *pneumothorax* from needle puncture of the lung. It has resulted also from failure to use a three-way stopcock or inadvertently turning the stopcock lever in the improper direction. Although the pneumothorax is usually small, occasionally the lung may be torn so as to require a tube thoracostomy for decompression. Breaks in sterile technique may lead to an *empyema,* particularly in the presence of recurrent accumulations of fluid or air. Fortunately, these are infrequent and almost nonexistent if a single thoracentesis is permanently effective.

Pleural shock is a nebulous term referring to sudden syncope or even death following a thoracentesis. Air embolism, the air entering the pulmonary veins to proceed directly to the left side of the heart and thus to the coronary or cerebral vessels, may have accounted for some of these episodes. Should this occur, the patient should be placed on his right side with his head dependent, to keep the air in the left ventricle until it can be absorbed, rather than ejected into the aorta to enter the coronary or cerebral vessels. Other cases have resulted from excessive fluid withdrawal when the mediastinum has become fixed, as with a malignant tumor. Rapid fluid removal allows shifting of the heart and mediastinum with resultant kinking of the superior and inferior venae cavae and diminished cardiac return. Treatment of this may require reinjection of sterile fluid to maintain fairly normal hemodynamics.

Bronchoscopy

Although bronchoscopy is an extremely valuable measure for both diagnosis and therapy, it is not without its attendant complications. The principal complications reported have been those of the anesthesia. As most bronchoscopies are done under local anesthesia, the dangers of toxic reactions to the topical agents must be considered, for convulsions, syncope, and even cardiac arrest have occurred.[42] In our own experience, however, in over 3000 consecutive bronchoscopies and bronchograms there was only one serious toxic manifestation. We find it important to use adequate preoperative medication, a minimum quantity of dilute topical anesthetic (e.g., 0.5 per cent tetracaine) and to switch to another topical agent at the first manifestation of toxicity. General anesthetics are attended by the danger of ventilatory insufficiency. This insufficiency can be avoided by using a ventilating bronchoscope to maintain respiratory volume during the apnea of curarization. Undoubtedly the use of general anesthesia and full relaxation affords the easiest and most satisfactory method for bronchoscopy.

The second complicating factor concerns trauma, which ordinarily should be minimal or non-existent. At times, however, when the patient is uncooperative or presents physical obstacles such as a short, thick neck or long, strong teeth, there may be trauma to the teeth or perforation of the pharynx leading to mediastinitis. In addition, trauma to the tracheobronchial tree may give rise to bleeding or bronchospasm. Bronchospasm following bronchoscopy is relatively common, particularly in patients with chronic bronchitis or a tendency toward asthma. Bronchoscopic biopsies which can include pulmonary or bronchial vessels or even the wall of an impinging aortic aneurysm can give rise to massive bleeding with exsanguination or respiratory obstruction. Too forceful biopsies have likewise produced perforations of the trachea or major bronchi, with a resultant mediastinal emphysema or pneumothorax.

The surgeon generally uses the rigid and flexible bronchoscopes in a complementary fashion — in combination in most diagnostic instances and often separately in therapeutic instances to take advantage of each one's unique qualities. For example, in the aforementioned situation in which trauma from use of the rigid endoscope would be highly likely, then only the flexible endoscope would be used. When aspiration of large volumes of blood or pus is anticipated, the rigid endoscope would be used first or used alone.

Endoscopy in patients with fragile cardiac status must be accorded the same importance as a major operation, from initial preoperative management and anesthetization to solicitous post-procedure monitoring.

Chylothorax

Injuries to the thoracic duct may occur at any point along its course in the chest or left side of the neck. It enters the chest through the esophageal hiatus of the diaphragm to ascend between the azygos vein and the aorta on the anterior surface of the vertebrae. At about the fifth dorsal vertebra it crosses to the left side of the mediastinum and enters the left subclavian vein near its junction with the left internal jugular vein. Although in most cases chylothorax occurs spontaneously owing to obstruction with a malignant process such as lymphoma, in many cases it follows injury to the thoracic duct with esophagectomy, cardiovascular procedures, and surgery in the left supraclavicular region.[46]

Diagnosis is based on aspiration of the characteristic milky fluid with fat globules and a creamy layer that separates on standing. Chyle is alkaline in reaction, has no odor or the odor of ingested food, has a specific gravity exceeding 1.012, and contains fat up to 4 gm. per dl. and protein averaging 3 gm. per dl.

Symptoms are due to pressure effects of the accumulating fluid and the nutritive deficiencies due to the massive losses of fat (60 to 70 per cent of all absorbed fat) and protein. As the chyle is bacteriostatic, infection rarely supervenes, and it causes a minimal sterile inflammatory response.

Immediate *therapy* is directed toward removal of the chyle and maintenance of the patient's nutrition. A high-protein, low-fat diet supplemented with vitamins should be given, and the chyle can be refed through an indwelling gastric tube. Intravenous administration has not been sufficiently free of risk to justify its use. Most thoracic duct fistulas will close spontaneously if the lung is kept expanded by a large-caliber thoracostomy tube attached to water-seal drainage.

Conservative measures should be abandoned before signs of deterioration appear. Interruption of the thoracic duct causes no embarrassment of nutrition, since there are adequate lymphatic collaterals. Surgical ligation is most easily accomplished at the level of the diaphragm through a right thoracostomy incision, though a left-sided approach may be preferable for a left chylothorax if complications are present or a decortication is required. Chylothorax from accumulations in the neck rupturing into the pleura can be treated by ligation of the duct in either the neck or the chest. Surgical ligation of the duct has been uniformly curative.

Bibliography

1. Adriani, J., and Phillips, M.: Use of the endotracheal cuff: Some data pro and con. Anesthesiology *18*:1, 1957.
2. Anscombe, A. R.: Pulmonary Complications of Abdominal Surgery. Chicago, Year Book Medical Publishers, 1957.
3. Ashbaugh, D. C., Petty, T. L., Bigelow, D. B., Harris, T. N., and Waddel, W. R.: Continuous positive-pressure breathing (CPPB) in adult respiratory distress syndrome. J. Thorac. Cardiovasc. Surg. *57*:31, 1969.
4. Beecher, H. K.: The measured effect of laparotomy on the respiration. J. Clin. Invest. *12*:639, 1933.
5. Berson, W., and Adriani, J.: "Silent" regurgitation and aspiration during anesthesia. Anesthesiology *15*:644, 1954.
6. Bredenberg, C., Taylor, C., and Webb, W. R.: Thrombocytopenia altering the pulmonary hemodynamic response to intravenous endotoxin. Surg. Forum *28*:186, 1977.
7. Bosher, L. H., Jr.: A review of surgically treated lung abscess. J. Thorac. Surg. *21*:370, 1951.
8. Bowden, L., and Schweizer, O.: Pneumothorax and mediastinal emphysema complicating neck surgery. Surg. Gynecol. Obstet. *91*:81, 1950.
9. Churchill, E. D.: The reduction in vital capacity following operation. Surg. Gynecol. Obstet. *44*:483, 1927.
10. Clendon, D. R. T., and Pygott, F.: Analysis of pulmonary complications occurring after 579 consecutive operations. Br. J. Anaesth. *19*:62, 1944.
11. Cotton, B. H., and Birsner, J. W.: Surgical treatment of pulmonary coccidioidomycosis. J. Thorac. Surg. *38*:435, 1959.
12. Culver, G. A., Makel, H. P., and Beecher, H. K.: Frequency of aspiration of gastric contents by the lungs during anesthesia and surgery. Ann. Surg. *133*:289, 1951.

13. DeTakats, G., Fenn, G. K., and Jenkinson, E. L.: Reflex pulmonary atelectasis. J.A.M.A. *120*:686, 1942.

14. Forbes, G. B., Salmon, G., and Herweg, J. C.: Further observations on post-tracheotomy mediastinal emphysema and pneumothorax. J. Pediatr. *31*:172, 1947.

15. Green, A., and Berkowitz, S.: An anesthesiologist's program for the prevention of postoperative pulmonary complications. New York J. Med. *52*:1871, 1952.

16. Harrison, R. W., et al.: Cardiopulmonary reserve five to fifteen years following fifty per cent or more reduction of lung volume. Surg. Forum *7*:209, 1956.

17. Henry, J. N., McArdle, A. H., Scott, H. J., and Gurd, F. N.: A study of the acute and chronic respiratory pathophysiology of hemorrhagic shock. J. Thorac. Cardiovasc. Surg. *54*:666, 1967.

18. Keller, C. A., Scramel, R. J., Hyman, A. L., and Creech, O., Jr.: The cause of acute congestive lesions of the lung. J. Thorac. Cardiovasc. Surg. *53*:743, 1967.

19. Kurzweg, F. T.: Pulmonary complications following upper abdominal surgery. Am. Surg. *19*:967, 1953.

20. Lamy, M., Fallot, C., and Koeneger, C.: Pathologic features and mechanisms of hypoxemia in A.R.D.S. Am. Rev. Respir. Dis. *114*:267, 1976.

21. Luisada, A. A.: Therapy of paroxysmal pulmonary edema by antifoaming agents. Proc. Soc. Exp. Biol. Med. *74*:215, 1950.

22. Macklin, M. T., and Macklin, C. C.: Malignant interstitial emphysema of the lungs and mediastinum as an important occult complication in many respiratory diseases and other conditions. Medicine *23*:281, 1944.

23. Modig, J.: Post-traumatic pulmonary microembolism. Pathophysiology and treatment. Ann. Clin. Res. *9*:164, 1977.

24. Moersch, H. J.: Bronchoscopy in treatment of postoperative atelectasis. Surg. Gynecol. Obstet. *77*:435, 1943.

25. Murakami, T., Wax, S. D., and Webb, W. R.: Pulmonary microcirculation in hemorrhagic shock. Surg. Forum *21*:25, 1970.

26. Neohren, T. H., Lasry, J. E., and Legters, L. J.: Intermittent positive pressure breathing (IPPB) for the prevention and management of postoperative pulmonary complications. Surgery *43*:658, 1958.

27. Neuhof, H.: Acute putrid abscess of the lung. Surg. Gynecol. Obstet. *80*:351, 1945.

28. Palmer, K. N. V., and Sellick, B. A.: Effect of procaine penicillin and breathing exercises in postoperative pulmonary complications. Lancet *1*:345, 1952.

29. Peters, R. M.: Work of breathing following trauma. J. Trauma *8*:915, 1968.

30. Piper, D. W.: Respiratory complications in the postoperative period. Scott. Med. J. *3*:193, 1958.

31. Powers, J. H.: Vital capacity: Its significance in relation to postoperative pulmonary complications. Arch. Surg. *17*:304, 1928.

32. Rudy, N. E., and Crepeau, J.: Role of intermittent positive pressure breathing postoperatively. J.A.M.A. *167*:1093, 1958.

33. Saldeen, T.: The microembolism syndrome. Microvasc. Res. *11*:227, 1976.

34. Shields, R. T., Jr.: Pathogenesis of postoperative pulmonary atelectasis: Experimental study. Arch. Surg. *58*:489, 1949.

35. Stringer, P.: Atelectasis after partial gastrectomy. Lancet *1*:389, 1947.

36. Swank, R. L., and Smedal, M. I.: Pulmonary atelectasis in stuporous states: A study of its incidence and mechanism in sodium amytal narcosis. Am. J. Med. *5*:219, 1948.

37. Thoren, L.: Postoperative pulmonary complications: Observations on their prevention by means of physiotherapy. Acta Chir. Scand. *107*:193, 1954.

38. Walters, W., Gray, H. K., Priestly, J. T., and Waugh, J. M.: Advances in the surgical treatment of cancer of the stomach. Proc. Staff Meet. Mayo Clin. *27*:39, 1952.

39. Webb, W. R.: Pulmonary complications of nonthoracic trauma: Summary of the National Research Council Conference. J. Trauma *9*:700, 1969.

40. Webb, W. R.: Clinical evaluation of a new mucolytic agent, acetylcysteine. J. Thorac. Cardiovasc. Surg. *44*:330, 1962.

41. Webb, W. R.: Modern concepts of empyema thoracis. Med. Times *85*:1250, 1957.

42. Webb, W. R.: Fundamentals of cardiac resuscitation. Mississippi Doctor *32*:312, 1955.

43. Webb, W. R., and Campbell, G. D.: The use of the endotracheal tube in pulmonary edema. J. Thorac. Surg. *28*:222, 1954.

44. Webb, W. R., Johnston, J. H., Jr., and Geisler, J. W.: Pneumomediastinum: Physiologic observations. J. Thorac. Surg. *35*:309, 1958.

45. Wichert, P., and Kohl, F. V.: Decreased dipalmitoyllecithin content found in lung specimens from patients with so-called shock lung. Intensive Care Med. *3*:27, 1977.

46. Woodhall, J. P.: Traumatic chylothorax: Case report and general discussion. Surgery *42*:780, 1957.

8

CARDIAC ARREST AND RESUSCITATION

James R. Jude

The treatment of cardiopulmonary arrest has undergone a great change in the last decade. No longer is it absolutely necessary for the surgeon to perform an emergency thoracotomy with direct compression of the heart in order to reinstitute circulation when cardiac action has ceased. The technique of external cardiac compression has provided an alternative to direct cardiac massage. A simplified and more readily applicable technique is thus available, and when combined with rapid methods of recognition by the anesthesiologist and surgeon, it has permitted the tragic complication of cardiac arrest to be more adequately treated.[12]

DEFINITION AND HISTORICAL ASPECTS

What was once termed cardiac arrest is now generally more properly called cardiopulmonary arrest. This is the sudden and unexpected cessation of functional circulation and ventilation from whatever cause. In view of the fact that during most surgical procedures the respirations are well controlled by the anesthesiologist, the term car-

diac arrest alone is still applicable. Under such circumstances ventilation is usually adequate, although the depth of anesthesia may be more profound than is desirable.

Cardiac arrest was one of the earliest important complications of the developmental era of surgery. It is interesting that it became recognized as a problem only after the introduction and use of general anesthetics. The first recorded cardiac arrest of this nature occurred in England in 1858 in a patient under chloroform anesthesia for the removal of a toenail.[3] There was no recovery. The open-chest method of cardiopulmonary resuscitation by direct cardiac massage, which was first used successfully by Igelsrud[15] in 1901, evolved from the research studies of Schiff[28] in the latter part of the nineteenth century. This direct cardiac massage technique was the one generally applied by surgeons in and near the operating theater until the introduction of external cardiac compression, by Kouwenhoven and co-workers, in 1960.[19] Interestingly, this latter technique had been applied successfully in the late nineteenth century by König[16] and Maas.[21]

The surgeon is interested in how to pre-

James R. Jude was born in Minnesota and educated at the College of Saint Thomas and the University of Minnesota Medical School. His training in general and thoracic surgery was obtained at Johns Hopkins under Dr. Alfred Blalock, where he remained on the staff until assuming the position of Head of Thoracic and Cardiovascular Surgery at the University of Miami. Since 1971 he has been in the private practice of thoracic and cardiovascular surgery in Miami, Florida. He has received wide recognition for the development of the closed technique of cardiopulmonary resuscitation. His research interests continue in this area and in coronary artery disease.

vent and treat, if necessary, the sudden and unexpected cessation of cardiac activity that might occur during the induction of anesthesia, during the operative procedure, or during postanesthesia awakening following the surgical operation. Although sudden and unexpected cessation of circulation and ventilation may occur also on the surgical wards either preoperatively or postoperatively, this will be less common in the experience of the surgeon, though such sudden cardiopulmonary arrest is common in their respective areas for the internists. The incidence of surgical sudden death under the influence of anesthesia varies greatly from hospital to hospital throughout the United States, and on an average may be expected to occur in about one in 1800 administrations of general anesthesia.[6, 13] In an average-sized hospital with 200 to 300 beds one would expect to see at least two or three cardiac arrests in the operating theater or environs each year.

Sudden cessation of functional cardiac output can occur in any of three forms of cardiac action or inaction. These consist of (1) *asystole,* in which the heart is mechanically entirely flaccid and without electrical activity, (2) *electromechanical dissociation,* in which there is coordinated but poor electrical activity of the heart without any significant degree of mechanical contraction sufficient to deliver adequate cardiac output for the maintenance of life, and (3) *ventricular fibrillation,* which is the condition in which there is chaotic, vigorous mechanical and electrical activity of the myocardium, which is, however, entirely incapable of any degree of cardiac output. Of these three types of cardiac arrest, those most commonly seen in the operating theater are asystole or electromechanical dissociation. Ventricular fibrillation may be the primary type of cardiac arrest, or may result with direct open-chest cardiac massage from irritation of the myocardium by the compressing hand. In the postoperative period, during which hypoxia may occur, the most common type of cardiac arrest is again asystole or electromechanical dissociation. After cardiac surgery, however, the most common type of cardiac arrest is ventricular fibrillation because these patients are prone to develop ventricular arrhythmias.

ETIOLOGY OF CARDIAC ARREST

Cardiac arrest as a complication of surgery may be due to a multiplicity of factors. The most common are hypoxia from insufficient ventilation and overdosage of, or idiosyncrasy to, the anesthetic agent. Generally such a cardiac arrest occurs as either asystole or inefficient mechanical contractions known as electromechanical dissociation. Under appropriate conditions of hypoxia or hypercapnia, asystolic cardiac arrest may occur as a reflex reaction to vagal stimulation during the intubation of the trachea or during the surgical procedure by traction on the mesentery. Such an arrest may be reversed spontaneously by stimulation of the heart by a blow on the precordium or intermittent firm pressure against the diaphragmatic surface of the heart through the diaphragm. Unreplaced blood loss may produce profound cardiovascular shock and functional cardiac arrest in asystole or cardiac electrical activity without life-sustaining cardiac output. Preoperative electrolyte imbalance may cause sudden cardiac arrest under anesthesia, owing to relatively minor degrees of hypoxia or hypercapnia, as for example with hyper- or hypokalemia. Air embolism to the heart occurring during operative procedures around the internal jugular vein or insufflation of the fallopian tubes may cause an air lock in the right atrium and ventricle with functional cardiac arrest. An all-too-common problem is that of coronary vascular insufficiency with myocardial ischemia or myocardial infarction resulting in either cardiac power failure and functional cardiac arrest or inefficient arrhythmias such as ventricular tachycardia or fibrillation. In the postoperative period, irritability of the myocardium secondary to electrolyte imbalance, operative cardiac procedures, hypoxia, or hypercapnia may result in any of the three types of cardiac arrest.

OBJECTIVES OF CARDIOPULMONARY RESUSCITATION

Sudden loss of cardiac output results in lack of oxygen supply to all tissues of the body. Initially, aerobic metabolism may continue for a few minutes until the oxygen level of the arterial blood in the organs is depleted, but there then results an anaerobic metabolism rapidly leading to the development of metabolic acidosis. This, together with the oxygen deprivation, causes tissue damage and ultimately cellular death. The changes in the tissues are reversible for a period of time, some as little as 4 to 6 minutes. Beyond this time the tissues most sensitive to oxygen lack, located in the *central nervous system,* become irreversibly damaged so that even though circulation may be reestablished, they remain partially or totally incapable of normal function.

The initial purpose of cardiopulmonary resuscitation is to continue artificially the functioning of the oxygenation system of the body. Thus by artificial ventilation oxygen is supplied to the lungs, and by artificial circulation the oxygenated blood is distributed to the tissues. The ventilatory system is readily reestablished by the anesthesiologist. Circulation is artificially produced by cardiac compression. For a successful result cardiopulmonary resuscitation must therefore by initiated quickly to support the oxygenation system of the body, prevent cellular death, and preserve total function of the body. Time is thus available to apply definitive pharmacologic and electrical therapy that may reinstitute spontaneous cardiac and respiratory activity.

RECOGNITION OF CARDIAC ARREST

Successful outcome in the treatment of the complication of cardiac arrest is dependent upon its immediate recognition followed by rapid action to remedy the situation. Any delay in realizing that there has been sudden loss of circulation may result in an irreversible change in the central nervous system. Indeed, the lack of immediate recognition and procrastination on the part of the surgeon for verification or in the hope that true cardiac arrest has not occurred have been the main reasons for inferior and unsuccessful treatment of cardiac arrest.[8] In general it is the anesthesiologist who is the first to recognize that cardiac action has weakened or suddenly totally failed. This evidence is acquired by frequent and almost continuous checking of an arterial pulse and pressure in addition to observation of signs in depth of anesthesia. In most anesthesia situations today, wherein respirations are controlled, the lack of respiratory activity cannot be used as an indication of cardiac arrest. The anesthesiologist will always monitor the patient's electrocardiogram; this is an aid in determining the sudden presence of cardiac arrest or of arrhythmias that might lead to either asystole, ventricular fibrillation, or ineffectual contractions. It must be remembered, however, that there may be coordinated electrical activity without adequate cardiac output to sustain life. Recognition could best be facilitated by a method of continuously determining cardiac output, but a simple method is not available to date. There are available techniques that continuously determine arterial pulsations in the ear, finger, or nasal septum by photoelectric cells and give some indication of effective circulation. Most of these, however, are not convenient enough to be used on every patient, and indeed many are inaccurate under certain circumstances. An indwelling arterial pressure cannula can give a continuous arterial pulse reading on an oscilloscope (TV) and should be used in all patients undergoing complicated cardiac operations and in those surgical patients at high risk for other reasons such as advanced age, possible blood loss, or cardiac instability. There is also increasing employment of a pulmonary artery catheter (Swan-Ganz) for continuous monitoring of left heart pressures.

In general it can be said that close monitoring and observation of vital signs and cardiac electrical and hemodynamic data by the anesthesiologist will prevent cardiac arrest or at least provide the first indication of factors or conditions leading to, or the actual onset of, the complication of cardiac arrest.

The surgeon himself must at all times be concerned with the possibility of cardiac arrest. The circumstances may be such that he will be able to realize that cardiac action has ceased at an even earlier moment than the anesthesiologist. Such would occur in surgical procedures on or near the heart or large arterial vessels. Also the sudden cessation of any bleeding of the tissues might give evidence of circulatory arrest.

The surgeon must be ready to verify

within a few seconds the anesthesiologist's suspicion of a possible cardiac arrest. In general this can be readily accomplished by palpation of a major pulse in some area of the operative field. Thus in the abdomen the abdominal aorta can be palpated, or even the heart through the diaphragm. At times, however, the heart may feel active because of ventricular fibrillation, and yet there will be no cardiac output. If an apparent cardiac arrest occurs just before the operative incision is to be made, the incision itself can be begun, and the absence of bleeding will indicate that circulatory arrest is most likely present. Similarly, in the performance of the emergency left thoracotomy for open-chest cardiac massage the absence of bleeding in the chest wall, intercostal muscles, and subcutaneous tissues would be positive confirmation of the actual presence of circulatory arrest.

Because of the dangerous consequences of procrastination and delay in initiation of artificial circulation, it must be considered that any time there is a question of cardiac arrest and a major pulse is not readily palpable, the emergency procedures of cardiac massage must be initiated. It is for this reason that the non-invasive external resuscitative measures have gained so much application not only outside the operating room by non-surgeons, but also by surgeons in the operating theater itself. It must be remembered that even after confirmation of cardiac arrest it still would take 30 to 60 seconds to perform a thoracotomy and begin artificial circulation by direct cardiac massage. External cardiac compression, on the other hand, can be begun immediately.

METHODS OF RESUSCITATION

MAINTENANCE OF VENTILATION. When cardiac arrest occurs under anesthesia, ventilation is not a problem because of the presence of the anesthesiologist, who will have available the proper equipment for adequately ventilating the lungs with oxygen. This can usually be accomplished with a face mask and bag or direct tracheal intubation if this has not already been done. All anesthetic gases should be flushed from the lungs as quickly as possible. This will eliminate one of the possible causes of the

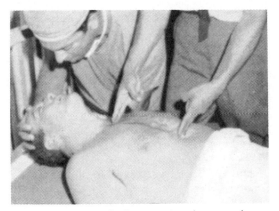

Figure 8–1 Outside the operating theater and anesthesia room, ventilation is initially provided by mouth-to-mouth or -nose artificial respiration, as shown. The position of the sternum for external cardiac compression is readily located.

sudden cardiac arrest and also will remove explosive gases, if used, in case electrical countershock becomes necessary. If the complication of sudden cardiopulmonary arrest occurs in the postoperative recovery room, immediate emergency ventilation may be accomplished by the nurse or physician present by any of the expired air techniques such as mouth to mouth, mouth to nose, or a self-inflating bag and face mask.[7] Generally anesthesiologists are close to this area and can continue the ventilatory resuscitative effort. They can continue with the face mask and bag or perform tracheal intubation and provide positive pressure oxygen by that means.

The methods of artificial ventilation are essentially the same whether compression is performed by the open-chest or closed-chest cardiac compression technique.

ARTIFICIAL RESUMPTION OF CIRCULATION. Two equally effective methods of providing circulation artificially are available. These are closed-chest cardiac compression[11, 14, 22] and open-chest cardiac compression.[31, 32] It has been definitely shown by many investigators that both techniques are beneficial in their effectiveness in providing circulation,[23] although open-chest cardiac compression may be effective in certain situations in which the closed-chest method is unsuccessful or contraindicated.[30]

The ease of use of each method is not equal, however, for simplicity and rapidity of onset of application is much greater with *closed-chest cardiac compression*. This technique is based upon the principle of compression of the heart between the lower part of the sternum and the thoracic vertebral column, thereby forcing blood out into the systemic and pulmonary circulations.[23] Some recent studies suggest that increase in intrathoracic pressure may force blood from the lungs into the circulation.[2, 26] Repeated rhythmic compression at the rate of 60 to 80 times a minute will provide a cardiac output of at least 30 to 40 per cent of normal, which is apparently adequate to maintain the viability of the central nervous system and other organs for as long as 2 or 3 hours. *Open-chest cardiac compression* (massage) is based upon the principle of directly squeezing the heart in the palm and fingers of the hand so as to force blood into the systemic and pulmonary circulations. Again the cardiac output produced of at least 30 to 40 per cent of normal is sufficient to maintain viability of the central nervous system and other vital centers.

The advantages of external cardiac compression over open-chest cardiac compression are as follows: (1) It is always available, and it can be applied without any hesitancy or procrastination; no irreversible damage is done to the thorax. It can be used even when only the possibility of cardiac arrest is present. (2) It can be performed through the surgically draped thorax so as not to contaminate the operative field. (3) Damage

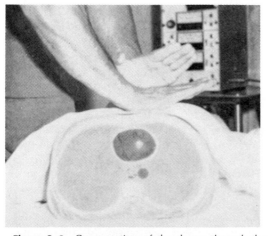

Figure 8–2 Cross section of the thorax through the lower part of the sternum. The heel of one hand with the opposite hand over it is applied over the lower half of the sternum. The fingers do not touch the chest wall.

to the myocardium is much less than with direct handling of the heart by the hand and fingers. The serous membranes of the pericardium protect the heart from contusions and other damages that occur when direct cardiac compression is carried out.

The advantages of open-chest cardiac compression are as follows: (1) Observation of the heart permits determination of the exact type of cardiac arrest and whether or not electrical defibrillation will be necessary. (2) Intracardiac injection of drugs is exact and simpler when the heart is under direct observation.

Disadvantages of external cardiac compression are as follows: (1) The exact type of cardiac arrest must be determined by the use of an electrocardiogram rather than by direct observation. (2) Drugs must be injected either into an intravenous catheter or by transthoracic injection into the heart chamber by use of a long needle. (3) Generally fractures of the costochondral cartilages occur, and there is a possibility of fracture of the anterior angles of the ribs. Improper application of external compression may also cause damage to the liver, spleen, and other intra-abdominal organs.[5] (4) Effectiveness of attempts at external defibrillation must be determined by observation of the electrocardiogram rather than by direct observation of the heart.

Disadvantages of open-chest cardiac compression are as follows: (1) There is a delay in application. (2) A scalpel must be available and an emergency left thoracotomy performed. (3) Risk of infection is increased because of the generally unsterile nature of the emergency thoracotomy. (4) Integrity of the pleura is interrupted so that the lung collapses and the filling phase of the heart is partially compromised. (5) Damage to the myocardium in the form of contusions or perforation by the fingers may occur from the direct contact.[1] (6) Asystole may be converted to ventricular fibrillation by the direct irritation of the hypoxic myocardium.

SPECIFIC INDICATIONS FOR ONE TECHNIQUE OR THE OTHER.   When a thoracotomy has already been performed as for a heart or lung operation, then obviously open-chest cardiac compression is the choice. It is also the method to be used in those cases in which cause of the cardiac arrest is possibly intrathoracic. Such causes would be tension pneumothorax or perforating wounds with hemorrhage within the thorax. Closed-chest cardiac compression is specifically indicated in those cases in which there would be even brief delay in obtaining necessary equipment for making the thoracotomy to perform open-chest cardiac compression. Also in those cases in which there is any question that cardiac arrest is actually present, the closed-chest technique is indicated.

In all other cases of the complication of sudden cardiac arrest either closed-chest or open-chest cardiac compression can be carried out. When performed properly, either should result in total cardiac resuscitation and a normal functioning of the central nervous system, barring complicating factors.

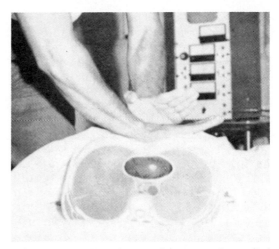

Figure 8–3 Firm downward pressure is applied, squeezing the heart against the vertebral column at a rate of 60 to 80 per minute.

TECHNIQUES OF CARDIAC COMPRESSION

Closed-Chest Cardiac Compression. Closed-chest cardiac compression is performed by depressing the lower half of the sternum toward the vertebral bodies 1½ to 2 inches at a rate of 60 to 80 times per minute. The depression is held for about half a second and rapidly released. The exact degree of depression of the sternum is dependent upon the size of the patient and is correspondingly less for the thin one and the child than the large or emphysematous adult. The exact location of the pressure point is the lower half of the sternum only, and not the thorax or ribs to either side. This point can be located through the operative field drapes if the cardiac arrest occurs during the actual operation and there

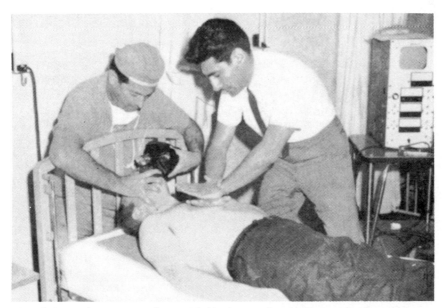

Figure 8–4 Ventilation with oxygen may be provided by face mask and self-expanding bag as soon as available. The surgeon positions himself with his body above the patient. An electrocardiogram is taken to determine the type of cardiac arrest.

is no need to retract the drapes for exposure of the chest wall. If the heart is found to be in ventricular fibrillation, then exposure of the skin of the chest wall will be necessary for external electrical defibrillation.

In the actual procedure of cardiac compression the heel of one hand is placed on the lower half of the sternum, the surgeon standing to either the right or left of the patient. The opposite hand is placed over the first hand, and the surgeon uses his body weight to push the sternum posteriorly toward the vertebral column. It is best to lower the table to the lowest point or to stand on a footstool to place the weight of the surgeon over the patient. The anesthesiologist or some other person such as the nurse should be able to palpate a carotid or femoral pulse with each cardiac compression. If circulation is adequate, the pupils of the eye should constrict or remain in a constricted state, provided the plane of anesthesia has already been lightened.

OPEN-CHEST CARDIAC COMPRESSION. For the performance of open-chest cardiac compression an emergency left anterior thoracotomy is performed in the fourth or fifth intercostal space. Since this is an emergency, this is generally performed without use of any antiseptic preparation.

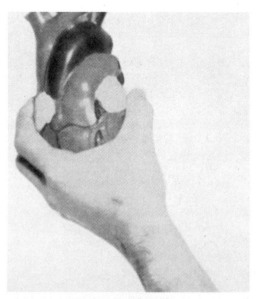

Figure 8–5 Method of application of direct cardiac compression. The heart is grasped with the left or right hand and squeezed from apex to base at a rate of 60 to 80 per minute.

The ribs are then pulled apart with the hands and the left or right hand is introduced; the heart is grasped in the hand through the pericardium and rhythmically squeezed. Although compression may be carried out with the pericardium intact, this is not nearly as satisfactory or as efficient as when the pericardium is widely opened. With the pericardium open the left hand is introduced anteriorly to the heart, the fingers going around posteriorly to the right of the heart. The palm of the hand overlies the right and left ventricles, the thumb extending around the left side of the heart. A milking action is carried out from the apex toward the base of the heart in order to squeeze out blood into the systemic and pulmonary circulations. The hand is then totally relaxed to allow venous filling. This performance is continued rhythmically 60 to 80 times a minute. In infants and small children two fingers of the right hand may be introduced behind the heart and used to compress the heart against the posterior sternum area. The opposite hand may be placed on the chest wall opposite the sternum for counterpressure. For patients with very large hearts, it may be necessary for both hands to be introduced into the thorax and the heart squeezed between them.

A rib spreader should be placed in the thoracotomy wound as soon as possible in order to spread the ribs and prevent their pressure on the wrist of the surgeon.

DETERMINATION OF THE EXACT NATURE OF THE CARDIAC ARREST

Cardiac arrest may exist in (1) asystole, (2) ventricular fibrillation, or (3) very faint or weak mechanical cardiac action, but with electrical complexes (electromechanical dissociation). Irrespective of the exact type of cardiac arrest, the initial resuscitative measures are the same: ventilation with oxygen and cardiac compression by the internal or external technique. To provide more definitive therapy, in order to resume spontaneous cardiac action, the exact nature of the cardiac arrest must be known.

Open thoracotomy with direct cardiac compression permits the exact nature of the cardiac arrest to be determined by direct observation of the heart. *Asystole* would be evident by a totally still and quiet heart without any mechanical contractions. *Ventricular fibrillation* would be evident by rapid or slow waves or uncoordinated mechanical activity passing over the entire surface of the heart. *Electromechanical dissociation* would be evident by the presence of weak but coordinated contractions incapable of producing cardiac output. An electrocardiogram must be made to determine the type of cardiac arrest when closed-chest cardiac compression is being performed. *Asystole* is evident by a straight line electrocardiographic tracing, *ventricular fibrillation* by erratic, totally uncoordinated fluctuations of the tracing, and *electromechanical dissociation* by poor but coordinated electrical complexes without objective evidence of cardiac output.

PHARMACOLOGIC THERAPY

VASOCONSTRICTOR DRUGS. Every effort must be made to provide the best possible

TABLE 8 1 PHARMACOLOGIC AGENTS IN CARDIAC RESUSCITATION (INTRAVENOUS DOSES)

Vasoconstrictors	
Epinephrine	0.5 mg.
Phenylephrine	2.0 mg.
Mephentermine	45.0 mg.
Cardiotonic agents	
Epinephrine	0.5 mg.
*Isoproterenol	0.1 to 0.2 mg.
Calcium chloride	1.0 gm.
Antacid drugs	
Sodium bicarbonate	3.75 gm.
Tris(hydroxymethyl)aminomethane (THAM)	9.00 gm.
Vasopressors (titrate as IV drip)	
Epinephrine	1 to 2 mg./250 ml. 5% G/W
Dopamine HCl	400 to 800 mg./250 ml. 5% G/W
Dobutamine HCl	250 to 500 mg./500 ml. 5% G/W
Cardiac depressants	
Lidocaine	75 mg.
Quinidine gluconate	150 mg.
Procainamide	150 mg.
Cerebral dehydrating agents	
Urea	40 gm.
Mannitol	25 gm.
Furosemide	40 mg.

*Must be used with peripheral vasoconstrictor

circulation to the entire body and specifically to the tissues most sensitive to hypoxia and those that must have good circulation for spontaneous activity to be resumed. Thus circulation to the central nervous system and the myocardium, respectively, must be kept optimal as far as possible. Although an increase in perfusion to the carotid and coronary arteries will be obtained by cross-clamping of the descending aorta during open-chest cardiac compression, a physiologic direction of arterial blood to the organs supplied by these vessels will also be caused by the use of peripheral vasoconstrictor drugs. Thus the use of epinephrine in 0.5 mg. aliquots will cause peripheral vasoconstriction and the selective direction of blood to these more vital centers. This pharmacologic mechanism will be equally effective with either open-chest or closed-chest cardiac compression. The epinephrine should be injected directly into the bloodstream through either an indwelling intravenous drip or by intracardiac injection inside the left or right ventricle of the heart. Duration of action of epinephrine is approximately 3 to 5 minutes, and injections should be repeated at these intervals.

CARDIOTONIC DRUGS. Spontaneous cardiac contraction can be stimulated by the use of a cardiotonic drug,[24] and the most readily available and efficient drug is also epinephrine in doses of 0.5 mg. every 3 to 5 minutes. Epinephrine has thus a dual role. Other drugs, such as isoproterenol hydrochloride, might also be used, but a vasoconstrictor would have to be used in addition, since isoproterenol hydrochloride has a peripheral vasodilatory effect.

Calcium chloride, 0.5 to 1.0 gm., injected directly into the bloodstream also has a cardiotonic effect and is of special value when there is present some weak electrical and mechanical myocardial activity. This dose should be repeated every 5 to 10 minutes. Cardiac contraction, cardiac output, and arterial blood pressure are improved by its use.

ANTACID DRUGS. The low cardiac output developed by either the internal or external technique of artificial circulation, together with the period of total cardiac arrest preceding the initiation of cardiac compression, causes a rapid development of anaerobic metabolism and metabolic acidosis. In order to allow the return of normal function of the myocardium and a good response to endogenous and exogenous catecholamines, the blood pH must be maintained at somewhat near its normal value.[25] For this reason antacid drugs such as sodium bicarbonate or THAM should be injected into the bloodstream at approximately 8- to 10-minute intervals. In general, sodium bicarbonate is the most readily available antacid, and 50 ml. containing 3.75 gm. (44.6 mEq.) is given every to 8 to 10 minutes or titrated to the arterial pH. Use of an antacid is of vital importance and may prevent what might otherwise be a total failure in resuscitation or a prolonged period of hypotension after cardiac action has been resumed.

VASOPRESSOR AGENTS. After resumption of spontaneous cardiac activity, arterial blood pressure may remain low and necessitate the continued use of vasopressor drugs. Epinephrine can be used as an intravenous drip diluted 1 to 2 mg. of epinephrine in 250 ml. of 5 per cent G/W and titrated to obtain adequate arterial pressure of 90 to 100 mm. Hg. Also, dopamine hydrochloride (400 to 800 mg. in 250 ml. of 5 per cent G/W) or dobutamine hydrochloride (250 to 500 mg. in 500 ml. of 5 per cent G/W) can be used as a titrated intravenous drip.

DRUGS TO DECREASE CEREBRAL EDEMA. If cardiac action is resumed, but for some reason there was some delay in the initiation of artificial circulation and ventilation or if the artificial circulation and ventilation were inadequate, there may have resulted some central nervous system tissue damage with the result that the patient might not immediately awaken. There will then develop edema of the damaged central nervous system tissues; this edema must be prevented to avoid further damage by compression against the calvarium. Urea can be given intravenously in doses of 40 gm. immediately and at 6 hours. Other diuretics such as furosemide may also be employed.

There is some evidence that the use of glucosteroids may be of some value in the prevention of cerebral damage following hypoxic insults.[20] It has been suggested that barbiturate loading may prevent or ameliorate brain damage after global ischemia. General application will depend upon clinical trials currently under way.[4, 27]

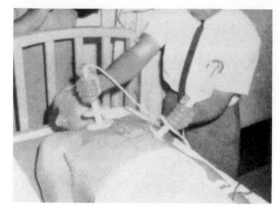

Figure 8–6 Method of external cardiac defibrillation. One electrode is placed over the base of the heart (right second intercostal space parasternally) and the other over the apex of the heart (below the left nipple). The discharge shock must be controlled by the surgeon.

TREATMENT OF VENTRICULAR FIBRILLATION

Ventricular fibrillation requires special treatment in order to resume spontaneous cardiac function. The only efficient method currently known is that of total electrical depolarization of the heart to allow spontaneous coordinated electrical action.[17, 18] Electrical defibrillation can be executed by either the external or internal technique. This is best accomplished by direct-current capacitor devices. In the external method of defibrillation large, 3-inch diameter electrodes are placed on the chest wall at the base of the heart (the right first or second intercostal space, parasternally) and at the apex of the heart (below the left nipple). The shock is then delivered between these two electrodes with 100 to 400 watt-seconds delivered over a period of 4 to 6 milliseconds. The electrical shocks are repeated as necessary to accomplish defibrillation or to treat recurrent fibrillation.

When open-chest, direct-contact cardiac defibrillation is to be carried out, two large paddle-shaped electrodes, dipped in saline solution, are placed one on the right side of the heart over the right atrium and the other on the left side of the heart over the left ventricle. The electric shock is then delivered between these electrodes with 20 to 60 watt-seconds delivered over 4 to 6 milliseconds.

Electrical defibrillation may not be successfully accomplished unless the quality of the myocardial fibrillatory activity is such that the heart is vigorously active. This requires a well-oxygenated myocardium that has maximal tone. The proper conditions for defibrillation are provided by the circulation of oxygenated blood through the myocardium and the use of cardiotonic pharmacologic agents such as epinephrine. Weak fibrillatory activity is not readily converted. When there is an irritable focus in the heart that causes persistence or recurrence of ventricular fibrillation, the focus must be depressed by the use of cardiodepressant drugs. Lidocaine hydrochloride should be used in doses of 50 to 100 mg. intravenously or directly into the blood inside the heart. Quinidine gluconate or procainamide hydrochloride can also be employed in aliquots of 100 to 240 mg. intravenously. Defibrillation attempts should be repeated after use of such drugs and when the fibrillatory quality is vigorous.

CLOSURE OF THORACOTOMY

The emergency thoracotomy performed for open-chest cardiac massage must be closed under conditions that are as sterile as possible. The thoracic cavity should be irrigated voluminously with saline solution to wash out any possible bacterial organisms in the contaminated area. An intercostal cath-

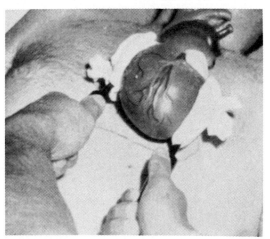

Figure 8–7 A superimposed view of the method of direct cardiac defibrillation. Electrodes are soaked in saline and applied over the right atrium and left ventricle.

eter should then be placed in the posterior thoracic gutter and attached to underwater drainage. The ribs are approximated with pericostal catgut. All bleeders that were not evident on the opening of the chest because of the circulatory arrest should be clamped and tied with 00 catgut. Wide spectrum antibiotics such as sodium cephalothin should be given after closure of the chest to help prevent the development of an empyema or wound infection.

POSTRESUSCITATIVE CARE

After cardiac resuscitation, the patient's vital signs including arterial blood pressure and electrocardiographic activity should be constantly monitored. Generally this necessitates that the patient be observed in an intensive care unit or recovery room. Steps should be taken to prevent the development of cardiac arrhythmias or hypotension that might lead to a recurrent cardiac arrest. Proper attention must also be directed to fluid intake and output and electrolyte balance.

If there is any remaining respiratory embarrassment, the patient should be maintained on a respirator. The endotracheal tube can be replaced by a tracheostomy if the mechanical respiration is to be prolonged over 72 hours. A portable chest x-ray should be taken to check for pneumothorax and expansion of the lungs.

All patients who have had a cardiac arrest must be observed closely in the postrecovery period for evidence of possible permanent cardiac damage, especially if direct cardiac compression was performed. The patient must also be observed for slowness in regaining central nervous system activity indicating some degree of cerebral hypoxia. If found to be present, it should be treated by methods directed at preventing further cerebral edema with the adverse effect of compression of the brain against the calvarium, and additional central nervous system damage. Urea or other diuretics can be given immediately and after 6 hours. There is some question whether or not a rebound edema phenomenon might occur with this method. Total-body hypothermia has been shown to prevent the development of further cerebral edema and thereby protect the brain.[33, 34] It has made it possible to salvage some of the patients who have had border-line cerebral hypoxic episodes. Total-body hypothermia to 32 to 33° C. should be produced immediately if the patient does not totally awaken and should be continued for 72 to 96 hours unless the patient shows signs of return of central nervous system function during this period. There has been some recent evidence that glucosteroids may be of beneficial effect to the central nervous system that has suffered hypoxic damage.

If brain damage has been severe, the patient will exhibit, in addition to coma, other signs of a decerebrate state, including Cheyne-Stokes breathing, decerebrate rigidity, convulsions, hyperthermia, diabetes insipidus, and bradycardia. In irreversible cases the coma deepens, blood pressure falls, oliguria develops, and spontaneous respirations become less frequent. Over a period of 72 to 96 hours the patient generally worsens markedly or shows signs of improvement. It is rare for a patient to survive with severe neurologic defects.

TERMINATION OF OPERATION AND REOPERATION. When sudden cardiac arrest occurs during an operative procedure, all efforts should be directed immediately toward reestablishment of spontaneous cardiac activity. Thereafter the operation should be terminated as soon as a proper point can be reached — for example, a colostomy rather than bowel anastomosis or drainage rather than gallbladder resection.

Reoperation can generally be safely undertaken with all safeguards and monitoring in effect in 48 hours, if the patient's recovery of cardiac and central nervous system function is complete.[10] Clearance should be obtained by cardiology and neurology consultation. Myocardial infarction should be ruled out. Anesthesia selection must be made with extreme care.

CONCLUSION

Cardiac arrest will always be a complication in medicine. Its appearance is all the more tragic in surgery in which the association of an operative procedure — elective or emergency — has led to its development. The total resuscitation rate has shown an over-all improvement with earlier recognition and initiation of therapy.[9, 11, 13] The techniques outlined should be so well known by every surgeon that he or she can apply them without fear or hesitancy. This is not only a moral, but also a legal, responsibility.[29]

Bibliography

1. Adelson, L.: A clinicopathologic study of the anatomic changes in the heart resulting from cardiac massage. Surg. Gynecol. Obstet. *104*:513, 1957.
2. Babbs, C. F.: New versus old theories of blood flow during CPR. Crit. Care Med. *8*:191, 1980.
3. Beecher, H. K.: The first anesthesia death, with some remarks suggested by it in the fields of the laboratory and the clinic in the appraisal of new anesthetic agents. Anesthesiology *2*:443, 1941.
4. Brievik, J., Safar, P., Sands, P., et al.: Clinical feasibility trials of barbiturate therapy after cardiac arrest. Crit. Care Med. *6*:228, 1978.
5. Clark, D. T.: Complications following closed-chest cardiac massage. J.A.M.A. *181*:337, 1962.
6. Degerli, I. U.: The treatment of sixteen cases of cardiac arrest. Resuscitation *1*:247, 1972.
7. Elam, J. O., Brown, E. S., and Elder, J. D., Jr.: Artificial respiration by mouth-to-mask methods. N. Engl. J. Med. *250*:749, 1954.
8. Green, T. A.: Heart massage as a means of restoration in cases of apparent sudden death, with a synopsis of forty cases. Lancet *2*:1708, 1906.
9. Greenberg, H. B.: The results of resuscitation with external cardiac massage or direct cardiac massage in eleven surgical patients. Angiology *14*:529, 1963.
10. Hanks, E. C., and Papper, E. M.: Reoperation after resuscitation from cardiac arrest. Surg. Gynecol. Obstet. *119*:997, 1964.
11. Jude, J. R., Kouwenhoven, W. B., and Knickerbocker, G. G.: External cardiac resuscitation. Monogr. Surg. Sci. *1*:59, 1964.
12. Jude, J. R., and Elam, J. O.: Fundamentals of Cardiopulmonary Resuscitation. Phiadelphia, F. A. Davis Company, 1965.
13. Jude, J. R., Bolooki, H., and Nagel, E.: Cardiac resuscitation in the operating room: Current status. Ann. Surg. *171*:948, 1970.
14. Jude, J. R., and Nagel, E. L.: Cardiopulmonary resuscitation 1970. Mod. Concepts Cardiovasc. Dis. *39*:133, 1970.
15. Keen, W. W.: Case of total laryngectomy (unsuccessful) and a case of abdominal hysterectomy (successful) in both of which massage of the heart for chloroform collapse was employed with notes of 25 other cases of cardiac massage. Ther. Gaz. *28*:217, 1904.
16. König, F.: Lehrbuch die allgemeinen Chirurgie. Göttingen, 1883, pp. 60–61.
17. Kouwenhoven, W. B., and Kay, J. H.: A simple electrical apparatus for the clinical treatment of ventricular fibrillation. Surgery *30*:781, 1951.
18. Kouwenhoven, W. B., Milnor, W. R., Knickerbocker, G. G., and Chestnut, W. R.: Closed-chest

defibrillation of the heart. Surgery *42*:550, 1957.

19. Kouwenhoven, W. B., Jude, J. R., and Knickerbocker, G. G.: Closed chest cardiac massage. J.A.M.A. *173*:1064, 1960.

20. Long, D. M.: The ultrastructure of cerebral edema and its response to glucosteroid administration. Med. Bull. Univ. Minnesota *336*:339, 1965.

21. Maas, Dr.: Die Methode der Wiederbelebung bei Herztod nach Chloroformeinathmung. Berl. klin. Wchnschr. *12*:265, 1892.

22. Oliver, G. C., Jr., Gazetopoulos, N., and Davies, D. H.: Effect of closed chest cardiac massage on the aortic pulse during ventricular fibrillation. Lancet *1*:1303, 1964.

23. Pappelbaum, S., Lang, T.-W., Bazika, V., Bernstein, H., Herrold, G., and Corday, E.: Comparative hemodynamics during open vs closed cardiac resuscitation. J.A.M.A. *193*:659, 1965.

24. Pearson, J. W., and Redding, J. S.: The role of epinephrine in cardiac resuscitation. Anesth. Analg. *42*:599, 1963.

25. Pierce, E. C.: Significance and management of acidosis occurring in conjunction with cardiac resuscitation. J. Tenn. Med. Assoc. *56*:321, 1963.

26. Rudikoff, M. T., Freund, P., and Weisfeldt, M. L.: Mechanisms of blood flow during cardiopulmonary resuscitation. Circulation *56*(Suppl. 3):97, 1977.

27. Safar, P.: Introduction: On the evolution of brain resuscitation. Crit. Care Med. *6*:199, 1980.

28. Schiff, M.: Über direckte Reizung der Herzoberflache. Arch. ges. Physiol. *28*:200, 1882.

29. Standards and guidelines for cardiopulmonary resuscitation (CPR) and emergency cardiac care (ECC). J.A.M.A. *244*:453, 1980.

30. Stephenson, H. E., Jr.: Pathophysiological considerations that warrant open chest cardiac resuscitation. Crit. Care Med. *8*:185, 1980.

31. Stone, H. H.: Cardiac massage: A report of 148 cases. Am. Surg. *27*:495, 1961.

32. Turk, L. N., and Glenn, W. W. L.: Cardiac arrest: Results of attempted cardiac resuscitation in forty-two cases. N. Engl. J. Med. *251*:795, 1954.

33. White, R. J.: Preservation of cerebral function during circulatory arrest and resuscitation: Hypothermic protective considerations. Resuscitation *1*:107, 1972.

34. Williams, G. R., Jr., and Spencer, F. C.: The clinical use of hypothermia following cardiac arrest. Ann. Surg. *148*:462, 1958.

9

COMPLICATIONS OF SURGERY THAT INVOLVE THE VENOUS SYSTEM

Robert M. Miles

Venous thrombosis (phlebothrombosis), thrombophlebitis, and thromboembolism all refer to intravenous coagulation and its effects, which are the principal venous complications of surgery. Although these terms are sometimes used synonymously, by definition thrombophlebitis implies venous thrombosis associated with a large inflammatory and possibly infectious element, and thromboembolism or thromboembolic disease indicates the association of pulmonary embolism. The incidence of pulmonary embolism associated with thrombophlebitis is relatively small when compared with that associated with phlebothrombosis, presumably because of adherence of the clot to the vein wall as a result of the inflammatory reaction. In phlebothrombosis, which is accompanied by little such inflammation, the symptoms are few, and since the clot is loosely if at all attached to the vein wall, embolism to the lungs is more likely.

The process may occur in any location, but as a surgical complication the deep veins of the lower extremities and pelvis have been most frequently involved and the superficial veins of the legs to a lesser extent. More recently, with the advent of long-term continuous infusion and central venous pressure procedures by means of the intravenous plastic catheter, thrombophlebitis of the veins of the upper extremities and neck has become more common. Pulmonary embolism is much more commonly associated with venous thrombosis of the lower extremities and pelvis than with that of the upper extremities. The cause of this is unknown. It is generally accepted,[29] and borne out by the studies of Coon and Coller,[19] that the sources of pulmonary emboli are the lower extremities in about 80 per cent of cases, the pelvis in 10 per cent, and the heart in 5 per cent, and in approximately 5 per cent the source is unknown.

INCIDENCE

Postoperative venous thrombosis and pulmonary embolism occur much more frequently than is generally appreciated and, together, they account for one of the most common and potentially disabling and lethal complications of surgery. From the following reports on incidence the problem can be seen to be of such magnitude that all

Robert M. Miles is a Tennessean who received his college and medical education at the University of Tennessee. He served as an intern and took residency training at the John Gaston Hospital and the Kennedy Veterans Hospital in Memphis. As Director of the Surgical Research Laboratory at Kennedy, he became deeply interested in the pathophysiology and surgical management of venous thromboembolism. As a result of his detailed and prolonged investigations, the extensively used Miles caval clip was developed. Dr. Miles has been an officer of many surgical societies, and his teaching and administrative talents have been widely recognized.

who invade the body surgically should be familiar with all aspects of these complications.

The true incidence of venous thrombosis and pulmonary embolism is only now being established. In the past statistics were not accurate since they were based only upon studies of patients who had died from thromboembolic disease and of those relatively few patients (approximately 10 per cent)[20] in whom clinical diagnosis could be made. Recently, however, with the development of scanning with iodine-125 fibrinogen and other sophisticated non-invasive diagnostic techniques, a much more valid picture of the true magnitude of the problem has begun to unfold.

Whereas in 1958 Anlyan and associates[5] predicted that deep vein thrombosis would develop in approximately three of every 100 surgical patients, Atkins and Hawkins (1965)[7] and Kakkar and associates (1969),[54] using iodine-125 fibrinogen and scanning techniques, found the actual incidence to be from 30 to 60 per cent. However, symptoms were present in only half of these patients. In the United States, it is estimated that 50,000 to 200,000 patients die yearly from pulmonary embolism and that non-fatal embolism occurs in about 600,000 patients.[20, 64, 95, 107]

The incidence of findings of embolism at autopsy ranges from approximately 18 to 63 per cent.[45, 74] The incidence of pulmonary embolism following surgery was found by Allgood and associates,[2] using pulmonary scans, to be 14.1 per cent, while Kistner and co-workers[55] reported a 52 per cent incidence in patients with venographically proven lower limb venous thrombosis. In 75 per cent of these patients there were no symptoms and pulmonary embolism was unsuspected. Morrell and Dunnill,[74] in necropsy studies of lungs, found pulmonary emboli in 62.8 per cent of patients dying after surgery, and of these deaths, 43 per cent were due to embolism itself.

Although the greater numbers of cases shown by these statistics probably reflect refinement in diagnostic techniques, it is also possible that an actual increase in the incidence of thromboembolic disease is taking place; for example, Hartman[47] reported the necropsy incidence of pulmonary embolism in Germany to have been 4.3 per cent in 1915, 9 per cent in 1938, and 18.2 per cent in 1965.

EPIDEMIOLOGY

Studies have shown that patients with certain conditions have thromboembolic complications more frequently than do other patients[6, 19] and should be regarded as being in the high-risk category whenever surgery is considered. The conditions that have been indicted are previous episode of thrombosis or embolism, heart disease (increase of risk of three and one-half-fold), myocardial failure or atrial fibrillation (tenfold increase), malignant disease (fourfold increase — prostate and pancreas most common), leg trauma (eightfold increase), obesity (twofold increase), immobility (from whatever the cause, such as operation, fracture, paralysis, or serious medical illness), blood types A, B, and AB,[51] ileostomy for ulcerative colitis (thromboembolic complications develop in one-third of the patients),[26] middle and older age, and operations on the great vessels and blood vessels of the legs.

Whether or not oral contraceptives predispose to thromboembolic disease is still open to debate. Our experience impresses us that there is an increased incidence and we agree with earlier reports[41, 65] on retrospective studies that there is an increased incidence of thromboembolic disease in women who are taking the "pill." Drill,[33] however, in a large prospective study, suggests that there is no actual increase in incidence in this group.

Despite some reports to the contrary, Coon and Coller,[19] in reviewing 606 instances of pulmonary embolism in 4391 autopsies over a 10-year period, found no difference in incidence related to sex or seasons. They found the incidence of embolism to be twice as high in surgical as in medical patients and more common after gynecologic surgery (32 per cent), general surgery (28.8 per cent), and urologic surgery (21.6 per cent). Embolism was almost twice as common in obese as compared to non-obese females, but there was no difference between obese and non-obese males. Surprisingly enough, with relation to surgery, the highest incidence occurred within the first 24 hours postoperatively. This is at variance with the experience of those, including ourselves, who have observed it more commonly approximately 7 days after surgery.

Patients with a past history of thromboembolic disease deserve special emphasis since they are generally considered to be at highest risk. Coon and Coller[19] refer to Barker's report of 46 such patients who underwent hysterectomy. Thirty-one (67 per cent) had pulmonary emboli postoperatively, and of these, 15 (50 per cent) died; that is, the over-all postoperative mortality rate from pulmonary embolism was approximately 30 per cent.

PATHOGENESIS AND NATURAL HISTORY

The very nature of surgery is conducive to all basic etiologic factors involved in intravenous coagulation — stasis, trauma, and hypercoagulability (Virchow's triad), as well as infection. These factors combine to cause thrombosis at sites of intimal damage or in areas of pooling such as behind the valve cusps.[85]

Hunter and co-workers[49] in autopsy studies found evidence that thrombosis began in the small veins of the muscles of the calf and foot and extended into the femoral veins. Thrombi, when found, were usually multiple and present bilaterally. This concept is supported by the work of Frykholm[38] and more recently by the iodine-125 fibrinogen scanning studies of Kakkar and co-workers.[54] Others, including Sevitt[94] and Mavor and Galloway,[61] believe peripheral venous thrombi may not be of serious clinical importance and that pulmonary emboli usually arise from thrombi forming de novo in the larger veins of the thigh and pelvis. More recently Shoobridge[97] in morphologic studies suggested that the thrombus may form as a single uniform entity through the entire length of a vessel segment.

The majority hold with the former opinion and believe the process probably begins as a platelet-coralline thrombus and propagates into a proximal tail that may occlude the vessel, causing further stasis, inflammatory reaction, and propagation, or break off and cause an embolus to the lungs.

Intraoperatively, prolonged lying on the operating table in a relaxed, hypotonic muscular state is associated with reduced velocity of venous blood flow, with stagnation, particularly if the lower extremities are in a dependent position or constricted by a restraining belt.

The traumatic effect of the instrument tray on the shins and toes and the utilization of the patient's thighs for an auxiliary instrument table may also be contributory. Hypotensive episodes associated with hemorrhage may aggravate the whole cycle and increase the likelihood of thrombosis. Flanc, Kakkar, and Clarke[37] showed that thrombosis occurred during the operation in approximately 50 per cent of patients in their study series.

In addition, the inherent trauma of surgery and resulting hypercoagulability state contribute to the initiation of thrombosis. The observations of Flanc and associates[37] on the effect of intensive prophylactic measures designed to prevent stasis in the leg veins before, during, and after operation surprisingly showed no significant effect on the incidence of thrombosis as determined by iodine-125 fibrinogen scanning, except in the elderly. This suggests that hypercoagulability may be the most important etiologic factor; anticoagulants were not used in the study.

Infection is already present in many surgical patients, and recently Altemeier and associates[3] have discovered atypical bacterial or "L" forms in cultures from patients with thromboembolic disease. This finding suggests an etiologic relationship with anaerobic Bacteroides. Appropriate antibiotic therapy in these patients reduced markedly the amount of heparin required for adequate anticoagulation.

Postoperatively, the immobility of patients occasioned by pain and the commonly employed reversed-N position, with the head elevated and the thighs and knees flexed, causes venous pooling in the iliofemoral segment as well as in the foot and calf veins and contributes to venous stasis and subsequent thrombosis.

Venous thrombi, once formed, can lead to several possible conclusions. Undoubtedly the most common and happiest is resolution caused by normal fibrinolytic mechanisms. In studies on the natural history of postoperative deep venous thrombosis,

Kakkar and associates[54] and Flanc and coworkers[37] showed that spontaneous lysis of deep venous thrombi occurred in almost one-third of their patients and that an average of 5.9 days was required for complete lysis. The second eventuality is thrombus persistence with or without propagation, associated with varying degrees of venous obstruction manifested by clinical signs and symptoms. In 65 per cent of those developing thrombosis, thrombi could be demonstrated for more than 72 hours. In 47 per cent the process remained limited to the calf and in 22 per cent thrombi extended into the popliteal and femoral veins. In 20 per cent of these patients pulmonary embolism occurred but only one of them exhibited leg signs. In all too many instances (approximately 80 per cent)[20] the process is "silent" and the thrombus does not sufficiently obstruct the major veins or cause enough inflammatory reaction to produce symptoms until a portion of it breaks off and is embolized to the lungs where, if it is large enough to obstruct the pulmonary arteries sufficiently, it may cause sudden death or symptoms that are related to the degree of obstruction and to whether or not pulmonary infarction occurs. Fortunately, most emboli are too small to cause symptoms and are completely lysed by the fibrinolytic mechanism within 3 to 7 days; however, chronic pulmonary hypertension with its associated morbidity and mortality may develop as a residual effect of pulmonary arterial damage either from a non-fatal massive embolism or repeated episodes of small embolizations.

In many cases of venous thrombosis, however, enough venous obstruction or inflammation (phlebitis) occurs to produce symptoms, which, if recognized, may lead to prompt diagnosis and appropriate treatment.

Still, even though the acute attack subsides, venous valves in the involved areas are irreparably damaged as a result of thrombosis and recanalization and are rendered incompetent, with resulting venous stasis and chronic venous hypertension whose sequelae depend upon the extent of the thrombotic process. This postphlebitic syndrome is manifested by varying degrees of pain, edema, brawny induration, pigmentation, and ulceration. The natural history of this syndrome is one of exacerbations and remissions with gradual progression of the disease.

DEEP VEIN THROMBOSIS

SYMPTOMS

It should be emphasized that venous thrombosis is reportedly "silent" — completely without symptoms — in 30 to 50 per cent of the cases, and leg signs may be absent in up to 75 per cent of patients having pulmonary embolism.[49, 54, 55] Despite these reports, in this author's experience the incidence of silent significant disease is not this high. Although there may be no subjective symptoms, in many instances suggestive signs, if tested for, will be present. Unexplained tachycardia and anxiety frequently accompany venous thrombosis and should serve to alert the surgeon to the possibility. Most important is the routine checking for leg signs in all postoperative patients. In high-risk patients the lower extremities should be monitored by ultraso-nography, plethysmography, or iodine-125 fibrinogen scanning at frequent intervals. Frequently Homan's sign is positive and calf tenderness or tenderness along the course of the femoral vein is present even in the absence of subjective symptoms.

In the patients presenting symptoms, three recognizable symptom complexes may be produced, depending upon the degree of venous obstruction and associated phlebitis. Any of these may arise de novo or develop by progression from one type to the other and give rise to pulmonary embolism.

The first symptom complex is associated with minimal thrombosis with little inflammatory reaction involving the small veins of the feet and calf muscles; sometimes there is obstruction of the popliteal vein. This process may or may not cause symptoms, which if present usually consist of calf pain and tenderness, with pain precipitated by dorsiflexion of the foot (Homans' sign) or by manual compression of the calf muscles. Prominence of superficial veins in the lower leg is sometimes seen. This is usually unaccompanied by alteration of the vital signs, edema, discoloration, or changes in peripheral arterial pulses.

The second, and more easily recognized, entity is caused when there is enough thrombosis to obstruct the iliofemoral venous segment. This is commonly referred to as iliofemoral thrombosis or thrombophlebitis, phlegmasia alba dolens, or "milk leg." Classic symptoms are pain, edema involving the thigh as well as the distal extremity, pale discoloration of the extremity, distention of the superficial veins (caused by deep venous obstruction), and slight diminution of temperature of the lower limb. Homans' sign is positive and calf tenderness and tenderness along the course of the femoral vein are usually present. Peripheral arterial pulses are usually present but may be diminished when compared with the uninvolved side owing both to edema and to arterial vasospasm.

The third and severest degree is known as phlegmasia cerulea dolens. This is due to massive venous thrombosis of the lower extremity with involvement of the internal as well as the external iliac vein and occasionally the inferior vena cava. This catastrophic limb- and life-threatening condition was first described in 1929 by Tremolières and Veran,[103] who referred to it as "blue phlebitis" because of the characteristic blue discoloration of the massively swollen lower extremity. This cyanosis is caused by diminished arterial blood flow secondary to arterial vasoconstriction or frank collapse of the arterial wall, brought about by increased tissue pressure secondary to edema, which in turn accounts for the absence of arterial pulses in the extremity.[16] This has been mistaken for arterial embolism and has been called pseudoembolic phlebitis.[45]

The extremity is cold, tightly distended, and excruciatingly painful, with pain and tenderness frequently involving the low abdomen. Tachycardia, tachypnea, slight temperature elevation, and hypotension with varying degrees of clinical shock may be associated.

DIAGNOSIS

Acute phlebothrombosis or thrombophlebitis can usually be diagnosed easily by the symptoms already mentioned when they are present. However, in borderline cases the diagnosis may be difficult, and in the "silent" type the diagnosis may be impossible unless routine screening procedures are used. In all too many cases, sudden, fatal, massive pulmonary embolism occurs in what appeared to be a normally convalescing postoperative patient.

Several measures have been helpful in diagnosis of "silent" phlebothrombosis. A high index of suspicion should be maintained by the surgeon in regard to patients in the high-risk category referred to earlier. Routine examination for calf tenderness and search for the cause of unexplained alterations in the vital signs, particularly tachycardia and hyperpnea, are occasionally rewarded by discovery of the diagnosis. These patients for unknown reasons occasionally complain of a sense of impending disaster. This must never be treated lightly, and any patient with this complaint should be thoroughly examined with the possibility of venous thrombosis kept in mind.

The following specific diagnostic modalities have been used extensively and may be helpful in these cases.[75, 81]

SCANNING WITH RADIOACTIVE FIBRINOGEN. Human fibrinogen labeled with iodine-125[1, 54] or iodine-131[76] is given orally to patients after previous blocking of the thyroid gland by sodium iodide. Radioactivity over the legs is monitored 2 hours later and periodically afterwards if desired. Both legs can be monitored in about 10 to 12 minutes. An increase in the percentage value of 20 or more represents deep vein thrombosis. In comparison with phlebography, accuracy rates as high as 92 per cent have been reported.[54] The chief drawbacks to the technique are its unreliability above the inguinal ligament,[71] the necessity of blocking the thyroid gland, and some risk of hepatitis.

DOPPLER ULTRASONOGRAPHY. The ultrasonic velocity detector is used over the leg veins to detect absence of spontaneous flow signals normally heard over the common femoral, superficial femoral, and popliteal veins. Absence of signals after the limb has been compressed distal to the point being examined to augment flow is interpreted as indicating occlusion of that venous segment. This bedside technique can be performed in approximately 10 minutes. Strandness and Sumner[101] report its accuracy as 93 per cent as correlated with venography; Milne and co-workers,[71] on the other hand, found it no more valuable than clinical examination. The technique is more helpful in patients with obstruction in the iliofemoral and femoropopliteal venous segments. Its chief drawbacks are that venous occlusions in the small veins of the calf cannot be evaluated by this technique and the validity of interpretation depends greatly upon observer skill.

IMPEDANCE PLETHYSMOGRAPHY. This bedside technique is based on the fact that thrombosis alters the rate and degree of venous volume changes in the legs in response to physiologic obstruction and release by the Valsalva maneuver or a pressure cuff upon the thigh. Despite enthusiastic reports by Wheeler and associates,[108, 109] who observed only three false-positive and three false-negative results in 101 instances, and by Gazzaniga and associates,[40] high incidences of false-positive results have been reported by others.[28, 32] Disadvantages are its inaccuracy in detecting clots in small calf veins and non-occlusive small thrombi in larger veins and the requirement of an understanding by the user of the physiological principles upon which the test is based.

VENOGRAPHY. The direct visualization of the deep veins of the legs by radiopaque media remains the most reliable method of diagnosis and the standard against which all the newer non-invasive techniques are measured. Figure 9–1 shows a large thrombus with a free-floating tail in the superficial femoral vein in a patient with equivocal symptoms, and Figure 9–2 reveals the presence of multiple small thrombi in the lower leg veins with extension into the popliteal vein in a relatively asymptomatic patient. Our experience compares with that of Dale and Lewis,[24, 57] who found the procedure to be reliable and innocuous, without untoward effect on existing thrombosis and not productive of pulmonary embolism. In addition, the author and others[82] have found it suitable for use in outpatients.

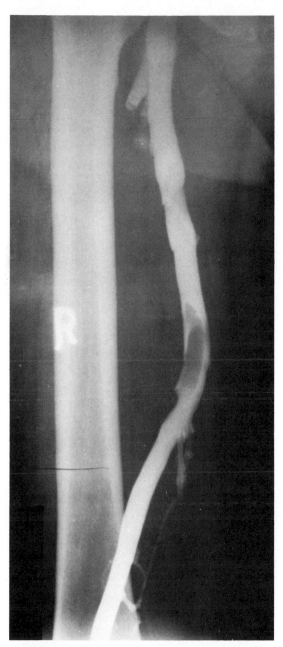

Figure 9–1 Right femoral venogram, showing large, loosely attached thrombus in a patient with equivocal signs and symptoms.

Each of these diagnostic techniques has its limitations. Although venography is the most reliable, it may not be as well suited for mass screening, serial monitoring, and detection in the "silent" cases since it is invasive, expensive, and time-consuming. The non-invasive techniques for which there is current enthusiasm lend themselves well for serial testing and mass screening; however,

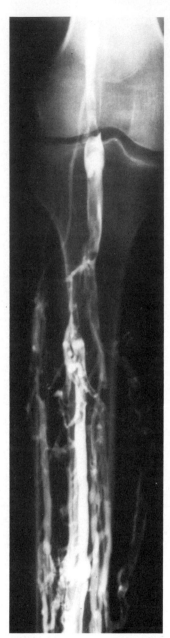

Figure 9–2 Venogram revealing multiple small thrombi in calf and lower leg veins with extension into popliteal vein.

these too require specially trained personnel for performance and interpretation and, in the author's opinion, require venographic confirmation of the diagnosis in asymptomatic patients before anticoagulant therapy is instituted. All factors considered, venography seems to be more available for general use.

PREVENTION

GENERAL MEASURES.   Undoubtedly, many cases of thrombophlebitis may be prevented by measures designed to avoid the primary etiologic factors associated with phlebothrombosis — stasis, trauma, infection, and hypercoagulability.

Important measures in the prevention of stasis of the blood in the lower extremities are routine leg exercises preoperatively and postoperatively, early ambulation, passive dorsiflexion of the feet at short intervals or intermittent stimulation of calf muscles during surgery, elevation of the foot of the operating table during surgery and of the foot of the bed postoperatively, and avoidance of constricting restraints on the lower extremities and pressure and trauma from the operating team and table during the procedure.

Interestingly enough, Flanc and associates,[37] utilizing such measures intensively before, during, and after surgery, found no significant difference in the incidence of thrombosis as determined by iodine-125 fibrinogen testing except following major operations in the elderly; however, the spontaneous clot dissolution time in patients so treated averaged 2.6 days as compared to 5.9 days in untreated controls. This is in conflict with reports of Tsapogas and associates,[104] who observed significantly fewer cases of venous thrombosis (4 per cent) after similar prophylactic measures as compared to a 14 per cent incidence in a control group. Light elastic antiembolism stockings have been used extensively for prevention of thromboembolic complications;[50] however, graded compression elastic hose are probably more effective.[10] There is also recent enthusiasm for the use of automatic intermittent compression cuffs intra- and postoperatively and there are reports of their efficacy in preventing thromboembolism.[22] However, further validation and a determination of their cost effectiveness seem desirable before their use is strongly endorsed.

The importance of observance of Halsted's principles to minimize operative trauma and of the judicious use of aseptic technique and appropriate antibiotics for prevention of infection cannot be overemphasized. Adequate fluid and blood replacement to prevent hypervolemia and hypotension are also valuable.

ANTICOAGULANTS. Heparin in low doses and dextran are being used extensively in an effort to prevent phlebothrombosis by decreasing coagulability or factors contributing to the coagulation mechanism.

The rationale for low-dose heparin prophylaxis rests upon the presumption that antithrombin III, a naturally occurring inhibitor of factor X, is enhanced by heparin, and, when heparin is given before any tissue trauma activates factor X, only small doses are needed to prevent thrombosis.[65] The same doses given once tissue trauma has taken place are ineffective against activated factor X.

Nicholaides and co-workers[78] give 5000 units of heparin subcutaneously 2 hours preoperatively, and then every 12 hours after operation for 1 week. With this regimen only 0.8 per cent of the test group of patients were found to have thrombosis when rated by iodine-125 fibrinogen scanning, as compared to 24 per cent of the control group. Despite this and other enthusiastic reports[52] low-dose heparin is associated with significant increases in intraoperative blood loss and wound hematomas and, for this reason, may not be the ideal prophylactic agent.[39, 100]

Dextran, either low-molecular-weight dextran (M.W. 40,000) or dextran 75 (M.W. 75,000), theoretically may aid in preventing venous thrombosis by decreasing platelet adhesiveness and increasing perfusion of smaller vessels. Atik and co-workers[6] have reported success in reducing the incidence of pulmonary embolism and phlebothrombosis in surgical patients and in patients with hip fractures with use of this polysaccharide. They give 500 ml. of 6 per cent dextran (M.W. 75,000) in 5 per cent dextrose in distilled water daily beginning the day before operation and continuing for 3 days postoperatively, and then every other day until the risk is reduced. Brisman, Parks, and Haller,[15] on the other hand, using essentially the same regimen, observed no significant difference.

Warfarin has also been used in an effort to prevent thromboembolism after surgery[91, 92] but has never been popularly accepted because of the high incidence of hemorrhagic complications and little de-monstrable evidence of its advantage over other methods. The value of antiplatelet agents, such as aspirin, remains an unsettled issue, and until more convincing evidence is available they cannot be recommended as effective.[100]

In general, the surgeon is leery of using anticoagulants in the surgical patient because of the danger of hemorrhage.[59] Because of this, in high-risk patients we prefer dextran prophylactically until 3 or 4 days after operation, at which time heparin is started and is usually continued a week or 10 days.

TREATMENT

CONSERVATIVE THERAPY. When the diagnosis of deep venous thrombosis (exclusive of phlegmasia cerulea dolens) is made or strongly suspected, conservative therapy is instituted initially and is usually effective. This consists of the following measures:

1. Heparin, 12,000 to 15,000 units intravenously, is given immediately, and then 24,000 units every 24 hours by continuous infusion or 5000 units every 4 hours by intermittent injections. This regimen provides immediate anticoagulation by inhibition of thrombin in the coagulation mechanism. Its prime purpose is to prevent further coagulation and thrombus propagation and to permit maximal dissolution of thrombi by normal fibrinolytic mechanisms. It is doubtful that heparin itself has any thrombolytic effect upon existing thrombi. Prior to initiation of heparin therapy a prothrombin time, an APTT, and a platelet count are performed to rule out any existing coagulation defects. Appropriate monitoring by APTT determinations is mandatory in full dose heparin therapy.[31]

2. Elevation of the lower extremities insures the best possible venous drainage of the legs, discourages further thrombosis, and minimizes edema.

3. Intermittent warm wet compresses to the lower extremities seem to help not only by making the patient more comfortable but also by decreasing the edema.

4. Broad spectrum antibiotics are given in severe cases and in those associated with a marked febrile or leukocytic response, for even though most cases are inflammatory,

only in some cases are cultures positive. Demonstration of atypical bacterial and "L" forms has been reported by Altemeier and associates.[3] Specific antibiotics are given in those cases in which there is proven culture sensitivity.

5. Anti-inflammatory agents such as phenylbutazone (Butazolidin), acetylsalicylic acid, and steroids are usually not given unless there is considerable associated inflammation evidenced by redness, heat, and local tenderness. Whenever these agents are used, their propensity to cause gastric ulceration and massive gastrointestinal hemorrhage should be remembered. For this reason we rarely employ these drugs in the postoperative patient.

The fibrinolytic agents streptokinase and urokinase can effectively dissolve thrombi if they are employed within 3 days of onset. Prompt improvement in symptoms can be expected and valvular damage and its serious sequelae can be avoided in many cases. However, their use is contraindicated for 10 days postoperatively because of hemorrhagic complications,[12] and for this reason their general use in surgical patients is not recommended. However, thrombolytic therapy in non-surgical patients appears promising, and the reader is referred to the encouraging reports of Kakkar[53] and Bell[12] and their respective associates on the use of streptokinase and urokinase in treatment of both deep venous thrombosis and pulmonary embolism. Chief drawbacks are hemorrhage and allergic and febrile reactions. The latter two are minimized when urokinase is used. The cost of these agents, however, should be considered. Although there has been some recent reduction in price, they are still quite expensive, particularly urokinase.

This regimen (exclusive of fibrinolytics) is generally followed by improvement within 6 to 8 hours, with diminution of edema and pain.

Femoral Venous Thrombectomy. If iliofemoral thrombosis (phlegmasia alba dolens) is of short duration (less than a week) and does not respond promptly, or if more limited degrees of thrombosis progress to involve the iliofemoral segment, or in the case of phlegmasia cerulea dolens, femoral venous thrombectomy should be performed. Any anticoagulant effect is reversed, and the operation is performed under local or general anesthesia. Important technical aspects of thrombectomy are as follows:

1. Preoperative reversal of anticoagulation with vitamin K_1 oxide, 25 mg. intravenously, will usually bring an elevated prothrombin time to normal when warfarin (Coumadin) or related drugs have been used. Since the effect of heparin is short-lived, discontinuance of this agent is usually sufficient to bring the coagulation time to normal before surgery. However, if necessary, its effect can be neutralized by protamine sulfate intravenously; 1 mg. protamine neutralizes about 90 units of USP heparin.

2. Adequate control of the femoral vein and its branches proximal and distal to the phlebotomy site is necessary.

3. Suction with a right-angle tube or catheter is used to remove proximal thrombus; care must be taken not to dislodge it accidentally. Good backflow usually indicates adequate thrombectomy; however, valves in femoral or iliac veins may interfere. Our anatomic studies have shown an average of one valve per side, with the most common location being approximately 2 cm. above the saphenofemoral junction.[68] This valve can be reached frequently and collapsed by inserting a curved Kelly clamp proximally when checking for backflow. We have been hesitant to use the balloon catheter for proximal thrombectomy for fear of accidental dislodgment of the thrombus, with resultant pulmonary embolism. Because of this danger we recommend prior application of a vena caval clip whenever the balloon catheter is to be used for this purpose (Fig. 9–3).

4. We believe that, after a reasonable attempt at proximal thrombus removal, prolonged and traumatic efforts to obtain good backflow are inadvisable. They are usually unrewarding and may convert a relatively minor procedure into a major one with considerable blood loss and other complications.

5. Distal thrombus expression by tightly wrapping a sterile Esmarch bandage from base of toes to groin has been quite satisfactory. Many times thrombi with an aggregate length of approximately 50 cm. have been recovered.

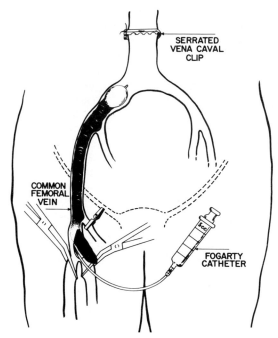

Figure 9–3 Fogarty balloon catheter thrombectomy of right femoroiliac venous segment with ancillary use of serrated vena caval clip to prevent pulmonary embolism. Note control of veins entering area. A large-caliber suture or one-eighth inch umbilical tape is also used proximal to venotomy for proximal control.

6. Ancillary clipping of the vena cava is recommended when thrombectomy is performed in patients who have had an associated embolus, when the thrombus extends into the vena cava, and in instances of incomplete proximal thrombectomy.

7. Anticoagulation is again instituted with 7500 units of heparin intravenously immediately after venotomy, and the venotomy site is liberally irrigated with dilute heparin solution (1000 units heparin per 100 cc. saline) just before closure.

Heparin administration is continued postoperatively, the foot of the bed is elevated, and elastic bandages from base of toes to groin are used whenever the patient is out of bed. The sitting position with the knees and thighs flexed is avoided during early convalescence. Anticoagulation is continued for 7 to 10 days with heparin and then with Coumadin for an indefinite period.

The question of how long to continue anticoagulants is controversial, but from our observations Coumadin is continued in most patients for about 6 to 8 weeks by most physicians. Despite the paucity of material on the subject of recurrence of thromboembolism, the excellent report of Coon and Willis[21] suggested that although the duration and intensity of anticoagulant treatment affected frequency of recurrence during hospitalization, there was no evidence that it influenced later recurrence. They found risk to be very high immediately after hospital discharge and to decrease gradually to a plateau after 3 years. The study suggests the continuance of oral anticoagulants for ambulatory patients for at least 4 months, and longer in patients with past history of venous thrombosis or pulmonary embolism who are at greater risk for recurrence.

The value of venous thrombectomy has been a controversial issue. Initial enthusiasm prompted by the work of Mahorner[60] and Haller[46] was dampened by reports by Lansing and Davis[56] and Barner and associates[9] suggesting such a high incidence of rethrombosis as determined by venography that the value of thrombectomy was open to question. This was followed by a wave of conservatism in which heparin and elevation were the mainstays of treatment. Although there are intermittent enthusiastic reports of success with thrombectomy such as that of Edwards and associates[35] and others,[58] most therapists still agree that initially anticoagulant therapy is the treatment of choice.

PULMONARY EMBOLISM

SYMPTOMS

Unfortunately, pulmonary embolism is asymptomatic in the vast majority of instances. Coon and Willis,[20] in analyzing 606 necropsy patients with pulmonary embolism, found that 80 per cent had had no suggestive signs or symptoms, only approximately 10 per cent had had leg signs, and in only 7 per cent was a definite diagnosis made prior to death. The classic triad of symptoms of pulmonary embolism — chest pain, dyspnea, and hemoptysis — had been found in only 3 per cent of the patients.

The exhibition of symptoms depends upon the size, location, and number of emboli in the pulmonary arterial tree, the degree of obstruction produced, and whether or not pulmonary infarction occurs. Accordingly, symptoms may vary from none at all with small emboli to sudden substernal pain, severe dyspnea, and circulatory failure with massive emboli. Four symptom complexes may be recognizable within this spectrum:[25]

ACUTE COR PULMONALE. When emboli obstruct more than 60 per cent of the pulmonary arterial tree, the increased pressure usually causes acute dilatation and failure of the right ventricle. This results in an increase in its filling pressure and causes an increase in right atrial and central venous pressure.

The chief symptoms are anxiety, dyspnea, substernal pain, and collapse. Examination will reveal loud P_2 sounds, distended neck veins, and hepatomegaly with tenderness. Tachypnea, tachycardia, cyanosis, and hypotension are often present. Electrocardiographic signs of right ventricular strain are produced and chest x-ray may reveal enlargement of the right ventricle and pulmonary conus.

SHOCK OR CARDIOVASCULAR COLLAPSE. Massive pulmonary embolism may present as acute circulatory failure due to shock or cardiac arrest. Usually, however, this state is preceded by acute cor pulmonale, and this may be the key to prompt diagnosis. In those with shock, the central venous pressure is frequently elevated higher than 15 cm. H_2O. The electrocardiogram here also may facilitate the diagnosis by showing evidence of right ventricular strain rather than myocardial infarction.

PULMONARY INFARCTION. This complication of pulmonary embolism, although well known, is one of the less frequent and is present in fewer than one-third of the cases; however, mortality rates as high as 65 per cent have been reported.[62] Clinically dyspnea, pleuritic chest pain, and hemoptysis or cough are present. Signs include fever, tachycardia, tachypnea, friction rub (infrequently), and splinting. Leukocytosis, an elevated lactic dehydrogenase level, and the classic wedge-shaped density on chest x-ray (Fig. 9–4) are frequently associated.

MISCELLANEOUS. Mild dyspnea, chest discomfort, low-grade fever, unexplained tachycardia, increase in respiratory rate, and syncopal attacks[83] may signal repeated episodes of small emboli. Frequently they mimic bronchopneumonia and postoperative atelectasis. They may cause intensification of symptoms of chronic lung disease, such as asthma or bronchiectasis. In some cases of heart disease they may precipitate failure; in others, unusual resistance to digitalis may be observed.

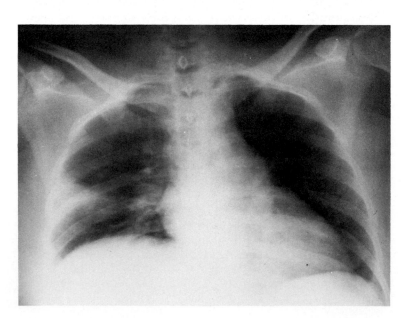

Figure 9–4 Chest x-ray revealing classic peripheral wedge-shaped density of pulmonary embolism and infarction. Pleuritic pain, hemoptysis, and dyspnea were also present.

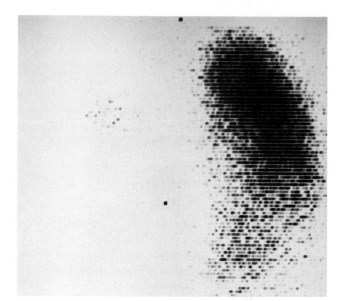

Figure 9–5 Pulmonary scan revealing multiple perfusion defects due to pulmonary emboli. Note almost complete obstruction on right due to massive embolus as well as defect in left costophrenic angle region.

DIAGNOSIS

The diagnosis of pulmonary embolism is considered in any postoperative patient presenting the symptoms just described or in whom sudden unexplained dyspnea, cyanosis, shock, tachycardia, chest pain, or cor pulmonale develops.

The chest x-ray may show no significant findings in the case of small emboli without infarction, or it may show areas of "emptiness" or hyperlucency with decreased lung markings (Westermark's sign) in early segment or massive pulmonary embolism. The characteristic peripheral wedge-shaped density caused by segmental infarction (see Fig. 9–4) is seen in only one-third of the cases. Although ventilation-perfusion pulmonary scanigrams (Fig. 9–5) may be of benefit, particularly if positive in the patient with a normal chest film, it should be remembered that this technique reveals only decreased pulmonary perfusion, which may be caused by other conditions. On the other hand, a negative scan usually rules out pulmonary embolism.

The most reliable diagnostic technique in the doubtful case is direct pulmonary angiography, which usually demonstrates all but small peripheral emboli. Figure 9–6 shows

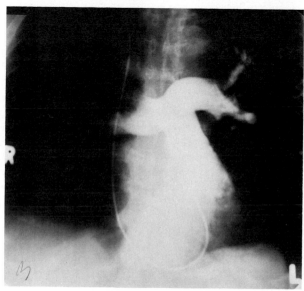

Figure 9–6 Pulmonary angiogram in patient with massive multiple pulmonary emboli with almost complete obstruction bilaterally.

obstruction of most of the major pulmonary arteries by emboli. A normal pulmonary angiogram excludes significant pulmonary embolism.

Pulmonary embolism must be differentiated diagnostically from any entity that causes chest pain, particularly acute myocardial infarction and heart failure.

The electrocardiogram may show no abnormalities in pulmonary embolism, but in many cases there is evidence of right ventricular strain with depression of S-T segments in leads 2 3 aVF, V_2, and V_3 as well as inversion of T waves in V_1 through V_3.[93] Serial electrocardiograms serve to rule out myocardial infarction.

Chest x-rays in different planes, bronchoscopy, and bronchography are helpful in ruling out other pulmonary problems such as idiopathic pleurisy, pneumonitis, bronchiectasis, and malignant disease.

Laboratory findings are not very helpful in diagnosis. Elevated lactic dehydrogenase with normal serum glutamic oxaloacetic transaminase and a normal serum bilirubin suggests pulmonary infarction. Arterial blood gases, however, may be helpful — P_{O_2} and P_{CO_2} are usually decreased and rarely is the P_{O_2} normal.

The central venous pressure is usually elevated, and if it is low, massive pulmonary embolism can usually be ruled out.

TREATMENT

Treatment is instituted immediately once the diagnosis is made or cannot be definitely ruled out.

BASIC SUPPORTIVE AND SYMPTOMATIC TREATMENT

Oxygen should be given by nasal catheter, by mask, or, if necessary, by endotracheal tube to counteract the low P_{O_2}, and its effect is monitored by frequent blood gas determinations. Ventilatory assistance is given if necessary. A large-caliber intravenous catheter is placed in either the subclavian or internal jugular vein for fluid administration and central venous pressure monitoring. If hypotension is present, isoproterenol (4 mg. in 1000 ml. of 5 per cent dextrose in distilled water) is given. It has the added

advantage of its inotropic cardiac effect and also causes bronchodilatation and vasodilatation. If there is no response, dopamine or a vasopressor agent such as levarterenol or metaraminol is used instead. Morphine or meperidine hydrochloride (Demerol) may be helpful for control or pain of apprehension. Antibiotics are given prophylactically.

DEFINITIVE TREATMENT

Treatment directed at the embolism itself is designed either to prevent additional embolizations and permit autolysis by the individual's own fibrinolytic mechanisms or to lyse or extract existing emboli.

PREVENTION OF RECURRENT EMBOLISM. Fortunately most initial embolisms are not massive or fatal and it remains for additional episodes to cause death, serious infarction, or debilitating, chronic pulmonary hypertension. It is estimated that approximately 25 to 30 per cent of first embolic episodes are fatal, and many times even in these cases death is probably caused by emboli additional to an original asymptomatic embolus. For this reason the prevention of recurrent embolism may be the most important aspect of treatment. Methods of prevention include both medical and surgical modalities including administration of anticoagulants and fibrinolytic agents and surgical interruption of the vena cava to prevent the passage of emboli to the lungs.

ANTICOAGULATION. Anticoagulants have become the cornerstone of therapy for pulmonary embolism. Utilizing these agents the mortality rate has been reduced from over 50 per cent to approximately 8 per cent.[31, 87, 95] Consequently the initial treatment of pulmonary embolism should include basically the anticoagulants. Despite this, it should be remembered that anticoagulants serve only to arrest the thrombotic process and prevent further thrombosis, permitting the patient's own fibrinolytic system to lyse existing thrombi or emboli. They do not significantly affect existing thrombi or emboli or prevent recurrent embolization from them.

Heparin is the anticoagulant of choice; its effect is immediate and easy to control. The technique of heparin administration has been described under treatment of deep venous thrombosis. Some investigators, however, use higher doses than those described above in the treatment of pulmonary embolism, on the ground that they may effectively help associated bronchospasm and reduce mortality.[23, 102]

SURGICAL INTERRUPTION OF THE INFERIOR VENA CAVA. Successful results with anticoagulant therapy have reduced significantly the need for procedures and devices designed to prevent recurrent embolism by completely or partially occluding the inferior vena cava. However, in many patients anticoagulants are either contraindicated, ineffective or complicated, and some reports indicate rates of recurrent embolism as high as 30 to 75 per cent with 15 to 55 per cent mortality.[8, 47, 74, 87] In addition, an untold number of the remainder will probably have repeated embolic episodes with resultant chronic pulmonary hypertension and become pulmonary cripples. For these reasons there remains a definite place in the therapeutic armamentarium for caval interruption, which has shown protective rates as high as 95 per cent against recurrent embolism and mortality rates under 10 per cent[67] (Table 9–1).

Indications for vena caval interruption of some type are as follows:

1. Recurrent embolism occurring during anticoagulant treatment.

2. When anticoagulant therapy is contraindicated, ineffective, unduly complicated, or impractical.

3. In chronic recurrent pulmonary embolism.

4. In conjunction with pulmonary embolectomy.

5. Prophylactically in selected high-risk patients.

6. Non-occlusive thrombosis of the iliac or femoral vein.

7. Septic embolism.

Two basic types of procedures are available for this. Complete vena caval ligation, which was originated by Homans[48] and popularized during the early and mid-1940's by Ochsner and DeBakey,[79] is still preferred by many.[80] However, because of the high incidence of disabling stasis sequelae and problems with acute hypotensive episodes following complete ligation, several methods of partial caval occlusion have been developed. The common rationale of these methods is to prevent passage of emboli but at the same time to permit some blood flow so that the resulting complications are avoided. Among the many techniques available are the suture plication of Spencer,[98] Moretz[73] slotlike clip, the harp-string suture grid of De Weese,[30] and the author's serrated Teflon clip (Fig. 9–11C, D, E).[66] We prefer the last-named, since its application is relatively simple and quick and is followed by fewer instances of recurrent embolism than application of the Moretz clip.[69] When compared to caval ligation, use of the serrated Teflon clip is, in our experience, followed by significantly fewer stasis sequelae and acute hypotensive episodes and is equally efficacious in prevention of recurrent embolism.[67] On the other hand, caval ligation is indicated instead of partial occlusive methods in patients with septic embolism from the pelvis or lower extremities.

A number of intracaval devices have been devised that can be inserted under local anesthesia via the internal jugular vein. Two of the more popular ones, the Mobin-Uddin umbrella[72] and the Kim-Ray Greenfield filter,[44] are shown in Figures 9–7 and 9–8. However, insertion of these is a blind procedure, and some difficulty with positioning and filter migration has been reported.[44, 106] Aldelston and associates[1] have recently reported a 12 per cent incidence of recurrent embolism after insertion of the Mobin-Uddin umbrella, and at autopsy they found inferior vena caval occlusion in 6 of 7 patients and thrombi on the cardiac side of the filter in 4 and in the pulmonary artery in 1. At the time of this writing, one of our patients has such an umbrella residing in the right ventricle to which it embolized after what was thought to be a precise, uneventful placement in the vena cava, just below the right renal vein.

Although such complications occur relatively infrequently the potentiality is ever-present, and when they occur a more

TABLE 9–1 LONG-TERM RESULTS IN 121 VENA CAVAL CLIPPINGS*

Intraoperative hypotension	0
Acute thrombophlebitis (post-op)	15.0%
Disabling edema	7.8%
Recurrent embolism	2.4%
Clip patency	76.0%
Mortality	8.2%

*Data from Miles, R. M., and Elsea, P. W.: Clinical evaluation of the serrated vena caval clip. *Surg. Gynecol. Obstet. 132*:581, 1971.

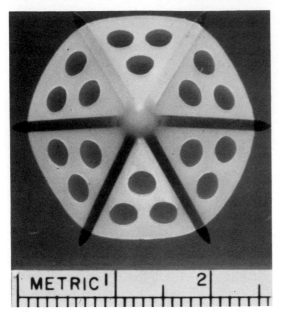

Figure 9–7 The Mobin-Uddin intracaval umbrella for prevention of pulmonary embolism. This device can be inserted under local anesthesia via the internal jugular vein and may be indicated in the desperately ill patient.

serious problem is created than was originally present.

These complications are practically impossible with clips or ligatures, since they are extraluminal and may be applied precisely under direct vision. All things considered, we believe that clipping or ligation should be the standard technique for most patients requiring caval interruption and that intracaval devices should be utilized only in patients too critically ill to warrant a general anesthetic.

Preoperative Preparation. Regardless of which operative method is chosen, any anticoagulant being used is discontinued and the anticoagulant effect is reversed by either vitamin K_1 oxide or protamine.

A large-bore (No. 16) Angiocath or needle is introduced into an upper extremity vein, or a central venous pressure apparatus is placed in the subclavian or internal jugular vein for pressure monitoring and possible infusion of blood. Although blood has rarely been necessary, it is advisable to have 1500 ml. of cross-matched blood available should inadvertent hemorrhage occur.

Technique of Clip Application. The serrated Teflon clip requires general or high spinal anesthesia and is usually applied via the retroperitoneal approach, which is better tolerated by the seriously ill patient. The transperitoneal approach is required, however, when the technique is used as an ancillary to another abdominal procedure, or in cases of pelvic thrombophlebitis when the gonadal veins must also be ligated.

Our recent study of the anatomy of the inferior vena cava and the lumbar veins suggests that the optimal sites for caval clipping (or ligation) are the 3-cm. segment

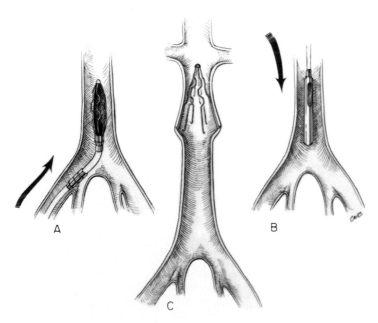

Figure 9–8 The Kim-Ray Greenfield metal springlike intracaval filter for prevention of pulmonary embolism. This device can be inserted under local anesthesia via the femoral vein *A,* or from above down via the internal jugular vein *B. C,* The device in situ showing the tiny hooks which hold it in place within the vena cava. (Reproduced with permission from Greenfield, L. J.: Pulmonary Embolism: Diagnosis and Management, in Ravitch, M. M., et al. (eds.): CURRENT PROBLEMS IN SURGERY. Copyright © 1976 by Year Book Medical Publishers, Inc., Chicago.)

just proximal to the caval bifurcation when the retroperitoneal approach is used and the 1-cm. segment just beneath the right renal vein when operating transperitoneally.[68] The sites were selected because of the relative paucity of lumbar veins in these areas, which simplifies the procedure and renders it less hazardous from the standpoint both of hemorrhage from accidental avulsion of an unexpected lumbar vein and of the relative exposure afforded by the two approaches. In addition, in most cases there are enough lumbar veins to discourage proximal thrombosis and, with the right gonadal and right renal, to afford adequate collateral circulation following interruption at these sites (Fig. 9–9).

Retroperitoneal Approach. An incision is made from a point in the midline approximately 4 cm. above the umbilicus to the right axillary line midway between the costal margin and the iliac crest (Fig. 9–10). The anterior rectus sheath is incised transversely, but the muscle is not divided (Fig. 9–11).

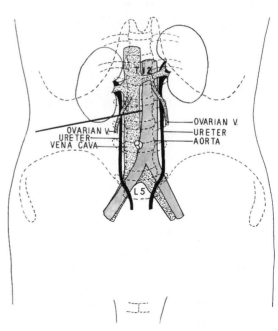

Figure 9–10 Diagrammatic sketch showing relationships of inferior vena cava including surface markings and location of incision (black line in right upper quadrant) for vena caval clipping via the retroperitoneal approach. This incision affords better exposure to the lower portion of the cava than to the subrenal segment despite the suggestion of illustration. It is extremely difficult and hazardous to attempt vena caval clipping in the subrenal segment via the retroperitoneal approach. The general tendency is to make the incision too low — this has caused the right common iliac vein to be clipped or ligated mistakenly in some cases.

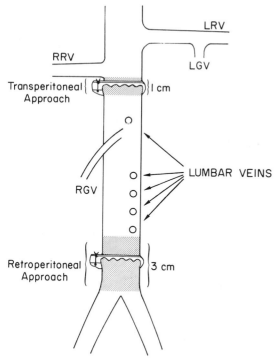

Figure 9–9 Diagrammatic sketch of inferior vena cava demonstrating optimal sites for caval clipping and mean number and most common location of lumbar veins in 100 necropsy dissections. The 1 cm. segment just below the right renal vein is preferred when the transperitoneal approach is used and the 3 cm. area just above the bifurcation when the retroperitoneal approach is employed.

The lateral muscles are split in gridiron fashion, and the retroperitoneal space is entered. The peritoneum and contained viscera are reflected by "walking" them to the left with the fingers, care being taken to include the right gonadal vein and right ureter with the peritoneum. The psoas muscle is first visualized, and then the fatty lymphatic sheath about the inferior vena cava. A deep heart-shaped or Deaver retractor is placed over a pad and used to hold the peritoneum off the cava (Fig. 9–11*B*) and other padded retractors are placed above and below. If the peritoneum is reflected properly there should be practically no bleeding, and it is unusual to have to clamp or tie a vessel in this area of the dissection. The pericaval lymphatics are opened and the plane between them and the adventitia of the cava is entered. Lumbar veins are carefully avoided. An appropriately curved clamp (usually a large right-angled clamp) is

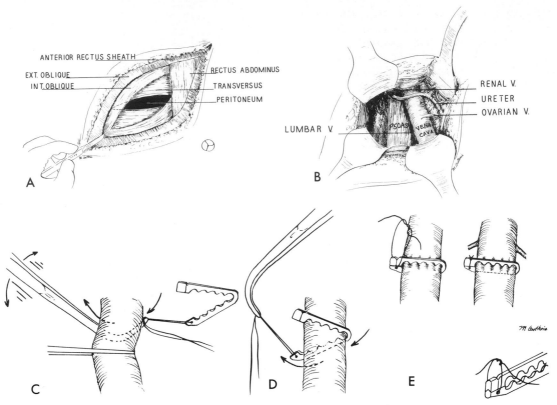

Figure 9–11   Technique for vena caval clipping via the retroperitoneal approach.

A, Incision for retroperitoneal vena caval clipping — medial end of incision is actually not as high as in illustration. Note that the anterior rectus sheath has been incised, but the rectus muscle is not divided. The external oblique muscle is incised and the internal oblique and transversus are split in gridiron fashion. In many cases the external oblique is split rather than incised.

B, The retroperitoneal space is entered and the peritoneum with the right gonadal vein and ureter is reflected medially to expose the inferior vena cava.

C, A right-angled clamp is passed behind the cava, with care being taken to avoid lumbar veins, and an eighth-inch umbilical tape is passed for use as a retractor and for distal control if inadvertent hemorrhage should occur. The clamp is again passed behind the cava and used to grasp both ends of a 0 silk suture which has been passed through the opening in the lower jaw of the clip.

D, The clip is then slipped in place from left to right by traction on the suture.

E, The jaws of the clip are now approximated by tying down the silk suture in the notch on the upper jaw of the clip — a surgeon's knot is used to avoid slipping after the first throw.

carefully passed behind the cava until it exits on the left. This should pass easily. If it does not, it should *not* be forced for fear of avulsing an unseen posterior lumbar vein; rather, the clamp should be removed and passage attempted at a slightly different level. When the clamp has been passed successfully it is used to grasp a one-eighth inch umbilical tape which is passed around the cava for use as a retractor and to afford distal control. The clamp is again passed behind the cava and used to grasp both ends of a 0 silk ligature that has been passed through the aperture in the lower jaw of the clip (Fig. 9–11*C*). The silk ligature is now

drawn behind the cava and used to facilitate slipping the clip on the cava from left to right (Fig. 9–11*D*). The clip is now approximated by tying the ligature down in the groove on the upper limb of the clip (Fig. 9–11*E*). A surgeon's knot is used to avoid slipping after the first throw. A silver or tantalum clip is applied to the knot for x-ray visualization unless other clips have been necessary for hemostasis. The tape is removed, the retroperitoneal space is irrigated with sterile saline, and the wound is closed in layers with interrupted O Ethiflex sutures.

Transperitoneal Approach.   The clip may

be easily applied through almost any mid- or upper abdominal incision (see Fig. 9–12, inset). We believe that when clipping is done prophylactically in conjunction with another abdominal procedure in embolus-prone patients, it is advisable to apply the clip first for immediate protection unless exigencies of the situation demand otherwise.

The duodenum is mobilized by the Kocher maneuver, and it and the head of the pancreas are retracted to the left to expose the vena cava immediately beneath at the level below the renal vein. The clip is applied here with the technique already described (Fig. 9–12).

When this route is used in case of embolism from pelvic thrombophlebitis, in addition to applying the clip at the subrenal level (which is above the caval entrance of the right gonadal vein and consequently protects from embolism via this source), the transverse mesocolon is placed at tension and a transverse incision is made in its base near the ligament of Treitz. The left renal vein is exposed and the left gonadal vein which enters from below is doubly ligated

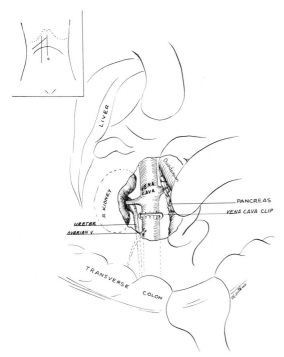

Figure 9–12 Transperitoneal exposure of the vena cava for clipping. This may be performed through almost any type of upper abdominal incision (inset) and affords excellent exposure of the subrenal segment.

and divided just distal to the renal vein. In this way routes of embolism from the pelvis as well as the lower extremities are blocked.

Technique of Caval Ligation. If caval ligation is the operator's preference and in cases of septic embolism in which caval ligation is indicated instead of clipping, the procedure may be carried out through either approach and with the same general technique. The cava is ligated in continuity with two eighth-inch umbilical tapes placed 1 cm. apart. In studies on recanalization of the cava we found that placement of single heavy catgut or silk ligatures was followed by recanalization of the cava to a degree that would permit passage of lethal-sized emboli.[70] However, when a segment of the cava approximately 1 cm. in length was obliterated by multiple ligatures, gross recanalization did not occur. The cava should not be severed — this is unnecessary and technically dangerous.

Postoperative Management. Reanticoagulation with heparin to discourage additional thrombosis and acute flare-ups of existing thrombophlebitis is desirable as soon as possible after clipping. However, because of the possibility of hemorrhage into the recently dissected retroperitoneal space, heparin is withheld for several days. We believe dextran is less dangerous from this standpoint and give 500 ml. of 6 per cent dextran 75 intravenously daily for the first 3 days. Then heparin is given for 5 to 7 days, and then it is replaced by Coumadin, which is continued indefinitely. The foot of the bed is elevated and early ambulation is encouraged, with the legs wrapped from toes to groin in elastic bandages.

Long-term follow-up studies have shown the serrated Teflon clip to be at least 95 per cent effective in preventing recurrent embolism and to be associated with disabling stasis sequelae in only 8.4 per cent of patients.[67] Acute flare-ups of thrombophlebitis have occurred in approximately 15 per cent. The mortality rate has been approximately 8.2 per cent, but only one patient has been lost who was not moribund at the time of clipping.

FIBRINOLYTIC AGENTS. There is great enthusiasm among medical therapists for streptokinase and urokinase which have recently been released by the Federal Drug

Administration for use in treatment of pulmonary embolism. They have been shown to cause dissolution of emboli in about 50 per cent of patients if used within 2 or 3 days of onset of symptoms while the embolus is still "fresh." Mortality and recurrent embolism rates of less than 10 per cent have been claimed. However, their use is complicated by hemorrhage in 30 to 45 per cent,[14, 105] and significant allergic and febrile reactions are associated with the use of streptokinase in particular. In addition, as mentioned above, urokinase is almost prohibitively expensive.

Although these agents may be of value in non-surgical patients, their use in postoperative patients is extremely limited, since they are contraindicated within 10 days of operation because of hemorrhagic complications.

PULMONARY EMBOLECTOMY. The direct removal of the embolus from the pulmonary artery was proposed by Trendelenburg in 1908, but it remained for Kirschner in 1924 to perform this procedure successfully with survival of the patient.[11] Sharp[96] performed the first successful embolectomy under cardiopulmonary bypass in 1961, and many successful embolectomies have been performed since then. However, because the mortality rate is approximately 50 per cent, and because most patients will survive without embolectomy if additional embolic episodes can be prevented, this procedure is reserved for the patient in whom other methods have failed or in whom continuous vasopressive support is necessary for blood pressure maintenance.

Beall and Cooley[11] demonstrated that temporary peripheral femoral cannulation under local anesthesia will permit decompression of the right heart and safer induction of endotracheal anesthesia and surgical exposure. Total cardiopulmonary bypass is then instituted for safer, more complete pulmonary embolectomy, which entails direct embolus removal through a longitudinal pulmonary arteriotomy, the use of the Fogarty catheter, the opening of both pleural cavities, and milking of both lungs to obtain satisfactory embolectomy. In addition, as soon as the general condition permits, some type of partial caval interruption should be performed. With this method survival rates of approximately 70 per cent have been achieved.[13]

Since the mortality rate with thoracotomy embolectomy, even with bypass techniques, remains high, better methods are needed. One promising innovation is an ingenious device developed by Greenfield, Reif, and Gunter.[43] This consists of a catheter with a vacuum cup tip (Fig. 9–13) that can be introduced via the femoral vein under local anesthesia and passed through the right heart into the pulmonary tree from which emboli are retrieved. Greenfield has used this device with simultaneous insertion of

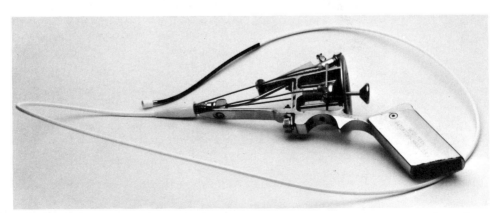

Figure 9–13 The vacuum cup–tipped catheter developed by Greenfield, Reif, and Gunter.[43] This catheter is introduced via the femoral vein and passed through the right heart into the pulmonary arterial tree from which emboli are retrieved. (Reproduced with permission from Greenfield, L. J.: Pulmonary Embolism: Diagnosis and Management, in Ravitch, M. M., et al. (eds.): CURRENT PROBLEMS IN SURGERY. Copyright © 1976 by Year Book Medical Publishers, Inc., Chicago.)

the vena cava filter in 22 patients and reduced the operative mortality from 40 to 17 per cent. Successful extraction of emboli was accomplished in 86 per cent of the patients with an overall survival rate of 14 (64 per cent).[42]

Chronic recurrent pulmonary embolism with pulmonary hypertension manifested by severe respiratory insufficiency has emerged as a distinct entity and is probably more common than is generally recognized. This problem has been attacked surgically by Sabiston and associates,[90] who achieved good results at up to eight years with extensive pulmonary embolectomy combined with inferior vena cava ligation in 5 of 6 such patients. Although the number is small, the importance of this concept in therapy for this condition, previously considered hopeless, cannot be overemphasized.

MISCELLANEOUS VENOUS COMPLICATIONS

SUPERFICIAL THROMBOPHLEBITIS OF THE LOWER EXTREMITIES

This condition usually occurs as a postoperative complication in patients with varicose veins and may be localized to one or more varices or may involve any part or all of the saphenous vein. It was also a common complication earlier when the saphenous vein at the ankle was routinely used for venous cutdown for fluid administration via cannula or catheter.

Clinically this condition presents as a painful, tender, reddened nodule or cord in the subcutaneous tissue along the course of a vein or as a cluster of such areas in superficial varices. Usually the patient is afebrile, but a low-grade fever may be present. Deep venous thrombosis may also be present and should be ruled out by diagnostic tests if possible.

Treatment in limited and mild cases consists of rest, elevation, and warm wet compresses. In more extensive cases and in those with proximal progression, heparin and antibiotics are used. If progression continues despite heparinization, proximal ligation and division at the saphenofemoral junction are performed. Although the incidence of pulmonary embolism is small, the author has seen several deaths from this complication of superficial thrombophlebitis.

In some cases the inflammatory process becomes subacute and will not subside; in these cases complete excision is performed along with the usual stripping procedure in the case of varicose veins.

PELVIC THROMBOPHLEBITIS

Pelvic thrombophlebitis may occur after gynecologic or other pelvic operations in which thrombosis appears within the veins of the uterine wall or pelvis and gradually propagates to include both the uterine and ovarian veins. Progression into the hypogastric and common iliac veins may occur, with extension into the inferior vena cava. Pulmonary emboli may originate from any of these sites.

The situation is much more serious whenever these thrombi become infected, and infection is especially likely in cases of septic abortion. This is known as suppurative pelvic thrombophlebitis and may cause generalized sepsis or septic pulmonary embolism.

Diagnosis may be difficult since there are no characteristic physical findings to differentiate the condition from pelvic cellulitis with which it is most commonly confused.[84]

Suppurative pelvic thrombophlebitis is characterized by shaking chills caused by showers of infected emboli and septic spiking fever with peaks as high as 105° to 106° F. Blood cultures may show anaerobic streptococci. A sustained tachycardia is present which varies little with temperature excursions. Pain and discomfort are not prominent symptoms. Septic shock frequently occurs.

In pelvic cellulitis the pelvic floor is stony hard and the uterus and adnexa are bound down in a fixed mass that cannot be differentiated by palpation, whereas tenderness alone is present in pelvic thrombophlebitis. The temperature is generally sustained and the pulse tends to parallel it. Chills are usually absent, and septic shock and pulmonary embolism are less likely. Symptoms of non-infected pelvic thrombophlebitis differ little from those of pelvic cellulitis. Venography may be helpful in diagnosis when the iliac veins are involved and occasionally thrombi may be visualized in the internal iliac veins by using the Valsalva maneuver.

Treatment consists of adjustment of antibiotics to maximal dosage, intensive supportive treatment, shock therapy, and anticoagulants unless contraindicated (in nonsuppurative cases). Ligation of the inferior vena cava and ovarian veins is indicated in the septic type,[18] rather than partial caval interruption procedures such as clipping, because of the danger of septic embolism.

INTRAVENOUS CATHETER THROMBOPHLEBITIS

The introduction of the plastic intravenous catheter has facilitated and revolutionized intravenous therapy and has made possible long-term parenteral therapy, hyperalimentation, and continuous central venous pressure monitoring. This method is not without complications, however, the most common of which is thrombophlebitis (Fig. 9–14), which may give rise to sepsis,

pulmonary embolism, and bacterial endocarditis.

It is generally believed and has been shown experimentally[77] that a bland thrombus usually forms on or about the catheter and this may become infected by bacteria that either invade the vein from the skin via the catheter itself or come from some remote site by way of the bloodstream.[34] The vein about the catheter may become thrombosed, inflamed, and infected and may give rise to sepsis or to propagation of the thrombus and embolism. Peters and others[86] report the formation of fibrin sheaths about these catheters in 60 to 100 per cent of cases, depending upon the anatomic site of introduction. These sheaths appear to originate either at the sites of insertion or at the catheter tip and surround the catheter for varying distances. They are more extensive when the catheter is placed in antecubital and hand veins than when the subclavian vein is used. However, the authors observed that whenever the catheter was misplaced retrogradely into the jugular vein, complete sheath formation occurred, with obstruction of the jugular vein. The fate of 4 to 8 inches of clot and sheath after removal of the catheter is uncertain, but they have been observed (by venography) in situ for 10 minutes after removal of the catheter.

The reported incidence of positive catheter cultures varies from approximately 9.5 per cent[17] to 41 per cent,[34] with the in-

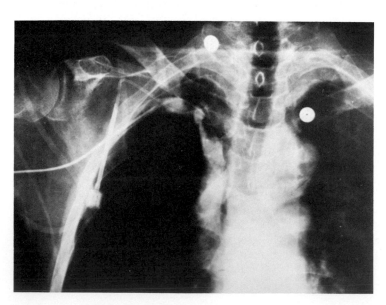

Figure 9–14 Venogram showing catheter thrombophlebitis involving the right subclavian and innominate veins. (Courtesy of Dr. George Blackburn, New England Deaconess Hospital).

cidence of significant infections being about 16 per cent.[36] Druskin and Siegel[34] point out, however, that although 30 per cent of these patients had clinical evidence of phlebitis, it bore no relationship to the duration of the catheter in situ or to the presence of or absence of bacterial growth from the catheter tip. Stein and Pruitt[99] reported that suppurative thrombophlebitis at catheter sites occurred in 4.6 per cent of burn patients, and, in these, a latent period of 2 to 10 days was observed between the removal of the cannula and the appearance of thrombophlebitis.

A variety of organisms have been cultured from these catheters. The organism most frequently found by Druskin and Siegel[34] was *Staphylococcus albus* (coagulase-negative), while in Altemeier and associates'[4] series Serratia was the most common. Pruitt and associates[88] found cultures in general to reflect the surface flora of the patient.

Important preventive measures are aseptic technique for catheter insertion, utilization of a large-caliber vein such as the subclavian or internal jugular rather than an antecubital vein, local antibiotic ointment about the puncture site, and removal of catheters within 48 hours if possible. When catheters must be left in place for long periods of time, as in hyperalimentation, the site should be changed every 4 or 5 days. If this cannot be done, then dressings about catheter sites should be changed every 3 or 4 days with reapplication of antimicrobial ointment. Peters and co-workers[86] report that all infected catheters (14 per cent) in their series had been in place more than 48 hours, and McDonough and Altemeier[63] have observed subclavian vein thrombosis in 4 patients who had long-term subclavian vein catheters. Qureshi and Lilly[89] report a similar case in which a central venous pressure catheter was placed in the inferior vena cava via the left cubital vein. Use of heparin-coated catheters probably does not alter the incidence of thrombosis; however, the addition of 100 units of heparin to each 1000 cm. of solution may inhibit thrombus formation. Although Silastic catheters are less likely to cause thrombosis, there have been reports of thrombosis even with Silastic catheters.[88]

Treatment of catheter thrombophlebitis entails removal of the catheter, local application of warm wet compresses, elevation, type-specific antibiotic therapy in cases of extensive involvement, and heparin in cases that are extensive or progressive. In patients with subclavian vein thrombosis, venous thrombectomy has been advocated but is frequently unsatisfactory because of rethrombosis and inability to achieve complete thrombectomy.

Suppurative thrombophlebitis implies intraluminal suppuration and sepsis, which is accompanied by mortality rates as high as 60 to 80 per cent.[88]

The reader is referred to the excellent report of Pruitt and associates[88] who reviewed 193 burned patients with suppurative thrombophlebitis. Multiple veins were involved in approximately 15 per cent and local signs of infection were present in less than half (35 per cent). The most frequent clinical presentation in patients without local signs was recovery of a positive blood culture in a clinically septic patient. Establishment of the diagnosis mandates exploration, culture, and excision of involved veins plus administration of appropriate antibiotics. In the absence of local signs all previously cannulated veins should be carefully examined and explored for the presence of pus or thrombi, which, if found, should be smeared and cultured and checked for sensitivity to antibiotics. Excision of the involved veins should include the thrombophlebitic segment plus proximal normal vein until it joins the next larger order of veins. Even with such aggressive treatment, only 30 (40 per cent) of 75 patients survived.

Suppurative thrombophlebitis of the central veins is more difficult to diagnose, and the diagnosis must be made on venogram and positive culture. Treatment includes systemic antibiotics in maximum dosage, Fogarty catheter extraction in some, and heparin, if pulmonary embolism has occurred.

Pruitt emphasizes the prophylactic value of utilizing a vein underlying unburned skin to obtain access to the venous system, and strict cannula intravenous line asepsis must be observed to minimize intracannular contamination. The period of intravascular residence for an individual cannula in burn patients should be no longer than necessary and should be limited to a maximum of 72 hours.

In instances of non-suppurative superficial or saphenous thrombophlebitis with proximal extension, anticoagulants are used. If progression continues, proximal vein ligation at the saphenofemoral junction is performed.

Bibliography

1. Adelston, J., Steer, M., Glotzer, D. T., Skillman, J., Simon, M., and Salzman, E. W.: Thromboembolism after insertion of the Mobin-Uddin caval filter. Surgery 87:184, 1980.
2. Allgood, R. J., Cook, J. H., Weeder, R. J., Speed, H. K., Whitcomb, W. H., and Greenfield, L. J.: Prospective analysis of pulmonary embolism in the postoperative patient. Surgery 68:116, 1970.
3. Altemeier, W. A., Hill, O. E., and Fullen, W. D.: Acute and recurrent thromboembolic disease: New concept of etiology. Ann. Surg. 170:547, 1969.
4. Altemeier, W. A., McDonough, J. J., and Fullen, W. D.: Third day surgical fever. Arch. Surg. 103:158, 1971.
5. Anlyan, W. G., DeLaughter, G. D., Fabrikant, J. I., Sullenberger, J. W., and Weaver, W. T.: Management of acute venous thromboembolism. J.A.M.A. 168:725, 1958.
6. Atik, M., Hanson, B., Isla, F., and Harkess, J. W.: Pulmonary embolism: A preventable complication. Ann. Surg. 34:888, 1969.
7. Atkins, P., and Hawkins, L. A.: Detection of venous thrombosis in the legs. Lancet 2:1217, 1965.
8. Barker, W. F.: The management of venous thrombosis and pulmonary embolism. Surgery 45:198, 1959.
9. Barner, H. B., Willman, V. L., Kaiser, G. C., and Hanlon, C. R.: Thrombectomy for iliofemoral venous thrombosis. J.A.M.A. 208:2442, 1969.
10. Barnes, R. W., Brand, R. S., Clarke, W., Hartley, N., and Hoak, J. D.: Efficacy of graded-compression antiembolism stockings in patients undergoing total hip arthroplasty. Clin. Orthop. 132:61, 1978.
11. Beall, A. C., Cooley, D. A., and DeBakey, M. E.: Surgical management of pulmonary embolism. Dis. Chest. 47:382, 1965.
12. Bell, W. R., and Meek, A. G.: Guidelines for the use of thrombolytic agents. N. Engl. J. Med. 301:1266, 1979.
13. Berger, R. L.: Pulmonary embolectomy for massive embolization. Am. J. Surg. 121:437, 1971.
14. Blackman, J. R., and other principal investigators: Urokinase pulmonary embolism trial — Phase I Results — A Cooperative Study. J.A.M.A. 214:2163, 1970.
15. Brisman, R., Parks, L. C., and Haller, J. A.: Dextran prophylaxis in surgery. Ann. Surg. 174:137, 1971.
16. Brockman, S. K., and Vasco, J. S.: The pathologic

17. Cheney, F. W., Jr., and Lincoln, J. R.: Phlebitis from plastic intravenous catheters. Anesthesiology 25:92, 1964.
18. Collins, C. G., Norton, R. O., Nelson, E. W., Weinstein, B. B., Collins, J. H., and Webster, H. D.: Suppurative pelvic thrombophlebitis. IV. Results. Surgery 31:528, 1952.
19. Coon, W. W., and Coller, F. A.: Some epidemiological considerations of thromboembolism. Surg. Gynecol. Obstet. 109:487, 1959.
20. Coon, W. W., and Willis, P. W.: Deep venous thrombosis and pulmonary embolism —prediction, prevention and treatment. Am. J. Cardiol. 4:611, 1959.
21. Coon, W. W., and Willis, P. W.: Recurrence of venous thromboembolism. Surgery 73:823, 1973.
22. Cotton, L. T., and Roberts, V. C.: Prevention of postoperative deep venous thrombosis by intermittent compression of the legs. In Bergan, J. J., and Yao, J. S. T. (Eds.): Venous Problems. Chicago, Year Book Medical Publishers, 1978.
23. Crane, C.: Diagnosis and treatment of pulmonary embolism. Surg. Clin. North Am. 46:551, 1966.
24. Dale, W. A., and Lewis, M. R.: Heparin control of venous thromboembolism. Arch. Surg. 101:744, 1970.
25. Dalen, J. E., and Dexter, L.: Pulmonary embolism. J.A.M.A. 207:1505, 1969.
26. Dennis, C.: Discussion of Allgood, R. J., et al., Surgery 68:116, 1970.
27. DeTakats, G.: Thromboembolic disease and oral contraceptives. J.A.M.A., 206:2742, 1968.
28. Deuvaert, F. E., Dmochowski, J. R., and Couch, N. P.: Positional factors in venous impedance plethysmography. Arch. Surg. 106:43, 1973.
29. DeWeese, J. A.: Venous and lymphatic disease. In Schwartz, S. I. (Ed.): Principles of Surgery. New York, McGraw-Hill Book Company, 1969, p. 785.
30. DeWeese, M. S., and Hunter, D. C.: A vena cava filter for the prevention of pulmonary embolism. Bull. Soc. Int. Chir. 17:17, 1958.
31. Deykin, D.: Indications and techniques for the use of heparin in the treatment of thromboembolism. World J. Surg. 2:39, 1978.
32. Dmochowski, J. R., Adams, D. F., and Couch, N. P.: Impedance measurement in diagnosis of deep venous thrombosis. Arch. Surg. 104:170, 1972.
33. Drill, V. A.: Oral contraceptives and thromboembolic disease. J.A.M.A. 219:583, 1972.
34. Druskin, M. S., and Siegel, P. D.: Bacterial contamination of indwelling intravenous polyethylene catheters. J.A.M.A. 185:146, 1963.
35. Edwards, W. H., Sawyers, J. L., and Foster, J. H.: Iliofemoral venous thrombosis — Reappraisal of thrombectomy. Ann. Surg. 171:961, 1970.
36. Erwin, P., Strickler, J. H., and Rice, C. O.: Use of polyethylene tubing in intravenous therapy for surgical patients. Arch. Surg. 66:673, 1953.
37. Flanc, C., Kakkar, V. V., and Clarke, M. D.: Postoperative deep vein thrombosis — Effect

and intensive prophylaxis. Lancet *1*:477, 1969.

38. Frykholm, R.: Pathogenesis and mechanical prophylaxis of venous thrombosis. Surg. Gynecol. Obstet. *71*:307, 1940.

39. Gallus, A. S., Hirsh, J., O'Brien, S. E., McBride, J. A., Tuttle, R. J., and Gent, M.: Prevention of venous thrombosis with small subcutaneous dosages of heparin. J.A.M.A. *235*:1980, 1976.

40. Gazzaniga, A. B., Pacelo, A. F., Bartlett, R. H., and Geraghty, T. R.: Bilateral impedance rheography in diagnosis of deep vein thrombosis of the legs. Arch. Surg. *104*:515, 1972.

41. Goddard, J. L.: Letter. Food and Drug Administration, U.S. Dept. Health, Education and Welfare. Washington, D.C., May 10, 1968.

42. Greenfield, L. J.: Intraluminal techniques for vena caval interruption and pulmonary embolectomy. World J. Surg. *2*:45, 1978.

43. Greenfield, L. J., Reif, M. E., and Gunter, C. E.: Hemodynamic and respiratory response to transvenous pulmonary embolectomy. J. Thorac. Cardiovasc. Surg. *62*:890, 1971.

44. Greenfield, L. J., Zocco, J., Wilk, J., Schroeder, T. M., and Elkins, R. C.: Clinical experience with Kim-Ray Greenfield vena caval filters. Ann. Surg. *185*:692, 1977.

45. Grégoire, R.: La phlébite bleue (phlegmasia cerulea dolens). Presse Méd. *46*:1313, 1938.

46. Haller, J. A.: Thrombectomy for acute iliofemoral venous thrombosis. Arch. Surg. *83*:448, 1961.

47. Hartman, H.: Fatal pulmonary embolism. German Med. Monthly *10*:314, 1965.

48. Homans, J.: Deep quiet venous thrombosis in the lower limb. Surg. Gynecol. Obstet. *79*:70, 1944.

49. Hunter, W. C., Sneeden, V. D., Robertson, T. D., and Snyder, G. A. C.: Thrombosis of the deep veins of the leg. Arch. Intern. Med. *68*:1, 1941.

50. Husni, E. A., Ximenes, J. O. C., and Goyetti, E. M.: Elastic support of the lower limbs in hospital patients. J.A.M.A. *214*:1456, 1970.

51. Jick, H., Slone, D., Westerholm, B., et al.: Venous thromboembolic disease and ABO blood type. Lancet *1*:539, 1969.

52. Kakkar, V.: Current status of low-dose heparin in prophylaxis of thrombophlebitis and pulmonary embolism. World J. Surg. *1*:3, 1978.

53. Kakkar, V. V., Flanc, C., O'Shea, M. J., Flute, P. T., Howe, C. T., and Clarke, M. B.: Treatment of deep-vein thrombosis with streptokinase. Br. J. Surg. *56*:178, 1969.

54. Kakkar, V. V., Howe, C. T., Flanc, C., and Clarke, M. B.: Natural history of postoperative deep vein thrombosis. Lancet *2*:230, 1969.

55. Kistner, R. L., Ball, J. J., Nordyke, R. A., and Freeman, G. C.: Incidence of pulmonary embolism in thrombophlebitis of lower extremities. Am. J. Surg. *124*:169, 1972.

56. Lansing, A. M., and Davis, W. M.: Five year follow-up study of iliofemoral venous thrombectomy. Ann. Surg. *168*:620, 1968.

57. Lewis, M. R., and Dale, W. A.: Practical value of phlebography. South. Med. J. *73*:9, 1980.

58. Lindhagen, J., Haglund, M., Haglund, U., Holm,

J., and Schersten, T.: Iliofemoral venous thrombectomy. J. Cardiovasc. Surg. (Torino) *19*:319, 1978.

59. Macon, W. L., Morton, J. H., and Adams, J. T.: Significant complications of anticoagulants. Surgery *68*:571, 1970.

60. Mahorner, H., Castleberry, J. W., and Coleman, W. O.: Attempts to restore function in major veins which are the site of massive thrombosis. Ann. Surg. *146*:510, 1957.

61. Mavor, G. E., and Galloway, J. M. D.: Iliofemoral venous thrombosis — Pathological considerations and surgical management. Br. J. Surg. *56*:4, 1969.

62. May, I. A., Samson, P. G., and Mittal, A.: Surgical management of patients with complications of pulmonary infarction due to nonseptic pulmonary emboli. Am. J. Surg. *124*:223, 1972.

63. McDonough, J. J., and Altemeier, W. A.: Subclavian vein thrombosis secondary to indwelling catheters. Surg. Gynecol. Obstet. *133*:397, 1971.

64. McNamara, M., Takaki, H. W., and Yao, J.: Venous diseases. Surg. Clin. North Am. *54*:1201, 1977.

65. Meeker, C. I.: Use of drugs and intrauterine devices for birth control. N. Engl. J. Med. *280*:1058, 1969.

66. Miles, R. M., Chappell, F., and Renner, O.: A partially occluding vena caval clip for prevention of pulmonary embolism. Am. Surg. *30*:40, 1964.

67. Miles, R. M., and Elsea, P. W.: Clinical evaluation of the serrated vena caval clip. Surg. Gynecol. Obstet. *132*:581, 1971.

68. Miles, R. M., Flowers, B. F., Parsons, L., and Benitone, J. D.: Some surgical implications of the anatomy of the cava-iliofemoral system. Ann. Surg. *177*:740, 1973.

69. Miles, R. M., Richardson, R. R., Wayne, L., Elsea, P. W., Stewart, S. B., and Duncan, D.: Long-term results with the serrated Teflon vena caval clip in the prevention of pulmonary embolism. Ann. Surg. *169*:881, 1969.

70. Miles, R. M., and Young, J. M.: Recanalization of the vena cava: An experimental study. Surgery *33*:849, 1953.

71. Milne, R. M., Griffiths, J. M. T., Gunn, A. A., and Ruckley, C. V.: Postoperative deep venous thrombosis: Comparison of diagnostic techniques. Lancet *2*:445, 1971.

72. Mobin-Uddin, K., Collard, G. M., Bolooki, H., et al.: Transverse caval interruption with umbrella filter. New Engl. J. Med. *286*:55, 1972.

73. Moretz, W. H., Rhode, C. M., and Shepherd, M. H.: Prevention of pulmonary embolism by partial occlusion of the inferior vena cava. Am. Surg. *25*:617, 1959.

74. Morrell, M. T., and Dunnill, M. S.: The postmortem incidence of pulmonary embolism in a hospital population. Br. J. Surg. *55*:347, 1968.

75. Moser, K. M., Brach, B., and Dolan, G. F.: Clinically suspected deep venous thrombosis of the lower extremities — A comparison of venography, impedance plethysmography and ra-

diolabeled fibrinogen. J.A.M.A. *237*:2195, 1977.

76. Nanson, E. M., Palko, P. D., Dick, A. A., and Fedoruk, M. A.: Early detection of deep venous thrombosis of the legs using I_{131} tagged human fibrinogen. Ann. Surg. *162*:438, 1965.

77. Nejad, M. S., Klaper, F. R., Steggerda, F. R., and Gianturco, C.: Clotting on the outer surfaces of vascular catheters. Radiology *91*:248, 1968.

78. Nicholaides, A. N., DuPont, P. A., Desal, S. T., et al.: Small doses of subcutaneous sodium heparin in preventing deep venous thrombosis after major surgery. Lancet *2*:890, 1972.

79. Ochsner, A., and DeBakey, M.: Intravenous clotting and its sequelae. Surgery *14*:679, 1943.

80. Ochsner, A., Ochsner, J. L., and Sanders, H. S.: Prevention of pulmonary embolism by caval ligation. Ann. Surg. *171*:923, 1970.

81. O'Donnell, T. F., Abbott, W. M., and Darling, R. C.: D.V.T. or not D.V.T. — That is the question. Surgery *79*:606, 1976.

82. O'Donnell, T. F., Abbott, W. M., Athanasoulis, C. A., Millan, V. G., and Callow, A. D.: Diagnosis of deep venous thrombosis in the out-patient by venography. Surg. Gynecol. Obstet. *150*:69, 1980.

83. Oster, M. W., and Leslie, B.: Syncope and pulmonary embolism. J.A.M.A. *224*:630, 1973.

84. Parsons, L., and Sommers, S. C.: Gynecology. Philadelphia, W.B. Saunders Company, 1962, pp. 551–553.

85. Paterson, J. C., and McLachlin, J.: Precipitating factors in venous thrombosis. Surg. Gynecol. Obstet. *98*:96, 1954.

86. Peters, W. R., Bush, W. H., McIntyre, R. D., and Hill, D.: The development of fibrin sheath on indwelling venous catheters. Surg. Gynecol. Obstet. *137*:43, 1973.

87. Pollak, E. W., Sparks, F. C., and Barker, W. F.: Pulmonary embolism — An appraisal of therapy in 516 cases. Arch. Surg. *107*:66, 1973.

88. Pruitt, B. A., McManus, W. F., Kim, S. H., and Treat, R. C.: Diagnosis and treatment of cannula related intravenous sepsis in burn patients. Presented before the Southern Surgical Association, December, 1979.

89. Qureshi, G. D., and Lilly, E. L.: Complications of CVP catheter insertion in cubital vein. J.A.M.A. *209*:1906, 1969.

90. Sabiston, D. C., Wolfe, W. G., Oldham, H. W., Wechsler, A. S., Crawford, F. A., Jones, K. W., and Jones, R. H.: Surgical management of chronic pulmonary embolism. Ann. Surg. *185*:699, 1977.

91. Salzman, E. W., Harris, W. H., and DeSanctis, R. W.: Anticoagulation for prevention of thromboembolism. N. Engl. J. Med. *275*:122, 1966.

92. Salzman, E. W., Harris, W. H., and DeSanctis, R. W.: Reduction in venous thromboembolism by agents affecting platelet function. N. Engl. J. Med. *284*:1287, 1971.

93. Scully, N. M.: A new look at pulmonary embolism. Surg. Clin. North Am. *50*:343, 1970.

94. Sevitt, S.: Venous thrombosis and pulmonary embolism — Their prevention by oral anticoagulants. Am. J. Med. *33*:703, 1962.

95. Sharma, G. V. R. K., and Sasahara, W. A.: Diagnosis and treatment of pulmonary embolism. Med. Clin. North Am. *62*:239, 1979.

96. Sharp, E. H.: Pulmonary embolectomy: Successful removal of a massive pulmonary embolus with the support of a cardiopulmonary bypass. Ann. Surg. *156*:1, 1962.

97. Shoobridge, M.: Do massive clots form instantly? Med. World News. Oct. 10, 1970, p. 16.

98. Spencer, F. C.: An experimental evaluation of partitioning of the inferior vena cava to prevent pulmonary embolism. Surg. Forum *10*:680, 1959.

99. Stein, J. M., and Pruitt, B. A., Jr.: Suppurative thrombophlebitis — A lethal iatrogenic disease. N. Engl. J. Med. *282*:1452, 1970.

100. Strandness, D. E.: Prevention of deep venous thrombosis in general surgical patients. Contemp. Surg. *14*:55, 1979.

101. Strandness, D. E., Jr., and Sumner, D. S.: Ultrasonic velocity detector in diagnosis of thrombophlebitis. Arch. Surg. *104*:180, 1972.

102. Thomas, D. P.: Treatment of pulmonary embolic disease. N. Engl. J. Med. *273*:885, 1965.

103. Tremolières, F., and Veran, P.: Syndrome d'oblitération arterielle du membre inférieur droit apparu au cours d'une phlébite superficielle et profonde avec embolies pulmonaires. Effet thérapeutique de l'acetylcholine. Bull. Méd. Paris *43*:1101, 1929.

104. Tsapogas, M. J., Goussous, H., Peabody, R. A., et al.: Postoperative venous thrombosis and effectiveness of prophylactic measures. Arch. Surg. *103*:561, 1971.

105. Urokinase-Streptokinase Embolism Trial. Phase 2 Results. J.A.M.A. *229*:1606, 1974.

106. Von Gizycki, A. C., Gannon, P., and Tassel, R. V.: Distal migration of vena cava filter. J.A.M.A. *224*:529, 1973.

107. Wessler, S.: Prevention of venous thromboembolism by low-dose heparin. Mod. Concepts Cardiovasc. Dis. *65*:105, 1976.

108. Wheeler, H. B.: Impedance testing for venous thrombosis. Arch. Surg. *106*:762, 1973.

109. Wheeler, H. B., Pearson, D., and Mullick, S. C.: Impedance phlebography: Technique, interpretation, and results. Arch. Surg. *104*:164, 1972.

10

COMPLICATIONS OF ANESTHESIA

John E. Forestner*

Surgery and anesthesia have developed as parallel specialties, mutually dependent on each other for continued scientific progress in their separate but closely related spheres. As the length, complexity, and invasiveness of surgical procedures have grown steadily in recent decades, the benefits of these extensive operations are being offered to patients whose disease involvement would have contraindicated surgery and anesthesia only a few years ago. The role of anesthesia in adapting to the challenges of surgical innovation has been essential in assuring maximum survival and minimum morbidity for such patients under our care.

Improvements in anesthetic techniques, based on research conducted by basic scientists, surgeons, and anesthesiologists, have radically altered the practice of anesthesia over the last 30 years. In pharmacology, the use of newer, volatile anesthetic agents, narcotics, muscle relaxants, and vasoactive agents deserves mention. The importance of fluid management in the perioperative period has become generally recognized, and effective respiratory support methods

for the intraoperative and postoperative period have been developed. Also, the wider utilization of laboratory data and physiologic parameters measured with invasive monitoring has markedly improved survival rates in surgery and critical care.

As a result of these significant advances, today's patient often expects that no harm will come from pharmacologic therapy or physiologic monitoring during surgery. Unfortunately, each innovation in surgical therapy entails some risk of complications, and anesthesia has been implicated in a substantial portion of these perioperative complications. It is generally accepted that the risk of morbidity and mortality from surgery is roughly correlated with the preoperative physical status of the patient.[1, 16] However, a large percentage of perioperative complications related to *anesthesia* occurs in previously healthy individuals undergoing relatively minor procedures. The causes of cardiac arrest associated with anesthesia reported in several series would suggest that the majority of these episodes are preventable, are due to human error, and are unrelated to the severity of patient disease.[6, 27, 33] While it is unlikely that even the most careful patient observation will en-

*This chapter was contributed by Dr. Hamilton S. Davis in the previous edition.

John Edward Forestner grew up in southern Illinois near St. Louis and received his undergraduate and medical degrees from Northwestern University in Chicago. He completed several years of surgery training at the University of Mississippi and subsequently completed a residency in anesthesiology at the University of Texas Southwestern Medical School in Dallas. After a teaching fellowship in pediatric anesthesia in Dallas and two years in the Army, he returned to the University of Mississippi as Director of Pediatric Anesthesia. He has since moved to Atlanta, where he is an Assistant Professor in the Pediatric Section of the Department of Anesthesiology at the Emory University School of Medicine.

tirely prevent anesthetic morbidity and mortality, the central importance of vigilant monitoring must be stressed from the outset. Furthermore, because complications are so frequently associated with innovations in surgery and anesthesia, a critical risk-benefit assessment is essential before new techniques can be generally accepted or specifically applied.

As important as it is to recognize and treat complications occurring during the course of anesthesia, this alone will not guarantee avoidance of anesthetic morbidity and mortality. In addition, the anesthesiologist must anticipate and prevent problems before they occur. Accordingly, throughout the discussion to follow, the *prior prevention, early detection,* and *proper treatment* of anesthetic complications will be discussed in turn.

Just as it is appropriate to divide the perioperative period into three time segments, the discussion will be divided into three sections: *the preoperative period,* the time to anticipate problems and begin preventive measures; the *operative period,* during which the stresses of the anesthesia-surgical experience are interrelated; and the *postoperative period,* the time when the therapy for significant anesthetic complications will be initiated or maintained.

PREOPERATIVE PERIOD

Anticipation of complications requires a careful pre-anesthetic evaluation of each patient by the responsible anesthesiologist. A thorough review of the chart and the available past medical history is followed by a personal interview that should include a physical examination appropriate to the circumstances. A tentative anesthetic plan is then decided upon and discussed with the patient (see Counseling and Informed Consent, below). Occasionally information obtained on the preoperative visit will indicate that additional laboratory tests are needed to complete the patient's work-up. Prophylactic measures may also be undertaken at this time to lessen or prevent complications later. Important considerations that significantly affect the choice of anesthetic technique will be discussed under four headings: the general medical condition of the patient, the cardiovascular system, the res-

piratory system, and the medications the patient is using.

General Medical Condition

Examination of the patient and review of the medical history may reveal important factors that can affect anesthetic management and suggest problems to be anticipated.

MENTAL STATUS. Moderate to severe depression of the sensorium may be caused by drugs, metabolic disease, increased intracranial pressure, cerebrovascular insufficiency, or in extreme instances, cardiovascular collapse. As evidence of severe cerebral malfunction, depression of sensorium suggests that serious complications may be expected under anesthesia, particularly when the reason for the problem is obscure. Appropriate consultation and diagnostic tests should be sought to determine the cause, and attempts to treat the disorder should be made prior to surgery if morbidity is to be minimized.

To the opposite extreme, the anxious, hysterical, belligerent, mentally retarded, or juvenile patient may be detected on the preoperative visit, and can be reassured and heavily sedated prior to anesthesia. Even with adequate preoperative medication these patients may still be poor candidates for conduction anesthesia.

THE AIRWAY. Difficulties with airway control may be anticipated in obese patients and in patients with prominent incisors, a high narrow maxilla, or receding chins. The mobility of the cervical spine and the temporomandibular joint must be carefully assessed by having the patient rotate his head from side to side and open his mouth as wide as possible. Induction of general anesthesia may cause relaxation of muscles and overlying soft tissues surrounding the airway, especially the tongue. In patients with poor skeletal mobility and small upper airways, this relaxation may lead to upper airway obstruction, and difficulty in attempts to re-establish the airway may then be compounded by this anatomic restriction, especially during endotracheal intubation. Conduction anesthesia should be considered under these circumstances, when it is appropriate to the surgical procedure and not contraindicated by obesity, childhood, or other factors. For procedures not compatible with regional techniques, blind nasal intubation or fiberoptic nasal intubation should be considered, after adequate sedation, so the airway can be secured before induction of general anesthesia.[26]

Loose teeth, removable dentures and bridges, and intra-oral infections should be carefully searched for and noted. It is often advisable to have extremely loose teeth extracted prior to surgery, rather than risk losing them in the upper airway and having to locate then intraoperatively. Removable dental prostheses should be left in the room before the patient goes to surgery. Dentures may be useful in facilitating airway maintenance in the edentulous patient, but they complicate endotracheal intubation and may be damaged or misplaced during removal and storage.

Extensive intra-oral infections, e.g., oropharyngeal cellulitis, can be extremely hazardous. Ludwig's angina and peritonsillar abscess are two such conditions that predispose to loss of the airway during anesthetic induction, distort the anatomy, and interfere with attempts to re-establish the airway. If possible, the infection should be controlled with antibiotics prior to surgery. If incision and drainage are necessary and the extent of airway obstruction is moderate to severe when the patient is first examined, *the airway must be secured before the patient is rendered unconscious.* Four alternatives should be considered: awake oral intubation with topical anesthesia, blind awake nasal intubation, fiberoptic nasal intubation, or elective tracheostomy with local anesthesia. Most of these patients are febrile, dehydrated, and exhausted, so sedation must be given sparingly and with close monitoring.

PHYSICAL STATUS. The nutritional status should be readily apparent and can be a significant indicator of increased risk of complications. Obese patients have increased perioperative respiratory complications, and technical difficulties can be anticipated with endotracheal intubation, venipuncture, and conduction anesthesia. Malnourished patients are typically anemic with contracted circulating blood volumes, and they have critical deficiencies of carbohydrates, proteins, and electrolytes. Circulatory instability and exaggerated cardiovascular depression owing to anesthetic agents should be anticipated.

Hypothermia presents no problem unless it is excessive. Hyperthermia is always undesirable, because it results in increased oxygen and anesthetic requirements, metabolic acidosis, and central nervous system irritability, particularly in children. Elective procedures should be postponed until the cause has been diagnosed and treated. If emergency surgery is imperative, vigorous steps must be taken to cool the patient before anesthesia.

METABOLIC DISEASES. Careful preoperative assessment should be made of patients with diabetes mellitus, adrenal cortical insufficiency, and porphyria.

The patient with maturity-onset diabetes mellitus controlled with oral hypoglycemic agents seldom has any difficulty during elective surgery; but hyperglycemia and ketosis may occur under stress, which increases insulin requirements, so it is usually advisable to discontinue the oral drug and regulate the blood sugar with parenteral insulin. Several days of observation of the diabetic patient preoperatively may be required to assess the adequacy of control with insulin. While several regimens are recommended for the day of surgery, it would seem most prudent to give less than the usual amount of insulin before surgery, while infusing generous amounts of glucose and checking the serum glucose level at frequent intervals to guide therapy.[24] The physician who normally manages the patient's disease can often be quite helpful during the perioperative period and should be consulted.

Emergency surgery is hazardous in the diabetic patient unless ketoacidosis is reasonably controlled. In an emergency, the diabetic is frequently dehydrated and febrile, with a variable but usually increased insulin requirement. Again, frequent monitoring of serum glucose and electrolytes during initial treatment and throughout surgery is mandatory if the extremes of hyperglycemia and hypoglycemia are to be successfully avoided.

Any patient who has received systemic glucocorticoid therapy for four days or longer during the preceding six months may potentially develop circulatory instability from iatrogenic adrenal cortical insufficiency due to the stress of surgery.[35] Supplemental corticosteroids should be administered prophylactically to any patient with a history of recent steroid therapy, whether or not they exhibit symptoms of adrenal insufficiency before operation.

Porphyria is a rare inherited disorder of porphyrin metabolism that is significant in anesthetic care because certain drugs, particularly barbiturates, may be lethal when administered to patients with this disease. Neurologic symptoms are common, so conduction techniques are usually avoided.

NEUROLOGIC CONSIDERATIONS. History of familial dysautonomia, neuromuscular dystrophies, myasthenia gravis, or other neurologic disease should indicate consultation with the patient's neurologist for assistance in perioperative management. Careful evaluation of baseline respiratory function in these patients is essential, because of the high probability of postoperative respiratory failure. In patients with recent burns or trauma or progressive neurologic disease with muscular atrophy, the depolarizing muscle relaxant succinylcholine may cause excessive potassium release from muscle tissue and resulting cardiac arrest. High-risk patients should be detected preoperatively, and the use of this drug should be avoided. (See Muscle Relaxants, below.)

Patients who are being considered for conduction anesthesia should be carefully examined for neurologic deficits during the preoperative physical examination, and if any abnormalities are detected, they should be carefully documented on the chart prior to the block. If such deficits have not previously been diagnosed, some explanation for the problem should be sought. The conduction technique must clearly be of benefit to be justified in the presence of prior neurologic damage, and careful documentation and patient counseling will be important in reducing the risk of subsequent litigation. A good example of the use of conduction anesthesia in the patient with prior neurologic damage is the paraplegic patient with a history of autonomic dysreflexia, in whom spinal or epidural anesthesia may protect against the typical severe hypertensive responses seen in such individuals.[32]

Obesity or anatomic deformity in the area of intended regional block would be considered relative contraindications to conduction anesthesia because of associated technical problems. Systemic anticoagulation or infection in the area of the injection is considered an absolute contraindication to regional techniques because of the complications that may result.

THE FULL STOMACH. The patient with a full stomach, who presents as an emergency or with bowel obstruction, is at high risk of regurgitation and aspiration of stomach contents into the trachea during induction of and emergence from anesthesia. The aspiration pneumonitis that may result is one of the most feared anesthetic complications, and one that has a high associated mortality. Attempts to empty the stomach preoperatively are generally ineffective in emergency patients, so those at risk of aspiration must be noted preoperatively and special precautions taken to protect the airway during anesthesia. (See Emergency Surgery, below.)

THE SURGICAL HISTORY. Previous surgical procedures and associated anesthetic experiences should be discussed with the patient. Any pleasant or unpleasant recollections should be examined, especially as they may affect patient preferences or the choice of anesthetic technique by the anesthesiologist.

Specific information about drug allergies should be obtained and offending drugs avoided. While true allergies to anesthetic drugs are rare, hepatic or renal damage may follow the administration of halogenated hydrocarbons in susceptible individuals, so that one should ask about previous exposure to the volatile anesthetic agents halothane,[20] enflurane,[8] or methoxyflurane,[19] and any postanesthetic symptoms that were noted. Any adverse renal or hepatic reaction contraindicates subsequent use of that agent in that patient. The fact that unexplained fever followed prior administration of an anesthetic agent is in itself insufficient reason to withhold the agent if good indications for its use are present.[11] There is not sufficient support at this time for the concept of a specific minimum time interval that should elapse between exposures to an anesthetic to minimize the risk of reactions.

One should also be alert for a history of previous unusual responses to muscle relaxants in patients or their families. Of particular interest is prolonged apnea following succinylcholine, which may represent chemical or hereditary plasma cholinesterase deficiency which causes delay in metabolism of the drug. Succinylcholine should be avoided in these individuals, and their families should be questioned about similar difficulties that may have occurred in relatives. (See Muscle Relaxants, below.)

As part of the family history, questions about anesthetic difficulties with high fevers and sudden death during surgery should be asked. Malignant hyperthermia, a recently recognized and rare but highly lethal complication associated with administration of general anesthesia to susceptible persons, can be avoided only through awareness of a history of familial incidence of the disease. (See Malignant Hyperthermia, below.)

CARDIOVASCULAR SYSTEM

Computer analysis of both prospective and retrospective data has demonstrated that certain clinical indicators correlate well with the risk of cardiovascular complications in the perioperative period. A study of 1001 patients over 40 years of age defined nine significant risk factors and weighted them according to their relative contributions to overall cardiovascular morbidity and mortality.[13] The two most heavily weighted preoperative predictors of cardiovascular complications were a history of myocardial infarction in the previous six months, and uncontrolled congestive heart failure as evidenced by an S_3 gallop or jugular venous distention seen on the preoperative physical examination. Less heavily weighted were two significant factors related to cardiac rhythm: the presence of greater than 5 premature ventricular contractions per minute documented at any time before operation, or a rhythm other than sinus or premature atrial contractions, seen on the last preoperative electrocardiogram. Also important, but of less predictive value, were such factors as age greater than 70; clinically significant valvular aortic stenosis; emergency surgery; thoracic, abdominal, or aortic surgery; and abnormal laboratory results suggestive of pulmonary, renal, or hepatic dysfunction. Multifactorial combination of these indices was shown to be highly

predictive of cardiovascular complications in individual patients from the series. While a rough correlation could be shown between this Goldman Index and the physical status classification of the American Society of Anesthesiologists, the former was much more successfully predictive of specific cardiovascular mortality in the study group. (See Assessment of Physical Status, below.)

Another attempt to predict cardiovascular complications in 566 peripheral vascular surgical patients defined six risk factors. An equation relating these factors to the incidence of complications was generated, and the equation had a high predictive reliability when used prospectively.[7] These factors in descending order of importance were angina pectoris, a history of myocardial infarction, congestive heart failure, arrhythmia, an abnormal electrocardiogram, and a history of cerebrovascular accident. The study emphasized that these factors predicted cardiovascular morbidity and mortality even after control of symptoms was attempted prior to surgery, but the effect of preoperative medical therapy on outcome was not assessed.

It has been pointed out that these risk assessment schemes should have good predictive accuracy when applied to the series from which they were derived and that validation will depend on further prospective analyses.[23] Nevertheless, they serve to underline those cardiovascular risk factors that must be detected during the preoperative visit, evaluated, and if possible, treated. Control of angina, congestive heart failure, and arrhythmias should be attempted in consultation with a cardiologist prior to surgery, and the resulting benefit to be derived in lessened morbidity and mortality cannot be seriously questioned.

Risk factors that cannot be controlled by therapy, such as age, debility, and recent myocardial infarction, must be carefully weighed in the decision to proceed with anesthesia and surgery. Purely elective surgery should be deferred until 6 months after a documented myocardial infarction. After 6 months, the perioperative reinfarction rate can be expected to stabilize at around 5 per cent and remain at that level for several years, so further temporizing would not seem justified.[30] A reinfarction rate of 27 per cent in the first 3 months and a 69 per cent mortality associated with reinfarction serve to emphasize the grave risk of unnecessary surgery in patients with recent transmural myocardial infarction.

All patients with cardiac symptoms and all patients above an arbitrarily set age at which the incidence of cardiovascular disease becomes significant (age 35 is a commonly accepted limit) should have a preoperative electrocardiogram. Careful consideration must also be given at this time to the need for invasive cardiovascular monitoring during surgery and afterward, and the anesthesiologist must be prepared to counsel the patient about the advantages and risks involved (see Invasive Monitoring, below).

Prevention of anesthetic morbidity related to the peripheral circulation will require assessment of fluid status, the blood hemoglobin level, and the presence of hypertension or hypotension. Also of concern are obliterative diseases of the cerebral or pulmonary vasculature that may pose particularly serious risks.

HYPOVOLEMIA. Decreased circulating blood volume from hemorrhage, dehydration, or starvation may impair the ability of the patient to compensate for anesthetic-induced cardiac depression or vasodilatation, and serious hypotension may follow. Every attempt should be made to restore an adequate blood volume before induction of anesthesia.

THE HEMOGLOBIN LEVEL. The anemic patient compensates for a reduced blood oxygen–carrying capacity by increasing cardiac output and plasma volume. Evidence from animal studies suggests that while anesthesia seems to reverse this compensation, it is well tolerated with no signs of peripheral acidosis or myocardial failure after reduction of the hematocrit to levels of 20 per cent or below.[15] Wide experience with the chronic anemia of renal failure has demonstrated that anesthesia can be performed with minimum risk of complications related to the low hemoglobin level. In children, however, data have been presented that relate an increased risk of cardiac arrest to uncorrected preoperative anemia.[27] The presence of increased oxygen consumption during childhood or with fever, or the suggestion of potential airway difficulties would prompt serious consideration of correction of anemia before surgery. The arbitrary

imposition of a limit of 10 gm./dl. of hemoglobin required before induction of anesthesia would not appear to be supported by available evidence.

When time permits, attempts should be made to improve severe degrees of anemia through appropriate iron therapy. When this fails in elective situations, or in emergencies, packed red blood cells are probably indicated before anesthesia and operation if the hemoglobin is less than 7.0 to 8.0 gm./dl. Such transfusions must be given slowly to avoid precipitating congestive heart failure. The particular problems of sickle cell disease will be discussed in the section on anesthetic management. (See Sickle Cell Disease, below.)

Polycythemia causes an increase in blood viscosity and is associated with a high incidence of thrombotic and hemorrhagic complications during and after surgery. Phlebotomy can be used with plasma volume supplementation to reduce red cell mass prior to surgery in patients with primary polycythemia, in the case of emergencies, or when the disease has not been responsive to long-term medical therapy such as radioactive phosphorus. Repeated venesection, however, only further stimulates the bone marrow and can be harmful in altering the compensatory balance achieved in secondary polycythemia associated with cyanosis.

HYPERTENSION. It is generally held that essential hypertension must be controlled pharmacologically prior to elective surgery, and that therapy must be maintained up until the day of surgery so that labile vasomotor responses will be minimized. This opinion has been examined by a prospective study of 676 patients over 40 years of age, which showed little variation between tightly controlled and uncontrolled moderate hypertensive patients, when indices of blood pressure stability during anesthesia and perioperative cardiovascular complications were evaluated.[12] Mild hypertensives either with or without treatment were apparently not at increased risk of perioperative cardiovascular morbidity when they were carefully managed in surgery. It was concluded from the study that elective surgical procedures in the absence of ideal hypertensive control should not subject patients to increased risk of complications provided that the diastolic blood pressure is stable and 110 torr or less, and provided that the systolic blood pressure is maintained above 66 per cent of the waking values throughout the procedure. Patients with more severe hypertension are at higher risk of precipitous falls in blood pressure and resulting myocardial and cerebral ischemia. In the essential hypertensive patient with diastolic pressures over 110 torr, preoperative control is still unquestionably of benefit.[25]

HYPOTENSION. Hypotension related to shock, hypovolemia, cardiac failure, or drug depression should be investigated and treated before anesthesia. Excessive premedication is frequently the cause. Patients who normally have a low blood pressure will seldom encounter difficulty with a well-managed anesthetic.

CEREBROVASCULAR DISEASE. Even short periods of hypoxia or hypotension can result in cerebral ischemia or infarction in patients with compromised cerebral circulation, and prolonged somnolence or permanent neurologic deficit may then occur. Consideration should be given to surgical correction of accessible carotid artery lesions prior to elective surgery in other anatomic regions.

PULMONARY HYPERTENSION. Obliterative disease of the pulmonary arterial circulation can be caused by conditions that produce persistent elevations of the pulmonary blood pressure or flow; it can occasionally be primary without apparent cause. This must be recognized before induction of anesthesia because the cardiac output is relatively fixed, and the right ventricle may be in failure. Cardiac reserve is thus limited, and hypoxemia may result from increasing imbalance between ventilation and perfusion that follows anesthetic induction. These patients tolerate only the most careful induction using limited amounts of anesthetic agents.

RESPIRATORY SYSTEM

The incidence of respiratory complications after anesthesia and surgery, 5 to 10 per cent in an unselected population, has not changed appreciably in the last half century, despite better understanding of the pathogenesis, prevention, and treatment of pulmonary complications.[21] Willingness to accept patients at increased risk of respiratory morbidity as candidates for surgery has of course been an important factor in maintaining this level of complications in the face of great advances in pulmonary medicine. Symptoms of pulmonary complications in the postoperative period include sputum production, fever, rales, rhonchi, clinical or radiologic evidence of atelectasis and consolidation, and, at the worst, frank respiratory failure requiring ventilatory support. Because preoperative evaluation and therapy have been effective in decreasing these postoperative respiratory complications, the pre-anesthetic visit is considered essential if adequate preparation is to be undertaken.

Risk factors clearly associated with increased respiratory morbidity would include the site and duration of surgery, age, obesity, smoking history, and the presence of dyspnea or productive cough in the preoperative period. Careful questioning of the patient may indicate that considering the above risk factors, further laboratory investigation of pulmonary reserve is indicated, and that preoperative therapy may be helpful in decreasing complications.

While bedside maneuvers such as testing the ability to hold the breath for 30 seconds or the ability to extinguish a match at 6 inches with the mouth widely open may suggest respiratory abnormalities, much more sensitive and predictive tests are available. Arterial blood gas analysis and spirometric pulmonary function tests can be obtained in most hospitals, can be performed at the bedside if necessary, and should be obtained in *every patient* with significant respiratory symptoms. Results of these tests serve two important functions: when they are abnormal, they are highly predictive of respiratory morbidity after surgery, and they establish baseline values for the patient's usual level of respiratory performance. Pulmonary function tests would appear to be the most sensitive available predictors of respiratory complications related to anesthesia.[31]

Reduction of ventilatory volumes is a significant factor in producing respiratory morbidity. The incidence of complications after upper abdominal and thoracic surgery can be directly related to the extent of reduction in the vital capacity seen during recovery. The effectiveness of cough is reduced at low lung volumes, and the sigh mechanism is depressed by narcotics given for pain, so a higher risk of pulmonary morbidity would be anticipated after upper abdominal or thoracic surgery than after more superficial procedures. Restricted ventilatory volumes in the obese patient or those associated with infection of the respiratory tract, abdominal distention, or skeletal malformations of the thorax, lead frequently to atelectasis and pneumonitis after anesthesia and surgery.

Detection of preoperative respiratory tract infections is an indication for appropriate cultures and antibiotic therapy. Surgery should be deferred when possible to allow time for treatment. The acutely or chronically infected airway is extremely irritable, and an increased incidence of coughing, laryngospasm, and bronchospasm should be anticipated during anesthesia under these circumstances. Appropriate aerosol and systemic bronchodilator therapy may be needed to open small airways, thus mobilizing secretions and partially correcting deficits in oxygenation. Maximum benefit from such treatment is desirable before surgery, and confirmation of therapeutic benefit should be sought with appropriate repeat testing. Warm aerosol therapy, positive pressure breathing, chest physical therapy, and incentive spirometry will help mobilize secretions in both acutely and chronically infected patients. Preoperative training in these maneuvers to increase ventilatory volumes and to aid in the clearance of secretions has been shown to increase their effectiveness in the postoperative period, and use of these maneuvers can reduce the incidence of respiratory morbidity by over half.[34] Skilled assistance from the respiratory therapist is invaluable in this regard.

The incidence of pulmonary complications in cigarette smokers is from 2 to 6 times the normal rate. If the patient can stop smoking several weeks in advance of surgery, there may be a slight improvement in respiratory status. There are indications, however, that stopping the habit just prior to surgery may increase secretions and have a deleterious effect.[5] Thus we have stopped recommending abrupt discontinuation of smoking when the patient enters the hospital, because anxiety is increased, patient compliance is poor, and the benefit is dubious.

The preoperative electrocardiogram may show signs of right ventricular hypertrophy or strain indicative of cor pulmonale, and digitalization may be necessary prior to surgery if cardiac reserve is compromised. The chest x-ray should be checked for infiltrates or hyperinflation, indicating possible sources of intraoperative difficulties.

The fact that the preoperative arterial blood gas values are normal is no assurance of adequate pulmonary reserve. However, the pulmonary function tests can be an excellent guide to respiratory reserve and can help predict ventilatory complications perioperatively. The forced vital capacity, a measure of lung volume that indicates possible restrictive disease, can be combined with the timed forced expiratory volume, a measure of ventilatory performance that indicates airway obstruction, to allow rough prediction of respiratory morbidity. The Miller nomogram (Fig. 10–1) is a useful predictor of ventilatory problems in the postoperative period, particularly of acute respiratory failure.[17] Severe combined obstructive and restrictive disease may indicate that the risk of anesthesia and surgery in a patient is prohibitive and should be under-

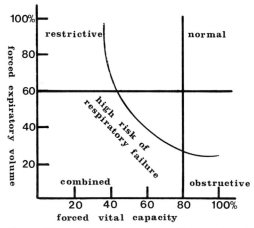

Figure 10–1 The Miller nomogram[17] relates the risk of postoperative respiratory failure to the patient's performance on a combination of two pulmonary function tests prior to surgery. A substantial percentage of those patients in the high risk area will require postoperative ventilatory support.

taken only when there is imminent threat to life. This relationship of respiratory morbidity to an index of combined pulmonary function test results has been summarized by Shapiro[29] in a useful rule: For an upper abdominal procedure in a patient with normal cardiovascular, hepatorenal, and central nervous systems, if the forced vital capacity (expressed as a per cent of the predicted value) combined with the forced expiratory volume over 1 second (expressed as a per cent of the vital capacity) add up to less than 100 per cent, there is a 50 per cent incidence of acute ventilatory failure in the first postoperative day, which will require committing the patient to ventilatory support. Significant disease in other systems will increase the chance of respiratory morbidity even more and should be taken into consideration of over-all risk.

Specific estimation of pulmonary reserve in candidates for pulmonary resection or pneumonectomy may require specialized split pulmonary function testing using a double lumen endotracheal tube. Balloon occlusion of the pulmonary artery on the side to be resected may be combined with these split lung functions, with and without exercise, to increase the predictive ability of these tests.[2] This is a controversial area, however, and generalization as to risk assessment in such patients is difficult on the basis of available data.

In summary, the preoperative respiratory evaluation should cover the history and manifestations of pulmonary disease in the patient, and appropriate testing will facilitate the estimate of risk and guide preoperative respiratory therapy. The judicious use of regional anesthesia techniques when appropriate may be of advantage in patients with significant pulmonary disease. Intraoperative monitoring of arterial blood gases will be indicated in most patients with respiratory disease undergoing surgery, and the choice between spontaneous and controlled ventilation during and after surgery will be primarily determined by the preoperative pulmonary assessment. Again the anesthesiologist must be prepared to counsel the patient with respiratory disease about the necessity of preoperative tests, the relative risk of pulmonary complications, and the possibility of postoperative ventilatory support when appropriate.

MEDICATIONS

Drugs the patient is taking before surgery may interact with anesthetic agents and may have potentially harmful effects during surgery, and should be carefully evaluated beforehand. With each drug the benefit of continued therapy must be weighed aganst the risk of drug-related complications under anesthesia. Most anesthesiologists now recognize the benefits of maintaining antihypertensive and psychopharmacologic therapy up until the time of operation, and the drugs that must be stopped in advance are probably limited to the anticoagulants and the monoamine oxidase inhibitors in current practice. Awareness of the intra-operative complications to be expected from various drugs and their proper treatment when they occur should justify proceeding cautiously with anesthesia under most circumstances.[18]

ANESTHETIC POTENCY. Most drugs known to potentiate the action of anesthetic agents have obvious sedative effects. Preoperatively administered antihistamines, narcotics, barbiturates, benzodiazepines, and prior-ingested ethanol all decrease the maintenance levels of volatile anesthetic agents needed for adequate anesthesia. The antihypertensive agents reserpine and methyldopa (Aldomet), the phenothiazines, and chronic amphetamine use are said to decrease anesthetic requirements by depleting catecholamines in the central nervous system. The butyrophenone major tranquilizers haloperidol (Haldol) and droperidol (Inapsine) block central dopaminergic transmission, an effect possibly related to their anesthetic potentiation. L-Dopa (Dopar, Larodopa) used in parkinsonism causes generalized central nervous system depression and has corresponding anesthetic effects. Maintenance of anesthesia with normal levels of agents may result in severe physiologic depression in patients taking these drugs, and the cautious anesthesiologist will restrict dosages accordingly.

Only a few drugs increase anesthetic requirements to any extent. Acutely administered amphetamines release previously stored catecholamines, while cocaine blocks the neuronal re-uptake of these neurotransmitters, and both will decrease the effectiveness of normal anesthetic dosages as a result. The monoamine oxidase inhibitors used in the treatment of depression interfere with the intramitochondrial metabolism of catecholamines and similarly increase required anesthetic levels. However, their cardiovascular side effects are more significant as anesthetic complications. (See below.)

MUSCLE RELAXANT INTERACTIONS. Potentiation of muscle relaxants by other therapeutic drugs can result in prolonged paralysis, unless precautions are taken to avoid certain relaxants in specific situations, or if titration of relaxants is guided by use of the peripheral nerve stimulator. The ions magnesium, used for toxemia of pregnancy, and lithium, a popular drug for treatment of manic-depressive neuroses, potentiate muscle relaxants of both the depolarizing and non-depolarizing classes. Certain antiarrhythmic drugs and antibiotics are also known to potentiate the non-depolarizing relaxants d-tubocurarine and pancuronium, and prolonged paralysis has been frequently reported in patients treated with aminoglycoside antibiotics who have been curarized in surgery. Usually such weakness responds to intravenous calcium, but temporary controlled ventilation may be necessary.

The action of the depolarizing muscle relaxant succinylcholine is terminated with hydrolysis by serum pseudocholinesterase, and drugs that lower cholinesterase activity may extend the duration of action of succinylcholine markedly. Echothiophate eyedrops (Phospholine Iodide) used in the treatment of glaucoma, the ankylating chemotherapeutic agents Cytoxan and Thiotepa, and organophosphorus insecticides all significantly prolong the duration of succinylcholine, and the potentiating effects of these drugs may extend for several weeks after discontinuation. It is usually simple to avoid the use of depolarizing agents in patients taking these drugs and to utilize curare or pancuronium if relaxation is desired.

CARDIOVASCULAR EFFECTS. Weak potentiation of injected vasopressors is occasionally caused by reserpine or the tricyclic antidepressants amitriptyline (Elavil) and imipramine (Tofranil). Occasional ventricular arrhythmias seen in patients using these drugs should respond to normal doses of antiarrhythmic agents.[28] Similar pressor

sensitivity may also be seen in patients abusing cocaine or treated with various oxytocics. The most severe reactions to injected pressors are seen with the monoamine oxidase inhibitors: phenelzine (Nardil), nialamide (Niamid), isocarboxazid (Marplan) and pargyline (Eutonyl). Indirect-acting pressors will have exaggerated effects and can produce severe hypertension and arrhythmias. Comatose reactions and hypotension have been reported as idiosyncratic responses in patients taking MAO inhibitors who are given narcotics, particularly meperidine. For these reasons, the MAO inhibitors must be discontinued for 2 weeks preoperatively and other antidepressant therapy substituted.

Hypertensive patients treated with diuretics should be watched for hypotension on anesthetic induction, related to their contracted fluid volume. Potassium levels below 3.5 mEq/l. resulting from diuretic therapy may potentiate arrhythmias and digitalis toxicity and should be corrected before surgery. Withdrawal of the antihypertensive drug clonidine (Catapres) before surgery may cause abrupt rebound hypertension 12 hours after the last dose, so therapy should be maintained orally up until the morning of surgery, or other antihypertensive agents should be substituted several days preoperatively.[3] The latter will be necessary if oral medications will be stopped for several days postoperatively, because no parenteral form of the drug is now marketed.

Patients on phenothiazines or haloperidol (Haldol) may have mild unexpected hypotension owing to the alpha adrenergic blocking properties of these drugs. This hypotension should respond to appropriate fluids or small amounts of pressors.

L-Dopa therapy contraindicates use of droperidol (Inapsine) or the combination drug Innovar, which contains droperidol, because of possible neuromuscular rigidity and pulmonary edema that may result from an interaction between the drugs at central dopaminergic synapses. Severe cardiovascular depression and arrhythmias have been reported in patients taking L-dopa who are anesthetized with halothane. The half-life of L-dopa is short, however, so the risk of such complications will be minimized by stopping the drug the night before surgery.[28]

Beta adrenergic blockade with propranolol used for control of hypertension and angina should be continued up to the day of surgery. Initial reports of severe cardiovascular depression noted in patients on propranolol under anesthesia have been counterbalanced by reports of acute hypertensive crises and myocardial infarction associated with its withdrawal, and extensive experience in anesthetizing patients taking the drug has shown that complications are minimal with careful management.[9, 28] The controversy over whether large doses of beta blockers should be tapered preoperatively is still unsettled.

STEROIDS. Appropriate supplementation of glucocorticoids should be given to any patient with depressed hypothalamic-pituitary-adrenocortical function from any cause. One regimen is to inject 25 mg. of hydrocortisone intravenously at induction of anesthesia for major surgery. This should be followed by 100 mg. of hydrocortisone infused every 24 hours until oral intake resumes and surgical stress has subsided.[14]

DIGITALIS. If there is any doubt concerning adequacy of digitalization, appropriate therapeutic levels can be confirmed by serum assays available in most hospitals. Administration of digitalis on the morning of surgery is omitted in most cases, but this and prophylactic digitalization of the elderly or of candidates for pneumonectomy remain subjects of controversy.

ANTICOAGULANTS. Appropriate clotting studies should be obtained in all patients on anticoagulants to aid in assessment of their effects. Heparin may be acutely reversed by protamine sulfate if surgery must proceed in an emergency, but time is usually sufficient for heparin effects to subside without therapy. Vitamin K in patients taking coumarin derivatives may take several days to restore normal values, so in addition to AquaMephyton, therapy with fresh frozen plasma or clotting factor concentrates may be appropriate if time is short. Conduction anesthesia is contraindicated when clotting function is abnormal. General anesthesia and surgery appear safe in patients on minidose heparin prophylaxis for pulmonary embolic disease, but the safety of conduction anesthesia in these patients has not been proven.[43]

DRUGS OF ABUSE. The first principle in dealing with patients with a history of drug abuse is to prevent and treat withdrawal in the perioperative period.[4] Multiple drug use should always be suspected, and problems associated with drug abuse that can influence the conduct of anesthesia should be searched for, e.g., venous thromboses, pulmonary microemboli, hepatitis, tetanus, and subacute bacterial endocarditis.

Chronic narcotics abusers should be given generous amounts of opiates to prevent withdrawal and cover pain. Their own estimates of their daily drug requirements can be useful in setting the dosages of narcotics to be administered. These patients typically have low resting blood pressures, and withdrawal can cause severe hypertension and diffuse adrenergic discharge. Under anesthesia, withdrawal may be manifested as hypotension that can be reversed by administration of additional opiates. Abrupt withdrawal caused by injection of even minuscule doses of narcotic antagonists can be fatal, so naloxone (Narcan) and pentazocine (Talwin), which also has opiate antagonist properties, should be carefully avoided in active narcotics abusers. In patients with remote histories of opiate abuse who are not currently using drugs, narcotic anesthetic techniques should probably be avoided. Relapsed heroin users frequently develop peripheral neuropathies, and conduction anesthesia is probably best avoided.

Sedative-hypnotic drug abuse is common in the population, and patients regularly ingesting such drugs as diazepam (Valium) or secobarbital (Seconal) are frequently dependent on the drugs without fully appreciating the extent of their habits. When the drug is stopped at the time of admission for elective surgery, the hyperexcitability of the central nervous system that is building up may be evident as anxiety or tremulousness on the preoperative visit. A careful drug history and proper maintenance of sedation with appropriate hypnotic agents will prevent seizures and cardiovascular instability related to withdrawal in the perioperative period. The risk of seizures with aspiration, apnea, and possible central nervous system damage makes sedative-hypnotic withdrawal probably the most dangerous drug abuse related problem in the operative period, Cross-tolerance to the thiobarbiturates must be expected in these patients, and larger doses of thiopental may be required at induction of anesthesia.

No clear withdrawal syndromes have been described for the amphetamines, hallucinogens, marijuana, or cocaine, and these stimulant drugs appear to produce psychologic dependence alone without physiologic dependence. The acute cardiovascular effects of these drugs may appear as potentiation of vasopressors or predisposition to arrhythmias under anesthesia, but the incidence of such complications is small, and these drugs appear to pose minimal problems during anesthesia. The physical status of chronic users should be carefully assessed, however, and doses of anesthetic agents should be reduced when appropriate. LSD is reported to inhibit cholinesterase and may potentiate the action of succinylcholine.

The acutely intoxicated alcoholic may be belligerent and uncooperative, and sedation often increases the agitation seen in these patients, so conduction anesthesia may be a poor option for anesthetic management. In the chronic alcoholic and in the barbiturate addict, the danger of withdrawal must be lessened with proper sedation, fluid therapy, temperature control, and close observation for seizures prior to surgery. The mortality rate of delirium tremens in patients subjected to anesthesia and surgery remains considerable, and surgery should not be undertaken without careful preoperative evaluation and attempts to adjust fluids, electrolytes, and sedative control. Chlordiazepoxide (Librium) and diazepam (Valium) are the sedative agents of choice in withdrawal and may be given intravenously or intramuscularly. Under anesthesia, fever may be the only evident symptom of acute withdrawal when seizure activity is suppressed. Along with the adrenergic excitability and hypermetabolism, myocardial irritability and failure related to alcoholic cardiomyopathy may be anticipated in chronic severe alcoholics. However, the incidence of alcoholic polyneuropathies in these patients would weigh heavily in a consideration of regional anesthesia for surgery. A carefully conducted light general anesthetic with endotracheal intubation is usually preferable.

ASSESSMENT OF PHYSICAL STATUS

After consideration of all factors noted on the preoperative visit, the anesthesiologist assigns a physical status classification to the patient. This classification is related *only* to the physical condition of the patient before surgery and is *not* influenced by the extent of the anticipated surgery or the risk of complications per se. Of course, correlation is high between the physical status classification and the incidence of complications or death from anesthesia and surgery.[1, 16] The surgeon should be familiar with this classification system and note the value assigned by the anesthesiologist as his or her estimate of problems to be anticipated in surgery.

Class 1 A normally healthy patient
Class 2 A patient with mild systemic disease
Class 3 A patient with severe systemic disease that limits activity but is not incapacitating.
Class 4 A patient with an incapacitating systemic disease that is a constant threat to life
Class 5 A moribund patient who is not expected to survive for 24 hours with or without operation
E Emergency cases are designated by addition of the suffix E to the classification number.

COUNSELING AND INFORMED CONSENT

A sympathetic forthright discussion of the anesthetic plan, with a clear description of alternative methods available and possible complications, is required by the implied contract between the patient and his anesthesiologist. A frank approach to the patient, in language he can understand, increases cooperation, reduces apprehension, and promotes trust. Above all, the patient's preferences should ultimately determine the final choice of technique.

Meticulous full disclosure of risk can increase anxiety and can be needlessly time consuming, so which complications are discussed must depend on the judgment of the anesthesiologist. Legal decisions have generally supported the loosely defined legal requirement that the patient must be told what *a reasonable man* would disclose under the circumstances. The local standard of care rule, based on the usual and customary medical practice in the area, has not consistently been judged applicable in litigation on informed consent. Dornette defines an incidence of significant permanent complications (0.1 to 1 per cent) and of moderate transient complications (1 to 10 per cent) that would indicate that a specific complication should be discussed with the patient.[10] Thus, before procedures commonly performed without significant morbidity, a discussion of such unlikely outcomes as death or permanent physical damage would neither be appropriate nor required. The anesthesiologist must ultimately judge the extent of disclosure necessary, and the discussion should be documented in the chart prior to surgery.

PREMEDICATION

The goal of preoperative medication is to produce tranquility and increase patient cooperation, while helping prevent harmful physiologic effects of anesthetic induction. Inadequate or improper sedation can produce an agitated or delirious patient, while oversedation on the ward without adequate observation is a source of serious anesthetic complications. The safe use of premedicants is learned from experience, but morbidity can be minimized by understanding a few simple principles about sedative drugs.

Narcotics provide excellent sedation, but nausea, vomiting, hypotension, and respiratory depression may follow their injection before surgery. Antiemetics, like promethazine (Phenergan) and droperidol (Inapsine), can be added to the narcotic to control nausea, but potentiation of opiate effects can occur, so narcotic dosage should be reduced accordingly. Hypotension is usually mild after narcotic premedication and can be counteracted with fluids or pressors when appropriate. Severe respiratory depression seldom follows premedicant doses of narcotics in healthy patients, but when it occurs, it can be counteracted with naloxone (Narcan).

Sedative-hypnotic drugs such as the benzodiazepines and barbiturates can produce dysphoria and combativeness in children or in the elderly, which cannot be pharmacologically reversed and can make anesthetic induction most unpleasant. One advantage of sedative-hypnotic drugs, however, is that they can be given orally with a sip of water, 90 minutes before induction of anesthesia, to patients who would prefer to avoid an injection. Adequate sedation is obtained without increasing the volume of stomach contents or the risk of aspiration.

Major tranquilizers used as premedicants, droperidol (Inapsine) and chlorpromazine (Thorazine), will frequently produce dysphoria when given alone and are usually combined with narcotic sedation to prevent this effect. Hypotension due to the alpha adrenergic blocking properties of these phenothiazines and butyrophenones should be anticipated and will respond to fluids and pressors. Both oversedation and dysphoria due to these agents will be corrected by intravenous injection of physostigmine (Antilirium), a central nervous system cholinesterase inhibitor.

The combination drug Innovar is a popular but problematic premedicant. The use of the short-acting potent narcotic fentanyl (Sublimaze) with the long-acting droperidol in this combination can have undesirable side effects if anesthesia is not induced promptly, when dysphoria ensues as narcotic effect subsides. This is easily avoided by using a longer acting narcotic in combination with the droperidol.

The use of atropine in premedication produces a dry mouth, blurred vision, and inadequate vagal blockade one hour after injection to prevent bradyarrhythmias during anesthetic induction. While drying of airway secretions is often desirable in children, it is of dubious benefit in asthma or chronic obstructive lung disease, and it can be a source of significant patient discomfort. The tachycardia that results from atropine may be harmful in patients with ischemic heart disease or with fixed cardiac outputs due to aortic or mitral valve stenosis. The routine use of atropine in premedication is thus yielding to a more selective approach. Airway secretions can be decreased when appropriate with small doses of atropine, scopolamine, or glycopyrrolate (Robinul), to reduce the incidence of breathholding and laryngospasm due to secretions around the glottis during inhalational induction. If delirium from the central anticholinergic effects of atropine and scopolamine occurs, it can be reversed with intravenous physostigmine salicylate (Antilirium). Glycopyrrolate offers the advantage of also reducing the volume and acidity of the gastric contents in patients at risk of vomiting and aspiration. Even more effective in this regard is the new drug cimetidine (Tagamet), but it must be given for one full day preoperatively if adequate prophylaxis is to be obtained. Intravenous injection of metoclopramide (Reglan) promotes gastric emptying in emergency patients but should not be used in cases of mechanical bowel obstruction.

Premedication must be injected at least 45 minutes to 1 hour prior to induction if adequate effect is to be obtained. If oral premedication is ordered, care must be taken to allow 90 minutes for adequate absorption. If the patient already has an intravenous infusion running, slow injection of one-half to two-thirds of an appropriate intramuscular dosage of the desired premedicants should produce adequate sedation.

THE OPERATIVE PERIOD

All anesthetic agents and methods have inherent hazards. It is beyond the scope of this discussion to consider the detailed pharmacology and toxicology of the individual *agents* except as they relate to particular complications under consideration. This discussion will be organized into three sections dealing with complications of general anesthesia, conduction anesthesia, and those related to special situations.

GENERAL ANESTHESIA

Safe conduct of general anesthesia first requires application of proper *monitoring devices* prior to induction. After *induction* of anesthesia and control of the airway, *maintenance* is begun with inhalational or intravenous agents, and the patient is *positioned* for operation. Following surgery *emergence* from anesthesia is carefully managed in the operating room and recovery area. Complications of general anesthesia particular to each of these phases will be discussed, with particular emphasis on their prevention, detection, and management.

Complications of Monitoring

BASIC MONITORING. It has become standard for the non-invasive monitoring devices used for following the pulse, blood pressure, and electrocardiogram to be applied to the patient prior to anesthetic induction. The cardiorespiratory effects of all anesthetic agents and airway maneuvers make this mandatory in all patients regardless of their preoperative physical status. At a minimum, a precordial stethoscope, blood pressure cuff, and electrocardiographic monitor will allow detection of unwanted deterioration of vital signs when it occurs and facilitate prompt application of corrective measures.

Because the blood pressure is the most reliable guide to the adequacy of anesthesia, inaccurate assessment of blood pressure may lead to underdosage or overdosage with anesthetic agents. To prevent such misinterpretation the blood pressure cuff should cover two-thirds of the upper arm or have a width equal to 0.4 times the circumference of the upper arm, which should provide reliable indirect measurement of arterial pressure. When the Korotkoff sounds are indistinct, as in the child or the obese individual, the use of the Doppler ultrasound probe for the detection of return to flow distal to the cuff may be necessary.

A crude but essential auditory assessment of the rate and force of cardiac contractions, as well as the respirations, can be maintained with the precordial stethoscope during anesthetic induction. If endotracheal intubation is performed, auditory monitoring can be continued with an esophageal stethoscope during the procedure. This is especially useful because indirect blood pressure measurement is intermittent, and the electrocardiogram may be slow to reflect acute changes in perfusion pressures. Thus, the audible heart tones are the only continuous basic monitoring modality that can provide immediate warning of dropping blood pressure caused by anesthetic depression or surgical manipulation. While the method is non-quantitative and subjective, beat-to-beat monitoring cannot be maintained otherwise without resort to invasive techniques.

Continuous observation of cardiac rate and rhythm has become standard in the last decade with use of the oscilloscope electrocardiogram. Arrhythmias can be an important indicator of hypoxia, hypercarbia, or myocardial decompensation under anesthesia, and changes in the S-T segment can be diagnostic of ischemia, particularly with intraoperative use of the V_5 precordial lead.[71] The simultaneous use of electrocardiographic monitors with electrosurgical units has raised the possibility of current-induced arrhythmias and electrical burns as complications of basic monitoring. The use of isolated power sources for these devices has not entirely eliminated the risk of current leakage, and if the patient is not properly grounded to the electrocautery, severe burns may occur at the point of application of the EKG electrodes. Fortunately, arrhythmias resulting from improperly functioning electrical equipment are extremely rare, but special care must be taken during endoscopy using radiofrequency current cautery or in the presence of cardiac pacing electrodes connected to temporary external pacemakers. *Prevention* of burns and electric current leakage requires regular equipment checks, the use of maximum-sized grounding pads applied as close to the surgical incision as possible, and placement of monitoring electrodes as far from the active cautery as is practical.[97]

Temperature monitoring devices are usually applied after induction for measurement of skin or core temperature, to allow detection of the common inadvertent hypothermia caused by the cold operating room environment when anesthesia has blocked the normal thermal conservation mechanisms of the body, and to facilitate early detection of the rare but potentially lethal malignant hyperthermia (see below). Probes may be applied to the skin or inserted into the mouth, nose, or rectum; tympanic membrane probes may lead to ear trauma and are less frequently used at this time.

Before lengthy operations or prior to surgery with a high anticipated blood loss, a urinary catheter should be inserted after induction. This will prevent overdistention of the bladder and allow for adequate assessment of fluid management during surgery.

Use of these basic non-invasive monitors will cause few complications while providing essential information about the physiologic state of the patient during anesthesia and surgery. For extensive procedures in high-risk patients, more invasive monitoring methods may provide certain advantages, but the complications associated with percu-taneous vascular cannulation should discourage its excessive and indiscriminate use.

INVASIVE MONITORING. Complications of invasive cardiovascular monitoring will be discussed under sections on intra-arterial, central venous, and pulmonary arterial pressure monitoring. When invasive methods are required for extensive surgical procedures in relatively low-risk patients, it may be preferable to insert the monitoring lines after induction of anesthesia. However, when the indication for invasive monitoring is the poor physical status of the patient, such monitoring should be established prior to induction, with the use of local anesthesia and appropriate sedation. In experienced hands this can be accomplished safely in the awake patient without increasing anxiety or producing cardiovascular instability.[99]

Intra-arterial Monitoring

The value of continuous direct arterial pressure monitoring in the poor-risk patient cannot be disputed. With the added advantage of repeated arterial blood gas and blood chemistry determinations, percutaneous arterial cannulation has become indispensable in anesthesia practice. The sites most commonly used for cannulation are peripheral arteries: the radial, dorsalis pedis, and superficial temporal arteries. More central cannulation of the femoral, brachial, or axillary arteries risks thrombosis and distal gangrene and is used only when more peripheral cannulation cannot be achieved.

Temporal artery cannulation has been used most frequently in infants and children, and owing to the abundant blood supply of the scalp, ischemic complications are infrequent. Distal ischemia in the extremities after cannulation of the radial or dorsalis pedis arteries is occasionally noted and may result in discoloration or frank gangrene. This is seldom a problem if adequate collateral circulation to the hand or foot can be demonstrated before arterial puncture is attempted by doing an Allen test for ulnar cross-circulation in the hand or by checking posterior tibial collateral flow in the foot.[76, 104] If adequate collateral circulation is not demonstrable, an alternative artery should be used for monitoring.

When distal ischemia is noted immediately after percutaneous arterial cannulation, acute local vasospasm should be suspected. A short interval should be allowed for resolution of symptoms, and treatment with sympathetic block or intra-arterial papaverine may be considered. Persistent distal ischemia should be considered an indication for prompt removal of the cannula.

Use of a continuous heparinized flush solution helps maintain the patency of the arterial line, and in this way the cannula can be used for several additional days of monitoring in the intensive care unit. Vigorous flushing of arterial lines with excessive amounts of solution is to be carefully avoided since significant arterial embolization can be produced.

The incidence of occlusion of the radial artery after percutaneous cannulation has been shown to be related to the size, material, and shape of the catheter, and duration of cannulation. The risk of arterial thrombosis seems to be minimized with the use of parallel-wall 20 Ga Teflon catheters, and with a duration of cannulation of 3 days or less; increasing the diameter or prolonging the duration of cannulation risks a higher resultant morbidity.[39, 76] An occlusion rate of 10 per cent is still noted when all known risk factors are minimized, so the collateral circulation is essential in prevention of distal ischemic complications. Nearly all of these occlusions are transient, however, and the artery will usually recanalize within one month of removal of the cannula, with restoration of near normal blood flow to the hand.

Other miscellaneous complications of arterial puncture should be mentioned. Local hematoma is frequent, especially when several arterial puncture attempts are required to cannulate the vessel, but this usually resolves without significant morbidity. Radial artery aneurysm or arteriovenous fistula may occur uncommonly and will require surgical closure or resection. Sterile technique must be observed for insertion and maintenance of the cannula if infection is to be prevented. Finally, the cannula and monitoring lines must be prominently labeled to distinguish them from the intravenous lines, so that inadvertent injection of intravenous medications may be avoided. Certain drugs that may be innocuous when injected into veins can cause distal arteritis and occlusion if injected intra-arterially. Red tape flags on the arterial lines at injection ports and at the site of cannulation have proven useful in our clinical practice in preventing such mishaps.

Central Venous Monitoring

Pressures in the right atrium and superior vena cava are an excellent guide to the intravascular fluid volume and reflect the filling pressure of the right and left ventricles in most healthy individuals. In conditions where functional disparity exists between the right and left ventricles, only a pulmonary artery occlusion pressure obtained with a Swan-Ganz catheter will adequately monitor left ventricular end-diastolic pressure.[61] Despite this limitation the central venous catheter has proven its usefulness for monitoring and for rapid fluid infusion and can serve as a point of central venous access for insertion of the pulmonary artery catheter when this seems necessary. The ideal approach for percutaneous cannulation of the central veins would combine simple technique and a low incidence of complications with a high rate of successful central placement. Unfortunately, those techniques with high reliability also have relatively high morbidity, and their continued use requires that potential complications be anticipated so they may be promptly detected and properly treated.

Insertion of long central venous cannulas through percutaneous puncture of the brachial veins at the elbow has little or no significant reported morbidity, but the rate of unsatisfactory catheter placement outside the thorax is 25 to 40 per cent in several series. Cannulation of the external jugular vein with Seldinger J-wire insertion of a longer central venous catheter has been reported to be 96 per cent successful with no associated morbidity, and this technique is being widely adopted.[41] Large diameter central venous cannulas for pulmonary artery catheter insertion may be difficult to pass through the external jugular route, however, and many practitioners continue to prefer the internal jugular and subclavian routes despite their admittedly higher associated complication rates.

Percutaneous puncture of the subclavian vein by the infraclavicular route is the central approach most favored among surgeons. A surprisingly high malposition rate (up to 33 per cent has been reported) may be seen when the catheters pass up the internal jugular veins.[59] Complications occur in as many as 11 per cent of punctures, with the incidences of pneumothorax (6 per cent) and subclavian artery puncture (0.8 per cent) being worthy of note.[65] Pneumothorax usually can be treated with observation, but the possibility of tension pneumothorax under anesthesia should be constantly kept in mind, and tube thoracostomy may be necessary on occasion, especially when high peak inspiratory pressures are noted during controlled ventilation. Bleeding from the subclavian artery may be profuse, and it may be difficult to apply external pressure to the site of inadvertent puncture. It is also important to consider occult intrathoracic bleeding following attempted subclavian vein puncture in the differential diagnosis of unexpected hypotension occurring later during anesthesia. With even a minimal risk of bleeding involved, subclavian puncture is contraindicated in patients with abnormal coagulation mechanisms.

Most anesthesiologists prefer cannulation of the right internal jugular vein as a direct route into the superior vena cava. Percutaneous puncture in the neck, directed toward the thoracic inlet, involves needle probing near the carotid artery, pleura, thoracic duct (on the left side), and various neurologic structures traversing the neck. Complications of internal jugular puncture may then result from needle injury to these structures, or from the local effects of hematoma or infiltrated fluid.

The standard approach involves puncture of the internal jugular vein below the junction of the sternal and clavicular heads of the sternocleidomastoid muscle. An alternative technique uses a more medial approach slightly above the muscle lateral to the carotid artery.[59] The most common complication to be expected is carotid artery puncture. Resultant bleeding can usually be stopped with local pressure, and significant morbidity is rare. The incidence of carotid artery puncture can be minimized by careful localization of the carotid pulsation fol-

lowed by needle probe only in a lateral direction. Use of a small 22 gauge finder needle may help in localizing the vein without risking puncture of the carotid artery with a larger intravascular cannula. As with subclavian puncture, this approach is best avoided in patients with coagulopathies.

Pneumothorax may result when puncture is attempted near the clavicle, but the incidence can be minimized if an effort is made to stay high in the neck. In my personal series, no pneumothoraces have been encountered in the last 300 internal jugular punctures, with the point of percutaneous needle insertion at least halfway up the neck between the clavicle and mandible.

Neurologic damage to the sympathetic chain may result in a transient Horner's syndrome that should be expected to resolve in several weeks. More extensive damage to cranial nerves and the brachial plexus has been reported owing to infiltration of drugs and intravenous solutions into the neck that went undetected for several days. Infrequently, the infusion of fluids through malpositioned catheters may cause hydrothorax or pericardial tamponade, and these complications may also follow late erosion of the catheter through vascular structures several days after insertion. Free aspiration of blood from the catheters after central insertion should rule this complication out, at least acutely.

Damage to lymphatics on the left side of the neck may result in lymphocutaneous fistula or chylothorax, and the nutritional or fluid deficits that result may be potentially lethal. This should be easily avoided by attempting only right internal jugular punctures or by remaining high in the neck whenever jugular puncture is performed on the left side.

Pulmonary Artery Pressure Monitoring

The measurement of the pulmonary artery occlusion pressure as an estimate of left atrial pressure can be obtained by passing a balloon-tipped flow-directed catheter across the heart into a peripheral wedge position in the pulmonary circulation. The Swan-Ganz catheter may be the only method for assessing left ventricular filling pressures in patients with severe cardiorespiratory dysfunction. Most pulmonary artery catheters are also equipped with thermal sensors that allow measurement of core temperature and thermodilution cardiac outputs, from which peripheral resistance values can be computed. Mixed venous blood can also be sampled directly from the pulmonary artery for determination of venous oxygen saturation to be used in the shunt calculation and to allow estimation of peripheral oxygen consumption. Finally, the catheter can have pacing electrode capability for both ventricular and sequential atrioventricular pacing. With all these possible functions, the Swan-Ganz catheter has become an indispensable tool in surgical anesthesia and intensive care.

The complications of pulmonary artery catheterization are quite limited considering the relative invasiveness of the technique.[83] As the catheter passes across the heart, endocardial stimulation may cause premature ventricular contractions that are usually transient and rarely progress to more serious ventricular arrhythmias. If these are persistent they usually will respond to intravenous lidocaine in a standard antiarrhythmic bolus of 1 mg./kg. Pressure on the conduction system in the septum from the adjacent catheter may cause an acute right bundle branch block that is apparent on the EKG monitor but is seldom of any hemodynamic significance.[95] In patients with antecedent left bundle branch block, catheter-induced right bundle branch block can result in complete heart block with decreased cardiac output. In this situation the catheter should probably not be used.

Endocarditis and valvular damage have been reported after prolonged insertion and should be minimized by early removal of the catheter. Pulmonary artery rupture and infarction have occurred when the balloon has been over-inflated, kept in too peripheral a location, or left in a permanently wedged position. The balloon should be deflated between wedge pressure determinations so that a clear pulmonary artery trace is seen on the oscilloscope, to minimize the chance of pulmonary artery occlusion or rupture. The catheter does act as a thrombogenic foreign body in the circulation. Formed clots can be seen on the exposed catheter inside the heart at operation, and the platelet count can be shown to be de-

creased by half after catheter insertion. The clinical significance of this appears to be minimal, because neither embolic damage nor coagulation deficit can be regularly demonstrated early following insertion of the catheter.[66]

Complications of Anesthetic Induction

The induction of anesthesia is the culmination of the process of patient evaluation, equipment preparation, and preliminary monitoring. This is for many patients the most crucial portion of the surgical procedure, during which they are administered drugs that depress consciousness and weaken airway reflexes, and that can potentially depress respiratory and cardiovascular function. During induction the anesthesiologist takes responsibility for monitoring of physiologic homeostasis as he or she tests the patient's cardiorespiratory reserve under the challenge of anesthetic medications. Three important factors in induction will be discussed: the effects of intravenous medications used to depress the sensorium, the management of the airway during induction and maintenance of anesthesia, and the adjunctive use of muscle relaxants.

LOSS OF CONSCIOUSNESS. Loss of consciousness is usually achieved with injection of small doses of short-acting thiobarbiturates. Inhalational inductions are usually reserved for small children, who will be upset by an intravenous injection, and for older patients with severe airway difficulties. Anesthesia can be maintained after intravenous induction with continued intravenous medications or with the inhalational agents that will be discussed under the section on anesthetic maintenance. The intravenous agents used for induction include the barbiturates, narcotics, benzodiazepines, butyrophenones, and phencyclidines. Technical errors associated with the injection of intravenous agents will also be discussed.

Barbiturates

Injection of the short-acting thiobarbiturates Pentothal (thiopental) or Surital (thiamylal), or the oxybarbiturate Brevital (methohexital) will cause loss of consciousness within 30 seconds when full anesthetic doses are given. In the elderly or hypovolemic patient, or when heavy preoperative sedation has been given, the barbiturates are most safely given in reduced incremental doses, because circulatory depression may result from vasodilatation and direct myocardial depression. Any patient who may potentially require rapid fluid infusion should have multiple large bore catheters in place before any depressant medications are given. Increased fluids may be required to cover slumps in the blood pressure after thiopental, and pressors may be added in small dosages until blood levels of the barbiturates subside and the vital signs return to normal levels, usually within 3 to 5 minutes. The acute respiratory depressant effects of the barbiturates may result in apnea, breathholding, or upper airway obstruction, which may require supportive measures. (See below.)

Narcotics

Occasionally, narcotics will be infused for anesthetic induction in patients who are expected to tolerate barbiturates poorly. Large doses of narcotics are injected over several minutes until the patient no longer responds to stimuli, and adjuvant drugs such as diazepam are frequently given at the same time to assure amnesia. The narcotics most often used are morphine and fentanyl (Sublimaze). Both are respiratory depressants; apnea and respiratory acidosis are to be expected and ventilatory control will be necessary after narcotic induction. Respiratory depression can be reversed, if desired, with naloxone (Narcan) in titrated doses. The narcotic reversal effect of naloxone is transient and recurrent respiratory depression should be anticipated, which may require additional therapy. Rapid infusion of narcotics may also result in chest wall muscle stiffness, known as the "wooden chest" syndrome. This can be quite upsetting to the semiconscious patient, but when the sensorium is seriously depressed, it may render ventilatory support measures ineffective. The stiffness can be reversed with intravenous naloxone, or with muscle relaxants in the unconscious patient.

Circulatory depression is seen frequently after initial injection of morphine but rarely after incremental dosages of fentanyl. Histamine release from the morphine is thought to produce vasodilatation, and the hypotensive effect may be compounded by limited ganglionic blocking effects of the drug. Neither fentanyl nor morphine has direct myocardial depressant effects. Circulatory depression from the narcotics will recover rapidly after fluid infusion, and pressors are seldom indicated. Slow incremental injection of the narcotics with careful monitoring will prevent most serious side effects of these drugs.

Benzodiazepines

The benzodiazepine diazepam (Valium) depresses consciousness and produces amnesia without significant cardiovascular effects. Upper airway obstruction and depression of respiration should be expected after intravenous injection; support of the airway and ventilatory control may be necessary. Minor phlebitis can occur owing to local vascular irritation; pain on injection of the drug can be blocked with prior slow injection of lidocaine through the same intravenous line.

Butyrophenones

Droperidol (Inapsine) is a butyrophenone major tranquilizer that has marked sedative and antiemetic effects. It is combined with the narcotic fentanyl in the preparation Innovar. The drug produces prolonged potentiation of the narcotics, so dosages of opiates must be reduced after administration of droperidol to lessen the possibility of respiratory depression. In common with the other antipsychotic drugs, it has alpha adrenergic blocking properties that may produce hypotension after injection; this hypotension should respond promptly to fluid infusion. Dysphoria may result when adequate additional sedation is not maintained in the non-psychotic individual. Finally, stiffness and abnormal posturing may result from extrapyramidal side effects of droperidol, similar to that seen after large doses of other major tranquilizers. Treatment with benadryl or benztropine (Cogentin) is rapidly effective in reversing the neuromuscular abnormality; no further droperidol should be given to the patient. Somnolence or dysphoria from droperidol may respond to intravenous physostigmine (Antilirium).

Phencyclidines

Ketamine is a phencyclidine derivative that produces rapid amnesia and analgesia after intravenous injection. The advantage of the drug lies in the sympathetic stimulation that it produces of the cardiovascular system, which makes maintenance of blood pressure more reliable in the hypovolemic patient. An occasional patient will have excessive hypertension and tachycardia after ketamine; this can be partially blocked by the prior administration of diazepam or the intraoperative injection of droperidol.[101] Minimal respiratory depression occurs, but increased airway reflexes and laryngospasm may be a problem. Copious airway secretions stimulated by ketamine can be prevented by premedication with an appropriate antisialagogue. Hallucinations and delirium may also occur in adults, which can be controlled with sedation and observation of the patient in a quiet isolated area.

Technical Problems

The pH of sodium Pentothal solution is around 11, and the alkalinity of the solution is very irritating to tissues if it is infiltrated into subcutaneous tissue or muscle. The patient will report immediate pain, and local blanching of skin may be seen. Frank necrosis of muscle or fat may develop after several days if large doses of Pentothal are injected, and skin slough may follow. Injection of local anesthetic solution for pain relief and dilution of the barbiturate is advised. Infiltration is prevented if thiobarbiturates are injected only through rapidly running intravenous lines, and if injection is stopped immediately when the patient reports severe pain in the area of injection.

If barbiturates, diazepam, or Demerol are inadvertently injected into an artery, the immediate response seems to be a transient arterial spasm as the patient experiences severe burning pain in the distribution of the artery. Blood flow is soon restored, but a progressive arteritis develops that leads to late occlusion of the vessel in 6 to 10 days. Resulting gangrene may lead to eventual loss of digits or areas of skin. The ability of the drug to produce arteritis seems related to its fat solubility. The fat-soluble drugs Pentothal and diazepam produce severe arterial damage, while ketamine and local anesthetics that are less lipid-soluble produce no apparent spasm, arteritis, or ischemia.[73]

Immediate therapy is necessary to increase the blood supply to the threatened area and to prevent deposition of fibrin on the damaged intima. Vasodilatation and pain relief can be obtained initially with brachial plexus block using a long-acting local anesthetic. Systemic heparinization should then be maintained for at least 10 days to retard thrombus formation; repeated axillary blocks can be performed just before heparin bolus injections to minimize the risk of bleeding. The arm should be elevated to minimize swelling. The immediate intra-arterial injection of heparin, papaverine, Priscoline, or lidocaine has been recommended, but the mechanism of injury appears to be cytotoxic rather than vasospastic, and the only effective intra-arterial injection in the rabbit ear model is Decadron 1 mg./kg., injected within 30 minutes of injury. When combined with continued systemic steroid therapy for 4 days, significant reduction in tissue loss was achieved.[45] The usefulness of steroids in human arterial injury remains unproven.

Because therapy is of dubious benefit and the outcome is a medicolegal disaster, prevention of intra-arterial injection of drugs is essential. Most reported instances involve use of 5 to 10 per cent solutions of Pentothal, with induction injections performed using free needles and syringes in the antecubital fossa of the arm. Infiltration of Pentothal in this region has also led to median nerve injury. Intra-arterial injection into an occasionally seen aberrant radial artery on the dorsum of the wrist has been reported several times. Because occasionally an intravenous line may be unknowingly inserted up an artery, many anesthesiologists take the precaution of a 2 cc. test dose injection of Pentothal prior to administration of the full dose, so that the injection may be stopped if the patient reports distal severe pain. If Pentothal is injected only in 2.5 per cent solution into a freely running intravenous line, and if the injection is discontinued promptly when indicated, the rare but catastrophic complication of intra-arterial injection of Pentothal may be prevented.

AIRWAY MANAGEMENT. With loss of consciousness tissues may collapse around the airway owing to loss of supporting muscle tone. Resulting upper airway obstruction will prevent maintenance of ventilation, even in the presence of normal respiratory drive. Stridor or chest wall retractions after induction are indications that the patency of the upper airway must be improved. The most common cause of upper airway obstruction is the tongue resting on the soft palate and posterior pharyngeal wall when the patient is supine (Fig. 10–2). In this situation, simple extension of the head can open the pharynx to allow respiration through the nasal passages. The "jaw thrust" (Fig. 10–3) may be applied if extension of the head is not sufficient, and this maneuver can be performed with the hand grasping the fitted anesthesia mask and mandible simultaneously. Positive pressure can be applied to the airway when a tight mask fit is maintained over the face, and this may further expand the upper airway to correct obstruction.

If obstruction still persists, an oropharyngeal or nasopharyngeal airway may be inserted (Fig. 10–4). Bleeding may result, particularly with insertion of the nasopharyngeal airway, and stimulation of protective reflexes by the artificial airways in light planes of anesthesia may compound airway obstruction by causing coughing, breathholding, or laryngospasm. Anesthesia must be deepened under these circumstances, positive pressure applied to the airway, and if all else fails, rapidly acting muscle relaxants injected to break the laryngospasm and allow ventilation.

In certain patients all maneuvers described to restore airway patency will fail. Endotracheal intubation must then be attempted before hypoxia and cardiac arrest occur. In those patients in whom the airway cannot be maintained by mask, positive pressure, and artificial mechanical airways, it is

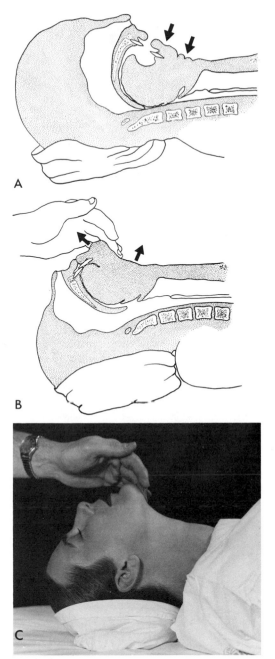

Figure 10–2 Unconscious patient, supine. *A,* Diagram showing how base of tongue and soft palate drop back against pharyngeal wall to obstruct airway. *B,* Diagram showing how extension of the head on the neck clears this obstruction. *C,* Photograph illustrating this extension.

quite likely that endotracheal intubation will also be technically difficult. These patients can be identified preoperatively and fall into certain clinical categories that deserve special consideration. *Any patient in the following*

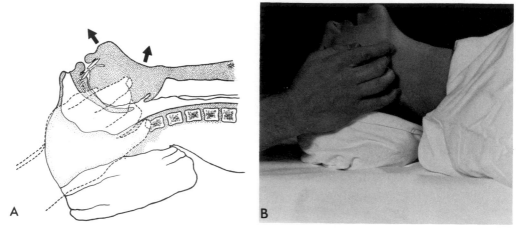

Figure 10–3   Unconscious patient, supine. *A,* Diagram showing how pushing the mandible forward from the angles clears the obstruction of the airway by the base of the tongue. *B,* Photograph illustrating the method.

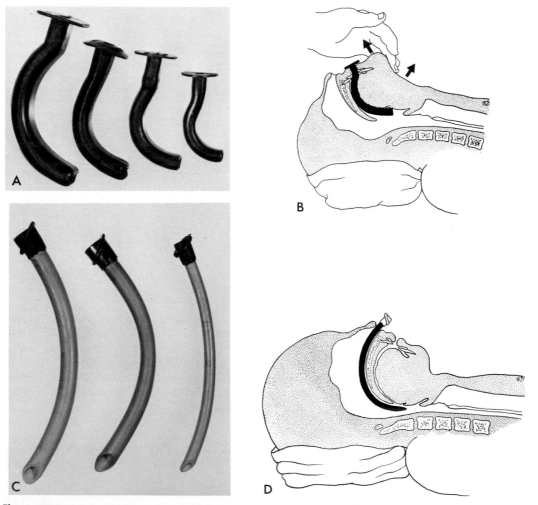

Figure 10–4   Mechanical airways. *A,* Rubber oropharyngeal airways, various sizes. *B,* Diagram showing oropharyngeal airway in place with base of tongue pushed forward. *C,* Rubber nasopharyngeal airways, various calibers. *D,* Diagram showing nasopharyngeal airway in place with base of tongue pushed forward.

groups should be considered at high risk for airway obstruction after induction of anesthesia and should not undergo intravenous or inhalational anesthesia induction, unless pre-anesthetic evaluation suggests that the airway can be easily maintained or controlled by the above methods.

Bull Neck. A short, thick neck often blocks visualization of the larynx by the sheer bulk of the tissues.

Receding Chin. A common test is a distance of less than 2 fingerbreadths between the thyroid notch and the anterior edge of the mandible. The high anterior glottis associated with difficult intubations should be anticipated.

Stiff Neck. Patients with cervical arthritis, "poker-spine," or Marie-Strümpell's disease cannot move the cerival spine or atlanto-occipital joint when mobility is required to facilitate exposure of the glottis. Patients in body casts or halo traction may present similar difficulties.

Temporomandibular Joint Fusion. Inability to open or sublux the mandible will make laryngoscopy difficult if not impossible.

Upper Airway Trauma. The fractured mandible, with or without extensive soft tissue trauma around the upper airway, fills the pharynx with blood and secretions and may so distort and obscure the anatomy as to make intubation impossible. Severe lacerations of the tongue and cheeks may present similar difficulties. The possibility of extension of soft tissue trauma during laryngoscopy should also be considered a real danger, when rough edges of the fractured mandible are exposed and abnormally mobile.

Inflammatory Edema. Acute epiglottitis, Ludwig's angina, or intra-oral cellulitis may so distort tissues that the glottis is difficult to locate and identify.

Neoplasms. The airway may be compromised, particularly with laryngeal tumors, so that even minimal sedation will rapidly obstruct respiration. Attempts at intubation may cause bleeding from friable tumor tissue, and laryngospasm is common.

Displaced Larynx. Certain tumors, particularly huge thyroid masses, can result in such displacement of the trachea and the larynx that visualization is extremely difficult.

Acromegaly. The massive jaw and tongue of the acromegalic patient may make direct laryngoscopy virtually impossible.

Again it is important to emphasize that such patients must be carefully evaluated, and most anesthesiologists will elect to achieve control of the airway before induction when they feel that they may be unable to control the airway adequately under anesthesia. The alternatives for airway control would include:

1. awake oral intubation with topical anesthesia under sedation

2. awake blind nasal intubation with topical anesthesia under sedation

3. direct fiberoptic visualization of the larynx through the nose or the mouth with a flexible fiberoptic laryngoscope or bronchoscope, and intubation using the endoscope as a stent for the endotracheal tube[86]

4. preliminary tracheostomy under local anesthesia with sedation.

The patient with a full stomach (e.g., acute trauma or bowel obstruction) is at risk of aspiration of stomach contents during awake intubation attempts, and oversedation or topical anesthetization of the glottis will decrease reflex protection of the upper airway. Because of the risk of aspiration such adjuvant techniques should be restricted or deferred entirely during intubation in these patients. Although this may seem unnecessarily cruel, to risk aspiration would be misguided humanitarianism in the extreme.

When difficult intubations are encountered after induction of anesthesia, morbidity can be expected to increase. Certainly damage to upper airway structures may be a relatively small complication compared with hypoxic destruction of the central nervous system. Certain tricks are utilized by the experienced anesthesiologist, however, to facilitate intubation under difficult conditions and to reduce the need for overpowering the airway with forceful distortions of the anatomy. The usefulness of the intubating stylet should be emphasized, and the availability of a wide choice of laryngoscope blades in the operating room is essential. Frequent adjustment of head position and external laryngeal pressure may serve to bring the glottis into view. Lastly, the use of the intubating pillow should be stressed; by causing extension of the cervical spine and flexion of the atlanto-occipital joint, it shortens the distance between the upper incisors and the glottis and facilitates exposure, especially when the straight laryngoscope blade is used.

After prolonged attempts at direct orotracheal intubation, if the airway is unsatisfactory during intermittent mask ventilation, and if attempts at blind nasal intubation are unsuccessful, a decision must be made between abandoning the anesthetic and awakening the patient, or controlling the airway by surgical tracheostomy. If hypoxia develops despite attempts to ventilate, cardiac arrest may occur before tracheostomy can be performed, and permanent brain damage can result. Acute cricothyroid puncture may be accomplished with a large intravenous cannula that can be connected to an oxygen source through a 3.5 mm. endotracheal tube adaptor to supply minimal oxygenation until tracheostomy can be performed.

Hypoxic cardiac arrest from loss of the airway, with subsequent death or permanent neurologic damage, is unquestionably the most disastrous and feared complication of anesthesia. The fact that caution and experience may minimize, but not completely eliminate, the risk of this complication is an imponderable problem each anesthesiologist must face daily in his or her work.

Traumatic Complications

Difficult intubation secondary to the conditions noted above or as a result of inexperience or ineptness can lead to varying degrees of trauma.

NOSE, LIPS, TEETH, PHARYNX.   Any of the structures in the pathways between the mouth (or nares) and the larynx can be traumatized either by intubation or by laryngoscopy. Teeth or dental restorations can be broken. Mucous membranes may be lacerated, abraded, or contused with varying degrees of swelling and bleeding. The mucosa may actually be penetrated, and perforation of the pyriform sinus by a laryngoscope blade may be followed by subcutaneous emphysema after application of positive pressure ventilation to the upper airway.

LARYNX.   Trauma to the larynx may occur as a result of laryngoscopy, but this more commonly follows the actual insertion of the endotracheal tube. Abrasion or contusion of the internal laryngeal structures can lead to edema and airway obstruction, particularly in the cricoid region in children where the trachea is narrowest. Rarely, a vocal cord has been avulsed by an extremely rough

intubation. Prolonged pressure and movement of the endotracheal tube in situ may ulcerate the mucosa over the arytenoid cartilages and lead to chronic ulceration.

Management of laryngeal edema includes careful observation for progressive obstruction after extubation, use of high humidity inhalation, intravenous corticosteroids, and adequate intravenous hydration. These methods usually clear symptoms of obstruction within several hours, but hoarseness may persist for several days. Occasionally, progression to impending complete obstruction may be seen. Tracheostomy or reintubation of the trachea will be necessary to preserve respiration. Granulomas may require surgical removal by an otolaryngologist and will frequently reoccur. The incidence of postintubation granulomas seems to be decreasing with the use of disposable endotracheal tubes.

TRACHEA.   Pressure of the endotracheal tube on the wall of the trachea may cause ischemia and sloughing of discrete portions of the mucosa below the cords. Most often tracheal damage occurs at the site of the endotracheal tube cuff. Overinflation of the cuff can cause significant ischemia of the mucosa, and resulting tracheal stenosis with chronic airway obstruction may be a serious complication of prolonged endotracheal intubation. Diffusion of nitrous oxide into the cuff during surgery can increase cuff pressure and further compound morbidity. When periods of hypotension occur, ischemic damage may be increased and the possibility of tracheal stenosis may be even greater. The use of high-volume low-pressure endotracheal tube cuffs and frequent deflation of the cuff both in surgery and in the intensive care period will minimize tracheal damage, but tracheal stenosis requiring surgical resection may still be seen.

Physiologic Airway Complications

In addition to traumatic difficulties, endotracheal intubation can result in mechanical impediments to ventilation that must be detected and treated.

INADEQUATE TUBE DIAMETER.   Too small a tube may increase airway resistance markedly, particularly in children. This leads to reduced tidal volume, hypercarbia, and fatigue. The vigorous inspiratory efforts necessary to overcome this resistance may result in pulmonary edema. Providing a tube that fits the glottis without an excessive leak will allow for a maximal internal diameter with minimal resistance to ventilation.

TUBE OBSTRUCTION. The lumen of the tube may become blocked by kinking, secretions, blood, or overinflation of the cuff. The resultant reduction of the internal diameter of the tube leads to the same physiologic disturbances as are seen with the inadequate sized tube. An unsuccessful attempt to pass a catheter through the tube is diagnostic. If adjustment of the tube does not relieve the obstruction, it may need to be removed and replaced by a fresh tube. This is particularly likely to occur in children with purulent respiratory tract secretions, as in cystic fibrosis.

ENDOBRONCHIAL INTUBATION. Insertion of too long a tube may lead to the inadvertent intubation of the right main-stem bronchus, with exclusion of the opposite side. This often leads to obstruction of the right upper lobe bronchus as well, and resultant hypoventilation and ventilation/perfusion mismatch may lead to asphyxia as well as massive atelectasis of the unventilated lungs. Ventilations must always be checked by auscultation on both sides after endotracheal intubation; in the small child, breath sounds may be conducted across the thorax so that ventilation sounds adequate over a non-ventilated thorax. Diagnosis of endobronchial intubation in such small children requires a chest x-ray. Correction of endobronchial intubation is achieved by withdrawing the tube a few centimeters until ventilation is adequate and equal over both sides of the chest.

MUSCLE RELAXANTS. During induction of anesthesia, maintenance of continuous ventilation or insertion of the endotracheal tube can be facilitated by rendering the patient flaccid with intravenous muscle relaxants. The patient becomes apneic and ventilation must obviously be controlled until the effects of the muscle relaxants subside, if hypoxia and hypercarbia are to be prevented. Prolonged respiratory depression due to the relaxants frequently occurs associated with gross overdosage or electrolyte imbalance and may necessitate postoperative mechanical ventilation. The assessment of postanesthetic respiratory function is an essential aspect in the prevention of complications in the recovery period, especially in patients receiving muscle relaxants during anesthesia, and will be reviewed in the section on postoperative care.

The most commonly used muscle relaxants are the short-acting succinylcholine (Anectine) and the longer-acting *d*-tubocurarine or pancuronium (Pavulon). The alternative agents gallamine (Flaxedil) and dimethyltubocurarine (Metubine) are available but are less commonly used. Complications particularly related to use of the first three drugs will be discussed, and problems arising from pharmacologic reversal of non-depolarizing agents are reviewed. For a more complete discussion of the complications of muscle relaxants, the reader is referred to the review by Walts.[100]

Succinylcholine

Succinylcholine is a rapidly acting depolarizing muscle relaxant of short duration. The patient shows chaotic muscle fasciculations within a minute after intravenous injection, and subsequent flaccid relaxation can be expected to last several minutes. Succinylcholine is the most widely used of the muscle relaxant drugs, and although complications with its indiscriminate use are common, observance of certain precautions can minimize the incidence or severity of the following problems.

RESPIRATORY OBSTRUCTION. Complete relaxation of the musculature surrounding the upper airway may lead to soft tissue obstruction, which usually can be overcome with positive pressure.

POSTFASCICULATORY PAIN. Fasciculations may be violent enough to produce significant postoperative muscle discomfort; associated myoglobinemia is probably of minimal clinical significance. Postfasciculatory pain can be blocked by pre-treatment with small doses of non-depolarizing relaxant such as curare or pancuronium, but because this decreases the effectiveness of succinylcholine, a larger dose of the depolarizer must be injected to achieve relaxation.

INCREASED INTRAGASTRIC PRESSURE. Fasciculations are said to increase the intragastric pressure and predispose to regurgitation of stomach contents, especially in emergency patients. Reducing the strength of fasciculations with curare pre-treatment may also prevent this problem.

INCREASED INTRAOCULAR PRESSURE. Succinylcholine causes prolonged contracture of the extraocular muscles, which is probably responsible for the transient rise in intraocular pressure seen following its use. In patients with open eye injuries, such pressure changes can lead to extrusion of vitreous through the delicate structures of the anterior eye, so here succinylcholine must be avoided. Large doses of pancuronium can be administered to provide relaxation without dangerous intraocular pressure rises; the disadvantage of prolonged paralysis that follows is accepted under these circumstances.

MYOTONIA. Generalized neuromuscular rigidity after succinylcholine injection may interfere with ventilation, and associated masseter spasm can make intubation impossible. This phenomenon strongly suggests the possibility of occult neuromuscular disease and has been associated with both myotonic and Duchenne's dystrophies and with familial malignant hyperpyrexia. The anesthetic is commonly abandoned when myotonia occurs in the patient with no diagnosed neuromuscular disease, to allow a neurologic investigation to be performed. Succinylcholine is generally avoided in patients with diagnosed muscular dystrophies.

MALIGNANT HYPERTHERMIA. Succinylcholine has been implicated as a prime triggering agent for malignant hyperthermia, a highly fatal familial disease related to stress and anesthesia. (See below.) Succinylcholine is contraindicated in patients with a known predisposition to the disease or in relatives of such patients.

BRADYCARDIA. Vagal potentiation causes cardiac slowing, seen commonly after repeated injections of succinylcholine in adults. In children with higher vagal tone the first dose of the drug may produce bradycardia or asystole, and this is usually prevented with prior administration of atropine. Whenever slowing occurs it may be treated specifically with atropine.

HYPERKALEMIA. Hyperkalemia with subsequent ventricular fibrillation and asystole is seen predictably in patients with recent immobilization after burns or trauma and can be noted as late as 4 to 6 months after injury. Relaxation should be achieved in these patients with the non-depolarizing blocking agents that do not cause excessive potassium release from depolarization of muscle cell membranes in susceptible patients.

PROLONGED APNEA. Excessive duration of succinylcholine action is seen, when decreased metabolism of the drug is present, due to quantitative or qualitative defects of pseudocholinesterase, the enzyme that breaks down succinylcholine in the plasma to terminate the action of the drug. In patients with advanced hepatic disease, prolonged action of succinylcholine owing to deficient plasma pseudocholinesterase synthesis by the liver may be seen. Patients who use echothiophate eye drops (Phospholine) or who have been exposed to organophosphorus insecticides will have most of their pseudocholinesterase inactivated and will have a predictable prolongation of succinylcholine action.

Certain patients have a genetically determined defect in the synthesis of plasma cholinesterase that leads to a qualitatively atypical enzyme that is unable to metabolize succinylcholine. This occurs in approximately 1 in 4000 patients, and paralysis may persist for 4 to 6 hours after a single dose of succinylcholine in these individuals. Mechanical ventilation may be necessary, so succinylcholine should probably be avoided when such problems can be anticipated by careful questioning of the patient preoperatively. Non-depolarizing relaxants may be carefully utilized and reversed in these patients without complications.

DUAL BLOCK. Prolonged infusion of succinylcholine, even in normal individuals, can cause paralysis resembling that caused by curare that will not subside for several hours after discontinuing the drug. Restriction of the dosage and duration of succinylcholine infusion will prevent this complication, and use of the more predictable non-depolarizing relaxants is preferred for longer surgical procedures. Dual block may respond to reversal with anticholinesterase drugs, but this may increase the paralysis when residual succinylcholine is still present. Dual block must initially be treated with mechanical ventilation, combined with sedation of the agitated patient who is aware of the paralysis; anticholinesterase therapy should be considered later to shorten the duration of ventilatory support.

Succinylcholine is an important and essential drug that makes anesthesia easier and safer; this formidable list of complications is not intended to discourage use of this valuable agent but rather to further its appropriate and intelligent utilization.

Non-depolarizing Relaxants

Pancuronium and *d*-tubocurarine are long-acting non-depolarizing neuromuscular blocking agents. Considerations relating to the respiratory effects of paralysis are essentially the same as with succinylcholine. Most of the other complications of succinylcholine do not occur with use of the non-depolarizing drugs. Overdosage with curare and pancuronium leading to prolonged paralysis is the most common complication of their use. Even restricted dosages of these non-depolarizers may produce excessively long neuromuscular blockade in patients with myasthenia or in patients treated with magnesium sulfate or certain antibiotics. The potentiation of relaxant effect by volatile inhalational anesthetics should also be taken into consideration in the calculation of relaxant dosages. Titration of these drugs guided by the peripheral nerve stimulator will help prevent such overdosage from the non-depolarizing agents. The effects of antibiotics or magnesium sulfate can be opposed by calcium; and in myasthenics careful regulation of anticholinesterase therapy may make the use of non-depolarizing relaxants in small amounts safe and helpful.

Complications that distinguish between curare and pancuronium in clinical use relate to the cardiovascular and respiratory effects of these agents. Curare causes histamine release that can lead to peripheral vasodilatation and hypotension and occasionally to bronchospasm. A generalized histamine flush of the skin can be seen, which is harmless, but hypotension may require rapid fluid infusion and pressors for correction when severe. Drops in blood pressure after curare injection seldom persist longer than 5 to 10 minutes and should respond promptly to corrective measures or

to stimulation from airway intubation or surgical incision. Halothane, aminophylline, or steroids can be used to reverse histamine-related bronchospasm.

While pancuronium has no significant effect on the lower airway (it is the relaxant of choice in asthmatics), its cardiovascular effects are almost the opposite of curare. Increases in blood pressure, pulse rate, and cardiac output, possibly related to cardiac vagal blockade, are seen soon after injection. While this may be of advantage in the hypovolemic patient, the increased work demanded of the heart under this stimulation can aggravate myocardial ischemia in the patient with compromised coronary blood flow. Pancuronium should be used carefully in such situations, and tachycardia associated with ischemic EKG changes should be treated with injection of propranolol or nitroglycerine.

Reversal of Neuromuscular Blockade

Depolarizing block is self-limited and does not require reversal. The effects of non-depolarizing blockers can be reversed with anticholinesterase agents that produce increases in cholinergic tone at the motor end plate to facilitate conduction and stimulate contraction. The most commonly used anticholinesterases are neostigmine (Prostigmine) and pyridostigmine (Regonol or Mestinon), which have a duration of action of several hours, and edrophonium (Tensilon), which lasts around 20 minutes. Besides improving neuromuscular conduction, these drugs also stimulate parasympathetic nerve endings. The main complications of relaxant reversal relate to these parasympathetic side effects or to underdosage of anticholinesterase agents with resultant reparalysis.

UNDERDOSAGE. The anticholinesterases do not remove the muscle relaxants from their site of action; they merely overwhelm relaxant effects until metabolism and excretion of the drugs terminate their action. Inadequate doses of reversal drugs may result in a transient return of strength that may lead to a false sense of security. Recurarization in the recovery room after extubation may lead to respiratory insufficiency in the obtunded patient. Proper doses, experience, and the use of the peripheral nerve stimulator will help prevent this complication. When it occurs, careful observation in the recovery room may allow prompt administration of additional anticholinesterase. The patient grossly overdosed with relaxant cannot be adequately reversed even with maximal doses of reversal drugs and should be mechanically ventilated after surgery until signs of neuromuscular recovery suggest that pharmacologic reversal may be successful.

PARASYMPATHETIC EFFECTS. Bradycardia or asystole, excessive secretions, and bronchospasm can follow administration of anticholinesterases. This effect can even be therapeutically of benefit, as when Tensilon is used to treat paroxysmal atrial tachycardia. Routine administration of anticholinergic drug along with the anticholinesterase should prevent these side effects. Atropine is the drug most commonly used for this, and additional doses may be required in the recovery room because late bradycardia is common. Secretions may still be a problem during acute reversal with atropine and neostigmine, so the use of glycopyrrolate (Robinul) has been recommended because it seems to decrease release of secretions after anticholinesterase administration better than does atropine. Glycopyrrolate also produces less acute tachycardia than atropine and has a longer duration of action, so supplemental injections may be unnecessary in the recovery room. Bronchospasm is rare but may require therapy if severe. Reversal is usually deferred in asthmatics or patients with significant bronchospastic disease to avoid this difficulty.

Complications of Patient Positioning

Anesthesia is usually begun with the patient supine, and changes in positioning appropriate to the location of the surgical incision, adjusted according to the surgeon's preferences, are accomplished after anesthesia is established. While positioning is essentially a surgical topic, it is appropriate to discuss resulting complications under the section on anesthesia. Depression of spontaneous movement and normal protective reflexes can make some positions quite damaging under anesthesia. The an-

esthesiologist is also responsible for monitoring the physiologic effects of positioning and for taking corrective measures at his disposal. Finally, the anesthesiologist is able to inspect the entire patient during surgery and need not focus attention primarily on the surgical field. Thus, the anesthesiologist is more likely to detect problems that may arise with positioning, and he or she should be able to avoid complications due to incorrect positioning or to acute effects of changes in position. Problems in this area will be discussed under effects on *ventilation, circulation, the peripheral nerves,* and *miscellaneous structures.* The complications of specific surgical positions are reviewed extensively in a recent book devoted entirely to this one subject.[77] Without discussing each individual position in detail, certain generalizations about the detection and prevention of morbidity related to positioning can be made, under the above physiologic classifications.

VENTILATION. Shifting the patient from the supine position alters the anatomic relationship of the soft tissues around the upper airway under anesthesia to produce respiratory obstruction. The difficulty of endotracheal intubation is also increased when attempts are made in an unaccustomed or unfavorable position. To prevent loss of the airway under such circumstances it is advisable to control the airway with an endotracheal tube prior to changes in position. Maintenance of anesthesia by mask is generally safe only in the supine or lithotomy position during short cases.

Care must also be taken that patient movement does not force the endotracheal tube down the right main-stem bronchus to exclude the left lung from ventilation. This can result from flexion, extension, or lateral rotation of the head under specific circumstances, or from external pressure caused by taping or the weight of tubings or adaptors. Breath sounds should be checked bilaterally after the patient is in the final position for surgery and the tube withdrawn and resecured in a position in which respirations are adequate over both lung fields.

In general, the effects of positioning on ventilation will be immediately obvious to the anesthesiologist, and he can make adjustments in patient position to maximize respiratory function before the patient is draped for surgery. Even after optimal posi-

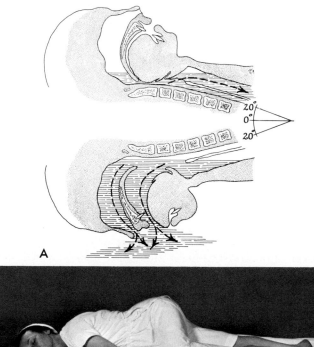

Figure 10–5 Positioning the unconscious patient. *A,* Upper diagram shows patient supine with tongue dropped back and the 20-degree downward tracheal slope favoring aspiration into lungs (fluid level and arrow). Lower diagram shows patient prone with tongue forward and the 20-degree upward tracheal slope and gravitation of fluid out of nose and mouth (arrows), making aspiration into lungs unlikely. *B,* Anterior view of recommended position. *C,* Posterior view of recommended position.

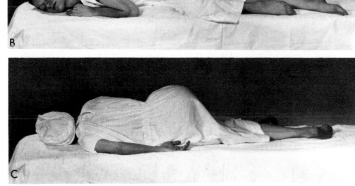

tioning, respiratory functional deficits will persist in many positions, but these deficits can be overcome with increases in ventilatory pressures, volumes, and oxygen concentrations, and the effects of these manipulations can be assessed with arterial blood gas analysis.

The most significant effects on ventilation caused by changes in position are related to decreases in compliance with resulting restriction of lung volumes. Deficits in respiratory volumes have been demonstrated in the awake patient after assuming various surgical positions, and even greater decrements can be shown in these positions under general anesthesia. For example, the lithotomy position decreases the vital capacity 18 per cent in the awake patient, but this seems to correspond to only a minimal 3 per cent deficit in tidal volume under anesthesia when non-obese individuals are placed in lithotomy position. When the effects of this position are combined with steep Trendelenburg tilt, however, a 20 per cent decrease in tidal volume can be expected owing to the weight of the abdominal viscera against the diaphragm. Thus, while the lithotomy position alone would cause few problems, the addition of Trendelenburg position would be expected to cause considerable respiratory embarrassment. This should be detected by changes in compliance, as judged by the hand on the breathing circuit bag, or by changes in peak inspiratory pressures with delivery of consistent tidal volumes either manually or by mechanical volume ventilator. Prevention of respiratory complications secondary to such decreased ventilatory volumes would involve use of assisted or controlled respiration, increased oxygen percentages in the inspired gas mixtures, and endotracheal intubation when steep Trendelenburg position is used.

Problems of decreased respiratory compliance with the patient in the prone position are readily demonstrated. Rolls should be placed under the chest and iliac crests to allow the abdomen to hang free and to minimize respiratory compromise. Again some estimate of compliance may be obtained by observation of ventilating pressures under anesthesia, and excessive pressures should prompt a reassessment of the position and adjustment of the chest rolls when indicated. Increases in ventilatory pressures and volumes may be needed to overcome changes in compliance and assure adequate respiration in the prone position, and during lengthy procedures the results of ventilatory management should be confirmed with arterial blood gas analyses.

Ventilatory volumes are actually improved under anesthesia in the sitting position owing to the decreased pressure of the abdominal contents on the diaphragm. The lateral decubitus position, particularly with elevation of the kidney rest, causes decreases in tidal volume of 14 per cent under anesthesia, which may produce significant respiratory compromise. This can be improved slightly by placing the kidney rest at the crest of the ilium, rather than above it, but some urologists feel that this provides less adequate surgical exposure of the kidney in this position. Ventilation in this position should be controlled in most cases, the FI_{O_2} increased, and arterial blood gas measurements obtained, because of the high incidence of respiratory abnormalities to be expected.

CIRCULATION. Most changes in position involve placing portions of the body in more dependent positions, which can lead to pooling of blood, decreased venous return, inadequate cardiac output, and lowered blood pressure. In the normovolemic awake patient such shifts will be physiologically compensated for, but general anesthesia blocks these acute compensatory mechanisms, which depend for the most part on peripheral vasoconstriction for their effec-

tiveness. In the hypovolemic patient, changes in position under anesthesia can be extremely hazardous, and fluid replacement may be indicated prior to placing the patient in certain high-risk positions. It is essential that the blood pressure be checked immediately after any position change. Decreases in pressure should be treated promptly with fluids and pressors, and placing the patient temporarily back in the supine position should be considered when correction of cardiovascular instability is not rapidly successful.

Occasionally dependent pooling of blood volume can be used to clinical advantage, as in the use of head-up position with peripheral tourniquets in pulmonary edema. Elevation of the legs in a hypovolemic patient can acutely shift as much as 10 per cent of the circulating blood volume centrally, and this can be an effective temporary corrective measure, when hypotension is related to volume deficits and not to inotropic depression of the heart. The Trendelenburg position has been traditionally used in this situation, but because the combination of low blood pressure and high cerebral venous pressure may compromise cerebral perfusion, caution is indicated in its application. Elevation of the legs with the patient supine seems equally effective, without requiring lowering the level of the head.

Acute hypotension can be expected frequently after lowering the legs from the stirrups used for the lithotomy position. To prevent this hypotension the legs are usually lowered slowly to allow for gradual shift of volume and to permit increased fluid infusion to be accomplished. Leg wraps and anti-embolism stockings may also help prevent hypotension owing to dependent positioning of the legs and may be helpful in supporting the pressure when patients are removed from the lithotomy position. Occasionally when the blood pressure drops during lowering of the legs, pressors or re-elevation of the legs will be indicated temporarily while fluid volume is supplemented. Patients on diuretics or patients who have had blood loss during surgery are particularly at risk for this complication.

Impeded venous return owing to pressure on the inferior vena cava or femoral veins can lead to signficant hypotension. The most frequently encountered example of this is the supine hypotensive syndrome seen in late pregnancy, when the gravid uterus collapses the inferior vena cava against the lumbar vertebrae. Subsequent hypotension can endanger both the mother and fetus unless lateral pressure is applied to the uterus to prevent venous pooling in the legs. Pressure on the vena cava and femoral veins can also produce hypotension in the improperly positioned prone patient and can cause engorgement of the collateral vertebral venous plexus in the epidural space, increasing the possibility of undesirable bleeding during and after back surgery. So that inferior vena caval flow will be unimpeded, care should be taken to leave the abdomen and inguinal regions free of excessive pressure during use of the prone position in surgery.

The lateral decubitus position with the kidney rest elevated may cause marked circulatory changes, especially when the kidney rest presses the inferior vena cava against the spine with the legs dependent. The blood pressure must be carefully watched while the patient is placed in this position, and fluid supplements and pressors may be necessary to support the blood pressure on occasion. Again, this complication may be partly preventable if the kidney rest is placed under the iliac crest, but the surgical exposure may be insufficient for some surgeons using this support location.

In the lateral decubitus position, the humerus may rotate to place undue pressure on the brachial vessels and the brachial plexus around them, and not only circulatory compromise but permanent neurologic damage as well may result. This can be prevented by placing a roll under the chest wall next to the axilla, so that the dependent shoulder does not bear the entire weight of the chest. The pulses should be checked distally in the dependent arm after positioning to confirm that compression has not interfered with the circulation to the arm. If pulses are present it can be reasonably assumed that excessive pressure is not being applied to the brachial plexus, provided that the shoulder has not been overly extended past 90 degrees.

Air embolism is a potentially catastrophic complication associated with the sitting position used frequently in neurosurgery. However, it can be anticipated any time the operative site is 4 inches or more above the right atrium after positioning. Air embolism has been associated with a wide variety of operations in the head and neck and has even been reported during pelvic node dissection in the Trendelenburg position. The column of blood between the heart and the surgical field can suck air into the venous circulation whenever the veins do not normally collapse with negative pressure, and if this siphon delivers a large quantity of air to the heart, the right ventricular outflow tract becomes unable to pump blood to the lungs. The condition can be rapidly fatal, even when adequate treatment is begun promptly.

Prevention of air embolism involves avoiding the surgical positions associated with this complication whenever possible. In this connection the risk of the sitting position should never be minimized. If the complications of the position are to be accepted to gain the advantages of the surgical exposure to be obtained, then emphasis must be placed on detection and treatment of air embolism when it occurs.

Effective treatment of air embolism requires adequate preparation beforehand. A long central venous catheter should be inserted, with position of the tip in the right atrium confirmed by x-ray before surgery. The balloon-tipped pulmonary artery catheter has also been used for sitting cases, with the catheter port placed in the right ventricle or pulmonary outflow tract. This allows for immediate aspiration of air from the vicinity of the catheter tip whenever air embolism is suspected. Air in the line confirms the diagnosis, and its removal may improve the pumping ability of the right ventricle.

Minimal air embolism often occurs undetected, with little or no apparent physiologic effect. The classic "mill-wheel" murmur requires a significant amount of air to be present in the right ventricle, and when this is detected through the esophageal stethoscope, cardiovascular instability should be anticipated. Two other means of detection have proven their clinical usefulness. The precordial Doppler probe, when aimed at the right atrium, can detect as little as 0.5 cc. of air entering the right ventricle. This is the most sensitive means of diagnosing air embolism, and the use of the precordial

Doppler has become mandatory for surgery in the sitting position. The partial pressure of carbon dioxide in the end-tidal air will decrease when pulmonary blood flow is suddenly impaired, and this can be used as an indicator of substantial cardiac dysfunction due to air embolism. The infrared determination of exhaled carbon dioxide is relatively insensitive but can serve to confirm the diagnosis of air embolism when it is suspected. Intra-arterial monitoring is also useful in continually assessing cardiac performance, as well as ventilatory function, and is used routinely for surgery in the sitting position.

When the diagnosis of air embolism has been made, an attempt to stop further air entry into the venous circulation should be made by flooding the surgical field with clear fluid, and a rapid inspection by the surgeon may reveal the site of air entry. All nitrous oxide should be discontinued, because it will tend to increase the size of volumes of air in the circulation and because 100 per cent oxygen is indicated during periods of low cardiac output. If the drop in blood pressure is significant and prolonged, the patient should be placed in the Durant position (left lateral decubitus with the right atrium up), to favor accumulation of air away from the right ventricle and pulmonary conus. When all else fails, inotropic agents may be required to stimulate myocardial contractility in an attempt to forcefully eject air into the peripheral pulmonary circulation; needle aspiration of the right heart has been described but should seldom be necessary. Right thoracotomy with aspiration of air from the right heart and cardiac massage rarely may be required.

It is generally advisable to counsel patients who are candidates for a procedure in the sitting position of the risk of air embolism and the difficulties involved in adequate treatment of severe cases. As a potentially lethal complication of benign positioning maneuvers, it is usually unexpected by patients and their families and deserves mention during the preoperative visit.

PERIPHERAL NERVE INJURIES.   As many as 11 per cent of all peripheral nerve palsies reported are due to improper positioning under anesthesia.[81] The peripheral nerves are vulnerable to injury from excessive pressure or stretch. A typical postoperative paresis usually involves pressure over a nerve where it passes under the skin over a bony prominence. The ulnar nerve at the elbow, the lateral femoral cutaneous nerve crossing the inguinal ligament, and the common peroneal nerve passing over the head of the fibula are relatively unprotected and susceptible to injury. These nerves should be padded appropriately in various positions and protected from pressure applied by hard surfaces or sharp edges. The common peroneal nerve injury results in foot drop and cutaneous anesthesia over the leg and foot and most frequently results from the lateral decubitus position or from the use of stirrups in the lithotomy position.

Injuries to the brachial plexus are usually related to stretch from extreme arm extension on armboards during surgery, and a high percentage of these injuries occurs following sternotomy during open heart surgery. The armboard when used should never allow extension of the arm past 90 degrees above the body. It is perhaps preferable to have the arms at the patient's side during surgery to prevent such injuries, but most anesthesiologists will find sacrificing ready access to the arms unacceptable.

Peripheral nerve palsies can be prevented by careful attention to the proper positioning and padding of the patient. Peripheral nerve injuries when they occur can be expected to heal in varying periods of time depending on the extent of disruption of the nerve fiber. Some may take several months to recover, but the usual course is several weeks to full restoration of function. Neurologic consultation should be sought to document the damage and follow recovery. Physical therapy may be helpful in preventing muscle atrophy during prolonged recovery.

MISCELLANEOUS INJURIES.   Pressure may be exerted by the weight of the body on various anatomic structures to produce ischemia, necrosis, and gangrene. The crushed, folded ear lobe under the weight of the head is a good example. Also, the male genitalia can be subjected to extreme pressure when the patient is placed prone over hard surfaces. Careful inspection of all vulnerable structures, especially the eyes, ears, and genitalia, after positioning and frequently throughout surgery, will help prevent such complications.

The eyes are especially prone to injury. During anesthesia, the conjunctival reflex is obtunded, the orbicularis oculi is relaxed, and the eyelids may be separated, thus allowing damage to the eye that ranges from a benign conjunctivitis to ulceration of the cornea. The former heals quickly with no sequelae, while the latter can lead to infection, scarring, and impaired vision. Prevention requires careful protection of the eyes during anesthesia with the use of suitable ophthalmic ointment and routine taping of the eyelids. When head drapes are placed over the eyes, traction on the eyelids should not be allowed to expose the cornea or conjunctiva. Conjunctivitis should clear in 6 to 12 hours after application of antibiotic or steroid ointment and an eyepatch. Failure of epithelialization is usually due to infection by either herpetic virus or bacteria. Persistence of symptoms or obvious severe initial damage deserves immediate ophthalmologic consultation. The extent and nature of ulceration are usually determined by slit-lamp examination and fluorescein staining.

Complications During Anesthetic Maintenance

Through the maintenance phase of an anesthetic that appears stable and satisfactory, complications that deserve consideration may arise in various physiologic systems. Some of these difficulties may be prevented by careful management, or detected by close monitoring and expeditiously treated. Other problems are more subtle and may become apparent only in the postoperative period. Most of these complications relate to the effect of inhalational anesthetic agents on various physiologic systems, or they are caused directly by surgical manipulations. The complications of anesthetic maintenance will be divided into sections on *cardiovascular, respiratory, renal,* and *central nervous system* effects during anesthesia.

CARDIOVASCULAR EFFECTS. Cardiovascular complications caused by the inhalational anesthetic agents are related to changes in myocardial contractility, systemic vascular resistance, and cardiac rhythm. The commonly used inhalational agents nitrous oxide, halothane (Fluothane), enflurane (Ethrane), and the newer agent isoflurane

(Forane) all depress myocardial contractility in a dose-related fashion. This has variable effects on cardiac output, depending on accompanying changes in systemic vascular resistance. Nitrous oxide increases systemic vascular resistance to compensate for decreased contractility, so while the blood pressure is minimally affected by 40 per cent nitrous oxide in oxygen, the cardiac output is decreased by 40 per cent.[57] While nitrous oxide is considered a relatively weak anesthetic agent, its myocardial depressant effects can be considerable in debilitated patients with vasoconstriction that is insufficient to maintain the arterial pressure.

Circulatory depression from halothane is partly mediated by depression of vasomotor centers in the brainstem and by decreased catecholamine output from the adrenal medulla and peripheral adrenergic terminals. The primary cause of decreased arterial pressure is direct myocardial depression, however, possibly owing to the disruption of calcium metabolism in the myocardial contractile mechanism. Limited decreases in systemic vascular resistance are also produced by halothane, and the total loss of cardiac output can be as high as 50 per cent during maintenance with a 2 per cent concentration in healthy individuals. The effects of enflurane are essentially the same as those seen with halothane. The depression from both agents seems to abate partially over several hours and will be corrected transiently by the intravenous administration of calcium.[85] The new agent isoflurane also depresses the blood pressure, but because the peripheral resistance is markedly reduced by the drug, the cardiac output is maintained at near normal levels.

The potential complications associated with the use of any of these inhalational agents, and particularly isoflurane, in the hypovolemic patient or in the presence of decreased myocardial reserve should be obvious. Hypotension is frequent during inhalational anesthesia, even in the most healthy patients. It can be prevented somewhat by volume support prior to surgery, and by restriction of inhaled concentrations, because of the relationship between anesthetic dose and cardiovascular depression. When blood pressure or pulse rate is inadequate during anesthesia, the concentration of anesthetic agent should be decreased, or the agent should be discontinued entirely if depression is severe. The increased infusion of fluids is usually appropriate, and surgical stimulation may help restore normal vital signs. Further therapy with atropine and calcium may also be helpful at this time.

Pressors should be carefully chosen because of the known potential for dysrhythmias when catecholamines are injected during the use of volatile anesthetic agents, especially halothane. Because the bulk of the blood pressure decrease is due to inotropic depression rather than to peripheral vasodilatation, a centrally acting non-catecholamine adrenergic stimulant is to be preferred to a direct-acting peripheral vasoconstrictor.[67] Ephedrine in low doses (5 to 10 mg.) is ideal for this purpose and should be immediately available when volatile agents are in use. Because nitrous oxide alone, without other volatile agents, is unlikely to predispose to dysrhythmias, the use of catecholamines for cardiovascular support during nitrous oxide anesthesia is relatively safe.

Dysrhythmias are frequently encountered during the use of all the volatile anesthetic agents, but they are most commonly seen during the use of halothane. Atrioventricular conduction is depressed by all agents, and nodal rhythms, nodal and ventricular premature contractions, and ventricular bigeminy occur frequently. Mechanisms that have been implicated in causing halothane-related arrhythmias are delayed conduction, alteration in the conduction pathway, varying degrees of conduction block, and re-entrant mechanisms. Hypercarbia and associated catecholamine release have also been described as predisposing to dysrhythmias during halothane maintenance. This increased incidence of rhythm abnormalities is most likely due to the sensitization of the myocardium to the arrhythmogenic effects of the catecholamines that halothane produces. Halothane sensitizes the myocardium to a much greater extent that either enflurane or isoflurane, but precautions are indicated with the use of injected catecholamines in surgery when anesthesia is maintained with any of these agents.

Dysrhythmias may potentially compound the cardiovascular depression already established during maintenance of anesthesia with a volatile agent. They should therefore be treated as soon as they are detected. The common nodal rhythm seldom affects the blood pressure significantly and is usually just noted and observed without requiring therapy. When a patient seems to need the atrial kick to maintain blood pressure, differences in systolic pressure of 20 torr are occasionally seen as sinus rhythm and nodal rhythm alternate. If treatment of nodal rhythm is considered necessary, atropine or low doses of succinylcholine may be effective in restoring a sinus rhythm.[60]

Ventricular ectopic contractions and bigeminal rhythm under halothane anesthesia seldom progress to ventricular tachycardia or fibrillation, but therapy is indicated because of the decreased cardiac output that is usually present. If the dysrhythmia is possibly related to catecholamine release under light anesthesia, the concentration of agent may be increased cautiously. Because hypoventilation or hypoxia may also be causative, an arterial blood gas analysis can be obtained, and the level of ventilation and oxygenation increased appropriately. Hypokalemia may also be implicated in causing arrhythmias, especially in patients on preoperative diuretic therapy. Small bolus injections of 1 mEq. of potassium chloride will often acutely suppress ventricular dysrhythmias and indicate that further potassium supplementation may be necessary while serum electrolyte determinations are obtained. Pharmacologic suppression of ventricular dysrhythmias may be achieved by injection of lidocaine, 1 mg./kg. If this is ineffective, propranolol may be injected in increments of 0.25 mg., up to a total of 5 mg. Finally, switching from halothane to a less arrhythmogenic agent, e.g., enflurane or isoflurane, is always an option when dysrhythmias are intractable.

When catecholamines are injected for hemostasis during procedures on the head and neck, the total dose of epinephrine must be carefully controlled to prevent arrhythmias due to myocardial sensitization. With halothane, epinephrine should be restricted to 1.5 μg./kg. in any 10-minute period, with no more than 4.5 μg./kg. injected in any hour.[72] When enflurane is in use, twice this amount is probably safe. For isoflurane, safe compatible levels of epinephrine have not been established; however, it is known to be nearly as safe as enflurane in this regard, so a level of 3.0 μg./kg. in any single injection should result in no dysrhythmias.[69] The use of a 1:200,000 dilution of epinephrine is recommended, because adequate vasoconstriction can be thus obtained, while the volume of local anesthetic solution that can be safely injected can be maximized.

RESPIRATORY EFFECTS. Complications of anesthesia related to the respiratory system may be due to anesthetic-induced respiratory dysfunction or to mechanical problems with the anesthesia equipment.

Anesthesia and Respiration

The respiratory stimulation produced by diethylether kept the arterial carbon dioxide partial pressure at normal levels until deep surgical anesthetic planes were reached. Much the opposite is seen with the inhalational anesthetic agents currently in use, which all produce central medullary depression of respiratory drive. In unstimulated patients breathing halothane or isoflurane, the arterial carbon dioxide will reach 45 torr with minimal surgical anesthesia, while with the more depressant enflurane, a level of 60 torr will result. This respiratory depression will be increased by higher concentrations of anesthetic agents or by premedication with opiates and will be opposed by surgical stimulation. The ultimate effect of this depression is primary respiratory acidosis and secondary hypoxemia, resulting from decreased alveolar ventilation.

Assessment of alveolar ventilation under anesthesia depends ultimately on measurement of the arterial carbon dioxide level, because the effects of anesthetic agents and equipment on dead space may make respiratory volume measurements unpredictive. However, a rough estimate of the patient's ventilatory exchange should allow an early decision as to whether adequate spontaneous respiration can be safely maintained during anesthesia. If there is any possibility of significant respiratory depression, ventilation should be controlled or the concentration of anesthetic agents decreased.

Besides depression of respiratory drive by anesthesia, alveolar ventilation can be re-duced by surgical positioning, intra-abdominal retraction against the diaphragm, or external pressure, to produce a restrictive ventilatory defect under anesthesia. This may further compound hypercarbia, and the reduction in ventilatory volumes will usually be an obvious indication for controlled respiration.

Hypoxemia is a frequent and usually preventable result of suboptimal anesthetic management. Early detection by visual inspection and blood gas analysis will permit corrective measures to be taken before acidosis, arrhythmias, and cardiac arrest develop.

Hypoxemia is most commonly a result of the blockage of diffusion of oxygen to the alveoli, caused by abnormalities of the peripheral airways. Atelectasis of portions of the lung is frequent during anesthesia and is related to decreased effectiveness of cough or sigh. The peripheral airways can also be blocked by mucus, blood, stomach contents, or foreign bodies, and bronchospasm as well may physically close the airway. In a similar fashion, pulmonary edema may cause bubble formation and mucosal edema proximal to the alveoli that can collapse the airway and block distal diffusion of oxygen. There is also a normal tendency of the terminal bronchioles in the dependent portions of the lungs to collapse during tidal respiration, and general anesthesia seems to increase the extent of this small airway closure.

Perfusion of these hypoxic alveoli decreases the oxygen saturation of arterial blood, and a shunt develops that can be demonstrated as a drop in the arterial oxygen partial pressure. Muscle relaxants and controlled ventilation may aggravate the problem by shifting ventilation to nondependent portions of the lung that are relatively underperfused. There is also a compensatory mechanism in the pulmonary circulation that involves vasoconstriction in the pulmonary blood supply to underventilated alveoli, to decrease intrapulmonary shunting by diverting blood flow to more oxygenated lung segments. Inhalational anesthetics block this hypoxic pulmonary vasoconstriction and on that basis may increase the hypoxic effects of atelectasis.

The prevention and treatment of hypoxemia during anesthesia involves increasing the inspired oxygen concentration and applying positive pressure to the airway. Hypoxemia owing to mismatch of ventilation and perfusion in the lungs can be reversed with hyperoxygenation. The other causes of hypoxemia all involve airway collapse and will be treated primarily with application of distending airway pressure.

Physical blockage of the airway by mucus or blood should be treated with humidification of the inspired gases, and bronchospasm when severe should be treated with aminophylline and steroids. Deepening the level of inhalational agents is often therapeutic in reversing bronchospasm and should be tried. The use of epinephrine or terbutaline with halothane is absolutely contraindicated, and even aminophylline must be injected slowly and with care when this agent is being administered. The same precautions are probably worthwhile with enflurane and isoflurane, despite their greater compatibility with catecholamines.

Distending airway pressure can be applied intermittently or constantly to reverse hypoxemia owing to airway collapse. Intermittent manual sighs can be given to prevent or reverse atelectasis during anesthesia, but to be effective positive pressure should be applied frequently and in a sustained fashion. One recommendation is that a 30 cm. H_2O plateau be maintained for 20 seconds 4 times each hour. More sustained distending airway pressure may be applied with the use of PEEP (positive end-expiratory pressure) valve devices or with manual compression of the breathing bag. A continuous 5 cm. H_2O pressure maintained throughout the respiratory cycle can be applied, and the resulting correction of hypoxemia can be assessed with blood gas analysis. The level of pressure maintained may need to be raised if hypoxemia persists.

Distending airway pressure may decrease arterial blood pressure, because central venous return is impeded by raised mean intrathoracic pressure. This may require temporary return of distending airway pressure to lower levels until hypovolemia can be corrected with fluid infusion. Another complication of PEEP is expansion of respiratory dead space, which may occasionally lead to hypercarbia. Full control of respiration or use of intermittent mandatory ventilation techniques may be necessary to control hypercarbia when this occurs.

The postoperative use of distending airway pressure and supplemental oxygenation increases the possibility of pressure trauma to the lungs, primarily seen as pneumothorax, and of oxygen toxicity due to prolonged exposure to high oxygen concentrations. Restriction of distending airway pressure and inspired oxygen concentration to supposedly safer levels that will be less likely to cause these complications may not be compatible with survival in extremely severe respiratory failure, and a minimal respiratory morbidity seems inevitable despite optimal management. These techniques have become indispensable in critical care, but their application requires acquaintance with the complications associated with their use and preventive measures that may be taken. The reader is referred to more extensive reviews of respiratory management for further information.[64]

A final complication of anesthetic maintenance related to the respiratory system may occur when nitrous oxide is discontinued. At this time nitrous oxide outflow into the alveolus proceeds 30 times faster than nitrogen uptake, so resulting dilution of oxygen in the alveolus can produce systemic hypoxemia. If the system is left open to air after nitrous oxide is stopped, either by turning off the nitrous oxide flow or by disconnecting the endotracheal tube from the system, severe hypoxemia can result with its attendant complications. This diffusion hypoxia can be prevented by administering 100 per cent oxygen for the first few minutes after nitrous oxide is discontinued. The contention that 100 per cent oxygen may promote absorption atelectasis in the alveoli has been proposed, and there may be some advantage to the use of 90 per cent oxygen in this situation to prevent iatrogenic increases in intrapulmonary shunt. The existence of this phenomenon is still argued, however, and a much greater problem is certainly posed by diffusion hypoxia, which must be treated.

Mechanical Problems with Anesthesia Equipment

Morbidity and death may follow mechanical failures in anesthesia systems. Certain portions of the apparatus seem especially accident prone, and complications to be expected may be due to poor equipment design, improper use of apparatus, or failure of worn out or inadequately maintained equipment. Whatever the factors involved, the net result is asphyxia or uneven anesthesia.

HYPOXIC GAS MIXTURES. The administration of hypoxic gas mixtures may rarely occur from improper setting of flowmeters by the anesthesiologist. Malfunction of the flowmeters may also be a cause, but this should be detected during equipment maintenance. Failure of the oxygen supply due to depletion of reservoir tanks or from connection of oxygen lines to non-oxygen sources may also be encountered. Such complications are not beyond the ability of the anesthesiologist to detect or prevent. The first line of defense is the oxygen analyzer, which is not routinely used in most institutions, but which helps guarantee that adequate concentrations of oxygen are present in the breathing circuit. Color coding of connectors and gas tanks, combined with pin index and diameter index safety connectors, should help eliminate most problems related to incorrect pressurized gas supplies. Special precautions are now being taken in recently built hospitals to check oxygen lines carefully for plumbing faults, after several suits were filed involving hypoxic damage due to incorrect gas connections in new facilities. Finally, the fail-safe systems in present anesthesia apparatus will guarantee that anesthesia gases will not flow when the oxygen source is not pressurized. However, these fail-safe systems will deliver hypoxic gas mixtures to the breathing system if they are purposely or inadvertently dialed in by the person giving the anesthetic.

Fail-safe systems are therefore no substitute for vigilance or for the oxygen analyzer. Newer fail-safe flow systems are available that will deliver no less than a 20 per cent oxygen concentration during anesthesia; when these are more widely in use, this should add a further element of safety.

INACCURATE CONCENTRATIONS OF AGENT. System leaks are a common cause of uneven anesthesia and inefficient positive pressure breathing. The system should be checked before use to confirm that it will maintain positive pressure during assisted or controlled ventilation. During the use of spontaneous respiration, inordinately high concentrations of agent required for adequate anesthesia may suggest that air mix is occurring somewhere in the system, usually from leaks around the mask or at the seal of the carbon dioxide absorber cannister. Malfunctioning vaporizers may occasionally deliver excessive concentrations of agent. Following the physiologic response of the patient to the agent, rather than relying on the concentration of the vaporizer dial, will help prevent problems related to overdosage from this cause. Regular maintenance of vaporizers is necessary to prevent morbidity related to malfunction, and this would also require that any vaporizer suspected of malfunction should be removed from use immediately and checked by competent personnel, before anesthetic overdosages result.

INCREASED RESISTANCE TO BREATHING. Resistance to breathing depends upon flow rate, gas viscosity and density, length and diameter of tubings, and the valves in the circuit. Resistance is further increased by regions of turbulence created by valves, acute angles, or constrictions. There is a definite, if small, resistance to breathing through a soda lime absorber. The sum of all these factors is the total resistance to gas flow within each circuit. This will be determined by proper choice of anesthetic circuits for particular patients, to minimize the resistance to breathing to be imposed upon the patient's ventilatory apparatus. With modern equipment applied to vigorous adults, the total resistance of any breathing circuit is negligible. Exceptions may be seen in the small child or the adult with severe muscle weakness, in whom the use of standard adult breathing circuits may produce progressive fatigue and hypoventilation. Resistance should be minimized by using apparatus of maximum diameter with minimum corners and valves that may produce turbulence. Endotracheal tubes of maximum internal diameter will also produce minimum resistance to flow, especially important in pediatric patients.

EXCESSIVE DEAD SPACE. Apparatus that significantly contributes to dead space increases the possibility of hypercarbia and respiratory acidosis. Increased respiratory exchange will be necessary to produce the same level of carbon dioxide in the blood, and the work of breathing is increased. Exhaustion and asphyxia may be expected to follow. The dead space of anesthesia equipment is increased by the use of masks or excessively long or large connectors between the y-piece of the breathing circuit and the endotracheal tube. The endotracheal tube itself can be used to significantly decrease the dead space, usually by 40 to 50 per cent, by excluding the entire upper airway. Circle systems depend on valves for proper functioning. If the valves malfunction and permit bi-directional flow of gas in the system, rebreathing may occur with resultant hypercarbia and hypoxia. Care should always be taken to note where the source of fresh gas flow is supplied to the patient and to establish where the dead space begins. Excessive gas volumes between this point and the alveoli should be eliminated, to minimize the work required to assure adequate ventilation.

INEFFECTIVE CARBON DIOXIDE ABSORBERS. Soda lime absorbers may be inefficient, exhausted, or turned off. Carbon dioxide will then accumulate and respiratory acidosis may produce hyperpnea, flushing, sweating, tachycardia, and a rising blood pressure. This complication is unlikely to occur when flows above 5 l./min. of fresh gas are supplied to the system, because the bulk of carbon dioxide elimination is accomplished by the waste gas flow from the system. With lower gas flows, however, carbon dioxide accumulation may be significant when the cannister is non-functional, and early detection and adjustment of the absorber will be needed to correct the problem.

The answers to all these problems lie in the areas of improved engineering and preventive maintenance. Better equipment is being produced that will assure a safer anesthetic and decreased complications related to equipment problems. The availability of comprehensive texts dealing with anesthesia equipment function and maintenance should also be an important factor in increasing the general knowledge of anesthesia apparatus and expected malfunctions to be encountered.[55]

RENAL EFFECTS. Maintenance of anesthesia with halothane or narcotics causes a decrease in urine production and a shift from positive to negative free water clearance, due to decreases in renal blood flow and glomerular filtration rate. In the unstimulated patient prior to surgical incision, this is related to increases in renal vascular resistance that are seen even with halothane anesthesia. Surgical incision causes release of antidiuretic hormone and activation of the renin-angiotensin system to release aldosterone from the adrenal, all of which may further limit urine formation. Renin-angiotensin activation can be decreased, however, if the patient is given adequate fluids during surgery.[97] After surgery renal vasoconstriction subsides while aldosterone and antidiuretic hormone levels return to normal. During high spinal anesthesia with renal sympathetic blockade, renal hemodynamics and urine output are practically normal, but the effects of surgical manipulation under conduction anesthesia are not established.[53]

This tendency toward oliguria during anesthesia and surgery is compounded by the shift of substantial amounts of fluid from the intravascular space to the interstitium in areas subjected to surgical trauma. When oliguria or anuria occurs during surgery, the most common cause is prerenal, and increased infusion of crystalloid is indicated. This is particularly true in the trauma case, the vascular surgical patient, or with any patient who has excessive bleeding or heavy fluid requirements intraoperatively. These patients will usually benefit from rapid fluid infusion while central venous pressure is monitored. If this does not increase the urine output to at least 1 ml./kg./hr., then the possibility of *acute renal failure* or *transfusion reaction* must be considered.

The appearance of pink-tinged urine, even when other signs of transfusion reaction are not noted, such as cardiovascular instability or clotting abnormalities, strongly suggests that transfusion of incompatible blood has occurred. Immediate treatment involves heavy fluid infusion and injection of sodium bicarbonate to produce a metabolic alkalosis, which increases the solubility of acid hematin released in the kidney by hemolysed red blood cells. If urine output is not immediately responsive to therapy, diuresis should be induced with mannitol,

12.5 to 25 gm. or furosemide (Lasix), 10 to 80 mg. given intravenously.

The differential diagnosis of oliguria caused by prerenal factors (hypovolemia or hypotension) and that caused by acute renal failure usually requires a trial of osmotic or loop diuretics. Hypotension following trauma or during surgery may set into action those mechanisms, still poorly understood, that cause acute renal failure in the perioperative period. A prolonged decrease in the blood pressure strongly suggests the diagnosis of acute renal failure when oliguria follows; because the treatment of prerenal oliguria is entirely the opposite of that for acute renal failure, an attempt must be made to restore urine output or confirm the alternative diagnosis as early as possible.

Fluid deficits must be corrected, and the bladder catheter and urinary collecting bags should be carefully checked before diuretics are injected. In the normovolemic patient with oliguria, mannitol 12.5 to 25 gm. or furosemide 10 to 80 mg. may be given, and urine output observed for one hour. Mannitol should not be used in the hypervolemic patient, because it may acutely expand intravascular volume and precipitate acute pulmonary edema. Furosemide would be preferred in the patient with a high central venous or pulmonary capillary wedge pressure. If no response to diuretics is seen, a second dose of mannitol can be considered, but gradually increasing doses of furosemide in the range of 1 to 10 mg./kg. are usually preferred in attempting to restore urine flow. Maintenance of restored urine output may require continued injection of Lasix or mannitol. The patient who remains anuric should be placed on restricted fluids while being maintained as normovolemic as estimates make possible. Temporary hemodialysis or peritoneal dialysis may be required; a nephrologist should be consulted, intraoperatively if possible, when the patient remains unresponsive to diuretics during the perioperative period.

The cost of acute renal failure in permanent morbidity and mortality is widely recognized, and its prevention entails rapid transport of trauma patients by trained personnel, with early therapy of fluid deficits *en route*, if indicated by hypotension or shock. In preoperative and intraoperative care, the generous infusion of crystalloid is also essential, and the wide use of central venous and pulmonary capillary wedge pressure monitoring will make this fluid therapy safer and more effective.

CENTRAL NERVOUS SYSTEM EFFECTS. Because the blocking of conscious perception of pain is the goal of general anesthesia, the primary target for all inhalational and intravenous anesthetics is obviously the central nervous system. During maintenance of anesthesia, the use of unnecessarily high concentrations of agents may not seriously depress physiologic processes in individuals with good functional reserve, but this will lead to gross overdosage and prolonged emergence. This can be prevented with use of minimal concentrations of agents that will still provide stable and adequate anesthesia.

Certain specific effects of anesthetics on the central nervous system will be discussed because of complications such as seizures, hypothermia, and reflex activity with which they can be associated.

Tonic-clonic movements associated with electroencephalographic seizure discharges are occasionally seen during the use of enflurane. Hyperventilation and deep anesthesia, with enflurane concentrations of 3.5 per cent or more, seem to predispose to convulsive activity, and increases in cerebral oxygen consumption have been shown to occur during these seizures in both dogs and humans. There is no evidence that hypoxic damage occurs during enflurane seizures or that cerebral function is subsequently altered after anesthesia, but convulsive activity is best prevented by avoiding hypocarbia with enflurane and by restricting the percentage to 3 per cent or less.[78]

Reflex activity under anesthesia is most often stimulated by surgical manipulation, and usually involves vagal efferent responses that result in sinus bradycardia or nodal escape rhythms. Children with their high vagal tone have especially active reflex responses in surgery. Traction reflexes due to pulling on the pleura or the mesentery of the bowel, or from distention of the perineum are occasionally encountered in both adults and children. The most frequently encountered response of this type is the oculocardiac reflex, which is triggered by pressure on or around the eye or by traction at surgery on the extraocular muscles, particularly the medial rectus. After atropine premedication (0.01 mg./kg. I.M.) 60 per cent of children will still show evidence of cardiac slowing during strabismus surgery. This can be decreased to 28 per cent with intravenous atropine (0.005 mg./kg.) or completely blocked with retrobulbar injection of local anesthetic, which should be considered in especially sensitive patients.[68, 93] Retrobulbar block itself may cause oculocardiac reflex, so caution is indicated.

Oculocardiac reflex is detected through electrocardiographic monitoring of all eye surgery patients, whether they are anesthetized or only sedated. Atropine should be administered preoperatively I.V. or I.M. to provide protection. If slowing is noted during surgical manipulation, the surgeon should be asked to immediately stop all stimulation on the field. Cardiac rhythm will usually return to normal shortly thereafter. If it does not, atropine may be given intravenously, but careful monitoring should be maintained during injection, because ventricular ectopic dysrhythmias may follow its use. The reflex seems to attenuate with time, and deep anesthesia appears to be protective, so the recommendation has been made to deepen anesthesia and withhold atropine because of the possible dysrhythmias. Many senescent patients undergoing eye surgery will tolerate bradycardia poorly, so preventive measures with atropine and retrobulbar block can be strongly recommended.

Autonomic hyperreflexia is an especially hazardous phenomenon seen in patients with spinal cord injuries above the mid-thoracic level. Surgical stimulation or bladder distention causes intense reflex vasoconstriction below the level of cord transection, and sudden severe hypertension may follow. Arrhythmias, cardiac decompensation, or intracranial hemorrhage is a significant complication to be anticipated. Pretreatment of patients with a suggestive history using phenoxybenzamine (Dibenzyline) may decrease the severity of resulting hypertension.[90] The reflex arc may be completely blocked with spinal anesthesia, but a reluctance to employ subarachnoid injection in patients with spinal cord injuries is certainly understandable. The risk of morbidity from severe hypertension makes this option more reasonable, and if the technique is planned, the patients must be carefully counseled beforehand concerning the irreversible nature of their injuries, and the necessity for preventing rises in blood pressure.[32] If the patient is given a general anesthetic, hyperreflexia is treated with phentolamine (Regitine) or nitroprusside (Nipride), and the protection of deep levels of anesthesia should be maintained from the start.

Hypothermia under anesthesia is caused in part by depression of thermal regulating centers in the hypothalamus. Shivering is blocked by general anesthetics and muscle relaxants, and metabolic heat production is also reduced. The use of cold, dry anesthetic gases increases evaporative heat losses in the lungs, and peripheral vasodilatation makes the patient nearly poikilothermic. In a cool operating room, a reduction in body temperature to the range of 32° to 34°C. is not uncommon when preventive measures are not taken. Children have a high surface area to body mass ratio and cool quickly to dangerously low temperatures. Hypothermia below 30° C. produces cardiac dysrhythmias and prolonged emergence from anesthesia.

Hypothermia may be utilized therapeutically to decrease the oxygen consumption of cerebral and myocardial tissue during threatened ischemia, but in general its effects are deleterious during anesthesia, and heat loss must be minimized if possible. The prevention and treatment of hypothermia involve essentially the same measures. The ambient temperature in the operating room may be raised, and heating blankets applied. Infused fluids and blood should be warmed, and a heated humidifier may be added to the anesthesia circuit. External heating lamps or radiant heaters are useful in adults as well as children, but precautions need to be observed to prevent iatrogenic burns.

COMPLICATIONS DURING EMERGENCE FROM ANESTHESIA

Complications associated with emergence from anesthesia are to be expected from the moment agents are tapered or discontinued. As pain begins to stimulate the cardiovascular system, increases in blood pressure and pulse rate can stress the heart to cause S-T segment changes in the electrocardiogram, arrhythmias, or myocardial failure, particularly in patients with ischemic disease. Sudden blood pressure changes may also result in bleeding and tissue disruption in the surgical incision that increase the risk of later infection or functional impairment.

The cardiovascular effects of emergence from anesthesia may be exaggerated in the hypertensive patient, but previously established control of the blood pressure with antihypertensive drugs in the severely hypertensive patient may lessen the extent of the hypertension and associated morbidity during emergence.[25] Therapy may also be started or maintained intraoperatively with hydralazine (Apresoline), methyldopa (Aldomet), or sodium nitroprusside (Nipride). The effects of myocardial ischemia may be minimized during emergence with propranolol (Inderal) or various nitrates. However, the mainstay of therapy is adequate analgesia with titration of narcotics, to achieve a careful balance between patient comfort and potential respiratory depression.

Pharmacologic reversal of depressed sensorium, narcotics, or muscle relaxants may also contribute to morbidity at this stage. Bradycardia after anticholinesterases can depress cardiac output and blood pressure and may require additional anticholinergics for effective treatment. Analeptics like doxapram (Dopram) provide sympathetic stimulation as they increase the level of responsiveness and, as a result, can produce hypertension and tachycardia. Naloxone (Narcan) used to reverse narcotic effects also produces similar cardiovascular stimulation related to the sudden perception of pain; the likelihood of vomiting after this drug should prompt caution and discourage removal of the endotracheal tube.

Acute pain during emergence frequently causes dysphoria and agitated behavior; and stimulation by monitoring and infusion lines, Foley catheters, chest tubes, and most importantly, the endotracheal tube, may add to the patient's confusion. The patient who is thrashing madly about can dislodge essential monitoring and support devices that may be needed in the postoperative period. Combativeness may also endanger the patient physically by threatening to disrupt the results of delicate surgical procedures. Analgesic and sedative drugs will be helpful in controlling such behavior, but again the balance between extremes of respiratory depression and undersedation may be difficult to attain and must be carefully maintained until the patient is again rational.

The essential decision must be made at this stage concerning the level of postoperative respiratory support to be required. In those patients who will benefit from mechanical ventilation, heavy narcotic, relaxant, and sedative regimens may be properly maintained into the intensive care period. Some patients will be committed to ventilatory support based on their clinical behavior in the recovery period. In general if there is the least doubt about the patient's ability to maintain oxygenation or eliminate carbon dioxide after anesthesia, they should remain intubated until they have been observed in the recovery room for an appropriate period. Premature extubation risks not only the complications of hypoxia and hypercarbia but adds to this the potential problems of the second intubation itself.

Most recovery rooms have formal criteria for extubation and discharge of patients, to be used as guidelines for anesthesiologists and nursing personnel under their direction. Extubation requires that the patient be able to maintain the airway, generate a normal tidal volume, and have some inspiratory reserve to allow for coughing to clear secretions. Performance criteria that reasonably assure this level of ventilation are widely accepted and include the ability to generate a minimum vital capacity of 10 ml./kg. and to sustain a negative inspiratory force of -20 cm. H_2O for 5 seconds. The patient who is responsive in the operating room and fulfills these criteria or who is agitated and should be expected to have adequate respirations may be extubated in surgery and moved to the recovery room while being administered supplemental oxygen by face mask. Extubation of all other patients should be deferred until they have been fully evaluated, and the move to the recovery room should include respiratory assistance with supplemental oxygen and a device for positive pressure breathing. The patient with regular respirations who can generate a tidal volume of 5 ml./kg. with the endotracheal tube in place can be safely allowed to breathe spontaneously with humidified oxygen-enriched air supplied with a **T**-piece. Patients who cannot meet this performance criterion should be placed on a mechanical ventilator or manually assisted until their tidal volume improves.

Occasionally, some patients meet these performance criteria but still have hypercarbia due to high dead space to tidal volume ratios or hypoxemia because of severe ventilation/perfusion imbalance. Cardiovascular instability can cause hypoxemia during periods of low cardiac output and is another indication for continued ventilatory control despite adequate respiratory volume performance, until the vital signs are stabilized. Blood gas analysis should be used to assess the ventilatory sufficiency of all patients in whom there is any suspicion of malfunction and will aid in detecting individual exceptions to the above generalizations.

The complications encountered during the move from the operating room to the recovery area are not inconsiderable. The shift from the operating table to the transport cart may cause hypotension, and essential monitoring or infusion lines may be dislodged in the process. The danger of such complications persists on the journey to the recovery area. The labile patient should be monitored en route with a precordial or esophageal stethoscope, or in extremely unstable situations, with portable electronic EKG and pressure monitors. It may be desirable to carry a supply of appropriate pressor and antiarrhythmic drugs, as well as a laryngoscope, especially if the route is long or involves elevator transport.

In the recovery room the greatest danger to the patient is the reoccurrence of respiratory depression from narcotics or muscle relaxants. The maximum risk is not reached immediately after arrival of the patient, but later, when reversal drug effects subside, the patient has settled and appears calm, and more recent arrivals distract the attention of nursing personnel. The prevention of recovery room disasters involves constant vigilance; apnea, hypoxia, and resultant permanent neurological damage, occurring in a previously healthy person under obser-

vation in the recovery area, may be interpreted by the courts as *res ipsa loquitur,* evidence of negligence.

Recovery room discharge criteria usually include evidence that the patient is awake, responsive, physiologically stable, able to summon help, and likely to tolerate appropriate doses of analgesics on the ward without incident. Failure to meet any of these standards puts the patient at risk of complications on the ward, and special precautions are indicated when patients must be discharged who do not fully meet local criteria. It is wise for the anesthesiologist responsible for discharging each patient to document on the chart that the patient meets the established discharge criteria at the time the final check is performed. A cursory review of the postoperative orders may be useful, especially in teaching hospitals in which the house staff is responsible for dosages of postoperative narcotics. A rapid call to the responsible physician by the anesthesiologist who suspects that an analgesic dosage is excessive may allow reduction of the dose and prevent problems later.

CONDUCTION ANESTHESIA

Conduction methods include topical, local, regional, vertebral, and intravenous regional anesthesia. With conduction anesthesia, the advantage of having an awake, cooperative patient with relatively stable vital signs must be balanced against some definite drawbacks. Most local anesthetic agents excite and then depress the central nervous system as plasma levels increase during absorption, and all eventually depress the cardiovascular system as well. To some anxious patients, being awake may be a disadvantage during surgery, and injections may not always be easily tolerated. For the surgeon and anesthesiologist, more technical facility and time are necessary for effective anesthesia than with general anesthetic techniques. Despite these negative aspects, the use of conduction techniques is achieving wider acceptance among patients and greater use by anesthesiologists.

Complications of regional techniques are most frequently due to one of three factors: toxic effects of the anesthetic agents, physiologic effects of nerve block, and anatomic trauma caused by the injecting needle. Above all, the principles of safe use of local anesthetics and proper therapy for these complications must be understood by surgeon and anesthesiologist and continually applied during conduction anesthesia.

Complications of Topical and Local Anesthesia

Mechanisms of adverse reactions with either topical or local methods are similar and relate primarily to allergic or toxic responses to local anesthetic drugs. The broad principles discussed here will similarly pertain to clinical use of the local anesthetics in the blocks discussed later.

ALLERGY TO LOCAL ANESTHETICS. A history of allergy to "caine" drugs may be reported by a patient with a true systemic anaphylactic reaction in the past that was due to local anesthetic agents. This is often difficult to distinguish, however, from toxic reactions to local anesthetics following absorption of excessive doses of agents or after inadvertent intravenous injections in vascular areas. Similarly, the systemic effects of epinephrine added to the injection to prolong local anesthetic action may be interpreted by patients as an allergic drug reaction. While such a history should not be entirely dismissed, true anaphylaxis following injection of local anesthetics is probably extremely rare.[50]

The first local anesthetics were of the ester type: cocaine, procaine (Novocaine), tetracaine (Pontocaine), chloroprocaine (Nesacaine), and benzocaine. They are metabolized by plasma pseudocholinesterase to break the ester linkage and produce para-aminobenzoic acid, a very allergenic substance in certain individuals. All the ester type agents can cross-react to produce allergic responses in susceptible persons, as will methylparaben, a chemically related preservative used in local anesthetic solutions. Dermal sensitivity to esters was common among dentists when these drugs were widely used, and skin testing has been performed to detect allergic responses to local anesthetics in patients with suspicious histories. In sensitive individuals, injection of ester-linked local anesthetics may rapidly

produce cardiovascular collapse, syncope, laryngeal edema, and generalized urticaria. Because most anaphylactic reactions to local anesthetics have occurred after the injection of esters, the incidence of these reactions has declined with the introduction of amide-linked local anesthetic agents over the last 25 years.

Amide-linked local anesthetics would include lidocaine (Xylocaine), mepivacaine (Carbocaine), bupivacaine (Marcaine), etidocaine (Duranest), prilocaine (Citanest), and dibucaine (Nupercaine). These agents undergo metabolic degradation in the liver and produce no allergenic metabolites. Since their almost universal adoption in clinical practice, they have produced only a handful of documented anaphylactic reactions. These usually begin with a generalized urticarial rash, slow in onset, which allows time for aggressive therapy to be started before severe symptoms appear.[51]

Prevention of allergic reactions would start with a careful history of local anesthetic exposure and avoidance of esters or amides, when appropriate, in patients with previous reactions. While amide local anesthetics may be safely used in patients with documented allergies to esters, care should be taken to use solutions free of methylparaben preservatives. *Treatment* of true anaphylaxis will require injection of epinephrine, supplemental oxygen, and ventilatory support measures as appropriate. Steroids and antihistamines may also decrease the severity of the reaction when administered during the acute episode or if given prophylactically beforehand.

TOXICITY OF LOCAL ANESTHETICS. The concentration of local anesthetics in the blood increases progressively as absorption occurs from the point of injection. The rate of absorption and the resulting peak level of the agent in the plasma are determined primarily by the vascularity of the site of injection, the use of vasoconstrictors in the local anesthetic solution, and the total dose of the agent. Toxic levels of local anesthetic can be reached after rapid absorption or following inadvertent intravascular injection during regional block. The major toxic complications involve central nervous system excitation, usually seizures, which may lead to death from asphyxiation or to permanent neurologic damage.

The first signs of dangerously increasing plasma levels of local anesthetic after injection of lidocaine or procaine may be reported by the patient as sedation, analgesia, facial tingling, tinnitus, or a metallic taste in the mouth. This is an urgent indication for measures to prevent grand mal seizures, which may follow shortly. This preconvulsive aura may not be seen with the other amide local anesthetics bupivacaine, mepivacaine, etidocaine, or prilocaine. With these drugs patients may suddenly convulse following only transient clouding of the sensorium. If central nervous system depression progresses still further, respiratory and cardiovascular depression may ensue as convulsive activity subsides and eventually may lead to cardiac arrest.

Treatment of central nervous system toxicity is based on the observation that the seizure activity arises in the temporal lobes and that measures that suppress cortical seizures may be ineffective. Anticonvulsants of the phenytoin type are useless and may actually enhance local anesthetic seizures. The use of succinylcholine to suppress objective signs of seizure activity causes no improvement in electroencephalographic patterns, and while it is effective in facilitating oxygenation with positive pressure ventilation during convulsions, it does not treat the underlying neuronal hyperactivity that promotes cerebral hypoxia. The most effective therapeutic measures include hyperventilation, which raises the convulsive threshold for local anesthetic toxicity, and intravenous injection of diazepam (Valium) in an initial dose of 0.1 mg./kg. These two measures will aid in *prevention* of seizures when instituted with the first symptoms of impending toxicity reported by the patient, who may at that time still be capable of voluntary hyperventilation. Should seizure activity occur despite therapy, appropriate respiratory support and further increments of diazepam may be necessary. Manifestations of developing cardiovascular toxicity should then be watched for carefully (see below).

Barbiturates can be used to suppress seizure activity, but central nervous system depression and apnea may result after the doses of drug necessary to achieve control. In addition, the barbiturates and local anesthetics may have synergistic depressant effects on the cardiovascular system. Diazepam seems to produce maximum seizure protection with minimum physiologic disturbance and is at present the preferred drug for control of local anesthetic seizures.[52, 75]

Cardiovascular toxicity due to local anesthetic drugs is usually not a problem clinically until plasma levels of these drugs are attained that are toxic to the central nervous system. Lidocaine at levels effective in controlling arrhythmias has no appreciable effect on myocardial contractility, but as convulsant levels of lidocaine are approached, hypotension may develop owing to a combination of peripheral vasodilatation and negative chronotropic and inotropic effects of the drug. If the plasma concentration increases still higher, further depression of the myocardium and conduction system may lead to complete atrioventricular dissociation or cardiac arrest. Such effects will be more likely during massive accidental intravascular injections of local anesthetics and will require rapid administration of fluids, vasopressors, inotropes, and possibly insertion of a temporary cardiac pacemaker.

An interesting toxicologic problem is encountered with the infrequently used local anesthetic prilocaine (Citanest). The drug is metabolized to ortho-toluidine in the liver, and this byproduct in turn produces methemoglobinemia, which can interfere with oxygen transport by the blood. Restriction of prilocaine to total doses below 600 mg. should prevent the development of dangerous levels of methemoglobin.

The effect of epinephrine absorption presents a picture that may superficially resemble central nervous system toxicity from local anesthetic agents, but that, upon closer scrutiny, shows diagnostic differences. Epinephrine reactions do result in restlessness, pallor, and the appearance of collapse and may lead to loss of consciousness followed on rare occasions by convulsions, but beyond this the similarity ceases. Quite unlike local anesthetic overdosage are the characteristic initial alertness, anxiety, palpitations with substernal pressure sensations, perspiration, dyspnea, and most importantly, elevated pulse rate and blood pressure, often with severe headache and nausea. Later the epinephrine reversal phenomenon may result in a lowered blood pressure and a shocklike picture; this should be remembered when the patient is encountered some time after onset of epinephrine-related symptoms.

The critical phase of these reactions is usually reached and passed rapidly, so results will depend on rapid diagnosis and immediate treatment. First, oxygen therapy should be started at once, regardless of the cause of the reaction; positive pressure assistance or controlled ventilation should be used if respiratory depression is apparent, with an ordinary mask and self-inflating bag connected to a source of oxygen. Second, blood pressure and heart rate should be observed. If the blood pressure is relatively low with a normal or slow pulse, and in addition, if the patient is stuporous, one is dealing with either a local anesthetic overdosage or, in rare instances, an allergic reaction. The patient's legs should be elevated to augment venous return, and a standard vasopressor and intravenous diazepam should be readied. If positioning does not improve the blood pressure, the vasopressor should be titrated intravenously to a desired response. If increasing restlessness and motor activity presage convulsions, small doses of diazepam are usually effective in suppressing seizures. If thiopental is readily available, small doses of that can also be used, but diazepam is preferred.

If the blood pressure and pulse rate are elevated, the patient is reasonably alert, and adrenalin-containing local anesthetic solution was used, it is almost certainly an epinephrine reaction. The patient should be reassured and sedated carefully with diazepam. Epinephrine is rapidly destroyed, so

TABLE 10–1 SUGGESTED MAXIMUM SAFE DOSES OF TOPICAL ANESTHETIC AGENTS (SINGLE APPLICATION)*

	Concentration	Maximum Dose (mg.)	Maximum Dose (mg./kg.)
Cocaine	4–10%	160	2
Dibucaine	0.2–1%	40	0.5
Lidocaine	2–4%	200	3
Tetracaine	1–2%	80	1

*These doses and concentrations should be reduced for extremes of age and debility.

the reaction will be relatively short in duration. Use of phentolamine (Regitine), chlorpromazine (Thorazine), or sodium nitroprusside (Nipride) titrated to lower the blood pressure would be logical, but symptoms will usually have subsided by the time the drug is prepared.

The minimal equipment and drug requirements mandatory for any area in which conduction anesthesia is being used are a source of oxygen and apparatus to administer it by positive pressure, nasopharyngeal and oropharyngeal airways, a good source of suction with suction catheters, a standard vasopressor, diazepam, epinephrine, an antihistamine, a glucocorticoid preparation, a laryngoscope, and a selection of endotracheal tubes.

Treatment is a poor substitute for *prevention*. Anyone who regularly uses these admittedly toxic local anesthetic drugs must observe the safe maximum concentrations and doses to avoid complications. (See Tables 10–1 and 10–2.) Caution in applying these agents to inflamed surfaces, careful

TABLE 10–2 SUGGESTED MAXIMUM SAFE DOSES OF LOCAL ANESTHETIC AGENTS (SINGLE INJECTION)*

	Concentration	Maximum Dose (mg.)†	Maximum Dose (mg./kg.)†
Bupivacaine (Marcaine)	0.125–.75%	225	3
Chloroprocaine (Nesacaine)	0.5–3%	1000	14
Etidocaine (Duranest)	0.5–1.5%	400	5.5
Lidocaine (Xylocaine)	0.5–2%	500	7
Mepivacaine (Carbocaine)	0.5–2%	500	7
Prilocaine (Citanest)	0.5–3%	600	8.5
Procaine (Novocaine)	0.5–2%	1000	14
Tetracaine (Pontocaine)	0.1–0.25%	100	1.5

*These doses and concentrations should be reduced for extremes of age and debility.

†Maximum dose refers to administration with epinephrine 1:200,000. For injection of plain anesthetic solution not containing vasoconstrictors, allowable dosage should be reduced by 25 per cent.

restriction of total dosages, and the use of no greater than 1:200,000 concentrations of epinephrine in local anesthetic solutions will help reduce plasma levels of these drugs and thus prevent toxic reactions. Finally it should be mentioned that oral, intramuscular, or intravenous premedication with diazepam should help allay anxiety and simultaneously reduce the incidence of convulsions after injection of local anesthetics for conduction block.

MISCELLANEOUS COMPLICATIONS OF LOCAL INFILTRATION. Fine-gauge needles may be broken and lost under the skin, an embarrassing complication that can be avoided by using disposable needles that are designed to prevent such breakage.

Sudden collapse from inadvertent intravascular injection of local anesthetic solutions must be treated rapidly and effectively when it occurs, according to the principles outlined in the section on toxicity. This can be avoided by frequent aspiration for blood return during injection in highly vascular areas and by constant movement of the needle during local infiltration.

The value of adding proper concentrations of vasoconstrictors to injected anesthetic solutions to reduce their absorption and prolong their anesthetic effect is unquestioned. However, concentrations greater than 1:200,000 of epinephrine are of no advantage and increase the chances of systemic reactions due to the vasoconstrictor. Until local vasoconstrictors are developed which have minimal systemic effects, such as the vasopressin derivatives now under investigation, careful restriction of epinephrine in local anesthetic solutions will be necessary. One final precaution with vasoconstrictors involves local infiltration of epinephrine solutions into the fingers, toes, nose, ears, or penis, which may cause tissue necrosis in these areas in which collateral circulation may at times be inadequate. Skin sloughs may result, so vasoconstrictors are not to be used.

Careless technique, such as injection through contaminated areas of skin or mucous membranes or injection of contaminated anesthetic solutions, may result in infection and possible sloughs. This can be avoided by meticulous technique during preparation and injection of properly sterilized solutions.

Complications of Regional Anesthesia

Regional anesthesia necessitates accurate placement of local anesthetic agents in proximity to nerves. Deeper needle injection is necessary than for local infiltration, and the technique requires knowledge of the anatomy, patience, and skill. The inherent dangers of toxic reactions are increased because of the more frequent entry into highly vascular areas and the subsequent risk of intravascular injection. Needling can also directly damage deep structures such as nerves, blood vessels, and viscera, particularly in those areas in which they are relatively fixed to unyielding skeletal landmarks.

Treatment of needle damage is symptomatic in most instances. *Prevention* is based upon knowledge of the anatomy, gentleness, frequent aspiration, and the use of x-ray confirmation and the peripheral nerve stimulator to aid in the accurate location of specific nerves. While transient paresthesias are a useful guide to accuracy of needle placement, continued pain or sensations down the nerve distribution would suggest that the nerve itself has been skewered, and the needle should be withdrawn quickly to prevent permanent damage. Under no circumstances should the injection of local anesthetic proceed in the presence of intense persistent paresthesias, because of the hazard of permanent neurologic damage following placement of solution *into* the nerve itself. Repositioning the needle should result in cessation of paresthesias, with the needle still close enough to the nerve to guarantee good block after injection of local anesthetic.

Again, it should be emphasized that regional blocks should not be performed in patients on anticoagulant therapy, as discussed in the section on patient medications (see above).

Complications following commonly performed regional blocks will be specifically discussed for the individual nerve blocks in turn.

STELLATE GANGLION BLOCK. The stellate ganglion is blocked by injection of anesthetic anterior to the transverse process of either the sixth or seventh cervical vertebra. The needle is inserted at a point above the clavicle between the carotid artery and the trachea, and complications can be expected related to the numerous anatomic structures traversing the anterior cervical region at that point. The block is actually applied to the entire cervical sympathetic chain on one side and impedes ipsilateral sympathetic outflow to the head and upper extremity. It is indicated for diagnosis and treatment of reflex sympathetic dystrophy in pain clinic work and to produce therapeutic vasodilatation in the arm when blood supply is compromised.

Complications of stellate ganglion block are frequent but mostly benign.[79] Pneumothorax occurs in 1 per cent or less of cases and is suggested by chest or shoulder pain after the needle is inserted. Complete collapse of the lung is uncommon; usually no more than a 10 per cent pneumothorax results, and this should be followed until it resolves spontaneously. *Prevention* involves using a strict medial approach to the transverse process to avoid the pleura. *Treatment* may require tube thoracostomy when extensive collapse of the lung is seen, but this is seldom indicated.

Subarachnoid injection of anesthetic solution may occur when the needle is inserted between the transverse processes. Complete spinal block will result, requiring respiratory support and vasopressor infusion. *Prevention* requires careful attention to the use of the skeletal landmarks for the block, and the injection of a small test dose of the drug before the full dose of local anesthetic is given. Another result of insertion of the probing needle between the transverse processes may be the intravascular injection of local anesthetic. This can be particularly dangerous when the needle is placed in the vertebral artery, because even a small quantity of local anesthetic can produce immediate severe convulsions. *Prevention* again requires careful use of landmarks and injection of a test dose.

Hoarseness and difficulty in swallowing, due to transient palsy of the recurrent laryngeal nerve, may be seen after stellate ganglion blocks in 5 to 8 per cent of cases. These problems will resolve with subsidence of the block. Partial brachial plexus palsy may also be encountered in 5 per cent of these blocks, and a small number of patients will experience phrenic nerve block with resultant diaphragmatic paralysis on that

side. These effects are usually temporary and harmless, but in individuals with pulmonary disease, respiratory compromise should be watched for. Bronchospasm is mentioned as a complication of stellate ganglion block but is said to be extremely rare, and perhaps related to drug allergy, when it occurs.[79]

Bilateral stellate ganglion block is dangerous because of the potentially disastrous consequences of the complications of simultaneous bilateral nerve blocks in the neck. Bilateral phrenic or recurrent laryngeal nerve blocks or bilateral pneumothoraces can cause severe respiratory problems; and the possibility of total inhibition of sympathetic cardioaccelerator fibers should be taken into account, because it may result in severe bradycardia due to vagal predominance.

In summary, care with landmarks for needle insertion, routine use of a test dose of anesthetic, and avoidance of simultaneous bilateral blocks are essential if morbidity is to be minimized in the performance of stellate ganglion blocks.

INTERSCALENE BLOCKS OF THE CERVICAL PLEXUS OR BRACHIAL PLEXUS. Supraclavicular block of the brachial plexus by walking the needle off the first rib has an inordinately high complication rate: pneumothorax (1 to 6 per cent), stellate ganglion block (70 to 90 per cent), and phrenic nerve block (40 to 60 per cent). This has been replaced in clinical practice by techniques involving injections higher in the neck, into the groove between the anterior and middle scalene muscles, to block the segmental nerves at the point at which they leave the vertebral column to form the cervical and brachial plexi.[102] Interscalene cervical plexus block is performed at the C_4 level, while interscalene brachial plexus injection is lower at C_6. Success with the block is high if paresthesias are elicited or if motor response to electrical nerve stimulation is used to confirm needle placement. Pneumothorax is extremely rare after high cervical needling; complications of neck injection, as seen after stellate ganglion block, may be expected infrequently and should be evaluated and treated as described under that block. These complications would include intra-arterial injection, especially of the vertebral artery; subarachnoid injection; phrenic, vagus, and recurrent laryngeal block; Horner's syndrome; and cervical hematoma. While these complications are even *less* likely after the axillary approach to the brachial plexus, the interscalene technique has the advantage of providing anesthesia in areas of the upper arm, shoulder, and neck that the infraclavicular approach does not reach. *Prevention* of complications requires gentleness, frequent aspiration, careful attention to anatomic detail, and maintenance of a slight caudad and dorsad tilt of the needle toward the transverse process of the appropriate cervical vertebra. Avoiding the use of simultaneous bilateral blocks is again advised owing to the danger of bilateral complications, and because potentially toxic volumes of anesthetic solution are needed to perform two blocks.

AXILLARY BLOCK. The brachial plexus surrounding the brachial artery is readily blocked at the point at which it leaves the axilla, crossing the border of the pectoralis major muscle. A single injection of anesthetic solution can be made after a single paresthesia is produced during superficial probing of the fascial compartment near the brachial pulse. Through-and-through puncture of the artery as a guide to the location of the plexus sheath has decreased in popularity because it does not increase the success rate of the block and may increase morbidity. Complications of axillary block would include toxic reactions from rapid absorption or intravascular injection of anesthetic solution, with or without epinephrine; axillary hematoma, with occasional obliteration of the radial pulse; and direct needle trauma to nerve tissue. *Prevention* of these problems involves gentle needle technique, aspiration before injection, the use of a test dose of anesthetic, and avoiding puncture of the brachial vessels.

INTERCOSTAL BLOCK. The proximity of the intercostal nerve, artery, and vein increases the possibility of intravascular injection with this block. When the injection is done near the posterior angle of the rib, it is also remotely possible that a lateral dural cuff may be entered and a subarachnoid injection performed, resulting in an unexpected spinal block. Pneumothorax after puncture of the underlying pleura should occur in less than 0.5 per cent of blocks done by experienced hands. Careful control of the needle tip as it passes the lower rib

margin and repeated warnings to the patient to expect stinging sensations during the injection and not to move should prevent pleural entry. Pneumothorax is usually limited in extent and is treated symptomatically while following the chest x-ray until resolution.

Absorption of local anesthetic is rapid through the intercostal neurovascular bundle. Plasma levels of lidocaine and mepivacaine after intercostal block are 30 to 50 per cent higher than after use of similar doses for epidural or axillary block.[98] Because the risk of toxicity is high, pretreatment with diazepam, addition of epinephrine to the anesthetic solution, and restriction of total dosage are advised when multiple blocks are indicated.

PARAVERTEBRAL SYMPATHETIC BLOCK. One may easily overshoot the desired depth in this block and, depending on the side, enter either the inferior vena cava or the aorta. Systemic reaction to injected agent or bleeding may result. One *prevents* intravascular injection by careful technique, including use of depth markers, aspiration, test dose, and if available, x-ray verification of needle position. Systemic reactions are *treated* as described earlier. These blocks are contraindicated in patients with abnormal clotting functions because of the risk of bleeding. Hemorrhage must be watched for and treated with transfusions and exploration if severe.

PERIPHERAL NERVE BLOCKS. Nerve blocks of peripheral branches of the brachial plexus are usually performed at the elbow and the wrist. In the lower extremity the sciatic, femoral, and lateral femoral cutaneous nerves can be individually blocked, and for surgery of the foot ankle block is coming into wider use. Complications of these techniques are infrequent. Direct needle trauma to the nerves is avoided by gentle technique and by not giving injections whenever constant paresthesias or pain is produced. When infection is noted in the region of the intended block, needle probe of the area or local injection should not be performed, lest spread of the infection be promoted. More proximal regional block may be attempted, but not when tenderness, adenopathy, or possible metastatic disease is detected.

Peripheral ischemia can result when vasoconstrictors or large volumes of anesthetic solution are injected into distal parts of the extremities, especially the digits. Should obvious ischemia result after such a block, for example in the arm, the extremity should be immediately elevated to reduce swelling and venous engorgement. The intra-arterial injection of vasodilators such as phentolamine (Regitine), reserpine, or papaverine at the level of the brachial artery may be helpful. Stellate ganglion block should be considered, to be *followed* by systemic heparinization to reduce thrombosis.

Complications of Intravenous Regional Anesthesia

Injection of a relatively large volume of a dilute local anesthetic solution into the empty venous system of an extremity isolated from the general circulation by an inflated tourniquet will produce effective anesthesia of the limb. The hazard exists, however, of a systemic toxic reaction either through inadvertent leakage past a faulty tourniquet or release of a large amount of drug at the end of the procedure. Mild toxic symptoms like tinnitus, dizziness, or dysarthria often occur after tourniquet deflation; very rarely, loss of consciousness, convulsions, and acute cardiovascular collapse may follow. Lidocaine and bupivacaine have been widely and safely utilized in intravenous regional anesthesia; chloroprocaine, because of a high incidence of phlebitis and peripheral neuritis, and etidocaine, which causes prolonged residual motor block, are contraindicated.[58] Proximal injection of local anesthetic near the tourniquet, with competent venous valves distally, may result in intravascular pressures that exceed tourniquet occlusion pressure, and immediate symptoms may then result from central injection of toxic amounts of the drug.

Prevention of toxic reactions requires a reliable tourniquet, premedication with diazepam or barbiturates, peripheral injection of the anesthetic solution, and restriction of the dose of local anesthetic (3 mg./kg. of lidocaine as 0.5 per cent solution or 1.5 mg./kg. of bupivacaine as 0.25 per cent solution are usually satisfactory). Tissue fixation of the local anesthetic in the extremity increases with time, and after procedures of short duration, an increased incidence of toxicity is seen following deflation of the tourniquet. Alternating 15 seconds of deflation with 2 minutes of inflation for several cycles may prevent toxicity by allowing redistribution of the drug before high plasma levels are attained in such situations. *Treatment* of reactions is similar to that previously described for managing systemic toxicity of local anesthetic drugs.

COMPLICATIONS OF VERTEBRAL CONDUCTION ANESTHESIA

Injection of local anesthetic agents into the subarachnoid or peridural spaces produces vertebral conduction block extending over multiple cord segments. In varying degrees, the function of all nerve components, including motor, sensory, and autonomic, is interrupted, with alteration of associated physiologic processes.

SPINAL ANESTHESIA. Subarachnoid anesthesia is usually produced with a single needle injection into the cerebrospinal fluid around the cauda equina. Fractional techniques involving multiple injections through indwelling subarachnoid catheters are seldom used. The large needles used for catheter placement cause excessive dural trauma, with a correspondingly high risk of postlumbar puncture headaches; and the incidence of meningeal infection seems to be greater as well. The prolonged block achieved with fractional techniques can also be obtained with continuous epidural techniques, which have less morbidity, so continuous spinal anesthesia has for the most part been abandoned.

Complications of spinal anesthesia are related to technique, sympathetic block, and motor block.

Technical Complications

The incidence and permanent significance of various technical complications of spinal anesthesia can be summarized from several large reported series.[82, 84] The major technical complications to be discussed are backache, infection, chronic adhesive arachnoiditis, headache, cranial nerve palsy, and peripheral nerve palsy.

BACKACHE. Significant pain at the site of lumbar puncture is reported postoperatively by 2.7 per cent of patients. Needle trauma to ligaments, periosteum, or dura should be suspected, and irritation or pressure from local bleeding may occasionally be implicated. Improper positioning during surgery and postoperative immobilization may be the real causes for low back discomfort that is nonetheless blamed on the spinal block. Many patients with postoperative backache will admit to a history of previous low back problems, probably a good enough reason to avoid the block *before* the fact.

Prevention involves use of small needles, atraumatic technique, and a willingness to abandon block attempts early if difficulties arise. Early mobilization may also be of help. *Treatment* is symptomatic, with narcotics and diazepam given for pain and muscle spasm, local heat applied to painful areas, and early mobilization.

INFECTION. Meningitis after subarachnoid block is exceedingly rare. With the exception of the rare patient with systemic bacteremia, infection strongly suggests faulty sterile technique either with the equipment used or in the performance of the block. *Prevention* requires meticulous technique, with skin cleansing, use of sterile gloves, and careful preparation of equipment. Disposable kits with guaranteed sterility, containing non-contaminated local anesthetic solution and with markers enclosed to confirm sterility, are apparently effective in assuring the minimal incidence of this complication we now see.

CHRONIC ADHESIVE ARACHNOIDITIS. This is an inflammatory process involving the spinal cord and meninges, causing ascending motor and sensory loss and frequently resulting in chronic respiratory paralysis and death. Almost certainly a form of chonic chemical meningitis, it is probably related to detergent-contaminated syringes used during spinal anesthetics or to antiseptics in which glass ampules of anesthetic solution were stored, which could leak into the ampules through small cracks. By gas or steam sterilizing of the drugs with the spinal trays and by meticulous rinsing of all needles and syringes after each cleaning before packing the trays, this complication was essentially eliminated a decade ago. The use of disposable spinal anesthesia trays also helps assure that this rare but dreaded complication will not recur.

HEADACHE. Postlumbar puncture cephalgia occurs in 3.5 per cent of patients when 25 Ga or 26 Ga needles are used for the dural tap. A higher incidence is reported in females, in younger patients, and when larger diameter needles are used. Leakage of cerebrospinal fluid from the dural puncture site causes the brain to settle against the tentorium and stretch pain-sensitive structures, resulting in headache. The pain is positional, worse when the patient is sitting or standing, and relieved by lying down. Mild discomfort usually resolves in 5 days or less, but the pain can be severe enough in some individuals to be incapacitating.

Postspinal headache is prevented by use of atraumatic technique and small gauge needles (25 Ga or smaller). Treatment involves analgesics, recumbency, and hydration. Tight abdominal binders and nursing the patient in the prone position may also be of benefit. If severe symptoms persist, most headaches will be cured by injection of 10 cc. of freshly drawn autologous blood into the epidural space.[54] This epidural blood patch lasts longer and is more effective than the epidural saline injections used in the past, which provided only transient relief and often had to be repeated.

CRANIAL NERVE PALSY. When the brain sags owing to loss of supporting cerebrospinal fluid, the cranial nerves may be stretched and injured. The abducens is the most vulnerable cranial nerve in its long intracranial course, and diplopia from sixth nerve palsy can be expected in about 1 in 1000 subarachnoid blocks, usually associated with moderate to severe cephalgia. In most instances abducens palsy will resolve without therapy before the patient is discharged from the hospital,[84] but ophthalmology consultation is advised because of the infrequent need for surgical correction.

PERIPHERAL NERVE PALSY. Transient peripheral nerve weakness or sensory deficit in the distribution of the cauda equina can be demonstrated in 0.4 per cent of patients, probably owing to direct needle trauma to the nerve roots. These deficits usually will resolve before discharge, with the incidence of permanent nerve palsy somewhere around 1 per 5000 spinal anesthetics. These deficits are not clearly associated with traumatic lumbar puncture; however, paresthesias are often reported in these patients at the time of injection of anesthetic solution, a normally painless procedure when the needle is free in the subarachnoid space.[84] In patients with previous neuropathy related to lumbar disc disease, some exacerbation of nerve root injury may follow spinal anesthesia, so subarachnoid block is wisely avoided. Any peripheral nerve palsy following spinal anesthesia should be carefully examined and documented by a neurologist. No therapy has been shown to be of much benefit in this situation.

Sympathetic Block

The most important physiologic effect of spinal anesthesia is the result of blocking the preganglionic sympathetic fibers traversing the subarachnoid space, which interrupts vasoconstrictor impulses to the peripheral vascular bed. The sympathetic block extends several segments above the level of skin analgesia or motor blockade. As the block ascends, sympathetically mediated compensation for hypovolemia or position changes may become ineffective. Vasodilatation follows, with reduced peripheral resistance, venous return, and cardiac output. The net effect is usually hypotension. If the sympathetic block includes the upper four thoracic segments, bradycardia results from interruption of cardioaccelerator impulses. The drop in blood pressure sometimes causes nausea, presumably due to medullary ischemia.

The hypotension may be sudden and profound, with reduced perfusion of heart and brain. Ability to withstand this hypotention will vary with the previous state of the circulatory bed, brain, and heart. Arteriosclerotic patients tolerate it poorly, as do those with hypovolemia or anemia. The immediate effect of severe hypotension is respiratory depression from medullary ischemia, accompanied by loss of consciousness. Death or serious morbidity may follow if the hypotension is not corrected promptly.

Hypotension is treated immediately with rapid fluid infusion of isotonic saline or balanced salt solution through an intravenous line that should be inserted in all patients undergoing spinal anesthesia. Oxygen should be administered at the same time. Early in the block before the local anesthetic is fixed to the nerves, hyperbaric solutions may shift and raise the level of the block to unintended levels, so Trendelenburg position should be used cautiously. The patient is probably best kept flat and still when the pressure drops soon after injection.

Poor response to fluid infusion is an indication for pharmacologic therapy, especially in the elderly patient or in the presence of ischemic heart disease. If mild hypotension is noted, accompanied by the bradycardia often observed during subarachnoid block, atropine in small doses is usually effective in restoring the pressure. With a normal heart rate and more severe hypotension, positive inotropic or chronotropic stimulation or peripheral vasoconstriction may be preferred. Usually a small bolus dose of ephedrine, phenylephrine, or methoxamine will raise the pressure to acceptable levels. Increased fluid infusion should be continued, and repeated doses of pressors may be necessary to maintain perfusion until intravascular volume is increased. Correction of the blood pressure will usually restore the sensorium and respiration, and nausea, when present, should subside.

In late pregnancy the uterus may compress the vena cava when the patient is in the supine position and impede venous return from the lower extremities to produce hypotension. Spinal or epidural anesthesia seems to increase the possibility of this supine hypotensive syndrome. Maternal hypotension must be treated promptly because of the danger of fetal hypoxia. Lateral uterine displacement usually restores the central venous return and blood pressure to normal, but until this is corrected oxygen therapy is indicated. If needed, ephedrine is the pressor of choice in pregnancy, because it produces the most favorable balance between pressor effect and uterine perfusion.

Somatic Motor Block

Motor blockade from spinal anesthesia can extend to variable levels depending on the dose of drug used. The effect this may have on respiratory function is a most significant cause of complications. Paresis of the thoracoabdominal musculature impairs cough and clearance of secretions. Significant intercostal paralysis impedes the ability to generate a normal sigh, and coupled with loss of sensation of the chest wall, gives many patients the feeling they cannot breathe adequately despite objective evidence to the contrary. Patients with heavy secretions or diminished respiratory reserve are thus at high risk of pulmonary morbidity during and after spinal anesthesia; but a well-conducted low spinal anesthetic may be preferable to the alternative general technique. High spinal blocks in such patients are probably best avoided.

Occasional hyperinflation using the anesthesia circuit and mask applied to the patient's face will assist the patient in generating a sigh volume to cough and clear secretions. An alternative method is to supplement the block with light general endotracheal anesthesia, which allows suctioning of secretions and hyperinflation of the lungs.

If the anesthetic level reaches the high cervical cord, the diaphragm may become paralyzed when the phrenic nerve is blocked. Quite often the patient has been coughing or moving about excessively, and then develops progressive dyspnea with marked dysphoria. Injection of amnesics followed by endotracheal intubation and respiratory support will be required. This should be differentiated from hypotension-related apnea, which is much more common. This is caused by stagnant hypoxia of the medullary respiratory center and not by respiratory muscle paralysis, and usually responds to treatment with fluids and pressors.

Suction should always be ready in case of regurgitation and aspiration of stomach contents, a constant threat under spinal anesthesia. Sedation and poor cough increase the risk of this complication, and nausea from spinal hypotension may predispose to vomiting as well. The debilitated patient with bowel obstruction is a particularly poor candidate for high spinal anesthesia because of the risk of aspiration during abdominal exploration, and general anesthesia is preferred.

Motor block also decreases venous return to the heart by decreasing skeletal muscle tone to promote peripheral pooling of blood volume. Resulting hypotension is indistinguishable from that due to sympathetic block, with which it combines, and should be treated similarly with fluid supplements and vasopressors.

PERIDURAL ANESTHESIA (EPIDURAL AND CAUDAL TECHNIQUES). Peridural anesthesia carries with it most of the complications of subarachnoid anesthesia, as well as a few of its own. Basically the same anesthetic effects are produced without puncturing the dura to enter the subarachnoid space. Much larger volumes of local anesthetic solution than those used for subarchnoid block are injected into the epidural space (10 to 40 ml.), and potential for systemic toxicity from direct intravenous injection or rapid absorption is correspondingly increased, especially when the rich vascularity of the epidural space is taken into consideration. Toxic reactions are treated according to the principles outlined in the section on local and topical anesthesia above.

Vasomotor block can produce hypotension as with subarachnoid block, but slower onset of sympathetic paresis during peridural anesthesia allows homeostatic vascular reflexes to compensate to decrease the incidence and severity of blood pressure changes. The complications of motor paralysis are potentially the same as with spinal anesthesia, but the concentration of local anesthetic can be reduced to produce autonomic and sensory block alone without complete motor loss. Morbidity due to effects of motor paralysis can thus be lessened along with the risk of systemic local anesthetic toxicity.

The peridural space is entered through the sacral hiatus with the caudal technique or between the spinous processes of the lower three lumbar vertebrae in the lumbar epidural technique. Anesthetic solution can be injected through a needle in the peridural space that is then removed — a single-shot technique; or a small plastic catheter can be inserted through a large beveled needle for the continuous peridural methods. Most complications of peridural anesthesia can result from either the single-shot or continuous techniques, but the use of the indwelling catheter has become more common because subsequent injections can be used to adjust anesthetic spread and to extend the duration of block, and even to provide postoperative analgesia. Complications are probably more frequent and serious with the continuous technique. Morbidity related to needle trauma, subarachnoid injection, and infection will be discussed for both methods, and the problem of catheter breakage during continuous techniques will be reviewed.

Trauma

Trauma to nerve tissue and blood vessels in the peridural space is probably more severe with the large needles used for continuous techniques, and complaints of low back discomfort are frequent but transient after continuous caudal or epidural blocks. Paresthesias during needle advancement or catheter insertion should suggest potential for nerve trauma. The position of the needle, or needle and catheter together, must be adjusted until paresthesias cease, before the technique can be completed. If paresthesias continue, the needle should be removed and another placement attempted. The catheter must always be removed with the needle *as a unit;* withdrawing the catheter through the needle risks shearing the catheter off in the epidural space. Permanent damage to nerve roots or spinal cord is extremely rare with current techniques for peridural anesthesia and should be evaluated and treated as outlined for spinal anesthesia.

Bleeding may follow injury to the epidural vessels, and the resulting epidural hematoma can produce symptoms of cord compression that will require laminectomy for relief. Usually the patient with an epidural hematoma has only minor back pain that can be treated with analgesics. As the hematoma resolves, it can provide an excellent nidus for infection. Thus, unexplained fever several days after epidural block should prompt antibiotic therapy to prevent an epidural abscess from developing. Most epidural hematomas have occurred in the past in patients on anticoagulant therapy, but they can form spontaneously in patients with normal clotting functions. Again, it must be emphasized that systemic anticoagulation contraindicates peridural techniques.

Subarachnoid Injection

Dural puncture during peridural techniques should be seen in less than 1 per cent of cases in experienced hands.[43] With the large needles used for catheter insertion, severe cephalgia can result, sometimes immediately, as fluid drains with the needle in place. The block should be abandoned at that level, and perhaps entirely, although some opinion favors a second attempt at another interspace. Treatment of headache is the same as outlined for subarachnoid block.

The greatest danger lies in undetected dural puncture followed by anesthetic injection. Massive spinal block after subarachnoid injection of the large volumes used in peridural anesthesia produces cardiorespiratory collapse and prolonged unconsciousness due to the effects of the local anesthetic. A test dose of 2 to 3 cc. of local anesthetic will produce a limited spinal block if injected after dural puncture, and the technique can then be converted to a continuous spinal method or discontinued. The test dose should be used before *each* dose of peridural anesthetic solution, because total spinal block has occurred on the second or third injection through an epidural catheter that had functioned normally on the initial injections. Erosion of the catheter through the dura is assumed to be responsible, and even the remote possibility of this complication would indicate that the test dose must be used for *each* injection.[43]

Infection

Peridural abscesses can occur, as well as superficial infections of the skin and underlying tissues. Implicated in many such cases are the prolonged use of indwelling catheters for analgesia, and caudal techniques with their high likelihood of fecal contamination. The incidence of infection can be reduced by preferential use of lumbar epidural block, especially in obstetrics, and by removing any epidural catheter after 3 days. Symptoms of back pain and fever that suggest possible epidural abscess can be treated with analgesics and antibiotics, but if neurologic deficits develop in rare instances, decompression with surgical laminectomy may be indicated.

Catheter Complications

Continuous peridural catheters can be sheared off during placement or may become brittle and break off later during use, so the markings on the end of all catheters removed after block should be carefully checked to confirm that they are intact. Newer materials used in catheters, such as Teflon, make such spontaneous breakage less likely. If the break occurs just under the skin, the catheter fragment can usually be removed under local anesthesia. When a catheter tip is sheared off in the epidural space or caudal canal, in the vast majority of instances no complications should result. The foreign body is well tolerated, and the difficulties encountered in locating the catheter remnant at laminectomy would indicate that surgery should be deferred unless significant symptoms develop. The patient should be advised that part of the catheter remains in the spine but that complications due to this are unlikely.[43]

Knotting up of catheters in the epidural space is caused by insertion of excessive lengths of catheter past the needle tip and can be avoided by advancing no more than 4 cm. during placement.

SPECIAL PROBLEMS

It has been the intent of this chapter to proceed through the details of a normal induction of anesthesia, discussing the complications to be expected from each phase of the procedure. Certain problems in anesthetic practice deserve particular consideration, either because they will be encountered frequently by the anesthesiologist or because while they are fairly rare, they pose a serious threat of death or severe morbidity whenever they occur. In the first category the problems of emergency surgery, the patient with increased intracranial pressure, the problems of sickle cell disease in black patients, and complications associated with the use of methylmethacrylate cement in orthopedic surgery will be considered. In the category of rare but sinister problems, malignant hyperthermia and pheochromocytoma will be discussed. Finally, the use of hypotensive anesthesia for control of blood loss in surgery will be discussed, with particular emphasis placed on the new vasodilator sodium nitroprusside.

Consideration of complications of particular subspecialties of anesthesiology is beyond the scope of this chapter. Excellent recent reviews of complications in obstetric,[89] pediatric,[91] neurosurgical,[49] and cardiac[70] anesthesia are available, and the interested reader is encouraged to consult them.

Emergency Surgery

The patient who enters the hospital after trauma will often be poorly evaluated and inadequately prepared for emergency surgery. The medical history may be incomplete, and the intravascular volume status is frequently uncertain. Anesthetic induction and maintenance under these conditions are much more likely to produce serious complications than induction during elective surgery.

The patient for emergency procedures, whether admitted from the emergency room or brought to surgery from the ward, should always be assumed to have a full stomach. Often a meal was eaten just prior to injury, but even if several hours have elapsed since the last ingestion of food, the effects of pain, stress, or sedation on gastric emptying may keep the stomach full for many hours. The parturient in labor has a particularly high gastric residual volume. This increases the risk of vomiting and regurgitation during anesthesia, to be followed by pulmonary aspiration of vomitus if the airway is unprotected. Because the pulmonary aspiration syndrome still carries a high mortality, even with the considerable advances in respiratory management in the past decade, general anesthesia for emergency surgery is conducted so the airway is protected at the earliest possible moment after consciousness is lost.

Alternatives to general anesthesia in the trauma patient are available that avoid the risk of aspiration. When no neurologic injury or spinal trauma is present, regional block can be considered for surgery on the extremities, but caution should be observed in the possibly hypovolemic patient. Because excessive sedation during regional block may obtund protective airway reflexes, dosages of such drugs as diazepam or the barbiturates should be reasonably restricted.

The airway may also be controlled before

loss of consciousness by awake endotracheal intubation through the nose or mouth. After intubation, general anesthesia can be induced without fear of aspiration. The use of topical anesthesia during this maneuver may make it more tolerable to the patient, but will prevent glottic protective reflexes, and will increase the possibility of aspiration if the patient vomits during endoscopy or blind nasal passage of an endotracheal tube. The use of local anesthesia and more than minimal sedation for awake intubation is therefore unwise, and the associated discomfort makes this method for airway control unacceptable to most patients. The airway *must* be controlled *before* induction of general anesthesia in any trauma patient in whom injury to the airway may complicate standard intubation techniques. If there is any question about the ability to rapidly control the airway with standard techniques, either an awake intubation or a preliminary tracheostomy under local anesthesia should be elected. This doubly prevents postinduction asphyxia and aspiration and cannot be too strongly recommended.

For patients with easily controllable airways, the technique for rapid sequence induction of anesthesia has been generally adopted to provide loss of consciousness followed as soon as possible by protection of the airway from aspiration. Prior to rapid sequence induction (or "crash" induction, a regrettable term still widely used), the patient is pre-oxygenated to fill the airway with a high oxygen concentration. A pretreating small dose of non-depolarizing muscle relaxant is injected (3 to 4.5 mg. of tubocurarine) to block fasciculations caused by succinylcholine, which may increase the intragastric pressure and favor regurgitation.

Loss of consciousness is produced by rapid intravenous injection of thiopental, 4 to 5 mg./kg., or in the hypovolemic patient, ketamine, 1 to 2 mg./kg. Immediately following the induction agent, succinylcholine, 1.5 mg./kg., is injected to produce a flaccid patient ready for endoscopy and intubation. To prevent regurgitation before the airway is controlled, digital pressure should be maintained on the cricoid cartilage to press its flat posterior surface toward the cervical spine to occlude the underlying esophagus. This Sellick maneuver should be applied as soon as consciousness is lost and the fingers

not removed until the airway is controlled and sealed. Before intubation, the use of positive pressure ventilation with oxygen applied to the upper airway by mask must be avoided, because of the possibility that gas may be blown into the stomach and increase the risk of regurgitation. After the patient is flaccid, laryngoscopy and intubation should be rapidly accomplished and the airway protected by inflation of the cuff on the endotracheal tube. This entire rapid sequence induction maneuver is easily accomplished in less than a minute in most instances.

When aspiration occurs despite these precautions, a severe chemical pneumonitis may result if the pH of the aspirated fluid is below 2.5. Intense bronchospasm occurs immediately with wheezing prominent over the affected portions of the lungs. The aspirated fluid diffuses rapidly to the periphery, so bicarbonate lavage to acutely neutralize acidity in the bronchi seems to be ineffective. The pH of a fluid sample should be analyzed, but immediate therapy should not await the result of the determination. As much of the fluid should be suctioned from the airway as is possible and respiratory supportive therapy begun immediately. Arterial blood gas values should be followed from the start; supplemental oxygen and controlled ventilation may be needed for several days, and distending airway pressure is often necessary to maintain ventilation and oxygenation. Atelectasis, superinfection, and resulting hypoxemia frequently complicate the course of aspiration pneumonitis and contribute to mortality.

The role of steroids in the treatment of aspiration pneumonitis is controversial. Large doses of steroids given just before or at the time of aspiration may lessen the duration and severity of symptoms.[92] The benefit of steroids given more than 5 minutes after the pulmonary insult is probably minimal.[103] The attitude that large doses of steroids will not hurt and may help in the treatment of aspiration is widely used to justify the administration of costly megadoses of steroids, even hours after the acute lung insult. The fact that steroids impede wound healing and inhibit immune responses must be considered, and their use in surgical patients should be based only on strong indications of benefit to be obtained.

The fact that the effectiveness of steroids in pulmonary aspiration has not been consistently demonstrated should temper enthusiasm for their use.

If solid particles are present in the aspirated gastric contents, an attempt at bronchoscopic removal is indicated. Smaller food fragments may lodge in the peripheral bronchial tree to cause atelectasis, distal pneumonitis, and local foreign body granulomas. Steroids again appear to be of little benefit in solid particle aspiration, and therapy consists mostly of supportive respiratory care and antibiotics when indicated for superinfection.[103] Prophylactic antibiotics are usually withheld; the airway secretions should be cultured at frequent intervals, and Gram stains of purulent secretions should be done to facilitate a choice of appropriate antibiotic coverage, while the results of culture and sensitivity determinations are pending.

Aspiration of stomach contents and acute asphyxiation during induction of anesthesia from loss of the airway remain the most serious potential complications of anesthesia. Their incidence can be minimized with appropriate preventive measures, but it is unlikely that the risk of their occurrence will ever be entirely eliminated.

The Patient With Increased Intracranial Pressure

Increased intracranial pressure should be suggested by headaches, vomiting, or excessive somnolence noted during the preoperative evaluation. The eye grounds should be checked for evidence of papilledema to confirm the diagnosis. Attempts must be made prior to anesthesia to control elevated intracranial pressure, because herniation of the medulla and death may result from acute rises in intracranial pressure occurring during induction. These sustained increases in intracranial pressure are especially likely following endotracheal intubation or surgical stimulation under light anesthesia. Anesthetic agents can also promote vasodilatation to increase intracranial pressure. This is true of nitrous oxide, halothane, enflurane, and isoflurane and can also follow the administration of vasodilators such as sodium nitroprusside. Hyperventilation prior to the introduction of inhalational anesthetic agents seems to limit the extent of the pressure rise; after acute lowering of the Pa_{CO_2}, the volatile agents can be used to deepen anesthesia prior to endotracheal intubation.[36] Large doses of barbiturates also acutely lower the intracranial pressure and may decrease pressure responses to airway maneuvers under anesthesia.[88]

Because the effects of anesthesia are so hazardous in patients with increased intracranial pressure, attempts at prior control are mandatory. Steroid therapy with dexamethasone (Decadron) may be used when several days of preparation are possible. When less time is available, mannitol or furosemide diuretics are rapidly effective in lowering intracranial pressure; at the same time, intravenous fluids should be restricted unless the arterial pressure is unstable. Bolus injection of thiopental, 4 to 5 mg./kg., is also acutely effective in lowering the intracranial pressure and is the preferred immediate therapy for severely increased intracranial pressure in previously intubated patients.

Intracranial pressure monitoring has proven indispensable in patients with head trauma, postanoxic cerebral edema, tumors, and in children with Reye's syndrome. To establish monitoring, intraventricular catheters can be placed operatively, or screw bolts can be inserted percutaneously at the bedside.[80] Direct connection to physiologic transducers produces a continuous record of the intracranial pressure and provides instant warning of acute rises that may prompt rapid pharmacologic therapy with the above drugs. This new monitoring modality facilitates prevention, detection, and treatment of dangerous rises in intracranial pressure and is effective in decreasing the complications of neurosurgical anesthesia.

Sickle Cell Anemia

Approximately 1 in every 400 American blacks has sickle cell anemia, due to the presence of homozygous hemoglobin S within the erythrocyte. The aggregation of this hemoglobin S inside the red cells can lead to the typical sickle-shaped deformity that predisposes to hemolysis and clumping of erythrocytes in the circulation. Symptoms are due to multiple infarcts of the lungs, kidneys, abdominal viscera, and skeletal structures; corresponding deficiencies in organ function can complicate anesthesia, and the effects of anesthetic agents can themselves predispose to further vascular occlusions. The sickling tendency is related to the percentage of Hgb S in the red cells, and to hypoxia, acidosis, or hypothermia in any part of the circulation. If unfavorable conditions are not corrected, the erythrocytes will sickle irreversibly and produce additional infarcts. Patients with sickle cell anemia come to surgery frequently with cholecystitis, hepatic abscess, osteomyelitis, aseptic necrosis of the femoral head, splenic hemolytic disorders, and priapism. Preventive therapy before surgery is designed to decrease the concentration of Hgb S, and in combination with intraoperative management, it attempts to reduce the factors that predispose to the sickling of red cells.

Preoperative evaluation should include a close examination for signs of acute painful sickle cell crisis. Pain from infarction of bowel or bone is treated with acetaminophen (Tylenol) and will usually subside after the infusion of 2 to 3 ml./kg./hr. of 1/4 normal saline with 30 mEq/L. of sodium bicarbonate added.[46] Oxygenation and acid-base status need to be assessed with arterial blood gas analysis, and acidosis should be rapidly treated with calculated doses of bicarbonate. Supplemental oxygen should be given, and pneumonitis, which is often detected, should be treated with appropriate antibiotics. Systemic anticoagulants predispose to hemorrhage into fresh infarcts and are not recommended. Congestive heart failure may be related to cor pulmonale from repeated pulmonary infarction or related to the anemia itself. Renal functional deficiencies are also common and should be detected in the routine laboratory results. Attempts to compensate preoperatively for cardiopulmonary or renal deficiencies are necessary if morbidity is to be minimized in sickle cell disease.

Preoperative lowering of the percentage of hemoglobin S is now widely advocated as a means of reducing the morbidity of anesthesia and surgery in patients with homozygous sickle cell disease. This can be achieved rapidly in emergencies with a two-volume exchange transfusion using fresh whole blood.[62] Over several days, hypertransfu-

sion can achieve the same result. One regimen is to infuse 10 ml./kg. of packed, washed erythrocytes every 12 hours. After 3 cycles, a hematocrit of 38 to 40 per cent with Hgb S less than 20 per cent of total hemoglobin should be reached. The chance of serious complications due to sickling seems to be reduced as long as the Hgb S remains below 40 per cent of the total hemoglobin.

During anesthesia, conditions that favor hypoxia, acidosis, and hypothermia should be carefully avoided. The FI_{O_2} should be kept at 0.5 or above, and deep levels of anesthesia with sluggish peripheral blood flow must not be maintained. An adequate blood volume is necessary at all times. For extremity surgery the pneumatic tourniquet is absolutely forbidden, an essential fact that is regrettably neglected by many surgeons and anesthesiologists. Metabolic acidosis must be rigorously controlled; iatrogenic metabolic alkalosis is considered therapeutic by some researchers, but respiratory alkalosis that induces increased peripheral vasoconstriction and oxygen consumption is obviously not advisable. Excessive heat loss must be prevented by standard measures, and shivering on emergence from anesthesia should be avoided if possible.

Postoperatively it is important that infections be detected and treated promptly, that adequate hydration be maintained, and that supplemental oxygen be given for several days, particularly following upper abdominal surgery. Prevention of sickling by the above measures should help prevent complications of infarction during surgery and afterward. Cerebral thrombosis is a particularly feared morbid event in sickle cell anemia, and prevention of just this one potential complication would justify the extensive preventive measures outlined above.

The Use of Methylmethacrylate Cement in Orthopedic Surgery

Total hip replacement procedures are becoming common even in community hospitals, and the complications of methylmethacrylate cement are being encountered regularly in anesthesia practice. Placement of both the femoral and acetabular prostheses in this procedure requires preparation of fresh methylmethacrylate cement from the liquid monomer and powdered polymer that are mixed together on the sterile field. Half the patients on whom the cement is used will demonstrate some drop in blood pressure during its application, and a decrease in oxygenation is commonly seen as well. This drop in arterial pressure is thought to be caused by the peripheral vasodilating effect of methacrylate monomer absorbed from the cement as it is applied. While the decrease in pressure is usually transient and limited in extent, cardiac arrest in the poor-risk or hypovolemic patient is occasionally seen.

Prevention of complications during use of methylmethacrylate requires that consideration be given to avoiding use of the drug in patients who will not tolerate hypotension or tachycardia after vasodilatation. The blood volume must be adequately supported prior to use of the cement, and there may be some advantage to distal venting of the shaft of the femur to prevent excessive rises in intramedullary pressure. Finally the recommendation that the cement be allowed to set temporarily before application to allow evaporation of monomer from its surface deserves mention.[40]

Pheochromocytoma

Anesthetic technique for excision of pheochromocytoma is governed by three primary considerations. First, a deep level of anesthesia is preferred during endotracheal intubation and surgical manipulation to minimize the physiologic effects of stimulation. Second, the hypertensive and arrhythmogenic effects of circulating catecholamines can be blocked by the appropriate antagonists. Third, it should be possible to avert catastrophic falls in blood pressure at the time of excision of the tumor by volume loading, withdrawal of anesthetic agents, and if necessary, pressors.

Recent pharmacologic and technical advances have greatly reduced the risk of surgery in patients with pheochromocytoma. An operative mortality of over 50 per cent in the 1940's has now been decreased to less than 3 percent in recent years, partly owing to better preoperative preparation and partly owing to improvement in intraoperative management.[44] Patients with

unsuspected pheochromocytomas who are anesthetized without specific preparation before surgery have morbidity and mortality rates comparable to those seen decades ago, a fact that demonstrates the importance of preoperative pharmacologic management with this tumor.

Prior to surgery, phenoxybenzamine (Dibenzyline) is administered orally in increasing doses until blood pressure is controlled. The total daily dose seldom exceeds 200 mg. Propranolol (Inderal) is used primarily to control arrhythmias, although some cardiologists use it routinely in all patients with pheochromocytoma prior to surgery. Control of catecholamine effect is confirmed with return of plasma volume to the normal range and a lowering of the hematocrit, while the blood pressure returns to normal or slightly elevated levels, and the severity of paroxysmal hypertensive episodes diminishes. It is recommended that both drugs be discontinued 12 hours prior to surgery. It may be necessary to taper propranolol over several days when high dosages are being administered. While the half-life of low doses of propranolol is from 2 to 4 hours, higher levels may persist in patients taking higher cumulative doses. Minimal beta adrenergic blockade is preferred in patients taking propranolol at the time of removal of the tumor. Phenoxybenzamine has a half-life of 24 hours once it is bound to the receptor, and adequate adrenergic blockade should persist through surgery.

Multiple large infusion lines should be placed prior to induction, and an intra-arterial monitoring catheter inserted under local anesthesia. Patients with a history of myocardial failure or with a high possibility of a catecholamine-induced myocardiopathy will also benefit from monitoring with a Swan-Ganz catheter; this can also be used to confirm an elevated wedge pressure after fluid-loading prior to excision of the tumor.[44]

Pentothal is safe for rapid intravenous induction, but immediate intubation with succinylcholine may lead to dangerous arterial pressure rises with possible intracranial bleeding. Coughing may also raise the blood pressure, so the patient should be flaccid and deeply anesthetized with a volatile anesthetic agent prior to laryngoscopy and endotracheal intubation. Enflurane and the new agent isoflurane seem the best agents for producing deep anesthesia without sensitizing the myocardium to the arrhythmogenic effects of the catecholamines released by pheochromocytomas.[47, 74] Flaccidity may be produced with the non-depolarizing muscle relaxant pancuronium, which has minor tachycardic and hypertensive side effects, but which is not associated with the marked hypertension seen with pheochromocytoma after succinylcholine and tubocurarine. Lidocaine may also be used to suppress the hypertensive response to intubation, while at the same time serving to control arrhythmias.

Despite adequate pressure control, tumor manipulation invariably causes rapid increases in blood pressure, and ventricular arrhythmias can be superimposed on the basal supraventricular tachycardia as a result of increased blood pressure and direct excitation of the myocardium by catecholamines. Control of the hypertension is necessary to restore stability. This can be achieved with alpha adrenergic blockade using phentolamine, 2.5 to 5 mg. intravenously, titrating to the desired blood pressure. The pressure should remain controlled for 5 minutes after each dose, but after several doses tachyphylaxis may be observed, at which time a sodium nitroprusside infusion may become necessary. Any agent used for hypotensive effects must be rapidly effective and rapidly dissipated; besides phenoxybenzamine any long-acting, fixed agents would be undesirable during anesthetic maintenance. The action of such agents must be terminated by the time the vascular pedicle is divided and levels of circulating catecholamines begin to subside.

Ventricular arrhythmias occurring as a result of pressure elevation should be treated primarily with hypotensive agents. If they do not resolve when lower pressures are attained, a bolus of lidocaine or propranolol may be injected. As the dissection of the tumor proceeds, the surgeons are asked to warn in advance of the time the vascular pedicle is divided, so the inhalational anesthetic can be tapered, and fluid loading can be accomplished. Replacement with whole blood and heavy loading with plasma or albumin solutions are used at this time to drive the pulmonary wedge pressure up to levels approaching 10 mm. Hg. This volume

expansion is essential to prevent hypovolemic hypotension as the vascular bed expands following removal of the tumor. In the apparently normovolemic or hypervolemic patient after volume expansion, any blood pressure drop of a substantial degree can be assumed to be due to myocardial insufficiency, and while this possibility is remote, the pulmonary capillary wedge pressure can be helpful in suggesting that central inotropic agents may be more useful than direct peripheral vasoconstrictors in this situation. If the wedge pressure falls as the arterial pressure drops, appropriate therapy would be peripheral direct alpha adrenergic agonists such as norepinephrine (Levophed) or phenylephrine (Neo-Synephrine) titrated by slow intravenous infusion. Further volume loading can also be continued until normal perfusion pressures are reached. If the pulmonary wedge pressure increases as the blood pressure drops, dopamine or epinephrine infusion is probably indicated. After an optimal blood pressure is obtained, weaning from both inotropic and vasoconstricting drugs can be guided by further monitoring of the wedge pressure. In most cases the pharmacologic support of the cardiovascular system can be decreased and discontinued within 6 to 12 hours.

The chief complications of pheochromocytoma surgery are due to uncontrolled hypertensive responses, which may lead to acute intracranial bleeding or myocardial decompensation; or they can be due to uncontrolled hypotensive episodes with cardiac arrest, caused by relative hypovolemia after catecholamine release by the tumor ceases. Close monitoring, judicious fluid management, and appropriate use of vasodilators or pressors will prevent these complications, when combined with adequate preoperative control with phenoxybenzamine, and maintenance of deep anesthesia with volatile agents.

Malignant Hyperthermia

Malignant hyperthermia is a genetically determined syndrome involving paroxysmal hypercatabolic reactions of skeletal muscle, set off by stress or exposure to triggering agents. The mortality of individual episodes was reported as 70 per cent when the syndrome was first described, but aggressive therapy and early detection have lowered this to 30 per cent or less.[42]

Symptoms of malignant hyperthermia may occur during anesthetic induction or at any time thereafter throughout surgery and the recovery period. Rigidity in response to succinylcholine given for endotracheal intubation is highly suggestive of possible developing malignant hyperthermia. Rigidity developing during anesthesia is seen in 75 per cent of instances of malignant hyperthermia, but the primary symptom is fulminant progressive fever, with temperature increases as fast as 1° F. every 5 minutes. Along with fever, hypermetabolism results in combined respiratory and metabolic acidosis. Hypoxemia and tachyarrhythmias may be observed quite early in the course of MH, even before a marked temperature rise is apparent. Without aggressive attempts at cooling the patient, the fever may go as high as 41° C., with rapid progression to pulmonary edema and death.

If control of the acute hyperthermia is achieved, other side effects of the syndrome may require therapy. Muscle destruction results in myoglobin release, and renal damage can occur even when proper preventive measures are carried out. Permanent neurologic deficits can remain after the resolution of fever, and hemolysis, thrombocytopenia, and disseminated intravascular coagulopathy should be expected in a high proportion of the cases.

The incidence of the syndrome is between 1 in 15,000 and 1 in 50,000 general anesthetics, and approximately a third of the cases occur in children below the age of puberty. The syndrome is inherited as a mendelian dominant trait with incomplete penetrance and variable expressivity, which means that some individuals in an affected family may never develop fever under anesthesia. However, any patient with a familial history of malignant hyperthermia should be considered at risk for developing the syndrome and should receive appropriate evaluation and preparation for surgery.

Certain physical abnormalities that require anesthesia and surgery are common in MH-susceptible patients, possibly related to a subclinical myopathy these patients may have in common. Strabismus and ptosis, inguinal hernias, scoliosis, lumbar disc problems, and clubfeet are examples of musculoskeletal problems common in MH-susceptible patients. Many of these individuals have large bulky muscle groups but demonstrate poor coordination that may predispose to trauma during athletic activity. Muscle and connective tissue diseases are diagnosed in two-thirds of all patients with documented malignant hyperthermia, with elevated serum CPK levels in 80 per cent of individuals in some families carrying the disorder.

Much of our knowledge of the metabolic defect in malignant hyperthermia comes from study of a similar disorder in certain species of pigs (such as Landrace or Poland China swine). A defect in muscle intracellular calcium balance, with decreased re-uptake of the ion at subcellular binding sites, seems to disrupt excitation-contraction coupling and lead to hypercatabolism. Excessive oxygen consumption, carbon dioxide production, dissipation of energy as heat, and extreme acidosis follow. The current theories of the pathogenesis of MH are comprehensively reviewed by Gronert,[63] along with an excellent correlation with recommended therapy at this time.

Drugs used in anesthesia may act as triggering agents to set off hyperthermic episodes in susceptible patients. The general anesthetic agents ether, halothane, and enflurane are examples, as are the depolarizing muscle relaxant succinylcholine and the amide local anesthetics (lidocaine, mepivacaine). To avoid triggering MH in susceptible patients, balanced anesthetic techniques are recommended using Pentothal, fentanyl, diazepam, nitrous oxide, and pancuronium — all agents with little or no triggering properties.[87] When regional anesthesia is appropriate to the procedure, only the ester local anesthetics should be used (procaine, Nesacaine, tetracaine, or cocaine).

In patients who have survived previous episodes of MH or who have relatives with a history compatible with the syndrome, the use of dantrolene sodium, a hydantoin derivative with direct relaxant effects on the muscle fibers, may be a helpful prophylactic measure before surgery. The drug can be given orally for 3 days before surgery, 25 mg. q.i.d. for the first day, 50 mg. q.i.d. on the second, and 100 mg. q.i.d. on the third.

On the day of surgery an oral dose of 2 mg./kg. 4 hours before induction of anesthesia is recommended.[87] There may be occasional liver toxicity from dantrolene therapy, so hepatic enzyme levels should be followed during its use.

Temperature should be monitored in all patients under anesthesia because one in every three episodes of MH occurs in a patient with a negative family history for the disorder. Whenever an excessive rise in temperature is detected, all anesthetic agents should be stopped, and surgery should be cancelled or finished as quickly as possible. An arterial cannula should be inserted, 100 per cent oxygen should be administered, and the patient should be hyperventilated through an endotracheal tube. Arterial blood gas results should be assessed, and metabolic acidosis treated aggressively with sodium bicarbonate. Serum potassium, glucose, and calcium levels should be checked and followed closely at frequent intervals throughout the episode. Arrhythmias may be treated with procainamide as necessary, but the arterial pressure should be watched closely during infusion. Urine output should be closely monitored and maintained with fluid infusion and diuretics if necessary.

Active cooling should be commenced with ice packs, iced intravenous fluids, and cold saline lavage of open body cavities or of the stomach. Cooling by femoral-femoral extracorporeal perfusion with a heat exchanger has also been utilized, but this may not be readily available in most hospitals.

Specific pharmacologic therapy with intravenous dantrolene is now possible, and this has proven effective both in humans and in swine in reversing the progress of established malignant hyperthermia. The dosage of 1 to 2 mg./kg. intravenously is recommended initially, with cumulative doses up to 10 mg./kg. given until fever is controlled. Dantrolene therapy should be maintained for 72 hours after the episode, because reoccurrence of fever and acidosis is occasionally seen after initial response to therapy.

Muscle soreness, highly elevated CPK levels, renal damage, and neurologic deficits should be carefully searched for in survivors. Relatives of susceptible patients should be alerted to the danger of anesthesia to members of the family, and they should be urged to mention the history of hyperpyrexia during anesthesia to the anesthesiologist, if they are ever scheduled for surgery.

It is impossible at this time to absolutely predict MH susceptibility prior to surgery in individual patients by using a simple inexpensive screening test. Because episodes occur sporadically in patients without a history of MH in their families, it is impossible to prevent the occurrence of malignant hyperthermia at this time. Despite adequate care to minimize the morbidity and mortality related to the syndrome, the complications are so severe that litigation may frequently result. The fact that an episode of malignant hyperthermia has occurred, however, should not be the issue in a malpractice suit, because it is most often beyond the control of the anesthesiologist or surgeon involved. Issues in litigation that *are* important involve failure to monitor temperature intraoperatively, failure to elicit a family history of hyperthermia, failure to discontinue anesthesia and institute prompt therapy, and failure to defer the surgical procedure. Evidence of any of the above lapses may be interpreted as negligence and weigh heavily in malpractice suits involving malignant hyperthermia.

Considering the low incidence of the syndrome in the practice of anesthesiology, the disorder has received an inordinate amount of attention in the anesthesiology literature in the 20 years since it was first described. Attention to thermal monitoring, rapid detection of fever, and newer pharmacologic therapy with agents like dantrolene have improved survival in MH. Certainly, the continued mortality rate of 30 per cent makes this one of the deadliest of anesthetic complications, and the emphasis in the literature is probably warranted on this basis.

Deliberate Hypotension

Hypotensive anesthetic techniques are utilized to deliberately lower the blood pressure in a controlled fashion, so that blood loss will be minimized. Decreased blood loss reduces transfusion requirements and presumably lowers the risk of related hepatitis. Surgery may also be facilitated because of decreases in bleeding on the surgical field, so that anatomic exposure is improved and operative time is shortened.[56] Reductions in blood loss and operative time have been reported with hypotensive techniques, but a decrease in the incidence of hepatitis remains to be demonstrated.[94]

Deliberate hypotension utilizes volatile anesthetic agents, vasodilators, and ganglionic blockers, singly or in combination, to reduce the mean arterial pressure by as much as 30 per cent. Patients must be chosen carefully to prevent increases in morbidity or mortality from the technique itself. Contraindications would include a history of cerebrovascular accident or transient ischemic attacks, myocardial infarction in the past 3 years, angina, congestive heart failure, renal failure, severe hypertension (blood pressure greater than 170/110), respiratory disease with carbon dioxide retention, or severe adrenal insufficiency or diabetes.[94]

Certain physiologic effects of decreased perfusion must be carefully watched for during hypotensive techniques. Increased dead space and shunting during deliberate hypotension can result in hypercarbia and hypoxia in patients allowed to breathe spontaneously.[38] Respirations should be controlled throughout and blood gas values followed closely during lowering of the blood pressure. If the systolic pressure falls below 80 torr, the urine flow may cease in some patients; a bladder catheter should therefore be inserted so urinary output may be monitored. Respiratory or renal dysfunction should be an indication for abandoning the technique and restoring pressures to normal levels for the patient during the remainder of the surgical procedure.

Deep halothane anesthesia can be used to lower the pressure; however, the myocardial depression from deep halothane may not be desirable in many patients. Usually short-acting intravenous agents are used to lower the pressure without requiring halothane maintenance with high concentrations. The two most commonly used intravenous hypotensive agents are trimethaphan (Arfonad), a ganglion blocking drug, and sodium nitroprusside (Nipride), a direct-acting vasodilator.

Trimethaphan is a ganglionic blocking drug that may also have limited direct vasodilating and histamine-releasing effects.

When infused at a rate of 1 to 4 mg./min., it will produce hypotensive effects lasting for 10 to 15 minutes after a stable infusion is discontinued. Tachyphylaxis is frequently encountered with trimethaphan, and the drug must occasionally be replaced by nitroprusside when it becomes ineffective.

Sodium nitroprusside is a direct vasodilating agent that is rapidly metabolized so that its effects dissipate in 2 to 5 minutes after it is discontinued. It is an extremely potent vasodilator; 1.5 μg./kg./min. usually produces a sufficient hypotensive effect at the beginning of an infusion to achieve control of pressure to the desired level. Changes in vascular resistance combined with peripheral pooling of blood may result in a compensatory tachycardia during the use of nitroprusside. When this strongly opposes the induced hypotension, tachycardia can be blocked with intravenous propranolol so that the desired drop in pressure can be attained.

During initial infusion, tachyphylaxis may develop slowly or rapidly, or marked resistance to the drug may be seen from the outset. Resistance to the effects of sodium nitroprusside is always an indication that toxicity of the drug is developing owing to the release of cyanide during metabolism of the vasodilator in the circulating red blood cells. If developing resistance to the drug is also accompanied by increasing metabolic acidosis, increased venous oxygen tension, and a decreased arteriovenous oxygen content difference, the presumed diagnosis of cyanide toxicity is strongly supported.

Sodium nitroprusside dosage may need to be restricted to as little as 5 μg./kg./min. during short infusion to minimize cyanide release; however, in most patients twice this dosage level seems to be reasonably safe.[96] If more hypotensive effect is needed, the use of trimethaphan as an alternative should be considered. The maximum infusion of sodium nitroprusside every 24 hours during prolonged therapy has not been established. Regular acid-base monitoring is obviously mandatory because metabolic acidosis may be the initial indicator of cyanide-related nitroprusside toxicity. As soon as indications of nitroprusside toxicity are apparent, the infusion must be immediately stopped and therapeutic maneuvers begun to treat cyanide effects.

Free cyanide may be bound by methemoglobin in the circulation, so initial therapy with sodium nitrite, 5 mg./kg. injected over 3 to 4 minutes, is recommended. This oxidizes hemoglobin to methemoglobin to bind free cyanide before it can bond to and poison the subcellular cytochromes. Cyanide can then enter the liver, where it is detoxified by the rhodanase enzyme system to produce thiocyanate. Rhodanase requires thiosulfate as a substrate; and sodium thiosulfate can be injected in a dosage of 150 mg./kg. over 15 minutes to speed up cyanide metabolism. The thiocyanate formed in the liver is then excreted by the kidney; adequate renal function is necessary or thiocyanate may be retained to produce thyroid depression and drowsiness, its major toxic effects.

Vitamin B_{12_a}, hydroxycobalamin, has been used to bind cyanide to produce cyanocobalamin, which is non-toxic. This has been prophylactically injected at a rate of 25 mg./hr. during sodium nitroprusside infusion, with a demonstrable reduction in blood cyanide levels and toxicity.[48]

Deliberate hypotension can be produced safely without undue complications in well chosen patients who are carefully monitored. It is not a technique to be casually or haphazardly employed. Anyone using deliberate controlled hypotension should be familiar with the complications of the hypotensive agents and with the specific contraindications to the use of the method outlined above.

POSTOPERATIVE PERIOD

The perioperative period is assumed to end when the patient leaves the postanesthesia recovery area. The risk of immediate anesthetic complications has for the most part subsided, and the patient has regained awareness, physiologic stability, and enough self-sufficiency to recuperate without constant nursing attention. Recovery discharge does not imply, however, that the risk of all anesthetic complications is past. Significant morbidity can result from anesthesia-related processes set off during surgery, which may not become apparent until noted days afterward on the ward. The most common of these are *postoperative pul-monary complications,* which are primarily related to the physical status of the patient and the type of surgery performed, but which deserve some consideration here because of the anesthesia-related respiratory management required to prevent or treat them. *Hepatic or renal toxicity from the volatile anesthetic agents* usually appears later in convalescence but is directly related to the duration and extent of intraoperative exposure to certain agents. While the renal effects of exposure to methoxyflurane and enflurane seem well established, considerable controversy surrounds the possible diagnosis of halothane hepatitis, which will be discussed. Finally, the phenomenon of *awareness of intraoperative events* by the lightly anesthetized patient may be uncovered during postoperative visits by the anesthesiologist or surgeon. The psychological problems involved and their treatment need to be outlined for the physicians providing care to such patients.

A last area of some concern is related not to anesthetic complications in patients but to the effects of *occupational exposure to trace amounts of anesthetic agents* on personnel working in the operating room environment. A review of current evidence on behavioral and reproductive effects should be of interest to anesthesia, surgery, and nursing personnel. Attempts to control this exposure by scavenging of overflow gases will also be discussed.

Respiratory Complications

Postoperative respiratory complications can be expected in 5 to 10 per cent of patients after anesthesia; 90 per cent or more of these complications will present as a complex of atelectasis, retention of secretions, and pneumonitis. The incidence of respiratory morbidity after surgery increases with age, obesity, and smoking; these complications will be slightly more frequent after longer operations and, as would be expected, they are considerably more frequent when patients have symptoms of acute or chronic respiratory disease prior to surgery.

Following surgery that does not enter the thorax or abdomen, pulmonary complications are usually due to pre-existing respiratory disease or to prolonged immobilization. The effects of inhalational or intravenous agents dissipate rapidly and ventilatory function is usually restored to preoperative levels within 12 hours after surgery.

The risk of respiratory complications increases markedly when the surgery enters the abdomen or chest, and the relative incidence of morbidity is directly related to reductions in the vital capacity seen after various surgical incisions. Splinting is greater with upper abdominal or sternal splitting incisions, when reductions of 50 to 75 per cent in the vital capacity are seen. Lower abdominal and intercostal incisions reduce the vital capacity to a smaller extent, 30 to 50 per cent. The vital capacity is better preserved when transverse rather than vertical incisions are utilized, and the incidence of atelectasis will be reduced as a result.[21]

Splinting causes restriction, limits the sigh mechanism, and predisposes to atelectasis. Maximum changes in vital capacity after abdominal and thoracic surgery do not occur until 12 to 18 hours after anesthesia, which for most patients is long after discharge from the recovery room.[105] Resulting maximum respiratory impairment will therefore not be encountered until on the ward, late in the operative day. Thus respiratory morbidity should be carefully watched for, and this will require several ward visits during the afternoon and night after operation.

The process of atelectasis leads to stasis, retained secretions, and eventually to pulmonary infection, if left uncorrected. Pulmonary arteriovenous shunting past collapsed alveoli in atelectatic areas results in hypoxemia, an expected postoperative complication of abdominal and thoracic procedures; this hypoxemia is usually mild and can be easily corrected by administration of supplemental oxygen for 2 to 3 days, until splinting subsides. Hypercarbia is seldom encountered and should be seen only in patients with significantly increased risk of respiratory morbidity owing to pre-existing disease or in patients heavily medicated with narcotics.

Maneuvers to increase respiratory volume will help reverse atelectasis and prevent progression of symptoms. Narcotic analgesics in small doses will lessen splinting and facilitate cough, without producing excessive carbon dioxide retention in most patients. In the presence of heavy retained secretions, preoperative bronchial hygiene for several days may lessen the severity of respiratory dysfunction after surgery. In the postoperative period, aerosol therapy, chest physiotherapy, IPPB, and incentive spirometry have all been advocated as effective in reversing atelectasis and restoring vital capacity. Conflicting reports concerning the benefit to be obtained from these individual therapeutic approaches make any preference for one technique over another dubious. All serve to increase ventilatory volumes, and aggressive therapy in this regard using any one or several modalities of respiratory therapy should be of help in lessening morbidity. Recent evidence seems to favor the use of incentive spirometry over IPPB, as long as aerosol medications are not required by the patient. Equipment and personnel requirements for utilization of incentive spirometry are relatively small; this is perhaps the main reason for its increasing application in postoperative respiratory care.

Assessment of risk and prophylactic respiratory care before surgery are helpful in preventing anesthesia-related pulmonary morbidity. Again, it should be emphasized that ward care over several days of the early postoperative period may be necessary to prevent, detect, or adequately treat pulmonary complications in high-risk patients.

Toxicity of Volatile Anesthetic Agents

The inhalational volatile anesthetic agents were long considered to be inert drugs. Inhaled, absorbed, and then exhaled unchanged by the organism, they were thought to be unable to interact with the enzyme systems of the body responsible for metabolizing drugs given orally or intravenously. Clear evidence to the contrary has accumulated over the last two decades, however, especially regarding the halogenated agents now most widely used. The use of radioactive labels has made possible quantitative estimates of the extent of metabolism of the volatile anesthetics, and the percentage of these agents recovered as urinary metabolites rather than as exhaled agent is now known to be considerable. As much as

50 per cent of administered methoxy-flurane, and 15 to 20 per cent of halothane can be recovered as metabolic breakdown products, produced by microsomal degradation of the agents in the liver. A lesser degree of metabolism has been demonstrated for enflurane (2.4 per cent) and isoflurane (0.3 per cent).

The amount of metabolism appears related to genetic factors, to induction of drug metabolism by other medications like barbiturates or hydantoin drugs, and by the ability of the organism to store the anesthetic agent in fat and release it slowly for hepatic metabolism, because the efficiency of the metabolic process is maximal when subclinical concentrations of agent are maintained in the circulating blood. Products of the metabolism of anesthetic agents are known in some instances to produce damage to organ systems, most notably to the kidney, and are also suspected of producing hepatic damage. This toxicity of the inhalational anesthetics will be evident only in the late postoperative period and may be missed entirely unless severe, because clinical symptoms are minimal and the laboratory determinations necessary to make the diagnosis may not be closely followed.

Renal Toxicity

The mechanism of nephrotoxicity due to methoxyflurane (Penthrane) is now clearly established. Non-oliguric renal failure, with high urine output poorly controlled by vasopressin, occurs with some frequency after prolonged anesthesia using this agent. Renal tubular damage directly caused by fluoride ion released from methoxyflurane metabolism is thought to be responsible. High serum fluoride levels can lead to oliguric renal failure after methoxyflurane exposure in susceptible patients, but this is fairly uncommon. Clinical serum fluoride levels as low as 30 μM./l. have been shown to produce renal functional deficits after anesthetic exposure; the duration and severity of renal dysfunction are clearly related to the dosage and duration of anesthesia with methoxyflurane.[117, 118]

Prolonged postoperative analgesia is seen in patients anesthetized with methoxyflurane, and it does not sensitize the myo-cardium to catecholamine effects, so it is quite compatible with epinephrine injected for hemostasis. Despite these definite clinical advantages, because of the liability of renal toxicity, methoxyflurane is seldom used in current clinical practice.

Fluoride ion is also released from the metabolism of enflurane, another halogenated volatile anesthetic. Peak fluoride levels after enflurane anesthesia are considerably lower and decline more rapidly than levels after methoxyflurane, possibly because enflurane is relatively less fat-soluble. In patients with normal preoperative renal function, no apparent damage is caused by the amount of fluoride ion released during enflurane anesthesia.[111] In patients with compromised renal function,[116] or who are taking enzyme-inducing drugs,[112] caution is advised with the administration of enflurane for long procedures. Pre-existing renal dysfunction may delay fluoride excretion, while the already damaged kidney may be more susceptible to fluoride-induced nephropathy as well. Increased metabolism of enflurane due to enzyme induction will also increase peak serum fluoride levels and make toxicity more likely. Enflurane is becoming widely used in anesthetic practice, and in many centers it has totally replaced halothane in daily use. In the particular circumstances mentioned above, however, its nephrotoxic potential should not be discounted or forgotten.

Hepatic Toxicity

Scattered sporadic reports of unexplained jaundice following halothane anesthesia began appearing shortly after the drug was first used clinically. Patients typically developed fever, right upper quadrant pain and tenderness, mild jaundice, eosinophilia, and elevated serum liver enzymes suggestive of hepatitis, several days into the postoperative period. Some patients progressed to massive hepatic necrosis and death. The National Halothane Study was organized to investigate the possible clinical relationship between halothane, postoperative jaundice, and massive hepatic necrosis.[108] The incidence of massive hepatic necrosis after halothane anesthesia was around 1 in 10,000, but 90 per cent of these were satisfactorily explained on the basis of severe hypoxia, shock, or trauma to the liver. Only around 1 in 100,000 cases involving halothane anesthesia was followed by massive hepatic necrosis, which would be compatible with the clinical picture described today as halothane hepatitis.

Originally, the occurrence of rashes, arthralgias, and eosinophilia in suspected cases suggested an allergic origin. The fact that most cases occurred after a repeated exposure to the drug suggested that sensitization could be a mechanism involved in the hepatotoxic reaction, and this appeared to be confirmed by reports of positive challenge tests with halothane in many "allergic" individuals. Numerous objections were raised, however, to the sensitization concept of halothane hepatitis. A small but consistent percentage of cases occurs in patients following their first exposure to the drug. Also, it was noted that halothane hepatitis almost never occurred in children, a group certainly not exempt from manifestations of allergy to other drugs. Finally, the observation was reported that post-halothane hepatitis appeared to be more common within 1 month of prior anesthesia, no matter what the agent for the first procedure had been.[120]

The mechanism is probably not allergic but is thought at this time to involve formation of toxic reductive metabolites of halothane in the liver, owing to shunting of halothane from the normal oxidative pathway to an abnormal reductive mechanism. There is probably a genetically determined susceptibility that explains the occurrence of the clinical syndrome after both single and multiple exposures. Liver biopsies and autopsy specimens demonstrate centrilobular necrosis indistinguishable from that due to infectious hepatitis or from that due to jaundice following exposure to various hepatotoxins.

Certain risk factors are clear after 20 years of clinical observation. Halothane hepatitis is most likely to occur in obese, middle-aged females following their second exposure to halothane. There is no clear evidence that a minimum time between repeated exposures to halothane will prevent hepatitic responses. While it has been claimed that 3 to 12 months should elapse between exposures to halothane, this is based on anecdotal rather than on broadly based statistical evidence. The diagnosis of halothane hepatitis remains one of *exclusion,* to be assigned only after hypoxia, trauma, transfusion, viral infection, and other hepatotoxins have been ruled out as causes of jaundice. It is significant that many devil's advocates who were long unwilling to accept halothane hepatitis as a clinical entity are now convinced by the weight of the evidence in its favor. The incidence is admittedly small, and the benefits of halothane in many clinical circumstances should not be lost because of the remote chance of hepatotoxicity. However, a massive shift from halothane to enflurane is occurring in clinical practice for this very reason. At this time enflurane does not appear to be significantly hepatotoxic, but a few scattered reports of hepatitis after its use have been published, and this should deserve watching in the next few years.

The only basis for prediction of potential hepatotoxicity in an individual patient is the previous occurrence of jaundice and enzyme elevations after exposure to halothane. This should be sufficient to contraindicate its use again in the same patient for any subsequent operation. The occurrence of fever, eosinophilia, or other various symptoms after anesthesia does not support a diagnosis of halothane hepatitis and should not be considered a contraindication to future use of the drug.

An animal model has recently been developed in which halothane exposure has been combined with a hypoxic reductive atmosphere to produce centrilobular necrosis. This may prove a useful investigative tool to help elucidate the role of reductive intermediates in this process.[119] Treatment at this time remains supportive and symptomatic, because no specific therapy for the clinical syndrome has been proposed.

Awareness Under Anesthesia

The lightly anesthetized but paralyzed patient may become transiently aware of intraoperative events and later, in the postoperative period, may remember bits of conversation, discomfort, or anxiety. Postanesthesia recall is particularly likely after cardiac surgery or trauma surgery when the individual patient will not tolerate deep anesthesia. Most commonly it is seen after caesarean section, when injected doses of intravenous agents are intentionally restricted to avoid drug-related depression of the newborn.

The incidence of awareness seems to be higher with the use of balanced nitrous oxide–narcotic anesthetic techniques than with the use of potent volatile anesthetics.[113] When fear of possible toxicity leads to avoidance of the volatile anesthetic agents, care must be taken to provide adequate doses of analgesic or amnesic supplements. The alcoholic or the chronic narcotic or sedative abuser will require increased amounts of intravenous agents to maintain adequate anesthesia and prevent recall. For the trauma patient or during cardiac surgery, incremental doses of scopolamine or diazepam will provide amnesia without causing significant physiologic side effects.

The parturient is a particularly difficult problem, because heavy intravenous supplements and a high concentration of nitrous oxide that may be harmful to the newborn cannot be given until after the umbilical cord is clamped. It has been a standard practice in some institutions to counsel patients prior to caesarean section under general anesthesia that there may be some awareness prior to delivery of the baby but that this is necessary for the safety of the newborn and that discomfort to the mother should be minimal. The effect of frank preoperative counselling in this situation should help prevent psychologic problems during recovery.

Awareness without recall is a frequently observed anesthetic phenomenon. Wrinkling of the brow, hand movements, tearing, and other purposeful movements are indications that anesthesia should be deepened to prevent unwanted physiologic stimulation and to block memory as well. Even with potent volatile anesthetic agents there may be some memory record of intraoperative events, especially if these involve serious threats to patient survival;[115] but studies purporting to demonstrate this have involved later recall of events elicited under hypnosis and have not been consistently reproduced during attempts to repeat these studies. Still, many anesthesiologists wisely refrain from flippant conversation or derogatory comments directed at patients under anesthesia, because of the possibility of later unconscious or conscious negative responses that may result.[113]

Patients who experience awareness under anesthesia later recall a feeling of helplessness and loss of control that can be overwhelming. They often report confusion about whether they should have been aware, or whether perhaps this represents a failure of effort or cooperation on their part. Patients are often reluctant to discuss their symptoms because of the fear they may be considered insane. A stereotyped postoperative traumatic neurosis often results, with anxiety, repetitive nightmares, and preoccupation with death as prominent features.[106] The link between this anxiety neurosis and intraoperative awareness is often not apparent to the patient; but a detailed discussion may allow this association to form, and the patient should then be able to settle those fears that may be quite threatening to him. Symptoms usually resolve after a careful explanation that the patient was indeed awake and that this is to be expected with the anesthetic technique employed. The reluctance of patients to discuss intraoperative awareness would suggest that it probably occurs more frequently than is recognized. A relaxed explanation helps prevent more prolonged psychological reactions, which should follow in less than 10 per cent of patients who exhibit symptoms of anxiety neurosis due to awareness.[114]

Operating Room Pollution by Trace Anesthetic Gases

Overflow of waste gases from anesthetic equipment may contaminate the operating room atmosphere to cause exposure of anesthesia, surgery, and nursing personnel to trace amounts of nitrous oxide and volatile anesthetic agents. This is reported to be associated with an increased spontaneous abortion rate in female operating room personnel, as well as a higher involuntary infertility rate in the same group. Birth defects are also increased in incidence in children of exposed anesthesia personnel, and cancer rates and hepatic disease may also be higher in this group. No specific cause for these effects has been determined, but the association with exposure to trace anesthesia gases in the operating rooms may well be the determining factor.[109]

Cognitive skills may also be affected by trace anesthetic gases. Reaction time and reasoning ability have been variably affected by trace amounts of halothane and nitrous oxide in several studies.[107, 110] Despite the conflicting results, these studies are also cited as evidence that control of trace anesthetic pollutants is necessary in the operating rooms. This can be achieved with scavenging devices that capture and evacuate overflow anesthetic gases to lower the concentration of trace gases to 10 per cent of the unscavenged level. A dose effect has not been demonstrated, however, with the effects of these trace gases, and it remains to be proven that these scavenging devices decrease the incidence of complications of anesthetic pollution of the operating rooms as described above.

Owing to the compelling evidence that operating room pollution is harmful, the Occupational Safety and Health Administration has set standards for maximum levels of nitrous oxide (25 ppm.) and halothane (0.5 ppm.) that are acceptable in the surgical suite. These levels as designated can be maintained only with low total gas flows combined with excellent scavenging devices. These regulations do not have the power of law and are only recommendations at this time. It is probably wise, however, to check the operating rooms for the concentrations of anesthetic agents in the air during surgery, and attempts to scavenge overflow gases and minimize exposure to all personnel would seem warranted by the evidence currently available.

Bibliography

PREOPERATIVE PERIOD

1. Beecher, H. K., and Todd, D. P.: A study of deaths associated with anesthesia and surgery based on a study of 599,548 anesthetics in ten institutions. Ann. Surg. 240:2, 1954.
2. Benumof, J. L.: Anesthesia for thoracic surgery. American Society of Anesthesiologists Annual Refresher Course Lectures, Lecture 209, 1980.
3. Brodsky, J. G., and Bravo, J. J.: Acute postoperative clonidine withdrawal syndrome. Anesthesiology 44:519, 1976.
4. Caldwell, T. B.: Environmental and behavioral disorders. In Katz, J., and Kadis, L. B. (Eds.): Anesthesia and Uncommon Diseases. Philadelphia, W. B. Saunders Company, 1973, pp. 487–531.
5. Chodoff, P., Margand, P. M., and Knowles, C. L.: Short term abstinence from smoking: Its place in preoperative preparation. Crit. Care Med. 3:131, 1975.
6. Cooper, J. B., Newbower, R. S., Long, C. D., and McPeek, B.: Preventable anesthesia mishaps: A study of human factors. Anesthesiology 49:399, 1978.
7. Cooperman, M., Pflug, B., Martin, E. W., and Evans, W. E.: Cardiovascular risk factors in patients with peripheral vascular disease. Surgery 84:505, 1978.
8. Cousins, M. J., Greenstein, L. R., Hitt, B. A., and Mazze, R. I.: Metabolism and renal effects of enflurane in man. Anesthesiology 44:44, 1976.
9. Cullen, B. F., and Miller, M. G.: Drug interactions and anesthesia: A review. Anesth. Analg. 58:413, 1979.
10. Dornette, W. H. L.: Informed consent and anesthesia. Anesth. Analg. 53:832, 1974.
11. Dykes, M. H. M.: Unexplained postoperative fever: Its value as a sign of halothane sensitization. J.A.M.A. 216:641, 1971.
12. Goldman, L., and Caldera, D. L.: Risks of general anesthesia and elective operation in the hypertensive patient. Anesthesiology 50:285, 1979.
13. Goldman, L., Caldera, D. L., Nussbaum, S. R., Southwick, F. S., Krogstad, D., Murray, B., Burke, D. S., O'Malley, T. A., Goroll, A. H., Caplan, C. H., Nolan, J., Carabello, B., and Slater, E. E.: Multifactorial index of cardiac risk in noncardiac surgical procedures. N. Engl. J. Med. 297:845, 1977.
14. Kohler, H.: A rational approach to dosage and preparation of parenteral glucocorticoid substitution therapy during surgical procedures. Acta Anaesthesiol. Scand. 19:260, 1975.
15. Loarie, D. J., Wilkinson, P., Tyberg, J., and White, A.: The hemodynamic effects of halothane in anemic dogs. Anesth. Analg. 58:195, 1979.
16. Marx, G. F., Mateo, C. V., and Orkin, L. R.: Computer analysis of postanesthetic deaths. Anesthesiology 39:54, 1973.
17. Miller, W. F., Wu, N., and Johnson, R. L., Jr.: Convenient method of evaluating pulmonary ventilatory function with a single breath test. Anesthesiology 17:480, 1956.
18. Muravchick, S.: Preoperative pharmacology and anesthetic risk. Int. Anesth. Clin. 18:11, 1980.
19. National Academy of Sciences — National Research Council Committee on Anesthesia: Special Report: The role of methoxyflurane in the production of renal dysfunction. Anesthesiology 34:505, 1971.
20. National Academy of Sciences — National Research Council Committee on Anesthesia: Summary of the national halothane study. J.A.M.A. 197:775, 1966.

21. Otto, C. W.: Respiratory morbidity and mortality. Int. Anesth. Clin. *18*:85, 1980.

22. Owens, W. D., Felts, J. A., and Spitznagel, E. L., Jr.: ASA physical status classifications: A study of consistency of ratings. Anesthesiology *49*:239, 1978.

23. Owens, W. D., and Spitznagel, E. L.: Anesthetic side effects and complications, an overview. Int. Anesth. Clin. *18*:1, 1980.

24. Pender, J. W., Fox, M., and Basso, L. V.: Diseases of the endocrine system. *In* Katz, J., and Kadis, L. B. (Eds.): Anesthesia and Uncommon Diseases. Philadelphia, W. B. Saunders Company, 1973, p. 104–144.

25. Prys-Roberts, C.: Hypertension and anesthesia — Fifty years on. Anesthesiology *50*:281, 1979.

26. Raj, P. P., Forestner, J. E., Watson, T. D., and Miller, R. D.: Technics for fiberoptic laryngoscopy in anesthesia. Anesth. Analg. *53*:708, 1974.

27. Salem, M. R., Bennett, E. J., Schweiss, J. F., Baraka, A., Dalal, F. Y., and Collins, V. J.: Cardiac arrest related to anesthesia, contributing factors in infants and children. J.A.M.A. *233*:238, 1975.

28. Schwartz, A. J., and Wollman, H.: Anesthetic considerations for patients on chronic drug therapy: L-DOPA, monoamine oxidase inhibitors, tricyclic antidepressants, and propranolol. A.S.A. Refresher Courses in Anesthesiology *4*:99, 1976.

29. Shapiro, B. A., Harrison, R. A., and Trout, C. A.: Clinical Application of Respiratory Care. 2nd Ed. Chicago, Year Book Medical Publishers, 1979, p. 463.

30. Steen, P. A., Tinker, J. H., and Tarhan, S.: Myocardial reinfarction after anesthesia and surgery. J.A.M.A. *239*:2566, 1978.

31. Stein, M., and Cassara, E. L.: Preoperative pulmonary evaluation and therapy for surgery patients. J.A.M.A. *211*:787, 1970.

32. Stirt, J. A., Marco, A., and Conklin, K. A.: Obstetric anesthesia for a quadriplegic patient with autonomic hyperreflexia. Anesthesiology *51*:560, 1979.

33. Taylor, G., Larson, C. P., Jr., and Prestwich, R.: Unexpected cardiac arrest during anesthesia and surgery — An environmental study. J.A.M.A. *236*:2758, 1976.

34. Thoren, L.: Postoperative pulmonary complications. Observations on their prevention by means of physiotherapy. Acta Chir. Scand. *107*:193, 1954.

35. Vandam, L. D., and Moore, F. D.: Adrenocortical mechanisms related to anesthesia. Anesthesiology *21*:531, 1960.

OPERATIVE PERIOD

36. Adams, R. W., Gronert, G. A., Sundt, T. M., and Michenfelder, J. D.: Halothane, hypocapnia and cerebrospinal fluid pressure in neurosurgery. Anesthesiology *37*:510, 1972.

37. Aronow, S., and Bruner, J. M. R.: Electrosurgery. Anesthesiology *42*:525, 1975.

38. Askrog, V. F., Pender, J. W., and Eckenhoff, J. E.: Changes in physiological dead space during deliberate hypotension. Anesthesiology *25*:744, 1964.

39. Bedford, R. F.: Long-term radial artery cannulation: Effects on subsequent vessel function. Crit. Care Med. *6*:64, 1978.

40. Bernstein, R. L.: Anesthesia for total hip replacement. *In* Zauder, H. L. (Ed.): Anesthesia for Orthopedic Surgery. Philadelphia, F. A. Davis, 1980, pp. 67–88.

41. Blitt, C. D., Wright, W. A., Petty, W. C., and Webster, T. A.: Central venous cannulation via the external jugular vein — A technique employing the j-wire. J.A.M.A. *229*:817, 1974.

42. Britt, B. A.: Malignant hyperthermia. Int. Anesth. Clin. *17*:VII, 1979.

43. Bromage, P. R.: Epidural Anesthesia. Philadelphia, W. B. Saunders Company, 1978, pp. 215–257 and 654–715.

44. Brown, B. R.: Anesthesia for pheochromocytoma. *In* Brown, B. R. (Ed.): Anesthesia and the Patient with Endocrine Disease. Philadelphia, F. A. Davis, 1980.

45. Buckspan, G. S., Franklin, J. D., Novak, G. R., Bennett, B. D., Lynch, J. B., and Dean, R. H.: Intraarterial drug injury: Studies of etiology and potential treatment. J. Surg. Res. *24*:294, 1978.

46. Burrington, J. D., and Smith, M. D.: Elective and emergency surgery in children with sickle cell disease. Surg. Clin. North Am. *54*:55, 1976.

47. Conner, J. T., Miller, J. D., and Katz, R. L.: Isoflurane anesthesia for pheochromocytoma: A case report. Anesth. Analg. *54*:419, 1975.

48. Cottrell, J. E., Casthely, P., Brodie, J., Patel, K., Klein, A., and Turndorf, H.: Prevention of nitroprusside-induced cyanide toxicity with hydroxycobalamin. N. Engl. J. Med. *298*:809, 1978.

49. Cottrell, J. E., and Turndorf, H.: Anesthesia and Neurosurgery. St. Louis, C. V. Mosby, 1980.

50. Covino, B. G.: Local anesthesia. N. Engl. J. Med. *286*:975, 1972.

51. de Jong, R. H.: Local Anesthetics. 2nd Ed. Springfield, Ill., Charles C Thomas, 1977, pp. 272–275.

52. de Jong, R. H., and Heavner, J. E.: Local anesthetic seizure prevention: Diazepam versus pentobarbital. Anesthesiology *36*:449, 1972.

53. Deutsch, S.: Effects of anesthetics on the kidney. Surg. Clin. North Am. *55*:775, 1975.

54. DiGiovanni, A. J., and Dunbar, B. S.: Epidural injections of autologous blood for postlumbar-puncture headache. Anesth. Analg. *49*:268, 1970.

55. Dorsch, J. A., and Dorsch, S. E.: Understanding Anesthesia Equipment: Construction, Care, and Complications. Baltimore, Williams and Wilkins, 1975.

56. Edwards, M. W., and Flemming, D. C.: Deliberate hypotension. Surg. Clin. North Am. *55*:947, 1975.

57. Eisele, J. H., and Smith, N. T.: Cardiovascular effects of 40% nitrous oxide in man. Anesth. Analg. *51*:956, 1972.

58. Finucane, B. T., McClain, D. A., and Smith, S.

R.: A double-blind comparison of etidocaine and lidocaine for IV regional anesthesia. Regional Anesth. *5*:17, 1980.

59. Fischer, J., Lundstrom, J., and Ottander, H. G.: Central venous cannulation: A radiological determination of catheter positions and immediate intrathoracic complications. Acta Anaesthesiol. Scand. *21*:45, 1977.

60. Galindo, A., Wyte, S. R., and Wetherhold, J. W.: Junctional rhythm induced by halothane anesthesia — Treatment with succinylcholine. Anesthesiology *37*:261, 1972.

61. Gallagher, T. J.: Monitoring. Int. Anesth. Clin. *18*:25, 1980.

62. Green, M., Hall, R. J. C., Huntsman, R. G., Lawson, A., Pearson, T. C., and Wheeler, P. C. G.: Sickle cell crisis treated by exchange transfusion. J.A.M.A. *231*:948, 1975.

63. Gronert, G. A.: Malignant hyperthermia. Anesthesiology *53*:395, 1980.

64. Hedley-Whyte, J., Burgess, G. E., III, Feely, T. W., and Miller, M. G.: Applied Physiology of Respiratory Care. Boston, Little, Brown and Company, 1976.

65. Herbst, C. A.: Indications, management, and complications of percutaneous subclavian catheters: An audit. Arch. Surg. *113*:1421, 1978.

66. Hoar, P. F., Stone, J. G., Wicks, A. E., Edie, R. N., and Scholes, J. V.: Thrombogenesis associated with Swan-Ganz catheters. Anesthesiology *48*:445, 1978.

67. Hug, C. F., Jr.: Pharmacology — Anesthetic drugs. In Kaplan, J. A. (Ed.): Cardiac Anesthesia. New York, Grune and Stratton, 1979, p. 9.

68. Jedeikin, R. J., and Hoffman, S.: The oculocardiac reflex in eye-surgery anesthesia. Anesth. Analg. *56*:333, 1977.

69. Johnston, R. R., Eger, E. I., and Wilson, C.: A comparative interaction of epinephrine with enflurane, isoflurane, and halothane in man. Anesth. Analg. *55*:709, 1976.

70. Kaplan, J. A. (Ed.): Cardiac Anesthesia. New York, Grune and Stratton, 1979.

71. Kaplan, J. A., and King, S. B.: The precordial electrocardiographic lead (V_5) in patients who have coronary artery disease. Anesthesiology *45*:570, 1976.

72. Katz, R. L., and Katz, G. J.: Surgical infiltration of pressor drugs and their interaction with volatile anesthetics. Br. J. Anaesth. *38*:712, 1966.

73. Knill, R. L., and Evans, D.: Pathogenesis of gangrene following intraarterial injection of drugs: A new hypothesis. Canad. Anaesth. Soc. J. *22*:637, 1975.

74. Kreul, J. F., Dauchot, P. J., and Anton, A. H.: Hemodynamic and catecholamine studies during pheochromocytoma resection under enflurane anesthesia. Anesthesiology *44*:265, 1976.

75. Maekawa, T., Sakabe, T., and Takeshita, H.: Diazepam blocks cerebral metabolic and circulatory responses to local anesthetic-induced seizures. Anesthesiology *41*:389, 1974.

76. Mandel, M. A., and Dauchot, P. J.: Radial arte-ry cannulation in 1000 patients: Precautions and complications. J. Hand Surg. *2*:482, 1977.

77. Martin, J. T.: Positioning in Anesthesia and Surgery. Philadelphia, W. B. Saunders, 1978.

78. Michenfelder, J. D., and Cucchiara, R. F.: Canine cerebral oxygen consumption during enflurane anesthesia and its modification during induced seizures. Anesthesiology *40*:757, 1974.

79. Moore, D. C.: Anterior (Paratracheal) Approach for Block of the Stellate Ganglion in Regional Block. 4th Ed. Springfield, Ill., Charles C Thomas. 1965, pp. 123–137.

80. Moss, E., and McDowall, D. G.: Monitoring of intracranial pressure. Int. Anes. Clin. *17*:375, 1979.

81. Nicholson, M. J., and McAlpine, F. S.: Neural injuries associated with surgical positions and operations. In Martin, J. T. (Ed.): Positioning in Anesthesia and Surgery. Philadelphia, W. B. Saunders, 1978, pp. 193–224.

82. Noble, A. B., and Murray, J. G.: A review of the complications of spinal anesthesia with experiences in Canadian teaching hospitals. Canad. Anaesth. Soc. *18*:5, 1971.

83. Pace, N. L.: A critique of flow-directed pulmonary arterial catheterization. Anesthesiology *47*:455, 1977.

84. Phillips, O. C., Ebner, H., Nelson, A. G., and Black, M. H.: Neurologic complications following spinal anesthesia with lidocaine: A prospective review of 10,440 cases. Anesthesiology *30*:284, 1969.

85. Price, H. L.: Calcium reverses myocardial depression by halothane. Anesthesiology *41*:576, 1974.

86. Raj, P. P., Forestner, J. E., Watson, T. D., Miller, R., and Jenkins, M. T.: Technics for fiberoptic laryngoscopy in anesthesia. Anesth. Analg. *53*:708, 1974.

87. Relton, J. E. S.: Anesthesia for elective surgery in patients susceptible to malignant hyperthermia. Int. Anesth. Clin. *17*:141, 1979.

88. Shapiro, H. M., Galindo, A., Wyte, S. R., et al.: Rapid intraoperative reduction of intracranial pressure with thiopentone. Br. J. Anaesth. *44*:506, 1972.

89. Shnider, S. M. (Ed.): Obstetrical Anesthesia. 2nd Ed. Baltimore, Williams and Wilkins Co., 1979.

90. Sizemore, G. W., and Winternitz, W. W.: Autonomic hyper-reflexia — Suppression with alpha-adrenergic blocking agents. N. Engl. J. Med. *282*:795, 1970.

91. Smith, R. M.: Anesthesia for Infants and Children. 4th Ed. St. Louis, C. V. Mosby, 1980.

92. Stewardson, R. H., and Nyhus, L. M.: Pulmonary aspiration: An update. Arch. Surg. *112*:1192, 1977.

93. Taylor, C., Wilson, F. M., Roesch, R., and Stoelting, V. K.: Prevention of the oculocardiac reflex in children, comparison of retrobulbar block and intravenous atropine. Anesthesiology *24*:646, 1963.

94. Thompson, G. E., Miller, R. D., Stevens, W. C., and Murray, W. R.: Hypotensive anesthesia

for total hip arthroplasty: A study of blood loss and organ function (brain, heart, liver and kidney). Anesthesiology *48*:91, 1978.

95. Thomson, I. R., Dalton, B. C., Lappas, D. G., and Lowenstein, E. L.: Right bundle-branch block and complete heart block caused by the Swan-Ganz catheter. Anesthesiology *51*:359, 1979.

96. Tinker, J. H., and Michenfelder, J. D.: Sodium nitroprusside, pharmacology, toxicology, and therapeutics. Anesthesiology *45*:340, 1976.

97. Tonneson, A. S.: Acute renal failure. Int. Anesth. Clin. *18*:107, 1980.

98. Tucker, G. T., Moore, D. C., Bridenbaugh, P. O., Bridenbaugh, L. D., and Thompson, G. E.: Systemic absorption of mepivacaine in commonly used regional block procedures. Anesthesiology *37*:277, 1972.

99. Waller, J. L., Zaidan, J. R., Kaplan, J. A., and Bauman, D. I.: Hemodynamic effects of vascular cannulation by residents. Anesthesiology *53*:S114, 1980.

100. Walts, L. F.: Complications of muscle relaxants. *In* Katz, R. L. (Ed.): Muscle Relaxants. New York, American Elsevier Publishing Co., 1975, pp. 209–244.

101. Wilson, R. D., Richey, J. V., Forestner, J. E., Hendrickson, M., Heriin, T. J., Norman, P. F., and Nigliazzo, A.: Cardiovascular effects of ketamine infusion. In Aldrete, J. A., and Stanley, T. H. (Eds.): Trends in Intravenous Anesthesia. Chicago, Year Book Medical Publishers, 1980, pp. 343–353.

102. Winnie, A. P.: Regional anesthesia. Surg. Clin. North Am. *54*:861, 1975.

103. Wynne, J. W., DeMarcok, F. J., and Hood, C. I.: Physiological effects of corticosteroids in foodstuff aspiration. Arch. Surg. *116*:46, 1981.

104. Youngberg, J. A., and Miller, E. D.: Evaluation of percutaneous cannulations of the dorsalis pedis artery. Anesthesiology *44*:80, 1976.

POSTOPERATIVE PERIOD

105. Ali, J., Weisel, R. D., Layug, A. B., et al.: Consequences of postoperative alterations in respiratory mechanics. Am. J. Surg. *128*:376, 1974.

106. Blacher, R. W.: On awakening paralyzed during surgery: A syndrome of traumatic neurosis. J.A.M.A. *234*:67, 1975.

107. Bruce, D. L., Bach, M. J., and Arbit, J.: Trace anesthesic effects on perceptual, cognitive and motor skills. Anesthesiology *40*:453, 1974.

108. Bunker, J. P., Forest, W. H., Jr., Mostell, F., et al. (Eds.): The National Halothane Study. A study of the possible association between halothane anesthesia and postoperative hepatic necrosis. National Institute of General Medical Sciences, Bethesda, Maryland, 1965.

109. Cohen, E. N., Brown, B. W., Bruce, D. I., et al.: Occupational disease among operating room personnel — A national study. Anesthesiology *41*:321, 1974.

110. Cook, T. L., Smith, M., Starkweather, J. A., Winter, P. M., and Eger, E. I.: Behavioral effects of trace and subanesthetic halothane and nitrous oxide in man. Anesthesiology *49*:419, 1978.

111. Cousins, M. J., Greenstein, L. R., Hitt, B. A., and Mazze, R. I.: Metabolism and renal effects of enflurane in man. Anesthesiology *44*:44, 1976.

112. Eichhorn, J. H., Hedley-Whyte, J., Steinman, T. I., Kaugmann, J. M., and Lassberg, L. H.: Renal failure following enflurane anesthesia. Anesthesiology *45*:557, 1976.

113. Eisele, V., Weinreich, A., and Bartle, S.: Perioperative awareness and recall. Anesth. Analg. *55*:513, 1976.

114. Guerra, F.: Awareness under general anesthesia. Guerra, F., and Aldrete, J. A. (Eds.): Emotional and Psychological Responses to Anesthesia and Surgery. New York, Grune and Stratton, 1980, pp. 1–8.

115. Levinson, B. W.: States of awareness during general anesthesia. Br. J. Anaesth. *37*:544, 1965.

116. Loehning, R. W., and Mazze, R. I.: Possible nephrotoxicity from enflurane in a patient with severe renal disease. Anesthesiology *40*:203, 1974.

117. Mazze, R. I., Calverley, R. K., and Smith, N. T.: Inorganic fluoride nephrotoxicity: Prolonged enflurane and halothane anesthesia in volunteers. Anesthesiology *46*:265, 1977.

118. Robertson, G. S., and Hamilton, W. F. D.: Changes in urine osmolality and urine fluoride concentrations following methoxyflurane anesthesia. Br. J. Anaesth. *46*:153, 1974.

119. Sipes, I. G., and Brown, B. R., Jr.: An animal model of hepatotoxicity associated with halothane anesthesia. Anesthesiology *45*:622, 1976.

120. Strunin, L., and Simpson, B. R.: Halothane in Britain today. Br. J. Anaesth. *44*:919, 1972.

11

MISCELLANEOUS COMPLICATIONS IN THE PREOPERATIVE AND POSTOPERATIVE PERIODS

C. Thomas Fitts
and John H. Davis

COMPLICATIONS OF TRACHEOSTOMY

The indications for tracheostomy have changed with the steady progression of knowledge concerning respiratory support in critically ill patients. The placement of an endotracheal tube by nasal or oral route is utilized as the preliminary emergency step in most airway problems excepting complete mechanical obstruction at or above the larynx. Accordingly the majority of tracheostomies are now done in the operating room electively in a patient who is well oxygenated with an anesthetist assuring continued oxygenation through a previously placed endotracheal tube. Good lighting, adequate instruments, and expert assistants then provide the remainder of the setting for a tracheostomy placed at the precise level one desires, with excellent hemostasis and a minimal liability of damage to adjacent structures. In a series of 378 consecutive unselected tracheostomies performed at the Medical University of South Carolina hospitals from 1962 through 1967, no early complications followed in 82 per cent, and no mortality was incurred in the operating room. Balancing this apparent success with the operative procedure, however, are recent reports from a number of clinics documenting an increase in the late complication of tracheal stenosis.

Charles Thomas Fitts was born in Tennessee and graduated from Princeton University and the University of Pennsylvania School of Medicine. Following his residency training at the University of Mississippi and important research experience at the Brooke Army Medical Center, he joined the surgical faculty at the Medical University of South Carolina where he is now Professor of Surgery. Dr. Fitts is broadly educated in the fields of general surgery, trauma, and transplantation immunology.

John Herschel Davis was born in Pennsylvania and received his medical training at Western Reserve University. His surgical education was acquired at the University Hospitals of Cleveland. An interest in research began when he was a medical student with Dr. William Holden and was continued at the United States Army Surgical Research Unit at the Brooke Army Medical Center, where he spent 3 years. He was a member of the United States Army Surgical Research Team in Korea, where he gained a broad experience in surgical physiology and trauma. After his military service he returned to the full-time staff of the University Hospitals in Cleveland, where he has been highly respected by the students as an inspiring and imaginative teacher. He is at present Professor of Surgery and Chairman of the Department, University of Vermont College of Medicine, and Surgeon-in-Chief of the Medical Center Hospital of Vermont.

OPERATIVE COMPLICATIONS

It is axiomatic that prevention of the complications that occur during or following tracheostomy is much more desirable and effective than their management. Those factors that will limit the occurrence of complications are the same for this operation as for any other. Good facilities and help ensure adequate hemostasis and exposure, which are absolutely necessary for accurate placement of the tracheostoma in the second or third cartilaginous ring. Placement more superiorly invites laryngeal stenosis, and placement more inferiorly makes exposure needlessly more difficult. (It should be noted here that in a large published series, cricothyroidostomy has been shown to be safe and practical. Certainly when the surgeon is familiar with the technique it has definite merit as an approach for true emergency situations.) Low placement increases the risk of the cannula entering the right or left mainstem bronchus or riding the carina, with constant irritation and spasmodic cough. In children especially, it also contributes to ease of dislodgment of the cannula. Neither the type of skin incision (vertical or transverse) nor the type of tracheal incision (oval window, rectangular window, flap, or vertical cut through two rings) would appear to contribute to complications as long as they are at the proper level. The size of the tracheostoma, however, should be such as to snugly accept the selected cannula. Too small an opening can result in frustrated forceful attempts to insert the cannula. On the other hand, too large an opening not only can contribute to delayed closure but allows an easy route for blood in the wound to reach the tracheal lumen. It is unfortunately not unusual for a small bleeder to make itself evident for the first time as a result of the coughing and straining induced by placement of the cannula. This is easily taken care of if the tube fits snugly in the stoma but can become difficult to manage if the blood is draining into the trachea with the resultant aspiration and paroxysms of coughing interfering with control of the bleeder. If this situation occurs and the cannula has a balloon cuff, the cuff should be inflated immediately to prevent additional blood from entering the distal pulmonary tree; then the bleeder can be methodically dealt with. If the cannula has no cuff, the best recourse is probably a small tonsil-tip suction used to give enough visualization temporarily while the corners of a Raytex sponge are tucked into the gap between the cannula and the overlarge stoma. After bleeding is controlled the sponge can be removed and a better-fitting tube selected. It is generally unwise to attempt to remove the cannula and replace it with either a larger or cuffed version until the bleeding is controlled. [In performing tracheostomy over an endotracheal tube, the endotracheal tube should never be withdrawn completely until the tracheostomy tube is securely in place below it. Ed.]

Esophageal Injury

Injury to the esophagus is not common but does occur, the incidence being higher in infants and children. In adults it probably occurs most commonly when the surgeon strays from the midline in an obese patient and places the tracheostoma too low, where the trachea angles sharply posteriorly. In this situation the surgeon may be deprived of the ability to palpate the trachea and accordingly may proceed too deeply. Here the esophagus can be injured by dissection in the medial border of the wound as the frustrated operator hunts for the bypassed trachea. The appearance of tiny mucoid bubbles in the wound is cause for alarm. A discovered injury should be repaired with two layers of fine interrupted nonabsorbable suture, and a small Penrose drain should be brought out from the site of injury through a stab wound laterally in the neck. Whenever the operator discovers that he has been dissecting posterior to the trachea, he should satisfy himself that the esophagus has not been injured even if he has not seen the telltale small mucoid bubbles. In children and infants the esophagus may also be injured at the time the trachea is incised to produce the tracheostoma. In infants especially, the trachea is so small and relatively elastic that pressure necessary to cut the anterior tracheal wall may depress the anterior wall onto the posterior such that completion of the stroke incises right through both walls and into the esophagus. To avoid injury, it is helpful to use a small sharp tracheal hook or even a simple suture to catch and fix the anterior wall, exerting mild outward traction to keep the anterior and posterior walls separated as the tracheostoma is made. An injury to the esophagus produced in this fashion is very difficult to identify and close, since the area has not been exposed. Therefore, it is probably wisest in this situation to treat the problem conservatively by simply giving the patient nothing by the mouth for several days postoperatively and administering antibiotics.

Injury to Blood Vessels

Injury to the carotid artery or jugular vein is also rare, but does occur. Again, it is almost impossible to produce this injury in the patient with normal anatomy unless the surgeon has strayed from the midline. Repairs should be made in the usual fashion, but in addition a careful attempt should be made to suture normal tissue over the repair in such a manner as to minimize the chances of tracheal secretions bathing the repair when the trachea is opened.

Subcutaneous and Mediastinal Emphysema

Subcutaneous and mediastinal emphysema may occur as a result of either inadvertent laceration of the pleural domes (more likely in children) or excessively tight closure of the skin allowing negative intrathoracic pressure to suck air into the wound with the flaplike action of the skin impeding egress. Whenever subcutaneous or mediastinal emphysema develops, the wound should be opened and covered loosely with Vaseline gauze, and a chest x-ray should be obtained. Significant pneumothorax is handled by the insertion of a chest tube attached to water-seal drainage.

Aspiration

Aspiration during tracheostomy can be lethal. The most common source is blood. It is absolutely foolhardy to open the trachea in a wound in which hemostasis is not good. At the first indrawn gasp blood is aspirated, paroxysms of coughing follow, and increased pressure in the neck veins, increased bleeding, loss of all visualization, cyanosis, and catastrophe may result. If an endotracheal tube is in place as it should be, the situation can be rescued by advancing the tube past the opening in the trachea and reinflating the balloon. This will stop further aspiration, and tracheal toilet can be carried out through the endotracheal tube and the bleeding can be dealt with. In the absence of a previously placed endotracheal tube it may be possible to retrieve the situation by using the sense of touch to occlude the opening in the trachea with a finger tip, to prevent further blood from entering and to allow the patient to cough out the remainder. Patients have also aspirated the piece of cartilage removed or other small objects in the field such as needles.

Selection of Cannula

Selection of a properly fitting tracheostomy tube is important. Some of the complications that occur from a tube too small or too large in diameter have already been discussed. Too short a tube is liable to dislodgment. A tube that is too long may impinge on the carina or actually enter one mainstem bronchus, thereby effectively occluding the other. The surgeon should always assure himself that this has not occurred before leaving the operating room. A tube with the wrong angle may abut on the tracheal wall and cause pressure necrosis with disastrous late complications to be discussed later, such as perforation of the trachea and/or erosion into a major vessel. A lateral film of the neck will usually reveal such threatening malpositions.

The balloon should be tested prior to insertion to be certain it has no leak and does not inflate eccentrically. Such eccentric inflation has been known to extend over the end of the tube and obstruct it. The balloon should be firmly cemented or fixed to the tube to prevent it from slipping partially or completely off the cannula with resultant tracheal obstruction.

In summary, it would seem appropriate to stress that most operative complications can be avoided or conveniently handled if the surgeon does the tracheostomy in the operating room over an endotracheal tube, is compulsive about staying in the patient's midline, does not open the trachea until hemostasis is secure, and chooses the cannula with care.

POSTOPERATIVE COMPLICATIONS

Infection

The most common postoperative complication listed in practically every collected series is infection. This can occur as a local wound infection with or without extension to the spaces of the neck and the mediastinum, as a purulent tracheobronchitis, or as pneumonia. The tracheostomy wound itself is probably contaminated in all cases, and therefore it is a standard and wise procedure to leave the wound open or at most place one skin suture at each end. The general success of this maneuver in the prevention of invasive wound infection is no excuse, however, for the frequent abandonment of even minimal further wound care. The gauze sponge in the wound and surrounding the stem of the tube should be carefully changed and replaced with a clean one as often as needed, and at least daily. In the presence of obvious purulent soaking of this dressing, saline-soaked gauze should be utilized and changed at least four times daily or more if necessary. This latter technique of frequent wet dressing changes will handle almost any local infection, unless of course the wound has been closed with sutures. These will have to be removed to initiate treatment of the infection, which they have practically guaranteed by their presence in the first place. Local infection can infiltrate along the fascial planes of the neck and result in mediastinitis. This very rarely occurs in a wound that has been left open and managed in the fashion described. The diagnosis of mediastinitis is suspected when a rise in temperature, pulse rate, and white blood cell count follows tracheotomy. The patient complains of substernal, epigastric, or shoulder pain, and if the pain persists and is increased by deep inspiration the diagnosis is relatively certain. Subcutaneous emphysema, tenderness, induration, and fullness in the lower neck region may be present but are not necessary to confirm the diagnosis. Roentgenograms may reveal widening of the mediastinum or anterior displacement of the trachea.

If the diagnosis of mediastinitis is made the wound should immediately be opened and cultured if this has not been done. Systemic antibiotic administration should be started on the basis of previous culture information if available, or simply broad spectrum coverage until such information is at hand. If the patient does not respond within 24 to 48 hours, one should suspect an undrained abscess in the mediastinum and consider formal surgical drainage under anesthesia.

Tracheobronchitis and pneumonia should be considered stages in a continuum that proceeds from initial colonization of the tracheal secretions with a pathogen to invasion of the tracheobronchial tree by that pathogen and thence to invasion of the pulmonary parenchyma with the production of pneumonia. A moderate amount of information has become available concerning this problem in recent years. At the present time the evidence is incontrovertible that in 80 to 90 per cent of patients who have tracheal intubation for 4 days or longer a pathogen will appear in the tracheal aspirate. Furthermore, in widely separated studies it has been consistently shown that gram-negative pathogens will predominate and that among these Pseudomonas will be most common, followed by Klebsiella and Proteus. These same organisms are also the most common offenders found when purulent tracheobronchitis or frank pneumonia develops. These organisms are almost always found in intensive care units in the connections, fittings, and tubes of respirators or other equipment if they are sought for. Accordingly, every effort should be made to insist on a routine that includes daily takedown, cleansing, and sterilization of respirators and the use of a separate new sterile suction catheter each time the patient's trachea is suctioned, together with the use of sterile gloves during the procedure. The problem has not been eliminated, however, even in units in which these and even more stringent measures are insisted on. It is the consensus of those physicians who have studied the problem that prophylactic antibiotic coverage is not helpful. Most of the safe broad spectrum antibiotics do not include the common offenders in their spectrum. Those antibiotics that do include them are slightly more toxic and carry the hazard of simply replacing one pathogen with another or a resistant form of the original. Therefore, at the present time the best advice would seem to be no antibiotic treatment for simple colonization without purulent tracheal secretions (tracheobronchitis) or radiologic evidence of pulmonary infiltrate (pneumonia). Specific antibiotic treatment should certainly be instituted if pneumonia is diagnosed. There does not seem to be good agreement on antibiotic therapy for tracheobronchitis without pneumonia — that is, a positive pathogen culture, purulent tracheobronchial secretions, and no evidence of pneumonia. Usually they are used in this situation and every effort is made to remove the tracheal cannula at the earliest conceivable time. The use of Pseudomonas immunization in high-risk populations should be advantageous in theory but has been found to be of no significant benefit in practice.

As a general measure, humidification of the air provided to a tracheostoma is essential to keep ciliary action intact and prevent crusting which can act as a foreign body or obstruction. Failure to provide this is an obvious invitation to infection. Tracheal suction is absolutely necessary but should be done gently with soft catheters; otherwise, trauma to the tracheobronchial mucosa invites local invasion by any pathogen present.

Obstruction

Obstruction can occur any time during the postoperative period. When it occurs in a patient with a tracheostomy tube in place the first maneuver is to suction the trachea. If this does not relieve the problem by aspirating a mucous or blood plug, or if the catheter meets an obstruction, then the balloon should be immediately deflated since it may have acted as the obstructing agent by prolapsing over the end of the tube, or it may even have slipped off entirely. If the obstruction still has not been relieved, then it is likely that either the cannula is out of the trachea or is obstructed by a tenaciously adherent inspissated plug. In either case prompt removal of the cannula with the neck hyperextended may be lifesaving.

Every patient with a tracheostomy should have a duplicate cannula complete with obturator at the bedside. Tracheostomy tubes can usually be changed with no difficulty 48 hours or later after placement, as a fairly well defined tract is present that tends to stay open, especially with the neck hyperextended. Some surgeons routinely place sutures in the edge of the stoma and leave them coming out of the wound so that the stoma can always be brought up into view if necessary when changing the tube. Another useful trick to avoid difficulty in routine changing of tubes is to place a catheter through the cannula into the trachea, remove the cannula over the catheter, leaving the catheter in the trachea, and utilizing it as a guide over which to place the new cannula.

Tracheoarterial Fistula

A dramatic and often fatal postoperative complication is tracheoarterial fistula. The great majority of such cases are due to direct erosion of the tracheostomy tube through the anterolateral tracheal wall and into the innominate artery. Other vessels reported to have been involved in such fistula formation on very rare occasions are the common carotid artery, inferior and superior thyroid arteries, and the right innominate vein. Fortunately this complication is rare. There is some evidence in the literature to support the contention that it is more likely to occur in patients with certain types of head injury in which hyperirritability and decerebrate posturing cause relentlessly repeated trauma to the same small area where the cannula tip impinges on the wall. Two important warning signs should alert one to the imminent likelihood of this disastrous complication. The first is vigorous pulsation of the tube and the second is a small brisk arterial hemorrhage that apparently stops of its own accord. If the physician does note vigorous pulsation of the tube with the arterial pulse, then the tube should be changed to a shorter flexible one in which the tip is certain to lie above the level of the original. It would seem a wise precaution to have a large intravenous line in place, blood cross-matched, and an operating room available at the time this is done since it is not inconceivable that release of the balloon pressure or removal of the tip may precipitate the emergency. If this occurs the balloon should be reinflated and the patient rushed immediately to the operating room where a median sternotomy is usually necessary to expose the bleeding site. A patient who has had a premonitory hemorrhage should probably be taken to the operating room as an emergency without further ado.

When massive hemorrhage does occur with or without the advance warning signs, there are two methods of immediate control. The first entails anterior traction on the tracheostomy tube in order to occlude the site of injury between the balloon and sternum. If this works, hemorrhage is controlled and the airway is secured. The next step should be the immediate insertion of an orotracheal tube down toward, but stopping above, the tracheostomy tube. The patient is then taken to the operating room where exposure of the injury through lateral extension of the tracheostomy wound and then downward extension to a median sternotomy is usually required. The purpose of the orotracheal tube is to establish an airway in case control of the bleeding point is suddenly lost. Establishment of an airway is accomplished by removing the tracheostomy tube while advancing the orotracheal tube into the trachea distal to the injury and inflating the balloon. At the same time, the hemorrhage can almost always be controlled by inserting a finger into the now empty tracheostomy wound, insinuating the finger between the trachea and the innominate artery, and compressing the artery between the finger and the posterior surface of the sternum. These maneuvers — simultaneous insertion of an orotracheal tube and pushing it distal to the site of injury while removing the original tracheostomy tube and gaining finger control — should be considered the cornerstone of the management of this dire emergency. At surgery, it is usually necessary to resect the portion of the innominate artery involved, preserving the connection between the right common carotid and the right subclavian arteries. The prognosis is grave.

This complication could probably be eliminated by the use of flexible tubes and a routine check using lateral x-ray of the neck to assure that the intratracheal portion of the tube is parallel to the long axis of the trachea. In addition every effort should be made to arrange respirator connections so as to allow the tracheostomy to move with the patient rather than having him pinned to the bed like a butterfly to a cork board.

Tracheoesophageal Fistula

Tracheoesophageal fistula is another late complication that is rare but frequently fatal when it occurs. In those reported cases in which etiology can be determined it is almost invariably thought to be due to pressure necrosis of the membranous posterior wall of the trachea secondary to overinflation of the cuff balloon. The problem can usually be recognized by the appearance of swallowed food or gastric contents in the tracheal aspirate. The diagnosis is confirmed by a contrast study since it must be differentiated from simple aspiration which is quite common in patients with tracheostomy. At the time the diagnosis is made, surgical treatment should be attempted with cervical esophagostomy, gastrostomy, and closure of the tracheal fistula. Because of the severe local infection and necrosis, the tracheal closure will probably fail more often than not, but this approach seems to offer the best chance of controlling the problem until the patient's general condition and the local infection improve enough to permit definitive repair of both trachea and esophagus.

Tracheopleural Fistula

Tracheopleural fistula secondary to cuff erosion has also been described, usually with a fatal outcome. This situation usually arises unheralded with the sudden development of bilateral pneumothoraces. Survival might be gained with immediate insertion of chest tubes bilaterally, removal of the tracheostomy tube, and replacement with an endotracheal tube through the orifice, with the cuff area placed below the site of perforation from the previous balloon. The patient could then be safely taken to the operating room for definitive repair.

Tracheal Stenosis

The late complication of tracheal stenosis has apparently become more common, as mentioned earlier, and an extensive literature on the subject has now been compiled. Clinical and experimental studies have confirmed that the most frequent cause is a cicatrix resulting from the healing of an area of circumferential pressure necrosis at the site of contact of the balloon cuff with the tracheal wall. The next most frequent cause is severe anterior deformity resulting from the healing of a tracheostoma in which either too large a segment of the trachea was removed or local invasive infection destroyed additional cartilage. In the majority of patients with a significant lesion, symptoms of upper respiratory tract obstruction will develop between 10 and 42 days after extubation, although they have occurred as early as 2 days and as late as 18 months after extubation. Any patient who has had a cuffed tube in place and exhibits dyspnea, difficulty in clearing secretions, or stridor after extubation should be suspected of having tracheal stenosis. Patients in whom wheezing stridor develops relatively late are especially prone to be diagnosed and treated as asthmatics. Confirmation of the diagnosis can usually be made by the air tracheogram revealed on a lateral neck film. Low obstruction may require laminagrams, and there are reports of tantalum inhalation being a successful and safe method for outlining the problem. Once the diagnosis has been confirmed, the patient should be referred to a surgeon experienced in surgery of the trachea. Symptomatic lesions do not respond well to conservative therapy, and tracheal resection with end-to-end anastomosis is the treatment of choice when possible. Acute obstruction that does not respond to tracheal suction is a most difficult emergency situation. Probably the best choice would be to attempt to insert a small bronchoscope through the stricture by direct vision; next best, a small non-cuffed endotracheal tube blindly forced through; and last, an emergency tracheostomy on the spot. Admittedly none of these maneuvers is without drawback, but any one of them is justified in the situation described since the patient will certainly die otherwise.

Attempts to minimize the tracheal damage done by the tube and cuff have resulted in a new generation of such devices. Several characteristics of the tube would seem to be important. One of these is the softness of the tube (and therefore less ability to transmit torque to the tip). A low-pressure, high-volume, uniformly distended cuff is desirable, as is the ability to monitor intracuff pressure. A predictable relationship of intracuff pressure and cuff to tracheal wall pressure, as well as a low cuff to tracheal wall pressure necessary to obtain minimal inspiratory leak, is desirable. Published data on these measurements are available for most of the commonly used tracheostomy tubes. This allows the physician to make a reasonable choice of which tube to use under particular circumstances. Regardless of which tube is chosen, the objective is the lowest possible pressure with minimal inspiratory leak. The cuff should be employed only as long as absolutely necessary.

COMPLICATIONS OF THORACENTESIS

PNEUMOTHORAX

Probably the most common cause of pneumothorax is needle aspiration during thoracentesis. Although some air may enter the pleural cavity through an open needle, this is probably an infrequent cause of the pneumothorax. A much more likely cause is puncture of the lung with the needle and air leak into the pleural space. Occasionally the needle puncture of the lung will cause a coughing spell, and this will force more air into the pleural space, thus permitting a tension pneumothorax to develop. Finally, air may enter the pleural space through the needle tract after the needle has been withdrawn. This situation may follow the use of a large needle but must indeed be rare.

The patient may have no symptoms, or there may be pain in the shoulder or abdomen and a heavy feeling in the chest. Physical examination and roentgenograms will confirm the diagnosis.

In most cases no treatment will be necessary, since the amount of trapped air will be small and will be absorbed in time. If the collapse is relatively complete, aspiration of the air and careful follow-up of the patient to determine whether there is any reaccumulation of air will be necessary.

When tension pneumothorax develops, immediate decompression by a needle is mandatory, and this may be followed by insertion of a thoracotomy tube connected to an underwater seal. The traumatized lung will heal in a few days, and the tube may be withdrawn.

EMPYEMA

The advent of antibiotics has greatly reduced this complication; however, it does occur on occasion. The pleura may become contaminated from the skin at the time the needle is introduced, but this must be a rare condition if aseptic technique is used in the procedure. A more common source of infection is entrance of the needle into an infected lung, permitting contamination of the pleural space. This may take place with acute inflammatory processes in the lung or with the more chronic forms of disease. Leaking of air and bacteria from the lung promotes the development of a pyopneumothorax. This is prevented by reexpanding the lung with water-seal drainage.

If for some reason contamination of the pleural cavity is suspected, a culture should be obtained and sent to the laboratory for identification of the bacteria and sensitivity studies. In the interim the patient should be started on a broad spectrum antibiotic. If a true empyema develops, the treatment consists in surgical drainage, antibiotics, and supportive therapy.

HEMORRHAGE

This rarely occurs from the needle striking the lung or other intrathoracic viscera. There may be injury to intercostal vessels. The more common mishap is for the needle to penetrate the diaphragm and tear the spleen or other intra-abdominal viscera. This usually follows too low a tap or a tap in the presence of a high diaphragm.

In most instances the bleeding will not only stop spontaneously but also will probably not even be recognized by patient or physician. If severe hemorrhage should occur, the vital signs will show evidence of hypotension, and surgical intervention will be necessary. Thoracentesis followed by paracentesis will usually indicate the location of the hemorrhage.

PLEURAL SHOCK

Any patient who has difficulty during thoracentesis is often labeled as having had pleural shock. A certain number of these patients for one reason or another faint during the procedure, but there is no organic reason for the sudden hypotension.

True pleural shock is a rare condition created when the aspirating needle penetrates the lung and a branch of the pulmonary vein at the same time, creating a fistula that permits air to leak into the pulmonary vein with resultant air embolism.

There is no known treatment for this condition except to support the patient, put his head down, and turn him on his side, with the left side up to trap the air in the left ventricle rather than allow it to escape into the coronary or cerebral vessels.

COMPLICATIONS OF PARACENTESIS

PERFORATION OF A VISCUS

Introduction of a needle into any of the body cavities always carries the risk of penetration into a viscus. In most instances little or no harm is done. Frequently paracentesis is performed in patients who have had previous acute or chronic intra-abdominal disease, which has predisposed the viscera to

adhesions, especially to the anterior abdominal walls. In the virgin abdomen the exploring needle is unlikely to penetrate most of the viscera, since they will be pushed away by the tip of the needle. The present widespread use of diagnostic paracentesis in acute trauma to the abdomen with few complications tends to support this thesis.

When for one reason or another the needle does penetrate a hollow viscus, the condition is unlikely to be serious unless the viscus is greatly distended and under pressure. Under these conditions leakage and peritonitis are likely to occur. The patient may experience sudden abdominal pain and the progressive signs and symptoms of peritonitis. Roentgenograms will usually confirm the diagnosis by the presence of free air in the abdomen. Antibiotics should be started immediately and supportive intravenous therapy given in the form of electrolyte solution. If there is any doubt in the physician's mind or if the signs and symptoms are progressive, surgical intervention may be necessary.

HEMORRHAGE

The exploring needle will under certain circumstances enter a large vessel with slight intra-abdominal bleeding, but serious blood loss probably occurs only if the needle tears the vessel. This may happen should the patient cough or retch at the time the needle enters the vessel. It is important that the exploring needle be held loosely so that it will move with the patient's movements and not tend to tear any of the abdominal contents. This is an extremely rare accident, and the treatment consists in supporting the patient's circulation and immediate exploration if there is evidence of progressive hypotension.

PLASTIC ADHESIVE PERITONITIS

Those conditions such as cirrhosis of the liver with ascites that demand repeated paracentesis may produce a low-grade chronic inflammation of the peritoneum that progresses to plastic adhesive peritonitis. This is frequently the forerunner of intestinal obstruction. Adhesions between one or more loops of bowel and the abdominal wall permit internal hernias, twists, or kinks to occur, which in turn produce various degrees of intestinal obstruction.

The production of adhesive peritonitis makes future paracentesis difficult, since adequate paracentesis requires access to the free peritoneal cavity to drain the fluid properly.

Scrupulous aseptic technique and infrequent paracentesis will help to prevent this complication, for which there is no treatment available.

PERSISTENT DRAINAGE

When a needle is used for aspiration, persistent drainage will not occur; however, the large trocars that are usually used to drain abdominal ascites may leave a hole large enough so that it will drain for many days, dependent upon the amount of fluid and pressure within the abdomen. Perhaps this should not be considered a complication, since it is accomplishing what was intended. If the procedure is done on an outpatient basis, it becomes a complication, since the patient is left with a draining fistula, which makes outpatient care difficult. Also, the presence of the draining fistula may permit the entrance of bacteria with subsequent peritonitis.

Treatment of the persistent drainage is closure of the tract by surgical means under local anesthesia. Careful closure of the skin will usually suffice to prevent external drainage. Some fluid may continue to leak into the abdominal wall, but this merely serves as a decompressing mechanism.

COMPLICATIONS OF GASTRIC DILATATION

Gastric dilatation is a common and serious complication of surgery. It frequently follows upper abdominal surgery, anesthesia of all types, blunt trauma to the abdomen, and fracture of the spine, to name but a few of the causes.

The initiating cause is probably reflex inhibition of the stomach by way of the autonomic nervous system so that secretions are not moved on down the intestinal tract. In most cases the patient has, in addition, a tendency to swallow air, and this is perhaps the most important aspect. Although it is difficult to prove that dilatation does not occur in the absence of air swallowing, it is true that a great deal of the dilatation is caused by air, and this can reach the stomach only by being swallowed. As the stomach begins to enlarge it hangs down across the duodenum and compresses it against the vertebral column, thus causing further obstruction to outflow of the gastric contents. A vicious cycle is initiated that will not ordinarily relieve itself.

The diagnosis is not clear-cut and is dependent upon a high index of suspicion on the part of the physician. The patient may complain of pressure in the epigastrium, hiccup, distention, or vomiting. Not infrequently the first sign may be hypotension and a rapid pulse noticed by the nurse while checking the vital signs.

The vomiting is usually not severe and is actually an overflow phenomenon of the gastric fluid running out of the patient's mouth. The fluid is usually dark, foul-smelling, and greenish brown, but does not appear to be fecal.

The upper part of the abdomen may be tympanitic, and there are no bowel sounds. A succussion splash may be elicited. X-ray examination will frequently confirm the diagnosis but is not necessary. A suction tube should be inserted through the nose into the stomach and the results observed. If dilatation exists, there will be a rush of air out of the tube, followed by fluid, often before the suction is applied. In severe dilatation as much as 3 to 5 liters of fluid may be aspirated.

FLUID AND ELECTROLYTE LOSSES

The dilatation itself is not the most serious aspect of the complication, although deaths from hypotension and reflex cardiac arrest have been reported. A more common sequel is the tremendous loss of fluid and electrolytes which occurs and leads to hypochloremic, hypokalemic alkalosis. If this is allowed to progress, secondary dehydration, hypotension, and death may result.

The stomach normally secretes about 2500 ml. of fluid per day with the following average electrolyte concentrations: sodium 50 mEq., chloride 105 mEq., and potassium 8 mEq. per liter.

If this condition goes unrecognized, the postoperative patient may lose several liters of fluid which are not replaced, and thus a severe dehydration occurs. In addition, there is electrolyte loss, most especially chloride, which produces hypochloremic alkalosis.

The relatively common use of a nasogastric tube after operation has probably prevented many cases of this complication in present-day surgical practice. When gastric dilatation does occur, the treatment is immediate decompression by means of a nasogastric tube and constant suction. The stomach should be kept at rest for at least 48 hours. When it is believed time to begin oral alimentation again, the tube can be removed and fluids given in small quantities. If these are tolerated, a gradual increase in oral intake can be instituted.

In addition to the decompression, a careful record of the patient's intake and output must be kept. The losses can thus be calculated for each 24-hour period and replaced volume for volume with the appropriate fluid. If the special fluids are not available, normal saline solution will suffice.

PERFORATION OF THE STOMACH

Occasionally the stomach will become overdistended, but the symptoms will not be sufficient to claim the physician's attention, and perforation will occur. This probably never occurs in the patient with a normal stomach but may occur with preexisting disease such as a peptic ulcer.

The onset of this complication, which fortunately is extremely rare, is sudden, severe, and often catastrophic. Severe abdominal pain and collapse may be the initial symptoms. The abdomen rapidly becomes tender in the epigastrium or throughout, and rigidity develops. There are no bowel sounds, and the patient's temperature begins to rise. X-ray films of the abdomen in the upright and lateral decubitus positions will almost always demonstrate free air in the peritoneal cavity. This may be difficult to interpret, however, if the patient has recently had abdominal surgery, since there is frequently free air in the abdomen for some days after the abdomen has been opened.

Treatment consists of immediate decompression, institution of fluid therapy to make up the losses, and surgical exploration with closure of the perforation.

ASPIRATION PNEUMONITIS

This rather subtle entity is a serious complication and probably causes many deaths following surgical procedures. The studies of Gardner suggest that aspiration of small amounts of food or liquid into the lungs is common in the postoperative state. The frequency of this complication is on the increase as more surgical procedures are performed on patients who are especially susceptible to aspiration. These would include the very young and the very old patient as well as those with bulbar paralysis, intoxication, and convulsions and those receiving emergency anesthesia. Although gastric dilatation is not necessary for aspiration to occur, it is frequently an important factor.

Aspiration rarely occurs in the alert, strong patient with a good cough reflex. It does occur rather frequently in three groups of patients: (1) the infant who is anesthetized and vomits during the phase of awakening from anesthesia. The cough reflex in the very young, especially if they are ill, may be weak or absent, thus permitting aspiration. (2) The strong, healthy patient undergoing elective surgery of prolonged duration without gastric decompression. The stomach dilates during the procedure, and as the patient awakens from anesthesia vomiting occurs with aspiration. Normally, the cough reflex would prevent this catastrophe, but the level of anesthesia is still deep enough to prevent adequate coughing. (3) The elderly patient or the patient with a chronic disease who is so weak that the cough reflex is diminished or absent. These patients may aspirate with or without the administration of anesthesia.

The aspiration of stomach contents is a serious complication because of the high acidity of the material. The inhalation of acid causes inflammation or a chemical pneumonia. If the amount aspirated is not enough to cause immediate asphyxiation, there is usually a latent period between the aspiration and the onset of respiratory distress. Within a few hours of the aspiration the respiratory rate increases, and a few fine rales may be heard over the lungs. Roentgenograms reveal extensive changes that resemble patchy pulmonary edema. This edema results from the intense inflammation that occurs in the delicate alveolar membrane. Cyanosis may occur in those patients with extensive involvement of the lungs.

Prevention is by far the easiest treatment of this condition. It is usually possible to prevent the aspiration by (1) awareness of the possibility because of the type of patient, (2) decompression of the stomach in this group of patients before or during operation, and (3) careful observation of the patient by competent personnel during the recovery period. This complication frequently occurs in the corridor on the way back to the patient's room from surgery and is best prevented by placing the patient in a recovery room or under professional supervision until he is fully awake.

If aspiration occurs, emergency measures are directed toward immediate reestablishment of the airway. The patient should be placed in the head-down position, and careful suction should be done. If immediate relief is not obtained, bronchoscopy or tracheotomy is necessary. No physician should be permitted to operate unless he is competent to perform good tracheobronchial suction, and tracheotomy or bronchoscopy. In emergencies such as this there is not time to summon qualified help. As soon as the tracheobronchial tree is clear and breathing is normal, a Levin tube should be inserted and constant suction applied to maintain decompression of the stomach.

Once the airway is established, or in those patients in whom no catastrophic event occurs, but the diagnosis of aspiration is made by a change in the vital signs and is confirmed by x-ray study, medical measures should be instituted. These consist in the administration of steroids, oxygen, and antibiotics. Hydrocortisone intravenously in doses of 300 mg. every 8 hours provides an effective pharmacologic dose. Oxygen is administered by face mask until it can be given by nasal catheter or endotracheal tube, or until a tracheotomy is elected. A broad spectrum antibiotic should be used, although it is difficult to prove the need.

Since these patients are on constant gastric suction, the antibiotics are given as a part of their intravenous drip.

Those patients with extensive involvement of the lungs should have an immediate endotracheal intubation with a cuffed tube, and assisted ventilation should be instituted.

Saline lavage of the tracheobronchial tree is particularly effective in patients who have aspirated gastric contents. Lavage with 50 ml. increments of normal saline followed by immediate suction will frequently clear the aspirated contents from the lung. A total of 200 to 400 ml. of saline is used. Positive-pressure ventilation with oxygen is an important part of tracheobronchial lavage and should be continued for at least 30 minutes afterwards.

Instruction in deep breathing is given as soon as the patient is able to manage his own airway. Blow bottles serve as a useful adjunct to deep breathing. When the patient is properly instructed in their use, the blow bottles provide him with an index of accomplishment. This makes deep breathing more understandable, and better cooperation is obtained from the patient.

COMPLICATIONS OF FECAL IMPACTION

Fecal impaction occurs primarily in certain groups of patients, but its incidence is on the increase as the surgical population grows older. In the hospital for chronic disease or in the rest home it is a trying complication and may be serious. It is also a serious problem in younger patients with congenital anomalies such as megacolon.

LOSS OF APPETITE

In some way our sense of well-being appears to be partially controlled by the ability to evacuate the colon. When fecal impaction occurs, this sense of well-being, as well as the appetite, diminishes. This is well recognized on geriatric services, and a diminution in appetite should arouse the suspicion of a fecal impaction. A rectal examination will confirm the diagnosis.

Fecal impaction is not limited to the very old patient but may occur in the very ill who are not moving about and are heavily sedated, in the patient with a neurologic lesion such as paraplegia, in the surgical patient after rectal or colon surgery, and in the pregnant woman. All these conditions and others lead to atony of the large bowel for varying periods of time, and if care is not taken fecal impaction may occur.

Prevention is the easiest form of treatment, and careful consideration should be given to the bowel habits of surgical patients.

Treatment of the diminished appetite is usually accomplished as soon as the impaction is relieved. The impaction may be relieved by enemas of oil instillation, provided the patient can retain the oil long enough to allow the impaction to soften and be expelled. Usually this method fails and more vigorous methods are necessary. These consist in manually removing the impaction by first breaking it up with the gloved finger and then instilling oil to permit the patient to expel the remainder. Often at the time the impaction is broken up the entire mass can be digitally removed.

Some unfortunate patients have been operated upon with a diagnosis of mechanical intestinal obstruction when fecal impaction was the true diagnosis. This should never be permitted and is one of the many reasons for routinely doing a rectal examination on all patients.

PARTIAL OBSTRUCTION

If the patient continues to eat in the presence of a fecal impaction, the colon becomes filled and a partial obstruction develops. This may permit the fluid content of the bowel to be expelled, but obstructs the evacuation of solid material. The physician is puzzled as to why the patient has diarrhea, and many studies may be done before a rectal examination is thought of. In any patient with diarrhea a rectal examination should be one of the first diagnostic studies performed. Obstruction that is allowed to progress may lead to moderate degrees of fluid deprivation and dehydration. Although this is uncommon, it has occurred. It is easy to believe that this complication cannot happen in your hospital, but the chances are that it has happened.

Treatment consists in removing the impaction, as already noted, and in replacement of the fluid deficits. A regimen of prevention should be instituted to prevent recurrence. This will vary to some degree with the type of patient, but a low-residue diet and one of the stool softeners such as mineral oil or Colace usually will be of value.

PERFORATION

There are instances on record in which the impaction is so complete that intestinal pressure rises behind the obstruction to levels that permit the bowel wall to burst. This usually occurs in the cecum, since the bursting pressure is lowest in this region of the colon. Although this more commonly occurs behind an obstructing carcinoma of the descending colon, it does occur behind a fecal impaction. Large bowel obstruction in the group of patients with fecal impaction may be insidious in its onset, and the patient may not complain a great deal. Perforation and an acute surgical condition of the abdomen may be the presenting symptoms. If immediate therapy is not instituted, death may result. The vital statistics of the United States for 1950 listed 172 deaths from fecal impaction among 4989 deaths from intestinal obstruction.

If complete obstruction without perforation has occurred, the treatment is removal of the impaction by the aforementioned methods. When it has progressed to this stage, however, colotomy may be necessary to remove the impaction.

If perforation has occurred, immediate surgical intervention with closure of the defect and proximal decompression is imperative. Supportive therapy such as fluids and antibiotics should be given. Most patients should recover, but they are frequently handicapped by a debilitated state before this complication occurs, and death may result.

COMPLICATIONS OF DIAGNOSTIC RADIOLOGY

EXCESSIVE EXPOSURE TO ROENTGEN RAYS

It is probably not possible to suffer overexposure to roentgen radiation during diagnostic radiology when relatively modern and safe equipment is being used. Some of the old equipment, which is now for the most part in museums, was of some danger if the patient had enough diagnostic irradiation. Generally speaking, modern equipment permits the patient to receive practically every diagnostic test known without the danger of excessive radiation as far as is known.

It is important, however, to keep in mind that there are many unknowns about radiation, and the rule should be adopted that no patient be subjected to any radiation that is not absolutely necessary for the diagnosis of his condition. When diagnostic tests are conducted, the equipment should be properly shielded, and the dosage and conditions should conform to the standards set by the National Commission on Radiation Protection. If these requirements are met, there will be no complications from diagnostic roentgenology.

There have been some reports on the danger of radiation during early pregnancy. Actually, the only concrete evidence that this is of danger is in experimental studies on animals in which the dosage, though low, exceeds that used for diagnostic purposes. These studies do show changes in the fourth or fifth generation after the radiation exposure. Although these studies may or may not apply to man, it will take a long time to determine their value, and most of the worries are merely speculation at present. As already stated, if there is a real indication for the radiation exposure, the patient should have the tests, since the disease or condition requiring diagnosis is much more likely to be harmful than the possible effects of the radiation.

SENSITIVITY TO CONTRAST MATERIALS

Many diagnostic techniques in radiology require administration of contrast materials either by mouth or by vein. There is little or no reaction rate from oral ingestion of the materials used in most hospitals.

The danger of mild to serious reactions following intravenous administration of contrast materials is always present. No figures cover all the materials available, but some idea of the *serious reactions* can be obtained from the statistics available on intravenous pyelography. In a collected series there were 31 deaths in 3,831,000 pyelograms, an incidence of one per 120,000 examinations. This mortality rate is about as low as with any agent we use in clinical medicine today.

In the past many institutions insisted upon routinely testing all patients for sensitivity to these agents before their administration. More recent studies, however, indicate that the tests are of little value, and the best screening is a good history about the patient's allergies and especially any sensitivity to iodine. If a history of allergy to iodine exists, a small intravenous test dose is administered with the necessary resuscitation equipment available. Although there is no question that death may occur from the use of these materials, this possibility is probably insignificant compared to the morbidity of the disease process that the diagnostic tests are trying to uncover. If the patient needs the examination, it should be done, with use of proper equipment and dosage, without fear of untoward consequences.

COMPLICATIONS OF ANGIOGRAPHY

The recent advances in the treatment of vascular disease by surgical means have necessitated an increased use of angiography. Although the technique is rather old, the recent impetus has come from the improved surgical techniques, which permit a direct attack on the diseased vessels. Although this diagnostic tool has been overused to some extent, it is of great value in diagnosing vascular disease, in precisely locating the lesion, and, perhaps most important, in giving some indication of prognosis before operative intervention. Many surgeons with a large clinical experience in cardiovascular surgery have decreased the need for angiography in their clinics, but it is still a useful tool and essential to the study of vascular disease.

The incidence of serious non-fatal and fatal complications is given as 1 per cent. It can be stated, however, that increased knowledge as to the cause of the complications makes most of them preventable. If the needle is carefully placed with a check of the position by the injection of 5 ml. of the contrast material and the taking of a roentgenogram, certain complications can be eliminated. Equally important are the concentration and total dose of the contrast material used. The authors usually use Renografin, the total dose not to exceed 300 ml. for the aorta or peripheral arteries. If it is injected properly, excellent contrast studies are obtained.

Keeping these two principles in mind will help diminish the possibility of complications.

Serious Non-fatal and Fatal Complications

RENAL DAMAGE. The most serious complication is damage to the kidneys, which has accounted for the majority of the deaths reported. In most of the cases preexisting renal disease was present. Since angiography may be necessary in patients with renal disease, an effort should be made to permit only the minimal amount of contrast material to enter the renal arteries. This is accomplished by injecting high above the renal arteries in the case of a suspected high lesion or well below them in terminal aortic or peripheral disease. Since most of the lesions do not involve the renal arteries, this is dependent upon proper placement of the needle and use of the minimal amount of contrast material.

Renal insufficiency is the most serious result of abdominal angiography. A study of renal function after injection of relatively large doses of contrast material at the level of the renal arteries or directly into them reveals hematuria, albuminuria, and an increase in the blood urea nitrogen. This may be transient and disappear in a few days or may progress to complete renal failure with recovery in 3 to 6 months or death. The treatment of renal failure, should it occur, is discussed elsewhere (Chapter 6).

NEUROLOGIC COMPLICATIONS. The second most common complication is transient or permanent neurologic damage. This is probably due to a high concentration of the contrast material reaching the spinal cord by way of the radicular arteries. These arteries take off from the aorta between the tenth thoracic and fourth lumbar vertebrae, being most common at the level of the second lumbar vertebra. The possibility of such a complication is increased when the aorta is occluded by disease or extraneous pressure. Transverse myelitis and a permanent paraplegia have been reported following aortography.

Proper placement of the needle and injection of a minimal amount of contrast material will generally eliminate this complication. If it should occur, the treatment is the same as for all cases of transverse myelitis.

HEMORRHAGE. There is probably some extravasation of blood at the site of needle puncture in almost every case. Generally speaking, the patient does not even complain of an ache or pain at the site of injection. Cases have been reported in which major hemorrhage caused the death of the patient or necessitated surgical intervention. In most cases this followed the penetration of an aneurysm by the needle, and it is understandable that this distended, diseased tissue is unable to close the needle hole. Since a clinical and roentgenologic examination of the region will in most instances outline the general level of an aneurysm, direct puncture can usually be avoided. It is probably unwise to puncture an aneurysm with a needle, although it has been done many times without complication.

Major hemorrhage after angiography will almost always require surgical intervention and correction of the defect. Because this will almost always require definitive vascular surgery, angiography should not be performed unless facilities are at hand for immediate repair of the lesion should trouble arise. All angiography should be done in a special x-ray unit in the surgical suite so that all facilities are immediately available.

GASTROINTESTINAL COMPLICATIONS. Difficulties may arise when contrast material is injected by accident or deliberately into the celiac axis or the superior mesenteric artery. The most serious complication is thrombosis of the artery. Subsequent infarction of the area supplied then occurs and necessitates immediate surgical intervention. Less severe complications are ileus following injection into the superior mesenteric artery or pancreatitis following injection into the celiac artery. Should these complications occur, conservative management will usually suffice.

OTHER COMPLICATIONS. Contrast material should never be injected unless there is a free flow of blood into the syringe. Occasionally the needle will not be completely in the vessel, and injection at this time deposits the material within the wall of the vessel. This may in turn promote a dissecting aneurysm, which demands immediate resection.

Since angiography is frequently done for occlusive vascular disease, there is always the possibility that a plaque will be separated from the vessel wall and act as an embolus to the vessel distally. If this occurs, immediate surgical intervention will usually be necessary, depending of course on the point of occlusion by the embolus.

Infection, pneumothorax, chylothorax, pleural effusion, and hemothorax have all been reported following angiography. In most instances these complications are not serious and should be treated conservatively. All these complications are discussed elsewhere in this volume.

COMPLICATIONS OF BRONCHOGRAPHY

This procedure has become routine in most hospitals that deal with the diagnosis and treatment of pulmonary disease.

Topically anesthetizing the larynx and bronchi is the usual procedure for bronchography. This introduces the hazard of reaction to the local anesthetic agent. Although there is no way to avoid this risk, a good history is the best way to detect possible sensitivity. The measures to be used in the prevention and treatment of such reactions are discussed in Chapter 10. When any anesthetic agent is administered, all drugs and equipment necessary for resuscitation should be at hand.

Perhaps the most serious complication is

the danger of overloading the pulmonary capacity of a patient who has preexisting pulmonary insufficiency and thus causing respiratory or cardiac failure or both.

A good history and physical examination, including clinical tests of pulmonary function, will prevent this complication. If the patient has a serious degree of pulmonary insufficiency, bilateral bronchography should not be attempted. Segmental or unilateral bronchograms should be taken, and if it is necessary to visualize the opposite lung, delay the second procedure about 1 week. This permits the opaque material to be cleared and any reaction to subside before visualization of the opposite side is undertaken.

In addition, the surgeon should be prepared to aspirate the opaque material immediately in the event that the pulmonary reserve is so low that adequate respiration becomes jeopardized. If only one side is visualized at a time, aspiration will rarely be necessary.

Most of the opaque media in use today contain iodine, and sensitivity to the material is not rare. Sensitivity testing by the sublingual or conjunctival route is not very satisfactory. Absence of a history of allergy, especially to iodine, is the best safeguard in preventing this complication.

Should a reaction occur, general measures such as support of the blood pressure, antihistamines, and maintenance of an adequate airway will usually see the patient through the acute episode.

It is extremely important for the surgeon to establish good rapport with patients undergoing bronchography. It not only makes the procedure less difficult but also helps to prevent serious complications. The procedure is done in a dark room where it is impossible to observe the patient for color, respiration, and so on. It is also impractical to feel the pulse as a guide. If good rapport has been established and the patient will cooperate and follow instructions, it is relatively easy to be sure that he is in no serious trouble. Failure of such a patient to heed an instruction is a good clue for the surgeon to turn on the lights and immediately check the patient. We have found this the most reliable way of avoiding serious trouble during the fluoroscopic part of the procedure.

The opaque material should be adminis-tered under fluoroscopic control. If the material fails to reach the periphery of the bronchial tree, it is likely that bronchospasm is occurring. An immediate check of the patient will confirm the diagnosis, and appropriate antispasmodics can be given. Aminophylline, epinephrine, and ephedrine are the agents usually given. Epinephrine (1 per cent) is as satisfactory as any and should be readily available.

Steroid therapy is commonly used today in the treatment of many patients with pulmonary disease. This has created a hidden hazard for the surgeon who performs bronchography. Frequently in a patient being maintained on steroids the sudden stress of a surgical procedure increases the requirement for the steroids. If they are not provided, vascular collapse may occur. A second situation is the patient on steroid therapy who is suddenly deprived of steroids and then subjected to the stress of bronchography. When vascular collapse occurs and the reason is obscure, the possibility of need for steroid therapy or an increase in the amount being given must be considered and immediate restoration provided.

BARIUM CONTRAST STUDIES

Examination of the gastrointestinal tract by means of barium contrast studies has become so routine in present-day medical practice that little thought is given to possible complications. Actually, complications are rare and are more easily prevented than treated.

Intestinal obstruction is sometimes difficult to localize, or for some reason the physician is interested in knowing the extent or level of the obstruction. Barium is introduced and a roentgenographic examination is made. In general, if the obstruction is in the stomach or small intestine, little difficulty due to the barium will ensue. If the obstruction is complete, the patient may vomit the barium, but this in itself is not harmful. If the obstruction is in the large intestine — even though it may be incomplete at the time of the examination — the barium may be retained, the water is absorbed, and a solid mass of barium remains to convert the partial obstruction to a complete one.

With a partial obstruction of the large

bowel, barium should be instilled cautiously. The barium is administered by means of an enema, and under fluoroscopic control it is easy to determine whether the contrast material will pass the obstruction with ease and what the likelihood of retention will be. If the lumen is small and there is little movement of the barium past it, the material should not be forced. If it moves past the obstruction and gives no evidence of returning, an immediate enema of water or an oil-retention enema may be given to maintain the liquid consistency of the material and encourage its passage.

Should complete obstruction ensue, the material should be removed at the time of elective surgical intervention, or it may become a large solid impaction that will have difficulty in passing the anastomosis and may thus complicate the postoperative course.

ASPIRATION OF CONTRAST MATERIAL. This is an unlikely complication except in the very young or the very old patient and is almost always secondary to impairment of the cough reflex. It is a danger in the roentgenologic diagnosis of congenital atresia of the upper intestinal tract, especially the esophagus. The diagnosis of tracheoesophageal fistula has often been attempted by oral administration of barium contrast material with subsequent aspiration of the material. Actually, the danger is apparently not as great as was formerly believed. Recent studies in dogs, in which barium has been deliberately placed in the bronchial tree, have shown no pathologic abnormalities in follow-up studies 6 months after the material was instilled. Although the barium itself is apparently not harmful, aspiration of any liquid material in the infant may lead to serious pulmonary complications and death. Since most of these children die because of pulmonary difficulties secondary to aspiration, administration of anything by mouth should be avoided. The diagnosis is made by history and ordinary roentgenograms, and confirmed by the attempt to pass a catheter into the stomach.

If a patient aspirates barium, the treatment is the same as for aspiration of any foreign material: immediate, careful tracheobronchial toilet that includes bronchoscopy when positioning and suction fail. The studies just discussed would apparently indicate that if some barium is retained, but the respirations are adequate, there is no danger from small amounts of the material remaining in the tracheobronchial tree.

PERFORATION OF THE INTESTINAL TRACT DURING CONTRAST STUDIES. Occasionally the rectum is perforated during the course of a barium enema. It is not always the fault of the radiologist, since many of these patients have a sigmoidoscopy just before the enema, and it is difficult to be sure who made the perforation. Any contrast material seen outside the intestinal tract at the time of fluoroscopy during the contrast study is evidence of perforation regardless of the cause, and immediate surgical intervention is usually necessary. It may be possible to proceed with the operation at this time, but more often the patient is not prepared and studies are not completed, so that definitive surgery is not advisable. This must be decided on an individual basis, but when such circumstances exist, the perforation should be closed and a proximal colostomy carried out. Some surgeons close the perforation and omit the colostomy, and the success of this procedure is relatively high. The safest course, however, is immediate proximal colostomy with the definitive procedure withheld until more favorable circumstances prevail.

COMPLICATIONS OF DRAINS

Drains are used for one of two purposes: either to prevent accumulation of fluid or secretions in a wound, or to permit escape of fluid, pus, or blood that has already accumulated. This discussion is limited to the complications occurring from drains placed for one of these two purposes. [Drains may also be placed for detection of any continued bleeding postoperatively. Ed.]

TISSUE REACTION

A drain placed in a wound of any type acts as a foreign body and will call forth the tissue response characteristic of all foreign bodies. The wound may in turn actually drain more material than one would expect, since part of the drainage is secondary to the drain itself. This extra drainage and the inflammatory response to the retained foreign body are rarely of serious consequence as far as is known. There is no treatment for the inflammatory response except to remove the drain as soon as possible.

It might be stated at this point that the indications for draining a wound are becoming fewer. When a drain is to be used, it should be selected to meet the following criteria: it should be soft so as not to erode the surrounding tissues, smooth so as not to permit fibrin to cling to it, and of a material that will not disintegrate and leave foreign bodies in the wound. The study and use of these principles may not prevent all the complications of drainage, but will most certainly reduce them.

SOURCE OF CONTAMINATION

Every surgical wound is contaminated to some degree; however, wounds are capable of handling the contaminating bacteria without difficulty. If hematoma, dead space, foreign material, or necrosis occurs in the wound, the minimal contamination present may develop into local or invasive infection. A drain is usually placed because of one of the foregoing possibilities, especially when the surgeon believes their likelihood to be great. It must be remembered, however, that the drain itself is a foreign body and permits rapid ingress of bacteria regardless of how carefully it is covered by dressings. For this reason it may cause the very thing it is designed to prevent. Careful dressing of the wound, using a no-touch technique, and removal of the drain as soon as feasible will reduce the possibility of contamination to a minimum.

DELAYED RETURN OF FUNCTION

A drain is placed to prevent premature closure of a wound surface and to prevent trapping of material beneath the surface. By the very act of preventing closure of the wound the return of function is delayed. This delay, however, is less than that which would occur if wound infection were allowed to develop with its attendant sequelae. In addition, drains delay function in a broader sense; e.g., a drain placed into the peritoneal cavity may provoke paralytic or mechanical obstruction and thus delay return of function of the bowel.

Treatment of this complication is basically preventive. A drain should be used only after careful consideration of its function in the particular wound and it should be removed as quickly as possible.

RETAINED FOREIGN BODY

As long as the drain is in place, a portion of it may become separated and be retained as a foreign body, causing secondary breakdown of the wound or necessitating reoperation for its removal. This can occur, for instance, when a T-tube is being pulled from the common duct. As the pull is increased, the tube may stretch and break in two. The portion in the abdomen disappears into the wound and cannot be reached, so that reoperation is necessary for its removal. Care should be taken to be certain that the drain is new and of good quality, that no lacerations have been made during manipulation, and that, if it is sutured in place, the suture has been removed before removal of the drain is attempted. If these precautions are taken, there is little likelihood of a piece of the drain remaining behind to cause trouble. Occasionally the entire drain will be lost in the wound. If there is any possibility of this, the drain should be properly tagged, usually with safety pins, to prevent it from slipping into the wound.

TISSUE NECROSIS

It must be remembered that a drain goes through soft tissues that are not accustomed to pressure. A drain that is too hard will tend to cause necrosis of the surrounding tissues as the pressure of motion and swelling occurs within the wound. The use of a soft drain in all cases will obviate this complication.

COMPLICATIONS OF IMMOBILITY — "PRESSURE SORES"

The largest organ in the human body is the skin, and its durability probably has no equal in nature. Provided its blood supply is not impaired and provided air can reach its surface, it will withstand almost unlimited trauma. Pressure of tremendous magnitude can be applied to the skin with little or no damage, provided the pressure is not maintained. A constant, steady pressure of only moderate intensity, however, can cause necrosis and sloughing of large areas of skin. Apparently in our daily activity, including sleeping, we move constantly enough to prevent the possibility of pressure necrosis. (In the numerous committee meetings of the modern medical center it is a wonder that more ischial ulcers do not occur.)

Any patient who for some reason is no longer able to move about is a candidate for pressure necrosis. This occurs most commonly on the hospital wards that deal primarily with the very old patient or patients with neurologic injuries that prevent movement. The recent wars have unfortunately provided many paraplegic patients in whom decubitus ulcers are a constant threat.

The cause of this complication would appear to be constant pressure against an area of skin. This causes a diminution of the blood supply to the area, with stasis and subsequent necrosis. In general this tends to occur over bony prominences such as the sacroiliac joints and the ischial tuberosities. The diminished nerve supply to these areas of the skin in patients with neurologic disease also is important in the causation. Skin with normal sensation will withstand more trauma than skin in which the sensation is diminished.

The prevention of "bedsores" is often difficult and requires careful and well balanced medical and nursing care. Regardless of the difficulty, prevention is infinitely easier and more satisfactory than correction of the established ulcer. The principles of prevention can be simply stated: avoid pressure by frequent motion or careful padding, scrupulous skin care, and maintenance of good nutrition.

The patient who is in bed and unable to move should lie on an air mattress, a sponge rubber mattress, or an oscillating mattress. The sheet should be smooth and free of wrinkles, and the patient should be moved at least every 2 hours to a new position. This is easily accomplished if a schedule is kept. Although this may seem unnecessary, the busy hospital of today requires a schedule or the patient may be forgotten for several hours as more pressing problems are met. If a schedule is kept and, in addition, everyone on the floor is instructed to turn the patient every time he goes by the bed, it becomes routine and is actually not very time-consuming. It can be as familiar as saying "hello" to the patient. The skin should be rubbed down with alcohol at least twice a day and powdered after the rub. Passive motion of the extremities on a scheduled basis and gentle massage of the muscles and skin help to promote better circulation. Pressure against the heel should be avoided by placing the heel in a soft rubber or cotton doughnut. Covering sheets should not be tucked in tightly, and though this upsets the routine of the neat ward, it is helpful to the patient unable to exercise his legs. The legs may rest on pillows part of the day, but prolonged pressure on the calves and thighs should be avoided to prevent the development of thrombophlebitis. The legs should be kept separated by pillows to prevent pressure from one leg against the other, and a foot board should be in place to prevent foot drop.

A Stryker frame is a valuable device in the care of such patients and should be used if available, but these devices are expensive and not available in many institutions.

TREATMENT.   If a decubitus ulcer develops and is not too large, the main effort should be to prevent enlargement of the ulcer and to promote healing. The small ulcer frequently occurs in the patient who is severely ill, but expected to recover in a few weeks. Such a patient often is receiving around-the-clock medical care to combat the disease process, but at the same time proper care of the skin may be ignored. This is especially true of the patient who is getting a constant intravenous infusion, and is so tied down by it that he remains flat on his back for hours to days at a time. Every effort should be made to keep the patient mobile even with the intravenous fluids running, and this can be done with a little thought. When circumstances permit, a patient can sit in a chair with an intravenous needle in place; he may even walk around carrying the intravenous solution. When movement or relief of the pressure can be accomplished and proper care of the surrounding skin is provided, the ulcer will usually heal spontaneously. This may require many days to several weeks, and the physician should not become impatient and resort to surgery too quickly. If no extension of the ulcer is occurring, every effort should be made to improve the local wound care and the patient's general nutrition. Spontaneous healing will frequently reward such efforts.

If the ulcer is large when it is first seen, then spontaneous healing, even though it may occur, usually is unsatisfactory because such healing is by scar. Scar over a pressure point or bony prominence rarely provides permanent healing, and recurrent breakdown is the rule. In these patients the initial effort should be to "clean up" the wound. Frequently the ulcer has a gangrenous slough on the surface, and this should be removed. Most often this can be done without anesthesia by careful débridement. There is no pain connected with removal of dead tissue. After débridement the local wound is dressed twice daily with sterile fine-mesh gauze against the wound and a heavy absorptive dressing over this. This type of dressing will absorb the drainage from the wound and at the same time serve as a protection. Topical antibiotics are of no value. Daily débridement may be necessary until the wound is clean. The ancillary measures mentioned earlier are instituted in addition to the local wound management.

When the wound is clean, the patient should be taken to surgery and the defects covered by full-thickness rotation skin flaps. At this time the bony prominences underlying the defects should be removed, so that no pressure point remains when the flap has been shifted. This is best accomplished by removal of the pressure point with an osteotome during the surgical procedure. This may mean removing part of the greater trochanter of the femur, the sacroiliac prominence, or the ischial tuberosity. Closure of the flaps and their attendant incisions is accomplished with fine stainless steel wire. Careful hemostasis is an essential part of the procedure. A bulky absorptive dressing is then applied with moderate pressure to prevent hematomas beneath the flaps. The patient is allowed to lie on the dressing, but for no longer than he would on normal skin. In other words, the same care must be given the postoperative wound as would be given in trying to protect against the formation of a decubitus ulcer initially.

Postoperative care consists of the usual supportive measures of fluids, adequate nutrition, and antibiotics. Patients are routinely given prophylactic antibiotics because the initial wound is contaminated, large areas of skin are handled during the procedure in an area where preparation is rarely satisfactory, bone is exposed and opened surgically and then buried, and finally because, although hemostasis is given careful consideration during the surgical procedure, the chance of small pockets of blood under the flaps remains high. These hematomas provide an excellent pabulum for bacterial growth. The antibiotics are given for 5 days and discontinued or replaced, depending on the clinical course. Aqueous procaine penicillin, 300,000 units, and dihydrostreptomycin, 0.5 gm., are given twice daily by the intramuscular route.

Once the sutures have been removed and the flaps are healed, the same routine as mentioned under prevention must be used to avoid recurrence of the ulcer even though the pressure points have been removed.

COMPLICATIONS OF PAIN

Pain is an interesting aspect of the complications of surgery because of its unique role. It is often a complication of the disease or trauma that necessitates surgical intervention, and it is also a complication of surgery. In addition, the management of pain in the preoperative and postoperative periods may produce complications. It is with this broad view in mind that this section is written.

PREOPERATIVE PAIN

Pain is one of the most common symptoms of disease or trauma that cause a patient to seek medical attention. It also serves to help the surgeon determine the cause and severity of the patient's condition, and thus, although it is a complication, it is also a signpost to correct diagnosis. Although the physician's task is to alleviate pain whenever possible, the administration of narcotics or anesthetic agents before adequate examination of the patient is mentioned only to be condemned. The physician should attempt to control the pain or at least to minimize it only after a satisfactory examination has been completed and a course of action determined. In general, this is accomplished by the use of narcotic drugs, such as morphine, administered in proper dosage and by the proper route.

The control of pain, especially that which follows trauma, may be obtained by other means, and these should take precedence over the use of drugs. It is discouraging to see large doses of narcotics given to a patient who is experiencing great pain following a fracture when simple splinting of the fracture may be all that is necessary to control the pain. Careful assessment of the forces causing pain may permit alleviation of the pain with little or no narcotic administration.

Fear is a large component of the sick or injured person and may intensify the pain sensation manyfold. A little time spent in explaining the situation to the patient, gentleness in handling the painful area, and a calm, deliberate manner may make previously "unbearable" pain tolerable. This can be illustrated by recalling a military surgeon and his approach to the dressing of burn wounds. He took a large group of patients with major burns who had been getting a general anesthetic for a change of dressing two or three times a week. He discussed the problem with them and gained their confidence with his manner and approach so that he was able to change their dressings daily without an anesthetic and frequently without any analgesic agent. All of us have had a similar experience in managing the minor trauma in children that makes up such a large portion of accident room cases.

If it is necessary to give the patient an analgesic, the type, dose, and route of administration must be carefully considered to avoid complications. The injudicious use of an analgesic agent may mask the advancing symptoms of a disease process such as peritonitis or may minimize the ability of the surgeon to assess the conscious level of the patient with a possible head injury. Assessment of the blood volume is also important at this time, since many of these agents will cause vascular collapse in the patient who has a diminished blood volume. Not infrequently a patient is admitted to the emergency room with a rapid pulse, but with a relatively stable blood pressure. His pain is intense and may well be stimulating compensatory vasoconstriction if there is an element of circulating volume deficit. If he is given an analgesic, the pain subsides, the vasoconstrictor mechanisms are blocked, and hypotension ensues.

Another complication may arise in choosing the route of administration of an analgesic for the patient who has an inadequate circulating volume. Occasionally one sees a patient with a diminished blood volume who has been given a subcutaneous or intramuscular injection of a narcotic with little or no relief of pain. Several more doses are given, and still no relief is obtained. When adequate tissue perfusion occurs, after restoration of adequate circulating volume, the several doses of the analgesic are rapidly absorbed, and acute respiratory depression occurs. If the patient with frank or impending shock requires an analgesic, it should be given slowly, intravenously, and in about two-thirds the usual dosage.

The complications of ill-timed or inappropriate dosage of preanesthetic medications are covered in Chapter 10.

POSTOPERATIVE PAIN

Incisional pain, the almost universal complication of surgery, is usually not severe and can be rather easily managed with minimal use of narcotics. The occurrence of severe pain usually indicates that something additional is taking place in the wound. The usual causes for this are tension, inflammation, pressure, or ischemia. In general, these are avoidable complications, and proper care in making and closing the wound will prevent their appearance. If one of these four factors does occur, the pain is treated by eliminating the offending factor and not

by giving large and frequent doses of narcotics. The single most common problem is
the tightly sutured wound. The tendency to
draw sutures tightly seems to be inherent,
and it is difficult to teach that apposition
and strangulation do not mean the same
thing. Proper wound closure is a vital part
of surgery and needs the same care on the
part of the surgeon as is required by the rest
of the procedure. Thus one main source of
postoperative pain is more easily prevented
than treated. If retention sutures are used,
they should not be pulled tightly, since their
purpose is to relieve tension on the suture
line, not to hold the wound together in a
water-tight closure.

Care to prevent hematoma formation and
postoperative infection must be a part of
good wound surgery. Careful hemostasis
using fine ligatures, plus irrigation and
drainage of the contaminated wound, will
help prevent undue pressure and inflammation in the postoperative period.

If the patient awakens from anesthesia
and complains of severe wound pain, or if
such complaints occur in the postoperative
period, immediate inspection of the wound
should precede the use of analgesic agents.

A second complication of the immediate
postanesthetic period is hypoxia wrongly
interpreted as pain. The patient is only
partially awake and begins to moan and
thrash about. He speaks of the incisional
pain and moans so loudly that a narcotic is
quickly administered to keep him quiet and
to relieve his pain. The real problem of
hypoxia goes undiagnosed. Vasomotor
mechanisms are further depressed by the
addition of a narcotic, and severe hypotension results. The patient who is already
hypoxic and now subjected to hypotension
is in serious jeopardy and certainly has had
his chance of survival greatly decreased. An
immediate evaluation of the patient's airway
is necessary to be sure that he is breathing
adequately, that his airway is open, and that
aspiration has not occurred. (The problem
of aspiration is discussed earlier.) Hypoxia
secondary to paralysis of the respiratory
muscles following the use of muscle relaxants during surgery is a relatively recent
complication. It is necessary to inspect the
chest and thorax to make sure that the
patient is breathing on his own and is using
his muscles of respiration satisfactorily.

Some patients appear to recover from anesthesia immediately postoperatively and
breathe quite well on their own. As time
passes, however, retained muscle relaxant,
especially in the patient with a low urinary
output, continues to act, and the muscles of
respiration weaken, so that he breathes only
with his diaphragm. This permits an inadequate exchange of air, and the patient
becomes hypoxic and hypercapnic during
this time. Once again, the administration of
a narcotic or even of oxygen without the
inspection of the respiratory musculature
will prevent a proper diagnosis and will not
permit satisfactory therapy to be instituted.
In some of these patients satisfactory diagnosis can be made by a test dose of the
short-acting anticholinesterase drug, edrophonium (Tensilon). When given intravenously, this agent frequently will combat the
residual effects of the relaxant agents, and
inspection over the next few minutes will
show an increase in the use of the patient's
respiratory musculature. This temporary
improvement with edrophonium must not
be interpreted as the end of the problem.
Frequently the respiratory effort will improve for a period of a few minutes, only to
relapse again into a paralyzed state with the
complications of hypoventilation. Neostigmine in combination with appropriate doses
of atropine should be substituted at this
point for its sustained action. If the patient
does not respond to adequate dosage of this
medication, he should be placed on a respirator and given assisted respiration until
his respiratory musculature is active again.
[Spontaneous hypoventilation postoperatively is such a hazard that the endotracheal
tube should be reinserted, with mechanical
ventilation, in most patients. Ed.]

The patient in the immediate postoperative period who is actually experiencing a
great deal of pain will require an analgesic
agent to make him comfortable. Once the
problem of hypoxia has been dispelled and
the cause of the patient's restlessness and
groaning is determined to be pain, an analgesic agent should be administered. The
patient in this case is in a twilight zone
between anesthesia and wakefulness, and
his vasomotor controls are somewhat more
tenuous than they would be under normal
circumstances. If, at this time, a standard
dose of an analgesic such as meperidine

hydrochloride is given, the patient may go into circulatory collapse. It is our practice to give a patient who is still emerging from anesthesia, but complaining of pain, half the standard dose of the narcotic that would successfully control the pain. If within 30 minutes to an hour the pain is not relieved, the remaining half of a standard dose of the narcotic is given. Once the patient is wide awake, the problem of hypotension following the use of analgesic agents is much less severe, and, in general, most patients tolerate them quite well. If one is dealing with patients in the older age group (above the age of 65), the use of analgesic agents must always be tempered and smaller doses utilized. The vasomotor system in an elderly patient, especially one who has been ill for some time, seems to be quite labile and subject to extreme changes following the use of analgesic agents.

The problem of postoperative pain has many unsolved aspects, but it would appear that if severe pain is prevented as the patient awakens from anesthesia and during the first 24 hours postoperatively, it is easier to control during the subsequent recovery. Therefore it is good practice to use a drug such as morphine to control the pain, give the patient a feeling of well-being during the first postoperative day, and minimize his difficulties. It would seem that when this is accomplished, there is less requirement for narcotics on subsequent days. The patient who receives little or no analgesia on the day of operation and is allowed to suffer a great deal of pain seems to become afraid of the pain and therefore requires more narcotics during the subsequent recovery phase.

The usefulness of morphine as an analgesic agent often appears to be overlooked. The horrors of drug addiction are known to every physician; too often he shies away from the use of morphine in the mistaken belief that meperidine hydrochloride is just as good an agent and has less addicting properties. Actually, for the average surgical patient who will be receiving narcotics for 3 or 4 days at the most, addiction is not a problem, and it is our belief that morphine is a more effective agent.

There are additional complications that occur when narcotics are used to control pain. These include urinary retention, constipation, and, on occasion, severe nausea and vomiting. Although they are complications of the control of pain, they must be considered complications of pain. These complications may be treated symptomatically and will disappear when the narcotics are withdrawn.

Bibliography

1. Brantigan, C. O., and Grow, J. B.: Cricothyroidotomy: Electing use in respiratory problems requiring tracheotomy. J. Thorac. Cardiovasc. Surg. *71*:72, 1976.
2. Bryant, L. R., Trinkle, J. K., Mobin-Uddin, K., and Griffen, W. O., Jr.: Interpretation of tracheal cultures in patients with intubation and mechanical ventilation. Am. Surg. *38*:537, 1972.
3. Cameron, J. L., Reynolds, J., and Zuidema, G. D.: Aspiration in patients with tracheostomies. Surg. Gynecol. Obstet. *136*:68, 1973.
4. Cooper, J. D.: Tracheo-innominate artery fistula: Successful management in three consecutive cases. Ann. Thorac. Surg. *24*:439, 1977.
5. Davis, H. S., Kretchmer, H. E., and Bryce-Smith, R.: Advantages and complications of tracheotomy, J.A.M.A. *153*:1156, 1953.
6. Dragstedt, L. R., Montgomery, M. L., Ellis, J. C., and Matthews, W. B.: The pathogenesis of acute dilatation of the stomach. Surg. Gynecol. Obstet. *52*:1075, 1931.
7. Galoob, H. D., and Toledo, P. S.: Comparison of five types of tracheostomy tubes in the intubated trachea. Ann. Otol. Rhinol. Laryngol. *87*:99, 1978.
8. Gardner, A. M. N.: Aspiration of food and vomit. Q. J. Med. *27*:227, 1958.
9. Grillo, H. C.: Surgery of the trachea. Curr. Probl. Surg. July, 1970.
10. Hubay, C. A., Keihn, C. C., and Drucker, W. R.: Surgical management of decubitus ulcers in the post-traumatic patient. Am. J. Surg. *93*:705, 1957.
11. Kenan, P. D.: Complications associated with tracheostomy: Prevention and treatment. Otolaryngol. Clin. North Am. *12*:807, 1979.
12. Kincaid, O. W., and Davis, G. D.: Abdominal aortography (Medical progress). N. Engl. J. Med. *295*:1067, 1958.
13. Linton, R. R.: Peripheral vascular disease (Medical progress). N. Engl. J. Med. *260*:272, 1959.
14. Mulder, D. S., and Rurush, J. L.: Complications of tracheostomy: Relationship to long-term ventilatory assistance. J. Trauma. *9*:389, 1969.
15. Pearson, F. G., and Andrews, M. J.: Detection and management of tracheal stenosis following cuffed tube tracheostomy. Ann. Thorac. Surg. *12*:359, 1971.
16. Simenstad, J. O., Galway, C. F., and MacLean, L. D.: The treatment of aspiration and atelectasis by tracheobronchial lavage. Surg. Gynecol. Obstet. *115*:721, 1962.
17. Wangensteen, O. H.: Intestinal Obstruction. Springfield, Ill., Charles C Thomas, 1955.

12

NUTRITIONAL COMPLICATIONS IN THE SURGICAL PATIENT*

Harry M. Shizgal*

Nutritional equilibrium is dependent on a balance between nutrient requirement and its intake. Disease, injury, and surgical operations are often associated with a decreased oral intake and an increased requirement for protein and calories. The magnitude and duration of these changes are proportional to the severity of the initiating traumatic event. The degree of the malnutrition that develops is directly related to the cumulative negative nutrient balance. A positive balance is likewise detrimental, resulting in the excessive accumulation of body fat. The obese individual is subjected to numerous social, psychological, and economic hardships and has a significantly shorter life expectancy.

Nutritional equilibrium is mandatory for the maintenance of maximum health and productivity. The infinitely complex biological processes that permit the normal activities of life function most efficiently in the normally nourished individual. The purpose of this chapter is to describe the prevention and treatment of nutritional disorders in the surgical patient.

NUTRITIONAL EQUILIBRIUM

The energy necessary for accomplishing the physical and chemical work of each human cell is derived from various processes of oxidation of special energy-rich fuels. During the process of photosynthesis, solar energy is captured and stored as chemical energy in various edible plants. This energy and the plant proteins are available for utilization by animals and man.

The daily quantity of energy necessary for maintaining the integrity of total cellular function has been termed basal metabolic rate (BMR) and is expressed in units of kilocalories per day. A predicted daily requirement for an individual can be obtained from standard BMR tables. A normal 70 kg. male has a basal daily requirement of approximately 1600 to 1800 kilocalories. The imposition of additional demands of me-

---

*This chapter was contributed by Drs. Stanley J. Dudrick and James H. Duke, Jr. in the previous edition.

Harry M. Shizgal is a Canadian who graduated from both college and medical school at McGill University. He took his surgical residency at Royal Victoria Hospital in Montreal and had extensive investigative experience in physiology, with particular emphasis on metabolic aspects of nutrition. Dr. Shizgal is an international authority in surgical nutrition, a member of the important surgical societies, and Professor of Surgery at McGill University.

chanical or chemical work raises the net daily requirement that must be met from either exogenous or endogenous sources.

The integrity of the body cell mass (BCM) requires a daily intake of amino acid substrate. Each of the different types of endogenous protein has a characteristic constant turnover rate of the amino acid components during normal health. The amino acids ingested in excess of those required for maintenance are metabolized through deamination of the amide fragment, and the remaining carbon skeleton is either oxidized, transaminated, or stored as fat. The amide fragment is either converted to urea, a major portion of which is excreted in the urine, or recycled to form one of the nonessential amino acids.

Stability of body weight usually implies, with few exceptions, a balance between intake and expenditure of nutritional substrate. In normal health, weight gain indicates an accumulation of energy-rich carbon molecules, predominantly in the form of fat. Some disease states are characterized by weight gain, the most common being those in which there is an imbalance in the mechanisms that maintain total body water integrity, as observed in ascites, pleural effusion, and anasarca. Weight loss associated with most disease processes reflects a change in body composition. Body weight determination is a relatively simple but gross quantitative measurement of body composition.

Normal Body Composition

The body cell mass (BCM) is the sum of all the cellular elements of the body. It includes the cells of both smooth and skeletal muscle, the viscera, nerve tissue, and the cellular components of those tissues with a sparse cellular population (cartilage, tendon, and adipose tissue). Skeletal muscle represents approximately 60 per cent of the BCM, while the viscera account for 20 to 30 per cent. The remainder is composed of red cells, the cellular mass of adipose and connective tissue, and the skeleton. The BCM is therefore the metabolically active component of body composition. It is that component which consumes oxygen, produces carbon dioxide, and performs all of the work. It is the living component of body composition and as such is the ideal reference parameter for the body's metabolic activity as assessed by oxygen consumption, carbon dioxide production, caloric requirement, and work performance.

The extracellular mass (ECM) surrounds and supports the BCM. Its major function is support and transport. It is not metabolically active, does not consume oxygen, and does not perform work. The fluid component of the ECM consists of plasma and interstitial and transcellular water. Transcellular water is extracellular water that is secreted into a well-defined space such as the lumen of the gastrointestinal tract and the cerebral, spinal, and joint spaces. The solid component of the ECM includes collagen, tendon, fascia, and the skeleton.

The sum of the BCM and the ECM is equivalent to the fat-free mass, i.e., the lean body mass (LBM) (Fig. 12–1). Total body weight is the sum of the LBM and body fat. Because the LBM is made up of both metabolically active and inactive components, it is

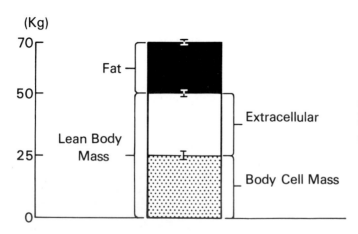

Figure 12–1 The body composition of 25 normally nourished volunteers. Body weight is the sum of body fat and the lean body mass. The lean body mass is composed of the body cell mass and the extracellular mass.

not an ideal parameter by which to assess the body's metabolic state or its nutritional state. In contrast, the BCM is an ideal parameter for this purpose, as it is a measure of the living, metabolically active portion of the body.

Uncomplicated Starvation

When the daily intake of calories and protein is equal to the amount required for maintenance, a zero balance is achieved, and the body weight remains stable. During a period of uncomplicated starvation, a negative balance for both calories and nitrogen develops, and a simultaneous decrease in body weight follows. The rate at which endogenous fuel is consumed during a period of food abstinence depends upon individual energy requirements and the efficiency of the adaptive mechanisms that attempt to limit the catabolism of protein components. Adaptation to total calorie and nitrogen deprivation is initiated immediately by the deficiencies of biochemical substrate.

Endogenous fuels are utilized to meet the daily energy requirements during periods of either partial or total starvation. The body stores of carbohydrate, in the form of muscle and hepatic glycogen, are minimal. In a normally nourished 70 kg. man, there are 150 and 75 gm. of glycogen in skeletal muscle and liver, respectively (Table 12–1).[8] These glycogen stores are depleted within the first 24 to 48 hours of total starvation.[3] Subsequently, the body relies on

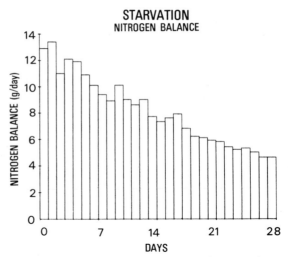

Figure 12–2 The daily urinary loss with uncomplicated normal starvation. (Adapted from: Owen, O. E., Felig, P., Morgan, A. P., Wahreu, J., and Cahill, G. F.: Liver and kidney metabolism during prolonged starvation. J. Clin. Invest. *48*:574, 1969.)

triglycerides from adipose tissue and amino acids from body protein. One of the primary functions of adipose tissue is to provide endogenous calories when exogenous nutrients are inadequate. However, a labile pool of body protein is unavailable for this purpose. All of the proteins broken down during periods of starvation serve either a structural or functional role. The major source of this protein is the skeletal muscles, although some protein is also made available from the viscera. This protein is converted in the liver to glucose, which is required by those tissues — principally the central nervous system — that rely on glucose as their primary fuel.

The normal unstressed individual adapts to starvation with an increased reliance on lipids as the major endogenous fuel and a consequent decrease in gluconeogenesis from protein. As a result, the daily urinary nitrogen loss decreases from 12 gm., early in starvation, to 5 gm. by the fourth week of starvation (Fig. 12–2).[41] This negative nitrogen balance can be converted to a protein loss, as 1 gm. of nitrogen is equivalent to 6.25 gm. of protein (Fig. 12–3). Because a labile pool of body protein does not exist, this protein loss represents a loss of BCM. Since 25 per cent of the BCM is protein, a 1 gm. loss of nitrogen represents 6.25 gm. of protein or 25 gm. of BCM. Thus, during the

TABLE 12–1 ENDOGENOUS FUEL CONSUMPTION OF NORMAL MAN*

Fuel	Kg.	Calories
Tissues:		
Fat (adipose triglyceride)	15	141,000
Protein (mainly muscle)	6	24,000
Glycogen (muscle)	0.150	600
Glycogen (liver)	0.075	300
Total		165,900
Circulating fuels:		
Glucose (extracellular fluid)	0.020	80
Free fatty acids (plasma)	0.0003	3
Triglycerides (plasma)	0.003	30
Total		113

*Adapted from Cahill, G. F., Jr.: Starvation in man. N. Engl. J. Med. *282*:688, 1970.

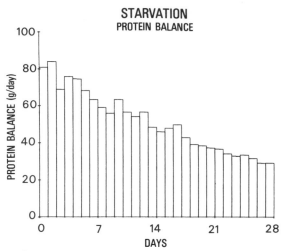

Figure 12–3 The daily net loss of body protein with normal uncomplicated starvation, calculated from the data plotted in Figure 12–2.

initial days of total starvation, the BCM decreases by 300 gm./day. With adaptation, this loss is reduced to 125 gm./day by the fourth week. Four weeks of total starvation in a healthy, normally nourished 70 kg. man results in a 5.7 kg. loss of BCM (Fig. 12–4), which represents 38 per cent of the skeletal muscle mass or 23 per cent of the BCM.

The adaptive mechanism to conserve protein requires several days to reach optimal efficiency. During this period amino acids are mobilized to a greater extent to meet energy requirements. The endogenous pro-

teins are energy poor and yield only 1000 kilocalories per kilogram and produce approximately 750 ml. water of hydration and about 135 ml. water of oxidation. A significant loss in weight is inevitable when a greater percentage of the endogenous energy is derived from protein. As fat is more actively utilized as the primary source of energy, the absolute weight of the tissues consumed to meet daily requirements decreases. When maximal adaptation has occurred, the protein-glucose interconversion contributes only a small but constant fraction to the total daily energy requirements.

The individual deprived of foodstuff can survive and sustain a significant loss in body fat stores until the gradual consumption of protein components exceeds the capacity to sustain life. The critical quantity of protein required for survival has not been determined in man. Not all proteins participate in the gluconeogenesis caused by starvation. Malnourished children were found to have severe depletion of total protein and noncollagen protein, while collagen protein was essentially unchanged.[43] At the point of death due to starvation, as much as 5 to 10 per cent of the body fat remains in the carcass.

Data confirming death secondary to absolute starvation are rare. Numerous reports of severe malnutrition in areas of natural and wartime famine have indicated that a loss of 35 to 45 per cent of body weight can be survived.[34, 37] Studley[53] first called attention to the significance of weight loss and postoperative survival. When preoperative weight loss was greater than 20 per cent of normal, the mortality rate was 33 per cent, in contrast to a 3.5 per cent mortality associated with less weight losses in patients with the same pathologic conditions.

NUTRITIONAL COMPLICATIONS IN THE SURGICAL PATIENT

Nutritional Complications Arising from Preexisting Disease

Most disease processes have the capacity to alter normal nutritional equilibrium if allowed to persist for a sufficient period of time. Insidious subclinical illnesses can gradually modify appetite, and consequent-

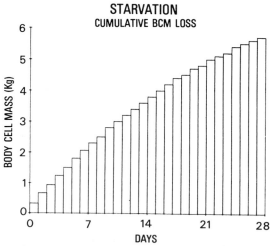

Figure 12–4 The cumulative loss of body cell mass with normal uncomplicated starvation derived from the data plotted in Figure 12–2.

ly patterns of intake, in a manner not readily apparent to the patient. More overt processes can directly impair ingestion, absorption, or assimilation. All of these processes share the common adverse effect of causing a reduction in total body protein, especially skeletal muscle. Precise determinations of changes in body composition are not available to all clinicians, but body weight can be an important, albeit gross, parameter of measurement.

IMPAIRED INGESTION DUE TO OBSTRUCTION

Obstruction to some portion of the gastrointestinal tract is probably the most common cause for inhibiting the adequate ingestion of foodstuff. The symptomatology of many types of alimentary tract obstructions is sufficiently insidious that a patient may be deteriorating gradually for months before actually becoming aware of his digestive impairment. Esophageal obstruction secondary to neoplasm is characterized by gradual changes in tolerance for solid food. Because of increasing discomfort and difficulty during swallowing, the patient with esophageal cancer gradually alters his daily intake in such a manner that an insidious, subclinical form of malnutrition erodes the BCM and energy reserve. These changes may not be clinically apparent in any parameter other than the change in weight. The true magnitude of the effect on body composition, especially on the BCM, is in no way evident from ordinary clinical or laboratory evaluation.

Gastric obstruction most commonly arises from either benign ulcer disease or a malignant lesion, both of which can adversely affect the patient's intake and initiate several nutritional deficiencies. Anorexia, a sense of epigastric fullness, and episodes of vomiting unfavorably affect adequate ingestion. When peptic ulcer disease has persisted for a sufficient time to cause obstruction of outflow, the quality and quantity of intake will inevitably be decreased. Weight loss and protein calorie malnutrition are the natural consequences. The characteristic weight loss associated with visceral malignant disease may reflect a systemic malfunction in nutrient utilization as well as in impaired inges-

tion. In gastric cancer, there is a significant correlation with disordered gastric mucosal function, the most outstanding example being the absence of intrinsic factor. The secondary complications of vitamin B_{12} deficiency are well recognized. Achlorhydria, another gastric mucosal derangement associated with gastric cancer, may be complicated by iron deficiency anemia or reflux alkaline gastritis, or both.

Hepatic and biliary tract diseases are associated with numerous nutritional complications. Obstruction within the biliary tract is caused primarily by cholelithiasis. It is usually an acute event that encourages the patient to seek medical attention promptly, and significant malnutrition from diminished intake is not a part of the usual clinical picture. Noncalculous obstruction of the intrahepatic or extrahepatic bile ducts, as observed in either sclerosing cholangitis or various forms of hepatitis, causes nutritional complications primarily by way of anorexia and abnormal assimilation secondary to hepatic dysfunction. Space-occupying lesions such as hepatocarcinoma or parasitic infestations such as echinococcosis or amebic abscesses evoke changes in intake and also alter proper assimilation of nutrients.

Obstructive lesions within the parenchyma of the pancreas secondary to inflammation, trauma, or neoplasia often result in significant malnutrition. Moreover, acute or chronic pancreatitis is frequently associated with a degree of hepatic insufficiency. The obstructive component of chronic pancreatitis, with or without pseudocyst formation, causes impaired ingestion secondary both to chronic pain and to anorexia. Injury to the pancreas is sometimes associated with subsequent subtle obstructive symptoms indistinguishable from those of any other form of chronic pancreatitis. Unless carcinoma of the pancreas is anatomically located to cause early obstruction of the biliary tree or gastric outlet, weight loss may be the only early evidence of its presence.

Nutritional complicatons arising from impaired ingestion often follow obstruction of the small bowel secondary to postoperative adhesions. Extrinsic pressure from fibrous bands, volvulus, or longitudinal rotation caused by unequal fibrotic contractile forces following previous episodes of peritoneal inflammation are the primary etiologic factors. Malrotation, parasitic infestation, foreign bodies, radiation enteritis, impaired arterial perfusion, and extrinsic pressure from the superior mesenteric artery or mass lesions are other causes for improper small bowel function. Primary small bowel tumors are unusual causes for partial or complete intestinal obstruction, although metastatic cancer is frequently implicated in this process.

Obstruction of the distal ileum is one of the most serious complications of regional enteritis. Fistula and abscess formation are frequently associated with this condition and serve to aggravate the obstruction. Patients who suffer from regional enteritis may have partial obstruction associated with diarrhea, nausea, vomiting, and abdominal pain. The chronic anorexia of these patients is probably caused by a combination of systemic toxicity and partial or complete bowel obstruction.

Adenocarcinoma is the most common cause of colonic obstruction. As with other malignant lesions, the attendant weight loss is due to the presence of anorexia and in part related to the abnormal utilization of available nutrients. With villous adenoma or villous adenocarcinoma, serious nutritional deficiencies can be provoked occasionally by excessive secretion and excretion of mucoprotein, water, and electrolytes, resulting in weight loss and severe muscle weakness. Postoperative adhesions, intermittent volvulus, and intussusception are causative factors in colon-mediated anorexia, vomiting, and attendant nutrient deficiencies. Ulcerative colitis is not a common cause of colonic obstruction unless it is associated with malignant disease or ileus caused by an acute severe exacerbation of the disease. The adverse nutritional effects of this disease are secondary to impairment of appetite, diarrhea, and systemic toxicity. Parasitic infestations of the colon, especially amebic colitis, can produce significant colon obstruction by formation of amebomas, most of which are located in the cecum.

IMPAIRED INGESTION DUE TO NEUROLOGIC DISORDERS

Impaired ingestion caused by neurologic disease is primarily manifested by ileus, dys-functional swallowing, or chronic constipation. Cerebrovascular accidents are the most common cause of dysphagia, regurgitation, and aspiration. Because patients with stroke are likely to be older, difficulties in maintaining adequate oral nutrition only serve to aggravate the nutritional deficiencies commonly found in the elderly, who tend to have poor dietary habits. The true magnitude of the malnutrition existent in such patients is rarely appreciated, measured, or documented. The unfavorable impact of the extreme nutritional depletion of a large percentage of aged stroke patients has not been challenged with adequate nutritional replacement during periods of rehabilitation. Most neurologic diseases impair nutritional equilibrium by impeding intake. Malfunction of colonic evacuation, secondary to the absence of the myenteric plexus, is most commonly manifested in children. The adult form of this disease process is well recognized but is not usually a cause of serious malnourishment.

IMPAIRED INGESTION DUE TO INTRINSIC TISSUE DISEASES

Connective tissue diseases, especially scleroderma, inhibit ingestion through impaired peristaltic activity. The esophagus is most commonly affected, although other portions of the alimentary tract can be involved. The basic defect in this disorder is an abnormality of submucosal connective tissue elements which, through fibrosis and contracture, inhibit motility. Overt weight loss and cachexia develop as ingestion is progressively impaired.

Regional enteritis is an affliction of the small bowel of unknown etiology that is characterized by a chronic transmural inflammatory process. As mentioned previously, obstruction can be a complication of this process when infection and fibrosis compromise the bowel lumen. Patients suffering from this disease frequently have serious nutritional deficiencies long before the surgical complications become manifest. Malaise, lethargy, and anorexia characterize any such inflammatory process, although the causes for these symptoms are not completely understood. Disordered peristaltic activity can cause uneasiness, pain, anorexia, and vomiting. The patient may have partial obstruction, or may have diarrhea due to excessively rapid transit. Many patients receive prolonged corticosteroid therapy, a complication of which is disordered nutritional status. The combination of steroid therapy and infection associated with abscesses and bowel perforations frequently compounds the existing nutritional aberrations in these patients.

Regardless of etiology, colitis causes sufficient discomfort to discourage normal food intake. Ulcerative colitis can be associated with severe malnutrition, not only because of the generalized malfunction of the intestinal tract but also because of the deleterious consequences of the often associated liver disease. Anorexia is a predictable consequence of an inflammatory disease of the large bowel which permits absorption of toxic substances. The medical therapy for this disease is likewise potentially detrimental to normal nutrition.

IMPAIRED DIGESTION AND ABSORPTION

The stomach is primarily a reservoir in which ingested foodstuffs are temporarily held, partially digested, and gradually passed into the small bowel for active degradation and absorption. Nutritional complications arising from gastric deficiencies are principally limited to vitamin B_{12} deficiency, iron deficiency, and an occasional protein-wasting syndrome associated with hypertrophic gastritis.

Since the pancreas is the major source of digestive enzymes, any condition that inhibits normal pancreatic exocrine function must inevitably affect digestion and subsequent absorption. Acute inflammation of the pancreas, whether caused by operative obstruction, cholelithiasis, alcoholism, or any other chemical, viral, or bacterial injury, will impose a serious stress upon metabolic integrity of the organism. During an episode of acute pancreatitis, the patient is not only in a state of self-imposed semistarvation because of abdominal discomfort and anorexia, but treatment is directed toward achieving bowel rest. Semistarvation is the inevitable result of this therapeutic approach. The healthy adult can tolerate a

period of such nutrient deprivation without serious harm for a limited period of time; however, if prolonged, severe malnutrition may develop. With chronic pancreatitis, nutritional deficiencies are common. Pain and intestinal tract malfunction aggravate anorexia. Incomplete digestion and absorption are commonly present, resulting in diarrhea.

Cholelithiasis and neoplasia are the most common causes for obstruction of both the bile duct and pancreatic duct. Failure to secrete the multifunctional pancreatic enzymes into the duodenum will cause severe malnutrition. The absence of bile salts produced in the liver will also prohibit normal digestion of lipids and therefore cause steatorrhea. The attendant weight loss is well documented.

Diseases of the liver, regardless of etiology, probably inflict the greatest single organ disturbances in nutritional status. Acute liver infection or injury can cause immediate interruption of enzyme system functions that can lead to death. Hypoglycemia, hypoproteinemia, hyperammonemia, hyperaminoacidemia, and the inability to detoxify hormones, metabolites, and certain medications are potential acute complications that seriously threaten survival. In chronic liver insufficiency, in which only marginal functional hepatic reserve remains, both absorption and assimilation of foodstuffs are reduced significantly. Under the most extreme circumstances, in which liver blood flow is impaired, as in cirrhosis or following construction of a portacaval shunt, protein metabolism is significantly impaired. The most ominous nutritional manifestation of inadequate hepatic function is that of hepatic encephalopathy, which occurs with only moderate amounts of protein ingestion. Maintenance of even minimal nutritional stability is difficult.

Most of the small bowel diseases contribute to nutritional deficiency by causing impaired absorption rather than impaired ingestion. A reduction in the total absorptive surface, which follows excision of a major portion of the small bowel as a result of some intra-abdominal catastrophe, causes severe nutrient deficiencies. The remaining small bowel mucosa in the duodenum or that portion of residual jejunum or ileum is initially inadequate in its capacity to meet nutritional requirements. With time the bowel undergoes hypertrophy that may become sufficient to maintain nutritional equilibrium. Diseases of the small bowel that impair absorption include regional enteritis, food allergies, excessive secretion (as in sprue), and parasitic infestation. The degree of diminished ability of the intestinal mucosa to function properly in a patient with regional enteritis is highly variable, but most closely related to the amount of small bowel involved and the severity of the inflammatory process. Under the most severe circumstances, especially after several resections have been performed and in which there is a limited amount of small bowel remaining, adequate absorption to maintain normal nutrition may become impossible.

Tropical and non-tropical sprue are characterized by weight loss, weakness, impaired glucose and fat absorption, chronic diarrhea, and steatorrhea. Digestion and absorption of all nutrients are impaired, and the result is a complex combination of several nutritional deficiency states.

IMPAIRED ENDOCRINE FUNCTION

Hypofunction of the pituitary gland is associated with an extremely complex variety of hormonal deficiencies that are in turn manifested in part by nutritional deficiencies. Diminished thyroid, adrenal, and gonadal function can alter every aspect of normal ingestion, digestion, absorption, and assimilation. There is diminished daily basal energy expenditure which is evident as reduced functional organ capacity.

Hyperfunction of the pituitary or adrenal gland is associated with the development of Cushing's syndrome. Whether the stimulus is derived from an accelerated production of corticotropin-stimulating factor, a functioning adenoma of the pituitary, or a functioning lesion within the adrenal cortex, the adverse nutritional effects are identical. Excessive cortisol secretion causes increased gluconeogenesis, which results in somatic protein catabolism, diabetes mellitus, and hypertension. This results in net protein catabolism, with a loss of BCM, accompanied by an increase in body fat.

When increased ACTH production is derived from ectopic sources, primarily oat-cell carcinoma of the lung, the classic

changes in body habitus may not occur. The chronic malnutrition associated with aggressive malignant lesions is usually sufficiently advanced to prevent the development of the usual endocrine-mediated changes.

Pheochromocytomas are functionally active tumors occurring in chromatin tissue that are characterized by the production of large quantities of catecholamines. Norepinephrine is uniformly secreted, and epinephrine is occasionally produced. Paroxysmal or constant hypertension is the most common symptom. Nausea, vomiting, abdominal pain, and weight loss occur regularly. In addition the resting metabolic rate is increased.

Thyrotoxicosis is the product of excess secretion of thyroid hormone caused by either a single adenoma, a toxic nodular goiter, or a diffuse toxic goiter. The symptoms of weight loss, increased appetite, and the sensation of being warm are the result of an increased energy expenditure caused by an elevation in the circulating thyroid hormone. Anorexia, common in elderly patients with this disease, aggravates the existing nutritional deficiencies.

Spontaneous hypothyroidism in the adult is rare, but it is a regular complication of the treatment of hyperthyroidism that includes surgical extirpation or radioactive iodine. The clinical symptoms include a generalized reduction in all system functions, manifested by lethargy, apathy, easy fatigability, and intellectual impairment. There is accumulation of body fat with an attendant weight gain. Functional capacity of both skeletal and cardiac muscle is altered. The response time and endurance for prolonged work is diminished. Symptoms of congestive heart failure are common manifestations of cardiac and hemodynamic impairment. Carefully administered thyroid hormone will effect a restoration of normal metabolic function.

Hypofunction of the endocrine portion of the pancreas, the islet cells, is the most common endocrine dysfunction with which man must cope. The abnormalities caused by decreased production of endogenous insulin represent only one aspect of the total disease process. Under normal circumstances, insulin has the capacity to enhance the transport of glucose into the cell and to potentiate protein synthesis. Diabetes mellitus is a much more complex entity than simply being an insulin deficiency. Every aspect of nutrition can be affected in this disorder. Intake may be excessive or significantly diminished, depending upon the patient's metabolic status. The abnormal utilization of available nutritional substrate in the patient with diabetes mellitus appears to be the major aberration and is probably responsible for the usual pathophysiologic picture.

Hyperfunction of the endocrine portion of the pancreas is much more unusual in its presentation. The most devastating cause of this abnormality is a functioning beta cell tumor. When excessive insulin is produced, the patient experiences episodes of hypoglycemia with all its attendant unpleasant effects, especially upon the central nervous system. Repeated attacks of severe hypoglycemia produce permanent central nervous system damage. Hyperfunctioning islet cells can be the cause for measurable hypoglycemia in patients who are especially sensitive to the delivery of a large carbohydrate meal into the small bowel. The reactive hypoglycemia can be managed by the regular ingestion of non-carbohydrate foodstuffs and does not cause a serious long-term nutritional abnormality. For the sake of completeness it should be noted that hypoglycemia can also be caused by deficiencies in liver function, but this condition has very specific characteristics that can be differentiated from those of pancreatic endocrine hyperfunction.

Parathyroid aberrations have nutritional implications because of the relationship of parathyroid hormone to calcium and phosphorus metabolism. Parathyroid hyperfunction can be caused by a parathyroid adenoma, hyperplasia of the parathyroid tissue, carcinoma of one or more of the parathyroid glands, or non-parathyroid ectopic neoplastic tissues. Osteitis fibrosa cystica, the exaggerated end-stage bony presentation of hyperparathyroidism, is rarely encountered in modern medical practice. This condition results from excessive osteoclastic activity with the resulting dissolution of cortical bone and subsequent cystic degeneration. An associated renal abnormality seems to be directly related to the duration and level of hypercalcemia. Renal calculi are commonly associated with this disease and have the potential of imposing subsequent kidney damage secondary to infection resulting from the attendant urinary tract obstruction. Peptic ulcer disease and pancreatitis are frequent complications of hyperparathyroidism. These patients complain of fatigability, depression, muscle weakness, anorexia, and constipation, along with the symptoms caused by ulcer disease or pancreatitis.

Hypoparathyroidism is most commonly caused by the inadvertent removal of the parathyroid glands during surgical treatment of hyperparathyroidism or thyroid disorders. The most obvious clinical manifestation of hypoparathyroidism is increased neuromuscular excitability caused by a decreased plasma concentration of ionized calcium. The resulting hypocalcemia is manifested by spasms in the fingers, wrists, elbows, legs, or feet. Convulsions may complicate the condition and may even be fatal.

Hyperfunction of ovaries is very unusual and is associated with excessive deposition of body fat. Hypofunction may also be associated with excessive weight gain. Testicular hypofunction is most directly manifested as abnormal development or maintenance of skeletal muscle tissue in the male. Hyperfunction is found in conditions of premature sexual development and an attendant premature development of secondary sexual characteristics.

The Malnutrition of Chronic Illness

The malnutrition that is associated with many chronic diseases is by far the most difficult to define quantitatively. In the majority of instances, by the time there is clinically observable weight loss, pallor, noticeable fatigability, or any one of the many other symptoms to indicate chronic illness, the etiological process has been active for a major portion of the natural history of that disease. In our highly industrialized western society, severe weight loss is most often associated with malignant disease. The relationship between the neoplastic process and the nutritional state is poorly understood. In the majority of patients, when the initial diagnosis of cancer is made, a slight weight loss may be present. However, at this stage most patients are not overtly malnourished. In a small minority of patients, severe cachexia is the presenting sign of an otherwise occult malignancy. The etiological factors responsible for the weight loss associated with cancer are clearly complex and multiple. Widely differing views and experimental results have been expressed in the literature. Weight loss may develop because of anxiety over the developing symptoms of anorexia, dysphagia, and gastrointestinal dysfunction, or possibly because of the metabolic demands of the malignant process. Generally, the deterioration of nutritional status parallels the increase in tumor mass. However, this is not true for all patients. The weight loss of patients with oat-cell carcinoma of the lung is rapid and out of proportion to tumor mass. The opposite is often true for patients with melanoma and breast carcinoma. These patients may have extensive metastatic disease without significant weight loss. Nevertheless, at some time during the treatment of patients with metastatic disease, malnutrition becomes a serious problem, especially since the various modalities of therapy, such as surgery, radiation, and chemotherapy, result in tissue injury and the consequent need for repair.

Progressive malnutrition also accompanies chronic failure of the liver, heart, kidney, and respiratory system. The etiological factors responsible for the malnourished state that develops with these chronic diseases are likewise poorly understood. Anorexia is commonly present and may play an important role. The nutrient requirements may also be increased, as in the patient with chronic bronchitis and emphysema whose work of breathing is significantly elevated. Congestive heart failure is characterized by a decreased cardiac output and an excessive accumulation of extracellular fluid. The resulting bowel edema may impair gastrointestinal function. The decreased oxygen-carrying capacity associated with both cardiac and respiratory failure may also impair the complex biochemical processes that are essential for the maintenance of nutritional equilibrium. The latter processes are undoubtedly affected in the patient with chronic liver disease who has experienced significant parenchymal damage.

THE RESPONSE TO INJURY

In the broadest sense, injury should be interpreted as any event that adversely af-

fects the functional cellular mass of an organism. Within this definition, it is acceptable to include mechanical, thermal, electrical, radiation, bacterial, and autoimmune forces as causes of injury. Many of the cells that receive the immediate impact of any damaging force are destroyed instantly. Those cells that survive seem to respond in a relatively uniform manner. There are both local and systemic responses. In the area of the injury an inflammatory response develops that is characterized by the accumulation of fluid and white blood cells. A complex neuroendocrine reflex is responsible for the systemic response. The integrated effect of these two major areas of response precipitates alterations in innumerable biological systems that create the clinical and laboratory findings known to follow an injury.

When the afferent impulses register the event of peripheral injury in the hypothalamus and brainstem, there is an immediate stimulus to release increased amounts of ACTH, cortisol, growth hormone (GH), and aldosterone. The release of some of the hormones is not entirely dependent upon the integrity of the nerve tracts. The quantitative release of ACTH and subsequent cortisol production is related to the magnitude of the injury. When adrenocortical function is insufficient for any reason, survival may be jeopardized. In addition, catecholamine release is stimulated by efferent impulses from the hypothalamus to the adrenal medulla. Several factors at the site of injury may also initiate a systemic response. Hypovolemia of any cause, whether it be hemorrhage or extracellular fluid sequestration, stimulates the increased release of renin, glucagon, antidiuretic hormone (ADH), epinephrine, norepinephrine, growth hormone (GH), aldosterone, and cortisol.[33]

Munro[40] classified hormones as being anabolic or catabolic according to their effects on somatic protein, especially skeletal muscle. Catabolic hormones have a tendency to mobilize protein, whereas anabolic hormones have the opposite effect. By this functional definition, insulin, growth hormone, androgens, and estrogen in low doses are anabolic, while glucocorticoids, thyroid hormone, progesterone, and estrogen in high doses are catabolic. The integrated sum of the effects of these hormones produces the familiar nutritional effects of the metabolic response to injury, which include increases in energy expenditure, metabolic rate, and urinary nitrogen excretion, and a loss of BCM, accompanied by a tendency to retain salt and water.

The biochemical balances that control metabolism of fats and carbohydrates are especially sensitive to the neuroendocrine stimuli evoked by an injury. Catecholamine secretion increases following almost any injury. Epinephrine stimulates glycogenolysis and inhibits insulin secretion.[44] Norepinephrine has a more pronounced effect than epinephrine in raising serum free fatty acid (FFA) levels through lipolysis.[9] Howard[32] drew attention to the relationship of decreased glucose tolerance and increased resistance to insulin as being proportional to the severity of the injury sustained. Allison[2] described two phases of insulin response to severe injury. In the immediate postinjury phase following a serious burn, the immunoreactive insulin (IRI) level did not change in response to a glucose load. As the acute effects of the severe injury passed, a second recuperative phase followed in which insulin resistance was evidenced by elevated IRI levels in association with relatively normal blood glucose concentrations. Subsequent data have shown a similar effect in other types of injury, and it is postulated that this is a result of the presence of an insulin antagonist stimulated by the neurohormonal response to the injury.[46] The serum FFA levels that are elevated after injury are strong insulin antagonists.[45] The glycogenolytic and lipolytic effects of catecholamines and the relative functional insulin insufficiency combine to contribute postinjury hyperglycemia.

The individual patient's response is dependent upon the age, sex, preinjury nutritional state, and the magnitude of the injury. The same injury will evoke a much greater increase in metabolic expenditure and nitrogen excretion in a well nourished young patient than in one who is elderly and poorly nourished. In contrast to the non-stressed starved individual, the traumatized patient is unable to increase his reliance on endogenous lipids and subsequently decrease the rate of gluconeogenesis from protein.[36] Furthermore, trauma causes an increase in both the resting metabolic rate and negative nitrogen balance. The

magnitude of the metabolic response is directly proportional to the severity of trauma. The resting metabolic expenditure increases by 10 per cent following uncomplicated elective operations, 10 to 25 per cent with multiple fractures, 20 to 50 per cent with major sepsis (e.g., peritonitis), and 50 to 125 per cent with a major thermal burn.[35, 36] The daily negative nitrogen balance is 10 to 15 gm./day following an uncomplicated operation of moderate severity, and 15 to 25 gm./day when injury is complicated with sepsis. With severe injury and sepsis (thermal burns), it may rise to 35 gm./day. These large nitrogen losses are indicative of an extensive erosion of the BCM. A nitrogen loss of 10 gm./day for one month represents a 7 kg. loss of BCM. In a normal 70 kg. man with a BCM of 25 kg., of which 15 kg. are skeletal muscle, this loss is equivalent to 47 per cent of the skeletal muscle mass or 28 per cent of the BCM.[49] A negative nitrogen balance of 30 gm./day for one week represents a 5.3 kg. loss of BCM. At this rate, in excess of 50 per cent of the BCM is lost by 2½ weeks. Thus, starvation and injury, especially when complicated with sepsis, result in a rapid erosion of the cellular mass.

The effect of severe malnutrition on body composition was demonstrated by determining body composition, using multiple isotope dilution, in 75 clinically diagnosed malnourished patients.[51] The majority had developed postoperative complications, and all had been referred for a course of total parenteral nutrition (TPN). Their body composition was characterized by a contracted BCM accompanied by an expansion of the extracellular mass (Fig. 12–5). Their mean body weight was 58.9 ± 1.8 kg., which was 16 per cent less than the mean body weight of 25 normal volunteers. However, the BCM of the malnourished patients was 14.7 ± 0.6 kg., while that of the normal volunteers was 24.7 ± 1.1 kg., a 40 per cent difference. Therefore, the body weight of the malnourished patients did not accurately reflect their nutritional state, primarily because of the expansion of the extracellular mass. The extracellular mass was 23 per cent larger in the malnourished patients than in the normal volunteers.

The effect of moderate injury and starvation was demonstrated by body composition measurements performed before and after

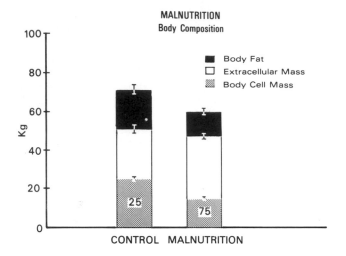

MALNUTRITION
Body Composition

Figure 12–5   The body composition of 75 malnourished patients compared to that of 25 normally nourished volunteers.

an elective operation of moderate severity in 19 normally nourished patients.[51] The majority of patients underwent either a gastrectomy or a colon resection. Body composition was determined preoperatively and on the fifth postoperative day (Table 12–2). Their body composition prior to surgery was normal. By the fifth postoperative day these patients had lost 1.8 ± 0.9 kg. of body fat and 3.2 ± 0.6 kg. of BCM, which is 13.9 per cent of their preoperative BCM. The resected specimen accounted for a portion of this loss of cellular mass. The decrease in the BCM was accompanied by a concomitant 2.4 ± 0.5 kg. expansion of the extracellular mass. As a result, the 3.9 per cent (2.6 ± 0.6 kg.) loss of body weight was not a good reflection of the 13.9 per cent decrease in their cellular mass. The body composition that developed following operation was consistent with the development of mild malnutrition.

Several recent studies have confirmed the hypothesis first proposed by Blackburn that the intravenous infusion of amino acids,

regardless of caloric intake, will prevent the postoperative catabolism of body protein.[5, 20, 26, 31] To assess the protein-sparing effect of amino acid solutions, body composition was measured in 38 patients, prior to and on the fifth postoperative day following elective surgery of moderate severity.[49] The majority of patients underwent either a gastrectomy or colon resection. Preoperatively, they were all normally nourished on the basis of a clinical examination. They were randomly divided to receive all of their postoperative intravenous fluids as either a 5 per cent glucose solution or a 5 per cent casein hydrolysate (Amigen, Travenol-Baxter Laboratories, Canada). In both groups electrolytes were administered as required to maintain electrolyte balance.

By the fifth postoperative day body weight had decreased significantly in both groups (Table 12–3). In patients receiving glucose, the postoperative body weight loss resulted from a loss of lean body mass and body fat. In contrast, weight loss in the patients receiving amino acids intravenously

TABLE 12–2   THE EFFECT OF MAJOR ELECTIVE SURGERY ON BODY COMPOSITION

	Normal Volunteers	Preoperative	Postoperative	Difference (kg.)	(%)
Body Weight (kg.)	70.4 ± 2.5	66.2 ± 1.9	$63.5 \pm 1.8^*$	-2.6 ± 0.6	-3.9
Body Fat (kg.)	20.2 ± 1.4	18.2 ± 1.6	$16.4 \pm 1.5^*$	-1.8 ± 0.9	-9.9
Lean Body Mass (kg.)	50.3 ± 1.9	48.0 ± 1.8	47.2 ± 1.6	-0.8 ± 0.6	-1.7
Extracellular Mass (kg.)	25.8 ± 0.9	24.9 ± 0.9	27.3 ± 0.9	2.4 ± 0.5	9.6
Body Cell Mass (kg.)	24.7 ± 1.1	23.1 ± 1.5	$19.9 \pm 1.4^*$	-3.2 ± 0.6	-13.9

*Significantly ($p < 0.05$) different from preoperative mean by a Student's paired t test.

TABLE 12–3   PROTEIN SPARING WITH I.V. AMINO ACIDS

| | Glucose | | | I.V. Amino Acids | | |
	Pre-Op	Post-Op	Difference	Pre-Op	Post-Op	Difference
Body Weight (kg.)	66.2 ± 1.9	$63.5 \pm 1.8*$	-2.6 ± 0.6	68.1 ± 3.9	$66.5 \pm 3.7*$	-2.0 ± 0.5
Body Fat (kg.)	18.2 ± 1.6	$16.4 \pm 1.5*$	-1.8 ± 0.9	20.0 ± 2.1	$15.9 \pm 2.4*$	-4.1 ± 0.8
Lean Body Mass (kg.)	48.0 ± 1.8	47.2 ± 1.6	-0.8 ± 0.6	48.2 ± 2.5	$50.3 \pm 2.4*$	$+2.1 \pm 0.8$
Extracellular Mass (kg.)	24.9 ± 0.9	27.3 ± 0.9	$+2.4 \pm 0.5$	25.3 ± 1.1	26.5 ± 1.3	$+1.2 \pm 0.6$
Body Cell Mass (kg.)	23.1 ± 1.5	$19.9 \pm 1.4*$	-3.2 ± 0.6	22.9 ± 1.5	23.8 ± 1.3	$+1.0 \pm 0.8$

*Significantly ($p < 0.05$) different from the preoperative mean by Student's paired t test.

resulted entirely from a loss of body fat. Their BCM remained normal following operation. The patients receiving the glucose-containing solutions experienced a significant ($p < 0.001$) loss of BCM. The postoperative loss of BCM was accompanied by an expansion of the extracellular mass — changes that are characteristic of mild malnutrition. Thus, the infusion of amino acids intravenously at a daily rate of 1.8 ± 0.2 gm./kg. body weight effectively prevented the malnutrition that developed in the control patients.

Blackburn and co-workers[5] attributed the protein sparing achieved with intravenous amino acids to the avoidance of glucose-containing solutions. In the absence of an adequate caloric intake, the average postoperative patient must rely on endogenous fuels to meet daily energy requirements. They postulated that the infusion of glucose increased the plasma insulin concentration, which in turn inhibited the mobilization of lipid and promoted gluconeogenesis from body protein to meet this caloric deficit. In support of this hypothesis, they reported an inverse correlation between both the plasma glucose and insulin concentrations and nitrogen sparing. A positive correlation was also present between nitrogen sparing and the plasma concentrations of both free fatty acids and ketone bodies. Subsequent studies have demonstrated that the protein sparing effects of amino acid solutions are a function of the amino acids themselves and are not affected by the additional infusion of either lipids or glucose.[20, 26] Protein sparing is therefore related to the infusion of the appropriate amino acids and not to the avoidance of glucose.

Physical trauma creates both immediate and long-term effects that are determined, for the most part, by the magnitude or severity of the injuring force. When the injuring force is of moderate degree and administered under well controlled conditions, as with elective surgery, the changes that result from this insult may only be detected at the hormonal level. There is no significant increase in energy requirements or nitrogen excretion following uncomplicated cholecystectomy. When the trauma imposed on the patient is of greater severity as with automobile injuries or major thermal trauma, a full spectrum of changes in calorie and nitrogen metabolism is produced. Infection from any cause further aggravates the metabolic status. Nutritional complications are derived not only from the excessive utilization of endogenous stores, but also from the inability of the patient to maintain an adequate intake. Food ingestion may be impaired because of generalized sepsis or because of an incompetent or malfunctioning gastrointestinal tract.

The most common perioperative process in which nutritional status must be given consideration is ileus, which is characterized by absence of normal peristaltic action within the bowel. Ileus is usually classified as being either adynamic or spastic. Adynamic ileus is the more common form and is associated with any condition that inhibits the neuromuscular function of the bowel. Any type of mechanical, chemical, or bacterial trauma to the bowel can initiate adynamic ileus. When adynamic ileus is precipitated by acute pancreatitis, retroperitoneal hematoma, or generalized peritonitis, a very prolonged period of disordered peristalsis and subsequent inhibition of normal intake must be anticipated and taken into account during medical and nutritional therapy. The causes for spastic ileus are less common. The hypertonicity of the bowel is usually associated with some metabolic derangement such as heavy metal intoxication or serious fluid and electrolyte aberrations. This form of ileus can be overcome fairly promptly with the proper therapeutic management of the primary disease process.

Bowel fistulas have always been associated with significant morbidity and mortality. Edmunds, Williams and Welch[17] found that the daily output of the fistula was the most accurate factor in prediction of closure and patient survival. The volume of the fistula drainage appeared to decrease progressively as the anatomic site of origin approached the rectum. MacFadyen, Dudrick, and Ruberg[38] have shown that with bowel rest and intravenous hyperalimentation these principles do not necessarily apply. Enterocutaneous fistulas are more successfully managed by this technique than internal fistulas. Before the institution of current practices in nutritional therapy, the complications of inadequate intake and assimilation were the primary causes of the rather high morbidity and mortality. Even if the patient was capable of ingesting food, there was little possibility of proper digestion or absorption, unless the fistula was located in the distal ileum or colon. The effects of semistarvation together with subsequent infection and inordinate losses of body fluid accelerated the depletion of endogenous nutrient sources.

Nutritional Complication Arising from Surgical Procedures

Any surgical procedure involving the gastrointestinal tract has the potential for causing nutritional complications. In most instances, the interval required for recovery of the gastrointestinal tract following elective operations is sufficiently brief to permit resumption of normal feedings and thereby avoid any serious nutritional deficiency.

Chronic obstruction of the esophagus imposes serious limitations on intake long before corrective surgical therapy is undertaken. The obstruction must be managed by either resecting the obstructed segment or performing some bypass procedure. Successful management will depend upon the nutritional status of the patient prior to the operation. The most common complication of an esophageal resection is anastomotic leak. Adequate preoperative nutritional preparation and postoperative bowel rest are the best means of reducing the incidence of this catastrophic complication.

Gastric surgery, for whatever indication, causes potential nutritional complications. A distal gastric resection can cause transient dumping in any patient who is fed a high-osmolar liquid meal. It is most unusual for the dumping process to cause severe enough symptoms to warrant surgical intervention. Successful techniques for managing the severe weight loss and malnutrition that occur in some patients have been reported by Herrington,[29] Buchwald,[7] and Rutledge.[47] Dietary discretion appears to be adequate for the majority of patients. Nutritional complications may also develop when a gastroenterostomy is created to restore gastrointestinal continuity. A partially obstructed or excessively long afferent loop of jejunum can be associated with chronic pain, vomiting, blind-loop syndrome, and malnourishment. If the efferent loop is partially obstructed, symptoms will usually be related to overdistention and poor drainage of the gastric pouch as well as reflux into the afferent loop. Alkaline reflux gastritis and esophagitis are well recognized entities associated with any procedure that obliterates the function of the pylorus. Vitamin B_{12} deficiency is also a recognizable complication secondary to the loss of intrinsic factor or blind-loop syndrome. The addition of vagotomy to an operative procedure imposes other potential complications. Diarrhea is a common early complication that usually disappears. Some evidence has suggested that there is an increased incidence of cholelithiasis and cholecystitis following vagotomy, although it remains unconfirmed. The cardinal manifestation of nutritional deficiencies that attend gastric surgery as complications is weight loss. The patients either are unable to eat, are unable to retain that which they do eat, lack the ability to absorb the nutritional substrate, or have excessively rapid transit through the gut.

Operations on the biliary tree do not usually have long-term nutritional complications unless infection or complete obstruction ensues. In the rare total biliary fistula, malabsorption of fat can lead to body wasting, and therapy with bile salts becomes mandatory. Operations on the duodenum and pancreas carry a higher risk of significant nutritional complications. Following the removal of a major portion of the pancreas, malabsorption and diabetes mellitus can occur. Substitutional pancreatic endocrine and exocrine therapy may be necessary. If severe, replacement therapy of both the endocrine and exocrine function should be instituted.

Hepatic resection is usually associated with a transient period of impaired liver function and the attendant suppression of biosynthetic capabilities. Because the hepatic parenchyma possesses the unique capacity for regeneration, most patients rapidly recover an acceptable functional liver mass.

The most serious and common complication following major small bowel resection is insufficient mucosal surface for adequate absorption. This occurs most commonly in patients who have survived a massive small bowel infarction due to either arterial or venous occlusion. Because of the inadequate absorption capability, malnutrition and inanition are inevitable.

Colon operations, including total colectomy, are usually associated with nutritional deficiencies. For the most part, resection of the diseased colon significantly improves the patient's capacity to eat and gain weight. However, with ileostomy or colostomy, obstruction or malfunction symptoms may at times result in a decreased oral intake.

Postoperative infection can cause significant nutritional impairment, over and above the potential nutritional complications secondary to the procedure itself. The severity of infection, the age of the patient, and the nature of the primary disease contribute significantly to the potential consequences.

Infection almost invariably results in an increased metabolic rate, which, in turn, increases the demand on endogenous resources. Anorexia is commonly present, and the function of the gastrointestinal tract is often impaired, especially with peritonitis and with wound dehiscence secondary to a serious wound infection.

Nutritional Complications Arising from Medical Therapy

Many of the myriad agents and combinations used in the chemotherapy of malignant diseases exert their effects as antimetabolites by interfering with cell division, protein synthesis, vitamin utilization, cell membrane structure and function, and so forth. Although these are favorable actions against the neoplastic cells, normal tissues are also adversely affected to varying degrees, and significant nutritional aberrations can result.

Exogenous steroid therapy is often employed for a wide spectrum of diseases that are characterized by some form of inflammatory process. Steroids classically invoke gluconeogenesis, resulting in a diabetogenic potential. These drugs will also seriously impair protein synthesis. The onset and magnitude of the malnutrition in these patients are insidious and frequently not well recognized until the patient experiences some stressful event. As in any patient with elevated serum levels of cortisone, there are increased susceptibility to infection, poor wound healing, and fluid and electrolyte imbalance.

Antibiotic administration may give rise to anorexia, nausea, vomiting, diarrhea, lethargy, malaise, and easy fatigability. Significant long-term nutritional complications arising from antibiotic administration fortunately are not common. On rare occasions, antibiotic therapy may result in impaired renal function that progresses to anuric renal failure, which, in turn, can precipitate enormous nutritional problems. Alterations in bowel flora, secondary to the administration of non-absorbable as well as systemic antibiotics, occasionally cause short-term but significant malfunction of the bowel. Cessation of antibiotic administration is usually associated with recovery.

RECOGNITION OF NUTRITIONAL COMPLICATIONS IN THE SURGICAL PATIENT

The presence of nutritional deficiencies is easily recognized by the average observer. The grotesque appearance of starving human beings in tortured captivity or among populations experiencing widespread starvation is well known and frequently is the first impression brought to mind at the suggestion of malnutrition. Almost any person has had the experience of witnessing massive weight loss in a friend or relative who is gradually deteriorating from systemic malignant disease. The astute observer can frequently recognize much more subtle changes in the body configuration and general countenance of a person with whom he is familiar. For the most part, these changes will result from a loss in facial muscle mass and tone as well as possible alterations in skin color. Anemia is one of the more common causes for the pallor associated with chronic disease and malnutrition, but others are possible. A person who is familiar with the patient may have a keener sense of change in the total body appearance than the physician who sees the patient for the first time.

A large number of patients seeking medical and surgical care for disease processes such as those described in previous sections of this chapter have incurred various degrees of clinical malnutrition that are not readily identified. The difficulty in recognizing these conditions has led to the widespread use of complicated schemes of nutritional assessment, based on biochemical and anthropometric measurements, often combined with a determination of cutaneous response to a battery of recall antigens.[6, 12, 24, 39, 42, 57] These measurements have for many years been performed in epidemiological surveys to assess a population's nutritional status and only recently have been applied to assess the nutritional state of the hospitalized patient. Serum albumin is frequently measured, as it is usually decreased with protein-calorie malnutri-

tion. The excretion rate of creatinine, a breakdown product of muscle, is a function of muscle mass, and therefore, the 24-hour creatinine excretion rate, expressed as a function of body height, may be determined to obtain a measure of the cellular mass. The weight/height ratio and the mid-arm muscle area are also measures of the BCM and therefore commonly used to determine the presence of protein-calorie malnutrition. Body fat is estimated by measuring the triceps skin fold. The major advantages of these measurements are that they are simple and inexpensive and provide quantitative and reproducible data. In addition, specialized equipment and highly trained personnel are not required.

As mentioned previously, these techniques have recently been applied clinically to assess the nutritional state of the hospitalized patient. The reliability of this approach was evaluated by simultaneously measuring body composition, serum albumin, serum total protein, mid-arm area, triceps skin fold, creatinine/height ratio, hand strength, and weight/height ratio in 216 patients.[19] The population consisted of both normal and malnourished patients and morbidly obese individuals before and after weight reduction surgery. The majority of malnourished patients were receiving TPN.

A statistically significant correlation (p < 0.001) existed between the serum albumin concentration and the BCM. However, the correlation coefficient was only 0.67 and the 95 per cent confidence limits about the regression were wide (Fig. 12–6). For a

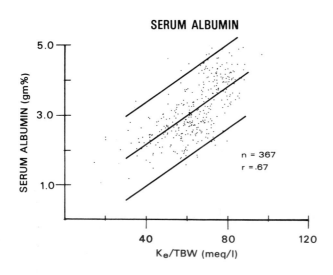

SERUM ALBUMIN

n = 367
r = .67

Figure 12–6 The serum albumin concentration, determined by serum electrophoresis correlated with the body cell mass, measured by exchangeable potassium (K_e) divided by total body water (TBW) to normalize the data for body size (n = 367). The correlation was statistically significant (p <0.001) with a correlation coefficient of 0.67.

TABLE 12–4   CORRELATION OF BIOCHEMICAL AND ANTHROPOMETRIC PARAMETERS OF NUTRITIONAL ASSESSMENT WITH BODY COMPOSITION MEASUREMENTS

Parameter (Dependent)	Body Composition Parameter (Independent)	n	r	Mean	95 Per Cent Confidence Limits
Weight/Height (kg./m.)	K_e	331	0.82	48.9	25.3 to 72.5
Triceps Skin Fold (mm.)	Body Fat	358	0.79	17.2	3.7 to 30.7
Mid-Arm Area (Sq. dm.)	K_e	358	0.68	0.54	0.10 to 0.98
Albumin (mg./dl.)	K_e/TBW	367	0.67	3.2	2.0 to 4.4
Total Protein (mg./dl)	K_e/TBW	367	0.62	6.6	5.0 to 8.2
Hand Strength (kp./sq. cm.)	K_e/TBW	86	0.45	0.41	0.03 to 0.79
Creatinine/Height (mg./m.)	K_e/TBW	331	0.37	7.1	−6.3 to 20.5

normal BCM, the regression predicted a serum albumin concentration of 3.8 gm./dl. with 95 per cent confidence limits of 2.6 and 5.0 gm./dl. In our institution the normal range for serum albumin, as determined by electrophoresis, is 3.5 to 5 gm./dl. Based on these criteria, our sample population consisted of a number of normally nourished individuals with a subnormal serum albumin, and malnourished individuals with a normal serum albumin. Similar results were obtained with the other parameters examined. Although all of the correlation coefficients were statistically significant ($p < 0.05$), the correlations were poor (Table 12–4). With all of the parameters, the 95 per cent confidence limits were wide. The best correlation ($r = 0.82$) was obtained with the weight/height ratio, and the worst ($r = 0.37$) with creatinine/height.

Data obtained by repeating the measurements in 179 patients permitted an assessment of the ability of the anthropometric and biochemical measurements to detect changes in body composition.[19] Sixty-nine patients were initially malnourished and experienced an improvement in their nutritional status, as indicated by an improvement in body composition. The anthropometric measurements did not reflect this improvement. Weight, mid-arm area, creatinine/height, and hand strength did not change significantly. The serum albumin and total protein concentration increased slightly. Neither the triceps skin fold nor total body fat changed. Similar data were obtained in 25 normally nourished individuals who became malnourished and in 42 malnourished patients whose nutritional state deteriorated.

The presence of a statistically significant correlation between each of the parameters evaluated and the nutritional state indicates that they accurately measure the mean nutritional state of a population. They are therefore useful in epidemiological surveys. The wide confidence limits and the failure to detect significant changes in the nutritional state demonstrate the lack of sufficient sensitivity and specificity. They are therefore of little value in assessing an individual's nutritional state.

Similar results were obtained when the nutritional state was evaluated by means of skin testing. A relationship between immune competence and the nutritional state was demonstrated in 257 hospitalized patients (459 studies) receiving TPN. These patients represent a population with a high incidence of malnutrition, in whom it is possible to measure accurately protein and caloric intake. Immune competence was assessed by skin testing with 5 recall antigens: purified protein derivative of tuberculin (PPD), mumps, candidin, trichophytin, and streptokinase-streptodornase. The patients were classified as normal, relatively anergic, or anergic if they reacted to at least two, one, or none of the recall antigens, respectively. Body composition measurements and skin testing were performed at the beginning and at 2-week intervals during TPN.

A relationship between the nutritional state and the response to skin testing was demonstrated. A deterioration of immune competence, as indicated by the development of relative anergy or anergy, was associated with a body composition characteristic of malnutrition. The difference in the body composition of the reactive and aner-

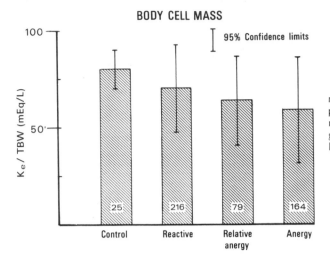

Figure 12–7 The mean body cell mass, as determined by total exchangeable potassium (K_e), expressed as a function of total body water (TBW) in 25 normal volunteers and in the reactive, relatively anergic, and anergic patients. The 95 per cent confidence limits for each group of patients are included.

gic patients was statistically significant (Fig. 12–7). In each group, there were wide 95 per cent confidence limits about the mean, indicating an overlap between the reactive and anergic patients. Thus, 93 (43 per cent) of the 216 reactive patients were malnourished, and 35 (21.3 per cent) of the 129 anergic patients had a normal body composition.

The reliability of skin testing to evaluate the nutritional state is similar to the reliability of the anthropometric and biochemical parameters. Because of the large variance associated with the response to skin testing, it is of little value in evaluating an individual's nutritional state. The presence of a statistically significant relationship between the response to skin testing and the nutritional state indicates that skin testing can be reliably employed in epidemiological surveys to determine a population's nutritional state.

Body composition measurements will accurately and quantitatively assess the nutritional state and determine the efficacy of nutritional support. The measurements are complex and time consuming and require specialized facilities and specially trained personnel. They are therefore not suitable for the routine clinical laboratory but are ideal for research purposes.

A good history and physical examination are often all that is needed to establish the requirements for nutritional support. In the majority of patients, the requirement for nutritional support is clinically obvious without the need to perform specialized measurements. The nature of and the length of nutritional support can also be established clinically. The patient with an obstructing esophageal carcinoma, a history of decreased food intake, and weight loss should be nutritionally repleted before undergoing a major surgical procedure. Nutritional repletion is indicated by weight gain, loss of edema, increased muscle strength, increased work capacity, an improvement in appetite, and a sense of well-being. In contrast, the presence of malnutrition and the need for nutritional repletion should not delay surgical intervention to drain an abscess, relieve bowel obstruction, or drain a septic biliary tract. On the other hand, the absence of malnutrition does not contraindicate nutritional support, especially for the patient in whom a prolonged inadequate oral intake is anticipated. Thus, nutritional support is indicated for the patient with an enteric cutaneous fistula even in the absence of malnutrition. For the vast majority of patients, a complete history and physical examination will provide all the information required to arrive at the appropriate decisions regarding nutritional therapy.

MANAGEMENT OF NUTRITIONAL COMPLICATIONS IN THE SURGICAL PATIENT

After the physician has determined a special need for nutritional supplementation, he or she is faced with the problem of determining the best possible method for administering this therapy. It has only been within the past decade that development of new techniques of enteral and parenteral feeding have allowed more choices for reasonable solutions to most of the nutritional problems encountered.[4, 13, 14, 27, 28, 55]

A consideration of the methods by which nutritional substrate can be administered involves two basic principles: the method of administration and the chemical composition of the regimen. The nutrient ration must be introduced into the patient either via the gastrointestinal tract or into the venous system. Nutritional support is best achieved by having a patient consume a balanced diet. However, this requires the presence of both a normal appetite and a normally functioning gastrointestinal tract. Manipulation of the appearance, preparation, and taste of the diet will substantially increase food consumption in the individual with a normal appetite but will only marginally affect the intake of the anorexic patient. An adequate oral intake is extremely difficult to achieve in the patient with severe anorexia. Tube feedings are employed in patients with a normally functioning gastrointestinal tract who, for a variety of reasons, have an inadequate oral intake. This includes patients who are comatose or anorexic or who have a mechanical obstruction of either the pharynx or the esophagus. The most effective tube feedings are commonly achieved through nasogastric or jejunostomy instillations. Intravenous feedings can be infused via peripheral or central veins. With the nutritional substrates currently available, a much greater quantity of calories and nitrogen-containing amino acids can be administered by the intravenous route.

The chemical composition of nutrient formulations can vary from that of simple cooked foods to that of an intravenous solution comprising all known elements required for growth, development, and tissue repair. For many decades, the primary method for meeting nutritional deficiencies in patients who could not otherwise ingest adequate quantities of food was some form of liquid tube feeding. For the most part, this was a milk-based formula to which was added a variety of fats, sugars, and vitamins.

The recent availability of free L-amino acids for parenteral use has promoted new approaches to nutritional therapy. It is now possible to maintain for many years patients who have lost gastrointestinal function and are totally dependent on parenteral nutrition.

NASOGASTRIC TUBE FEEDING

Because of ready access to the gastrointestinal tract through a nasogastric tube, it is frequently used as a feeding route. The advantages of this technique are that it avoids the necessity for a gastrostomy or jejunostomy, and the foodstuffs are digested and absorbed in a normal sequence. Nasogastric tube feeding is associated with serious and occasionally life-threatening complications. It should not be attempted in any patient who is obtunded for any reason or who otherwise has impaired pharyngeal reflexes. Reflux of gastric contents with a subsequent tracheobronchial contamination causes a potentially life-threatening pneumonitis. Because spillage of gastric content can occur around the inflated balloon, the presence of a cuffed endotracheal tube does not insure that gastric reflux will not occur.

Patients with chronic lesions in the proximal portion of the gastrointestinal tract are especially suited for nasogastric tube feedings. Chronic nutritional problems associated with oropharyngeal tumor management can be satisfactorily managed with a cervical esophagostomy.[25] Complications other than aspiration pneumonitis include pressure erosions of the nasopharyngeal and laryngeal tissues, obstruction, eustachitis, parotitis, and esophageal stricture. A variety of small (8 to 10 F) soft tubes have been developed that are extremely well tolerated by the majority of patients.

GASTROSTOMY FEEDING

Because of the previously described advantages of introducing foodstuffs into the stomach when there is gastrointestinal continuity, several gastrostomy techniques have been described and practiced to avoid a nasogastric tube. The risk of regurgitation and aspiration of gastric contents is not avoided with the use of a gastrostomy. The simplest temporary gastrostomy is fashioned by the introduction of a large catheter through the anterior gastric wall. The stomach is then approximated to the abdominal wall to prevent spillage into the peritoneal cavity. After removal of the catheter, the gastrostomy has a great propensity for spontaneous closure. If the catheter is accidentally removed it must be replaced immediately. Feeding should not be reinstituted until a radiopaque contrast study has verified the location of the catheter in the stomach. In those circumstances in which long-term tube feeding is indicated, a permanent gastrostomy, characterized by a mucosa-lined orifice from the skin to the gastric pouch, should be considered. By means of the Glassman technique,[22] as modified by Gibbon, Nealon, and Greco,[21] a mucosa-lined tract is created from the anterior stomach wall. An interposed jejunal loop has been used by others with some success.

JEJUNOSTOMY FEEDING

Nasogastric or gastrostomy feeding is contraindicated in the comatose or obtunded patient who continuously regurgitates gastric contents. Similarly, gastric feeding is contraindicated for the patient with a gastric or duodenal fistula. The long-term nutritional requirements of these patients can occasionally be achieved with jejunostomy feeding. The Witzel jejunostomy, which is a serosa-lined tunnel fashioned over a catheter that has been placed into the antimesenteric border of the jejunum, is most frequently employed. When the tube is removed, the tract generally closes rapidly. If reinsertion is desired, the location of the catheter tip within the lumen of the jejunum must be verified by water-soluble radiopaque substances before feeding is reinstituted. Tragic consequences due to the infusion of foodstuff into the peritoneal cavity have been reported when this precaution is not taken.

On rare occasions the permanent Roux-en-Y anastomosis is employed for feeding when the upper alimentary tract is chronically or permanently disabled. As with permanent gastrostomy, the mucosa-lined jejunum permits easy repeated entrance into the lumen of the bowel. The permanent jejunostomy has the advantage of minimizing gastric reflux in patients with diminished pharyngeal and laryngeal reflexes. The greatest limitation of chronic jejunostomy feeding is the relatively high incidence of attendant diarrhea.

ENTERIC DIETS

A wide variety of options are available for the patient who requires enteric tube feeding. These options vary from the blenderized diet prepared in the hospital's dietary department to the chemically defined diet. An enteric diet prepared by blenderizing cooked food is economical and will generally provide a completely balanced diet. There are, however, several serious deficiencies associated with its use. Its protein source is usually milk and therefore contributes to fecal residue, and it is not well tolerated by patients with lactose intolerance. These formulations tend to be viscous and therefore difficult to administer with small diameter tubes. They are generally contaminated with bacteria, and excessive delays from the time of preparation to administration or improper refrigeration will allow significant microbial proliferation that causes serious diarrhea. A number of commercial products are currently available that are similar to the blenderized diet, consisting of polypeptides, polysaccharides, and fat. These meal replacement solutions are generally not hypertonic, as their constituents are in a high molecular weight form. The commercial products generally provide a more complete diet, and since they are less viscous, they are easily administered with small tubes. Because they are bacteriologically sterile, they do not require refrigeration and can be administered at room temperature. In addition, the majority are low residue and lactose-free. These commercial products are generally inexpensive and should be used instead of the blenderized formulas produced by the hospital's dietary department.

The meal replacement formulas described above are generally well tolerated by the majority of patients who require enteric tube feeding. In contrast, a chemically defined diet is theoretically indicated for pa-

TABLE 12–5 COMPOSITION OF CURRENT CHEMICALLY DEFINED DIETS*
(Units/1000 KCal.)

	Vivonex 100	Vivonex High Nitrogen	W-T Low Residue Food	Flexical
Carbohydrates, gm.	226 Glucose, glucose oligosaccharides	210 Glucose oligosaccharides	226 Dextrin	155 Sucrose
Nitrogen, gm.	3.27 amino acids	6.67 amino acids	3.0 amino acids	3.5 protein hydrolysate and added amino acids
Protein, gm.	20.4	41.7	18.8	21.9
Fat, gm.	0.74 safflower oil and linoleic acid	0.44 safflower oil	0.74 safflower oil	34.0
Sodium, mEq.	57.6	35.5	55.7	15.7
Potassium, mEq.	29.9	17.9	30.0	38.9
Calcium, mEq.	22.1	13.3	27.8	26.0
Magnesium, mEq.	7.11	9.6	18.4	14.6
Iron, mEq.	0.19	0.11	0.34	0.02
Chloride, mEq.	71.2	52.2	85.0	34.3
Osmolarity: mOs./L.	1175	844	649	805

*All chemically defined diets contain standard additions of fat- and water-soluble vitamins for estimated normal daily requirements and essential trace elements. Vitamin B, C, and K should be supplemented to this diet program. (Adapted from: Nutrition Gap. Eaton Laboratories, Norwich, N.Y.; W-T Low Residue Food. Warren-Teed Pharmaceuticals, Inc., Columbus, Ohio; Flexical, Low-Residue Elemental Diet. Mead-Johnson Laboratories, Evansville, Indiana.)

tients who have a gastrointestinal tract with impaired digestive function. This includes patients with pancreatic insufficiency, short bowel, and inflammatory bowel disease.

All known elementary nutrients required for growth and support of life have been combined in varying concentrations to formulate the various chemically defined diets now available. The nitrogen-containing compounds are derived from free L-amino acids or the hydrolysates of complete proteins (Table 12–5). The chemically defined diets are characterized by (1) having zero residue, (2) requiring minimal or no digestion, (3) having the potential to maintain body weight, calorie balance, and nitrogen balance, and (4) having a disagreeable taste. Many attempts have been directed toward the elimination of the unpleasant taste, which prohibits the enthusiastic acceptance by the patient of this mode of therapy.

Some patients have been able to successfully ingest large quantities of a chemically defined diet for a sufficiently long time to achieve non-operative closure of bowel fistulas or significant improvement in inflammatory bowel disease.[15] Infusion of the chemically defined diet through nasogastric feeding tubes permits delivery of a large daily ration of nitrogen-containing compounds.[52] In developing countries in which hyperalimentation is not available, the infusion of chemically defined diets through nasogastric feeding tubes has proven successful in the chronic management of patients who have severe peritonitis secondary to typhoid perforations of the ileum or neglected perforated appendicitis.[16]

Much effort has been made to improve the taste of chemically defined diets. Recently diets have been produced in which the nitrogen source is derived primarily from short-chain peptides rather than from free amino acids alone. With such diets, the unpleasant flavor seems to be more easily masked and the opportunity exists to manipulate either the total nitrogen content or the osmolarity, as the clinical circumstances require. The chemically defined diet is of special value in outpatient management of disease processes in which it is desirable to completely eliminate roughage from the alimentary tract. Regional ileitis seems to respond favorably in some cases to such therapy. After the initial period of bowel rest has been achieved by a period of intravenous hyperalimentation, an outpatient trial of chemically defined dietary therapy is often a very practical and economical regimen.

There is a small but growing experience with the utilization of chemically defined diets for preoperative preparation of the large bowel. By this technique, positive nitrogen and calorie balance can be maintained while simultaneously taking advantage of this residue-free form of nutrition to completely clear the large bowel of all forms of particulate material. Reports have indicated that a substantial alteration in fecal content is achieved with preoperative preparation using an elemental diet, but no significant change in bacterial flora has been effected.[23]

Failure to achieve an adequate dietary intake with enteric tube feeding is generally due to the development of either gastric stasis or diarrhea. In the anorexic patient, enteric tube feeding often fails in spite of an intact G.I. tract, because of gastric stasis. To minimize the complications associated with enteric feeding, the following protocol should be followed. Prior to the infusion of any feeding, the proper placement of the feeding tube must be established radiographically. Initially, quarter strength formula is administered at room temperature using a continuous infusion pump. The initial rate is 50 ml./hr. The rate is increased by 25 ml./hr. each day until the required volume is achieved. Then the concentration is increased in a stepwise fashion each day, initially to half strength, then to three-quarter, and finally to full strength. It is important that enteric tube feeding be infused at a constant rate and not as a bolus, as this often produces diarrhea. If either diarrhea or gastric stasis develops, the infusion rate or the concentration is reduced. The presence of gastric stasis is determined by aspirating the stomach at hourly intervals. Aspiration of a large volume is indicative of stasis. Diarrhea may be precipitated by the instillation of tube feeding that is either hypertonic, too cold, or grossly contaminated with bacteria. Diarrhea is more common with the chemically defined diets, as opposed to the meal replacement diets, since the former generally contain far more osmotically active particles.

Intravenous Hyperalimentation

INDICATIONS

With the advent of total parenteral nutrition (TPN) it has become possible to meet nutritional requirements in patients in whom use of the gastrointestinal tract was impossible or ill advised. For the first time, the surgeon has been able to restore nutritional status to such an extent that operative intervention can either be avoided or undertaken with much greater confidence of success.

With the development of the capacity to administer intravenously all of the amino acids, calories, vitamins, minerals, and trace elements necessary for growth and development, favorable solutions have arisen to heretofore impossible clinical problems.

Many patients with disease processes that are either caused by or associated with a serious nutritional deficiency may profit from a period of repletion. If the nature of the disease process will permit delay, as in some cases of multiple gastrointestinal fistulas, several weeks or even months of nutritional supplementation may permit satisfactory surgical correction and postoperative recovery. On the contrary, in some disease processes a prolonged preoperative period of replenishment of nutritional substrate would not be in the best interest of the patient. Serious malnutrition in association with focal infection or large abscesses should not be corrected before drainage is effected in most cases. These deficiencies can be corrected more safely in the postoperative period. In some circumstances, after the patient has achieved sufficient improvement in nutritional status and function of the gastrointestinal tract, a less expensive and less complex technique for provision of nutritional substrate can be instituted. When an initial period of bowel rest in inflammatory intestinal disease has been the goal and has been achieved with TPN, an outpatient program with a chemically defined or low-roughage diet may be practical.

Intravenous hyperalimentation should not be expected to correct or alleviate clinical problems that are beyond the range of its capability. It is not a panacea for all disease processes that are associated with some form of malnutrition. A most difficult decision the physician faces is whether to institute TPN therapy in critically ill patients, with a hopeless prognosis, such as infants with total small bowel atresia or persons with incurable malignant disease in whom TPN is the only method of sustaining life. However, the malnutrition associated with malignant disease can be favorably altered with this technique. The proper utilization of TPN in association with chemotherapeutic agents can significantly improve the response to the antineoplastic therapy.[10] On the other hand, TPN cannot be expected to completely eradicate the nutritional deficiencies caused by the presence of unresectable or otherwise untreatable malignant lesions.

MacFadyen et al.[38] have reported spontaneous closure of 70.5 per cent of all gastrointestinal fistulas when TPN and bowel rest were used as the basic therapy. Another 21.8 per cent of the fistulas were successfully closed surgically after a preoperative period of nourishment with TPN. The overall mortality rate in this series of 78 fistulas in 62 patients was 6.45 per cent. On the other hand, the technique of TPN should not be expected to effect permanent closure of a fistula when there is an associated abscess, distal obstruction, foreign body, malignant lesion, visible everted mucosa, or epithelization of the fistulous tract.

Intravenous hyperalimentation is especially applicable to the correction of nutritional deficiencies caused by diseases that have prevented adequate intake. Obstruction of the gastrointestinal tract, as with carcinoma of the esophagus, prolonged ileus due to chronic peritonitis, single or multiple fistulas, or poor nourishment in the elderly are examples of states that will benefit from a course of adequate preoperative parenteral nutrition. The optimal length of time to be devoted to nutritional preparation prior to non-emergency surgery has not been absolutely determined. It is very common for the chronically malnourished patient to lose weight for several days following institution of TPN. This probably represents the mobilization and excretion of nutritional edema in the presence of an actual net gain in BCM.

Patients suffering from impairment in digestion or absorption may profit significantly from a brief or prolonged preoperative TPN program, depending on the nature of the disorder. Chronic pancreatic insufficiency renders a patient significantly malnourished because of the absence of adequate ingestion and digestion. These patients will often require a prolonged course of TPN prior to operation, while postoperatively they may readily tolerate oral intake. The patient who has lost virtually all of the small bowel because of a cataclysmic vascular accident will require TPN, while the remaining bowel becomes hypertrophied in surface and function to allow at least partial nutritional support from the oral intake of foodstuffs. During the first two months, these patients are maintained without any oral intake, while all nourishment is provided by the parenteral route. Throughout the third month, oral intake is gradually increased, first with fluids, electrolytes, vitamins, simple sugars, and proteins, and later with low-fat, high-protein nutrients, while the TPN is concomitantly reduced. Coconut oil can be given as a source of medium-chain triglycerides, and safflower oil can be given to provide essential fatty acids and vitamin E. Codeine, diphenoxylate hydrochloride (Lomotil), and anticholinergic agents help to reduce bowel motility and gastric hypersecretion. Supplementary calcium and liquid vitamins should be given by mouth. Sodium bicarbonate may be required for months to counteract the tendency to metabolic acidosis in these patients. Vitamin B_{12} and folic acid must be given intramuscularly for life in patients with less than 2 feet of bowel distal to the ligament of Treitz.

Chronic renal failure not only impairs a patient's sense of well-being and appetite but also causes aberrations within the protein-synthetic pathways. As an adjunct to the management of patients with renal failure, a special TPN formulation of essential L-amino acids and the other nonnitrogenous nutrients has been valuable in reducing blood urea nitrogen levels, and the frequency of dialysis. There is also an associated reduction in morbidity and mortality.[1] Blood urea is a readily available source of amide groups for the synthesis of nonessential amino acids. When all of the essential amino acids are available, the protein-synthetic mechanisms are capable of utilizing urea as a nitrogen source for the synthesis of non-essential amino acids. Moreover, less catabolism and urea production occurs when adequate protein substrates and calories are provided exogenously by vein. The net result is a reduction in total blood urea nitrogen. The nitrogen that had previously been derived via the mobilization of amino acids from protein is thus returned to the functional amino acid pool.

In the postoperative patient, the institution of TPN should be delayed for 1 to 2 days following operation, while the patient's condition is being stabilized. During this time specific attention is directed toward the correction of fluid and electrolyte imbalances that might otherwise be compounded by the administration of the hypertonic dextrose solution utilized with TPN therapy. Occasionally an otherwise relatively normal patient experiences a prolonged postoperative ileus. In most circumstances, the patient with normal nutritional balance prior to operation can support 5 to 7 days of semistarvation, receiving only glucose, vitamins, and electrolytes by vein, without significant ill effects. However, it is felt that if nasogastric suction and semistarvation are to be prolonged beyond 5 to 7 days, TPN therapy is warranted and should be instituted.

PROPER INSERTION AND MAINTENANCE OF THE TPN CATHETER. After extensive experience using a variety of sites for introduction of a catheter into one of the central veins, the infraclavicular subclavian vein access has been found to be most suitable. Complete freedom of both upper extremities, absence of an immobilizing neck dressing, ease of catheter insertion, and the short length of catheter required to reach the central vein are among the advantages of using this route. In some circumstances, the internal or external jugular vein can be utilized, but these catheterization sites have the disadvantage of causing some impedance to the movement of the neck. The insertion of long central venous catheters via such peripheral vessels as the saphenous, femoral, basilic, or cephalic veins is to be avoided because of the prohibitive risk of infection and thrombosis.

The proper insertion of the subclavian central venous feeding catheter is one of the procedures that must be accomplished with meticulous attention to detail if the long-range therapeutic goals are to be achieved without complications. In every instance, the patient should be placed in a true Trendelenburg position to assure maximal venous distention for ease of catheterization and positive central venous pressure to minimize the possibility of air embolus. After the chest has been properly shaved, it should be cleansed with a solvent such as ether or acetone. Using sterile gloves, the operator should prepare the entire hemithorax and shoulder with inorganic or organic iodine solution in the same manner as that utilized prior to a major operation. A rolled towel or sheet that is approximately 3 to 4 inches in diameter should be placed between the scapulae under the vertebral column. This facilitates maximal extension of the shoulders and improves the access to the subclavian vein. The operative field is draped with sterile towels, and the patient's head is rotated to the contralateral side. In the average adult patient, a 16-gauge, 8-inch-long polyvinyl catheter is inserted through a 14-gauge, 2-inch-long needle. The skin is anesthetized with 1 per cent lidocaine at a point below the midportion of the sigmoid curve of the clavicle. The periosteum and costoclavicular ligament are also anesthetized along the proposed path of insertion of the 14-gauge needle. The needle is attached to a 2- or 3-ml. syringe, is introduced through the skin, and is advanced virtually at a right angle to the lateral edge of the sternum. A fingertip pressed into the sternal notch provides an excellent target for directing the needle into the subclavian vein. While slight negative pressure is maintained within the syringe, the needle is advanced until the hub indents the skin. If venous puncture is not manifested by a prompt flashback of blood, the needle is withdrawn, redirected anteriorly or posteriorly a few degrees, and advanced again. When a free backflow of blood is obtained, the syringe is disconnected after the needle hub has been secured in place with a hemostat or needle holder. The catheter is then directed into the vein through the needle until the male portion of the catheter hub is seated firmly in the needle hub. The catheter must never be withdrawn from the needle if obstruction to the passage of the catheter occurs. Rather, the needle and catheter are removed as a unit to

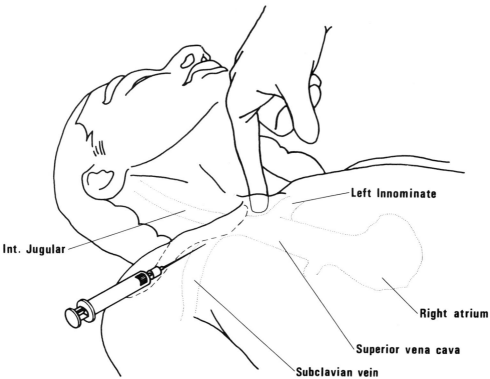

Figure 12–8   The 14-gauge needle is directed in a frontal or coronal plane toward a fingertip that is pressed firmly into the suprasternal notch. Accurate puncture of the subclavian vein is indicated by a flashback of blood in the syringe. (From Nyhus, L. M. (Ed.): Surgery Annual, 1974. Courtesy of Appleton-Century-Crofts, Publishing Division of Prentice-Hall, Inc., Englewood Cliffs, N.J.)

prevent laceration and embolization of the intravenous portion of the catheter, and another attempt at inserting the needle and catheter into the central vein must be made. After the catheter hub has been inserted securely in the needle hub, the combined unit is retracted until the needle point is outside the skin. At this moment, previously filled sterile intravenous tubing is connected to the catheter, and isotonic fluid is allowed to flow through the system. Confirmation of the central venous location of the catheter tip, and its patency, can be obtained by lowering the bottle to a level below that of the patient's heart and observing prompt backflow of blood into the catheter (Figs. 12–8 and 12–9).

It is imperative that the catheter be sutured to the skin at the point of entrance, and that a plastic clip be placed over the point of the needle to prevent laceration of the catheter. An optional suture may be placed to secure the catheter-or-needle connection. After an antimicrobial ointment

has been applied liberally to the point of entrance into the skin, the site is dressed with a small sterile bandage. The connection between the catheter and the tubing is secured with tape, as are all other connections in the infusion system (Fig. 12–10).

Immediate postcatheterization chest roentgenography is mandatory. Infusion of concentrated nutrient solutions should not begin until a responsible physician has viewed the roentgenogram to confirm the catheter's location in the superior vena cava and the absence of a pneumothorax (Fig. 12–11).

There are several potential complications attendant to insertion of a subclavian central venous catheter. Direction of the catheter tip into the wrong vein is probably the most common. Because of the venous anatomic configuration, the catheter can be directed inadvertently into either the internal jugular, external jugular, opposite subclavian, or innominate, azygous, intercostal, or internal mammary vein. The roentgenogram will

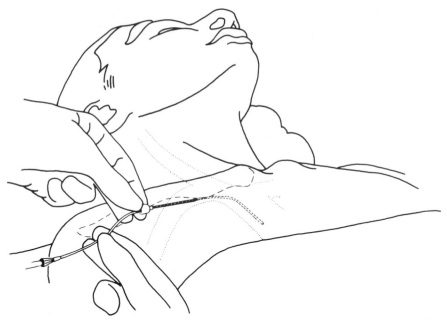

Figure 12–9 With the bevel of the needle directed inferiorly, a 16-gauge catheter is advanced into the superior vena cava. (From Nyhus, L. M. (Ed): Surgery Annual, 1974. Courtesy of Appleton-Century-Crofts, Publishing Division of Prentice-Hall, Inc., Englewood Cliffs, N.J.)

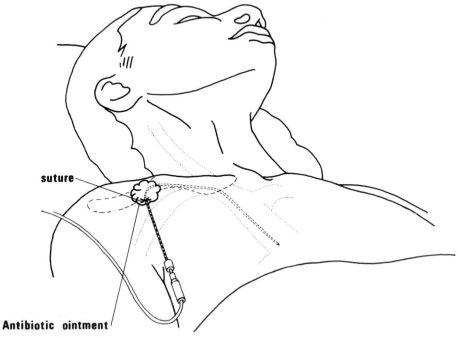

Figure 12–10 The catheter is sutured to the skin, and antimicrobial ointment is applied around the catheter at the skin entrance site. (From Nyhus, L. M. (Ed.): Surgery Annual, 1974. Courtesy of Appleton-Century-Crofts, Publishing Division of Prentice-Hall Inc., Englewood Cliffs, N.J.)

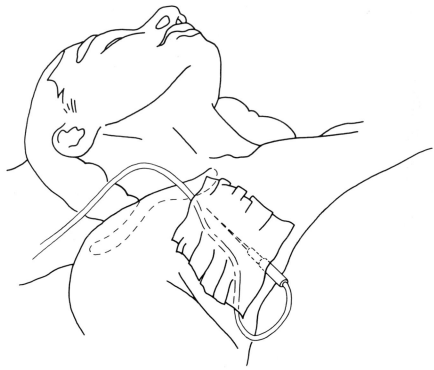

Figure 12–11   An occlusive water-repellent sterile dressing covers the catheter entrance site and secures the infusion tubing without interference of neck or arm motion. (From Nyhus, L. M. (Ed.): Surgery Annual, 1974. Courtesy of Appleton-Century-Crofts, Publishing Division of Prentice-Hall, Inc., Englewood Cliffs, N.J.)

alert the physician to an unacceptable location of the catheter. If the highly concentrated TPN solution is infused into one of these smaller veins, thrombophlebitis and occlusion are probable and may have serious consequences. When there is a propensity for the catheter to pass into veins of the shoulder or neck, it is recommended that the patient be instructed to maximally elevate (shrug) the shoulders after the catheter has been introduced a very short distance through the needle. With the change in anatomic relationships produced by this maneuver, the catheter will usually pass into the superior vena cava. Rotating the head in the opposite direction from which it had been placed may also help to achieve the same result.

The second most common complication of the insertion of a subclavian central venous catheter is pneumothorax. Many of the techniques previously described, such as extending the shoulders, maintaining a parallel relationship of the needle to the floor, and directing the needle toward the sternal notch, are designed to avoid this complication. Inexperience and poor knowledge of anatomic relationships are probably the primary causes for this complication. Pneumothorax must be treated with a small thoracostomy drainage tube placed in the second intercostal space in the midclavicular line. It is not necessary to remove the catheter if it is in the superior vena cava. Hemothorax is sometimes associated with a pneumothorax and should be managed in the same manner, unless there is excessive bleeding, which would require a posterior chest tube in the seventh intercostal space in the posterior axillary line. Laceration of the subclavian vein or subclavian artery is a potential complication with improper manipulation of the needle. Direct insertion and withdrawal of the needle without sweeping motions will virtually obviate any serious laceration. Incidental hemomediastinum has been reported at autopsy but has not been correlated with measurable morbidity. A brachial plexus injury is possible though highly improbable. Air embolus is a significant potential problem during insertion of the catheter or at any time when the infusion system is open. Placement of the patient in the Trendelenburg position at the time of catheterization and during infusion tubing changes will avoid this complication. Severing of the catheter with subsequent embolization to either a proximal venous site, right atrium, right ventricle, or pulmonary artery has been reported. These accidents usually result from transection of the catheter by the sharp needle point and are avoidable.

Routine management of the central venous lifeline should be as meticulous as that of the initial insertion. The dressings and all intravenous tubing between the catheter and the fluid reservoir should be changed at least three times a week. One well trained, well motivated person should be charged with the responsibility of these dressing changes. After the dressing has been carefully removed, the person performing the dressing change should don a pair of sterile gloves and proceed to clean the area around the catheter in ever-increasing concentric circles with an organic solvent such as ether or acetone. The skin is then cleansed with an iodine preparation in the same manner. An antimicrobial ointment is applied at the catheter entrance site, and a small, discrete dressing is applied. All tubing connections are retaped to prevent an inadvertent break in the system.

The rigid adherence to several practical safety rules is essential in order to prevent catheter related sepsis. The central venous feeding catheter is never used as a route for obtaining blood samples. It is never used as a site for monitoring central venous pressure except in an extreme emergency situation. Neither whole blood, plasma, nor medications are administered through the feeding catheter. The use of three-way stopcocks in the system is contraindicated. Every person charged with the responsibility of utilizing this route of nutrient infusion must recognize that the danger of contamination is ever-present in the multiple steps required for achieving adequate total parenteral nutrition.

When fever develops in a patient receiving TPN, catheter contamination must be suspected. Every reasonable effort must be made promptly to determine the etiology of the fever. Should no apparent cause be readily discerned, the bag or bottle of nutrient solution and the infusion tubing should be replaced. The patient's blood, the TPN bottle, and the tubing should be cultured aerobically and anaerobically and for fungus. If the fever persists for more than 4 to 8 hours, the catheter should be removed and the tip cultured. Depending upon the nutrition and fluid status of the patient, another catheter can be reinserted immediately or as indicated. It is preferable to insert the catheter in the other subclavian vein, but if necessary, the same site may be used again.

SELECTION AND REGULATION OF TPN SOLUTIONS. The amino acids in intravenous hyperalimentation fluids are derived either from casein or fibrin hydrolysates or are available as free L-amino acids. Protein hydrolysate solutions have been utilized as a means of providing intravenous protein substrates for several decades.[30] However, it was not until Dudrick et al.[14] demonstrated the efficacy of nutritional support provided entirely by the parenteral route that the great potential value of these solutions was realized. Protein hydrolysate solutions contain both free amino acids and short-chain peptides. Under conditions of stress some of the peptides are not utilized and are excreted in the urine.[54] Nevertheless, the TPN solutions formulated with nitrogen derived from protein hydrolysates have been very satisfactory in providing nutrient requirements. The opportunity of providing nutritional constituents in basic molecular form followed the development of techniques that allow production of large quantities of relatively inexpensive free L-amino acids. Both sources of nitrogen have continued to be valuable in various total parenteral nutrition techniques. Because TPN will promote protein synthesis, there is an immediate requirement for the cations and anions that predominate in intracellular water, such as magnesium, potassium, and phosphate. Extracellular cations and anions must be regulated and carefully followed as usual. The availability of acetate salts of both potassium and sodium allows the specific replenishment of either cation without providing excessive amounts of chloride. Vitamin supplementation is mandatory, and a single 5-ml. vial of MVI will provide sufficient quantities of most of the fat- and water-soluble vitamins to meet daily requirements. When more than 5 ml. of this vitamin preparation is administered daily, vitamin intoxication can occur. Vitamin K and folic acid should be administered in doses of approximately 10 mg. per week, and 1000 μg of vitamin B_{12} should be given every month.

TPN therapy should be instituted gradually over 2 to 3 days. Generally one-third of the calculated daily requirement is infused on the first day. This is increased by one-third each day so that by the third day the total requirements are being administered. For maximal safety and efficiency, the solution should be infused over the entire 24-hour period of each day. The maintenance of a constant flow rate is essential. An abrupt increase in the rate of administration is the most common cause of hyperglycemia, while hypoglycemia may develop when the rate is suddenly reduced drastically.

A successful TPN program can best be accomplished with the cooperation of a skilled pharmacist in a well equipped pharmacy. Because a mixture of amino acids and glucose will undergo the Maillard reaction to form glucosamines during the sterilization process, the individual solutions of amino acids and glucose must be mixed prior to their infusion. The mixing process is best accomplished using aseptic techniques under a laminar-flow, filtered air hood.[48] All the additives, including cations, anions, and vitamins, are mixed at the same time under these aseptic conditions. Even with these precautions, bacterial contamination is inevitable. The TPN solution must therefore be refrigerated prior to administration.

Meticulous daily attention to a variety of parameters will assure optimal results. Because the cations and anions of the extracellular fluid are most sensitive to rapid changes, serum electrolytes must be measured at least three times a week. Effective adjustments for any changes can be made by modifying the dosages of appropriate substances. Blood sugar, blood urea nitrogen, and serum creatinine determinations must also be made on a regular basis to evaluate the carbohydrate utilization and the capacity of the liver and kidneys to metabolize the infused nitrogen load. Serum constituents

that reflect intracellular function and concentration, such as phosphorus, calcium, magnesium, bilirubin, liver enzymes, and albumin, are usually measured once a week. Significant aberrations in any one or more of these components may require more frequent individual determinations of that particular metabolite.

Accurate daily weights serve as a valuable parameter in evaluating the entire process. After the initiation of a TPN program, the extremely malnourished patient may experience a weight loss of several pounds, which is secondary to mobilization and excretion of malnutritional edema. Rapid weight gain indicates a fluid overload and can be associated with symptoms of cardiovascular failure and excess interstitial pulmonary fluid.

Urine sugar and acetone determinations must be made every 6 hours. When a patient with diabetes mellitus receives TPN solutions, there may be a necessity for more frequent urine sugar and acetone evaluation. Blood sugar levels must be measured whenever urine sugar is 4+. Acute blood sugar elevations may be caused iatrogenically by suddenly increasing the flow rate. Hyperglycemia in a patient with diabetes mellitus or in an otherwise chronically ill patient should be carefully corrected with small doses of insulin until control has been attained. Thereafter, the addition of small quantities of insulin to the TPN solution will foster a more stable rate of carbohydrate metabolism.

The metabolic complications associated with TPN are all avoidable.[11] Hyperglycemia and glycosuria can usually be averted or corrected by manipulating insulin dosage and rates of TPN administration. Imbalance in serum levels of sodium, potassium, chloride, calcium, phosphorus, and magnesium can be identified and corrected. Hypertonic dehydration may occur as a result of inadequate monitoring of urine sugar and volume. Although these patients have hypernatremia, hyperkalemia, hyperchloremia, and hyperglycemia, there is an absolute deficiency both in water and electrolytes. While the hyperglycemia is being controlled, the administration of a slightly hypotonic electrolyte solution is indicated. As the carbohydrate aberration is brought under control through insulin administration, glucose infusion is reinstituted. Extremely cachectic, aged, or chronically ill patients are very sensitive to fluid overload. Early signs of congestive heart failure consisting of dyspnea, tachycardia, cough, distended neck veins, and rapid weight gain should suggest the presence of excess interstitial pulmonary fluid. Prompt administration of diuretics is the most effective management of this problem, but digitalization and the correction of intravascular hypovolemia may also be required. Temporary cessation of TPN is indicated until cardiovascular stability has been restored.

PROTEIN AND CALORIC REQUIREMENTS

The daily protein and energy requirements of the patient needing TPN remain controversial. As a result, we recently carried out a series of studies[50] to determine the caloric requirements of patients receiving TPN, the optimum amino acid concentration of TPN solutions, and the relative efficacy of carbohydrate and lipid as the major caloric source. The efficacy of TPN was evaluated by means of body composition studies performed at the beginning and at 2-week intervals during TPN.

Five hundred and thirty-three body composition studies were performed to evaluate 308 periods of TPN in 204 patients who received TPN for 4447 days. The patients were randomly allocated to receive one of the following three TPN solutions: 2.5 per cent crystalline L-amino acids (Travasol, Travenol-Baxter Laboratories, Canada) with 25 per cent dextrose; 5 per cent crystalline L-amino acids (Travasol) with 25 per cent dextrose; or a 10 per cent lipid emulsion (Intralipid, Pharmacia, Canada) infused with an equal volume of a solution containing 5 per cent amino acids (Travasol) and 25 per cent dextrose. Since the lipid emulsion and the hypertonic dextrose solution were infused at the same rate via a Y tube, the final solution administered contained 2.5 per cent amino acids, 12.5 per cent dextrose, and 5 per cent lipid. There were 102, 68, and 34 patients who received the first, second, and third TPN solutions, respectively. The number of patients in each group was unequal, since the study was performed in two stages. Initially, all patients referred for TPN were randomized to receive either the first or second solution. In the second stage of the study, patients were randomized between the first and third solutions. Each patient in the first two groups received 500 ml. of 10 per cent Intralipid twice a week to prevent the development of essential fatty acid deficiency.

The rate of change in the BCM was used to evaluate the efficacy of TPN. In a normally nourished individual, the BCM is not expected to increase, regardless of intake, except with a special exercise program designed specifically to increase muscle mass. Therefore, each group was subdivided according to the presence or absence of preexisting malnutrition, as defined by their body composition at the onset of each TPN period.

In the normally nourished patients, the BCM, as expected, did not increase with any of the three solutions. Body weight increased slightly, principally owing to an increase in body fat. Otherwise, their body composition remained unchanged. In the patients with preexisting malnutrition, TPN with each of the three solutions produced a significant improvement in body composition. Two weeks of TPN with 2.5 per cent amino acids and 25 per cent dextrose resulted in a mean increase in body weight of 1.1 ± 0.5 kg. (p < 0.5), principally owing to a 0.9 ± 0.3 kg. (p < 0.01) increase in BCM. Similar changes occurred in the malnourished patients receiving the 5 per cent amino acid solution and in those who received lipids. Increasing the amino acid concentration from 2.5 to 5 per cent did not affect the efficiency of TPN in this particular series of studies. Multiple linear regression was performed to account for the different caloric, protein, and lipid intake. The daily change in the BCM was correlated with the carbohydrate, lipid, and protein infused and with the nutritional state. This analysis was performed on a total of 212 TPN periods by combining the data obtained in the three groups of malnourished patients. This approach is possible, since the ratio of amino acid to non-protein calories and the ratio of lipid to carbohydrate calories were different in the three solutions.

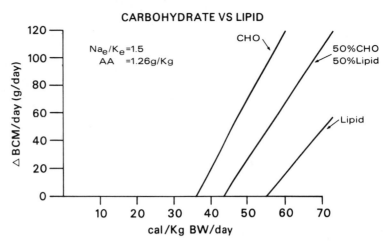

Figure 12–12 The relationship between the daily increase in the BCM and the non-protein caloric intake when the latter is either carbohydrate, lipid, or equally divided between lipid and carbohydrate. The amino acid infusion rate and Na_e/K_e were set at 1.26 gm./kg. body weight and 1.5 respectively. With the carbohydrate curve, the BCM is maintained with 36 cal./kg./day, while an infusion of 50 cal./kg./day results in a 69 gm./day increase in the BCM.

According to the resultant regression, the restoration of a depleted BCM is related to caloric intake and to the degree of malnutrition and is not affected by increasing the amino acid concentration from 2.5 to 5 per cent. In addition, carbohydrate calories are more efficient than lipid calories. This is demonstrated in Figure 12–12, where the daily change in the BCM is related to the non protein calories infused. Because the regression involves four independent parameters and one dependent parameter, a multidimensional space is required to plot the experimental data and the regression. A two-dimensional graph was obtained by setting some of the independent parameters constant. In Figure 12–12, Na_e/K_e is set at 1.50 (indicative of moderate malnutrition), and the daily amino acid infusion rate is set at 1.26 gm./kg. body weight, the mean amino acid infusion rate in the patients who received the 2.5 per cent amino acid solution. Under these conditions, when all of the non-protein calories are carbohydrate, the BCM is maintained with a daily infusion of 36 cal./kg. body weight, while 55 cal./kg. body weight are required with lipid. When lipid supplies 50 per cent of the non-protein calories, an infusion of 44 cal./kg. body weight is required to maintain the BCM. A daily infusion of 50 non-protein calories/kg. body weight results in a 69 gm./day increase in the BCM with the carbohydrate solution, and 16 gm./day when 50 per cent of the non-protein calories are lipid. In the depleted malnourished patient, carbohydrate calories are therefore more efficient than lipid

calories. An additional important consideration is that lipid calories are considerably more expensive than carbohydrate calories.

Doubling the amino acid concentration did not alter the repletion rate of a depleted BCM. In Figure 12–13, the daily change in the BCM is plotted against the caloric intake, with a daily amino acid intake of either 1.26 or 2.37 gm./kg. body weight, the mean amino acid intake of the malnourished patients receiving the 2.5 and 5 per cent solutions, respectively. All of the non-protein calories are in the form of carbohydrate. Increasing the amino acid concentration shifted the curve to the left. However, this apparent increased efficiency disappeared when the extra calories associated with the higher amino acid concentration were accounted for. In a recent review, Wilmore[56] pointed out that at any level of protein intake, nitrogen balance improves as the caloric intake is increased. With a constant caloric intake, nitrogen balance improves as the protein intake is increased. However, this latter relationship reaches a maximum such that a further increase in protein intake does not result in any further improvement in nitrogen balance. In the present study, the flat portion of the curve was probably achieved with the 2.5 per cent solution. As a result, increasing the amino acid concentration above 2.5 per cent had little effect on the rate at which a depleted BCM was restored.

The amino acid concentration of the solution has a significant impact on the cost of

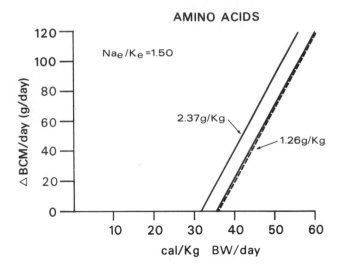

Figure 12–13 The two solid curves depict the relationship between the non-protein caloric intake and the daily increase in the BCM for amino acid infusion rates of 1.26 and 2.37 gm./kg./day, the mean rates achieved with amino acid concentrations of 2.5 and 5 per cent, respectively. The Na_e/K_e was set at 1.5. The broken curve results when the extra calories associated with the higher amino acid concentration are taken into account.

TPN. When this study was carried out, the amino acid concentrations of the commercially available TPN solutions varied from 2.5 to 4.25 per cent, representing a considerable variation in cost. With the 2.5 per cent solution, amino acids accounted for 81 per cent of the solution's costs. Increasing the amino acid concentration to 5 per cent resulted in an 84 per cent cost increase. Thus, considerable cost savings can be achieved by employing a 2.5 per cent amino acid solution and using glucose as the major source of non-protein calories. However, Intralipid should continue to be administered to prevent the development of essential fatty acid deficiency. This can be

achieved with 500 ml. of a 10 per cent solution twice a week.

The relationship between the restoration of a depleted BCM and the degree of malnutrition is illustrated in Figure 12–14. The daily change in the BCM is plotted against the caloric intake for increasingly more severe malnutrition, as indicated by the Na_e/K_e ratio. As the severity of malnutrition is increased, the caloric requirements for maintenance are decreased. Thus, with moderate malnutrition ($Na_e/K_e = 1.5$) the BCM is maintained with a caloric intake of 36 cal./kg. body weight. With severe malnutrition ($Na_e/K_e = 2.5$) 16 cal./kg. are sufficient for maintenance. With caloric intakes

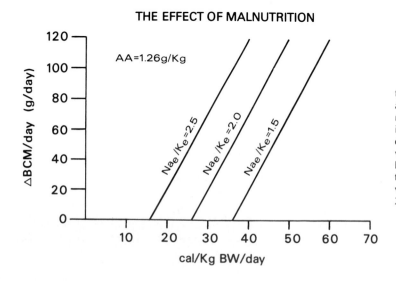

Figure 12–14 The relationship between the daily increase in the BCM and the non-protein caloric intake for malnutrition of increasing severity, as indicated by a larger Na_e/K_e ratio. The daily infusion of 50 cal./kg. body weight results in a daily increase in the BCM of 69.9 with moderate malnutrition ($Na_e/K_e = 1.5$) and 168 gm./day with severe malnutrition ($Na_e/K_e = 2.5$).

in excess of the amount required for maintenance, the restoration of the depleted BCM is more rapid in the more malnourished. Thus, with a daily infusion of 50 cal./kg. body weight, the BCM increases at a rate of 69 gm./day when $Na_e/K_e = 1.5$ and 168 gm./day when $Na_e/K_e = 2.5$. As the malnourished state is corrected, the daily increase in the BCM decreases continuously and becomes zero as the normally nourished state is achieved. This is consistent with the observation that in the normally nourished individual, there is no change in the BCM with TPN. These data also emphasize the importance of a knowledge of an individual's nutritional state when evaluating the results of nutritional therapy. This is true with both body composition measurements and nitrogen balance data. In the normally nourished individual, a prolonged positive nitrogen balance is impossible, except with a special exercise program designed to increase muscle mass. Thus, in evaluating the effects of nutritional support, it is imperative to differentiate the normally nourished from the malnourished individual. Otherwise, the data from the normally nourished will bias the data from the malnourished. It is also important to estimate the degree of malnutrition present, as this will affect the response to nutritional therapy.

The restoration of a depleted BCM is related to caloric intake and the degree of malnutrition but is not affected by increasing the amino acid concentration from 2.5 to 5 per cent. Elwyn et al. have reported a similar relationship.[18] In a group of depleted patients receiving TPN, they described a straight line relationship between nitrogen balance and the daily caloric intake. With the latter relationship and the mean values for the malnourished patients receiving the 2.5 per cent solution, a mean daily positive nitrogen balance of 45 mg./kg. body weight was obtained. This is equivalent to a daily increase in the BCM of 64 gm./day. Using the same data, our regression equation predicted a restoration rate of 69 gm./day. At this rate, two weeks of TPN would result in a 0.97 kg. increase in the BCM, which is the increase measured in the malnourished patients who received the 2.5 per cent solution.

The restoration of a malnourished individual is directly dependent on the caloric intake, provided the protein intake is adequate. There is no apparent advantage to increasing the daily protein intake to levels above 1.5 to 2 gm./kg. body weight. Carbohydrate calories are more efficient than lipid calories. These data also emphasize that correction of the malnourished state is relatively slow compared to the rate at which it develops. The normally nourished individual, during the first few days of starvation, breaks down more than 300 gm./day of BCM. A much more rapid breakdown occurs with trauma, especially when complicated with sepsis. However, in spite of large caloric intakes the BCM is only restored at a rate of 50 to 100 gm./day.

OVERVIEW

There is no pathophysiologic condition that can be endured or treated optimally when a patient is malnourished. The best therapeutic results with minimal complications are the surgeon's reward for the effort expended in maintaining the best possible nutritional status of patients throughout the diagnostic, preoperative, operative, postoperative, convalescent, and rehabilitation periods. Although a thorough discussion of all the nutritionally related complications in surgical patients could not possibly be accomplished within the confines of this chapter, it is hoped that a better awareness of and insight into the magnitude and importance of this crucial area have been attained by the reader.

Bibliography

1. Abel, R. M.: Improved survival from acute renal failure after treatment with essential L-amino acids and glucose. N. Engl. J. Med. *288*:695, 1973.
2. Allison, S. P., Hinton, P., and Chamberlain, M. J.: Intravenous glucose tolerance, insulin, and free fatty acid levels in burned patients. Lancet *2*:1113, 1965.
3. Benedict, F. G.: A Study of Prolonged Fasting. Washington, Carnegie Institute, 1915 (Publication No. 203).
4. Birnbaum, S. M., Greenstein, J. P., and Winitz, M.: Quantitative nutritional studies with water-soluble, chemically defined diets. II. Nitrogen balance and metabolism. Arch. Biochem. Biophys. *72*:417, 1957.

5. Blackburn, G. L., Flatt, J. P., Clowes, G. H. A., Jr., et al.: Protein sparing therapy during periods of starvation with sepsis or trauma. Ann. Surg. 177:588, 1973.

6. Blackburn, G. L., Bistrian, B. R., Maini, B. S., Schlamm, H. T., and Smith, M. F.: Nutritional and metabolic assessment of the hospitalized patient. J. Parent. Enter. Nutr. 1:11, 1977.

7. Buchwald, H.: The dumping syndrome and its treatment. Am. J. Surg. 116:81, 1968.

8. Cahill, G. F., Jr.: Starvation in man. N. Engl. J. Med. 282:688, 1970.

9. Carlson, L. A., and Liljedahl, S.: Lipid metabolism and trauma. Acta Med. Scand. 173:25, 1963.

10. Copeland, E. M., MacFadyen, B. V., Jr., and Dudrick, S. J.: The use of hyperalimentation in patients with potential sepsis. Surg. Gynecol. Obstet. 138:377, 1974.

11. Dudrick, S. J., and Copeland, E. M.: Intravenous hyperalimentation. In Nyhus, L. M.: Surgery Annual. New York, Appleton-Century-Crofts, 1973, pp. 69–95.

12. Dudrick, S. J., Herndon, B. L., Senior, J. R., and Rhoads, J. E.: Nutritional care of the surgical patient. Med. Clin. North Am. 48:1253, 1964.

13. Dudrick, S. J., Rhoads, J. E., and Vars, H. M.: Growth of puppies receiving all nutritional requirements by vein. Fortschritte der Parenteralen Ernahrung. Symposium of the International Society of Parenteral Nutrition in 1966. Locham bei Munchen, Pallas Verlag, 1967.

14. Dudrick, S. J., Wilmore, D. W., Vars, H. M., and Rhoads, J. E.: Long-term total parenteral nutrition with growth, development and positive nitrogen balance. Surgery 64:134, 1968.

15. Duke, J. H., Jr.: A dietary therapy for rectovaginal fistula. In Balanced Nutrition and Therapy. International Symposium. Nuremberg, April, 1970. Stuttgart, Georg Thieme Verlag, 1971.

16. Duke, J. H., Jr., and Yar, M. S.: Management of surgical nutritional complications in developing countries. In Balanced Nutrition and Therapy. International Symposium, Erlangen, Stuttgart, Georg Thieme Verlag, in press.

17. Edmunds, H., Jr., Williams, G. M., and Welch, C. R.: External fistulas arising from the gastrointestinal tract. Ann. Surg. 152:495, 1960.

18. Elwyn, D. H., Gump, F. E., and Munro, H. N.: Changes in nitrogen balance of depleted patients with increasing infusions of glucose. Am. J. Clin. Nutr. 32:1597, 1979.

19. Forse, R. A., and Shizgal, H. M.: The assessment of malnutrition. Surgery 88:17, 1980.

20. Freeman, J. B., Stegink, L. D., Wittine, M. F., et al.: The current status of protein sparing. Surg. Gynecol. Obstet. 144:843, 1977.

21. Gibbon, J. H., Jr., Nealon, T. F., and Greco, V. F.: A modification of Glassman's gastrostomy with results in 18 patients. Ann. Surg. 143:838, 1956.

22. Glassman, J. A.: A new aseptic double-valved tubogastrostomy. Surg. Gynecol. Obstet. 68:789, 1939.

23. Glotzer, D. J., Boyle, P. L., and Silen, W.: Preoperative preparation of the colon with an elemental diet. Surgery 74:703, 1973.

24. Goodhart, R. S., and Wohl, M. G.: The diagnosis of malnutrition. In Manual of Clinical Nutrition. Philadelphia, Lea & Febiger, 1964, p. 41.

25. Graham, W. P., and Royster, H. P.: Simplified cervical esophagostomy for long-term extraoral feeding. Surg. Gynecol. Obstet. 125:125, 1967.

26. Greenberg, G. R., Marliss, E. B., Anderson, G. H., et al.: Protein sparing therapy in postoperative patients. N. Engl. J. Med. 294:1141, 1976.

27. Greenstein, J. P., Birnbaum, S. M., Winitz, M., and Otey, M. C.: Quantitative nutritional studies with water-soluble chemically defined diets. I. Growth, reproduction, and lactation in rats. Arch. Biochem. Biophys. 72:396, 1957.

28. Greenstein, J. P., and Winitz, M.: Amino acids in nutrition. In Chemistry of the Amino Acid. New York, John Wiley and Sons, 1961.

29. Herrington, J. L.: Remedial operations for severe postgastrectomy symptoms (dumping). Ann. Surg. 162:789, 1965.

30. Holden, W. D., Krieger, H., Levey, S., and Abbott, W. E.: The effects of nutrition on nitrogen metabolism in the surgical patient. Ann. Surg. 146:563, 1957.

31. Hoover, H. C., Jr., Grant, J. P., Gorschboth, C., et al.: Nitrogen sparing intravenous fluids in postoperative patients. N. Engl. J. Med. 293:172, 1975.

32. Howard, J. M.: Studies on absorption and metabolism of glucose after injury. Ann. Surg. 141:321, 1955.

33. Hume, D. M.: Endocrine and metabolic responses to injury. In Schwartz, S. E., Lillehei, R. C., Shires, G. T., Spencer, F. C., and Storer, E. H.: Principles of Surgery. New York, McGraw-Hill Book Company, 1974, pp. 1–64.

34. Keys, A., Brozek, J., Henschell, A., Mickelsen, O., and Taylor, H.: The Biology of Human Starvation. Minneapolis, University of Minnesota Press, 1950.

35. Kinney, J. M., Long, C. L., Gump, F. E., and Duke, J. H., Jr.: Tissue composition of weight loss in surgical patients. Ann. Surg. 168:459, 1968.

36. Kinney, J. M.: Energy requirements of the surgical patient. In Manual of Surgical Nutrition. Committee on Pre- and Postoperative Care. American College of Surgeons, pp. 223–235. Philadelphia, W. B. Saunders Company, 1975.

37. Krieger, M.: Uber die Atrophie de Menschlichen Organe bei Inanition. Anat. Konstitutional 7:87, 1921.

38. MacFadyen, B. V., Dudrick, S. J., and Ruberg, R. L.: Management of gastrointestinal fistulas with parenteral hyperalimentation. Surgery 74:100, 1974.

39. Mullen, J. L., Buzby, G. P., Waldman, M. T., Gertner, M. H., Hobbs, C. L., and Rosato, E. F.: Prediction of operative morbidity and mortality by preoperative nutritional assessment. Surg. Forum 30:80, 1979.

40. Munro, H. N.: General aspects of the regulation of protein metabolism by diet and by hormones. In Munro, H. N., and Allison, J. B.: Mammalian Protein Metabolism. Vol. I. New York, Academic Press, 1964, pp. 381–481.

41. Owen, O. E., Felig, P., Morgan, A. P., Wahreu, J.,

and Cahill, G. F.: Liver and kidney metabolism during prolonged starvation. J. Clin. Invest. *48*:574, 1969.

42. Pearson, W. N.: Biochemical appraisal of nutritional status in man. Am. J. Clin. Nutr. *11*:462, 1962.

43. Picou, D., Halliday, D., and Garrow, J. S.: Total body protein, collagen, and noncollagen protein in infantile protein malnutrition. Clin. Sci. *30*:345, 1966.

44. Porte, D., Grabler, A. L., Kuzuya, T., and Williams, R. H.: The effect of epinephrine on immunoreactive insulin levels in man. J. Clin. Invest. *45*:228, 1966.

45. Randale, P. J., Garland, P. B., Hales, C. N., and Newsholme, E. A.: The glucose fatty-acid cycle: Its role in insulin sensitivity and the metabolic disturbances in diabetes mellitus. J. Lab. Clin. Med. *69*:256, 1967.

46. Ross, H., Johnston, I. D. A., Welborn, T. A., and Wright, A. D.: Effect of abdominal operation on glucose tolerance and serum levels of insulin, growth hormone, and hydrocortisone. Lancet *2*:563, 1966.

47. Rutledge, R. H.: Comments on Henley's remedial operation for dumping syndrome. Surgery *55*:762, 1964.

48. Serlick, S. E., Dudrick, S. J., and Flack, H. L.: Nutritional intravenous feeding. Bull. Parenteral Drug Assoc. *23*:166, 1969.

49. Shizgal, H. M., Milne, C. A., and Spanier, A. H.: The effect of nitrogen sparing intravenously administered fluids on postoperative body composition. Surgery *85*:496, 1979.

50. Shizgal, H. M., and Forse, R. A.: Protein and calorie requirements with total parenteral nutrition. Ann. Surg. *192*:562, 1980.

51. Shizgal, H. M.: The effect of malnutrition on body composition. Surg. Gynecol. Obstet. *152*: 22, 1981.

52. Stephens, R. V., and Randall, H. T.: Use of a concentrated balanced liquid elemental diet for nutritional management of catabolic states. Ann. Surg. *170*:642, 1969.

53. Studley, H. O.: Percentage of weight loss, a basic indicator of surgical risk. J.A.M.A. *106*:458, 1936.

54. Vinnars, E., Fürst, P., Hermansson, I. L., Josephson, B., and Lindholmer, B.: Protein catabolism in the postoperative state and its treatment with amino acid solution. Acta Chir. Scand. *136*:95, 1970.

55. Wilmore, D. W., and Dudrick, S. J.: Growth and development of an infant receiving all nutrients exclusively by vein. J.A.M.A. *203*:860, 1968.

56. Wilmore, D. W.: Energy requirements for maximum nitrogen balance retention. *In* Green, H. L., Holliday, M. A., and Munro, H. M. (Eds.): Clinical Nutrition Update: Amino Acids. Chicago, American Medical Association, 1977, pp. 47–58.

57. Young, G. A., Chem, C., and Hill, G. L.: Assessment of protein-calorie malnutrition in surgical patients from plasma protein and anthropometric measurements. Am. J. Clin. Nutr. *31*:429, 1978.

13

COMPLICATIONS OF SURGERY FOR CANCER OF THE HEAD AND NECK

Oliver H. Beahrs
and John E. Woods

Operations for cancer of the head and neck region can be limited, but most often they are extensive. The anatomy of the region is complex, involving many important structures and body systems. As a result, complications during surgery and the postoperative period may be many and varied. Being aware of the problems and taking certain preventive measures during and after the operation can prevent or reduce the seriousness of the complications. The operation involves removal of soft tissues, cartilage, and at times, bone. Most malignant tumors of the head and neck region, in addition to involving the tissue of origin, spread by infiltration to the immediately adjacent tissues and by embolization to the regional lymphatic structures. The primary tumor may be excised separately or may be removed en bloc with the regional lymphat-

ic nodes. Removal of the primary lesion may be by partial excision of the lip, by hemiglossectomy, by removal of a portion of the cheek, or by partial or total laryngectomy. The regional lymphatic structures (Fig. 13–1) are removed by a radical neck dissection, as originally described by Crile.[6] If the tissues are removed en bloc, especially when the hemimandible is removed, the procedure is considered a commando operation, as named by Martin,[14] or more commonly a composite or a combined operation. In addition to the oral pharynx, larynx, and accessory parts, surgery of the head and neck can involve the salivary glands, thyroid gland, skin, and other structures of the head and neck, along with the regional lymphatic nodes when indicated (Fig. 13–2).

Surgery in this region requires knowledge of the anatomy, the various operative proce-

Oliver H. Beahrs was born in Alabama, attended college at the University of California, and graduated from Northwestern University Medical School. He received his surgical training at the Mayo Clinic and was Head of the Section in General Surgery there, Professor of Surgery in the Mayo Medical School, member of the Board of Trustees of the Mayo Foundation, and Vice-Chairman of the Board of Governors of the Mayo Clinic. He is past president of the American Surgical Association and is a Regent of the American College of Surgeons. He is broadly versed in general surgery, but it is in the area of head and neck surgery that he has made many of his most important and widely recognized contributions.

John E. Woods was born in Michigan, spent his childhood and adolescence in Peking, China, attended Asbury College in Wilmore, Kentucky, and graduated from the University of Minnesota Medical School. He received his surgical and plastic surgical training at the Mayo Clinic and the Peter Bent Brigham Hospital, and he is currently Associate Professor and Head of the Section of Plastic and Reconstructive Surgery and Consultant in Head and Neck Surgery at the Mayo Clinic. His major clinical interest is in ablative and reconstructive surgery of head and neck cancer.

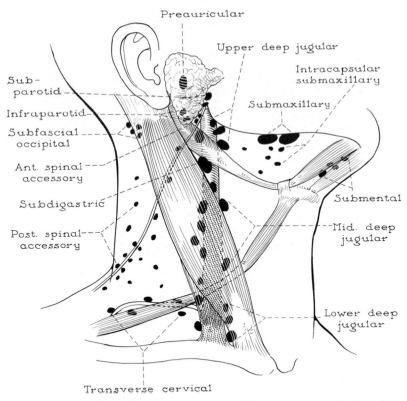

Preauricular

Upper deep jugular

Intracapsular
submaxillary

Submaxillary

Sub-
parotid

Infraparotid

Subfascial
occipital

Ant. spinal
accessory

Subdigastric

Submental

Mid. deep
jugular

Post. spinal
accessory

Lower deep
jugular

Transverse cervical

Figure 13–1 Purpose of a radical neck dissection is to remove en bloc the regional nodes into which primary cancer of the head and neck will spread. Accomplishing this exposes the patient to complications, some of which are serious (hemorrhage and airway obstruction). (From Beahrs, O. H., Gossel, J. D., and Hollinshead, W. H.: Technic and Surgical Anatomy of Radical Neck Dissection. Am. J. Surg. 90:490, 1955. By permission of Dun-Donnelley Publishing Corporation.)

dures, and the preventive measures to ensure not only that the best treatment is given but also that complications and iatrogenic injuries are minimized.[4]

The mortality rate from surgery for head and neck cancer is low, and most often death is related to local problems and not to problems associated with the opening of a body cavity, such as shock or electrolyte disturbances. Removal of the primary lesion alone is infrequently associated with death. The mortality rate for simple neck dissection is 1.5 per cent,[3] or lower, while that for bilateral radical neck dissection, either simultaneous or non-simultaneous, is 2.5 per cent.[1] When a composite or combined operation is done in one stage, the rate is 3 per cent.[19] About half of the deaths are due to local complications such as hemorrhage or airway obstruction, while the other half are related to systemic disease, most often cardiovascular or pulmonary conditions.

Although there are many complications

of head and neck surgery, the two most serious are hemorrhage and airway obstruction — the two complications most likely to lead to death.

HEMORRHAGE

Operative bleeding can be profuse, but it does not need to be so. The patient should be under a well controlled general anesthesia, and in a head-up (reverse Trendelenburg) position of about 30 degrees. If this is done, the systolic pressure most often will decrease to about 60 mm. Hg. Whether chemical agents should be used to reduce the blood pressure in head and neck surgery is open to question. Their use has not been necessary in our experience.

The surgical dissection should be along and in anatomic planes, and the major vessels to be sacrificed should be ligated in advance of their transection. During the

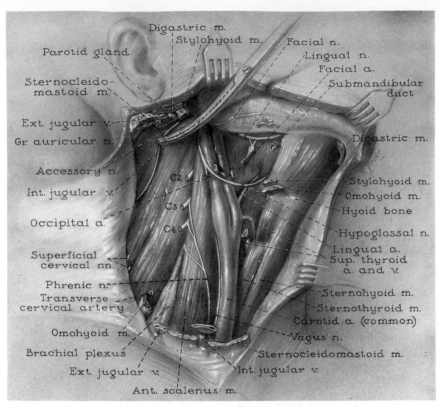

Digastric m.
Stylohyoid m.
Facial n.
Parotid gland
Lingual n.
Facial a.
Sternocleido-
mastoid m.
Submandibular
duct
Ext. jugular v.
Gr. auricular n.
Digastric m.
Accessory n.
Stylohyoid m.
Int. jugular v.
Omohyoid m.
Hyoid bone
C2
Occipital a.
C3
Hypoglossal n.
C4
Lingual a.
Sup. thyroid
a. and v.
Superficial
cervical nn.
Phrenic n.
Sternohyoid m.
Transverse
cervical artery
Sternothyroid m.
Carotid a. (common)
Omohyoid m.
Vagus n.
Brachial plexus
Sternocleidomastoid m.
Ext. jugular v.
Int. jugular v.
Ant. scalenus m.

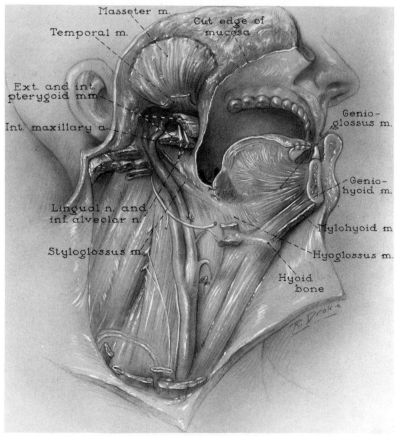

Masseter m.
Cut edge of
mucosa
Temporal m.
Ext. and int.
pterygoid mm.
Genio-
glossus m.
Int. maxillary a.
Genio-
hyoid m.
Lingual n. and
inf. alveolar n.
Mylohyoid m.
Styloglossus m.
Hyoglossus m.
Hyoid
bone

Figure 13–2 *See legend on opposite page*

procedure, if sponge pressure, tension, traction, and countertraction are used on the tissues, most oozing and minor bleeding can be easily controlled. Using these techniques not only will help control the bleeding but also will facilitate the anatomic dissection and the identification of structures not to be disturbed or sacrificed.

During the course of neck dissection, loss of blood should be less than 500 ml., and certainly no more than 1000 ml. Nevertheless, prior to the start of any operation on the head and neck, adequate intravenous needles should be in place for fluid replacement and infusion of blood. In bilateral simultaneous radical neck dissection, or in composite operations, blood loss can be 1000 to 2000 ml.; rarely should it be more. This amount is great enough that the blood should be replaced to maintain body blood volume and to prevent a postoperative decrease in blood pressure.

A massive loss of blood can occur quickly if the internal jugular vein is accidentally opened. Bleeding from this source can be quickly controlled by pressure exerted directly over the bleeding site. The vessel then can be isolated and ligated above and below the bleeding site. Other major hemorrhage can occur if the common, internal, or external carotid arteries are injured. Here again, direct pressure over the bleeding site will control blood loss while the vessel is isolated. If bleeding is from the external carotid artery, or one of its branches, then this vessel should be sacrificed. However, if the bleeding is from the common or the internal carotid artery, then the vessel should be repaired if this is technically feasible. Grafting a major vessel, especially if a composite operation is being done, leads to a significant risk of postoperative hemorrhage. Major arterial bleeding requires control of the vessel, both proximally and distally, because of retrograde blood flow when the vessel proximal to the bleeding site is occluded.

Prevention of hematoma or seroma formation in the operative site and subsequent infection is important in reducing the chance of hemorrhage during the postoperative period. The operative site can be drained either by Penrose drains or by pressure dressings but is best drained by negative suction, using one or two catheters (Hemovac-type drains). Thus, blood, serum, and exudate will not collect in the operative site, and viable surfaces will be allowed to approximate each other, sealing off the tissues. Infection, necrosis of skin flaps, uncovering of vessels, and the development of mucocutaneous fistulas will lead to inflammatory reactions that will erode arteries, which in turn will rupture and cause hemorrhage. Although local measures may control the bleeding, the wound should be explored and the vessel ligated above and below the bleeding point.

When the common or the internal carotid artery is ligated unilaterally, the risk of death is approximately 25 per cent and that of hemiplegia is great. Hemiplegia is due to slowly developing and creeping thrombus formation that extends to the circle of Willis. Pemberton and Livermore[15] found that ligation of major cervical vessels often can be safely done in older patients with systemically administered anticoagulants and local injection of heparin in the artery distal to the ligature.

In the event that carotid blowout occurs after surgery, prior preparation of nursing personnel as to management of this event may be lifesaving. Immediate pressure over the bleeding site allows local control. If the patient is then transfused up to a normal blood volume prior to ligation of the common carotid, the salvage rate is extremely good. The importance of prior transfusion cannot be overemphasized.

Figure 13–2 *Top,* Appearance of anatomy of neck after completion of standard radical neck dissection. Note the many exposed anatomic structures, especially carotid arteries that, if sacrificed or injured, could lead to morbidity and death. (From Roy, P. H., and Beahrs, O. H.: Spinal Accessory Nerve in Radical Neck Dissections. *Am. J. Surg.,* 118:800, 1969. By permission of Dun-Donnelley Publishing Corporation.)

Bottom, Radical neck dissection extended into a composite operation, with removal of part of the tongue and mandible. Here the operative site is exposed to infection and fistula formation. (From Masson, J. K.: Radical surgical treatment of intraoral carcinoma. Surg. Clin. North Am., *43:*1013, 1963.)

When the operation is intraoral, pharyngeal, or laryngeal, bleeding may occur postoperatively without visible evidence, because the blood may be swallowed. The hematocrit or the hemoglobin level should be determined daily after the operation, until the patient's condition has stabilized (usually 1 to 5 days).

Any significant amount of blood loss during or after the operation should be estimated and replaced by whole blood transfusions. If blood volume and blood components are maintained within the normal ranges, healing will likely proceed satisfactorily and other complications will be less apt to occur.

AIRWAY OBSTRUCTION

As with hemorrhage, airway obstruction requires prompt and immediate action if serious consequences for the patient are to be prevented. If the airway is not obstructed by the cancer, the first risks come during anesthesia and the operation.

There are three types of problems in the anesthetic management from the surgeon's point of view. First and most important is the possibility of airway obstruction. This may happen at any time as a result of an obstruction in the gas-carrying tubes that lead to the patient. The usual causes are kinking of the endotracheal tube, placement of the tube with the bevel against the wall of the trachea, and blocking of the tube by a plug of mucus or blood. The obstruction may be sudden, with cyanosis, decrease in blood pressure and pulse, and possibly death within 2 to 3 minutes. The obstruction may be partial with slowly developing hypoxia and delayed onset of the circulatory changes. Whether sudden or slow, the obstruction can cause irreversible brain damage, even if the patient recovers cardiopulmonary function.

Second, failure to administer blood by transfusion in sufficient amounts to maintain an adequate blood volume during the period of peak loss may be an obvious or sometimes insidious cause of exsanguination.

Third, the necessary cooperation between the surgeon and the anesthesiologist may fail. These two principals must work jointly as a team in the preoperative planning, in the execution of the operation, and in the immediate after-care of the patient. During the operation, each must continually keep the other informed of the details of technique. The surgeon must warn of the possible increase in bleeding and be prepared to delay the operation in order to inspect the endotracheal tube for patency. The anesthesiologist must notify the surgeon of any significant changes in blood pressure, pulse, or respiration. He must be alert for obstruction of the endotracheal tube and be ready to request the surgeon to halt the operation for inspection of the airway system.

Tracheal intubation for surgical procedures of the head and neck has almost entirely eliminated airway problems during the course of surgery, except those previously mentioned. If the airway is partially obstructed before operation, or if serious difficulty is anticipated in intubating the patient, elective tracheostomy must be considered before the anesthesia and operation are begun. If tracheostomy is necessary, it is best done under local anesthesia. Elective tracheostomy carries less risk to the patient than tracheostomy during or after the operation as an emergency procedure.

At the completion of the operation, elective tracheostomy should be considered under certain circumstances to prevent airway complications in the postoperative course. These include cases in which a composite operation or bilateral simultaneous or nonsimultaneous radical neck dissection has been done, swallowing or coughing is a problem, or debilitating conditions are present. Tracheostomy is indicated after radical excisions of the vallecula, the pyriform sinuses, and the base of the tongue, because bloody oozing and massive edema make normal swallowing and respiratory action impossible. In a radical neck dissection in which a tracheostomy is planned, the operative site must not be in continuity with the tracheostomy site, so that aspiration of any neck exudate into the tracheal stoma cannot occur.

Maintenance of an adequate airway is a critical problem for 48 hours after operation and a serious one for the subsequent 3 to 5 days. Postoperative airway obstruction may be sudden and complete. Death will result unless the airway is reestablished within 3 to 4 minutes. Obstruction is usually caused by aspiration of blood, vomitus, or mucus in the pharynx, posterior displacement of the tongue and epiglottis to block the glottis, external pressure from hematoma under the wound flaps, or a tightly constricting neck bandage.

This kind of obstruction may be prevented by frequent catheter aspiration through nose and mouth and frequent inspection of dressings for tightness and hematoma. Aspiration of the stomach by nasogastric tube routinely after operation is helpful to prevent vomiting. Placement of the patient on his side or in the sitting position keeps the tongue from falling posteriorly, but such placement is ineffective if the tongue and its supporting muscles have been severed from their mandibular attachments.

A significant contributory factor to airway obstruction in patients undergoing combined intra-oral surgery and neck dissection is intra-oral edema. It has been our experience that such edema may be significantly reduced or essentially prevented with the use of intraoperative intravenous methylprednisolone — 500 to 1000 mg. over 30 to 60 seconds. Repeat doses of 250 to 500 mg. may be given 2 or 3 times in the 24 to 48 hours after surgery.

Airway obstruction may be progressive, slow, and insidious, with little local change in the oral or neck wound and without subjective awareness by the patient. Objectively, the patient is restless, irritable, and yet drowsy, and usually has suprasternal skin retraction at inspiration. Soon he has a slight "crowing" at inspiration which becomes more pronounced. Within 8 to 10 hours after operation, the patient has dullness of sensorium and is irrational; this is followed by loss of cerebral and cardiac functions. Brain damage will be so severe that tracheostomy, artificial respiration, cardiac massage, and other measures to revive the patient will fail. Significantly, these changes take place without cyanosis and probably are due to the mild but cumulative effects of hypoxia, which are sufficient to cause death of brain cells when the hypoxia lasts for several hours. The mechanism is thought to be blockage of the laryngeal airway by swelling in the region of the true vocal cords. This type of edema more likely occurs in patients who have had trauma to

the vocal cords at intubation, recent upper respiratory tract infection, and previous operations or radiation exposure. When restlessness develops, a cause must be sought early before respiratory depression becomes irreversible. Sedatives should not be given because they may further reduce the respiratory exchange.

Airway obstruction is treated by tracheostomy as an emergency operation, performed under local anesthesia and in the operating room if time permits. The more rapid direct insertion of an endotracheal tube or a bronchoscope before the tracheostomy may be lifesaving if it can be accomplished without delay. Although an emergency tracheostomy is the most dramatic treatment of airway obstruction, even more significant are the recognition of the onset of hypoxia and a realization of its importance. Randall[16] reported on airway problems in head and neck surgery and stressed an educational program to anticipate and prevent postoperative respiratory tract complications. All persons — staff, nurses, and patients — must be aware of the emergency conditions of airway obstruction. In extreme circumstances, cricothyrotomy has been advocated as a lifesaving measure because of its rapidity and ease of performance.

Special attention must be given to the management of the airway in children, in whom an anatomic problem exists in addition to the difficulties of anesthesia. Eckenhoff[7] showed that the laryngeal opening in children is proportionately smaller than in adults. Consequently, slight edema of the true vocal cords, the presence of small quantities of blood, mucus, or vomitus in the larynx, or compression by a tight dressing is more likely to cause complete obstruction than in the adult. Children lack adult power in coughing and clearing the throat and often cannot cooperate in maintaining correct body position for efficient respiratory function. Tracheostomy should be resorted to if laryngeal obstruction is imminent. The premonitory sign is most often insidious inspiratory "crowing." Complete obstruction without warning is rare. Tracheostomy in children less than 2 years old, although lifesaving, injects a complication that may in itself be serious. First, tracheostomy is associated with a higher rate of pneumonia despite the use of antibiotics, and second, the tube must remain in place for several months to 1 year because the child cannot breathe through the normal route.

CAROTID SINUS REFLEX

In the radical neck dissection and in the supramyohyoid dissection, the common carotid artery bifurcation is exposed. In most patients, the blood pressure would not be appreciably lowered by manipulation of this anatomic region, but occasionally the sinus is hypersensitive and is affected by minimal mechanical stimulation. The blood pressure may decrease to levels of 50 to 60 mm. Hg and remain there for a few minutes.[18]

Obliteration of the carotid sinus reflex can be accomplished by the injection of 2 to 3 ml. of 1 per cent procaine into the areolar tissue at the carotid bifurcation, especially in the fork between the internal artery and the external carotid artery where the carotid sinus nerve lies. The procaine should be injected before the region is fully exposed, and another injection of procaine may be necessary as the vessels are cleared. The anesthesiologist should be made aware of the approaching dissection and injection in order to record blood pressures and to administer fluids and vasopressors as required.

The carotid sinus reflex almost always can be prevented by careful dissection in the region and by not applying undue pressure to the carotid vessels or to the bifurcation of the common carotid artery.

LATE POSTOPERATIVE TRACHEAL ASPIRATION

After the first postoperative week, when wound swelling and bleeding have largely subsided, and when the airway is adequate (with or without a tracheostomy), the patient may still be unable to swallow his saliva or liquid food. When the operation has been so extensive that the larynx cannot be covered by the epiglottis during swallowing, the condition may become permanent, and the patient can then be fed only by nasogastric tube or gastrostomy. The gastric tube may be placed through the lateral pharyngeal wall at the operation and brought out through the skin flap, with elimination of the hazards and discomfort of an indwelling nasopharyngeal tube. Laryngectomy is rarely necessary to eliminate tracheal aspiration.

Tracheal aspiration may occur after operations that do not result in an anatomic disturbance in the larynx and its adnexa. The aspirated fluid causes multiple foci of lung infection, followed by fever, cough, and debilitation. The chest roentgenogram shows little abnormality. The mechanism of aspiration cannot always be detected by the patient or the observer and may escape notice. It is seen commonly in older patients in whom a physical basis for its mechanism is difficult to establish, but when tracheal aspiration occurs in patients less than 50 years old, it is usually due to perilaryngeal edema which prevents adequate glottal closure. There is no specific means of preventing this complication, because it has multiple causes.

Treatment consists in feeding by nasogastric tube until the patient can swallow normally.

Although lifesaving, tracheostomy can cause complications. The skin flaps must be developed in such a manner that a communication does not exist between the primary operative site and the stoma. Such a communication may lead to wound contamination and infection, with fistula formation through the tracheal stoma.

Hemorrhage after tracheostomy is uncommon. Minor oozing and venous hemorrhage, which might occur, can be controlled with packing. Arterial hemorrhage results from operative injury to the thyroidea ima artery or erosion of the innominate artery by acutely curved tracheostomy tubes or tracheostomy tubes placed below the third tracheal ring. Hemorrhage from the innominate artery may result in death unless promptly treated. Recognition of impending arterial injury is possible if the tube is found to "bob" with the cardiac action. Removal of the tracheostomy tube before hemorrhage occurs is usually sufficient.

A definite schedule should be set for removal of the tracheostomy tube. Once the clinical state of the patient indicates that the danger of secondary hemorrhage has passed and that the laryngeal edema has decreased and frequent tracheobronchial aspiration is no longer necessary, the tube should be plugged for 24 hours. This provides a period of observation to ensure the adequacy of ventilation without the tracheostomy. At times, removal of the tracheostomy tube may be required to allow certain patients to swallow without aspirating. The tracheostoma rarely needs to be closed surgically.

AIR EMBOLISM

Although a potential hazard of head and neck surgery, air embolism rarely occurs. The use of general anesthesia and of the head-up position of the patient during the operation prevents air from passing into the general circulation even though bubbles of air occasionally can be seen in the exposed veins in the operative site. Air embolism during operation usually produces cardiac arrest because of accumulation of sufficient air bubbles in the pulmonary artery to block the outflow of blood. Prevention can be best accomplished by clamping the veins before dividing them; this avoids aspiration of air during inspiration. Successful treatment consists in the immediate lowering of the head of the table and turning the patient on his left side to allow the air to rise and settle in the apex of the right ventricle. The chest must be opened, the air aspirated, and circulation reestablished by manual pumping of the heart and later by electric shock until spontaneous beating resumes.[10]

EMPHYSEMA

Although uncommon after head and neck surgery, subcutaneous or mediastinal emphysema is most likely related to an air leak beneath the skin flaps near the tracheal stoma or elsewhere along the tracheobronchial tree. Routine postoperative roentgenograms will show a low percentage of this complication, because such emphysema is rarely obvious.

PNEUMOTHORAX

Pneumothorax occurs occasionally as a result of injury to the apex of the pleural reflection at the root of the neck during neck dissections. It is recognized by the ebb **and** flow of air through the wound and by the usual pulmonary signs observed by the anesthesiologist.[13] To prevent pneumothorax, care must be taken to avoid entering the pleura in operations at the root of the neck. Treatment consists in temporarily packing the region to make it airtight and inflating the lungs to provide expansion and obliteration of the trapped air. After operation, tight adhesive strapping over pads may be applied to the base of the neck. A large drainage tube is introduced into the thoracic cavity and led to a water trap as after thoracic operations.

LYMPH AND CHYLOUS FISTULAS

During radical surgery of the head and neck region, many lymphatic vessels are interrupted and the normal flow of lymph is altered. Lymph accumulates in the operative site, and its accumulation causes elevation of the skin flaps and leads to delay in healing. This delay is another reason for adequate drainage, preferably by a negative-suction catheter. Usually these lymphatic vessels seal off easily, and most often the extravasation decreases to a minimum within 2 to 3 days. Rarely, interruption of the right lymphatic duct in the lower neck may lead to prolonged lymphatic drainage. The opposite is true if the left duct (thoracic duct) is interrupted during surgery. The duct should be identified during the dissection in the left lower neck. Ligation of small contributory branches of the thoracic duct should not be attempted. The thoracic duct itself may arch as high as 6 cm. in the neck before angling downward again and entering the subclavian vein. If by intent or accident the duct is injured, repair should not be attempted because its wall is thin and friable. If there is continuity, the duct should be left alone; if continuity is interrupted, the duct should be ligated and tied off completely. Usually, no significant complication results. If the duct has been transected and the transection has not been recognized, a chylous fistula will develop.

Chyle will coagulate and, if not drained, will form a mass beneath the skin flaps; it is best removed manually. Direct drainage of the duct is preferred by opening the operative site directly over the duct; after a tract is well established, pressure dressings can be applied to the left lower area of the neck.

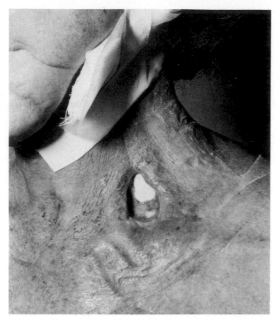

Figure 13–3   Chylous fistula plugged with polyvinyl mesh (Marlex). Defect in skin due to necrosis of skin flaps. Defect of this size usually heals without secondary surgical procedures. (From Gossel, J. D., Martin, W. J., and Beahrs, O. H.: Management of complicated chylous fistula following radical dissection of the neck. Surg. Clin. North Am., 35:1091, 1955.)

Often a plug of polyvinyl mesh (Marlex) or other material will be helpful (Fig. 13–3). Ligation of the duct can be attempted, but ligation is not often successful because this endangers adjacent structures. If the patient's condition is serious enough to justify ligation, transthoracic ligation of the thoracic duct can be considered.

The volume of fluid drained in 24 hours from the average fistula is about 1500 ml.; the flow stops after 1 to 3 weeks. In others, the amount in 24 hours may reach 6000 ml., and drainage may continue unless the duct is either ligated or plugged. The electrolytic composition of thoracic duct lymph is about the same as that of serum, except that there is less than 1 per cent protein in lymph. The fat content varies directly with the amount of fat ingested. Consequently, the effect on the body of a lymph fistula will be proportionate to the volume of fluid lost. An uncontrolled and uncompensated lymph fistula produces severe disturbances of fluid, electrolyte, and fat metabolism.

Management of the fluid and electrolyte imbalance requires great care to prevent hyponatremia and hypochloremia. Because some protein and 20 to 30 per cent of the ingested fat are also lost, malnutrition will soon occur. Frequent blood chemical analyses for sodium, potassium, chloride, carbon dioxide–combining power, blood urea nitrogen, and creatinine must be done to determine the daily intravenous requirements. Urinary levels of chloride and sodium should be measured once or twice to determine whether the body is conserving these substances. The lymph fluid draining from the neck should be collected on sponges and weighed hourly at the bedside, or if the fluid is removed by suction catheter, the amount should be determined and an aliquot analyzed for sodium, chloride, fat, and protein content.

In spite of the severe upset, the metabolic abnormality reverts to normal when the duct is ligated, provided sufficient fluid and electrolytes have been administered and the condition has not existed so long that the malnutrition has predisposed to intercurrent infection.

FACIAL EDEMA

After unilateral neck dissection, swelling occurs in the lower part of the face on the side of the operation. This is partly due to trauma of the surgery, but it is also due to interruption of the lymphatic vessels that drain this site. Within a few weeks, the swelling usually disappears and the face becomes bilaterally equal and normal. The findings are different after bilateral neck dissection. Cyanosis might first occur because of excision of the jugular system of veins. This most often disappears within 2 or 3 days, after which edema of the face becomes apparent. Sometimes the edema is severe, the swelling being so great that the eyes cannot be opened (Fig. 13–4). The edema is most pronounced at about 7 days after the operation, and then it subsides gradually over a period of several weeks. Most often after bilateral neck dissection the edema in the lower part of the face does not completely disappear, leaving the patient with a chipmunk-like appearance. Normal flow of lymph is rarely attained because subsequent surgery or infection in the operative site causes an increase or recurrence of

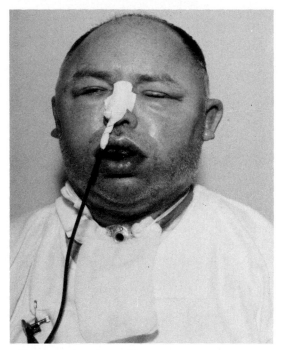

Figure 13–4   Edema of face and tongue. This frequently follows bilateral radical neck dissection (done in one or two stages). Severity of edema is basis for considering elective tracheostomy in most cases when both sides of neck are operated on.

lymphedema for a period after the trauma to the tissues.

Immediate postoperative edema, as in the case of intra-oral resections, may be diminished or significantly reduced by the use of intravenous methylprednisolone, as previously mentioned. This may also be helpful in minimizing the increase in cerebral venous pressure described below.

INCREASE IN CEREBRAL VENOUS PRESSURE

Increased cerebral venous pressure occasionally occurs during unilateral jugular vein ligation and often produces an immediate increase in cerebrospinal fluid pressure. The increase in intracranial pressure may be sustained for several days after operation; the increase is usually slight and occasionally accompanied by headache. Under normal conditions, outflow of blood from the cranial cavity takes place through the internal jugular veins. In unilateral vein ligation, the contralateral vein is large

enough to carry all the outflow with no more than a transient, harmless increase in intracranial pressure. Rarely, as shown by Woodhall,[22] one lateral sinus may be so narrow that cranial blood outflow is greatly reduced and intracranial pressure increases when the opposite vein is compressed. Additional venous channels exist in the vertebral veins, and in 12 to 24 hours these veins become sufficiently "adapted" for greater capacity.[9] Batson[2] has demonstrated that the cross-sectional area of the paravertebral system of veins in the neck is greater than that of the jugular system of veins. During this period immediately after operation, the critical increase in pressure may be fatal.[18, 20]

According to Royster,[18] symptoms of seriously increased intracranial pressure may be noted at operation and may be reflected in a slow pulse and high blood pressure. At the termination of operation, the patient may fail to regain consciousness, and the observer may note spasmodic contractions and irritability of muscles, irrationality, and finally, convulsions and death within 12 to 24 hours. When the pressure increase is moderate, emergence from anesthesia will be retarded and the sensorium dulled. On regaining full consciousness, the patient will experience severe headache, which will continue until the intracranial pressure is reduced. The headache will become worse when the patient assumes the recumbent position and will be improved when he elevates his head.

In our experience, increase in pressure of cerebrospinal fluid after unilateral neck dissection is rarely serious, and we have not seen intracranial complications except for one instance of bilateral blindness. A similar experience has been reported by Torti and Ballantyne.[21]

After bilateral radical neck dissection, we have seen no central nervous system abnormalities or abnormalities other than transient headache in some patients, even though cerebrospinal fluid pressures were increased for 24 to 48 hours (Fig. 13–5). Withdrawal of spinal fluid to reduce the temporarily elevated pressures to normal has not been necessary. However, an anomalous cerebral venous outflow can be detected before operation by the Queckenstedt test. If routes of flow through both jugular veins are patent, intracranial pressure

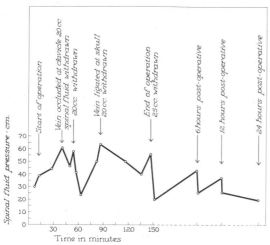

Figure 13–5 After sacrifice of jugular veins on second side when bilateral neck dissection is done, spinal fluid pressure increases during operation and for 24 hours after it. This causes headaches in some patients for short periods. (From Beahrs, O. H., and Jordan, G. L., Jr.: Bilateral radical cervical dissection for malignant lesions of the head and neck. Proc. Staff Meet. Mayo Clin. 27:449, 1952. By permission.)

should not increase to a dangerous level when one internal jugular vein is ligated. If the test indicates reduced cerebral outflow on the side opposite the expected ligation, an abnormal increase in intracranial pressure can be expected and may be prevented by withdrawing cerebrospinal fluid through an indwelling catheter inserted in the lumbar space before operation. The catheter is connected with a glass tube manometer, and the pressure is kept at a level not above 600 mm. by draining off fluid at intervals during operation. If the pressure increases above normal after the patient emerges from anesthesia, the catheter may be left in place for 24 to 48 hours for intermittent aspiration.

Practically, whether a bilateral neck dissection is done in one stage or in two stages makes little difference in mortality and morbidity.

FEVER

Fever is regarded as a reaction of the body to the trauma of operation. Infection of the wound, intercurrent disease, and other factors also must be considered when fever is evaluated. Oral temperatures as high as 100° F. (101° F. rectally) have been arbitrarily chosen as the basic response to a

major operation of the head and neck region, and when temperatures exceed 101° F., a complication must be sought as a cause.

INFECTION

Early primary invasive wound infection occurs infrequently with radical neck dissection. The usual type of infection becomes manifest about the fourth or fifth postoperative day. The predisposing cause is almost uniformly postoperative hematoma or seroma under the loosely attached skin flap. The organisms commonly found, staphylococci and streptococci, rarely delay healing. Infections are more frequent and severe when the oral cavity is entered and when the orocervical tissues have been previously infected or subjected to radiation.

Most often, infection can be prevented if careful wound toilet is performed, with attention to hemostasis and maintenance of neck flaps in contact with the deep wound surface.

Wound infection is treated locally by packing the infected areas of the wound or by inserting soft rubber drains and by applying compresses of physiologic saline solution at room temperature (hot compresses may cause necrosis of the ischemic flaps). Drainage is more effectively promoted if dressings are changed two or three times every day.

Systemic therapy with penicillin and a broad spectrum antibiotic should be started immediately. The wound should be cultured, and after the organisms have been identified and sensitivities determined, the antibiotic may be appropriately chosen.

MEDIASTINITIS

In patients with neck wound infections, mediastinitis can occur, but it usually responds to intensive antibiotic therapy. Most often, adequate drainage of the infected neck wound prevents mediastinitis from developing.

NECROSIS OF CERVICAL SKIN FLAPS

In neck dissection performed through the standard T-type incision, there are three large flaps. The upper flap, with the base at the cheek, is rarely affected by necrosis except at the very edge of the skin incision. The anterior and posterior flaps below may undergo necrosis, occasionally so extreme that both flaps are completely lost. Technically, the surgeon may carry the subcutaneous dissection too widely and too superficially, with damage to subdermal vessels, causing ischemia sufficient to result in necrosis of all or part of the flap. The surgeon must choose whether to keep the platysma muscle on the skin flap. If it is left on the reflected flap, the skin circulation is only slightly impaired, but there is a greater risk of cutting into the tumor. In the healing period, the skin flaps must be adherent to the underlying neck tissues, because nourishment is supplied by osmosis as well as by way of the remaining intact vessels of the flaps. The type of incision seems to have little relationship to the incidence of necrosis if the base of the flap is broad compared to its length.

Hematoma, infection, and previous exposure to radiation increase the incidence of necrosis of the skin flaps. If one or more of these is present, even a skin flap that is well supplied with blood may not survive. Again, attention to the details of wound toilet and emphasis on postoperative care are extremely important.

Management of necrotic flaps consists in removal of dead tissue once a line of demarcation has been definitely established, but this must be performed carefully over a period of several days if the necrotic skin overlies any part of the carotid artery system, for fear of damaging the blood supply to the adventitia of the artery or of dislodging a clot at a point of ligature. During the process of serially removing slough, the open wound surface should be covered with moist saline pads, which are changed three or four times daily. Once the dead tissue has been removed, a decision must be made whether to apply a split-thickness skin graft, to rotate an adjacent skin pedicle, or merely to allow the tissue to heal spontaneously. Use of the recently described pectoralis myocutaneous flap provides a means of vessel coverage that utilizes both muscle and skin with a non-irradiated blood supply and provides good healing. There is a slight disadvantage of imperfect cosmesis. A split-thickness graft may be used if the denuded area is large and the arterial wall and surrounding wounds are cleanly granulating. Contrarily, spontaneous healing may be so rapid that a graft will not be required.

In patients who have had previous radiotherapy or in whom the platysma muscle must be removed or in patients who do not want a vertical scar in the neck, two parallel incisions as described by MacFee[12] can be used. This approach avoids the placement of a vertical incision over the length of the carotid vessels, and thus will less likely expose them if any margin of the wound becomes necrotic.

RADIATION AND COMPLICATIONS

Tissue heavily irradiated for the treatment of cancer has been permanently and severely damaged, and healing of it takes place less readily. After incision, wound edges become necrotic and fail to heal, hematomas form readily, skin grafts do not take well, and oral tissues, particularly bone, may not heal. The surgeon who operates in a field previously exposed to radiation must consider this possible failure to heal as a calculated risk that will cause increased morbidity and occasionally death.

About one-third of patients who have had previous radiation therapy to the neck will have skin necrosis after radical neck surgery, whereas less than 10 per cent of patients without previous radiation to the neck will have necrosis. The real hazard with necrosis of the skin flaps is not the loss of skin but the exposure of the carotid arteries. Without viable cover for these arteries, the danger of ulceration and rupture of the arteries is real and the risk to life is great.

In heavily radiated head and neck tissues in patients undergoing combined resections, one of the chief threats to healing is infection secondary to breakdown of the intra-oral incisions. In such instances, the construction of a controlled fistula may prevent disastrous wound breakdown. Closure of the fistula may be later accomplished when neck healing is complete.

Postradiation edema of the airway structures also exposes the patient to airway obstruction; tracheostomy is needed more frequently in these patients than in those not treated by radiation. If elective tracheostomy is used whenever indicated, emergency tracheostomy is rarely necessary. The effect of radiation on bone often leads to osteonecrosis and formation of sequestrum even in the absence of infection or operation.

Dead bone has to be removed before the radiated or operative site will heal. The evidence is clear that irradiation influences the course of patients undergoing head and neck surgery by causing a greater degree of skin and bone necrosis and laryngeal edema sufficient to obstruct the airway.

Skin necrosis may be prevented by using extreme care in raising the skin flaps and by avoiding undermining that is too extensive. Little can be done to prevent bone necrosis. Tracheostomy by election or at the first sign of laryngeal edema is the only means of circumventing respiratory obstruction. Radiation exposure also may retard healing of primarily sutured wounds and wounds covered with skin grafts.

NEUROLOGIC COMPLICATIONS

Many sensory and motor nerves traverse the head and neck region. Some of these can be sacrificed during surgery without significant long-term functional morbidity, whereas removal of others leads to neurologic deficit of importance. Loss of the greater auricular nerve and other superficial cervical nerves results in numbness of the skin overlying and adjacent to the operative site. In most instances, a large measure of sensation will have returned in 6 to 12 months, but sacrifice of the greater auricular nerve results in some permanent numbness of the lower ear and parotid region.

Traumatic neuromas may develop at the ends of transected nerves. These can almost always be differentiated from nodules of recurrent cancer by their exquisite tenderness on palpation.

When parotidectomy is necessary and the facial nerve must be sacrificed, paralysis of the facial muscles on the affected side occurs. This leaves a severe cosmetic deformity that is distressing to the patient. Plastic surgery may bring improvement if the patient remains well. Of most importance is protection of the eye since the lower lid will not function. This can be corrected by blepharorrhaphy. In selected patients, a free nerve graft can be inserted between the proximal nerve trunk and the peripheral branches. This will give good to excellent results in approximately 70 per cent of patients.[5] If the proximal trunk of the facial nerve is not available, the use of hypoglossal or spinal accessory nerve transplant should be considered. When this is done, reeducation of muscle function is necessary.

During the standard radical neck dissection, the marginalis branch of the facial nerve should be protected where it passes over the anterior facial vessels. usually just below the lower border of the mandible. This will prevent weakness of the lower lip on the side of the operation. If the submandibular lymph nodes are metastatically involved, then this nerve should be sacrificed and the cosmetic defect accepted.

Clinical symptoms of the Frey syndrome, or gustatory sweating over the parotid and upper neck areas,[8] develop in about one-third of the patients undergoing surgical procedures that include parotidectomy. Flushing and sweating of the skin in the parotid region are noted mostly while eating. This complication is probably caused by irregular regrowth of fibers of the auriculotemporal nerve, previously stimulating the saliva gland, into the sweat glands of the overlying skin. For most patients, reassurance and explanation of the problem is sufficient. When the syndrome is severe, transecting the Jacobsen nerve in the middle ear should be considered; transection often will eliminate the symptoms.[11]

In the classic radical neck dissection, the spinal accessory nerve that is motor to the trapezius muscle is sacrificed. This leads to atrophy of the muscle, drooping of the shoulder, and difficulty in lifting the arm laterally over the head. Sacrifice of both spinal accessory nerves makes it difficult for the patient to put on a shirt or a coat. Many patients complain of discomfort and lameness in the shoulder. A study of selected patients in whom the spinal accessory nerve was preserved revealed no increase in the recurrence rate of cancer in the neck as compared to those in whom the nerve was sacrificed.[17] Thus, the spinal accessory nerve probably should be preserved in all patients except those in whom gross evidence of cancer is encountered in the process of dissecting the nerve free of adjacent soft tissues.

If the lingual nerve is resected, the ipsilateral side of the tongue becomes numb. Sacrifice of the hypoglossal nerve results in paralysis of the corresponding half of the tongue. On protrusion, the tongue will deviate to the side of the operation. The only untoward effect of sacrificing the vagus nerve on one side is paralysis of the corresponding vocal cord. Excision of the glossopharyngeal nerve results in difficulty in swallowing on that side of the throat, because of paralysis of the pharyngeal muscles. Injury of the phrenic nerve leads to paralysis of the hemidiaphragm, while trauma to the sympathetic nerve results in the Horner syndrome. Injury to the brachial plexus causes sensory or motor dysfunction (or both) in the upper extremity.

Except for the brachial plexus, any of the nerves mentioned justifiably can be sacrificed if in doing so the operation becomes definitive and offers the patient a chance of cure. Otherwise, the nerves should be protected and preserved.

MALNUTRITION

Malnutrition is present in many patients (50 per cent) with head and neck cancer because of poor dietary habits, difficulty and pain when eating, and loss of blood. Nutrition should be improved as rapidly as possible before operation to aid in preventing complications. The nutritional status of each patient must be determined by clinical observation and the usual laboratory tests. Enough days should be allowed before the operation for forced feedings and transfusions. If necessary, the program for feeding must be a diet of 3500 to 5000 calories, high in protein, taken by mouth or by nasogastric tube. Qualitative vitamin supplement of three to four times the daily normal requirement is given parenterally to ensure absorption. Preoperative weight gain is ideal, but not always possible. After operation, this regimen must be resumed within 2 to 3 days to maintain a positive metabolic balance, and it may be continued for 1 to 2 weeks or until the patient can satisfy his needs by a normal diet. In malnourished or wasted patients hyperalimentation for several days before surgery and in the immediate postoperative period is of great benefit.

Many patients with carcinoma of the oral cavity may be alcoholics, and delirium tremens may be a problem in the early postoperative or even preoperative period. Dietary correction of vitamin deficiencies and use of sedatives may be sufficient in many instances, but intravenous or oral administration of alcohol may be needed.

RECURRENCE OF CANCER

Recurrence of cancer of the head and neck region must be considered a complication if the primary treatment was considered adequate. In recurrence, the prognosis is poor; of all patients with head and neck cancers, 40 to 50 per cent survive 5 years. After radical neck dissection, 26 per cent of patients in a series of 615 had recurrence of the disease in the neck.[3] Approximately 30 per cent of the patients had recurrences of the primary lesion or the occurrence of a second primary lesion nearby. If recurrence is to be prevented or the incidence of recurrence reduced, treatment must be earlier and more aggressive. Ultimately, new knowledge regarding etiology of the disease or new modalities of management (or both) will become available and lead to improved results, less mortality, and fewer complications.

Bibliography

1. Barber, K. W., Jr., and Beahrs, O. H.: Bilateral radical dissection of the neck: Surgical treatment for carcinoma of mouth and larynx. Arch. Surg. *83*:388, 1961.
2. Batson, O. V.: Anatomical problems concerned in the study of cerebral blood flow. Fed. Proc. *3*:139, 1944.
3. Beahrs, O. H., and Barber, K. W., Jr.: The value of radical dissection of structures of the neck in the management of carcinoma of the lip, mouth, and larynx. Arch. Surg. *85*:49, 1962.
4. Beahrs, O. H., Gossel, J. D., and Hollinshead, W. H.: Technic and surgical anatomy of radical neck dissection. Am. J. Surg. *90*:490, 1955.
5. Beahrs, O. H., Judd, E. S., and Woodington, G. F.: Use of nerve grafts for repair of defects in the facial nerve. Ann. Surg. *153*:433, 1961.
6. Crile, G.: Excision of cancer of head and neck: With special reference to the plan of dissection based on one hundred and thirty-two operations. J.A.M.A. *47*:1780, 1906.
7. Eckenhoff, J. E.: Some anatomic considerations of the infant larynx influencing endotracheal anesthesia. Anesthesiology *12*:401, 1951.
8. Frey, L.: Le syndrome du nerf auriculo-temporal. Rev. Neurol. *2*:97, 1923.
9. Gius, J. A., and Grier, D. H.: Venous adaptation

following bilateral radical neck dissection with excision of jugular veins. Surgery *28*:305, 1950.

10. Groesbeck, H. P., and Cudmore, J. T. P.: Fatal air embolism during head and neck surgery. Paper delivered at meeting of Society of Head and Neck Surgeons, Washington, D.C., March 30, 1959.

11. Hunt, W., Joseph, D., Newell, R., and Hanna, H. H.: Gustatory sweating: Report of a case treated by tympanic neurectomy. Arch. Otolaryngol. *83*:260, 1966.

12. MacFee, W. F.: Transverse incisions for neck dissection. Ann. Surg. *151*:279, 1960.

13. Marchetta, F. C., and Sake, K.: Pneumothorax — Frequency following radical neck surgery. Paper delivered at meeting of Society of Head and Neck Surgeons, Washington, D.C., March 30, 1959.

14. Martin, H.: Radical surgery in cancer of the head and neck. Surg. Clin. North Am. *33*:329, 1953.

15. Pemberton, J. deJ., and Livermore, G. R., Jr.: Surgical treatment of carotid body tumors: Value of anticoagulants in carotid ligation. Ann. Surg. *133*:837, 1951.

16. Randall, P.: Adequate airway — A necessary precaution: Introduction of a routine for management and an evaluation of 100 cases of radical neck dissection. Plast. Reconstr. Surg. *20*:18, 1957.

17. Roy, P. H., and Beahrs, O. H.: Spinal accessory nerve in radical neck dissections. Am. J. Surg. *118*:800, 1969.

18. Royster, H. P.: The relation between internal jugular vein pressure and cerebrospinal fluid pressure in the operation of radical neck dissection. Ann. Surg. *137*:826, 1953.

19. Simons, J. N., Beahrs, O. H., and Woolner, L. B.: Tumors of the submaxillary gland. Am. J. Surg. *108*:485, 1964.

20. Sugarbaker, F. D., and Wiley, H. M.: Intracranial pressure studies incident to resection of the internal jugular veins. Cancer *4*:242, 1951.

21. Torti, R. A., Ballantyne, A. J., and Berkeley, R. G.: Sudden blindness after simultaneous bilateral radical neck dissection. Arch. Surg. *88*:271, 1964.

22. Woodhall, B.: Variations of the cranial venous sinuses in the region of the torcular herophili. Arch. Surg. *33*:297, 1936.

14

COMPLICATIONS OF THYROID AND PARATHYROID SURGERY

John S. Kukora and James D. Hardy

Surgical procedures on the thyroid and parathyroid glands are generally safe and well tolerated. Nonetheless, the occasional complication following such surgery may be life-threatening or at least permanently disabling. These complications derive from anatomic disturbances of the many vital structures associated with these glands in the neck or from metabolic and physiologic abnormalities caused by the disease processes of the glands or by their ablation. Since these complications occur so infrequently despite the high volume of surgery on these glands, no individual surgeon is likely to encounter a large experience with a particular complication. Yet, the astute clinician must be ever mindful of the potential for complications and be prepared for rapid intervention should a serious problem develop. Recent reports of increased thyroid malignancy,[5] along with increased longevity of renal dialysis patients with greater corresponding incidence of secondary hyperparathyroidism and increased dissatisfaction with the long-term results of radioactive iodine ablation of toxic goiter, will almost certainly lead to an increased frequency of surgery on these glands, and more patients will be exposed to potential surgical complications.

ANATOMIC COMPLICATIONS OF THYROID AND PARATHYROID SURGERY

SAFE TECHNIQUE

The exemplary work of Theodor Kocher during the last century in developing a safe technique for thyroidectomy resulted in a Nobel Prize and allowed continuing progress in thyroid surgery by his successors. In the United States, pioneer thyroid surgeons included Halsted, Crile, C. H. Mayo, and Lahey, among many others.

The importance of safe operative technique can hardly be overemphasized, for it is far better to prevent a complication than to treat it. A thorough knowledge of anatomy and pathophysiology is of paramount importance in order consistently to avoid

---

John Steven Kukora was born in Michigan. He received his college and medical school education at the University of Michigan and his internship and residency training at the University of Michigan Medical Center. He was elected to both Phi Beta Kappa and Alpha Omega Alpha. In 1979, Dr. Kukora joined the faculty of the University of Mississippi Medical Center, where he is Assistant Professor of Surgery. He has a deep interest in endocrine problems.

injury to the vital structures in the depths of the neck, and a gentle and skillful technique is required to preserve delicate and essential structures.

Descriptions of thyroidectomy technique are abundant.[8, 22] The best help for the young surgeon learning this procedure is careful review of neck anatomy and of the steps of the operation prior to assisting at or performing thyroid and parathyroid operations under the direction of a skilled surgeon.

Exposure of the Thyroid Gland

Good exposure of the thyroid gland is essential for consistently safe surgery. A transverse curvilinear cervical collar incision is made to the mid-mandible, centering the incision carefully on the midline as judged by a line from the center of the sternal notch to the mid-thyroid cartilage. The incision should extend to the medial border of each sternocleidomastoid muscle, and it is placed no lower than 3 cm. above the clavicle. It should follow a natural skin crease, if possible, to minimize cosmetic deformity. If the incision is made too low, the scar will have a tendency to widen and to migrate downward over the sternum, becoming unsightly. The incision is carried deep to the platysma muscle, and sub-platysmal flaps are elevated superiorly to the level of the notch of the thyroid cartilage and inferiorly to the sternal notch and clavicular heads. Ligation of venous branches during this dissection will prevent blood-staining from obscuring later dissection (Fig. 14–1).

The delicate areolar midline fusion fascia of the pre-tracheal strap muscles is then separated, obtaining careful hemostasis of small venous tributaries crossing the midline. These muscles are then retracted laterally, separating them from the thyroid gland by gentle finger dissection or gauze pledget dissection. Repeated re-application of small retractors during mobilization of these muscles aids substantially in their lateral retraction.

Some surgeons prefer to divide the strap muscles routinely to facilitate exposure of a difficult gland, especially one with a high-positioned superior pole, or when there is a very large goiter. We divide the strap muscles on the first side, where necessary, and occasionally on the opposite side as well; however, division of the strap muscles is usually not necessary. Even with large substernal goiters, excellent exposure often can be obtained with appropriate placement of the strap muscle retractors and by elevation and medial rotation of the thyroid lobe by the assistant. Of course, the strap muscles should be divided and removed en bloc if invaded by thyroid carcinoma. No complication should arise from bilateral division of these muscles, provided that secure hemostasis is obtained from their cut edges. It is important to dissect the strap muscles from the thyroid gland in the correct plane, in order to prevent bleeding from the surface of the gland or from torn muscle fibers

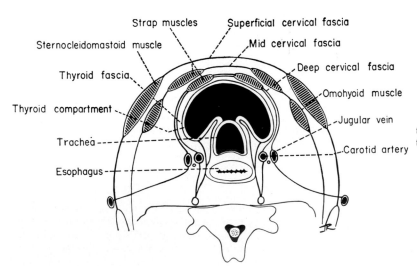

Figure 14–1 A cross section of the neck at the level of the thyroid gland.

when dissection strays. The middle thyroid vein is next encountered and ligated between mosquito hemostats with fine suture material.

Thyroid vessels should be ligated, when encountered, in order to prevent bleeding and vessel retraction later on in the event that hemostats become dislodged from these delicate vessels during further dissection. Vigorous spreading motions along the sides of vessels are to be avoided, since tearing of vessels is likely to ensue, causing blood-staining and obscuration of anatomic detail. The bleeding vessel must be ligated precisely to avoid injury to adjacent structures and in particular to the recurrent laryngeal nerve. The choice between silk, catgut, or synthetic-absorbable suture material will depend on the individual surgeon. Silk is the easiest to tie and does not tend to slip off the ligated vessel readily, but occasionally silk has a tendency to be extruded or "spit" from thyroidectomy wounds. We ligate pole vessels with silk but may employ catgut ligatures for other bleeders. We generally avoid use of electrocautery on or about the thyroid gland because of possible thermal damage to the recurrent laryngeal nerve and parathyroid glands. After division of the middle thyroid vein, the thyroid lobe is rotated medially on a longitudinal axis by means of a gauze traction sponge and the assistant's fingers. The use of a thyroid tenaculum is not recommended if the operation is being performed for suspected carcinoma, since malignant cells might be released into the wound.

These maneuvers are common to all initial approaches to the thyroid and parathyroid glands. Subsequent maneuvers depend on the specific operation to be performed and will be discussed individually.

Total Thyroid Lobectomy and Total Thyroidectomy

Total thyroid lobectomy is performed for suspected malignancy within the lobe, usually for a palpable, firm hypofunctioning nodule. Careful palpation for any nodules in the contralateral lobe is performed after mobilization of the strap muscles from the midline. The abnormal lobe is rotated medially as described previously. The superior pole of the lobe is usually mobilized first. This is facilitated by downward traction on the gland by the assistant and upward and lateral retraction of the strap muscles. The suspensory ligament of the isthmus and its vessels are ligated and divided. An avascular plane between the medial border of the superior pole and the cricothyroid muscle fascia is developed until the superior thyroid artery and vein branches are seen approaching the capsule of the gland. These are individually ligated between pairs of fine hemostats *close to the gland* to prevent injury to the external branch of the superior laryngeal nerve, a complication we shall discuss later. Occasionally, serious hemorrhage from a retracted and divided superior thyroid artery will occur. This should be controlled by finger pressure of the assistant, while the origin of the superior thyroid artery off the external carotid is exposed by the surgeon and ligated cleanly. Such an approach will prevent damage to the superior laryngeal or hypoglossal nerves that may follow attempts at blind clamping and mass ligation of the bleeding vessels.

Next, the location of the superior parathyroid gland should be sought. The gland is usually adherent to the areolar tissue investing the deep medial surface of the superior pole of the thyroid adjacent to the carotid sheath. The gland should be mobilized laterally and slightly downward by very delicate technique, avoiding any crushing of the gland by forceps and any upward traction away from the blood supply of the gland that enters it inferiorly. A superior anti-hilar approach to the superior parathyroid in reflecting it from the thyroid capsule will likely prevent any inadvertent division of its blood supply based on a branch of the inferior thyroid artery. At this point, the superior pole will have been completely mobilized to the point of firm attachment of the thyroid gland to the trachea.

Next, the lowermost branches of the inferior thyroid artery and vein are divided and ligated close to the capsule of the gland. A search is made for the inferior parathyroid gland, which often lies among these branches just deep to the inferior thyroid lobe. The parathyroid is carefully mobilized away from the thyroid gland, just as was the superior parathyroid. The blood supply to the inferior gland from the inferior thyroid artery usually approaches the gland from above.

At this point, the lobe must be mobilized from the trachea by dividing any remaining small branches of the inferior thyroid artery and sharply dissecting through the ligament of Berry, the fascial attachment of the lobe to the trachea. This part of the dissection poses the greatest threat of injury to the recurrent laryngeal nerve by traction, cutting, or crushing, and proper care must be taken (Fig. 14–2). The branching patterns and location of this nerve and its relation to other structures, especially the inferior thyroid artery and thyroid capsule, are widely variable and do not allow a useful categorization. More variability is encountered on the right side, with non-recurrence reported in 0.3 per cent of cases,[21] and a more common lateral position than on the left side.[14]

Most surgeons prefer to identify the recurrent nerve in the tracheoesophageal groove before ligating the medial branches of the inferior thyroid artery and to follow the nerve into the larynx, dissecting it away from the thyroid capsule before dividing the ligament of Berry. This should be performed by spreading a small hemostat in the direction of the nerve's course, using the most gentle dissection technique to prevent avulsion, cutting, or stretching of the nerve, or interference with its blood supply by excessive mobilization. Other experienced surgeons prefer careful division of the in-

ferior thyroid vessels as they enter the thyroid capsule near the ligament of Berry without specifically identifying and tracing the course of the recurrent laryngeal nerve.

The occasional nerve closely applied to the thyroid capsule or entering the substance of the thyroid gland will become apparent during the course of the meticulous capsular dissection, and it can be preserved. If tumor extension outside of the capsule or a large goiter has distorted the anatomy, then the nerve should be sought and traced. The majority of nerves positioned lateral to the capsule of the gland and the ligament of Berry are thus not specifically exposed and are spared any possible attendant injury during mobilization, nor will they be injured during mobilization of the inferior thyroid branches as they enter the gland or during sharp transection of the ligament of Berry. The incidence of recurrent laryngeal nerve injury appears to be less than 1 per cent in several large series, whether or not the recurrent laryngeal nerve was specifically traced.[16, 22] Thus, an individual preference for either technique appears justified, although the majority of surgeons will probably be best served by routine safe exposure of the nerve.

At this point, the entire lobe has been mobilized, with no residual thyroid tissue adherent to the trachea on this side. The isthmus is then divided in the midline between Kocher clamps and the remaining cut

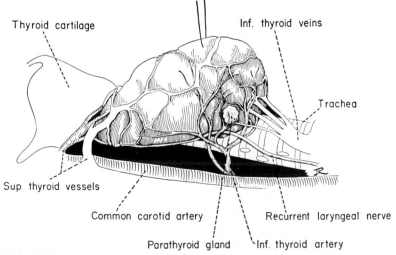

Figure 14–2 The recurrent laryngeal nerves usually bear a close anatomic relation to the inferior thyroid arteries. Modern thyroid surgery requires that the surgeon acquire the ability to identify, expose, and preserve these nerves when indicated.

end of the isthmus hemostatically secured with mattress sutures.

A frozen section of the nodule is obtained. If carcinoma is proven but the opposite thyroid lobe appears normal, a radical subtotal resection on that side should be performed. Some surgeons recommend total thyroidectomy, but total thyroidectomy may be associated with a higher overall complication rate than that of subtotal resection. However, if there is clinical evidence of involvement of the opposite lobe, total thyroidectomy is indicated. A search for metastatic nodal disease is undertaken in the tissues of the suspensory ligament and along the jugular chains, and involved nodes with papillary or follicular cancer are removed as encountered. An en bloc modified radical neck dissection is indicated if medullary or resectable anaplastic carcinoma is encountered, although the long-term results with anaplastic carcinoma are poor.

Again, total thyroidectomy exposes the patient to the greatest risks of bilateral recurrent laryngeal nerve palsy and permanent hypoparathyroidism. Leaving a small amount of tissue (1 or 2 gm.) on the contralateral side — i.e., a subtotal contralateral lobectomy — may decrease the likelihood of contralateral recurrent nerve injury or parathyroid devascularization and may well be the preferred procedure if the ipsilateral nerve is suspected of injury or involved by tumor or if there is uncertain viability of the ipsilateral parathyroids. However, the presence of bilateral carcinoma or multilocular carcinoma is best treated by complete thyroidectomy, as previously indicated. The implantation of parathyroid tissue into the sternocleidomastoid or forearm muscles may preserve function of these glands if they are inadvertently devascularized,[18] but in our opinion the uncertainty of viability after implantation highlights the importance of preserving the natural blood supply of one or more of these glands at the time of surgery.

An inadequate resection of the thyroid cancer decreases the likelihood of cure and exposes the patient to much greater risk of complications during re-operation to complete the inadequate initial resection.[4]

A frozen section for pathologic interpretation of any nodule in the thyroid is mandatory. Incisional biopsy of a thyroid nodule carries the risk of dispersing malignant cells and is to be condemned. Excisional biopsy of the nodule with a margin of 2 to 3 mm. of normal thyroid tissue and, at times, of the adjacent total lobe with the isthmus is the preferred method of establishing a histologic diagnosis.

Occasionally, the operative frozen section report is that of benign disease or is equivocal, but the permanent section report returns in several days as definite carcinoma. Thus, the patient should remain in the hospital until the permanent section report is returned, and should it reveal carcinoma, the patient is promptly returned for contralateral total or nearly total lobectomy before postoperative scarring progresses to the point that a repeat neck exploration becomes unduly hazardous.

Subtotal Thyroidectomy

Subtotal thyroidectomy is performed for symptomatic multinodular goiter or for Graves' disease. The operative exposure of the gland and procedure are exactly as those for total thyroidectomy, except that complete removal of all thyroid from the ligament of Berry is not performed and approximately 2 gm. of thyroid are left at this attachment bilaterally. This decreases the likelihood of direct damage to the parathyroid blood supply from inferior thyroid artery branches in the area and also of injury to the recurrent laryngeal nerve as it courses near the ligament of Berry; however, caution must be exercised during exposure not to stretch the nerve unduly. Considerably more than 2 gm. of tissue may be safely left if operation is performed for non-toxic goiter, but recurrent hyperthyroidism may appear if much more than 2 gm. are left during a sub-total thyroidectomy for Graves' disease.

Parathyroid Exploration and Parathyroidectomy

The initial approach to the parathyroids is best made through the same incision and exposure as for thyroidectomy, with rotation of the thyroid lobes medially after ligation of any middle thyroid veins. Careful dissection along the deep surface of the superior pole adjacent to the carotid sheath will usually disclose the location of the superior parathyroid. Similarly, a search near the medial branches of the inferior thyroid artery, or lower to the inferior pole of the thyroid lobe, or lower yet into the thyrothymic tract of the superior mediastinum will disclose the majority of inferior parathyroids. Every attempt should be made to preserve the blood supply of these glands as they are encountered, until all have been located. Special care should be used in the region of the recurrent laryngeal nerve to prevent injury. Commonly, a hyperplastic gland may be deceptively adherent to the thyroid, and its coloration may resemble that of the thyroid itself. Such a gland can be recognized by dissecting next to the thyroid capsule from the lateral posterior surface of the lobe to the medial posterior surface of the lobe, and cleaning this plane will lead to a free dissection of the parathyroid gland. The parathyroid dissection must be relaxed and never hurried, and care is needed to prevent blood-staining of the tissues, which severely impedes recognition of the parathyroids and recurrent nerves.

To minimize postoperative hypoparathyroidism or recurrent hyperparathyroidism, the following biopsy technique has worked well. If operating for primary hyperparathyroidism and an enlarged gland with three normal glands is found, the enlarged gland is removed and one or two of the normal-sized glands are biopsied, leaving unbiopsied those that have had the least mobilization or dissection near their blood supply. The glands are biopsied on the side away from the feeding artery. Frozen section is needed to confirm that the enlarged gland is hyperplastic or adenomatous and that the normal-sized gland is normal. The operation is then terminated.

If four normal or enlarged glands are found, two are biopsied to confirm hyperplasia and a 3½-gland parathyroidectomy is performed. If the pathology reports are normal, a diligent search must be undertaken for an ectopic fifth gland. This search may reveal an adenoma of the fifth gland. The presence of a fifth gland is not as rare as one might expect.

If three or fewer glands that appear normal are found, a careful search for an ectopic adenomatous gland is indicated. Any enlarged gland is always biopsied to confirm hyperplasia, and one or two of the smaller glands are biopsied to confirm normality.

The accessory maneuvers to find an ectopic parathyroid gland include careful search within the length of the carotid sheath, search along and posterior to the cervical esophagus in the prevertebral fascia, and exploration of the superior mediastinum through the neck with excision of the thyrothymic tract and thymectomy. Rarely, an ectopic gland may be found within a thyroid lobe, and as a last resort, with the finding of three normal glands, a thyroid lobectomy on the side of the missing gland is justified and may reveal the missing gland. We have found a number of adenomas that were almost encircled by thyroid tissue and very rarely a parathyroid adenoma that was completely within the thyroid lobe.

All parathyroid tissue should be appropriately identified, the site of the parathyroid glands remaining should be marked with a metal clip, and an accurate diagram should be drawn and added to the patient's chart to facilitate re-exploration later, if necessary.

All large glands should be palpated prior to excision and removed widely en bloc if a firm or gritty texture suggests the rare parathyroid carcinoma.

The current choices of operation for secondary hyperparathyroidism vary from total thyroidectomy, to 3½-gland resection, to total parathyroidectomy with autotransplantation of part of one gland in the forearm.[26] Our current choice is a total parathyroidectomy in patients who are not renal transplant candidates and 3½-gland resection in those who are.

The best opportunity for cure of hyperparathyroidism is at the original operation. Thoroughness of exploration and pathologic confirmation of the parathyroid tissue removed will decrease the need for repeated neck exploration and the attendant morbidity of a second procedure in a scarred operative field.

POSTOPERATIVE COMPLICATIONS

Postoperative Hemorrhage

As mentioned earlier, meticulous hemostasis must be secured along the way in performing safe thyroid and parathyroid surgery, not only to prevent blood-staining and obscuration of important structures in the neck but also to decrease the likelihood of postoperative hemorrhage. Vessels should be clamped and tied as they are encountered to prevent tearing and retraction that might necessitate clamp placement in proximity to easily injured structures, such as the recurrent laryngeal nerve. Holding sutures between the jaws of mosquito hemostats and using them as "passers" facilitates passing the suture around the tips of deeply placed hemostats. Should blood-staining occur, irrigation with saline often restores the visibility promptly. Blind clamping of vessels near the recurrent laryngeal nerve is to be avoided at all times.

At the completion of the operation the wound is irrigated briskly with saline to wash away superficial clots and disclose any unligated vessels. Hemostasis must be satisfactory at this point, for to close the wound without good hemostasis is to invite the hazard of respiratory tract compression by hemorrhage with resulting hypoxia, the most serious postoperative complication and the principal cause of death following thyroidectomy. The bleeding need not be of large volume to embarrass respiration, for the hemorrhage is deep to the tough cervical fascia. It is wise to use a drain in all except minor thyroid or parathyroid surgery. The drain can be removed at 24 hours, the cosmetic suture at the drain site tied down, and a good cosmetic result achieved.

Again, postoperative hemorrhage can be fatal because of rapid development of tracheal compression, and its recognition may be difficult or delayed (Figs. 14–3 and 14–4). Even the use of a drain, which usually reveals postoperative bleeding if present, does not guarantee that a potentially fatal hematoma has not formed, as the drain and tract may be occluded by clot, and thus bleeding can spread widely into the confines of the deep cervical fascia without external evidence. Any patient may be prone to develop postoperative hemorrhage, but markedly hypertensive patients are especially at risk of hemorrhage that is occasionally large enough to decrease significantly the circulating volume. Four hundred to five hundred ml. of blood may be confined

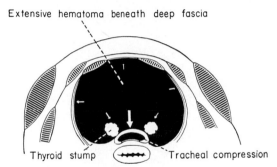

Figure 14–3 The tough cervical fascia, once closed, may prevent escape of blood, and the confined hematoma may produce serious and even fatal compression of the trachea and larynx.

within the deep cervical space and the superior mediastinum.

Diagnosis

The first sign of concealed hemorrhage may be repeated clearing of the throat or complaints of dysphagia or of smothering. There may be respiratory stertor or stridor or other noisy and labored respiration. If serious oozing is taking place and blood is emerging from between the skin flaps, it is usually best to move the patient immediately to the operating suite and there open the wound under local anesthesia and sterile conditions and ligate any bleeding points that can be found. If the patient must be given a general anesthetic for this exposure or if evidence of significant respiratory embarrassment develops, nasotracheal intubation using topical anesthesia should be performed while the patient is awake; this may be difficult if the larynx and trachea have been displaced by the clot. The use of thiopental (Pentothal) anesthesia here is hazardous, for sudden cessation of respiratory effort or laryngospasm may lead to cardiac arrest before intubation or tracheotomy can be accomplished.

It is important to realize that substantial hemorrhage deep to the cervical fascia may occur without producing outward physical signs, such as neck swelling, as the expansion of the hematoma is inward, compressing the pharynx and trachea. At the slightest evidence of suspicion of significant hemorrhage, the closest observation of the patient is required, either in the Recovery

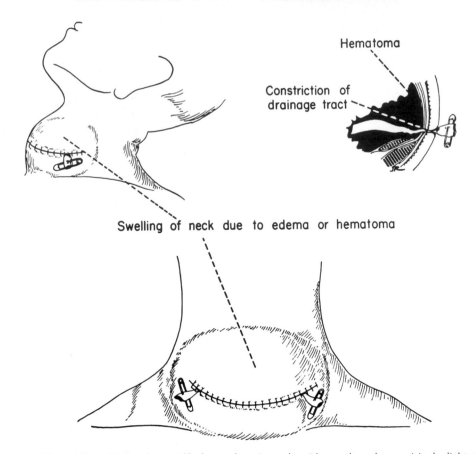

Hematoma

Constriction of drainage tract

Swelling of neck due to edema or hematoma

Figure 14–4 The swelling of the neck caused by hemorrhage into a thyroid wound may be surprisingly slight, compared with the relatively large volume of blood that is present. Even when a drain has been placed, deceptively little blood may appear on the dressings. This failure of blood to escape may be due to either excessively snug closure of the wound around the drain or obstruction of the drainage tract by clot. If it is necessary to evacuate the hematoma by reopening the wound postoperatively, a nasotracheal tube should perhaps be inserted to assure an adequate airway over the next 24 hours. The paramount consideration is to prevent asphyxia due to tracheal compression.

Room or the Intensive Care Unit where emergency tracheostomy can be performed through the recent thyroidectomy wound if indicated. If the patient must be reintubated for respiratory distress, the tube should be left in place for 24 hours and even then removed only with close monitoring.

Air Embolism

Air embolism is a potential hazard from any unligated, severed vein, especially from branches of the great venous trunks in the neck. Small volume air emboli are probably common occurrences with intravenous catheter placement during most surgical procedures and are rarely of any physiologic consequence, because they do not impair filling of the right side of the heart.

Massive air embolism is a serious development. The likelihood of its occurrence can be decreased by use of a cuffed endotracheal tube and positive-pressure ventilation during the administration of anesthesia, to increase intrathoracic pressure. Keeping the head of the operating table elevated 30 degrees is another useful precaution. Careful attention to the heart sounds by an esophageal or precordial stethoscope may alert the anesthesiologist to the classic loud gurgling murmur of intracardiac air before any decrease in cardiac output or change in vital signs occurs. If massive embolism should occur, the patient should be rolled to the left lateral decubitus position and the venous portal of air entry controlled. If persistent hypotension is present, an attempt should be made to aspirate the air through a small catheter placed in the superior vena cava and thence into the right heart via the internal jugular vein. Rarely, emergency thoracotomy and cardiac massage may be required if cardiac arrest occurs.

Airway Complications

Respiratory tract obstruction following thyroid and parathyroid surgery can be lethal and may be difficult to recognize. The causes include tracheal compression due to hemorrhage, laryngeal edema, recurrent laryngeal nerve damage, laryngotracheal displacement from a goiter that is not improved with surgery, and tracheal collapse because of unstable cartilaginous rings.

As discussed earlier, tracheal compression from postoperative hemorrhage occurs infrequently, yet it may cause a death every 3 to 4 years in hospitals with active surgical services. A sense of complacency develops in the staff caring for postoperative thyroid and parathyroid surgery patients based on the benign postoperative course of the overwhelming majority of such patients. This tendency, coupled with scarcity or subtlety of physical findings with early tracheal compression, makes it likely that the condition may go unrecognized until severe hypoxemia is present. Unfortunately, intervention then can be futile.

Respiratory obstruction, from whatever cause, tends to arise late in the evening of the day of surgery, usually after the patient has returned to his room from the close observation of the recovery room. Increasingly disturbed by dyspnea and progressive hypoxia, the patient may actually be given sedation for "restlessness" by the nursing staff — obviously a potentially disastrous action. Again, the patient with significant respiratory symptoms and signs should be moved back to the I.C.U. and, in most instances, a nasotracheal tube should be inserted to permit good pulmonary ventilation. With a safe airway secured, the precise cause of the respiratory difficulty can be diagnosed accurately and appropriate therapy initiated. If re-intubation is difficult and a genuine emergency exists, immediate tracheostomy must be performed, even before any attempt at removing clots or ligating bleeders in the wound, other than for exposure of the trachea itself. *A good airway is paramount.* Obviously, clinical judgment is an important guide to what should be done first, but unfortunately, the patient is usually seen first by inexperienced personnel who may not realize the gravity of the situation and the operating surgeon may be called too late.

If the respiratory obstruction was caused by hemorrhage, the operative area should be re-explored in the operating room, perhaps even under general anesthesia. Thereafter, the wound should be widely drained and the endotracheal tube left in place for at least 24 hours. Low-pressure cuffed endotracheal tubes or tracheostomy tubes should be utilized to decrease the likelihood of tracheal stenosis.

Tracheal instability caused by collapse of weakened cartilaginous rings from a longstanding goiter (tracheomalacia) should be suspected when preoperative airway obstruction exists with a goiter. All patients with large goiters, particularly those extending substernally, should have an experienced anesthesiologist present at the time of induction and should preferably be intubated while awake. If this intubation proves impossible, an isthmusectomy and tracheostomy under local anesthesia may be necessary to secure the airway prior to thyroidectomy. If a weakened trachea is observed during surgery, a tracheostomy should be performed with the tracheostomy tube extending through to below the weakened area to serve as a stent for several weeks until the tracheal wall regains stability. The weakening of the trachea is often recognized only postoperatively.

Laryngeal edema is seen as an increasingly rarer complication with modern anesthesia techniques but may follow a particularly difficult intubation or extensive manipulation of the larynx during surgery with an endotracheal tube in place. It is recognized by postoperative (usually prompt) stridor and must be differentiated from bilateral recurrent nerve injury (by direct or indirect laryngoscopy) or paratracheal hemorrhage. Mild cases of laryngeal edema may be treated by placing the patient in a high Fowler position (head and trunk elevated) and using humidified oxygen therapy. Inspiratory crowing sounds are ominous, and prompt re-intubation for progressive signs of airway obstruction is indicated before cardiac arrest occurs. An intravenous bolus of 100 mg. of hydrocortisone is frequently helpful in reversing mild laryngeal edema, as well as intermittent positive-pressure breathing therapy with 1 to 2 drops of 1:200,000 racemic epinephrine in 3 ml. of normal saline.

The key to success in handling airway complications is awareness of the problem. A policy of educating all staff caring for these patients to alert the responsible surgeon to any potential problem no matter how minimal will allow early intervention with greater likelihood of a successful outcome.

Recurrent Laryngeal Nerve Injury

Unilateral recurrent nerve injury can be mainly troublesome, whereas bilateral injury can be extremely serious. Fortunately, bilateral injury is extremely rare, occurring about once in every 30,000 operations.[6] Factors that increase the likelihood of injury include large goiters, invasive malignancy, and previous surgery in the area.

It has been our practice to perform indirect laryngoscopy on most patients prior to thyroid and parathyroid surgery, in order to assess the presence of preoperative cord paralysis that may be idiopathic or related to invasive neoplasm or previous surgery. The recognition of an already paralyzed cord on one side is helpful in operative decision-making regarding the extent of resection on the functional side, aside from the obvious increasing medicolegal significance of such information. Mirror laryngoscopy is safe and readily performed at the hospital admission work-up, at which time it becomes part of the patient's permanent record.

The recurrent laryngeal nerve is a branch of the vagus nerve sweeping around the aortic arch on the left and the subclavian artery on the right to ascend lateral to the trachea, usually in the tracheoesophageal groove, to penetrate the cricothyroid membrane deep to the fibers of the inferior laryngeal constrictor. It supplies motor innervation to all the intrinsic muscles of the larynx except the cricothyroideus and sensation to the mucous membrane of the larynx below the cords.

The course of the recurrent laryngeal nerve can vary considerably. It can often be found displaced along the anterolateral border of the trachea away from the usual location in the tracheoesophageal groove.[24] It bears no fixed relationship to the inferior thyroid artery, which it may cross either superficially or deeply, or among its branches. The nerve may branch into two or three or more trunks prior to perforating the larynx.[1] Indeed, it may not even recur (as is observed in 0.34 per cent of cases on the right side) but may pass directly from the vagus to the larynx and thus may be exposed to danger as inferior thyroid branches are ligated.[21]

Two useful maneuvers for ascertaining the position of the nerve include palpating it against the trachea in the tracheoesophageal groove or palpating the inferior cornu of the thyroid cartilage and realizing that the nerve usually passes obliquely toward the larynx about 0.5 cm. below the cornu.[25] During exposure of the nerve, delicate spreading motions should be made parallel to the nerve's likely course of travel. It should never be looped with a suture, elevated from its blood supply, crushed, or stretched.

At the end of the procedure, we commonly use the laryngoscope to examine cord function following removal of the endotracheal tube, realizing the imprecision of this exam in the presence of deep anesthesia. If a cord is clearly paralyzed and uncertainty exists about the integrity of the nerve, the neck should probably be re-explored then and the nerves examined, since the release of a ligature that includes a nerve may result in return of function;[11] or primary re-anastomosis of severed nerve ends may be indicated[19, 20] (though the authors have had no experience with this). Moreover, it is reassuring to know that the nerves were functioning immediately postoperatively should one or both subsequently become paralyzed because of local edema, which almost always resolves with time.

The surgeon may not be the only factor in postoperative cord paralysis, as local damage from the endotracheal tube is thought to be responsible for some cases of cord paralysis.[13]

Diagnosis

The diagnosis of unilateral cord paralysis is best made by endoscopy. The patient with such an injury may have a normal voice and no symptoms, although hoarseness and a breathy, ineffective cough and inability to phonate high-pitched sounds are commonly noted. The cord lies in a paramedian position on laryngoscopy. No airway problems are likely to be present or to ensue. The voice may gradually improve with time and a 6-month period of observation is undertaken. Return of nerve function from a reversible cause such as local pressure from edema will usually manifest itself by 6 to 8 weeks. If the cord is completely and permanently paralyzed, the paralyzed cord will gradually be drawn to the midline by fibrosis of the paralyzed laryngeal muscles, and the contralateral cord will gradually hyperadduct across the midline with improvement of phonation by better cord approximation.

The injection of Teflon paste lateral to the paralyzed cord is indicated to improve the quality of the voice if little or no spontaneous improvement has occurred after 6 to 12 months.[2] This procedure has been very successful in restoring satisfactory phonation.

Bilateral vocal cord paralysis is seen very rarely but can be devastating when it occurs. The patient usually has a component of respiratory obstruction that may be evidenced by labored breathing, intercostal retraction, and inspiratory stridor. The voice may be hoarse or almost non-existent, coughing may be ineffective, and high-pitched sounds may be impossible to phonate. Laryngoscopy reveals both cords in a paramedian position. When signs of airway obstruction from bilateral cord paralysis are noted immediately after surgery, the patient should be endotracheally intubated immediately and the area of the recurrent nerves in the neck re-explored to identify a treatable nerve injury. A tracheostomy is performed next and maintained until adequate unilateral or bilateral cord function is documented by periodic laryngoscopy. More potentially serious is the occasional case of bilateral cord paralysis without early signs of airway obstruction, in which the cords are not visualized postoperatively. The hoarseness in such a patient is likely to improve with time, as the cords approach the midline, because of intrinsic laryngeal muscle fibrosis, yet this apposition implies progressively severe airway obstruction that unfortunately may be recognized only when signs

of severe preterminal hypoxemia supervene. Immediate tracheostomy is advisable for this situation, but the problem should rarely occur if routine postoperative laryngoscopy is performed. If no return of cord motion occurs in bilaterally paralyzed cords in 6 to 12 months, closed or open arytenoidopexy and lateral fixation of one or both cords to the lateral larynx will open the airway and allow closure of the tracheostomy, although phonation will be impaired. A strap muscle transplant procedure that may allow some glottic motion has been proposed by Tucker.[23]

Superior Laryngeal Nerve Injury

The superior laryngeal nerve is a branch of the nodose ganglion of the vagus that divides into the internal and external branches. The external branch supplies motor innervation to the inferior pharyngeal constrictor and to the cricothyroid muscle. Because it lies among the branches of the superior thyroid artery, it is susceptible to injury during ligation of these vessels, unless each branch is ligated on the thyroid capsule as described earlier in the discussion of safe technique.[17] Injury to this nerve may produce no symptoms, but early voice fatigue and change in voice timbre with occasional hoarseness may develop. No specific therapy has been effective for this complication, which is preventable.

The internal branch of the superior laryngeal nerve penetrates the thyroid membrane and supplies sensory innervation to the superior larynx and part of the epiglottis. This branch may be prone to stretch injury from a large goiter or during its removal, resulting in a tendency to aspiration or difficulty in swallowing. In the occasional patient the dysphagia and pulmonary aspiration can be so severe as to require prolonged tube feeding.

Miscellaneous Anatomic Complications of Thyroid and Parathyroid Surgery

Other injuries to the anatomic structures in the neck and thoracic inlet are likely to occur during removal of large goiters or during node dissection for thyroid carcinoma.

A **Horner's syndrome** may be caused by interruption of the cervical sympathetic chain and its superior ganglion during dissection deep to the internal jugular vein.[4]

Esophageal perforation may occur and should be closed with two layers of suture and drained with a soft rubber drain, and broad spectrum antibiotic therapy should be initiated at once. Tracheal injury occurring during surgery should be repaired with interrupted silk sutures. The use of a tracheostomy tube to stent the site of tracheal repair may be elected in some cases.

Injury to the **thoracic duct** may result in a chylous fistula through the wound. These fistulas usually close spontaneously with time, but some may require ligation either in the neck or in the chest.

The **subclavian vein** or **artery** may be injured and result in massive hemorrhage during removal of a substernal goiter. The likelihood of such a complication is decreased by dividing all vessels on the thyroid capsule and rolling the gland carefully out from under the sternum, avoiding blind and blunt mobilization of the enlarged gland. Should a large vessel injury occur, bleeding can be controlled by finger pressure, and exposure of the vessel can be obtained if necessary either by resection of the clavicular head or by upper sternal split with incision laterally into the third intercostal space.

Pneumothorax may occur during a substernal dissection, especially while seeking a parathyroid gland. If a pleural tear is recognized during operation, it should be closed with a purse-string suture while the lungs are maximally inflated. At the end of the operation a chest roentgenogram is obtained to see if any pneumothorax is present. A chest tube is placed if necessary. Ordering a postoperative chest roentgenogram is a good idea whenever a substernal dissection is performed, even though no apparent pleural injury was sustained, as an occult pneumothorax will occasionally be detected.

Cosmetic and Infectious Complications

Care taken in careful cosmetic closure of the thyroid or parathyroid surgical incision is likely to be appreciated by the patient, as the wound is often exposed publicly. Care must be taken to assure that the scar will be symmetrical. The midlines of platysma muscle and skin flaps must be closed precisely on center to prevent redundancy or stretching of the scar. A carefully placed running intradermal stitch or interrupted sutures may be used to neatly coapt the skin edges. Interrupted sutures are best removed by the third postoperative day to prevent epithelialization of their tracts and a "railroad" scar.

The problems of scar thickening and migration downward over the sternum have been alluded to in our discussion of safe technique and are best prevented by making the incision about 3 cm. above the clavicle. Occasionally the scar will become adherent to the trachea and move when the patient swallows. This complication is most commonly seen following repeat operations in the neck. We feel that it is less likely to occur if the strap muscles are carefully reapproximated over the trachea and a secure closure of the platysma muscle layers of the flaps is effected, being careful to isolate the platysmal sutures from deeper sutures. Secure platysmal closure prevents widening of the scar with the passage of time.

The use of classic radical neck dissection for thyroid neoplasms is unnecessary and cosmetically mutilating. We favor a node-plucking procedure for metastatic differentiated thyroid neoplasms (papillary and follicular) and a modified radical neck dissection (with preservation of the sternocleidomastoid muscle) for medullary carcinoma. Rarely, a formal radical neck dissection may be indicated for a resectable anaplastic carcinoma.

We have alluded to the problem of suture extrusion from the wound in our discussion of vessel ligation technique earlier. To minimize this complication and yet assure the security of well-ligated thyroid arterial and venous branches, we prefer to use absorbable sutures for hemostasis in raising the flaps and separating the strap muscles and to use silk for ligating the deeper vessels, in which the sutures are less likely to extrude with the passage of time.

Infection is very rare in thyroid and parathyroid surgery. Should a wound become infected the sutures are removed from the skin and platysma layers until good external drainage is obtained. Culture of the infection is obtained, but antibiotics are rarely required. The wound is irrigated several times daily with saline and peroxide and packed with gauze until healed.

METABOLIC COMPLICATIONS OF THYROID AND PARATHYROID SURGERY

HYPERTHYROIDISM AND THYROID STORM

The signs and symptoms of the accelerated metabolic state of hyperthyroidism should be well known to every clinician, as they represent a classic state of altered endocrine feedback inhibition. For the surgeon, failure to control adequately the state of hyperthyroidism by administration of various anti-thyroid drugs prior to surgery subjects the patient to severe risks during the stress of surgery and anesthesia — risks that derive mainly from hyperthermia and altered cardiac function.

We favor preoperative thyroid suppression in thyrotoxic patients by administration of propylthiouracil, 150 mg. t.i.d. for about 4 to 8 weeks prior to surgery (or somewhat larger doses if needed), and then monitoring serum T_3 and T_4 and the resting pulse rate as indicators of return to a euthyroid state. When the patient is rendered euthyroid, he is administered Lugol's iodine solution 10 drops t.i.d. for 1 week prior to surgery. When the patient is admitted to the hospital, he is treated with propranolol in amounts of 10 mg. t.i.d., increasing the dose to as much as 1000 mg. daily if any resting tachycardia is observed. The end point of the propranolol therapy is to bring the resting pulse rate below 80, and the propranolol is discontinued by 48 hours postoperatively in the majority of patients.

We feel that this represents the optimal therapy for the thyrotoxic patient, rather than reliance on one agent alone. The Lugol's iodine is very helpful in decreasing the vascularity of the thyroid gland in patients with Graves' disease, and the propranolol is helpful in blocking the rampant beta-sympathetic hyperactivity of thyrotoxicosis. We prefer propylthiouracil to methimazole as the primary thyroid blocking agent because of its proven effectiveness and the fact that it blocks peripheral conversion of T_4 to the metabolically more active T_3.

The use of such a preoperative blockade should reduce the likelihood of perioperative thyroid crisis or thyroid storm to nearly zero, but nonetheless the condition may still arise. Thyroid crisis or storm may be seen more commonly in stressed patients with occult hyperthyroidism and unfortunately may be unrecognized. The symptoms include rapid and high temperature elevation in the absence of infection, plus nausea, vomiting, diarrhea, mental obtundation, and severe tachycardia.

The treatment of thyroid crisis must be immediate and definitive.[7] Oxygen is started by mask. The tachycardia is the best monitor of immediate therapy, and increments of intravenous propranolol 0.5 mg. should be given repeatedly, each over 3 to 5 minutes until a resting heart rate of 80 or less is obtained. The fever should be controlled by a cooling blanket and alcohol sponging. Salicylates are contraindicated for thyrotoxic hyperthermia. The patient must be placed in an intensive care facility, and careful EKG monitoring is essential. Intravenous crystalloid solution is indicated to replace fluid losses from the gastrointestinal tract and from the skin owing to hyperthermia. An intravenous drip of hydrocortisone, 100 mg. every 4 to 6 hours, is valuable if there is a component of adrenal exhaustion accompanying the storm. Any precipitating cause of the storm should be treated if possible. A dose of 1000 mg. propylthiouracil is administered orally and 200 mg. thereafter every 6 hours. Lugol's iodine may be started 3 to 6 hours after propylthiouracil administration.

RECURRENT HYPERTHYROIDISM

Recurrent hyperthyroidism should occur rarely if adequate subtotal thyroidectomy was performed for Graves' disease. We prefer to leave at most about 2 gm. of residual thyroid tissue on each side. This tends to produce a slightly higher incidence of postoperative hypothyroidism than if more gland were left, but the hypothyroidism is readily prevented or treated with thyroid supplementation and is preferable to recurrent thyrotoxicosis. Lifelong follow-up of these patients is necessary, as thyroid hypofunction or hyperfunction can develop insidiously long after surgery.

Should recurrent hyperthyroidism develop, it is preferable to treat the patient with propylthiouracil or to ablate remaining thyroid tissue with ^{131}I, rather than to perform a repeat thyroidectomy with the attendant increased danger to the recurrent laryngeal nerves and parathyroid glands.

HYPERTHYROIDISM AND PREGNANCY

Thyrotoxicosis may first become manifest during pregnancy and, if uncontrolled, can jeopardize the life and health of both mother and child.[12] Difficulty in recognizing the state of laboratory determinations occurs because of the variable levels of serum proteins during pregnancy that affect the measurable protein-bound iodine and T_3 and T_4.

Treatment is by judicious administration of propylthiouracil to control the clinical signs of thyrotoxicosis, rather than adjustment of a biochemical parameter. Overtreatment must be assiduously avoided to allow normal fetal thyroid development and to prevent cretinism. Exogenous thyroid hormone supplementation after control of thyrotoxicosis will prevent fetal hypothyroidism. Many of these women will revert to euthyroidism after delivery, and the medication can be discontinued. A close and regular cooperation between patient and physician is necessary to maintain tight medical control of thyrotoxicosis of pregnancy.

Surgery for thyrotoxicosis during pregnancy is best performed during the midtrimester, after establishing adequate dosages of propylthiouracil and Lugol's iodine and propranolol blockade. In our experience, this is the treatment of choice for extremely toxic patients or those who require large doses of propylthiouracil for control. Surgery at that time poses little threat to infant or mother in the presence of adequate blockade. Careful follow-up for hypothyroidism is necessary for the mother throughout the pregnancy.

HYPOTHYROIDISM AND POSTOPERATIVE THYROID SUPPRESSION

Hypothyroidism will occur regularly following total or nearly total thyroidectomy and in about 25 per cent of patients in long-term follow-up after subtotal thyroidectomy.[9] The onset of myxedema is usually within the first year after surgery in the majority of cases (87 per cent).[3] However, symptoms can occur up to 25 years after surgery and long-term follow-up of patients at risk is advisable.

The classic symptoms and signs of myxedema include hypothermia, cold intolerance, dry skin, hoarseness, fatigue, mental dullness, weight gain, and prolonged duration of tendon reflexes. These may be deceptively subtle and go unrecognized for a long while by both patient and physician. Recognition of the postoperative hypothyroid state depends on a clinical suspicion based on history and physical examination and confirmatory laboratory evidence of decreased levels of T_3 and T_4, elevated levels of thyroid-stimulating hormone, and low levels of protein-bound iodine. An elevated cholesterol level is frequently observed.

Treatment consists of administration of exogenous thyroid hormone. The current preference is for L-thyroxine (Synthroid) administered in doses of 0.05 mg. to 0.2 mg. daily, until a euthyroid state exists by clinical assessment and T_3 and T_4 measurements. Desiccated thyroid tends to cause elevated T_3 levels relative to T_4 levels and an increased tendency to T_3 toxicosis.[15]

Myxedema coma is usually associated with profound hypothermia, bradycardia, and low cardiac output with hypoventilation. Hyponatremia and inappropriate antidiuretic hormone secretion may be present. Treatment should consist of mechanical ventilation, fluid and salt restriction, and intravenous administration of 500 μg. of L-thyroxine. Intravenous hydrocortisone should also be given. The mortality for this severe state is high despite vigorous therapy.

Some observers recommend postoperative thyroid suppression for life following thyroid resections for non-toxic goiters or solitary adenomas. When thyroid suppression is elected, we use the same doses of L-thyroxine as those used for replacement therapy outlined previously and we titrate the dose to the clinical state of the patient and document suppression by periodic determination of thyroid-stimulating hormone levels.

HYPOCALCEMIA AND HYPOPARATHYROIDISM

Factors other than interference with the function of the parathyroid glands may be responsible for some of the hypocalcemia seen after thyroidectomy. These include a "hungry bones" syndrome in which rapid uptake of calcium into the bones occurs after removal of the hyperthyroid stimulation of bony resorption. Additionally, changes in circulating levels of thyrocalcitonin may affect the postoperative serum calcium levels.[27] These effects are usually transient and can be controlled by short-term exogenous calcium administration.

Transient or permanent hypoparathyroidism will be responsible for the most difficult cases of postoperative hypocalcemia. The complication will be seen least frequently when care is taken to identify all parathyroid glands and preserve their blood supply or to reimplant devascularized glands. The complications of permanent hypoparathyroidism can be expected to be about 2 per cent or less following total thyroidectomy if careful technique is utilized.[22]

The hypocalcemia of postoperative hypoparathyroidism usually becomes evident on the second or third postoperative day and is associated with hyperphosphatemia. The symptoms vary with the individual and include fatigability, weakness, circumoral numbness and tingling, paresthesias, muscle spasms and cramps, headache, nervousness, carpopedal spasms, and positive Trousseau and Chvostek signs. Rarely, respiratory paralysis and convulsions may be seen. The serum calcium value correlates poorly with the severity of symptoms, and other variables such as acid-base status and serum magnesium levels may modifiy the clinical manifestations.

Serum calcium values should be checked daily after thyroidectomy until the values have been shown to stabilize in a normal range. Mild laboratory evidence of hypocalcemia without symptoms is not an indication for treatment. Mild symptoms of hypocalcemia can be treated by oral calcium carbonate or calcium lactate tablets given every 4 to 6 hours in a total daily dose of about 10 to 12 gm. A low phosphate and low oxalate diet is started to increase calcium absorption through the gastrointestinal tract. If the hypocalcemia is still symptomatic on this regimen, vitamin D (calciferol) 100,000 units daily is started, realizing that its effects may not be noted for about 1 week after starting therapy. If this is ineffective, the dose can be doubled or dihydrotachysterol can be added. If this latter potent vitamin D substitute is used, the patient is given a loading dose of 1 mg./day for 3 days, and then dosage is reduced to 0.4 to 0.6 mg./day, and serum calcium is monitored bi-weekly to ensure adequate adjustment of the dose.

Rapidly progressive signs of tetany or severe signs of hypocalcemia require that the patient be placed in a I.C.U. setting in which EKG monitoring is available. An intravenous infusion of 10 ml. of 10 per cent calcium gluconate is started immediately and given over 5 minutes. Great care must be exercised if the patient has received digitalis, since this parenteral calcium therapy may lead to fatal cardiac arrhythmia. Further calcium gluconate can be administered by slow infusion, as needed to control the symptoms, at the same time the oral calcium and vitamin D therapies are started, as outlined previously.

After several months of oral calcium and vitamin D therapies the vitamin D is discontinued and the patient's serum calcium level observed over several weeks. If it is normal, then the daily dose of calcium can be reduced slowly until none is required. The patient should be followed carefully for a long time, as recurrent parathyroid insufficiency may be a future problem. The patient should not be considered to have permanent hypoparathyroidism, unless hypocalcemia requiring treatment persists for over a year.

Hypocalcemia may follow removal of a parathyroid adenoma until the remaining suppressed glands become functional. Oral calcium therapy usually suffices during the several weeks necessary for this to occur.

Permanent hypoparathyroidism following parathyroid exploration is more likely if more aggressive removal of parathyroid tissue (i.e., subtotal parathyroidectomy) than we have earlier outlined is practiced. While some authors routinely perform such extensive parathyroidectomy in all cases of primary hyperparathyroidism, we reserve 3½-

gland parathyroidectomy only for cases with proven polyglandular hyperplasia. In the majority of cases, removal of the adenoma and biopsy of a normal gland or two are ample treatment for the disease. Again, the technique of parathyroid autotransplantation may be useful in preserving function of the inadvertently damaged normal gland.[18]

In parathyroidectomy patients with secondary hyperparathyroidism, postoperative hypocalcemia is the rule rather than the exception following subtotal parathyroid resection. These patients require a period of observation in the hospital until their serum calcium can be controlled in the normal range with supplementary calcium gluconate orally and vitamin D or dihydrotachysterol therapy. Very often, increasing the calcium concentration in the hemodialysis buffer is helpful in preventing tetany during dialysis.

HYPERCALCEMIC CRISIS

Hypercalcemic crisis may occasionally be seen associated with a florid case of primary hyperparathyroidism, or it may appear postoperatively when a functioning parathyroid adenoma could not be found and thus removed at operation. More commonly though, severe hypercalcemia will be due to other causes such as disseminated malignancy or ectopic parathormone production.

As serum calcium values rise to over 16 mg./dl. the likelihood of severe central nervous system symptoms and renal damage is substantial. Symptoms of fatigue, muscle weakness, bone and abdominal pain, polydypsia and polyuria, anorexia, hypertension, and mental confusion may be present.

Hypercalcemia over 14 mg./dl. should be treated vigorously by calcium restriction, intravenous saline loading, and a forced diuresis of up to 6 l./day of urine, sustained by careful saline and furosemide administration. Should these measures fail to decrease the serum calcium, mithramycin in a dose of 25 μg./kg. body weight may be repeated weekly if necessary. These methods should allow return of the calcium to normal in the majority of such patients and allow for optimal preparation of the patient for an urgent rather than an emergency neck exploration, if primary hyperparathy-

roidism is the cause of the hypercalcemia crisis.

PERSISTENT HYPERPARATHYROIDISM

Persistent hyperparathyroidism following neck exploration for primary hyperparathyroidism may be the most troublesome complication with which the astute endocrine surgeon must deal. If it occurs following neck exploration that the surgeon has performed, he or she is likely to feel a sense of foreboding about the failed original procedure and a sense of doubt that he or she can find the adenoma on a repeat exploration. If a surgeon is seeing a patient operated upon by another surgeon, then he or she is uncertain of what was recognized or excised or devascularized at the original operation and fears that a re-exploration will be fraught with difficulty.

This complication is obviously better prevented than remedied. Assurance of the correct diagnosis initially is mandatory. No parathyroidectomy is likely to provide lasting benefit if the cause of hypercalcemia is other than primary hyperparathyroidism. The widespread availability of low-cost and reliable parathormone radioimmunoassay screens should guarantee accurate diagnosis in all patients prior to consideration of neck re-exploration.

At the time of the initial neck exploration the surgeon must be thorough, unhurried, and meticulous in the dissection to expose all parathyroid tissue. He or she must be prepared to search from the angle of the jaw to the superior mediastinum and as deep as the prevertebral fascia to find ectopic or accessory glands, if necessary. Supernumerary glands up to seven in number have been described.[8] Only when an adenoma and three normal glands have been found can the surgeon feel relatively secure. Nonetheless, the occasional presence of two or more adenomas with supernumerary glands or diffuse parathyroid hyperplasia with more than four glands can be pitfalls leading to incomplete removal of hyperfunctioning parathyroid tissue. The surgeon must be thoroughly aware of the anatomic variability in number and location of these glands and conduct the exploration accordingly.

Another frequent error at initial exploration is to fail to identify a true adenoma and mistakenly diagnose hyperplasia of the remaining glands, performing a subtotal parathyroidectomy. Of course, the hyperparathyroidism will not improve and subsequent removal of the adenoma will be very likely to cause permanent hypoparathyroidism unless a small portion of the adenoma can be transplanted to provide an autogenous source of parathormone.

Continuing symptomatic hypercalcemia following initial parathyroid exploration for true primary hyperparathyroidism justifies a repeat neck exploration.[10] The surgeon should study carefully the operative dictation and diagrams of the initial operation for assistance in planning a strategy for search. A pathologist's review of the previously resected parathyroid glands is often of great help. Exposure should be broad and bloodless, and initial search should be in the regions most likely to disclose an enlarged gland unobserved at the original operation. This should theoretically prevent devascularization of any remaining normal gland(s).

It may be helpful to invite a second skilled surgeon to participate in a parathyroid reexploration, to bring more expertise and observational prowess to confront the problem. Usually an adenoma will be found. If none is found, however, we prefer to close and perform formal mediastinal exploration at another time. There are two

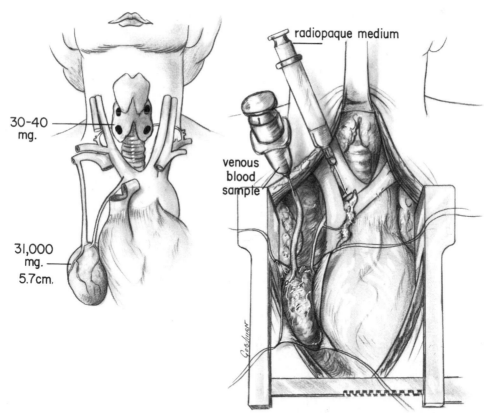

Figure 14–5 *Left,* Locations of the four cervical parathyroid glands and the intrathoracic parathyroid adenoma. A normal parathyroid gland weighs approximately 30 to 40 mg. It derives its blood supply from the inferior thyroid artery, which arises from the thyrocervical axis of the subclavian artery. The parathyroid adenoma derived its blood supply from a single relatively large anomalous artery which arose from the innominate artery. The venous drainage of the adenoma was likewise embodied in a single rather large vein which coursed in the general direction of the right subclavian vein. *Right,* At operation a generous blood sample was taken from the vein draining the large functioning parathyroid adenoma, and thereafter arteriography was performed by injecting radiopaque medium into the artery to the adenoma at its origin from the innominate artery. (From Hardy, J. D., Snavely, J. R., and Langford, H. G.: Low Intrathoracic Parathyroid Adenoma: Large Functioning Tumor Representing the Fifth Parathyroid. Opposite Eighth Dorsal Vertebra with Independent Arterial Supply and Opacified at Operation with Arteriogram. *Ann. Surg.,* 159:310, 1964.)

reasons for this. First, the blood supply of an undetected adenoma may have been disrupted by the second procedure, resulting in cure although this is unlikely. Second, if formal mediastinal exploration is needed we prefer to obtain parathyroid hormone samplings from many veins in the base of the neck and upper mediastinum to assist in localization of the adenoma.

MISCELLANEOUS COMPLICATIONS OF HYPERPARATHYROIDISM

Because hyperparathyroidism is a common feature of the multiple endocrine adenopathy states, it is good practice for the surgeon to make inquiries into the family history and past history of hyperparathyroid patients, especially those with multiglandular hyperplasia. Associations of hypertension, peptic ulcer disease, thyroid cancer, or pituitary-related problems may be an early clue to a patient with multiple endocrine adenopathy, which can be of great preventive value for the patient and other family members.

Hyperparathyroidism is known for its associated renal calculi, which can cause severe urinary tract infections in the postoperative patient. Furthermore, the tendency of patients with hyperparathyroidism to develop pancreatitis is well recognized, and abdominal pain in these patients should raise suspicion. Treatment of both these conditions is conventional.

Bibliography

1. Armstrong, W. G., and Hinton, J. W.: Multiple division of the recurrent laryngeal nerves. Arch. Surg. 62:532, 1951.
2. Arnold, G. E.: Further experiences with intrachordal Teflon injection. Laryngoscope 74:802, 1964.
3. Bartels, E. C.: Post thyroidectomy myxedema and the preoperative use of antithyroid drugs. J. Clin. Endocrinol. 13:95, 1953.
4. Beahrs, O. H., and Vandertoll, D. J.: Complications of secondary thyroidectomy. Surg. Gynecol. Obstet. 117:535, 1963.
5. Cancer Statistics, 1980. CA 30:23, 1980.
6. Colcock, B. P., and King, M. L.: The mortality and morbidity of thyroid surgery. Surg. Gynecol. Obstet. 114:131, 1962.
7. Dobyns, B. M.: Prevention and management of hyperthyroid stress. World J. Surg. 2:293, 1978.
8. Dozois, R. R., and Beahrs, O. H.: Surgical anatomy and technique of thyroid and parathyroid surgery. Surg. Clin. North Am. 57:647, 1977.
9. Edis, A. J.: Prevention and management of complications associated with thyroid and parathyroid surgery. Surg. Clin. North Am. 59:83, 1979.
10. Edis, A. J., Sheedy, P. F., Beahrs, O. H., et al.: Results of reoperation for hyperparathyroidism with evaluation of preoperative localization studies. Surgery 84:384, 1978.
11. Hawe, P., and Lothian, K. R.: Recurrent laryngeal nerve injury during thyroidectomy. Surg. Gynecol. Obstet. 110:488, 1960.
12. Herbst, A. L., and Selenkow, H. A.: Hyperthyroidism during pregnancy. N. Engl. J. Med. 273:627, 1965.
13. Holley, H. S., and Gildea, J. E.: Vocal cord paralysis after tracheal intubation. J.A.M.A. 215:281, 1971.
14. Holt, G. R., McMurray, G. T., and Joseph, D. J.: Recurrent laryngeal nerve injury following thyroid operations. Surg. Gynecol. Obstet. 144:567, 1977.
15. Jackson, I. M., and Cobb, W. E.: Why does anyone still use desiccated thyroid USP? Am. J. Med. 64:284, 1978.
16. Katz, A. D., and Bronson, D.: Total thyroidectomy. Am. J. Surg. 136:450, 1978.
17. Moosman, D. A., and DeWeese, M. S.: The external laryngeal nerve as related to thyroidectomy. Surg. Gynecol. Obstet. 127:1011, 1968.
18. Paloyan, E., Lawrence, A. M., Brooks, M. H., and Pickleman, J. R.: Total thyroidectomy and parathyroid autotransplantation for radiation-associated thyroid cancer. Surgery 80:70, 1976.
19. Peters, L. L., and Gardner, R. J.: Repair of recurrent laryngeal nerve injuries. Surgery 71:865, 1972.
20. Sato, F., and Ogura, J. H.: Neurorrhaphy of the recurrent laryngeal nerve. Laryngoscope 88:1034, 1978.
21. Stewart, G. R., Mountain, J. C., and Colcock, B. P.: Non-recurrent laryngeal nerve. Br. J. Surg. 59:379, 1972.
22. Thompson, N. W., Olsen, W. R., and Hoffman, G. L.: The continuing development of the technique of thyroidectomy. Surgery 73:913, 1973.
23. Tucker, H. M.: Human laryngeal reinnervation. Laryngoscope 86:769, 1976.
24. Wade, J. S. H.: Vulnerability of the recurrent laryngeal nerve at thyroidectomy. Br. J. Surg. 43:164, 1955.
25. Wang, C.: The use of the inferior cornu of the thyroid cartilage in identifying the recurrent laryngeal nerve. Surg. Gynecol. Obstet. 140:91, 1975.
26. Wells, S. A., Ross, A. J., Dale, J. K., and Gray, R. S.: Transplantation of the parathyroid glands: Current status. Surg. Clin. North Am. 59:167, 1979.
27. Wilkin, T. J., Paterson, C. R., Isles, T. E., et al.: Post thyroidectomy hypocalcemia: A feature of the operation or the thyroid disorder? Lancet 1:621, 1977.

15

COMPLICATIONS OF PULMONARY RESECTION

Paul C. Adkins, M.D.
and Benjamin L. Aaron, M.D.

Resection of a lung or a portion thereof carries with it certain attendant risks and potential complications. Some of these complications are common to any major surgical endeavor, and others are unique to this type of operative procedure. In order to manage adequately any complications resulting from pulmonary resection, one must be able to recognize these complications early and be familiar with all their ramifications. Consequently, the discussion in this chapter will be divided into those potential complications that should be recognized and addressed preoperatively, intraoperatively, and postoperatively.

PREOPERATIVE EVALUATION

The major problems that, if not recognized in the preoperative period, might preclude a successful outcome following pulmonary resection are (1) pulmonary insufficiency, (2) preexisting cardiovascular disease, or (3) unusual medical problems that compromise the patient's response. Consequently, these factors should be thoroughly evaluated prior to any operative procedure, except an emergency. Except for those associated with trauma, most pulmonary resections are elective, and the surgeon and the staff have sufficient time for adequate preoperative evaluation.

Pulmonary Insufficiency

Evaluation of pulmonary function begins with the surgeon's appraisal of the patient's history and performance. Knowing the patient's normal performance level, and observing the patient perform a few simple

Paul C. Adkins was born in New York City and received his college and medical school education at Johns Hopkins University where he was elected to Alpha Omega Alpha. At George Washington University and Hospital, where he was voted the outstanding surgical house officer in 1953 and was the recipient of the medical school yearbook dedication in 1961, he rose from Instructor in Surgery in 1954 to Professor of Surgery in 1966, and Chairman of the Department in 1970. He received many honors and was a most vigorous leader in thoracic surgery. His many contributions to books and periodical literature remain as evidence of his rich knowledge of thoracic physiology and surgical practice. Dr. Adkins died on August 13, 1980.

Benjamin L. Aaron, born in Jefferson City, Missouri, received his B.A. degree from the University of Missouri and his M.D. degree from the University of Texas Medical Center, Galveston, where he was elected to Alpha Omega Alpha. A career naval officer, he completed his internship and residency in surgery and thoracic surgery in naval hospitals, as well as fellowships in cardiovascular surgery at the Medical College of Virginia and the University of Alabama. Prior to his current position as Associate Professor of Surgery at George Washington University, he was Chief of the Thoracic Surgical Program at the Naval Hospital, San Diego.

clinical tests, usually gives the surgeon a fairly accurate grasp of what the patient will tolerate from the standpoint of resection. In order to confirm the evaluation and to document the nature and extent of the patient's pulmonary compromise, the surgeon should obtain appropriate pulmonary function studies such as vital capacity, maximum voluntary ventilation, FEV_1, and resting and exercise arterial gases. Removal of a destroyed lobe or lung will have little long-range effect on pulmonary function, whereas a pneumonectomy can be severely debilitating should it involve a significant amount of functional lung. In the presence of marginal pulmonary function, the demonstration by xenon ventilation-perfusion scan of decreased function in the lung containing tumor, as has been described in a high percentage of cases,[18] often will allow for a safe resection. In the presence of chronic obstructive pulmonary disease (COPD) or in the patient who is a heavy smoker with a significant amount of tracheobronchitis, it may well be worthwhile to defer the operation for a week or more in order to allow him to achieve maximal pulmonary function. We have found that cessation of smoking, use of incentive inspirometry with and without bronchodilators, and a very aggressive program of chest physical therapy have been extremely helpful in avoiding major postoperative pulmonary complications.

Cardiovascular Disease

A major problem area in the postoperative period in our experience has been cardiac arrhythmias and congestive heart failure. These are commonly associated with inadvertent hypoxia or hypotension and in some instances may occur in patients without known preexisting cardiovascular disease. Nevertheless, it is imperative that the surgeon be aware of the presence of any preexisting cardiovascular problems such as arrhythmias, coronary artery disease, or cerebral vascular insufficiency. The patient who has had a previous myocardial infarction has a markedly enhanced liability for a second fatal infarction, depending to a large extent on the length of time elapsed since the first infarction.[26]

Good cardiologic evaluation with appropriate invasive and non-invasive studies can be most helpful and beneficial in defining the nature and extent of the disease process, thus allowing for directed watchfulness throughout all phases of the operative and postoperative course. Digitalization is known to be effective in preventing postoperative supraventricular tachyarrhythmias in the elderly, especially following pneumonectomy, and this course should be considered.[17] Patients with carotid bruits can be evaluated by oculoplethysmography and the results factored into the patient's risk profile.

Unusual Medical Problems

Patients can present for pulmonary biopsy or resection with a host of preexisting medical problems. Inanition, anemia, thrombocytopenia, and leukopenia are seen in patients with chronic renal failure, those with chronic wasting diseases, and those who may be on various immunosuppressive regimens. Patients on chronic steroid therapy experience poor wound healing and are at some increased operative risk. Diffuse infiltrative lung disease with associated respiratory insufficiency is common to this group of patients and requires very astute management for a successful outcome.

The judicious use of blood components, including platelet therapy, antibiotics, hyperalimentation, and ventilatory support can provide the margin of safety for this difficult group of patients. The surgeon's goal — to establish an accurate diagnosis and thereby provide adequate control of the infection or other threat — while challenging, can be extremely satisfying when accomplished.

INTRAOPERATIVE COMPLICATIONS

Bronchoscopy may be necessary before pulmonary resection in patients with large amounts of secretions or blood in the tracheobronchial tree. The decision should be made before the induction of anesthesia and the procedures carried out either as soon as the patient is anesthetized or under topical anesthesia before induction. Bronchoscopy serves to clear the tracheobronchial tree and minimizes the possibility of intraoperative airway obstruction and atelectasis. If the disease process is such that continued flooding of the tracheobronchial tree may be anticipated during the operation — for example, in the presence of abscess, bronchiectasis, or a fluid-filled cyst — it may be wise to use some form of bronchial blockade such as a Robertshaw or Carlen's tube to prevent spillage of the material into the contralateral lung. There are several disadvantages in the use of these or other types of double-lumen tubes that should be remembered: introduction is technically difficult; there is a high resistance to air flow; and the lumens are long and narrow, rendering suctioning of the airway difficult. An alternative in selected circumstances is to use a single-lumen tube and place it in the opposite main-stem bronchus. Arterial blood pressure and electrocardiographic monitoring as well as frequent blood gas analysis have become the standard of practice and enable early correction of developing abnormalities. Systemic air embolism, a rare but dangerous complication of injury to the lungs involving the pulmonary veins, has been found to be related both experimentally and clinically to very high intra-airway pressures during the procedure.[11] The surgeon should be watchful in this setting for the scenario of the struggling patient and the struggling anesthesiologist, resulting in high applied airway pressures. Positioning of the patient for thoracotomy and placement of the grounding pad for the electrocautery, often relegated to a nurse or other circulator, are of paramount importance, and it behooves the surgeon to check these thoroughly to protect against pressure injuries to the ulnar nerve, brachial plexus, and other pressure points, and grounding leak burns.

The choice of incision should be tailored to the operation, and while certain simpler types of surgery can be carried out through an anterior, anterolateral, or even a median sternotomy incision, it is our view that the vast majority of pulmonary resection cases are best performed through a posterolateral thoracotomy incision. This approach affords maximal visualization of all the intrathoracic structures to be handled during a resection and thus minimizes problems arising from inadequate exposure. The use of electrocautery for hemostasis during division of the musculature of the chest wall reduces operating time and provides better hemostasis; it has proven to be quite satisfactory. We have not encountered any significant increase in the incidence of wound infections or dehiscence when the electrosurgical technique has been used. The pleural space may be entered through an intercostal incision or by means of a subperiosteal resection of a rib, depending upon the nature of the lesion to be resected and the patient's age. If an extrapleural dissection is anticipated, as in the case of pulmonary tuberculosis or a large peripheral tumor mass, rib resection allows for easier and better access. Patients over 55 years of age have decreased elasticity of the chest wall, and rib resection allows better exposure, minimizing the risk of fracturing a rib as the rib spreader is advanced. Rib fractures occurring at the time the pleural space is being entered are generally a result of the surgeon's impatience, and care at this time will reduce the amount of postoperative pain and prevent the problem of injury or tearing of the residual lung by a sharp rib fragment in the postoperative period. As the rib spreader is opened over a number of minutes, the muscle tension at each end of the incision should be checked and the size of the incision increased, if necessary, to allow further opening without undue tension. If an intercostal incision is being used and the ribs do not spread readily, a short segment of rib may be resected posteriorly to allow better exposure without creating a fracture.

Once the pleural space is entered, the surgeon must make an assessment of the degree of mobility of the lung. When pleural adhesions are especially dense, as perhaps in a case of chronic granulomatous disease or in the presence of a large superficial tumor mass, extrapleural dissection should be carried out. In this manner considerable blood loss may be avoided and mobilization of the lung or lobe is greatly facilitated. In the event that block resection of a segment of the chest wall is necessary, as in the case of neoplasm invading the rib cage, the chest wall should be resected at a point well away from the tumor mass with careful attention to exposure and ligation of the intercostal vessels.

In performing an extrapleural dissection for mobilization of the lung, especially on the right side, the esophagus is particularly vulnerable to injury, and the presence of a nasogastric tube will facilitate identification and separation of that structure from the lung. That portion of the esophagus just distal to the carina is the area most often injured, and fistulization is often the result of such injury because of the poor blood supply of the esophagus at this point.[9]

As the extrapleural dissection is carried posteromedially on the right, rarely is it necessary to free the upper mediastinal pleura in order to mobilize the lung. Usually the pleural space can be entered in the area of the superior vena cava, and injury to the latter is uncommon unless one is dealing with a right hilar lesion or extension from a right upper lobe lesion. Division and mobilization of the azygos vein will allow complete inspection and dissection of the superior vena cava. If necessary, a portion of that structure may be excised after application of a vascular clamp, and the defect closed with a continuous vascular suture.

Having mobilized the lung, dissection of the vessels can be carried out safely only if the surgeon has solid knowledge of the vascular anatomy and its variability. As pointed out by Reed and Allbritten,[21] the veins are less consistent anatomically than are the arteries and the arteries vary more than the bronchi. A guide to the location of the anterior trunk of the right pulmonary artery is a lymph node that usually sits between the anterior trunk and the superior pulmonary vein. On the left, the pleura overlying the hilar vessels should be incised carefully to avoid injury to the vagus nerve above the origin of the recurrent laryngeal nerve.

Hemorrhage most frequently occurs when one attempts to encircle an inadequately exposed vessel with a clamp in order to pass a ligature and divide the vessel. Bleeding from the branches of the pulmonary artery can usually be controlled by digital pressure while the dissection is completed. Bleeding from a tear in the main pulmonary artery, however, may be more difficult to control, and if a vascular clamp cannot be applied, intrapericardial encirclement of the main pulmonary artery can be accomplished while manual pressure is maintained. In those instances when a lobectomy is being performed and the hilar

dissection is difficult, it is wise to pass a tape around the proximal main pulmonary artery before dissecting the branches. If the proximal cuff is insufficient after the dissection, application of a vascular clamp proximally and ligation distally will allow closure of the vessel origin with a continuous vascular suture.

Gundersen[12] showed that in patients with a left upper lobe lesion involving the midportion of the left main pulmonary artery and in whom pneumonectomy would be hazardous because of poor pulmonary function, a segmental resection of the main pulmonary artery can be performed with an end-to-end anastomosis.

In performing a pneumonectomy, the pulmonary artery and, as dictated by the exposure, the superior and inferior pulmonary veins should be divided between vascular clamps and closed with a continuous vascular suture (Fig. 15–1). Chuang et al.[5] showed that in dogs a vascular suture technique is preferable to a ligature in the closure of the pulmonary artery stump. Ligature closure causes puckering of the stump and possible intimal damage, which may initiate thrombus formation. Thrombi developed in the stump in seven of nine dogs with pulmonary artery ligation. These investigators also pointed out the deleterious effect of a long vascular stump, which is usually found on the right.

Injuries to the pulmonary veins are usually less serious than arterial injuries, since the arterial branches have been divided prior to dissection of the veins and digital control is rendered easier by the resulting low flow and pressure. On the right side, the superior and inferior pulmonary veins join to form a common trunk in approximately 3 per cent of cases. On the left, a common venous trunk occurs in 25 per cent of the cases. If enough length cannot be obtained after the vein has first been tied distally, an intrapericardial dissection can be used.

Before the right upper lobe branches of the superior pulmonary vein are divided in performing a right upper lobectomy, the middle lobe vein should be identified. A single middle lobe vein is found in 52 per cent of cases; two veins are found in 36 per cent. In cases in which tumor invasion of the right upper lobe venous branches requires that an intrapericardial venous ligation be

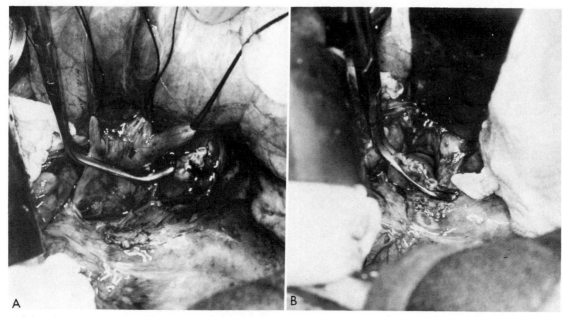

Figure 15–1 *A,* Division of left superior pulmonary vein after application of a Satinsky vascular clamp. *B,* Completed closure utilizing a continuous vascular suture.

performed, the middle lobe should be removed with the upper lobe, even though it is not involved with the disease process, to forestall hemorrhagic infarction of that lobe.

Not infrequently, the surgeon will find that the fissures between lobes are incompletely developed. In this case it may be necessary to divide lung parenchyma in mobilization of the lobe, but sharp or blunt dissection can lead to excessive air leaks and bleeding. In order to avoid this, it is helpful to divide the incomplete fissure between clamps and oversew the lung surface. In recent years we have found the use of the stapling device to be extremely helpful in the division of incomplete fissures and avoidance of postoperative air leakage (Fig. 15–2).

After the lobe or lung has been mobilized

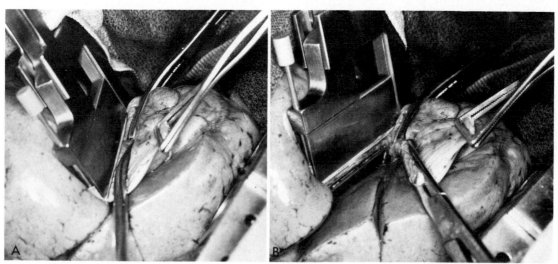

Figure 15–2 Division of the fissure between the right lower lobe utilizing the TA-55 autosuture.

and the vascular structures have been divided, only the bronchus remains to be transected. It is important to leave as short a bronchial stump as possible in order to avoid producing a pocket in which secretions may pool and chronic infections can occur. After the bronchus has been clearly defined and dissected free and the bronchial arteries have been ligated, a right angle clamp is placed across the bronchus and the anesthesiologist is requested to inflate the rest of the lung. This serves to insure that the correct bronchus is divided and that there is not some anomalous distribution of the bronchi.

Secure closure of an undiseased bronchial stump is necessary to avoid a postoperative bronchopleural fistula. Numerous suture techniques have been described to obtain a secure bronchial closure. At the present time, we prefer to use the bronchial stapling devices (Fig. 15–3), as they are efficient and provide secure closure of the stump.[24] However, these devices should be used only when the surgeon is quite sure that the bronchial stump is free of disease, since the lumen of the bronchial stump cannot be visualized when this technique is used. If there is any question regarding extent of tumor at the site of transection, the open technique, with interrupted non-absorbable sutures, should be used. In a left pneumon-

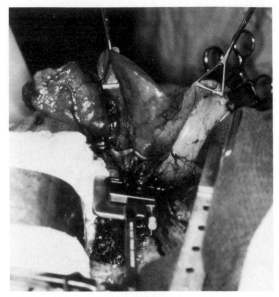

Figure 15–3 Division of the left upper bronchus utilizing the TA-55 autosuture.

ectomy, the suture technique of closure is preferred, as on this side the aorta interferes with proper positioning of the stapling device, which may leave an undesirably long bronchial stump (Fig. 15–4).

After removal of the specimen, the bronchial closure should be tested under water. Small air leaks are more likely to occur with

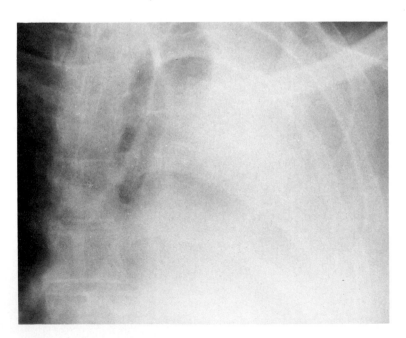

Figure 15–4 This long bronchial stump was left after left pneumonectomy in which the autostapler was used for bronchial division.

the suture closure techniques than with the stapling device and point to the need for another suture or closure of the needle hole with a transverse suture. Some surgeons routinely reinforce the bronchial line with surrounding pleura or pericardial fat. Regardless of the technique used to close the bronchus, the ends should be inspected for bleeding from bronchial vessels, and when encountered, the vessels should be individually ligated. Goldman[10] has shown that staple closure does not interfere with the bronchial blood supply.

Occasionally after removal of a lobe, difficulty may be encountered in expanding the remaining lung on the same side. This is usually due to the presence of mucoid secretions, intra-airway blood, a malpositioned endotracheal tube or, rarely, a tumor embolus so that the remaining bronchus is obstructed. If the lobe does not reinflate readily after adequate suctioning and a reasonable amount of pressure, intraoperative fiberoptic bronchoscopy may be carried out to establish the cause of obstruction and to remove the obstructing material. Rarely a bronchotomy may be necessary if the obstructing material cannot be removed by bronchoscopy.

POSTOPERATIVE COMPLICATIONS

Postoperative Bleeding

Bleeding from the chest, following a pulmonary resection, usually comes from one of three sources: the major vessels within the thorax; the chest wall or mediastinum; or the pulmonary parenchyma. Unless a pneumonectomy has been performed, it is standard practice to leave one or more tubes in the pleural space after a thoracotomy and to attach them to water-seal suction. In the first few hours after any thoracotomy there is some bloody or serosanguineous drainage, commonly amounting to less than 300 ml. If, however, there is abnormal bleeding within the thoracic cavity, this blood loss should be apparent from the amount of drainage through the chest tube or tubes. In addition, a clot of blood may remain within the pleural space and may be detectable by portable roentgenograms of the chest in the postoperative period.

Bleeding From Great Vessels

Although it is uncommon in the postoperative period, ligatures may slip off the pulmonary artery, its major branches, or the pulmonary vein and cause massive blood loss. This usually occurs when the stump of the vessel is short and ligatures alone have been used. The result may be catastrophic unless the diagnosis is made quickly and rapid hemostasis is obtained. Great vessel bleeding should be suspected in a patient in whom evidence of significant bleeding in the pleural space appears suddenly within 24 hours after pulmonary resection. There may be signs of hypovolemic shock, significant bleeding through the chest tube, or shift of the mediastinum to the opposite side. If it is apparent that there is massive bleeding in the pleural space and the situation is life-threatening, the thoracotomy incision should be reopened on the spot. If bleeding is coming from a major pulmonary vessel, there is rarely time to return the patient to the operating room. The color of blood within the pleural space may afford some clue regarding the source of the bleeding. Blood from the pulmonary artery is usually darker than that from a pulmonary vein, which is bright red. On this basis the probable site of bleeding should be examined immediately. In most instances, after evacuation of blood from the pleural space, it is possible to identify the source of bleeding and to control it with finger pressure. Once control has been obtained, finger pressure should be held until whole blood transfusions can be started and the hypovolemia can be corrected. Then a vascular clamp should be applied and the vessel secured with a running vascular suture. The patient may then be returned to the operating room for thorough irrigation of the pleural space, full expansion of the remaining lung, and closure of the thoracotomy incision under sterile conditions.

After pneumonectomy, a chest tube is not customarily inserted. Under these circumstances, massive intrapleural bleeding may be less easy to detect but should be suspected on the basis of systemic hypotension, tachycardia, and other signs of hypovolemia. In addition, rapid accumulation of blood within the pleural space will cause a shift of the mediastinum to the contralateral side, and this should alert one to the appropriate diagnosis. Again, bedside thoracotomy may be lifesaving. As in management of intraoperative hemorrhage, it may be necessary to open the pericardium and gain intrapericardial control of the pulmonary artery in order to stop the bleeding. After control of bleeding and blood replacement, the patient should be returned to the operating room for a thorough irrigation of the pleural space and closure of the wound.

Bleeding From Chest Wall and Mediastinum

Postoperative bleeding from the chest wall or mediastinum is far more common and less lethal than bleeding from major intrathoracic vessels. The source of such bleeding may be adhesions between the visceral and parietal pleura that have been divided during the course of the thoracotomy, the intercostal vessels or internal mammary artery, or mediastinal structures, particularly the vessel contained in the inferior pulmonary ligament. Adhesions between the lung and the parietal pleura associated with pulmonary tuberculosis are notoriously vascular, and extreme care must be taken to achieve hemostasis after dividing these adhesions at the time of pulmonary resection. Bleeding caused by unrecognized injury to the intercostal vessels or, less commonly, the internal mammary artery is most apt to occur during closure of the thoracotomy and may not be apparent until later. In most pulmonary resections of any magnitude such as lobectomy, it is common practice to divide the inferior pulmonary ligament, and the surgeon must take care to recognize and secure the vessel that always lies within this structure.

In the postoperative period, continued blood loss after the first two hours is indicative of either failure to achieve adequate hemostasis or an abnormality in clotting mechanism. Although clotting abnormalities are relatively uncommon following pulmonary resection, they should be ruled out by the performance of screening tests such as the partial thromboplastin time. If there is no evidence of a clotting abnormality and the blood loss continues at the rate of 200 ml. or more per hour for three consecutive hours, reexploration should be undertaken.

It is also important to obtain serial portable chest films to assess the amount of blood accumulating in the pleural space. In the event that blood loss is more rapid than 200 ml. per hour, exploration should not be delayed for three hours. We believe the important factor in postoperative care in the event of continued bleeding is a definitive point at which reoperation is obligatory. If not, there is a tendency to defer reexploration, continue transfusions, and further compound the clotting problem by adding a large amount of bank blood to the patient's circulation.

At the time of reexploration, after evacuation of clots from the pleural space and expansion of the lung, no obvious bleeding point may be apparent. A thorough search of the entire lung surface, chest wall, and mediastinum should be carried out. If the patient's blood pressure is within normal range and if, after observation for 20 or 30 minutes, no bleeding can be found, the lung is fully reexpanded and the chest is closed again. In our experience the majority of patients do not have further problems of blood loss when this course is followed. Only very rarely has it been necessary to return a patient to the operating room because of continued intrathoracic bleeding.

Atelectasis, Air Leaks, Subcutaneous Emphysema

After completion of a pulmonary resection, a portable chest roentgenogram should be taken as soon as possible to determine the degree of expansion on the operated side, the position of the mediastinum, the presence of fluid, and whether atelectasis is present. This should be done while the patient is still asleep so that any additional maneuver, such as insertion of chest tubes or bronchoscopy, can be readily performed. If there is radiologic evidence of residual atelectasis in the immediate postoperative period, intratracheal suctioning should be performed immediately to remove the offending secretion (Fig. 15–5). This is particularly important after a pneumonectomy; some surgeons routinely perform bronchoscopy before the patient is removed from the operating room.

Following extubation, the most common

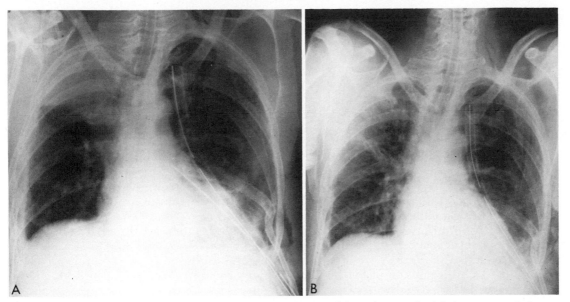

Figure 15–5 *A,* Immediate postoperative x-ray showing right upper lobe atelectasis after left thoracotomy. *B,* Repeat chest x-ray immediately after bronchoscopy, showing clearing of the right upper lobe.

cause of atelectasis is inability of the patient to clear secretions from the tracheobronchial tree because of inadequate cough and ventilation. Early elevation of the pulse rate and temperature usually signifies the presence of atelectasis. Routine nasotracheal suctioning (Haight maneuver) not only is effective in bringing about vigorous coughing immediately in most patients, but it also may encourage voluntary coughing in subsequent hours in patients who wish to avoid the unpleasantness of further suctioning. The use of incentive inspirometry coupled with insufflation of mucolytic agents, isoproterenol, and saline may help in loosening secretions. Nevertheless, in patients who cannot or will not cough effectively, mechanical removal of the secretions is necessary to avoid further atelectasis or pneumonia. Kirimli et al.[16] evaluated tracheobronchial suction techniques and concluded that a straight catheter seldom enters the left main-stem bronchus, regardless of the head position, and is less than optimal for tracheobronchial suctioning. A curve-tipped rubber catheter will enter the right side more often than the left, irrespective of the head position, but can be guided into the main-stem bronchus more often than can a straight catheter.

Bryant et al.[4] studied preoperative and postoperative lung scans in patients undergoing thoracic operations. They found that the presence of a significant degree of atelectasis or pleural effusion was associated with a significant reduction in blood flow distribution to the affected side and was capable of producing a non-functional lung or a physiologic pneumonectomy in the early postoperative period.

If two or three attempts at nasotracheal suctioning fail to expand the atelectatic area, bronchoscopy should be performed. The bedside use of the fiberoptic bronchoscope is less traumatic to the patient than the rigid bronchoscope and allows for instillation of normal saline and removal of retained secretions. However, in our experience, if the secretions are thick and tenacious, use of the rigid bronchoscope is more effective in removing them. In those patients in whom tracheobronchial secretions become a continued problem in the postoperative period, repeated bronchoscopies may be necessary to maintain a clear airway. In occasional instances in which secretions are a major problem and numerous bronchoscopies are necessary, a tracheostomy simplifies management. Suctioning of the tracheobronchial tree may be carried out frequently under sterile conditions, and the bronchoscope may be readily passed down through the tracheostomy stoma.

Following lobectomy, full reexpansion of

the remaining lung on the operated side is essential in order to obliterate the pleural space. After a lobectomy, two chest tubes should be placed, one at the apex of the pleural space, the other posteriorly at the base. These tubes are connected to water-seal drainage with a negative pressure of approximately −15 cm. of water. These tubes should be tested for patency and "milked" at frequent intervals while they are in place. Postoperative air leaks from raw parenchymal surfaces may last up to two weeks after resection. However, if the lobe is fully expanded and there is no residual air space, these leaks will almost always seal off. Chest tubes are not removed until (1) there is no residual air leakage, (2) fluid drainage is minimal, and (3) there is radiographic evidence of full reexpansion of the remaining lung. We have utilized various maneuvers to stop air leaks that have persisted beyond a few days. These include utilization of low suction or high suction depending on the amount of air leak, tube manipulation, the instillation of 500 to 1000 cc. of intraperitoneal air (Fig. 15–6), and lately, instillation of tetracycline in the pleural tube as a sclerosing agent. The effectiveness of these procedures may vary with the individual

case, but it is rare for a leak of the usual variety to persist following the use of such stratagems.

Obliteration of the pleural space is accomplished by expansion of the remaining lung, elevation of the diaphragm on the operated side, and some shift of the mediastinum to that side. Occasionally a small air cap will be left at the apex of the lung with no evidence of active air leakage. In our experience, this has not been a deterrent to a satisfactory recovery, and the space is usually obliterated by accumulation of some fluid and organization and fibrosis of the apex of the pleural space. Infrequently, particularly after an upper lobectomy for tuberculosis, the remaining lung will not fill the apical portion of the pleural space, and there will be a continued air leak. If this persists for a period of two weeks, despite implementation of the above maneuvers, consideration should be given to the performance of a "tailoring thoracoplasty." This involves subperiosteal resection of the upper three or four ribs, allowing the parietal pleura and accompanying chest wall musculature at the upper portion of the chest to drop down and cover the uppermost portion of the lung. This permits the apical pleura to fall in and obliterate the air space as well as cover the leaking lung surface, and it almost invariably stops the air leak.

There are occasions in the early postoperative period when differentiation between atelectasis and insufficient expansion of the remaining lung can be difficult (Fig. 15–7). Insufficient expansion occurs when tube drainage or applied suction is inadequate, usually in the presence of a significant shift of the mediastinum to the contralateral side, compression of the residual lung, and massive subcutaneous emphysema. Early development of a significant degree of mediastinal or subcutaneous emphysema should indicate that the tube drainage of the pleural space is inadequate; additional chest tubes should be inserted and attached to water-seal drainage in this circumstance (Fig. 15–8).

Following pneumonectomy, usual policy is to close the chest without water-seal drainage. At the conclusion of the operation, sufficient air should be evacuated from the pleural space to create a slight negative

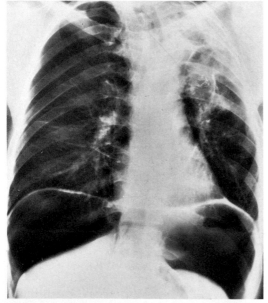

Figure 15–6 Intraperitoneal air displaces the diaphragm cephalad, thus reducing residual space in the thorax.

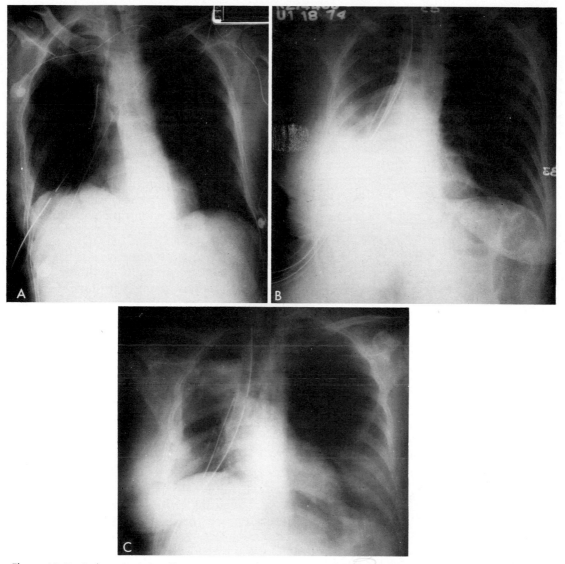

Figure 15–7 Atelectasis vs. insufficient expansion: *A,* Insufficient expansion seen on chest x-ray approximately 24 hours after right lower lobe lobectomy with single chest tube drainage. Note the absence of massive subcutaneous emphysema or mediastinal shift to the contralateral side. Placement of an anterior apical tube resulted in complete expansion. *B,* Chest x-ray 24 hours after right upper lobe lobectomy showing right middle and lower lobe atelectasis. The mediastinum has shifted to the side operated on. *C,* X-ray immediately after bronchoscopy, showing re-expansion and return of the mediastinal structures to the midline.

pressure. This may be done with a small rubber catheter left in the incision and removed after aspiration of the pleural space is accomplished. Alternatively, a syringe, needle, and three-way stop-cock may be used. In the postoperative period, repeated aspirations of air may be necessary to keep the mediastinum in the midline. Rapid accumulation of fluid within the pleural space may cause evacuation of the air, and some

degree of postoperative subcutaneous emphysema may be palpated in the area of incision. This is not unusual and needs no treatment if there is not undue shift of the mediastinum. Uncommonly, in the early period following pneumonectomy, there may be a shift of the mediastinum toward the operated side, usually the result of evacuation of too much air from the pleural space. The instillation of 200 to 300 cc. of

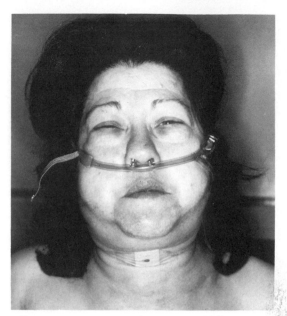

Figure 15–8 Massive subcutaneous emphysema secondary to air leakage.

air into the pleural space with a syringe and needle will usually return the mediastinum to its normal position.

On the other hand, drainage of the pleural space is called for after pneumonectomy in a patient with a destroyed lung and accompanying empyema. Under these circumstances, the mediastinum is usually fixed, and tube drainage of the pleural space may be desirable in view of the preexisting empyema. Usually, simple water-seal drainage without negative pressure is sufficient.

Cardiac Herniation and Torsion

Following closure of the incision after an intrapericardial pneumonectomy, herniation and torsion of the heart may occur when the patient is returned to the supine position. The onset of shock will be sudden and cardiac arrest may occur. In 60 per cent of cases the superior vena cava syndrome is also present, usually associated with right pneumonectomies. The onset in most cases occurs immediately after operation but may be delayed from 4 hours to 3 days after surgery. In most reported cases, the pericardial defect was left open. Coughing, nasotracheal suction, intermittent positive-pressure breathing, position change, and

negative intrapleural pressure can be contributing factors. Usually there is no time for an x-ray, but if taken, it will show marked shift of the heart to the operated side. Either side may be affected, and whereas herniation to the right usually reflects primarily caval obstruction, herniation to the left more commonly causes strangulation of the heart. The mortality is approximately 40 per cent.[1] Formerly, the method of prevention was wide excision of the pericardium, but this approach has been shown not to prevent herniation. Levin et al.[19] believed that the pericardial defect should be closed with a flap of pleura or fascia lata graft. They felt that fine prosthetic mesh would undoubtedly erode into the heart because of its constant motion. Dippel and Ehrenhaft[8] recommended simple suturing of the edges of the pericardial defect to the adjacent atrial or ventricular myocardium. This technique, however, proved to be inadequate in two of our patients as the sutures pulled free and herniation of the heart occurred soon after surgery. In two instances in which the pericardial defect could not be closed by direct suture, knitted Dacron graft material has been used to close the defect. Sheet Silastic is available and will work as well.

Lobar Torsion and Gangrene

Lobar torsion and gangrene occur as a result of intraoperative or postoperative 180-degree rotation on the bronchial and vascular pedicles or damage to the residual pulmonary vessels during lobar resection. Shuler[23] reviewed 31 of 40 cases of pulmonary gangrene resulting from torsion or intraoperative injury and found that in 25 cases either an air leak or incomplete expansion of the lung occurred. Consolidation or a honeycomb or ground-glass appearance was found on chest x-ray in only 9 patients. Fever was present in only 6 patients. Following right upper lobectomy, the middle lobe with a free minor fissure is free to rotate on its pedicle, unless the anatomic position prior to the lobectomy is preserved by suture of the middle lobe to the lower lobe. In addition, the marking technique of Irani and others[14] may be used to outline the middle lobe. The position of three sets of clips on postoperative x-rays is an excellent guide in determining the expansion and displacement of the middle lobe. If the area of the right middle lobe becomes opacified in the postoperative period and its expansion is questioned, torsion should be considered. Bronchoscopy will allow visualization of the lobar orifice, and pulmonary angiography will show the arterial and venous supply and the anatomic extent of the lobe. Pleural changes or fluid collection may prevent adequate x-ray visualization of the right middle lobe, which moves into the apex adjacent to the mediastinum.

Bronchopleural Fistula

Air leakage from the lung following lobectomy, segmental resection, or wedge resection is quite common during the first few postoperative days. This is usually due to small leaks from the parenchymal surface of the lung, and these will almost invariably seal, provided the lung is fully expanded against the parietal surface. The presence of a large air leak in the early postoperative period or continued air leak after 10 days should suggest the possibility of a bronchopleural fistula due to a defect in the bronchial stump. The main causes of this complication are technical errors in closure of the bronchus, closure of a diseased bronchus, and leaving an excessively long bronchial stump. Preoperative radiation as a predisposing factor is refuted by Williams and Lewis.[28] It may be confirmed by bronchoscopic visualization of the stump or the instillation of contrast material into the appropriate bronchus and demonstration of the communication with the pleural space.

In the presence of a bronchopleural fistula, it is imperative that continued tube drainage of the pleural space be maintained as a route of egress for the air. All efforts should be made to achieve obliteration of the dead space in the pleural cavity by maximal expansion of the remaining lung. If there is residual dead space, accumulation of fluid will usually occur with a resulting empyema complicating the bronchopleural fistula. If the air leak is not large and there is no residual pleural space, spontaneous closure of the fistula may occur, provided continued decompression with the tube

is employed and assuming that the bronchus is not seriously diseased. In the presence of an obviously large bronchial leak in the early postoperative period, consideration may be given to early reoperation and revision of the bronchial stump. If a bronchopleural fistula is associated with an empyema, open drainage of the empyema space with rib resection is essential. Once the empyema cavity has been adequately drained and is reasonably clean, consideration may be given to thoracoplasty to obliterate the space and allow closure of the bronchopleural fistula. In the presence of a chronic bronchopleural fistula associated with a diseased segmental or lobar bronchus, further pulmonary resection with closure of a healthy, more proximal bronchial stump may be considered.

Bronchopleural fistula occurring after pneumonectomy presents a significantly greater hazard than that following a lesser pulmonary resection. In the postpneumonectomy patient, the sudden onset of dyspnea associated with coughing up of large amounts of serous or serosanguinous fluid will indicate the presence of a bronchopleural communication. This most commonly occurs between the seventh and tenth day after operation. Since there is a danger of drowning from flooding of the remaining lung, the patient should be immediately positioned with the operative side down. Tube drainage of the pleural space on the side of the pneumonectomy should be instituted as rapidly as possible, with drainage of all the fluid that has accumulated in the pleural space. In some patients, a mild bronchial leak may occur with less dramatic onset. The diagnosis should be suspected when air bubbles appear in the pleural fluid on the operated side that were not present on the previous postoperative chest films or when the air fluid level is lower than in earlier postoperative films (Fig. 15–9). Bronchoscopy, bronchography, and sinography can be used in addition to serial x-rays to demonstrate a bronchopleural fistula. Since there is no pulmonary remnant to fill the pleural space following a pneumonectomy, empyema is an almost inevitable consequence of a bronchopleural fistula in the postpneumonectomy patient.

Management of this problem is difficult. In the rare case in which a bronchopleural

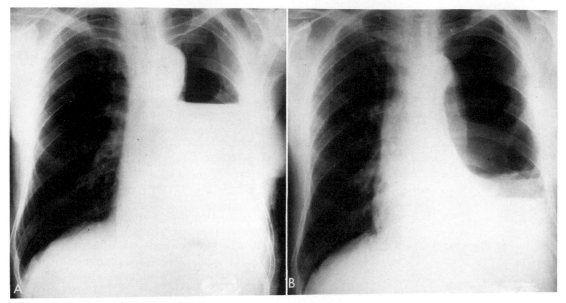

Figure 15–9 Bronchopleural fistula after pneumonectomy. *A,* Chest x-ray at time of discharge 9 days after left pneumonectomy for squamous cell carcinoma. *B,* Chest x-ray 16 days after left pneumonectomy, at which time the patient experienced the sudden onset of dyspnea associated with coughing of large amounts of serosanguineous fluid. Note the marked reduction in fluid level in the left hemithorax.

fistula occurs within the first 2 to 3 days after pneumonectomy, immediate reoperation and revision of the bronchial stump may be undertaken. In bronchopleural fistulas occurring later, revision of the bronchial stump will usually lead to continued air leak because of active bronchial infection. Consequently, complete drainage of the pleural space should be carried out. In some instances an intercostal muscle pedicle flap for closure of the bronchopleural fistula has been utilized with success.[13] Often, however, a persistent or chronic bronchopleural fistula involves convalescence extending over a period of years, necessitating drainage of the pleural space with subsequent multistage thoracoplasty to obliterate the space.

According to Boyd and Spencer,[3] the incidence of bronchopleural fistula following pneumonectomy should not exceed 3 per cent. Williams and Lewis[28] point out that pneumonectomy carries a threefold incidence of fistula over lobectomy, i.e., 4.58 versus 1.48 per cent. Demos and Timmes[7] have advocated management of early postpneumonectomy infection by evacuation of the hemothorax, intercostal muscle pedicle closure of the bronchopleural fistula, and daily postoperative instillation of broad spectrum antibiotics into the pleural space.

Malave and others[20] reviewed 52 cases of bronchopleural fistula, an incidence of 2.7 per cent following all types of pulmonary resections over a 12-year period. Fistula closure was accomplished in 61.9 per cent of the patients, although the majority underwent multiple procedures. The overall mortality was 23.1 per cent. Mortality was higher among patients in whom a bronchopleural fistula developed early after pulmonary resection than in those in whom the complication arose later. The majority of patients in this series had undergone resection for tuberculosis, involving an upper lobectomy and a wedge or segmental resection of the lower lobe. Common etiologic factors for bronchial leak in this series were believed to be endobronchial disease, drug-resistant organisms, concomitant illness, preoperative radiation therapy, and surgical technique. The authors concluded that in the presence of a diseased bronchus, early direct closure should not be undertaken.

Despite the variety of surgical procedures, all surgeons will agree that the nutritional status of the patient must be ideal. Even though patients may have an adequate oral intake, intravenous hyperalimentation may be used to prepare them for further surgery.

Empyema

Empyema may occur in the pleural space after pulmonary resection in the absence of a bronchopleural fistula. This is usually the result of a dead space within the pleural cavity, which is filled with blood or fluid. Subsequent contamination results in infection and development of a frank empyema. It may be associated with a transient bronchopleural fistula that closed spontaneously and may occur anytime after surgery, even years after a pneumonectomy.

The diagnosis of empyema after pulmonary resection is usually based on change in chest tube drainage from clear serosanguineous to cloudy or frankly purulent. Fever is usually present. In the postpneumonectomy patient, persistent fever may be the only finding when there is no bronchopleural fistula. Serial chest films may show a normal filling of the pleural space. Thoracentesis should be done to obtain material for culture and gram staining to establish a diagnosis and identify the offending organism. The presence of an empyema must be suspected in a patient in whom a wound infection develops after pneumonectomy. In later stages following operation, the pleural infection may present as empyema necessitatis.

The diagnosis of empyema may be readily made when pus is found in the pleural space, obtained either through drainage tubes or by thoracentesis. The initial management is adequate drainage of the pleural space. Surgical placement of new large-bore pleural tubes will be necessary in the early case with utilization of underwater seal, as the pleural space is still fluid. In the presence of pleural symphysis, tube placement is most readily accomplished by identifying the space both by x-ray and by aspiration, and then resecting a segment of a rib overlying the space. Upon entrance into the empyema space, its lowermost portion may be defined, and if necessary, another segment of rib may be resected to provide dependent drainage. A large tube should be placed in the thoracic cage at the most dependent portion of the empyema pocket. Daily irrigation should be carried out until the space is cleaned. Then if the pocket is of significant size and the underlying lung is not diseased, a form of decortication or resection of the empyema pocket with reexpansion of the lung may be carried out. If the underlying lung is not capable of reexpanding to fill the space, an alternative to long-term tube drainage is the creation of an Eloesser flap. This involves creating an adequate opening into the pocket by resection of one or more ribs, developing skin flaps immediately above and below the entrance to the empyema space, and suturing the skin to the parietal pleura. This procedure

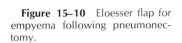
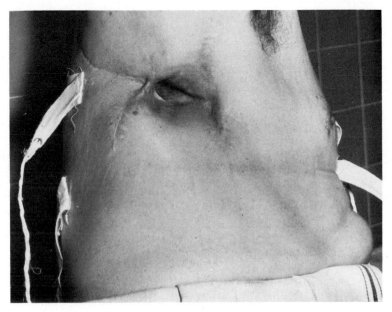

Figure 15–10 Eloesser flap for empyema following pneumonectomy.

creates an epithelialized surface that will stay open indefinitely (Fig. 15–10). We have found this to be far more comfortable and easier to manage than use of a tube if the empyema must be managed on a long-term basis.

Empyema following a pneumonectomy in the absence of a bronchopleural fistula creates a slightly different problem in that there is no lung to expand to fill the space. The classic method of management was drainage followed by staged thoracoplasty and total obliteration of the involved pleural space. As an alternative, in 1963 Clagett and Geraci[6] successfully treated 3 cases of postpneumonectomy empyema with open drainage by rib resection, daily irrigation with half-strength Dakin's solution, and definitive closure with instillation of 0.25 per cent neomycin in saline solution 6 to 8 weeks later. In 1972, Stafford and Clagett[25] reported on 18 patients treated by this method over a 12-year period. In 6 of 8 patients with empyema occurring in the early postoperative period, and 5 of 10 patients with late empyema, closure was successful after the first attempt. Zumbro et al.[29] noted that this procedure for the management of postpneumonectomy empyema is of value only in those patients with no evidence of a persistent bronchopleural fistula. Kärkölä et al.[15] had uniform success, however, in patients with fistulas as well.

Esophagopleural Fistula

This complication is an uncommon postoperative problem. It usually is a result of esophageal injury at the time of pneumonectomy on the right.[17] Extensive extrapleural dissection, especially on the right, and extensive lymph node dissection are probably the precipitating factors. Dumont and DeGraef[9] pointed out that the blood supply to the esophagus is segmental and that the part of the esophagus just below the carina has the poorest blood supply; this is the most common site of fistula formation. Takaro et al.[27] reviewed the reported cases of esophagopleural fistula in 1960 and found that 24 cases occurred after pneumonectomy for tuberculosis or suppurative pulmonary disease. The mortality rate was 49 per cent; the cure rate, 21 per cent. Benjamin and others[2] added 3 cases of esophagopleural fistula after right pneu-

monectomy for carcinoma to 3 other reported cases. Two cases occurred early in the postoperative period and one occurred 8 months later. They pointed out that the clinical picture may be confused with that of bronchopleural fistula and empyema but that a Gastrografin x-ray study is diagnostic. Esophagoscopy and bronchoscopy were performed in each case to rule out the presence of tumor. They recommended empyema drainage followed by direct closure of the fistula with protection by a flap of pleura. After the fistula healed, the empyema was closed by the Clagett method. Richardson et al.[22] reported 2 cases of postpneumonectomy esophagopleural fistula successfully treated with a one-stage procedure of intercostal pedicle flap closure of the fistula with an extensive thoracoplasty. The collapsed empyema space was then continuously irrigated with antibiotics.

The best treatment for this entity is prevention. The gastric tube will permit location of the esophagus. If the esophagus is injured at the time of pneumonectomy, the wound should be covered with a pleural flap or intercostal muscle pedicle and methylene blue should be instilled into the esophagus to determine the adequacy of closure.

Wound Infections

The incidence of wound infection following the posterolateral thoracotomy incision is approximately 1 per cent in most institutions. The major concern in the management of this problem should be prevention of extension of the superficial wound infection into the pleural space and creation of an empyema. This is particularly worrisome in the postpneumonectomy patient. The entire infected areas should be opened early and debrided. Subsequent packing and frequent irrigation should result in a clean granulating area that will close without residual dead space. With this method of management, it is rare to find a patient in whom empyema occurs in conjunction with the wound infection in the absence of a bronchopleural fistula.

Bibliography

1. Arndt, R. D., Frank, C. G., Schmitz, A. L., et al.: Cardiac herniation with volvulus after pneumonectomy. Am. J. Roentgenol. *130*:155, 1978.

2. Benjamin, I., Olsen, A. M., and Ellis, F. H., Jr.: Esophagopleural fistula, a rare postpneumonectomy complication. Ann. Thorac. Surg. 7:139, 1969.

3. Boyd, A. D., and Spencer, F. C.: Bronchopleural fistulas: How often should they occur? (Editorial). Ann. Thorac. Surg. 13:195, 1972.

4. Bryant, L. R., Spencer, F. C., Greenlaw, R. H., Prathnadi, P., and Bowlin, J. W.: Postoperative changes in regional pulmonary blood flow. J. Thorac. Cardiovasc. Surg. 53:64, 1967.

5. Chuang, T. H., Dooling, J. A., Connally, J. M., and Shefts, L. M.: Pulmonary embolization from vascular stump thrombosis following pneumonectomy. Ann. Thorac. Surg. 2:290, 1966.

6. Clagett, O. T., and Geraci, J. E.: A procedure for the management of postpneumonectomy empyema. J. Thorac. Cardiovasc. Surg. 45:141, 1963.

7. Demos, H. J., and Timmes, J. J.: Myoplasty for closure of tracheobronchial fistula. Ann. Thorac. Surg. 15:88, 1973.

8. Dippel, W. F., and Ehrenhaft, J. L.: Herniation of the heart after pneumonectomy. J. Thorac. Cardiovasc. Surg. 65:207, 1972.

9. Dumont, A., and DeGraef, J.: La fistule oesophago-pleurale, complication tardive de la pneumonectomie. Lyon Chir. 57:481, 1961.

10. Goldman, A.: An evaluation of automatic suture with UKL-60 and UKL-40 devices by pulmonary resection. Dis. Chest 46:29, 1964.

11. Graham, J. M., Beall, A. L., Jr., Mattox, K. L., et al.: Systemic air embolism following penetrating trauma to the lung. Chest 72:449, 1977.

12. Gundersen, A. E.: Segmented resection of the pulmonary artery during left upper lobectomy. J. Thorac. Cardiovasc. Surg. 54:582, 1967.

13. Hankins, J. R., Miller, J. E., and McLaughlin, J. S.: The use of chest wall muscle flaps to close bronchopleural fistulas: Experience with 21 patients. Ann. Thorac. Surg. 25:491, 1978.

14. Irani, B., Miller, J. E., Linberg, E., and Attar, S.: Use of radiopaque markings on middle lobe (or lingula) following upper resectional surgery. Ann. Thorac. Surg. 5:1, 1968.

15. Kärkölä, P., Kairaluoma, M. I., and Larmi, K.: Postpneumonectomy empyema in pulmonary carcinoma patients. J. Thorac. Cardiovasc. Surg. 72:319, 1976.

16. Kirimli, B., King, J. E., and Pfaeffle, H. H.: Evaluation of tracheobronchial suction techniques. J. Thorac. Cardiovasc. Surg. 59:340, 1970.

17. Kirsh, M. M., Rotman, H., Benrendt, D. M., et al.: Complications of pulmonary resection. Ann. Thorac. Surg. 20:215, 1975.

18. Lefrak, S. S.,: Preoperative evaluation for pulmonary resection: The role of radionuclide scanning. (Editorial). Chest 72:419, 1977.

19. Levin, P. D., Faber, L. P., and Carleton, R. A.: Cardiac herniation after pneumonectomy. J. Thorac. Cardiovasc. Surg. 61:104, 1971.

20. Malave, G., Foster, E. D., Wilson, J. A., and Munro, D. C.: Bronchopleural fistula —Present-day study of an old problem. A review of 52 cases. Ann. Thorac. Surg. 11:1, 1971.

21. Reed, W. A., and Allbritten, F. F.: The lungs: Suppurative and fungal diseases. In Gibbon, J. H., Sabiston, D. C., Jr., and Spencer, F. C. (Eds.): Surgery of the Chest. 2nd Ed. Philadelphia, W. B. Saunders Company, 1969, pp. 341–415.

22. Richardson, J. D., Campbell, D., and Trinkle, J. K.: Esophagopleural fistula after pneumonectomy. Chest 69:795, 1976.

23. Shuler, J. G.: Intraoperative lobar torsion producing pulmonary infarction. J. Thorac. Cardiovasc. Surg. 65:951, 1973.

24. Scott, R. N., Feraci, R. P., Hough, A., et al.: Bronchial stump closure technique following pneumonectomy: A serial comparative study. Ann. Surg. 184:205, 1976.

25. Stafford, E. G, and Clagett, O. T.: Postpneumonectomy empyema, neomycin instillation and definitive closure. J. Thorac. Cardiovasc. Surg. 63:771, 1972.

26. Steen, P. A., Tinker, J. H., and Tarhan, S.: Myocardial reinfarction after anesthesia and surgery. J.A.M.A. 239:2566, 1978.

27. Takaro, J., Walkup, H. E., and Okano, T.: Esophagopleural fistula as a complication of thoracic surgery: A collective review. J. Thorac. Cardiovasc. Surg. 40:179, 1960.

28. Williams, N. S., and Lewis, C. T.: Bronchopleural fistula: A review of 86 cases. Br. J. Surg. 63:520, 1976.

29. Zumbro, G. L., Jr., Treasure, R., Geiger, J. P., and Green, D. C.: Empyema after pneumonectomy. Ann. Thorac. Surg. 15:615, 1973.

16

COMPLICATIONS OF ESOPHAGEAL AND DIAPHRAGMATIC SURGERY

W. Spencer Payne,
Howard K. Leonardi,
and F. Henry Ellis, Jr.

A variety of surgical procedures are currently employed to correct or palliate pathologic conditions affecting the esophagus and diaphragm. Procedures performed for malignant conditions are, for the most part, extirpative in nature and require reconstructive maneuvers of varying complexity. Others are designed primarily to correct derangements in esophageal or diaphragmatic structure or function. Any of these procedures may be followed by troublesome or even tragic complications. Their occurrence will be minimized, however, if the surgeon has a thorough understanding of

W. Spencer Payne was born in St. Louis, Missouri, completed his undergraduate education at Haverford College, and received his medical degree from Washington University. Following residency training in general, thoracic, and cardiovascular surgery at the Mayo Clinic he joined the surgical staff at that institution in 1961. He now serves as Consultant in the Section of Thoracic and Cardiovascular Surgery at the Mayo Clinic and Professor of Surgery in the Mayo Medical School. Dr. Payne has published extensively on thoracic and esophageal surgical problems.

Howard K. Leonardi was born in Maine and graduated cum laude from Harvard Medical School in 1969. His extensive postgraduate training in surgery included the Harvard Service of the Boston City Hospital, the Aberdeen Royal Infirmary in Scotland, and the New England Deaconess Hospital. In 1977–78, he served as Chief Resident in Thoracic and Cardiovascular Surgery at the New England Deaconess Hospital, and he is now a member of the staff of the Overholt Thoracic Clinic. He has published significantly in the field of esophageal disease.

F. Henry Ellis, Jr., born in Washington, D.C., was elected to Phi Beta Kappa at Yale and to Alpha Omega Alpha at Columbia Medical School. He received his Ph.D. in Surgery at the University of Minnesota. After residency training in general and thoracic surgery at the Mayo Foundation, he joined the staff and became one of the most able members of that illustrious group, being advanced to full professor. In 1970 he became Chief of Cardiovascular Surgery at the Lahey Clinic and Lecturer in Surgery at the Harvard Medical School. In 1972 he became Chief of the Thoracic and Cardiovascular Surgical Training Program at the New England Deaconess Hospital, a Harvard Medical School–affiliated hospital, and in 1974 was promoted to the rank of Associate Clinical Professor of Surgery, Harvard Medical School. His works in thoracic and cardiovascular surgery are recognized throughout the world.

the normal anatomy and physiology of these organs, employs proper patient selection, and adheres to the basic principles of surgical technique. There appears to be a growing tendency in this country to try to improve esophageal surgical results by adding to the complexity of the operative procedure. The fact that the patient can usually survive these interventions is no brief for their use, and we would like to warn against the use of all but the simplest, most logical, and most physiologic procedures as far as possible.

The scope of this chapter does not permit a detailed discussion of normal esophageal physiology, the details of which are available elsewhere,[23, 67, 82] but there are some important considerations in esophageal and diaphragmatic surgery which warrant attention before consideration of some of the specific complications of various surgical procedures and their management.

GENERAL CONSIDERATIONS

Many operative procedures on the esophagus are undertaken for the relief of esophageal obstruction, and patients so afflicted obviously have not had an adequate oral intake of food. Restoration of proper nutrition preoperatively is usually necessary to avoid certain postoperative complications. From a practical standpoint, it is difficult to determine just how extensive the preparation should be and whether or not it should be applied to all patients. The heavy economic burden that may be imposed by a long period of hospitalization must be weighed against the uncertain advantages that may accrue to the patient.

It has been our practice to utilize preoperative preparation only in selected patients with esophageal obstruction. As a rule, the preparation has consisted of several days of hospitalization devoted to efforts to restore blood volume and fluid and electrolyte balance. Supplementary administration of vitamins includes adequate amounts of vitamin B complex and vitamins C and K. In some cases the patient's swallowing mechanism can be improved by forceful dilatation to provide a few days of adequate oral intake before operation. There is little doubt that oral feedings are far superior to any known form of intravenous feedings. In the obstructed, nutritionally depleted patient, however, intravenous hyperalimentation begun preoperatively and continued through the postoperative period until oral feeding is well established may assure early positive nitrogen balance and facilitate healing. Preoperative gastrostomy is rarely used for preoperative preparation of these patients, with the exception of patients who have congenital tracheoesophageal atresia and who are too ill to withstand immediate primary reconstruction.

Many patients with esophageal disease have associated pulmonary problems that may also require treatment before an operation is undertaken. The infant with congenital tracheoesophageal fistula is a good example. In such patients, operation can be delayed to permit resolution of the pulmonary inflammation. Regurgitation of retained food and secretions by patients with esophageal obstruction, particularly patients with esophageal achalasia, can lead to pulmonary complications requiring preoperative care. Esophageal aspiration should be performed on the morning of operation in all such patients. Chronic bronchitis and emphysema are frequent complications in older patients with esophageal obstruction. The preoperative use of expectorants, antibiotics, humidification, chest physiotherapy, and bronchodilators may simplify the postoperative course. Studies of lung volumes and mechanics, as well as of arterial blood gases, may facilitate assessment of associated pulmonary complications.

Careful attention to important anatomic details at operation helps to minimize postoperative difficulties. The close proximity of the esophagus and diaphragm to many vital structures necessitates care in dissection and handling of tissue to avoid injury to such structures as the heart, aorta, vena cava, azygos vein, and vagus, recurrent, and phrenic nerves, as well as the esophageal hiatus and the thoracic duct. Incisions across the esophageal hiatus are particularly to be avoided unless destruction of the sphincteric mechanism is a necessary part of the operative procedure. Diaphragmatic incisions can be designed to minimize unnecessary injury to branches of the phrenic nerve.[90]

There is widespread belief that the blood supply of the esophagus is precarious and that anastomotic leaks are a reflection of this anatomic fact. To be sure, this organ receives a segmental blood supply from the aorta, but the intramural vascular anastomoses, particularly in the proximal portion, are sufficient to permit adequate mobilization of this organ. We believe that anastomotic leaks are more often ascribable to poor nutrition of the patient, trauma due to the application of clamps to the stomach or esophagus, tension on the suture line, or impaired blood supply of the organ to which the esophagus is being joined rather than to devascularization of the esophagus itself. In esophagogastrostomy procedures, special care should be directed to preserving intact the right gastroepiploic artery, because more often than not it is this vessel that maintains the viability of the gastric pouch after extensive resective procedures.

The lack of a serosal covering deprives the esophagus of the protection afforded to intestinal anastomoses by the visceral peritoneum. There is a sturdy submucosa, however, which holds sutures well, so that, if accurately constructed, anastomoses are usually successful. Because of the serious consequences of an intrathoracic anastomotic leak, an extrathoracic site such as the cervical region or a subphrenic intra-abdominal site may be selected if the choice exists. Although the use of interrupted silk sutures for the mucosal row of esophageal anastomoses and esophagotomy closures has been advocated, continuous catgut is equally suitable, if not preferable. Care must be taken, however, to avoid pursestring narrowing of the anastomosis. Impairment of the blood supply is not likely to occur with proper suture technique. Of note are the recent successes reported with the use of stapling devices in the construction of esophagogastric anastomoses.[21, 28]

Above all, we wish to stress the importance of an accurate preoperative diagnosis and the proper selection of an operative procedure. Disregard of these important fundamentals may lead to serious consequences after esophageal and diaphragmatic surgery. A patient with moderate esophageal symptoms may be reduced to an esophageal cripple by replacing a minor disorder with a serious disabling illness of life-threatening nature.

SPECIAL PROBLEMS

ESOPHAGUS

Instrumentation

PERFORATION.   Perforation of the esophagus is the most common serious complication of esophageal instrumentation and may occur during esophagoscopy, gastroscopy, dilatation of the esophagus, tamponade for esophageal varices, or simple intubation of the esophagus for any reason. The number of such perforations appears to be increasing as an inevitable result of greater use of instrumentation in the diagnosis and treatment of esophageal conditions.[107, 121, 140] Although this is the most rapidly fatal perforation of the alimentary tract, survival can be expected in most cases of esophageal perforation if it is promptly recognized and treated.

Although there has been an increase in the number of instrumental perforations in the past 30 years, the actual incidence is relatively small, perforation occurring 1 to 5 times in every 1000 rigid endoscopic examinations; flexible fiberoptic esophagoscopy is considerably less hazardous than rigid endoscopy in this regard. Perforation after hydrostatic pneumatic dilatations for achalasia of the esophagus occurs approximately 10 to 15 times in every 1000 procedures. The risk with simple dilatation with a bougie is somewhat less.

Causative Mechanisms. The wall of the esophagus can be breached in a number of ways:[107] (1) simple penetration of the entire wall of the esophagus by the instrument; (2) simple splitting or rupture of the esophagus by exceeding its circumferential tensile strength; (3) mucosal tears that result in a localized inflammatory process that breaks down the wall of the esophagus; and (4) perforation through pressure necrosis.

Instrumental perforation can occur at any level in the esophagus; however, the sites of normal narrowing are the ones most frequently involved. The narrowest of these is at the esophageal introitus at the level of the cricopharyngeal muscle. The sudden narrowing, the changes in direction of the esophagus, and the tendency for a posterior transverse fold of mucosa at the cricopharyngeus to obscure the lumen and confound the endoscopist are thought to be responsible for the high incidence of instrumental perforations at this level. In addition, the posterior wall of the cervical esophagus can be injured by the crushing effect of a rigid instrument as it impinges on the prominent aspect of bodies of the hyperextended lower cervical vertebrae. Such an effect may be further accentuated by the presence of hypertrophic bony spurs on the anterior margins of these vertebrae and the presence of a cuffed anesthetic tube in the trachea.

The second common site is in the lower part of the esophagus, immediately above the narrowing where the esophagus passes through the diaphragm. The incidence of perforation at this level is contributed to by the increased occurrence of disease and the frequent need for biopsy and mechanical dilatation in this region.

Instrumental perforations in the middle third and in the abdominal part of the esophagus occur less frequently.

Prevention. Although all instrumentation procedures of the esophagus carry an inevitable risk of perforation, the actual occurrence of perforation should be infrequent.

Roentgenographic studies during ingestion of radiopaque medium should precede major esophageal instrumentation procedures. In the presence of certain conditions, such as diverticula, strictures, or achalasia, the introduction of instruments into the esophagus may be more safely accomplished over a previously swallowed and well-anchored thread, which serves as a guide. Although foreign bodies in the esophagus may cause perforation, this complication may not occur until attempts are made to remove them. Knowledge of special techniques and equipment for dealing with foreign bodies may avoid difficulty. Often, a duplicate of the foreign body is available for practice of grasping and removal techniques before the procedure is performed on the patient. The localization of radiopaque foreign bodies is greatly facilitated by radiographic studies. The use of proteolytic agents to remove impacted meat may result in severe reaction if perforation or impending perforation has occurred through pressure necrosis of the esophagus.[5] Removal by instrumentation is preferable under such circumstances. Often, esophageal injury during removal of a foreign body can be avoided by advancing the foreign body into the stomach, where it can be digested and passed or can be removed surgically.

Pathophysiology. Contamination of periesophageal spaces with corrosive digestive fluids, food, and bacteria leads to a diffuse cellulitis with localized or extensive suppuration. The site of perforation need not be extensive or impressive to produce local and systemic reaction. The consequent sequestration of body fluids into the neck, mediastinum, or adjacent pleural spaces, pericardium, or peritoneal cavity not only constitutes a major loss of body fluids, which contributes to the development of septic shock, but also, by its extent, may significantly interfere with normal cardiorespiratory dynamics.

Anatomic considerations are of primary importance in both the evolution of signs and symptoms and in the treatment of esophageal perforation. In the neck the extension of periesophageal infection depends, to a large degree, on the presence of fascial spaces and planes (Fig. 16–1). The spaces, pretracheal and retrovisceral, are formed by the fusion of pretracheal, prevertebral, and buccopharyngeal fascias with those of the carotid sheath.

Infections involve the pretracheal space from perforations of the anterior wall of the esophagus as well as from the lateral pharyngeal spaces and pyriform fossa.[107] Such inflammatory reactions may extend inferiorly into the mediastinum where the fascia gains attachment to the pericardium.

Involvement of the retrovisceral space, however, is the more common pathway for the spread of infection from perforations of the cervical esophagus to the mediastinum,

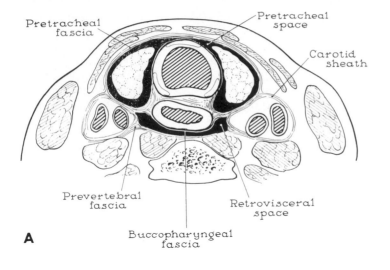

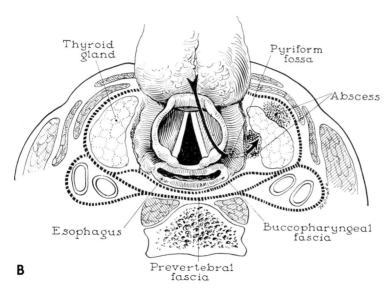

Figure 16–1 *A,* The retrovisceral space. This is more commonly affected in instrumental cervical esophageal perforations. *B,* The pretracheal space. This may be involved by instrumental injury to the pyriform fossa or anterior wall of the esophagus. (From Seybold, W. D., Johnson, M. A., III, and Leary, W. V.: Perforation of the esophagus: An analysis of 50 cases and an account of experimental studies. Surg. Clin. North Am. *30*:1155, 1950.)

since most perforations in this segment are in the posterior wall.

In the thoracic part of the esophagus, the spread of the inflammatory reaction from local perforation is dependent on the relationship of adjacent lung, pleura, or pericardium. The upper two thirds of the thoracic esophagus, although approximately in the midsagittal plane, lies in close proximity to the right pleural space. A short distance above the diaphragm, the esophagus deviates to the left to enter the esophageal hiatus and comes to lie adjacent to the left pleural space. Since perforations of the thoracic esophagus tend to penetrate through adjacent mediastinal pleura, the level of thoracic

esophageal perforations can be predicted with considerable accuracy on the basis of which pleural space is affected.

Symptoms. Esophageal perforation has rather characteristic clinical features that permit early diagnosis in most instances; yet it is apparent, from review of reported cases, that diagnosis is frequently delayed.

The symptoms of esophageal perforation depend largely on the level of the perforation and the location and extent of the inflammatory reaction. Pain, fever, and dysphagia are the most frequent early complaints.

In the cervical part of the esophagus, pain is the most frequent symptom. There may be a delay of minutes or hours between apparent perforation and the onset of this symptom. Pain is usually referred to the anterior part of the neck and "throat." Occasionally it may extend downward into the upper anterior region of the thorax. The pain is often aggravated by motion of the cervical part of the spinal column or by attempts to swallow. The patient characteristically moves his head with care, often supporting his occiput with his own hand when attempting to rise or lie down.

When the injury involves the thoracic part of the esophagus, the pain is usually substernal or epigastric or both. When the pleura is involved, the pain may be referred to one or both sides and may be accentuated by respiration or any motion of the trunk. Occasionally the pain is referred to the midline posteriorly between the scapulae. Diaphragmatic involvement produces typical referred shoulder pain.

When the esophageal perforation lies immediately above the diaphragm or in the subphrenic extrathoracic part of the esophagus,[125] the location and nature of the pain are often identical with those of a perforated peptic ulcer or other upper abdominal catastrophe.

Fever is the second most common reaction to perforation. In the early stages it is rarely accompanied by chills or temperatures above 102° F. (38.8° C.) Dyspnea is often a sign of pleural involvement, either by a thoracic perforation or by the mediastinal or diaphragmatic involvement of extrathoracic esophageal perforations. Rarely, dyspnea also may be seen as the result of partial airway obstruction by glottic edema or tracheobronchial aspiration. Hoarseness usually accompanies obstruction due to edema. In such cases tracheostomy may be urgently needed for adequate ventilation.

Dysphagia is a common symptom of all esophageal perforations. Localization of the distress may be of help in determining the level of perforation.

Physical Signs. Cervical tenderness is an early and constant feature of cervical esophageal perforation. It is usually maximal along the anterior border of the sternomastoid muscle. Often, pain can be accentuated by movement of the hyoid bone and larynx from side to side over the cervical vertebrae. Cervical crepitation may be minimal but is an almost constant sign. Swelling with obliteration of cervical landmarks usually occurs as a late sign of deep cervical infection, but actual redness, pointing, or presentation of a discrete cervical mass is unusual even in late cases. Splinting of cervical muscles may be minimal initially but later may produce nuchal rigidity.

The physical findings in thoracic perforations are usually limited to the thorax, although cervical crepitation may be a feature, but usually without cervical tenderness. Unilateral or bilateral accumulations of fluid and air in the pleural spaces may lead to tracheal deviation. Auscultation over the heart may elicit signs of mediastinal emphysema (Hamman's sign). Cardiorespiratory embarrassment with shock and cyanosis is more commonly seen early with thoracic and subphrenic esophageal perforations but may not be apparent until a late stage.

Physical findings indicative of an intraabdominal catastrophe, such as upper abdominal tenderness, guarding, and rebound, are usual with lower thoracic and subphrenic esophageal perforations. Since gas escaping from a ruptured hollow viscus does not follow fascial planes, cervical and mediastinal emphysema may be apparent with any level of esophageal leakage.

Roentgenographic Studies. Roentgenographic studies are of great assistance in diagnosis. Anterior, posterior, and lateral views of the cervical part of the spinal column often demonstrate pathognomonic signs of cervical perforation. Anterior displacement of the trachea, widening of the retrovisceral space, and, occasionally, widening of the superior mediastinum are seen (Fig. 16–2).

Widening of the superior mediastinum is a common sign in perforation of both the cervical and upper thoracic parts of the esophagus. Mediastinal emphysema and pleural effusion with or without pneumothorax may be present with thoracic or subphrenic esophageal injuries. Intrapulmonary abnormalities are uncommon. As mentioned previously, roentgenographic studies may be of aid in detecting the presence and location of associated radiopaque foreign bodies.

Roentgenographic studies with use of opaque medium are indicated to localize the site or sites of perforation and to detect

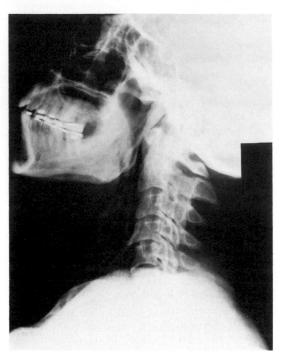

Figure 16–2 Lateral roentgenogram of cervical part of spinal column, demonstrating anterior displacement of the trachea by an anterior bulging of the retrovisceral space in a patient 2 hours after instrumental perforation of the cervical part of the esophagus. Note emphysema evident in tissue planes and hypertrophic bony spurs on the lower cervical vertebrae.

depends on roentgenographic demonstration as well.

Endoscopic procedures are rarely indicated in the diagnosis of esophageal perforations except when a foreign body is present. The larynx may be visualized with a mirror or laryngoscope, particularly if there is any suggestion of hoarseness or obstruction of the upper part of the airway. Rarely, a laceration may be seen on the posterior wall of the pharynx or esophagus.

Treatment. Although there is wide agreement that most perforations of the esophagus are best treated by immediate emergency surgical exploration, repair, and drainage, this is neither universally accepted nor always feasible.

Simple surgical exploration and drainage of the retrovisceral space or, on rare occasions, of the pretracheal space is the treatment of choice for cervical esophageal perforations (Fig. 16–4).[107, 140, 141] Suppuration extending as low as the fourth thoracic vertebra can be evacuated effectively by this route. The usually encountered early perforation may be disappointingly small and the

associated abnormalities (Fig. 16–3). The medium used should be non-irritating and, preferably, absorbable (iodized oil or one of the water-soluble iodinated compounds, such as one of the derivatives of diatrizoate [Gastrografin or Hypaque]). With subphrenic extrathoracic esophageal perforations there may be signs of mediastinal and cervical emphysema on radiographic examination, or free air even may be detected beneath the diaphragm. Gastrografin studies can almost always be carried out, and this examination should be done as part of the evaluation of all suspected esophageal perforations. While its accuracy in defining extravasation in the presence of cervical perforation has a high false-negative rate, it is extremely accurate in defining thoracic esophageal leak. Thus, the diagnosis of perforation of the cervical esophagus rests largely on clinical findings, while diagnosis of perforation of the thoracic esophagus

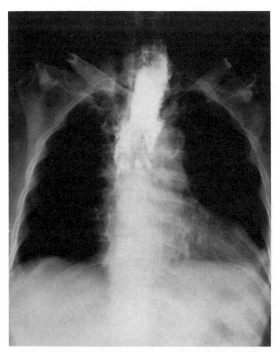

Figure 16–3 Extravasation of ingested contrast medium into neck and superior mediastinum is pathognomonic of a cervical esophageal perforation. In this patient the distal part of the esophagus failed to fill.

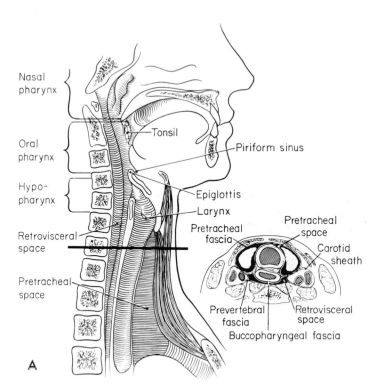

Figure 16–4 *A,* General scheme of pharynx, larynx, and cervical esophagus in sagittal section. Note retrovisceral and pretracheal spaces extending from neck into mediastinum. Insert is cross section of neck, indicating major fascial planes and spaces. Retrovisceral space usually is affected by perforations of cervical esophagus. Pretracheal space is affected by perforation injury of pyriform fossa and anterior aspect of esophagus. (From Payne, W. S., and Olsen, A. M.: The Esophagus. Philadelphia, Lea & Febiger, 1974.)

B, Technique of cervical mediastinotomy. Access to retrovisceral-prevertebral space is gained through low cervical incision by retracting sternomastoid muscle and cephalic vessels laterally and trachea and thyroid medially. Both pretracheal space and posterior mediastinum are accessible. Posterior collections as low as fourth thoracic vertebra are adequately drained through such an incision. (From Payne, W. S., and Larson, R. H.: Acute mediastinitis. Surg. Clin. North Am. *49*:999, 1969.)

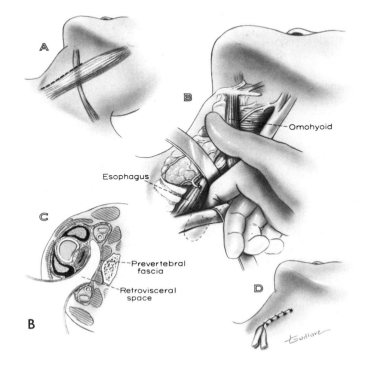

inflammatory reaction slight; however, occasionally major lacerations will be present and require suture closure with drainage of considerable retrovisceral and mediastinal collections. In early perforations of pharyngoesophageal diverticula, it may be possible to accomplish a one-stage resection,[106] but neglected lesions may require a two-stage procedure. While expectant supportive medical treatment of a cervical esophageal perforation can often be successful, it is now clear from Mayo Clinic data (Sarr and Payne, unpublished data) that morbidity and mortality can be avoided by early and prompt surgical drainage of the neck, irrespective of the initial severity of presenting signs and symptoms.

Instrumental perforations of the thoracic and subphrenic parts of the esophagus are often large and communicate freely with one of the pleural spaces. These perforations require surgical exploration, repair, and drainage. The upper two thirds of the esophagus is best approached transpleurally through a right midthoracotomy, and the lower third of the esophagus through a lower left thoracotomy. The rare subphrenic lacerations are best explored transabdominally.[125] Gastric decompression, either by nasogastric tube or, rarely, by gastrostomy, is indicated. On occasion, resection of the perforation and associated esophageal lesion will be required.[16, 84] However, the judgment to carry out extensive procedures must be tempered with an appreciation of the duration of perforation, the extent of contamination, the friability of tissues encountered, and most important, the patient's general status.

Of major concern are intrathoracic esophageal perforations diagnosed more than 18 to 24 hours after they occur, or those in which a fistula with acute suppuration develops after initial repair. Mortality is higher (80 per cent) unless infection can be confined by appropriate drainage of the pleural space and unless some sort of alimentation is resumed within a reasonable time.[141] Various procedures have been proposed for these desperately ill patients. Esophagogastrectomy with esophagogastrostomy, as proposed by Clagett[22] effects a satisfactory resolution provided tissues are not too friable. In many situations, however, the degree of inflammation defies such extensive dissection and reconstruction. Thal[128] has suggested using the gastric fundus to form a patch graft for all such perforations of the distal part of the esophagus. Woodward[137] has used a similar technique, except that he also wraps the entire distal portion of the esophagus with the fundus of the stomach.

Pericardial and diaphragmatic patch grafts have also been advocated to reinforce the closure of esophageal perforations.[92, 112] However, the benefits of such maneuvers are likely to be reduced by the concomitant contamination of the pericardial or peritoneal cavities. Of perhaps greater appeal are techniques that utilize thickened parietal pleura, lung, or an onlay intercostal pedicle graft to buttress the esophageal closure.[27, 48, 93]

Another approach to the dilemma of late esophageal perforation was originally suggested by Johnson and associates[70] and involved total esophageal exclusion by the creation of a cervical esophagostomy. The thoracic portion of the esophagus is closed proximal as well as distal to the perforation to prevent continued contamination. The mediastinum and pleural space are drained. Gastric decompression and subsequent alimentation are accomplished by tube gastrostomy. Esophageal replacement is carried out at a later date by colonic interposition.

More recently Menguy[88] and Urschel and associates[130] have modified this procedure by creating a diverting loop cervical esophagostomy with temporary occlusion of the thoracic esophagus distal to the perforation by applying a constricting Teflon band (Fig. 16–5). An additional modification suggested by Schwartz and McQuarrie[120] employs a Silastic rather than a Teflon band that is applied around the abdominal esophagus, thereby avoiding the insertion of a foreign body in an infected area. It appears that the Silastic material generates fewer adhesions than Teflon and is more easily removed once the patient's condition permits restoration of normal deglutition.

Abbott and associates[1] have described a special T-tube method for managing late postemetic esophageal perforations, while Berger and Donato[15] have reported success employing Celestin tube intubation in selected patients with esophageal disruptions. When this type of treatment was applied

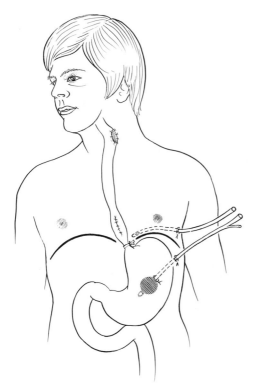

Figure 16–5 Another method of management of late esophageal perforations suggested by Menguy. Note temporary diverting cervical esophagostomy, tube drainage of pleural space, and feeding gastrostomy. Paulson has suggested temporary tape occlusion of distal esophagus to prevent reflux and continued contamination of mediastinum. After recovery, esophageal continuity is restored without need for esophageal replacement procedure.

correctly, no deaths, major complications, or strictures occurred.

Late localized cervical and mediastinal abscesses are uncommon complications after adequate early surgical treatment of perforations, but, when present, can be drained either by cervical mediastinotomy (see Fig. 16–4) or by posteroinferior mediastinotomy (Fig. 16–6). As a rule, the late development of empyema can be prevented by early and adequate closed intercostal tube drainage of the pleural space. The mediastinal pleura overlying the site of esophageal perforation should be left open at the time of surgical exploration and repair to allow free drainage into the adequately drained pleural space. When empyema occurs, it usually responds to appropriate open or closed drainage but, if not, thoracotomy may be required for pulmonary decortication.

Esophagopleural or esophagopleurocutaneous fistulas may occur as a complication of any esophageal perforation. If the esophagus is not obstructed distally and good drainage is provided, such fistulas invariably close with time, provided local infection, foreign body, malignant lesions, and epithelialization of the tract have been eliminated. In the presence of any esophageal fistula it is best to seek out and treat any factors that may contribute to chronicity. Generally, it is wise to carry out repeated esophageal dilatation over a previously swallowed thread during the healing stage of such chronic fistulas, even if no obstruction is demonstrated. With healing, cicatricial narrowing may occur.[129]

Tuttle and Barrett[129] stressed nutritional aspects of this complication and noted the difficulties attending long-term intravenous maintenance of patients after esophageal perforation. They stressed not only the desirability but also the feasibility of resuming early oral feeding, even in the presence of a fistula. If the fistula is not too large, most of the food passes to nourish the patient, adequate drainage providing egress for the remainder. Even with the availability of current parenteral hyperalimentation techniques, the value of oral or gastrointestinal feedings when feasible is to be stressed.

In 1943 Neuhof and Jemerin[98] demonstrated that surgical drainage alone resulted in a 60 per cent survival, whereas conservative non-surgical management resulted in an 84 per cent mortality. Later, Weisel and Raine,[134] Overstreet and Ochsner,[103] and Payne and Larson[107] reported greatly reduced mortality with early suture closure of esophageal perforations. In spite of a greater awareness of the problems and advances in available techniques, some more recent reports of series of esophageal perforations mention mortality rates of 10 to 30 per cent.[4, 83, 96, 129, 140, 141] A few surgeons have advocated conservative treatment of instrumental esophageal perforation.[81, 87]

Of special note is the report of Cameron et al.[19] who defined a small subgroup of esophageal perforations that is clearly amenable to conservative management. The criteria for selection of non-operative treatment include thoracic disruptions contained in the mediastinum with demonstrable drainage of the extravasation into the esoph-

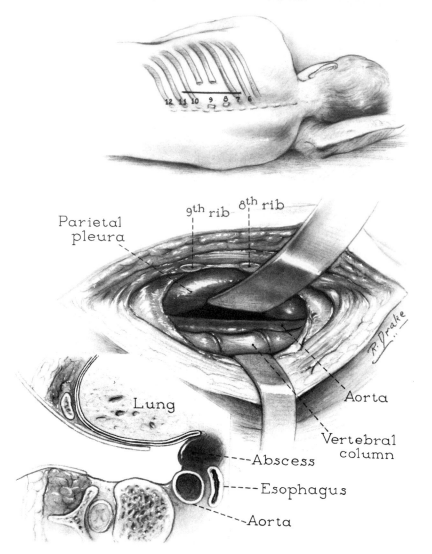

Figure 16–6   Posteroinferior mediastinotomy may be required for the extrapleural drainage of a mediastinal abscess. (From Seybold, W. D., Johnson, M. A., III, and Leary, W. V.: Perforation of the esophagus: An analysis of 50 cases and an account of experimental studies. Surg. Clin. North Am. *30*:1155, 1950.)

agus in a patient with minimal symptoms or signs of sepsis. With oral intake totally restricted and with the administration of antibiotics and parenteral hyperalimentation, the cavities contract and the esophageal leaks seal, permitting resumption of an oral diet in 1 to 5 weeks. This is an important subgroup to recognize. At the Mayo Clinic we have treated a subgroup of 10 esophageal perforations in this manner with success, and we feel that this constitutes a valid, definable exception to the dictum of surgical intervention for all instrumental perforations. Unlike the Hopkins' study, we have

tended to select for conservative management those perforations that are remote from the esophagogastric junction and certainly those that are not associated with gastroesophageal incompetence or more distal esophageal obstruction.

One of the important issues in the management of esophageal perforation is the question of when to resume oral intake after surgical repair. Early resumption of oral intake was once an essential aspect in recovery, but that no longer applies. Total parenteral alimentation now permits immediate and prolonged nutritional support.

At the Mayo Clinic we have felt that a repaired esophageal perforation is particularly vulnerable to breakdown if oral feedings are resumed too soon. Thus, we tend to keep patients on a regimen of nothing by mouth for 10 days to 3 weeks after repair and to carry out a Gastrografin contrast x-ray study at that point in time before considering resumption of diet by mouth. If there is no extravasation of contrast, liquids are resumed by mouth and diet is progressed. If there is confined extravasation and the patient is not septic, conservative management is continued until three to four weeks have elapsed. After that time the defect is either totally healed or has become so confined that oral feedings generally can be resumed without fear of disseminating infection. Complete resolution of the radiographic abnormality may require many weeks.

OTHER COMPLICATIONS. Dental injuries are not uncommon complications of endoscopic procedures. Diseased or normal teeth, restorations, and fillings may be broken or loosened. The chief danger of such complications is the possibility that, immediately or later, these dislodged fragments may become foreign bodies in the lower part of the respiratory or alimentary tract. Prolonged esophageal intubation for gastrointestinal decompression may lead to salpingitis of the eustachian tube with consequent otitis media, particularly in infants. Occasionally, laryngeal edema and esophageal erosions will occur after prolonged intubation. Gastroesophageal incompetence is not an infrequent consequence of esophageal intubation, with complicating mild to severe reflex esophagitis and occasional development of an esophageal stricture. Ketcham and Smith[74] described elective cervical esophagostomy as a substitute for the occasional long-term nasogastric or gastrostomy gavage. The procedure is particularly appealing not only because it eliminates the irritation and complications of a nasal tube and some of the inconvenience and risks of gastrostomy but also because it appears to eliminate the esophageal complications of longstanding intubation, if the tube is kept above the esophagogastric junction. After 6 or 7 days, a fistula tract is established that allows the patient to remove and replace the tube. When no longer needed, the tube is re-

moved, and the tract closes in 3 to 5 days. It should be stressed, however, that patients with thoracic esophageal perforation or fistulas between the esophagus and tracheobronchial tree tolerate gastric feedings by any route poorly, usually with reflux of gastric contents into the esophagus and thence through the fistula or perforation.

Tracheoesophageal and bronchoesophageal fistulas are serious but rare complications of esophageal perforation. Usually such communications develop with the spontaneous drainage of a postperforation collection into the tracheobronchial tree. Preferably, such collections are promptly diagnosed and drained before a fistula develops. Once it is established, prompt action should be taken to prevent continued tracheobronchial contamination. By direct surgical intervention it may be possible to excise and close a more chronic fistula and provide the necessary drainage and interposition of tissues to prevent recurrence.[139] As in the confined esophageal perforation, we have seen several instrumental perforations in the middle third of the esophagus that have been complicated by esophagobronchial fistula without sepsis. These have closed spontaneously with antibiotics, nothing by mouth, and parenteral alimentation, in a matter of one or two weeks. In the more acute septic patient it may not be possible to eliminate the communications effectively or completely, and only drainage of the local area may be possible. Defunctionalization of the esophagus in such a situation may require cervical esophagostomy and closure of the proximal and distal ends of the esophagus with feeding gastrostomy. Some type of reconstruction of esophagogastric continuity will be required later. Tracheostomy may be important in the management of such fistulas, particularly for elimination of secretions and prevention of esophageal spillage. Occasionally it may be possible to seal off the lower part of the respiratory tract from the continued contamination by placing a cuffed tracheostomy tube below the site of the fistulous communication.

Congenital Atresia of the Esophagus with Tracheoesophageal Fistula

One of the greatest challenges to the surgeon interested in esophageal disease is the infant with congenital atresia of the esophagus associated with tracheoesophageal fistula. The current survival rate for all types of surgical cases, including those with associated congenital anomalies (occurring in about 52 per cent of cases) and those infants who are premature (weighing less than 4 pounds [1.8 kg.]), is about 60 per cent.[63] It approaches 95 per cent, however, when one considers only those patients who have the usual defect (type C, Gross), who have no associated anomalies, and who weigh more than 6 pounds (2.7 kg).[56, 126] The high mortality rates in premature infants have prompted some surgeons to use staged procedures,[56, 64] although not all have found this approach successful.[57]

Waterston and associates[132] have effectively categorized these risk factors: Category A, nearly normal birth weight and no major pneumonia or other congenital anomalies; Category B, small or normal weight babies with moderate pneumonia or mild congenital anomalies; Category C, very ill, small babies with severe pneumonia or several anomalies. Richardson and associates[114] applying these criteria encountered survival in all Category A infants, 90 per cent in Category B, and 44 per cent in Category C. The late results were excellent in Categories A and B, while surviving Category C patients were all significantly impaired by associated anomalies.

To achieve good survival rates, postoperative complications must be minimized. Most surgeons would agree that the preoperative and postoperative management of these patients is of utmost importance and probably can best be accomplished with the help of expert nursing care on a pediatric surgical service. Early diagnosis of the condition and prompt referral for surgical therapy are important in minimizing the dangers of aspiration pneumonitis. When delay has occurred and pneumonitis exists, postoperative respiratory complications pose less of a problem if operation is delayed until the pneumonia has cleared. Early recognition and management of associated anomalies are also essential in minimizing postoperative complications.

Both early and late postoperative complications occur — the former consist of pulmonary complications, anastomotic leaks, and recurrent fistulas; the latter include anastomotic stricture, the aperistaltic distal esophageal segment, and tracheal stenosis.

EARLY COMPLICATIONS

Pulmonary Complications. Pulmonary complications account for 62 per cent of the deaths after repair of esophageal atresia.[63] The infant with this congenital defect should be placed in an Isolette in a moist atmosphere, and its head and chest should be kept elevated both before and after operation. Preoperatively, a small catheter should be placed in the proximal pouch to aspirate swallowed saliva, and careful attention should be directed to adequate tracheobronchial toilet. Consideration may also be given to performance of a gastrostomy at this time if gastric overdistention exists, for this in itself may interfere with diaphragmatic movement and lead to hypoventilation and hypoxia. This procedure might also benefit the right upper lobe pneumonitis encountered so frequently in these children, which is now thought to be the result of acid gastric reflux rather than of aspiration of swallowed liquids and saliva.

Choice of a thoracic incision that minimizes postoperative interference with ventilation is important, and some surgeons have advocated the use of an anterolateral incision with this in mind.[71] The posterolateral extrapleural approach, which includes removal of the posterior segments of three ribs, is unnecessarily detrimental to the infant's ventilatory efforts.

Postoperatively, the nasopharynx is suctioned frequently and the infant is turned from side to side as an aid to bronchial drainage. In a dyspneic, cyanotic infant, this may be required every few hours for a period of several days. The use of an infant laryngoscope and a fine catheter inserted into the trachea with suction applied has proven to be extremely effective in controlling postoperative secretions. When the secretions cannot be handled in this fashion, tracheostomy may be lifesaving, but it is a procedure not without complications and mortality in patients of this age.

Oral feedings are withheld for 5 to 7 days after operation and are offered cautiously to avoid regurgitation, aspiration pneumonitis, or even asphyxia. Nurses must be instructed to feed the child slowly while holding him in an upright position. After feedings, the child should be placed on his right side to prevent puddling of material in the gastric fundus.

The child should never be placed on his back. Frequent feedings of very small amounts are preferred, and the formula should be increased very slowly to avoid vomiting and its fatal consequences. Thickened feedings should be substituted early to aid in the prevention of postoperative stricture formation.

Anastomotic Leaks. Anastomotic leaks occur in approximately 17 per cent of patients and have been somewhat less frequent after the Haight type of repair in which both the muscularis and mucosa of the lower segment are anastomosed to the mucosa above, the muscle of the upper segment being brought down and over the suture line.[63] At operation, care should be taken to minimize mobilization of the distal segment. Extensive mobilization of the proximal segment is far safer because its intramural blood supply is better. When there is considerable distance between the segments, tension on the anastomosis can be lessened by inserting a nasogastric balloon catheter in the stomach and pulling it up.[59] Rather than creating a primary anastomosis under undue tension, it is preferable to exteriorize the proximal esophageal segment in the neck and to divide the fistula. Simple ligation of the fistula may result in a recurrence. Gastrostomy is done for feeding purposes, and reconstruction is carried out later. Such a planned staged procedure is essential when correcting esophageal atresia without fistula.

Approximately twice as many patients survive a leaking anastomosis if an extrapleural approach is used compared to when operation is done transpleurally.[63] When the transpleural approach is used, the use of a mediastinal pleural flap may minimize morbidity due to a leaking anastomosis.

Most leaks occur within 3 to 6 days after operation, and their prompt recognition is important if the patient is to be properly treated. Adequate drainage of the pleural space and mediastinum is essential, and this may require either rearrangement of the existing intrapleural catheter or insertion of additional catheters. A polyethylene nasogastric feeding tube or a gastrostomy tube may be inserted to maintain nutrition while the fistulous tract is healing. If the leak is a large one, resulting in pneumothorax and extensive pleural contamination, reoperation may be necessary to close the fistula. If this is impossible, the proximal segment may be exteriorized as a cervical esophagotomy, with closure of the distal part of the esophagus and gastrostomy. Under the circumstances, of course, a reconstructive operation will be required later if the patient survives. Although 21 per cent of the deaths after operation for congenital atresia of the esophagus with tracheoesophageal fistula result from anastomotic leaks[63] not all patients who have anastomotic leaks succumb. Prompt recognition and management along the lines discussed here may help to minimize the mortality rate for this complication. Occasionally, judicious dilatation of the anastomotic area may aid the healing of the fistula.

Recurrent Fistulas. Although rare, recurrent fistulas occur in a small percentage of patients after repair of esophageal atresia with tracheoesophageal fistula (Fig. 16–7). This complication, which may occur either early or late, should be considered in any

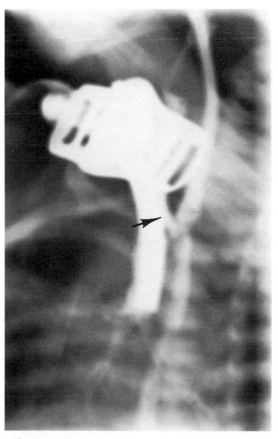

Figure 16–7 Ingested contrast medium outlining recurrent tracheoesophageal fistula 2 months after attempted primary repair. Arrow identifies fistula.

child who has repeated episodes of pneumonitis or of cyanosis and choking spells with feeding. It may be due either to a true recurrent fistula or to an overlooked second fistula from the proximal segment. If mobilization of the proximal segment is adequate, a second fistula will not be overlooked; but, regardless of the nature of the communication, once it is recognized, operation is necessary.

LATE COMPLICATIONS

Anastomotic Stricture. Narrowing of the anastomosis is a relatively common complication in those children who survive the early postoperative period. It is reported to occur in 35 to 50 per cent of cases[119] and has been identified any time from 2 to 15 weeks after operation. Although the Haight type of repair previously described has the lowest incidence of anastomotic leaks, it leads to more late strictures than do other techniques. Some surgeons recommend routine contrast roentgenography[65] and esophageal dilatation[54] prior to dismissal from the hospital to ensure that the anastomosis is of adequate size. Close attention to the clinical condition of the patient, however, may suffice, and parents should be alerted to the possible late development of this complication.

Esophageal dilatation is necessary when there is an anastomotic stricture (Fig. 16–8), and many infants require only one or two dilations to establish an adequate channel for the passage of food. When the stenosis is not severe, the passage of esophageal bougies over a previously swallowed thread is advocated. A very tight stricture may require esophagoscopy to pass filiform catheters of graduated sizes up to 12 or 14 French before placement of a string which will allow safe dilation with an esophageal bougie. Rarely, retrograde dilation through a gastrostomy will be required. These techniques are not without risk of perforation.

Retained foreign bodies must be included as another complication of a narrowed anastomosis. According to one report,[59] at least 15 per cent of patients were hospitalized at one time or another for the removal of retained foreign bodies, including oversized bites of meat (particularly wieners), apples, or various other objects. An obvious stenotic area may not be seen on the roentgenogram but the lodgment of these objects at the anastomosis may be related to the lack of distensibility of the organ at this site.

Abnormal Esophageal Motility. The frequency and severity of esophageal motility disturbances in patients with esophageal

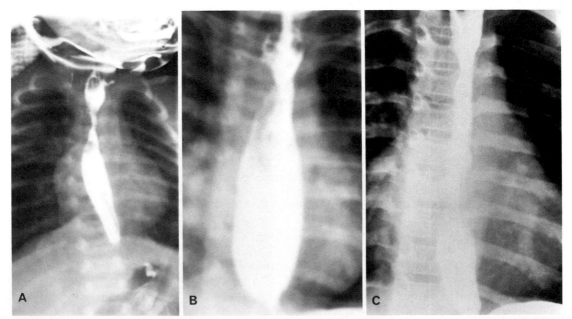

Figure 16–8 Anastomotic stricture after anastomosis of esophagus in patient with esophageal atresia, which has been well controlled by periodic dilatations. *A,* One month after operation; *B,* 18 months later; *C,* 8 years after operation.

atresia have been appreciated only recently and may prove to be a more common cause for postoperative dysphagia and respiratory complications than anastomotic strictures.[24, 53] While some investigators, notably Orringer et al.,[102] have observed normal esophageal motor function in children with repaired atresia, Werlin et al.[136] consistently demonstrated a long aperistaltic segment of thoracic esophagus in all their patients. Manometrically identifiable peristalsis occurred only in the cervical or distal esophagus or both.

The etiology of this motility disorder is unclear. It has been suggested that damage to the esophageal branches of the vagus nerve occurs during corrective surgery, although the findings of a negative Mecholyl test in one report[136] casts doubt on the role of simple denervation. The possibility also exists that a congenital defect of the esophageal nerve supply may be implicated. This speculation is supported by the observation that many children with tracheoesophageal fistula without atresia have esophageal motor dysfunction preoperatively.[102]

An additional, newly described motility disorder in esophageal atresia affects the lower esophageal sphincter and is characterized by transient, inappropriate relaxation of the sphincter.[136] It is likely that this functional abnormality explains the high incidence of gastroesophageal reflux in these children.

The parents should be instructed to feed these children in an upright position and to keep them propped up for a reasonable period after feedings. Training the child to sleep in a semisitting position may also minimize respiratory problems secondary to accumulation of salivary secretions in the lower esophageal segment. Such an accumulation leads to regurgitation with nocturnal cough and respiratory difficulties. Because of the lack of a normal esophageal peristaltic wave, ingested food enters the stomach under the influence of gravity.

Tracheal Stenosis. Stenosis of the trachea at the site of closure of the fistula is a serious complication which results from overzealous efforts to make the closure flush with the trachea. The symptoms are stridor, wheezing, dyspnea, and variable degrees of respiratory distress. Fortunately, this is a rare complication, particularly if care is taken during closure of the tracheal wall. Endo-

scopic treatment should consist of tracheal dilatation and removal of obstructing granulation tissue.[65] Tracheostomy is usually of little value, and reoperation may occasionally be required.

Esophagotomy

Opening the esophagus by means of a surgical incision is a common maneuver. The usual indications for esophagotomy are the excision of esophageal diverticula, ligation of bleeding gastroesophageal varices, and removal of mural and intraluminal benign tumors of the esophagus, as well as surgical management of granulomas, fistulas, foreign bodies, duplications, and cysts that may involve the esophagus. Cervical esophagotomy is occasionally performed as a temporary or permanent diverting procedure or as a substitute for gastrostomy or prolonged nasogastric intubation. The general principles involved in the management of esophagotomy are similar to those used in the management of lacerations and perforations of the esophagus.

LEAKAGE. Leakage is perhaps the most serious sequela of esophagotomy, and adequate drainage must be provided at the initial operation. The general principles for the management of this complication are outlined in the section dealing with perforation. The first prerequisite, however, in the prevention of this complication is adequate and precise watertight layer closure of esophageal incisions and, of course, avoidance (or prompt recognition and repair) of mucosal lacerations which may occur during the course of extramucosal excisions and esophagomyotomies.

Regardless of the adequacy of esophagotomy closure, disruption of the suture line is likely to occur if there is distal esophageal obstruction. Such associated obstructing conditions should be identified prior to esophagotomy and should be treated either prior to or at operation. Pulsion diverticula of the lower part of the esophagus will often recur or be followed by suture line leakage because a disturbance in esophageal motility frequently coexists. Therefore a concomitant long esophagomyotomy should usually accompany the excision of such a diverticulum.[31] Cricopharyngeal myotomy at the time of pharyngoesophageal diverticulectomy may provide further reduction of what is already a rather negligible incidence of leak and fistula formation after diverticulectomy alone.[135] Certainly, the use of myotomy alone for small diverticula avoids suture line complications completely.[43]

At the Mayo Clinic it has been our practice prior to feeding to study roentgenographically all patients in whom an esophagotomy is performed. This assures that a tight closure exists prior to feeding. If there is leakage, the routine for conservative management of esophageal perforation is followed and oral intake delayed until the leak either is healed or is confined, with a sufficient lapse of time so that contamination will not spread with resumption of oral intake.

OBSTRUCTION. The second principal complication of esophagotomy is narrowing of the esophageal lumen at the point of closure. This complication may be anticipated after overzealous attempts to excise completely the protruding mucosal sac during esophageal diverticulectomy. Minor obstructions produced in this manner are often compensated for spontaneously or may respond to a single dilatation. Others may cause severe obstructing strictures or suture line leakage or both. Often, obstruction can be avoided by performing the esophagotomy and its closure over an indwelling catheter of appropriate size.[106]

Once a stricture is recognized, preparation for esophageal dilatation should be made. The first and most important step is to introduce a thread into the esophagus, for use as a guide for subsequent dilatations. Although the esophagus should be threaded early, the time interval between operation and institution of dilatations may be of considerable importance. The level and type of the stricture and the presence of other local or systemic complications are important determinants. Generally, the minor obstructions that occur after esophagotomy or diverticulectomy can be dealt with safely, beginning 9 to 10 days postoperatively. With more severe problems, particularly those involving the thoracic part of the esophagus or requiring hydrostatic dilatation, at least 2 weeks should elapse before beginning such treatment.

The longer the stricture, the more difficult is its management. Although transverse closure of esophagotomy incisions may effectively reduce the length of a resultant stricture, attention to the direction of closure is less important than attention to the other factors previously outlined.

MISCELLANEOUS COMPLICATIONS

Although injury to neighboring structures is an inherent danger in the performance of any surgical procedure, during esophagotomy particular care must be exercised to avoid injury to the vagus nerve. Injury to this nerve may result in motility disturbances in either the esophagus or the stomach. Although "postvagotomy dysphagia" is a rare and often relatively benign complication,[7, 51] gastric atony and pylorospasm may require a gastric drainage procedure for control. Thoracic duct injuries should be recognized at the time of operation, and the duct should be promptly ligated. Chylothorax or other chylous fistulas are more likely to occur after esophageal resection for malignant lesions, but occasionally they occur after lesser surgical procedures on the esophagus. Their management will be discussed under the subsequent heading.

Esophagogastrectomy

An esophagogastric resection may be required for many conditions, but the most common by far is a malignant lesion of the esophagus or cardia. This is a major surgical undertaking even in a patient with benign disease, but when such a procedure is carried out for cancer, the patient usually is a poor surgical risk because of advanced age and associated pulmonary and cardiovascular disease. Furthermore, he usually has become debilitated because of inadequate oral intake of food and fluid for variable periods.

We have long advocated an aggressive surgical approach to esophagogastric malignancy, believing that resection and immediate reconstruction of gastrointestinal continuity whenever possible provides the most effective palliation at low risk and returns the patient to a relatively normal existence more rapidly than any other form of therapy. This approach has not been universally accepted, however, because of reported low operability rates and high mortality rates after resection. Although complications may occur after esophagogastric resection, we believe that their occurrence will be minimized by careful attention to preoperative, operative, and postoperative details of management.

As important as nutrition is to the management of patients undergoing esophageal resection, delaying operation in hopes of correcting weight loss or negative nitrogen balance is rarely indicated. Indeed, with current parenteral alimentation techniques, these efforts are better utilized in the postoperative period. This is not to say that the nutritional aspects should not be attended to preoperatively while diagnostic studies are under way, but it is a vain hope that depletions that have taken many weeks or months to develop can be significantly reversed in a reasonable period to justify delayed definitive surgical correction.

Reference already has been made to the advisability of a careful preoperative pulmonary program in patients with chronic obstructive lung disease and diminished pulmonary reserve and tenacious secretions. Anemia, hypoproteinemia, and decreased blood volume are corrected by means of transfusion and the administration of serum albumin. Vitamins, including generous amounts of ascorbic acid, are administered parenterally. Care must be taken with debilitated elderly patients to avoid overhydration and excessive administration of salt. Careful nursing care is particularly important in these patients because they are so susceptible to postoperative complications, which may be divided into the following general categories: (1) infection, (2) respiratory, (3) cardiovascular, (4) gastrointestinal, and (5) miscellaneous.

INFECTION. A leaking gastroesophageal anastomosis has been implicated in one third to one half of the deaths after esophagogastrectomy in large series of patients.[41, 78] The catastrophic consequences of an anastomotic dehiscence were markedly reduced by Nakayama[94] chiefly by avoiding, whenever possible, the performance of an intrathoracic anastomosis, preferring instead a cervical esophagogastrostomy. More recent series,[36, 109, 124] however, attest to the safety of an intrathoracic esophagogastros-

tomy, provided that proper attention is given to specific technical details including preservation of blood supply, avoidance of clamps in the stomach or esophagus, and avoidance of tension on the anastomosis. The use of an invagination or "ink well" technique to protect the anastomotic site may also play a role in preserving the integrity of the suture line. Emphasizing these technical details, Ellis and Gibb[36] reported an anastomotic leak in fewer than 6 per cent of 72 patients, the majority of whom underwent esophagogastrectomy for Stage III disease, with an overall hospital mortality in the series of 2.8 per cent.

Today, detecting a potential leaking anastomosis before it becomes a clinical problem is possible. At the Mayo Clinic, death from esophageal anastomotic leakage has been largely eliminated by performing a Gastrografin study of the esophagus prior to feeding. The details of this conservative management have been described in earlier sections of this chapter. This has been an important addition to the care of patients undergoing esophageal surgery but not a substitute for attention to technical details during operation.

Under ordinary circumstances a leaking anastomosis becomes apparent within the first week to 10 days after operation and may make its appearance insidiously with a low-grade fever associated with signs of inflammation and fluid accumulation in the pleural space on the side of the operation. If wide resection of a malignant lesion has required entry into the opposite pleural space, the first signs of a leaking anastomosis may be evident on the side opposite the one operated on. Occasionally a leak is heralded by the acute onset of pain in the chest mimicking a pulmonary embolus and may even be accompanied by a shocklike state requiring vasopressors for maintenance of blood pressure.

It is now our practice to leave the nasogastric tube in position on suction at least 4 to 5 days after the operation. On about the fourth or fifth postoperative day intestinal ileus usually resolves and is heralded by a spontaneous bowel movement. It is at this point that the Gastrografin x-ray study is performed. If there is no extravasation of the medium from the anastomosis, feeding by mouth is resumed, progressing from liquids to solids, and the chest drainage tube is removed. If, however, leakage is detected, a previously inserted subclavian central venous line is utilized for total parenteral alimentation, administering 2000 to 3000 calories per day. If the patient remains aseptic, this is continued for 10 days to 2 weeks and the x-ray contrast study is repeated. Diet may be resumed only when complete sealing is demonstrated or in the presence of a confined leak of 3 to 4 weeks' duration. Although the complication of a leaking anastomosis is a serious one with a high mortality rate, careful management of the patient with this potential complication improves the survival rate. In the absence of suspected leakage we have found it advisable to resume feedings as soon as possible. It is usually possible to return a patient to a general diet within a week to 10 days of operation. The head of the patient's bed is always kept elevated in the postoperative period to minimize reflux of gastric contents through the anastomosis.

If contamination of the pleural space occurs during the esophagogastrectomy, a pleural infection may develop postoperatively in the absence of a leak at the anastomotic site. Control of such an intrapleural infection may be achieved by the usual techniques of catheter drainage and even temporary open drainage of the thorax. Wound infections are common after resections of malignant lesions of the esophagus and cardia, and their management by the use of appropriate antibiotics, promotion of free drainage, and attention to the nutritional aspects of the patient is usually successful. When intraoperative wound contamination is recognized, we have found the closure of incisions with a subcutaneous catheter in place, as suggested by McIlrath and others,[85] a reliable means of minimizing wound infection.

RESPIRATORY COMPLICATIONS. Reference already has been made to the necessity for careful prophylaxis to avoid postoperative pulmonary complications. Bronchodilators, ultrasonic humidification, tracheal aspiration, and appropriate antibiotics all should be used. With proper preoperative selection of patients, tracheal intubation and respiratory support are rarely indicated. Intrapleural complications can be minimized by proper placement of intrapleural catheters for drainage after operation. The intrathoracic placement of the stomach may lead to respiratory embarrassment, particularly if the organ becomes distended with fluid and gas. The intraoperative placement of a nasogastric tube and its judicious removal postoperatively should eliminate these problems.

CARDIOVASCULAR COMPLICATIONS. Most patients undergoing esophageal resection are elderly; arteriosclerosis is common among them, and they are particularly susceptible to coronary occlusion and congestive heart failure. Therefore, prolonged enrichment of the oxygen content of inspired gas is advisable during the recovery period if blood gas studies indicate that the patient has decreased arterial oxygen tension while breathing room air. Cardiac arrhythmias are frequently encountered after operation, and the development of atrial flutter or fibrillation may be heralded by a sudden decrease in the patient's blood pressure, the cause of which may not be clear until an electrocardiogram has been obtained. Rapid digitalization of the patient is indicated under such circumstances, with special reference to acid-base balance, blood gases, and serum electrolytes.

A serious but rare vascular complication that occurs early in the postoperative period is hemorrhage. Bleeding may occur from many sources, including the anastomosis, an inadvertently lacerated spleen, or torn, short gastric vessels. The wide mediastinal resection required to remove bulky malignant lesions with considerable surrounding inflammation may result in mediastinal hemorrhage, particularly from esophageal arteries arising directly from the aorta. Care should be taken at operation to secure these esophageal branches of the aorta, which, if not properly controlled, may later lead to exsanguinating hemorrhage. Obviously, reoperation is required for control of bleeding when such a complication develops.

Rarely, bleeding may occur later in the postoperative period from a gastric ulcer that may bleed spontaneously or by secondary perforation into the aorta, resulting in an exsanguinating hemorrhage.[18] Such a complication has also been reported as a result of a leaking anastomosis.[77]

Other vascular complications include thrombophlebitis, pulmonary embolus, and cerebrovascular accidents, any of which may develop in seriously ill patients undergoing an operation of the magnitude of esophagogastrectomy.

GASTROINTESTINAL COMPLICATIONS. Delayed gastric emptying is a common sequela of bilateral vagotomy and always accompanies wide resection of the esophagus and cardia. For this reason a concomitant gastric drainage procedure should always be performed, if possible, at the time of esophagogastrectomy; sometimes, however, the location of the esophageal lesion or the build or condition of the patient prohibits it. In these cases, if symptoms of gastric retention develop postoperatively, they often can be relieved by a subsequent gastric drainage procedure, preferably of the Heineke-Mikulicz or Finney type.

Postvagotomy pylorospasm can lead not only to symptoms of gastric retention but also to another gastrointestinal complication of resections of the distal esophagus and cardia, namely, gastroesophageal reflux. The deleterious late effects of operative procedures that destroy the sphincter mechanisms are now well known.[11, 115] When possible, efforts should be made at operation to resect as much acid-bearing portion of the stomach as possible to minimize the acidity of the regurgitant stomach contents.[38] Efforts to fashion a valve-like anastomosis between esophagus and stomach after extensive gastric resection have not been universally successful.[79, 133] When esophagogastrostomy is effected high in the thorax, reflux is less often a problem. For lower esophageal anastomoses, however, gastroesophageal reflux is common. An effective surgical alternative is total gastrectomy with long-limb Roux-en-Y anastomosis.[105]

Although the amounts of gastric acid in elderly patients undergoing esophagogastrectomy for malignant lesions are often small, it is generally appreciated that the reflux esophagitis experienced after esophagogastrectomy is due less to acid-peptic reflux than to the erosive effects of alkaline biliary and pancreatic secretions. Irrespective of the exact chemical or enzymatic agents responsible, patients who have had resection of the esophagogastric junction are at risk of incurring significant reflux symptoms. They also should be told to sleep with the head of the bed elevated on blocks 8 to 10 inches (20.3 to 25.4 cm.. high to promote gastric emptying during recumbency and to minimize the possibility of gastroesophageal reflux. When regurgitant esophagitis has led to narrowing of the anastomotic area, esophagoscopy is essential to exclude the possibility of recurrent malignant disease. Bougienage may suffice to relieve the symptoms of esophageal obstruction. If the original resection was performed ,for a benign process and long-term survival is expected, occasionally a more aggressive surgical approach is required involving resection of the strictured area and either interposition of a segment of colon[99] or distal antrectomy with Roux-en-Y gastrojejunostomy.[52] It is also possible to effect a long-limb Roux-en-Y gastric drainage procedure after extensive proximal esophagogastrectomy.[122] We believe that these procedures are most effective for treatment of postesophagogastrectomy stricture that does not respond to the usual conservative measures. The occurrence of symptoms and complications of gastroesophageal reflux that develop as the consequence of operations that destroy or bypass the intrinsic esophageal sphincter should serve to emphasize a need for conservatism in the selection of operations in this region. Especially when dealing with benign disease, one should attempt to preserve the sphincter and, when this is not possible, to preserve sufficient fundus to make it possible to effect one of the competence-restoring procedures such as the Nissen or Belsey method.

Diarrhea, which may be debilitating, develops in some patients after esophagogastrectomy and is usually a consequence of bilateral vagotomy. Fortunately, this symptom usually subsides in time, but may require medication for symptomatic relief. Postoperative gastrointestinal symptoms related primarily to the lack of an adequate gastric reservoir include rapid filling and weight loss. Sometimes they can be managed by frequent small feedings. The dumping syndrome also may be encountered in patients who have had extensive resective procedures, particularly when a gastric drainage procedure has been performed. The usual advice for symptomatic relief of the dumping syndrome is often effective and includes elimination of carbohydrates and fluid intake at meals and a short period of recumbency after eating.

Nutritional disturbances may develop in patients who have had wide resection of the proximal part of the stomach. Increased loss of fat in the stool occurs,[108] and the loss of an adequate gastric reservoir with an inadequate oral intake makes it difficult for these patients to maintain their weight. Elimination of the intrinsic factor by resection of this type may result in a macrocytic anemia in long-term survivors.[116] Frequent small feedings of a diet high in protein and caloric content with supplementary vitamins, including B$_{12}$ when the patient has anemia, may provide some symptomatic benefit.

MISCELLANEOUS COMPLICATIONS. Various miscellaneous complications can occur after such extensive procedures as are involved in resections of the esophagus and cardia. These include urinary retention, anuria, and uremia, as well as fluid and electrolyte imbalance. No special comments are required here concerning the management of these complications.

Chylothorax is another complication that occasionally follows extensive resections in the mediastinum, particularly in its upper portions. Injury to the thoracic duct is responsible. If adequate drainage of the involved pleural space does not result in lessening of the chylous effusion within a few days, reoperation with ligation of the duct above the diaphragm as it enters the chest is mandatory. At the time of reoperation for chylothorax, abrasive pleurodesis should be effected to seal the pleural space and leaking lymphatic channels. Attention to the fundamentals laid down by Kausel and associates[72] will aid in identifying an accessory duct.

Interposition Procedures

Interposition of segments of colon or jejunum is occasionally indicated when esophageal resection or bypass is required for benign or malignant disease. Such operations have certain theoretical advantages over esophagogastrectomy because an adequate gastric reservoir is maintained and the dangers of reflux of gastric contents and acid-peptic digestion are minimized. When the proximal anastomosis is performed in the cervical region, the dangerous consequences of an anastomotic leak are fewer than when an intrathoracic anastomosis is made. Nevertheless, any or all of the complications just reviewed for esophagogastrectomy may occur. In addition, certain special problems that may develop after interposition procedures will be reviewed here briefly under the following headings: vascular complications, cervical fistula, obstruction, peptic ulceration, and pneumothorax.

VASCULAR COMPLICATIONS. The danger of impaired circulation to the interposed segment, whether jejunum or colon, is always a hazard of intestinal transplantation. The risk is greater when the jejunum is used because the anatomic distribution of the blood supply is such that when long segments are required, it is necessary to mobilize several loops of small intestine, thereby perhaps jeopardizing the viability of the proximal tip of the transplant. The colon is less subject to these hazards, and the more constant pattern of the circulation to the left colon makes it a more desirable substitute.[12] Obstruction to venous drainage may be more important than impairment of the arterial circulation as far as the development of gangrene of part or all of the interposed segment is concerned. Extreme care in handling of the transplant may minimize this occurrence, and torsion of or tension on the vascular pedicle must be avoided.

If more than a few centimeters of the transplant become necrotic, it may be necessary to reexplore, with excision of the gangrenous segment, establishment of a cervical esophagostomy, and esophageal reconstruction at a later date. When the gangrenous area is limited, it may occasionally be possible, by mobilizing the remainder of the transplant, to achieve adequate length for reanastomosis to the esophagus.

CERVICAL FISTULA. Since in many instances the proximal anastomosis will be carried out in the neck with the transplant lying substernally, mild degrees of vascular impairment may lead to another complication — cervical fistula. This, fortunately, is a far less dangerous complication than an anastomotic fistula developing within the thorax. If adequate drainage of the anastomotic region is provided when the bowel is joined, no serious consequences should ensue. Ultimate healing should occur, although in some instances there may be slight narrowing of the anastomosis. Without adequate drainage, a serious anterior mediastinitis may result, necessitating wide open drainage.

It is our practice to maintain oral feedings when the leak is small in order to improve the patient's nutrition and to promote healing. When total disruption of the anastomosis has occurred, feedings by a temporary gastrostomy tube are done, and reanastomosis is attempted at an appropriate time. If at the initial procedure there is any concern about the viability of the tip of the transplant, it and the proximal esophagus can be temporarily exteriorized, and thus one can be sure of anastomosing esophagus to viable bowel.

OBSTRUCTION. The problem of postvagotomy obstruction, which has already been discussed, may occur after interposition procedures as well as after the usual type of esophagogastrectomy. Interposition procedures may occasionally cause obstruction from other causes, which may be either functional or mechanical. Although at first glance the jejunum would seem to be an appropriate organ to use as an esophageal substitute because its caliber more nearly approaches that of the esophagus, it has proven to be less advantageous than the colon on several counts (one, its blood supply, has already been referred to above). Peristalsis in the transplanted jejunum is such that there is always some delay in the transit of food from the mouth to the stomach, particularly when long segments are used. This may lead to a feeling of fullness in the chest which requires the patient to eat very slowly. This sort of functional obstruction is far more pronounced if the transplant is inserted in an antiperistaltic direction, a technique that should under no circumstances be used.[111] These problems have not been observed with colon transplants.

Anastomotic strictures, either at the esophagocolonic or cologastric anastomosis, may cause mechanical obstruction to the passage of ingested food. They can easily be identified radiographically, and reoperation with revision of the anastomosis may occasionally be required. When an excessively long transplant has been used, obstruction may occur merely from the redundancy of the transplant; this occurs more commonly with jejunum than with colon. A mechanical obstruction may also develop at the subxiphoid region as the transplant emerges into the abdomen from its retrosternal position. An example of this is illustrated in Figure 16–9; reoperation with division of adhesions and enlargement of the aperture between abdomen and anterior mediastinum will correct the problem. If the vascular pedicle of a colon transplant is placed anterior to the stomach, pyloric obstruction may ensue, and so the retrogastric route should always be used.

PEPTIC ULCERATION. Although one of the purposes of using a segment of bowel to interpose between the stomach and esophagus is to avoid the dangerous complications of reflux esophagitis, peptic ulceration of

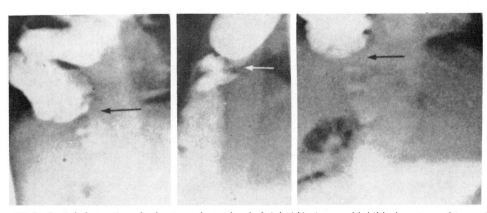

Figure 16–9   Partial obstruction of colon transplant at level of xiphoid in 4-year-old child who, at age of 1 year, had had esophageal reconstruction for esophageal atresia not amenable to primary repair. Arrows indicate point of obstruction.

the transplant itself may occur. It has been demonstrated experimentally that the proximal portions of the intestinal tract are more susceptible to peptic ulceration than the portions more distally located,[75] and instances of jejunitis from gastrojejunal reflux after interposition procedures have been reported.[49] There have also been a few instances of gastroduodenal ulceration after such procedures, the cause of which is not entirely clear.[9] The colon is also subject to this complication and may be no less susceptible to acid-peptic digestion than is the jejunum.[95] Both, however, are far more resistant to this complication than is the esophagus. One other complication of jejunal interposition procedures, which does not rightly deserve the name peptic ulceration, but which has led to minor problems in surgical patients, is the development of an alkaline esophagitis proximal to the esophagojejunal anastomosis.[13]

Whether inflammation of the interposed segment is due to reflux of acidic or alkaline juices, nonetheless the avoidance of obesity and constricting garments, the use of 8- to 10-inch (20.3 to 25.4 cm.) blocks under the head of the patient's bed, and administration of neutralizing agents by mouth are recommended.

PNEUMOTHORAX. The extensive retrosternal dissection required to interpose an intestinal transplant between the cervical part of the esophagus and the stomach may lead to an unrecognized pneumothorax. Much of this dissection must be done blindly and bluntly, and if time and care are not expended in the preparation of the retrosternal bed, one or both pleural spaces may be entered. If this is not recognized, the consequences may be catastrophic. It is our practice to obtain a thoracic roentgenogram immediately after the operative procedure so that the necessary steps can be taken to evacuate the pleural space if air is present.

Palliative Intubation of the Esophagus

Permanent esophageal intubation is being used more frequently than heretofore in the palliation of esophageal obstruction caused by malignant disease. Rarely it may be used for benign strictures. Palliative intubation has obvious advantages over more extensive procedures and over procedures that are less effective in returning function to the esophagus. Thus, various tubes and methods for their insertion have been developed since Symond's report[127] of the first successful application of this principle in 1885. In spite of advances, current methods are not without risk. Complications after permanent esophageal intubation may be attributed either to the method of introduction or to the presence of a prosthesis in an obstructed and diseased esophagus.[30]

Intubation may be accomplished through the mouth with or without preliminary esophageal bougienage, esophagoscopic control, or a previously introduced guide. Temporary gastrostomy may be used to insert, position, or anchor the tube. Management of complications from such instrumental procedures or incisions into the esophagus has been referred to previously. When they follow palliative intubation, their management poses certain specific problems.

PERFORATION. Esophageal perforation is the most frequent and serious complication of palliative intubation. It usually results from the passage of the prosthesis through the obstructing and necrotic lesion but may also result from pressure necrosis of more normal portions of the esophagus. Gastric erosions or actual perforation may occur in a similar manner with a long prosthesis that extends through the cardia into the stomach. False passage of a tube through the tumor, if recognized and corrected at the time it happens, rarely causes serious complications if the site of perforation is adequately bypassed by a snugly fitting tube. Perforations proximal to the prosthesis, however, pose a more serious problem, particularly if esophageal obstruction is not relieved.[30]

With most patients a rapidly fatal course will ensue if conservative measures alone are relied on. At best, a chronic esophageal fistula will result from attempts to drain contaminated spaces. Although the patient's poor prognosis and general condition may often preclude more aggressive management, some consideration should be given either to immediate resection of the obstructing tumor or to an esophageal exclusion procedure followed by a retrosternal colonic interposition. These approaches would be particularly applicable in patients in whom intubation is used to palliate benign strictures or in patients sustaining a perforation during a period of preoperative radiation.

OBSTRUCTION. Obstruction is the second most common complication of permanent esophageal intubation. It is usually due to the incrustation and impaction of ingested foods in the tube. This can be prevented by the use of a mechanically soft diet, liberal washing through of more solid foods with liquids, and the drinking of carbonated beverages to keep the tube clean. The ingestion of sips of hydrogen peroxide or proteolytic enzymes or esophagoscopy may be required to relieve such obstructions.[20] Malposition, dislodgement, and collapse or buckling of the tube are infrequent causes of obstruction and require removal of the tube and further palliation of esophageal obstructive symptoms. Esophageal intussusception[2] and mucosal prolapse[47] into a prosthetic tube are rare complications.

Severe bleeding or pain is unusual after palliative intubation and is related more often to the malignant lesion than to the prosthesis. Painful discomfort is not unusual with tubes in high cervical locations, however, and may require removal of the tube for relief. Heartburn may occur with prostheses in the lower part of the esophagus if they traverse the cardia. This gastroesophageal reflux may be controlled by a bland diet, antacids, and the use of a head-elevated bed.

Cardioplasty and Esophagomyotomy

Any incisional or excisional surgery performed on the esophagogastric junction will lead to a disturbance in the function of the lower esophageal sphincter. This disturbance is most noted after esophagogastrectomy and cardioplasties of the Wendel and Heyrovsky-Grondahl types,[11, 115] and the high risk of subsequent esophagitis has been well documented. One collective review of the results of cardioplasty disclosed that more than half the patients had poor results.[45] That such operations should still be advised is unfortunate and reflects a lack of understanding of the nature of esophageal achalasia.[3] The condition cannot be divided

into several different diseases with differing forms of treatment. "Megaesophagus" is merely a more advanced stage of the disease, and all stages are a reflection of the same disturbed motility and are amenable to the same treatment.

When a surgical method is to be used, extramucosal esophagomyotomy is the treatment of choice for esophageal achalasia because, if it is properly performed, it causes only minimal disturbance to the sphincteric mechanism. A modified esophagomyotomy is equally applicable in any stage of the disease, and we have not found any difference in the clinical results. We believe very strongly that ancillary procedures, such as gastric drainage procedures,[97, 131] vagotomy and pyloroplasty,[89] diaphragmatic fixation of the stomach,[10] and particularly interposition procedures,[91] are not only unnecessary but also harmful, and we can envision no clinical situation in which performance of a cardioplasty would be justified.

Esophagomyotomy, as now performed, differs markedly from the procedure originally described by Heller,[38] and differences in reported clinical results may reflect differences in surgical technique. Several technical points should be stressed, because if they are not observed, some of the complications to be discussed subsequently may result. A thoracic approach is preferred because it allows a direct attack on the region of disease — the distal part of the esophagus — without the necessity of major mobilization of the hiatal structures. Damage to the vagus nerve may lead to postoperative pylorospasm, which encourages gastroesophageal reflux. A long gastric incision adds nothing to the effectivenss of the operation in terms of reduction of sphincteric pressure. In fact, experiments have shown that there is a theoretical advantage to a relatively short myotomy restricted to the distal end of the esophagus, because, at least in the dog, after this procedure, gastroesophageal reflux did not occur.[86] The incision should pass onto the stomach only far enough to ensure complete division of all the encircling muscular fibers of the lower part of the esophagus.

If these principles are followed strictly, the complications to be discussed (particularly diaphragmatic hernia, reflux esophagi-

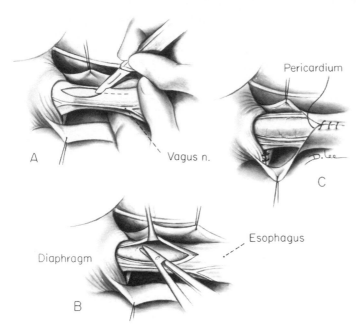

Figure 16–10 Modified Heller esophagomyotomy. After exposure of distal esophagus, an extramucosal incision (A) is made on anterolateral aspect of esophagus extending from esophagogastric junction to a point 8 to 10 cm. cephalad. Note in B that approximately 50 per cent of the circumference of the esophageal mucosal tube is freed of overlying muscularis to permit protrusion of mucosa through the myotomy. This is necessary to prevent healing of the myotomy and recurrence of achalasia. Myotomy is extended to esophagogastric junction and not onto stomach; thus reflux esophagitis after this procedure is avoided. C, Further competence is assured by restoration of esophagogastric junction to intra-abdominal position with suture narrowing of esophageal hiatus if necessary. Only if a frank sliding esophageal hiatal hernia is present should a formal repair be required. (From Ellis, F. H., Jr., Kiser, J. C., Schlegel, J. F., Earlam, R. J., McVey, J. L., and Olsen, A. M.: Esophagomyotomy for esophageal achalasia: Experimental, clinical, and manometric aspects. Ann. Surg. 166:640, 1967.)

tis, and esophageal obstruction) should be infrequent. Figure 16–10 contrasts the technique of modified esophagomyotomy with an extensively destructive procedure that will almost surely result in postoperative reflux esophagitis because not only has the esophageal hiatus been divided but also a major portion of the incision has been carried onto the stomach.

DIAPHRAGMATIC HERNIA. Extensive mobilization of the esophagogastric junction during performance of an esophagomyotomy will lead to disruption of the hiatal structures, and widening of the hiatus and disruption of the diaphragmaticoesophageal membrane may lead to a postoperative hiatal hernia. Care in elevating the distal part of the esophagus into the incision minimizes these dangers, but if wide mobilization is required for any reason or if a hiatal hernia is already present, the surgeon must reattach the diaphragmaticoesophageal membrane and narrow the diaphragmatic crus posteriorly to avoid the serious complications of a postoperative hiatal hernia. Frobese and associates[46] pointed out that the incidence of hiatal hernia after the Heller operation is significant and is probably due to lack of care in dealing with the supporting structures at the hiatus, either through operative alteration of the hiatus or disruption of the phrenoesophageal membrane. There is no more certain predisposing influence to gastroesophageal reflux than coexistence of a sliding esophageal hiatal hernia and an esophagomyotomy. McVey et al. have shown that reflux esophagitis invariably develops in dogs with this combined lesion.[86]

REFLUX ESOPHAGITIS. The incidence of symptomatic reflux esophagitis in reported series of patients undergoing Heller's operation is as high as 30 per cent.[68] When carefully sought, roentgenographic evidence of gastroesophageal reflux has been identified in 30 to 50 per cent of patients after esophagomyotomy.[32, 55] Because of such a high incidence of reflux, a significant postoperative incidence of esophagitis can be expected.

A marked reduction in the occurrence of gastroesophageal reflux has followed the use of the modified Heller myotomy. Recent reports by Okike et al.[100] and Ellis et al.[37] cite an incidence of postoperative gastroesophageal reflux of less than 3 per cent. Manometric evaluation of their patients after myotomy disclosed a marked diminution in the length and amplitude of the suprahiatal high pressure zone. Of note, however, was the partial retention of an increased pressure zone in the subhiatal segment, which undoubtedly explains the low incidence of postoperative reflux using this technique.

When esophagitis develops after myotomy, the usual measures for its control should be used. If a hiatal hernia coexists, it should be repaired. In the absence of a hernia, symptomatic control of gastric reflux can be effected in many patients by initiating a weight reduction program and advising the patient to follow an ulcer diet with antacids and to use a head-elevated bed at night.

If conservative measures fail to control reflux symptoms, an anti-reflux procedure will be required. It must be emphasized, however, that sphincter-enhancing operations performed in patients with esophageal aperistalsis may result in postoperative obstruction to swallowing. To avoid high normal sphincter pressures (20 to 25 mm. Hg), the Nissen operation can be modified by constructing a wrap of shorter length, 2 cm. rather than the usual 4 or 5 cm. On the other hand, the Belsey or Hill procedures may be more applicable in patients with ineffective esophageal peristalsis, since both operations are known to produce lower sphincter amplitudes (12 to 15 mm. Hg) than a total wrap. Regardless of the operation selected, intraoperative manometric calibration of the surgically created sphincter is recommended. In the presence of an esophageal stricture that no longer responds to bougienage, resection of the stricture, either with interposition of a segment of colon or distal antrectomy with a Roux-en-Y reconstruction, may become necessary.

OBSTRUCTION. Although more than 90 per cent of patients are benefited by a properly performed esophagomyotomy, there are a few in whom dysphagia continues in the postoperative period or in whom it develops later on. Roentgenographic evidence of esophageal dilatation, however, persists in many patients, but bears no relation to symptoms. The success or failure of the operation should not, therefore, be judged by the roentgenographic size of the esophagus.

When dysphagia persists in the immediate postoperative period, it is usually mild and probably represents an incomplete operation. We have found that the passage of graduated sounds up to 45 French will almost invariably relieve the patient of his dysphagia permanently. Presumably, residual constricting strands of circular muscle or fibrous tissue are torn by the bougienage. Reoperation in the early postoperative period has not been necessary.

When the obstruction to swallowing develops months or years postoperatively, it may represent the end-result of reflux esophagitis with stricture. Management of this problem has already been discussed. It may reflect also the development of scar tissue that has bridged the severed edges of esophageal muscle and so obstructed the esophagus. If, at esophagomyotomy, the esophageal muscle is freed from the mucosa for at least half its circumference, the mucosa will pout through the incision, and there will be little tendency for the cut muscular edges to become joined later. In the event that this very rare complication develops, reoperation should be done. In our experience, often the transabdominal esophagomyotomy is implicated in the late recurrence of obstruction due to achalasia. At reoperation through the thorax, the previous myotomy is usually not evident. A good result can be anticipated in such patients with a properly performed transthoracic procedure.[104]

One must not exclude the possibility that a totally new lesion has developed, and, for this reason, esophagoscopy must be performed before initiating therapy. There is now impressive evidence that carcinoma of the esophagus develops more readily in patients who have esophageal achalasia than in members of the general population not so afflicted.[33, 142]

PERFORATION. Occasionally the lumen of the esophagus is inadvertently opened during the esophagomyotomy. If recognized, the perforation can be closed with one or two interrupted, fine silk sutures, and nothing further need be done. If the perforation is not recognized, intrathoracic leakage of ingested food and fluids may occur. Esophageal x-ray using Gastrografin is indicated postoperatively prior to feeding to assure absence of leakage. Occasionally, of course, in spite of all efforts, it becomes necessary to reexplore, resuture the defect, and decorticate the lung.

ASPIRATION PNEUMONITIS. Ten per cent of patients with esophageal achalasia have clinical evidence of pulmonary complications due to aspiration before therapy is initiated.[6] Proper control of the infection, when present, is necessary before proceeding with operation. Preoperative aspiration of the dilated atonic sac of the esophagus should always be done on the morning of operation to minimize aspiration during anesthesia. The usual measures designed to combat postoperative pulmonary complications, which have been discussed earlier in the chapter, are initiated. Adrenal steroids may be helpful in the management of aspiration pneumonitis when acidic gastric juice has been aspirated. In patients with achalasia, however, gastroesophageal reflux is rare before treatment, and aspirated material is usually limited to the contents of the esophagus.

DIAPHRAGM

Most operations involving the diaphragm are for repair of herniations; yet various other operations require surgical manipulations of this structure. Whatever the procedure, an understanding of the anatomy and function of the diaphragm is essential to success. It is apparent that this structure is not merely a musculotendinous partition between the thorax and the abdomen (although this is an obvious and important feature); it also is vital to the dynamics of respiration and, to a lesser extent, to the dynamics of circulation and cardioesophageal function. There is a general awareness of the functional disturbances that occur after phrenic nerve injury in the neck and thorax in adults[29] as well as in children.[69] Merendino and associates[90] provided an excellent review of the intradiaphragmatic dis-

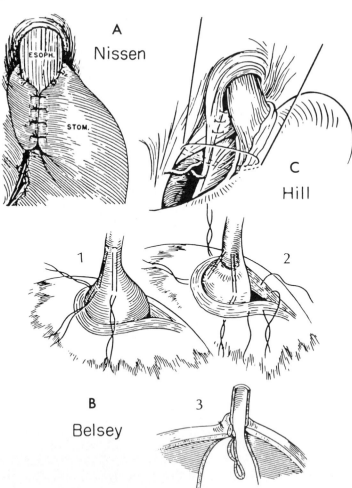

Figure 16–11 The operative procedures employed in the treatment of straightforward gastroesophageal reflux. *A,* Nissen fundoplication, *B,* Belsey Mark IV repair, *C,* Hill posterior gastropexy. (*A* from Ellis, F. H., Jr.: Gastroesophageal reflux: Indications for fundoplication. Surg. Clin. North Am. *51:*583, 1971. *B* from Payne, W. S., and Ellis, F. H., Jr.: Esophagus and diaphragmatic hernias. *In* Schwartz, S. I., Lillehei, R. C., Shires, G. T., Spencer, F. C., and Storer, E. H. (Eds.): Principles of Surgery. 2nd Ed. New York, McGraw-Hill, 1974, p. 1024. *C* from Payne, W. S., and Ellis, F. H., Jr.: Diaphragmatic hernia. *In* Ellis, F. H., Jr.: (Ed.): Lewis-Walters' Practice of Surgery. Vol. 5, Thoracic Surgery. Hagerstown, Maryland, Harper and Row, 1971, Chapter 15.)

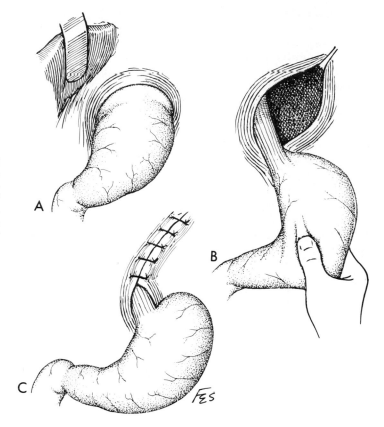

Figure 16–12 *A–C,* The surgical technique for the repair of a paraesophageal hiatal hernia. Reduction of the herniated stomach, and occasionally of other accompanying viscera, is accomplished by gentle inferior traction. Precise suture placement is facilitated by traction on the apex of the crural margin.

tribution of the phrenic nerves as they relate to the placement of diaphragmatic incisions and preservation of function.

Anti-reflux Operations and Esophageal Hiatal Hernia Repair

For all practical purposes, only two types of hernias involve the esophageal hiatus, the sliding hiatus hernia and the paraesophageal hiatus hernia. The anatomic and physiologic differences between these two hernia types have been described elsewhere[39] and will not be reviewed here.

In a sliding esophageal hiatus hernia, few, if any, symptoms are referable to the hernia itself. Symptoms, when present, typically are those of gastroesophageal reflux and reflect hypotension of the lower esophageal sphincter (LES). To be sure, hypotension of the LES occurs in many other situations than with a sliding hernia and may, in fact, be primary rather than secondary to the hernia. Surgery in these patients is designed to eliminate gastroesophageal reflux by re-

storing a normal LES mechanism. The operations currently employed for this purpose include the Hill posterior gastropexy, the Belsey Mark IV repair, and the Nissen fundoplication (Fig. 16–11). Each exerts its sphincter-enhancing effect by encircling a varying extent of distal esophagus with adjacent gastric fundus. The Allison repair, which enjoyed popularity in the past, emphasized an anatomic rather than a physiologic approach and now has few advocates.

In contrast to the sliding esophageal hiatus hernia, symptoms referable to the paraesophageal variety are common and include vague postprandial indigestion, substernal discomfort, nausea, retching without vomiting, and dyspnea. Abnormalities of LES function are rare in paraesophageal hiatus hernia, and therefore, the surgical correction of the condition strives to restore the normal anatomic relationships at the esophageal hiatus by reduction of the herniated viscera and suture narrowing of the patulous hiatus according to the technique of Collis (Fig. 16–12).

Complications of Anti-reflux Operations

RECURRENT REFLUX. Although the three sphincter-enhancing operations mentioned previously are widely employed to provide symptomatic relief of gastroesophageal reflux that is refractory to medical treatment, controversy persists concerning which of these procedures is most effective. Hill[60] himself reported the largest series of Hill repairs involving more than 500 patients and noted a 0.89 per cent incidence of recurrent reflux. Long-term follow-up results of the Belsey repair are less optimistic with recurrence rates ranging from 11 per cent to 33 per cent in various series.[14, 26] Recurrent reflux occurs more frequently after the Belsey procedure, presumably because important tethering sutures are placed in esophageal muscle, which is notoriously weak. Experience with the Nissen fundoplication reported by a variety of authors has been uniformly favorable with regard to reflux control. Ellis and associates[35] reported recurrence rates of less than 10 per cent with follow-up periods of up to 10 years. Similar results were recently reported by Rossetti and Hell[117] in a larger group of patients followed over the past 20 years.

Recurrent reflux symptoms are ascribable to partial or complete disruption of the fundoplication and generally occur within the first postoperative year. Manometric evaluation will invariably disclose a marked reduction in LES amplitude when compared with initial postoperative values. Disruption of the repair is most likely to occur when the wrap is constructed too tightly around the distal esophagus. The use of an intraluminal stent of adequate caliber, our preference being a 40 French mercury-filled bougie, is therefore advisable to prevent overzealous wrapping. Adequate mobilization of the upper stomach will also facilitate the construction of a tension-free wrap. Nasogastric intubation in the early postoperative period may be of benefit in preventing gastric distention, which would exert undue strain on the newly constructed repair.

If severe reflux symptoms recur, reoperation should be considered. Reconstruction of a Hill or Nissen repair can usually be accomplished without difficulty.[62] A disrupted Belsey repair, however, can be more difficult to revise and conversion to one of the other two repairs may be advisable.

DYSPHAGIA. Dysphagia may occur after each of the sphincter-enhancing procedures in the early postoperative period, presumably owing to edema at the operative site. This usually resolves without treatment. Persistent, disabling dysphagia may occur, however, particularly after a circumferential wrap of the Nissen variety. In some cases excessive tightness of the wrap has been implicated and is readily corrected by revision of the wrap over an intraluminal stent of adequate caliber.

In other patients the reason for dysphagia is more complex. Leonardi et al.[76] in a recent article classifying the causes of failed fundoplication noted that a prominent cause of disabling dysphagia was the improper application of the procedure in patients with previously unsuspected motility disorders characterized by aperistalsis of the esophagus. They emphasized the importance of preoperative manometric evaluation, particularly of the body of the esophagus, in order to avoid this pitfall.

Peptic stricture formation is a serious complication of chronic gastroesophageal reflux and is manifested primarily by symptoms of esophageal obstruction. While the anti-reflux procedures referred to earlier have been successful in modifying straightforward reflux, their efficacy is less certain in instances in which firm, panmural esophageal fibrosis has occurred. Some authors[61] have reported success with standard anti-reflux maneuvers performed around strictured segments, while others[35, 118] have been adversely impressed by the incidence of postoperative dysphagia.

More recently, the surgery for peptic esophageal strictures has involved separation of the strictured segment from the surgically created high pressure zone. Additional esophageal length is acquired by fashioning a gastric tube. The use of a stapling device facilitates this maneuver, which then enables the surgeon to construct a wrap of either the Nissen or Belsey variety around a healthy length of pliable tissue (Fig. 16–13). The same principle has been used by Evangelist

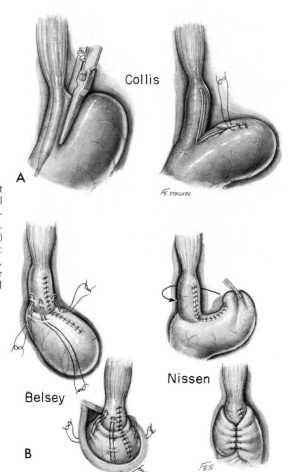

Figure 16–13 Operative procedure for the management of severe reflux esophagitis with panmural distal esophageal stricture. *A,* Esophageal lengthening is achieved by the performance of a Collis gastroplasty utilizing a stapling device. *B,* Fundoplication of either the Belsey (left) or Nissen (right) variety may then be constructed around the pliable gastric tube. (From Ellis, F. H., Jr., Leonardi, H. K., Dabuzhsky, L., Crozier, R. E., Cormack, J., and Gorrilla, M. A.: Surgery for short esophagus with stricture: An experimental and clinical manometric study. Ann. Surg. *188*:345, 1978.)

and associates[44] but without activating the stapling device. With an effective high pressure zone thus created, postoperative dilations of the strictured segment are performed until healing occurs.

GAS BLOAT SYNDROME. The gas bloat syndrome, characterized by an uncomfortable feeling of epigastric fullness, is usually attributed to the patient's inability to belch and has been emphasized by some clinicians, notably Woodward et al.,[138] in reviewing complications after the Nissen fundoplication. However, in Polk's[110] large experience with the Nissen procedure, gas bloat was one of the rarest postoperative complications.

The severity of the gas bloat syndrome tends to diminish with time, but occasionally it is severe enough to warrant reoperation.

Excessive tightness of the wrap has been implicated in the genesis of the syndrome, and its occurrence should be minimized if the wrap is loosely fashioned as recommended by the experimental work of Donahue and Bombeck.[25]

GASTRIC OBSTRUCTION. This complication is unique to the Nissen fundoplication and has been ascribed to the so-called slipped Nissen, a term used to describe the inferior displacement of the wrap from the esophagus above to the stomach below[101] (Fig. 16–14). Fixation sutures placed between the superior rim of the wrap and the diaphragmatic crus should eliminate such dislocation. We suspect, however, that the slipped Nissen usually occurs because the wrap is improperly fashioned around the upper stomach owing to inadequate mobili-

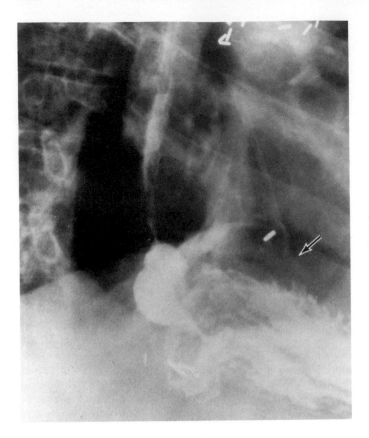

Figure 16–14 Roentgenographic appearance of a so-called slipped Nissen. Note that the fundic wrap (arrow) encircles the upper stomach rather than the distal esophagus.

zation of the distal esophagus. Whatever its cause, the resulting obstruction can be relieved only by reoperation and proximal relocation of the wrap.

PARAESOPHAGEAL HERNIA. The development of a paraesophageal hernia following antireflux procedures has been described in several series[8, 76] and underscores the importance of narrowing a patulous esophageal hiatus at the time of the initial operation. Should such a hernia occur, it is readily treated by transabdominal reduction of the herniated stomach and crural repair.

MISCELLANEOUS COMPLICATIONS. Other complications have been described following antireflux operations and include gastric ulceration,[17] gastric leaks resulting in fistulous communications with other viscera, such as bronchus or pericardium,[66] and esophagopleural or cutaneous fistulas. Fortunately, such complications are rare and are probably due to impairment of the blood supply of the gastric fundus or to the placement of deep necrosing sutures in the esophagus.

Complications of Paraesophageal Hernia Repair

RECURRENT HERNIA. A recurrent paraesophageal hernia is attributable to a technical deficiency in the original operation. Disruption of the crural repair may occur if sutures of inadequate strength are employed or if sutures are improperly placed. The latter event will be avoided if the crural margins are precisely identified. This is facilitated by grasping the apex of the widened hiatus with forceps and elevating it anteriorly. Serious consideration should also be given to the construction of a gastrostomy, with fixation of the gastric wall to the parietal peritoneum. This maneuver will encourage the stomach to retain an intraabdominal location and will reduce cephalad pressure by the stomach on the crural repair. Recurrence of the hernia is often a surgical emergency necessitating immediate reoperation.

GASTRIC PERFORATION. Gastric perforation is a grave complication of a strangulated paraesophageal hernia. Inadvertent gastric perforation may also occur during surgical attempts to reduce the suprahiatal stomach. Should reduction prove difficult, it may be facilitated by dividing the hiatal stricture or by employing a small decompressing gastrostomy. Rents in the gastric wall must be identified and carefully reapproximated to prevent serious and perhaps fatal fistula formation.

ESOPHAGEAL OBSTRUCTION. Excessive narrowing of the esophageal hiatus, resulting in postoperative obstruction to swallowing, is a rare complication of hiatal hernia repair. Its occurrence will be avoided if the patulous hiatus is narrowed sufficiently to allow the passage of an index finger between the esophagus and the crural repair.

MEDIASTINAL SEROUS CYST. After the herniated viscera is reduced, a peritoneally lined sac remains in the retrocardiac location. This sac should be excised completely to preclude the development of a fluid-filled cyst, which could impair deglutition or respiration or both.

GASTRIC ATONY. The return of gastric peristalsis is often slow following hernia repair, and a prolonged period of nasogastric intubation should be attempted. This likelihood lends further support to the use of a gastrostomy both for patient comfort and for intra-abdominal tethering of the stomach.

MISCELLANEOUS COMPLICATIONS. Current enthusiasm for the performance of ancillary procedures during hiatal hernia repair warrants special comment. The addition of vagotomy with gastric resection or pyloroplasty exposes the patient to disturbances of gastrointestinal function which, although rare, occur often enough to warrant caution in the use of these ancillary procedures except under special circumstances.[42, 113]

Injury of adjacent structures, particularly the phrenic and vagus nerves, during the course of esophageal hiatal hernia repair obviously is to be avoided. Subphrenic hematoma may follow unnoticed injury to the subphrenic vein or the spleen. The increased incidence of associated cholelithiasis, colonic diverticula, and duodenal ulcer should alert the surgeon to the possibility of postoperative complication from these conditions. Therefore, we favor operative exposure that permits assessment and treatment of associated conditions whenever possible.

Eventration and Congenital Hernias of the Diaphragm

The surgical treatment of eventration and large congenital hernias of the diaphragm is directed toward restoration of the diaphragm to its normal position to help stabilize the heart and mediastinum and to improve pulmonary function.[34, 123] Abdominal, thoracic, and combined approaches have been advocated. Plication of redundant tissue with or without incisions or excisions has been used successfully. Since dehiscence and recurrence may follow these repairs, some sort of prosthesis to fill defects or reinforce repairs may be used. These conditions or their recurrences are usually less significant in adults than in children or infants. In the latter, progressive, unrelenting respiratory embarrassment is usually fatal.

RESPIRATORY COMPLICATIONS. As with the larger congenital hernias of the diaphragm, eventration in the neonate may be associated with a hypoplastic lung. Efforts to reexpand the lung forcibly at the time of operation are usually fruitless and often lead to irreparable damage, with intractable postoperative pulmonary edema.[80] After the abdominal contents have been reduced it seems preferable to permit a pneumothorax and to allow the lung to reexpand spontaneously over ensuing days or even months. The empty space thus produced, although technically a pneumothorax, does not require treatment unless it increases in size.[123]

In pediatric practice, severe respiratory distress in the postoperative period can be avoided with large eventrations and hernias by intentionally creating a ventral hernia to provide residence for viscera reduced from the thorax. One of the difficult postoperative decisions in creating such a hernia may be in the timing of its repair. In adults it is usually feasible to acquire space preoperatively by appropriate weight reduction. In either age group, postoperative distention is to be avoided by appropriate gastrointestinal decompression. Assisted ventilation may be required even in the absence of this complication. Snyder and Greaney[123] noted the occurrence of a severe metabolic and respiratory acidosis in infants with large hernias and hypoplastic lungs. In their experience, administration of sodium bicarbonate may be needed postoperatively to correct the metabolic acidosis and support the patient until lung function becomes effective.

MISCELLANEOUS COMPLICATIONS. In the newborn, retention of the hernia sac after repair of a posterolateral diaphragmatic hernia may result in the formation of a cyst that may become as life-threatening as the untreated hernia.[73, 123] In the presence of this complication, simple aspiration seems to be the best course until definitive excision becomes feasible. Excision at the time of initial repair is, of course, preventive.

In the adult the route of repair of eventration and congenital hernias is less critical than it is in infants. In the latter the abdominal approach is preferable because of the high incidence of associated correctable intra-abdominal abnormalities, the greater ease of reduction and repair by this route, and, finally, the frequent need for the creation of a ventral hernia to accommodate reduced viscera. Attention to such details is, of course, important in the prevention of postoperative complications.

Bibliography

1. Abbott, O. A., Mansour, K. A., Logan, W. D., Jr., Hatcher, C. R., Jr., and Symbas, P. N.: Atraumatic so-called "spontaneous" rupture of the esophagus: A review of 47 personal cases with comments on a new method of surgical therapy. J. Thorac. Cardiovasc. Surg. 59:67, 1970.
2. Adams, C. L., and Enerson, D. M.: Obstruction of a Mousseau-Barbin tube from prolapsed esophageal mucosa. J. Thorac. Surg. 49:259, 1965.
3. Adams, H. D.: Amyenteric achalasia of the esophagus. Surg. Gynecol. Obstet. 119:251, 1964.
4. Alford, B. R., Johnson, R. L., and Harris, H. H.: Penetrating and perforating injuries of the esophagus. Ann. Otol Rhinol. Laryngol. 72:995, 1963.
5. Andersen, H. A., Bernatz, P. E., and Grindlay, J. H.: Perforation of the esophagus after use of a digestant agent: Report of case and experimental study. Ann. Otol Rhinol. Laryngol. 68:890, 1959.
6. Andersen, H. A., Holman, C. B., and Olsen, A. M.: Pulmonary complications of cardiospasm. J.A.M.A. 151:608, 1953.
7. Andersen, H. A., Schlegel, J. F., and Olsen, A. M.: Postvagotomy dysphagia. Gastrointest. Endosc. 12:13, 1966.
8. Balison, J. R., Macgregor, A. M. C., and Woodward, E. R.: Postoperative diaphragmatic herniation following transthoracic fundoplication: A note of warning. Arch. Surg. 106:164, 1973.
9. Bansmer, G., Bill, A. H., Jr., and Crystal, D. K.: Two cases of perforated peptic ulcer occurring as postoperative complications of esophagectomy with jejunal interposition. Ann. Surg. 149:586, 1959.
10. Barlow, D.: Problems of achalasia. Br. J. Surg. 43:642, 1961.
11. Barrett, N. R., and Franklin, R. H.: Concerning the unfavourable late results of certain operations performed in the treatment of cardiospasm. Br. J. Surg. 37:194, 1949.
12. Beck, A. R., and Baronofsky, I. D.: A study of the left colon as a replacement for the resected esophagus. Surgery 48:499, 1960.
13. Belsey, R.: Reconstruction of the esophagus with left colon. J. Thorac. Surg. 49:33, 1965.
14. Belsey, R.: Mark IV repair of hiatal hernia by the transthoracic approach. World J. Surg. 1:475, 1977.
15. Berger, R. L., and Donato, A. T.: Treatment of esophageal disruption by intubation: A new method of management. Ann. Thorac. Surg. 13:27, 1972.
16. Blalock, J.: Primary esophagogastrectomy for instrumental perforation of the esophagus: With a report of two cases. Am. J. Surg. 94:393, 1957.
17. Bremner, C. G.: Gastric ulceration after a fundoplication operation for gastroesophageal reflux. Surg. Gynecol. Obstet. 148:62, 1979.
18. Brookes, V. S., and Stafford, J. L.: Peptic ulceration and perforation of the stomach after oesophagectomy. Thorax 7:167, 1952.
19. Cameron, J. L., Kieffer, R. F., Hendrix, T. R., Mehigan, D. G., and Baker, R. R.: Selective non-operative management of contained intrathoracic esophageal disruptions. Ann. Thorac. Surg. 27:404, 1979.
20. Carter, R., and Hinshaw, D. B.: Use of the celestin indwelling plastic tube for inoperable carcinoma of the esophagus and cardia. Surg. Gynecol. Obstet. 117:641, 1963.
21. Chassin, J. L.: Esophagogastrectomy: Data favoring end-to-side anastomosis. Ann. Surg. 188:22, 1978.
22. Clagett, O. T.: Quoted by McBurney, R. P., Kriklin, J. W., Hood, R. T., Jr., and Andersen, H. A.[84]
23. Code, C. F., et al.: An Atlas of Esophageal Motility in Health and Disease. Springfield, Ill., Charles C Thomas, 1958.
24. Desjardins, J. G., Stephens, C. A., and Moes, C. A. F.: Results of surgical treatment of congenital tracheo-esophageal fistula, with a note on cine-fluorographic findings. Ann. Surg. 160:141, 1964.

25. Donahue, P. E., and Bombeck, C. T.: The modified Nissen fundoplication — Reflux prevention without gas bloat. Chir. Gastroenterol. *11*:15, 1977.

26. Donnelly, R. J., Deverall, P. B., and Watson, D. A.: Hiatus hernia with and without esophageal stricture: Experience with the Belsey Mark IV repair. Ann. Thorac. Surg. *16*:301, 1973.

27. Dooling, J. A., and Zick, H. R.: Closure of an esophagopleural fistula using onlay intercostal pedicle graft. Ann. Thorac. Surg. *3*:553, 1967.

28. Dorsey, J. S., Esses, S., Goldberg, M., and Stone, R.: Esophagogastrectomy using the auto suture EEA surgical stapling instrument. Ann. Thorac. Surg. *30*:308, 1980.

29. Drake, E. H.: Phrenicotomy of esophageal hiatus hernia. N. Engl. J. Med. *256*:487, 1957.

30. Duvoisin, G. E., Ellis, F. H., Jr., and Payne, W. S.: The value of palliative prostheses in malignant lesions of the esophagus. Surg. Clin. North Am. *47*:827, 1967.

31. Effler, D. B., Barr, D., and Groves, L. K.: Epiphrenic diverticulum of the esophagus: Surgical treatment. Arch. Surg. *79*:459, 1959.

32. Ellis, F., and Cole, F. L.: Reflux after cardiomyotomy. Gut *6*:80, 1965.

33. Ellis, F. G.: The natural history of achalasia of the cardia. Proc. R. Soc. Med. *53*:663, 1960.

34. Ellis, F. H., Jr.: Eventration (unilateral elevation) of the diaphragm. *In* Nyhus, L. M., and Harkins, H. N.: Hernia. Philadelphia, J. B. Lippincott Company, 1964, pp. 554–64.

35. Ellis, F. H., Jr., El-Kurd, M. F. A., and Gibb, S. P.: The effect of fundoplication on the lower esophageal sphincter. Surg. Gynecol. Obstet. *143*:1, 1976.

36. Ellis, F. H., Jr., and Gibb, S. P.: Esophagogastrectomy for carcinoma: Current hospital mortality and morbidity rates. Ann. Surg. *190*:699, 1979.

37. Ellis, F. H., Jr., Gibb, S. P., and Crozier, R. E.: Esophagomyotomy for achalasia of the esophagus. Ann. Surg. *192*:157, 1980.

38. Ellis, F. H., Jr., and Hood, R. T., Jr.: Experimental esophagogastrectomy: Relation of type of resection to development of esophagitis. Surg. Gynecol. Obstet. *98*:449, 1954.

39. Ellis, F. H., Jr., and Leonardi, H. K.: Surgery for esophageal hiatus hernia. Adv. Surg. *13*:263, 1979.

40. Ellis, F. H., Jr., and Olsen, A. M.: Achalasia of the Esophagus. Philadelphia, W. B. Saunders Company, 1969, p. 176.

41. Ellis, F. H., Jr., et al.: Carcinoma of the esophagus and cardia: Results of treatment of 1946 to 1956. N. Engl. J. Med. *260*:351, 1959.

42. Ellis, F. H., Jr., and Payne, W. S.: Motility disturbances of the esophagus and its inferior sphincter: Recent surgical advances. *In* Welch, C. E.: Advances in Surgery. Chicago, Year Book Medical Publishers, Inc., 1965, pp. 179–246.

43. Ellis, F. H., Jr., Schlegel, J. F., Lynch, V. P., and Payne, W. S.: Cricopharyngeal myotomy for pharyngo-esophageal diverticulum. Ann. Surg. *170*:340, 1969.

44. Evangelist, F. A., Taylor, F. H., and Alford, J. D.: The modified Collis-Nissen operation for control of gastroesophageal reflux. Ann. Thorac. Surg. *26*:107, 1978.

45. Fish, J., and Harrison, A. W.: Achalasia of the esophagus. A review. Am. Surg. *28*:545, 1962.

46. Frobese, A. S., Stein, G. N., and Hawthorne, H. R.: Hiatal hernia as a complication of the Heller operation. Surgery *49*:599, 1961.

47. Gooselaw, J. G., and Isaacson, P. G.: Partial intussusception of esophagus into a plastic prosthesis. Surgery *55*:248, 1964.

48. Grillo, H. C., and Wilkins, E. W., Jr.: Esophageal repair following late diagnosis of intrathoracic perforation. Ann. Thorac. Surg. *20*:387, 1975.

49. Grimes, O. F., and Stephens, H. B.: Surgical management of acquired short esophagus. Ann. Surg. *152*:743, 1960.

50. Guest, J. L., Jr., and Ellison, R. G.: The current role of mediastinotomy in diagnosis and management of poor risk patients. J. Thorac. Surg. *49*:1048, 1965.

51. Guillory, J. R., Jr., and Clagett, O. T.: Postvagotomy dysphagia. Surg. Clin. North Am. *47*:833, 1967.

52. Gunnlaugsson, G. H., Wychulis, A. R., Roland, C., and Ellis, F. H., Jr.: Analysis of the records of 1,657 patients with carcinoma of the esophagus and cardia of the stomach. Surg. Gynecol. Obstet. *130*:997, 1970.

53. Haight, C.: Some observations in esophageal atresias and tracheoesophageal fistulas of congenital origin. J. Thorac. Surg. *34*:141, 1957.

54. Haight, C.: Discussion. J. Thorac. Surg. *49*:31, 1965.

55. Hawthorne, H. R., Frobese, A. S., and Nemir, P., Jr.: The surgical management of achalasia of the esophagus. Ann. Surg. *144*:653, 1956.

56. Hays, D. M.: An analysis of the mortality in esophageal atresia. J. Dis. Child., *103*:765, 1962.

57. Hays, D. M., and Snyder, W. H., Jr.: Results of conventional operative procedures for esophageal atresia in premature infants. Am. J. Surg. *106*:19, 1963.

58. Heller, E.: Extramuköse Cardiaplastik beim chronischen Cardiospasmus mit Dilatation des Oesophagus. Mitt. a.d. Grenzbeg, d. med. u. chr. *27*:141, 1913.

59. Hertzler, J. H.: Congenital esophageal atresia: Problems and management. Am. J. Surg. *109*:780, 1965.

60. Hill, L. D.: Progress in the surgical management of hiatal hernia. World J. Surg. *1*:425, 1977.

61. Hill, L. D., Gelfand, M., and Bauermeister, D.: Simplified management of reflux esophagitis with stricture. Ann. Surg. *172*:638, 1970.

62. Hill, L. D., Ilves, R., Stevenson, J. K., and Pearson, J. M.: Respiration for disruption and recurrence after Nissen fundoplication. Arch. Surg. *114*:542, 1979.

63. Holder, T. M., Cloud, D. T., Lewis, J. E., Jr., and Pilling, G. P., IV: Esophageal atresia and tracheo-esophageal fistula: A survey of its members by the surgical section of the Ameri-

can Academy of Pediatrics. Pediatrics *34*:542, 1964.

64. Holder, T. M., McDonald, V. G., Jr., and Woolley, M. M.: The premature or critically ill infant with esophageal atresia: Increased success with a staged approach. J. Thorac. Surg. *44*:344, 1962.

65. Holinger, P. H., Brown, W. T., and Maurizi, D. G.: Endoscopic aspects of post-surgical management of congenital esophageal atresia and tracheoesophageal fistula. J. Thorac. Surg. *49*:22, 1965.

66. Ikard, R. W., and Jacobs, J. K.: Gastropericardial fistula and pericardial abscess: Unusual complications of subphrenic abscess following Nissen fundoplication. South. Med. J. *67*:17, 1974.

67. Ingelfinger, F. J.: Esophageal motility. Physiol. Rev. *38*:533, 1958.

68. Jekler, J., Lhotka, J., and Borek, Z.: Surgery for achalasia of the esophagus. Ann. Surg. *160*:793, 1964.

69. Jewett, T. C., Jr., and Thomson, N. B., Jr.: Iatrogenic eventration of the diaphragm in infancy. J. Thorac. Surg. *48*:861, 1964.

70. Johnson, J., Schwegman, C. W., and Kirby, C. K.: Esophageal exclusion for persistent fistula following spontaneous rupture of the esophagus. J. Thorac. Surg. *32*:827, 1956.

71. Johnson, P. W., and Snyder, W. H.: Problems with the surgery of esophageal atresia and fistula. Ann. Surg. *30*:501, 1964.

72. Kausel, H. W., Reeve, T. S., Stein, A. A., Alley, R. D., and Stranahan, A.: Anatomic and pathologic studies of the thoracic duct. J. Thorac. Surg. *34*:631, 1957.

73. Kenigsberg, K., and Gwinn, J. L.: The retained sac in repair of posterolateral diaphragmatic hernia in the newborn. Surgery *57*:894, 1965.

74. Ketcham, A. S., and Smith, R. R.: Elective esophagostomy. Am. J. Surg. *104*:682, 1962.

75. Kiriluk, L. B., and Merendino, K. A.: The comparative sensitivity of the mucosa of the various segments of the alimentary tract in the dog to acid-peptic action. Surgery *35*:547, 1954.

76. Leonardi, H. K., Crozier, R. E., and Ellis, F. H., Jr.: Reoperation for complications of Nissen fundoplication. J. Thorac. Cardiovasc. Surg. *81*:50, 1981.

77. Le Roux, B. T.: An analysis of 700 cases of carcinoma of the hypopharynx, the esophagus, and the proximal stomach. Thorax *16*:226, 1961.

78. Logan, A.: The surgical treatment of carcinoma of the esophagus and cardia. J. Thorac. Surg. *46*:150, 1963.

79. Lortat-Jacob, J. L., Maillard, J. N., and Fekete, F.: A procedure to prevent reflux after esophagogastric resection: Experience with 17 patients. Surgery *50*:600, 1961.

80. Lynn, H. B.: Personal communication.

81. Lyons, W. S., Serementis, M. G., deGuzman, V. C., and Peabody, J. W., Jr.: Ruptures and perforations of the esophagus: The case for conservative management. Ann. Thorac. Surg. *25*:346, 1978.

82. Mann, C. V., Greenwood, R. K., and Ellis, F. H., Jr.: The esophagogastric junction. Surg. Gynecol. Obstet. (Int. Abstr. Surg.), *118*:853,1964.

83. Mathewson, C., Jr., Dozier, W. E., Hamill, J. P.,

and Smith, M.: Clinical experiences with perforations of the esophagus. Am. J. Surg. *104*:257, 1962.

84. McBurney, R. P., Kirklin, J. W., Hood, R. T., Jr., and Andersen, H. A.: One-stage esophagogastrectomy for perforated carcinoma in the presence of mediastinitis. Proc. Staff Meet. Mayo Clin. *28*:281, 1953.

85. McIlrath, D. C., van Heerden, J. A., Edis, A. J., and Dozois, R. R.: Closure of abdominal incisions with subcutaneous catheters. Surgery *80*:411, 1976.

86. McVey, J. L., Schlegel, J. F., and Ellis, F. H., Jr.: Gastroesophageal sphincteric function after the Heller myotomy and its modifications. An experimental study. Bull. Soc. Int. Chir. *22*:419, 1963.

87. Mengoli, L. R., and Lassen, K. P.: Conservative treatment of esophageal perforation. Arch. Surg. *91*:238, 1965.

88. Menguy, R.: Near-total esophageal exclusion by cervical esophagostomy and tube gastrostomy in the management of massive esophageal perforation: Report of a case. Ann. Surg. *173*:613, 1971.

89. Merendino, K. A.: Important side-issues in the treatment of cardiospasm (Editorial). Arch. Surg. *73*:1047, 1956.

90. Merendino, K. A., Johnson, R. J., Skinner, H. H., and Maguire, R. X.: The intradiaphragmatic distribution of the phrenic nerve, with particular reference to the placement of diaphragmatic incisions and controlled segmental paralysis. Surgery *39*:189, 1956.

91. Merendino, K. A., and Thomas, G. I.: The jejunal interposition operation for substitution of the esophagogastric sphincter. Surgery *44*:1112, 1958.

92. Millard, A. H.: 'Spontaneous' perforation of the oesophagus treated by utilization of a pericardial flap. Br. J. Surg. *58*:70, 1971.

93. Moore, T. C., Goldstein, J., and Teramoto, S.: Use of intact lung for closure of full-thickness esophageal defects. J. Thorac. Cardiovasc. Surg. *41*:336, 1961

94. Nakayama, K.: Statistical review of five-year survivals after surgery for carcinoma of the esophagus and cardiac portion of stomach. Surgery *45*:883, 1959.

95. Nardi, G. L., and Glotzer, D. J.: Anastomotic ulcer of the colon following colonic replacement of the esophagus. Ann. Surg. *152*:10, 1960.

96. Nealon, T. F., Jr., Templeton, J. Y., III, Cuddy, V. D., and Gibbon, J. H., Jr.: Instrumental perforation of the esophagus. J. Thorac. Surg. *41*:75, 1961.

97. Nemir, P., Jr., and Frobese, A. S.: The modified Heller operation for achalasia of the esophagus. Surg. Clin. North Am. *42*:1407, 1962.

98. Neuhof, H., and Jemerin, E. E.: Acute Infections of the Mediastinum. Baltimore, Williams & Wilkins Company, 1943.

99. Neville, W. E., and Clowes, G. H. A., Jr.: Reconstruction of the esophagus with segments of the colon. J. Thorac. Surg. *35*:2, 1958.

100. Okike, N., Payne, W. S., Neufeld, D. M., Bernatz, P. E., Pairolero, P. C., and Sanderson, D. R.:

Esóphagomyotomy versus forceful dilation for achalasia of the esophagus. Results in 899 patients. Ann. Thorac. Surg. *28*:119, 1979.

101. Olson, R. C., Lasser, R. B., and Ansel, H.: The "slipped Nissen" (Abstract). Gastroenterology *70*:924, 1976.

102. Orringer, M. B., Kirsh, M. M., and Sloan, H.: Long-term esophageal function following repair of esophageal atresia. Ann. Surg. *186*:436, 1977.

103. Overstreet, J. W., and Ochsner, A.: Traumatic rupture of the esophagus (with a report of 13 cases). J. Thorac. Surg. *30*:164, 1955.

104. Patrick, D. L., Payne, W. S., Olsen, A. M., and Ellis, F. H., Jr.: Reoperation for achalasia of the esophagus. Arch. Surg. *103*:122, 1971.

105. Payne, W. S.: The long-term clinical state after resection with total gastrectomy and Roux loop anastomosis. *In* Smith, R. A., and Smith, R. E.: Surgery of the Oesophagus (The Coventry Conference). London, Butterworth & Co., Ltd., 1972, pp. 23–28.

106. Payne, W. S., and Clagett, O. T.: Pharyngeal and esophageal diverticula. Curr. Probl. Surg. April, 1965, pp. 1–31.

107. Payne, W. S., and Larson, R. H.: Acute mediastinitis. Surg. Clin. North Am. *49*:999, 1969.

108. Phillips, D. F., Wollaeger, E. E., Ellis, F. H., Jr., and Power, M. H.: Fecal excretion of fat and nitrogen after esophagogastrectomy in man. Surgery *49*:433, 1961.

109. Piccone, V. A., LeVeen, H. H., Ahmed, N., and Grosberg, S.: Reappraisal of esophagogastrectomy for esophageal malignancy. Am. J. Surg. *137*:32, 1979.

110. Polk, H. C., Jr.: Fundoplication for reflux esophagitis: Misadventures with the operation of choice. Ann. Surg. *183*:645, 1976.

111. Pories, W. J., Gerle, R. D., Sherman, C. D., and Hinshaw, J. R.: The danger of esophageal replacement with antiperistaltic loops of small bowel. Ann. Surg. *156*:68, 1962.

112. Rao, K. V. S., Mir, N., and Cogbill, C. L.: Management of perforations of the thoracic esophagus: A new technic utilizing a pedicle flap of diaphragm. Am. J. Surg. *127*:609, 1974.

113. Raphael, H. A., Ellis, F. H., Jr., Carlson, H. C., and Andersen, H. A.: Surgical repair of sliding esophageal hiatal hernia: Long-term results. Arch. Surg. *91*:228, 1965.

114. Richardson, J. V., Heintz, S. E., Rossi, N. P., Wright, C. B., Doty, D. B., and Ehrenhaft, J. L.: Esophageal atresia and tracheoesophageal fistula. Ann. Thorac. Surg. *29*:364, 1980.

115. Ripley, H. R., Olsen, A. M., and Kirklin, J. W.: Esophagitis after esophagogastric anastomosis. Surgery *32*:1, 1952.

116. Root, H. D.: Evaluation of operations for megaesophagus (cardiospasm). Surgery *43*:270, 1958.

117. Rossetti, M., and Hell, K.: Fundoplication for the treatment of gastroesophageal reflux in hiatal hernia. World J. Surg. *1*:439, 1977.

118. Safaie-Shirazi, S., Zike, W. L., and Mason, E. E.: Esophageal stricture secondary to reflux esophagitis. Arch. Surg. *110*:629, 1975.

119. Schultz, L. R., and Clatworthy, H. W., Jr.: Eso-

phageal strictures after anastomosis in esophageal atresia. Arch. Surg. *87*:120, 1963.

120. Schwartz, M. L., and McQuarrie, D. G.: Surgical management of esophageal perforation. Surg. Gynecol. Obstet. *151*:669, 1980.

121. Smith, C. C. K., and Tanner, N. C.: The complications of gastroscopy and oesophagoscopy. Br. J. Surg. *43*:396, 1956.

122. Smith, J., and Payne, W. S.: Surgical technique for management of reflux esophagitis after esophagogastrectomy for malignancy: Further application of Roux-en-Y principle. Mayo Clin. Proc. *50*:588, 1975.

123. Snyder, W. H., Jr., and Greaney, E. M., Jr.: Congenital diaphragmatic hernia: 77 consecutive cases. Surgery *57*:576, 1965.

124. Steiger, Z., Nickel, W. O., Wilson, R. F., and Arbulu, A.: Improved surgical palliation of advanced carcinoma of the esophagus. Am. J. Surg. *135*:782, 1978.

125. Strauch, G. O., and Lynch, R. E.: Subphrenic extrathoracic rupture of the esophagus: First reported case. Ann. Surg. *161*:213, 1965.

126. Swenson, O., Lipman, R., Fisher, J. H., and DeLuca, F. G.: Repair and complications of esophageal atresia and tracheoesophageal fistula. N. Engl. J. Med. *267*:960, 1962.

127. Symonds, C.: Quoted by Coyas, A.: Nouveau procédé d'intubation dans le cancer inopérable de l'esophage. Ann. Otolaryngol. *72*:639, 1955.

128. Thal, A. P.: A unified approach to surgical problems of the esophagogastric junction. Ann. Surg. *168*:542, 1968.

129. Tuttle, W. M., and Barrett, R. J.: Late esophageal perforations. Arch. Surg. *86*:695, 1963.

130. Urschel, H. C., Jr., Razzuk, M. A., Wood, R. E., et al.: Improved management of esophageal perforation: Exclusion and diversion in continuity. Ann. Surg. *179*:587, 1974.

131. Wangensteen, O. H.: Technique of achieving an adequate extramucosal myotomy in megaesophagus (achalasia, cardiospasms, dystonia). Surg. Gynecol. Obstet. *105*:339, 1957.

132. Waterston, D. J., Carter, R. E. B., and Aberdeen, E.: Oesophageal atresia: Tracheo-oesophageal fistula: A study of survival in 218 infants. Lancet *1*:819, 1962.

133. Watkins, D. H., Rundles, W. R., and Tatom, L.: Utility of a new procedure of valvular esophagogastrostomy in cases of brachyesophagus and stricture: Clinical and experimental studies of circumferential esophagofundopexy. J. Thorac. Surg. *38*:814, 1959.

134. Weisel, W., and Raine, F.: Surgical treatment of traumatic esophageal perforation. Surg. Gynecol. Obstet. *94*:337, 1952.

135. Welsh, G. F., and Payne, W. S.: The present status of one-stage pharyngo-esophageal diverticulectomy. Surg. Clin. North Am. *53*:953, 1973.

136. Werlin, S. L., Dodds, W. J., Hogan, W. J., et al.: Esophageal function in esophageal atresia. Dig. Dis. Sci. (in press).

137. Woodward, E. R: Discussion. Ann. Surg. *168*:549, 1968.

138. Woodward, E. R., Thomas, H. F., and McAlhany, J. C.: Comparison of crural repair and Nissen

fundoplication in the treatment of esophageal hiatus hernia with peptic esophagitis. Ann. Surg. *173*:782, 1971.

139. Wychulis, A. R., Ellis, F. H., Jr., and Andersen, H. A.: Acquired nonmalignant esophagotracheobronchial fistula: Report of 36 cases. J.A.M.A. *196*:117, 1966.

140. Wychulis, A. R., Fontana, R. S., and Payne, W. S.: Instrumental perforations of the esophagus. Dis. Chest *55*:184, 1969.

141. Wychulis, A. R., Fontana, R. S., and Payne, W. S.: Noninstrumental perforations of the esophagus. Dis. Chest *55*:190, 1969.

142. Wychulis, A. R., Woolam, G. L., Andersen, H. A., and Ellis, F. H., Jr.: Achalasia and carcinoma of the esophagus. J.A.M.A. *215*:1638, 1971.

17

COMPLICATIONS OF SURGERY OF THE HEART AND ADJACENT GREAT VESSELS

Derward Lepley, Jr.
Robert J. Flemma
and Donald C. Mullen

Application of surgical therapy to the heart and adjacent great vessels has expanded at a phenomenal rate in recent years. From its early beginnings in a few, relatively crude, closed procedures, cardiac surgery has entered an era in which the inside of the heart can be exposed for prolonged periods, defects can be corrected by numerous available techniques, and not just one but several valves can be replaced simultaneously. Definitive procedures for both congenital and acquired diseases of the great vessels also have been developed to the point that no area of the aorta and its major branches remains inaccessible to surgical attack.

As with any rapidly advancing area of medicine, knowledge from a multitude of disciplines has been integrated into the field of cardiovascular surgery. Anatomic variations in the heart and great vessels have required that a number of traditional concepts of embryology and anatomy be modified. Temporary radical alterations in the

Derward Lepley, Jr., received his college and medical education at Marquette University where he was elected to Alpha Omega Alpha. Following internship at the Wisconsin General Hospital and general and thoracic surgical residencies at the Wood Veterans Administration Hospital, he served as a National Heart Institute Research Fellow at the University of Minnesota. Returning to Milwaukee, he rapidly developed a strong cardiovascular surgical unit at the Medical College of Wisconsin, where he is now Professor and Chairman, Department of Thoracic and Cardiovascular Surgery. Dr. Lepley is a member of many important national committees and societies, and he is richly qualified to survey the major postoperative problems in cardiac surgery.

Robert J. Flemma took his medical school training at the University of Rochester, interned at Duke University, and completed the residency program there. He then served 2 years in the Burn Study Branch at Brooke Army Medical Center. He joined the faculty at Marquette University in 1970 and is Clinical Professor of Surgery at The Medical College of Wisconsin.

Donald C. Mullen attended Duke University Medical School and interned at Duke University Hospital, where he also completed his residency. He practiced cardiovascular surgery in the Sanger Clinic from 1969 to 1975 and since then has been Associate Clinical Professor of Surgery at The Medical College of Wisconsin.

circulatory system required during many of these operations have necessitated an intimate understanding of both normal and abnormal physiology of numerous organ systems. And, in addition to his role in developing cardiovascular operative techniques, the surgeon has become a part-time engineer in order to devise and successfully use currently available sophisticated equipment required for this sort of surgery.

As these operations have increased in magnitude and complexity, opportunities for complications to occur have become numerous. Many of these complications can be prevented by careful attention to detail. Others must be accepted as risks inherent in such surgery, and plans must be made for their management. Although review of all possible complications of operations on the heart and adjacent great vessels is not possible, it is the purpose of this chapter to discuss the more common complications to be expected and to suggest methods of prevention and treatment that have been useful to us.

SURGERY OF THE HEART

Until relatively recently heart surgery was limited to the management of cardiac trauma and the relief of constrictive pericarditis, both operations first performed successfully by Rehn. Although successful mitral commissurotomy was reported by Souttar as early as 1925, impetus for the current surgical attack on cardiac disease has resulted in large part from the pioneering efforts of Gross, who successfully ligated a patent ductus arteriosus in 1938, and of Blalock and Taussig, who reported an indirect approach for palliation of the tetralogy of Fallot in 1945. This was followed shortly by commissurotomy for rheumatic mitral valve stenosis by Harken, Bailey, and Brock. Successful clinical application of the pump oxygenator for open-heart surgery by Gibbon in 1954 paved the way for development of corrective operative procedures for the majority of congenital intracardiac defects and for subsequent development of caged ball cardiac valve prostheses by Starr and others. Few cardiac lesions remain today that are immune to surgical intervention, although, unfortunately, palliative procedures still are required under certain circumstances.

TECHNICAL CONSIDERATIONS

Closed Procedures

Although open-heart surgery has allowed innumerable advances in the operative therapy of cardiac disease, several closed procedures are still useful. In the field of congeni-

tal heart disease such procedures usually are designed to allow a controlled amount of admixing between the systemic and pulmonary circulations under circumstances in which definitive correction of the lesion is not possible or must be postponed until later. An example of the former category is the creation of an atrial septal defect in infants with transposition of the great vessels as described by Blalock and Hanlon (Fig. 17–1). In the latter category are shunt procedures, described by Blalock and Taussig (Fig. 17–2, *a*), Potts (Fig. 17–2, *b*), and Cooley (Fig. 17–2, *c*), which now are used when necessary to allow infants with conditions such as tetralogy of Fallot to survive until they reach larger size, at which time definitive open-heart surgery can be undertaken with far greater safety. Similarly, banding the pulmonary artery of an infant with a ventricular septal defect and severe pulmonary hypertension is used to allow postponement of open correction until a size is reached at which morbidity and mortality rates are more acceptable. These procedures should be planned in such a manner, however, so as not to complicate unduly the future definitive procedure, as is the case if a superior vena cava to pulmonary artery anastomosis is used for temporary palliation of patients with tetralogy of Fallot. In the past few years, principally as a result of the work of Subramanian and Barratt-Boyes of New Zealand, there has been a trend toward total correction of these defects in infants at a very early age. Deep hypothermia and extracorporeal circulation are combined to provide a safe means of

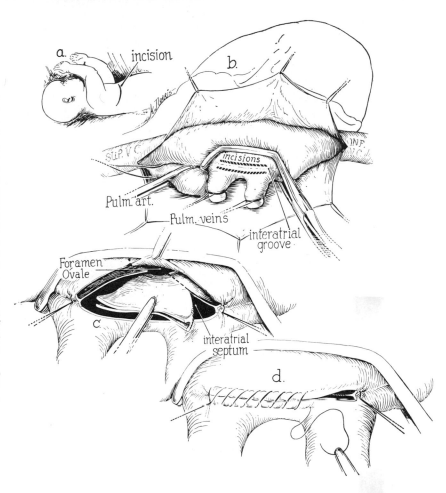

Figure 17–1 Drawings illustrating Blalock-Hanlon procedure for palliation of transposition of great vessels. *a,* Location of thoracotomy incision. *b,* Right pulmonary artery occluded to prevent overdistention of lung. Right pulmonary veins occluded distally and partial occluding clamp placed with one blade on left atrium behind pulmonary veins and other blade on right atrium. Dotted lines demonstrate locations of incisions into both atria. *c,* Atrial septum progressively teased out through combined incisions and excised back to foramen ovale. Sutures placed at both extremities of incisions before the atria are entered prevent slippage from partial occluding clamp. *d,* These sutures used finally to approximate right atrial wall above to left atrial wall below.

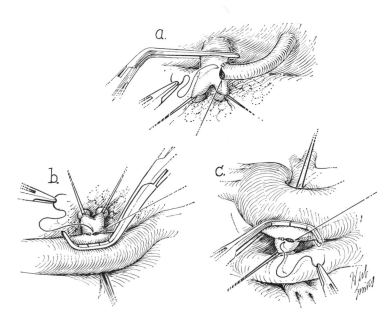

Figure 17–2 Drawings illustrating systemic-pulmonary artery shunt procedures. *a,* Blalock-Taussig anastomosis between subclavian artery and left pulmonary artery. *b,* Potts-Smith anastomosis between descending aorta and left pulmonary artery. *c,* Cooley-Hallman anastomosis between ascending aorta and right pulmonary artery.

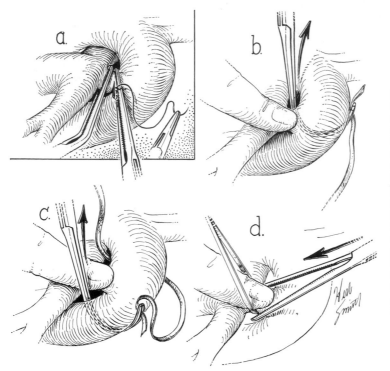

Figure 17–3 Drawings illustrating division and suture of patent ductus arteriosus. *a,* Technique of stepwise division and suture rather than complete division followed by suture, to ensure against slippage of ductus from clamps. *b,* Technique of controlling hemorrhage from posterior aspect of ductus by direct finger pressure. Parietal pleura divided lateral to aorta and umbilical tape passed around the aorta proximal to ductus. *c,* Other end of same umbilical tape passed around aorta distal to ductus. *d,* Umbilical tape, having been passed indirectly around ductus, now used to elevate ductus with finger still in place. Clamps then applied and ductus handled in usual manner.

carrying out total correction in these tiny hearts. Acceptable results have been obtained in correction of ventricular septal defect and tetralogy of Fallot, as well as of transposition of the great vessels and total anomalous pulmonary venous return. The secondary operation for total correction after banding of the pulmonary artery was associated with a very significant mortality rate in most surgeons' hands, and therefore early total correction even in the newborn and infants weighing as little as 3 kg. has a great deal of merit.

Some closed procedures for congenital heart disease are definitive, such as division and suture of a patent ductus arteriosus (Fig. 17–3). Closed operative procedures also are useful in certain patients with acquired heart disease. Pericardectomy for chronic constrictive pericarditis still finds useful application, although cases of this type have become relatively rare.

Since 1968, with the introduction of the direct approach to coronary artery disease using methods developed by Effler, Favaloro, and Johnson, there has been a huge increase in the number of patients operated upon for coronary arteriosclerosis, and these methods have produced probably the best results of any of the procedures designed for treatment of coronary arteriosclerosis. In 1971, vein bypass grafts were implanted in about 20,000 patients with coronary arteriosclerosis. Since we do not know the complete natural history of coronary disease, it is difficult at this time to make absolute determinations about the worth of direct coronary artery surgery. Nevertheless, we do know that patients with normal ventricles and without diffuse disease are able to undergo surgery with a low mortality rate — no more than 2 to 3 per cent. Ninety-six per cent of the patients who survive surgery are free of angina. In spite of a combined national study involving VA hospitals, Flemma, in 1979,[162] found that in comparing the medically treated group in the VA study with his own personal series of surgically treated patients, the long-term survival of the surgically treated patients with normal ventricles showed a statistically significant improvement over those treated medically by a wide margin. Those patients with bad ventricles had not nearly as significant an improvement or chance of increased survival, as would be expected. Rimm et al.,[160] in looking at the return-to-work data of the patients who underwent surgery,

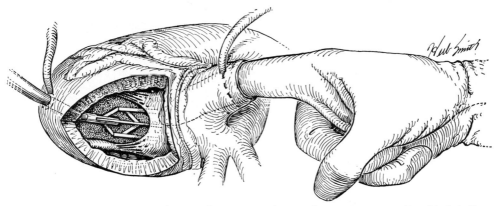

Figure 17–4 Drawing illustrating technique of transventricular mitral commissurotomy. Two-bladed dilator passed through stab wound in left ventricular apex and controlled by purse-string suture. Index finger in left atrium through atrial appendage used to guide dilator into stenotic mitral valve orifice and to evaluate progressive steps in commissurotomy.

showed that more than 90 per cent of the 50 to 55 year age group who had been working before surgery returned to their occupations following coronary surgery. Although the benefit of coronary surgery, now being performed on many thousands of people per year, is controversial in some quarters, it would appear that vein bypass surgery has been a major contribution in the treatment of coronary artery disease.

Closed mitral commissurotomy is still carried out by some surgeons, particularly with the use of the transventricular dilator (Fig. 17–4); however, this operation represents a closed procedure that violates most principles of surgery. In view of the fact that perfusion-associated morbidity and mortality have been reduced below 1 per cent, most surgeons now prefer to use complete cardiopulmonary bypass and perform open mitral commissurotomy. If valve replacement is required because of calcification or loss of substance of the leaflets or the chordae tendineae, it can be carried out at the same time. This method also avoids the danger of unrecognized thrombi in the atrium and subsequent dislodgment and embolism, which is a risk of the indirect procedures. Open commissurotomy has been reported by Reed et al.[171] to give good palliation for many years and is still the procedure to be used in those patients who have not had complete destruction of the mitral apparatus.

Heart block is a common complication in heart disease. It can be iatrogenically induced at the time of surgery either in clo-

sure of ventricular septal defects or in complete correction of tetralogy of Fallot. The original artificial pacemakers were external, connected by exteriorized wires to the heart. Then Chardack and Greatbatch designed the implantable unit that could be inserted transthoracically (Fig. 17–5). Electrodes were implanted directly into the heart and

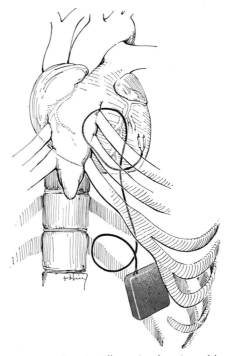

Figure 17–5 Drawing illustrating location of battery and component package of implantable cardiac pacemaker and course of myocardial leads. Slack in wire and wide loops used to prevent tension on wires or kinking.

brought out through the chest wall and attached to an implantable pacemaker buried in the abdominal wall, under the subcutaneous tissue of the abdominal wall, or under the pectoralis or rectus muscle. During the past 3 years, the transvenous approach has been used in increasing numbers of patients and the transthoracic approach has for the most part been superseded. The catheter is passed through a cephalic vein or an external jugular vein, through the superior vena cava, and into the right atrium and right ventricle, so that the electrode impinges near the apex of the right ventricle in the trabeculae. This procedure is much simpler since a thoracotomy does not have to be performed and only local anesthesia is necessary, but a great deal of care must be used to prevent damage to the electrode, to place the electrode correctly, and to prevent infection. A temporary pacemaker inserted through an arm vein can be used until the permanent transvenous pacemaker is placed and functioning. The implantable unit of the early days has been constantly improved upon so that the failure rate has been reduced to a minimum, and the electrodes also have been markedly improved so that breakage is uncommon, In recent years, because the incidence of conduction problems has been significantly high after valve replacement, we have been implanting permanent electrodes on the heart at the time of the original surgery. The electrodes are then buried under the skin in the left upper quadrant for future use, if needed. These are placed particularly in the older patient with mitral or aortic disease, in calcified valves with intrusion of the calcium into the wall of the ventricle, and in all tricuspid valve replacements.

Open-Heart Surgery

Successful open intracardiac repair of both congenital and acquired heart defects is dependent upon adequate extracorporeal perfusion with a pump oxygenator. Many and varied types of pumps and oxygenators have come into vogue, each with its own advocates. Innumerable agents are available for priming, and varying degrees of hypo-

thermia are used in conjunction with cardiopulmonary bypass. Each system has its advantages and disadvantages, and these must be weighed one against the other in selection of a method of open-heart surgery. In spite of such a conglomeration of systems, however, each appears to offer satisfactory support of the circulation for intracardiac repair, provided the team of surgeons, anesthesiologists, cardiologists, physiologists, nurses, and others, understands the method used and is prepared to deal with whatever alterations ensue in the patient's physiology.

The technique of extracorporeal circulation for open-heart surgery that functions best in our hands is illustrated diagrammatically in Figure 17–6. Blood from the superior and inferior vena cava is drained by gravity into the oxygenator column of the disposable plastic oxygenator, which has been primed either with 5 per cent glucose and water, 20 to 30 ml. per kilogram of the patient's body weight, or with Ringer's lactate and varying amounts of blood, depending upon the patient's hematocrit and the desire of the surgeon. The oxygen flow passes through a dispersion plate, forcing blood up the oxygenating column in tiny bubbles that provide exposure of a large surface area to oxygen. Gas exchange takes place, and then the blood enters a defoaming chamber (Fig. 17–6, *a*), where it comes in contact with a large surface area coated with antifoam. From here, the blood passes through a filter and into a reservoir (Fig. 17–6, *b*). Blood from the outlet of the reservoir then is returned by roller pump (Fig. 17–6, *c*) into a cannula, which is usually inserted into the ascending aorta just proximal to the innominate artery (Fig. 17–6, *d*).

Coronary sinus return and bronchial arterial flow are collected by a sump connected to negative pressure created by a roller pump. The sump is placed through the junction of the right superior pulmonary vein and interatrial septum (Fig. 17–6, *e*) and then passed into the left atrium and left ventricle. Any additional blood is collected by intracardiac aspirator. This blood also is collected through roller pumps into a disposable plastic cardiotomy reservoir (Fig. 17–6, *g*), again over a large surface area with defoaming agents through a filter into the base of the oxygenating column. When cor-

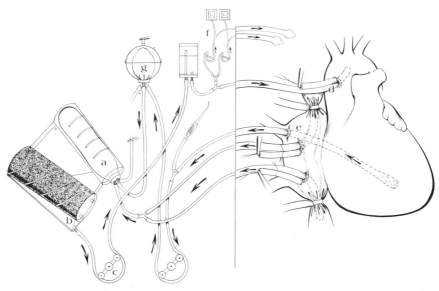

Figure 17–6 A commonly used method of carrying out open heart surgery using a pump oxygenator. The circuitry is described in the text. If hypothermia is used, water lines are connected to the two plugs in the drum in the center of the blood reservoir as seen in *b*.

onary perfusion is required, a separate line is used for each coronary artery. Roller pumps (Fig. 17 6, *h*) are used to maintain the pressure in each line at no more than 90 to 100 mm. Hg monitored by aneroid manometers and as much flow is delivered as possible without these pressures being exceeded. Throughout the procedure, extracardiac blood loss is replaced intravenously with banked acid-citrate-dextrose blood as needed. At the completion of bypass all blood remaining in the oxygenator and tubings is returned slowly to the patient, after which the oxygenator, cardiotomy reservoir, and all tubings are discarded.

Selection of chest wall and cardiotomy incisions is dependent upon the type of intracardiac repair planned. Uncomplicated septal defects are closed either by direct suture (Fig. 17–7*A, a*) or by patch (Fig. 17–7*A, b*), depending on the size and location of the defect. Complicated septal defects, such as are seen with tetralogy of Fallot, usually require patch closure of the defect in addition to correction of associated anomalies (Fig. 17–7*A, c*). Congenital defects such as total anomalous pulmonary venous drainage require even more complicated procedures for definitive repair (Fig. 17–7*B*). During the past 10 years, the devel-

opment of artificial valves for replacement of badly damaged cardiac valves has opened a new field in the surgical therapy of acquired valvular disease. These prostheses are used in almost all such patients who require operation (Figs. 17–8 and 17–9), with the exception of those with uncomplicated mitral stenosis, as previously mentioned, and children with congenital simple valvar, pulmonic, or aortic stenosis.

Coronary artery disease resulting in myocardial infarction followed by development of ventricular aneurysm is another acquired condition for which relief is available using extracorporeal circulation with a pump oxygenator. Excision of the major portion of such an aneurysm with restoration of left ventricular continuity by direct suture (Fig. 17–10) effectively relieves the paradoxical motion of these aneurysms, resulting in signficant increases in cardiac output. With this procedure, however, care must be exercised to prevent injury to the left coronary artery or to the mitral valve mechanism and to avoid excision of too much tissue, which might result in a left ventricle of inadequate volume. Deep bites into healthy muscle beyond scar can result in alteration of the geometry of the remaining ventricle, which results in poor ventricular function and

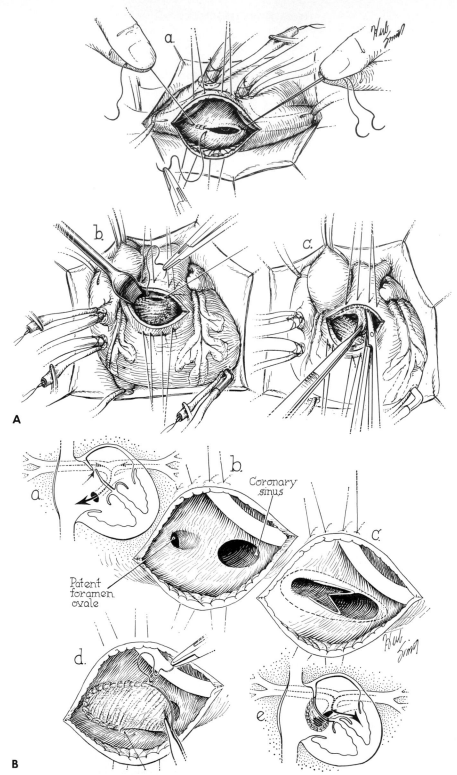

Figure 17–7 *A,* Drawings illustrating repair of septal defects. *a,* Primary suture of secundum type of interatrial septal defect. *b,* Patch repair of large interventricular septal defect. *c,* Complicated ventricular septal defect closed with patch. Associated anomaly, such as infundibular pulmonic stenosis, also corrected. *B,* Drawings illustrating correction of most common type of total anomalous pulmonary venous drainage. *a,* Pulmonary veins emptying into coronary sinus and subsequently into right atrium. *b,* Intracardiac location of patent foramen ovale and enlarged coronary sinus. *c,* Incision enlarging opening of coronary sinus. *d,* Patch used to enlarge size of left atrium and transpose coronary sinus opening into this enlarged chamber. *e,* Completed repair.

inability of the ventricle to contract properly.

Pulmonary embolectomy, described by Trendelenburg as early as 1908, and performed successfully by Kirschner in 1924, found little practical application until relatively recently. Addition of support by cardiopulmonary bypass during the procedure now allows successful pulmonary embolectomy in the majority of patients who otherwise would die of this unfortunate catastrophe (Fig. 17–11, *a*). Ready availability of the pump oxygenator using the described technique of priming without blood provides favorable circumstances for such an emergency operation. Even when the patient is moribund, partial cardiopulmonary bypass from the femoral vein to the femoral artery, instituted under local anesthesia, may provide sufficient resuscitation and support until preparation for definitive embolectomy can be completed (Fig. 17–11, *b*). However, with use of the sternal-splitting incision, the patient can be rapidly connected to the pump oxygenator if hemodynamic collapse has occurred. Using the ascending aorta for cannulation, and cannulation of the right atrium into both venae cavae can probably bring the patient out of jeopardy within a matter of minutes, at least as fast as by use of femoral-to-femoral bypass or other means of support until embolectomy can be performed.

Many other operative procedures, both open and closed, are available for rare forms of congenital and acquired cardiac disease. Others are now in the experimental stage and should soon become a part of routine clinical practice. Still others will be developed, and continued improvements will be made in those procedures now in current use, as advances have become a daily occurrence in this rapidly progressing field of cardiac surgery.

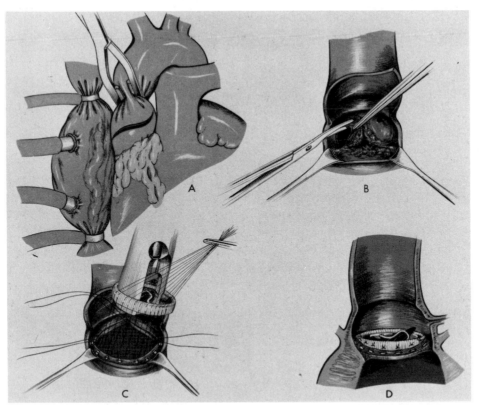

Figure 17–8 Method of replacing a valve in calcified aortic stenosis or in aortic insufficiency. The valve, including all calcium, is trimmed away completely and a Bjork-Shiley prosthesis is then used to replace it. Mattress sutures with pledgets of Teflon felt are placed from above downward through the remnants of the valve annulus and then up through the sewing ring as seen in C. D depicts a cross section as the valve is seated in place with the reinforced sutures with pledgets of Teflon felt.

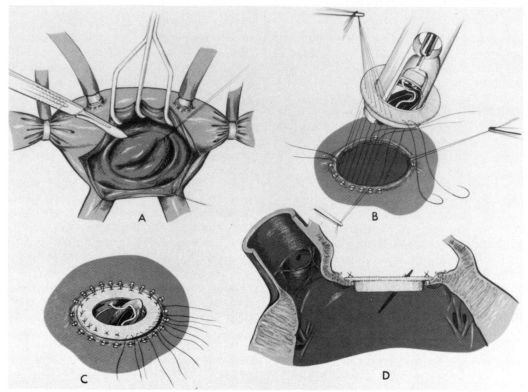

Figure 17–9 A method of replacing the mitral valve. The valve is removed in its entirety with its chordae and the tips of the papillary muscles as seen in A. In B, sutures are being passed through the remnants of the mitral annulus which are reinforced with pledgets of Teflon felt. Sutures are then passed up through the sewing ring as shown in B. In C, the valve is in place with the sutures tied, and in D, a cross-sectional view shows the relationship of the valve prosthesis to the aortic outflow tract. Note that by using this suturing method, all material from beneath the valve is pulled up behind the sewing ring.

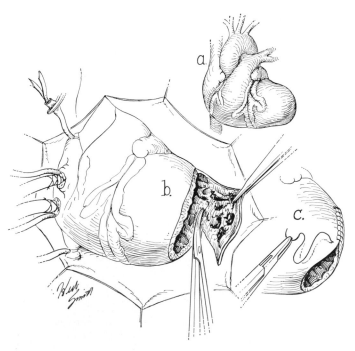

Figure 17–10 Drawings illustrating excision of left ventricular aneurysm. a, Usual location of aneurysm after myocardial infarction. b, Major portion of aneurysm excised, with caution to prevent damage to mitral valve mechanism or major coronary vessel, too great a reduction in left ventricular cavity size, or loss of laminated thrombus into ventricle from which it could embolize. c, Closure of left ventricle with continuous suture reinforced by interrupted sutures.

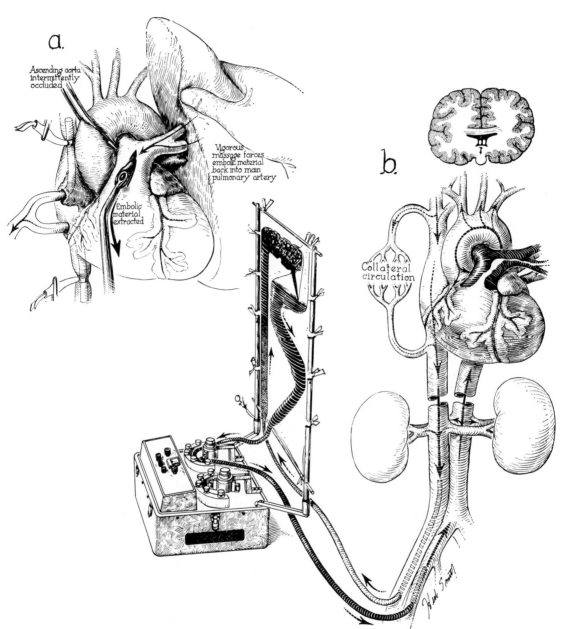

Figure 17–11 Drawings illustrating pulmonary embolectomy using temporary cardiopulmonary bypass. *a,* Technique of embolectomy during total bypass. Lungs are massaged toward hilar areas to express distally lodged emboli back into main pulmonary artery, from which they are extracted. *b,* Partial cardiopulmonary bypass from femoral vein to femoral artery for resuscitation prior to definitive embolectomy.

COMPLICATIONS

Extracorporeal Circulation

Numerous technical difficulties that may result in complications, both during and after operation, are associated with the use of extracorporeal perfusion for temporary cardiopulmonary bypass. Recent evidence suggests that many complications previously believed inherent to extracorporeal circulation actually are manifestations of the "homologous blood syndrome," associated with use of large quantities of fresh, heparinized blood to prime most types of pump oxygenators. These complications may be prevented by use of a system with a low volume that can be primed with some type of blood substitute, such as the described technique of priming with 5 per cent dextrose in distilled water or balanced electrolyte solution.

Other complications may be associated with necessary cannulations for connection of the pump oxygenator. Caution must be exercised in the passage of tapes around the venae cavae and aorta, especially in the presence of dense pericardial adhesions. Tears in these structures, unless properly managed, may result in massive hemorrhage and death of the patient. The most frequent site of such a tear is in the right branch of the pulmonary artery near its origin from the main pulmonary artery, occurring in the process of passing a tape around the ascending aorta. This complication can be avoided if the muscularis of the aorta is closely adhered to in scissors dissection, if a large curved hemostat is then used to dissect further around the aorta within the same plane, and if a large mixter clamp is ultimately passed through to pick up a tape to surround the aorta. Tears also commonly occur when instruments are passed about the superior and inferior vena cava. The right pulmonary artery is immediately adjacent to the superior vena cava and careful dissection in this area is mandatory to ensure that a clamp is passed around the superior vena cava in such a way that it does not tear the right pulmonary artery. Finger palpation of the tissues binding the superior vena cava through the area of the right pulmonary artery will usually determine how much dissection needs to be done.

Often finger dissection can be used to free up the superior vena cava. The inferior vena cava may be the source of complications owing to passage of an instrument into a greatly enlarged left atrium, and tears of the inferior vena cava itself may occur. If a tear occurs during the time of preparation for cannulation, a sponge can be readily placed in this area or the bleeding can be managed by finger control, since it is a low pressure system; the patient can then be placed on bypass and the rent repaired at a time when all blood can be returned to the pump oxygenator without massive blood loss. In most cases, catastrophic hemorrhage during surgery occurs in a low pressure system. Surgeons tend to use clamps in an attempt to stop hemorrhage in the venous system or right atrium, and this must be strictly avoided. In more than 90 per cent of the cases finger pressure is sufficient until control of the proximal and distal vessels can be obtained and direct suture with adequate exposure can be done with ease. In general, finger dissection and palpation is preferred to "peanut" or instrument dissection. It is best to cannulate the cavae before attempting to encircle these structures with tapes. This also has the advantage that in huge hearts, partial bypass can be instituted to empty the heart and thus facilitate the dissection so that tapes may be placed about these structures.

During retrograde cannulation of the femoral artery for return from the pump oxygenator, intimal dissection may be started unless caution is exercised. Occasionally it may be necessary to tack down thickened intima prior to cannulation or to use the opposite femoral artery or an external iliac artery to prevent such a complication. Rarely, a dissection may be produced in the common iliac artery or in the aorta itself by retrograde flow raising an atheromatous plaque, and with this complication one must depend on prompt recognition and management rather than prevention. Retrograde dissection usually manifests itself first by a fall in venous return to the pump oxygenator due to loss of blood into the retroperitoneal space. At times this may be recognized through the incision for femoral artery exposure; on other occasions an exploratory abdominal incision must be made on suspicion alone. Regardless of the cause

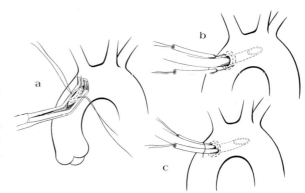

Figure 17–12 Two purse-string sutures are placed in the ascending aorta near the innominate artery. A Beck clamp is applied as depicted in *a* and an incision is made with a No. 11 blade and extended with a Potts scissors to about two-thirds the size of the cannula to be used. Homemade half-inch cannulas of polyvinyl chloride are used in our institution for this purpose. The Beck clamp is then released and the cannula is slid into position as depicted in *b* and then the purse-string sutures with tourniquets are tied to the cannulas *(c)*.

or stage in the operative procedure, however, once a retrograde dissection begins, it becomes mandatory to discontinue bypass temporarily and move cannulation for arterial return to the other femoral artery or even an accessible spot in the aorta itself, depending upon where the dissection begins and its extent. Failure to do so almost always results in death of the patient.

Most surgeons now prefer direct cannulation of the ascending aorta, as depicted in Figure 17–12. Two purse-string sutures are carefully placed in the ascending aorta just below the innominate artery; the muscularis of the aorta, and preferably the intima, should be picked up with the needle at the superior pole of the purse string. A Beck clamp (Fig. 17–12, *a*) is then placed tangentially on the aorta and an incision two-thirds the size of the cannula to be inserted is made in the aorta and the cannula is inserted as the Beck clamp is released (Fig. 17–12, *b*). Blood is allowed to rise freely in the cannula and then a clamp is placed. This latter maneuver precludes any chance of air being trapped in the cannula and thus the possibility of air embolization to the cerebral vessels. Currently, the usual practice is to insert a dilator after incision without clamping and the cannula is then inserted directly. This avoids the problems associated with putting a partial occluding clamp on a fragile, arteriosclerotic aorta.

Open-heart operations on the aortic valve require direct exposure of the coronary orifices, and unless the procedure is a very short one, such as commissurotomy for congenital aortic stenosis, some means of myocardial protection must be utilized. Coronary perfusion of either the left, right, or both coronary ostia is still carried out by

some surgeons, but this is not common now. For the past five years, the use of cardioplegia has become extremely popular to protect the myocardium. A cold solution with balanced osmolality, varying amounts of potassium ion, and, occasionally, other drugs, is used to perfuse the root of the aorta at the onset of the procedure; this solution is approximately 4° C. Immediate cardiac arrest is achieved, and the high energy phosphates are preserved throughout the entire procedure. Some surgeons feel that 90 per cent of the protection is afforded by the cold rather than by the cardioplegic agents. We are of similar persuasion and have not used cardioplegic drugs routinely; instead, we use cold Ringer's solution (4° C.) in the pericardial sac and into the left ventricle as a continuous infusion. On occasion, in long procedures and multiple valve replacement or procedures requiring long cross-clamp time, the right ventricle is also infused with the same solution. This can be readily achieved even in those patients having secondary surgery in which the chambers of the heart are not dissected free. A plastic catheter of size 14 gauge can be inserted easily into the left ventricle, even though it is not dissected free, by passing it through the anterior wall of the right ventricle and into the left ventricular cavity for constant infusion of cold solution. The same applies to the right ventricle if protection is needed there. Intermittently, Ringer's solution at 4° C. can also be dumped into the pericardial cavity to cover the entire heart. It would appear that good protection can be achieved if the septal temperature can be reduced to below 17°C., but it is seldom possible in the hypertrophied septum to drop the temperature below the level of 17° C., regardless of whether the solution is injected through the coronary system or through the methods described above.

Cannulation of the coronary orifices carries with it certain inherent dangers related to intimal damage produced by the cannulas themselves. One must guard against use of too large a cannula and avoid rough manipulation. Semirigid metal cannulas, which must be held by an assistant, appear to increase the incidence of intimal damage to the coronary arteries. We prefer flexible cannulas such as the Mayo cannula, a self-inflating balloon cannula that is extremely soft, if they are to be used at all.

In patients requiring longer clamp times, such as in double valve replacement or replacement of the aortic valve and ascending aorta, we use the following procedure: In double valves the aorta is clamped, the pericardial well constantly infused with 4° C. Ringer's solution, the left atrium opened, the mitral valve excised, and all sutures are placed through the mitral valve. Cold solution is poured directly into the left ventricle and the left atrium throughout this procedure. When all sutures have been placed through the artificial valve, attention is turned to the aortic valve which is completely excised and replaced with a proper prosthesis, the aorta resutured, air expressed, and the aortic clamp released. The mitral valve is then tied in place at leisure with coronary flow restored. Using this procedure, clamp time is reduced to no more than 70 to 90 minutes with good protection of the heart.

Should the intima at a coronary orifice be torn, meticulous repair is necessary, with double-armed, small vascular sutures passed through each side of the tear and tied on the outside of the vessel. If damage is great, a vein graft bypass should be carried out to that particular vessel without delay, since this offers good protection without a lot of wasted ischemia time.

In the past, a great number of complications occurred in the conduct of extracorporeal circulation because close attention was not paid to maintenance of homeostasis of the patient. It is our opinion that careful monitoring of extracorporeal perfusion — that is, by means of electrocardiogram, systemic arterial pressure, central venous pressure, urinary output, and electroencephalogram, as well as frequent analysis of blood gases with use of a nomogram — is required to maintain homeostasis. In the early days of extracorporeal circulation, when monitoring and frequent examination of blood gases and electrolytes were not done, it was common to find patients in severe metabolic acidosis at the completion of the operation; in a patient whose heart had marginal ventricular function this could cause death. Renal complications and pulmonary complications also were much more common, and the treatment of the low-output syndrome was practically routine. In using these methods over the past 5 years, the number of extracardiac complications occurring in the patient with abnormal physiology has been reduced to a minimum.

In recent years, many surgeons have used extensive hemodilution without regard for oxygen needs of the patient. It is not uncommon for perfusion to be carried out with a hematocrit of 17 (4 to 6 gm) of hemoglobin) although oxygen-carrying capacity is only one-half to two-thirds that required for adequate total perfusion. Oxygen debt and metabolic acidosis are the end results because actually the patient is underperfused. In addition, with this reduced carrying capacity, cold is likely to produce a "core" circulation (perfusing only the heart, brain, liver, and kidneys) without perfusing the peripheral circulation. Even at 30° C. (moderate hypothermia), over a prolonged period of time, metabolic acidosis may develop to an extreme degree with hypoperfusion.

One of the most frequent difficulties associated with cardiopulmonary bypass is a sudden decrease in venous return. Usually this is simply corrected by having an assistant, or even the surgeon, remove his foot from the venous line. At other times the venous line or one of the cannulas has become kinked within the operative field, or an assistant has become too vigorous with a retractor on one of the caval catheters, such as during repair of an atrial septal defect or during mitral valve replacement from the right side. If mechanical obstruction to venous return is ruled out, consideration should be given to the adequacy of circulating blood volume. At times a sudden extracardiac blood loss will go unrecognized by the anesthesiologist, such as blood lost into one of the pleural cavities or the mistaken use of one of the wall suckers rather than the intracardiac aspirator by a member of the operative team. Correction of this difficulty is by blood replacement. In the same category is retroperitoneal blood loss from retrograde dissection, which must be managed by blood replacement as well as changing cannulation for arterial return, as described previously. And, during relatively long perfusions using the described technique of priming with blood substitutes, we have found it helpful in maintaining venous return to add another 250 to 500 ml. of priming solution as perfusion progresses to replace amounts excreted by the kidneys with adequate attention to the hematocrit level.

Hemolysis associated with cardiopulmonary bypass is produced primarily in the intracardiac suction system. This can be minimized to some extent by running the roller pumps connected to sumps and intracardiac aspirators at a rate no greater than that needed to prevent extracardiac blood loss and to keep the operative field unobscured. Although red blood cells can stand a great deal of positive pressure, they are extremely sensitive to high negative pressure, and thus may be ruptured or traumatized with a great deal of negative pressure suction. The amount of blood passed through the intracardiac suction system with resulting hemolysis also can be reduced by intermittently occluding the ascending aorta during the intracardiac procedure to allow controlled coronary flow with decrease in coronary sinus return. This maneuver is especially helpful in patients with massive cardiomegaly associated with acquired valvular heart disease. If significant hemolysis should occur, whether from the extracorporeal perfusion, a hemolytic transfusion reaction, or any other reason, a mannitol-induced osmotic diuresis is usually effective in clearing the plasma. This can be accomplished by the intravenous injection of 12.5 to 25.0 gm. of mannitol, followed by the addition of 12.5 gm. to each 1000 ml. of intravenous solution given until plasma hemoglobin levels have returned to an acceptable range. More recently it has been our practice to use furosemide or ethacrynic acid to keep diuresis effective throughout the procedure. Should unquestionable anuria ensue for any reason, however, one should not continue in attempts to induce an osmotic diuresis with mannitol or other drugs, since the only result will be an increase in circulating blood volume and pulmonary and systemic circuit overload.

Hemorrhage

Both during and after surgery of the heart, hemorrhage can be a troublesome and even fatal complication. Bleeding from inadvertent tears in the heart and great vessels associated with preparations for cardiopulmonary bypass have already been discussed. Operative hemorrhage also may be a complication of closed cardiac procedures. The most dangerous type of hemorrhage during decortication of the heart for constrictive pericarditis is that from a major coronary artery, since measures used for control may result in occlusion of the coronary vessel. A similar problem exists during manipulation of the left atrial appendage for entry into the atrium, such as during transventricular mitral commissurotomy, since injury to the left coronary artery may occur as it courses along the base of the appendage. If a major coronary vessel is injured, every effort should be made to repair the vessel itself by means of fine vascular sutures rather than controlling hemorrhage by large sutures that encircle it, or to insert a vein graft if these methods fail.

Attempts to remove too large a portion of the atrial septum when performing the Blalock-Hanlon procedure may result in invagination of the atria with creation of a defect in the opposite atrial wall and should be guarded against. Another pitfall that may occur during this procedure is slippage of the atrial walls from the partial occluding clamp at one end of the combined incisions into the right and left atria. This can be prevented easily by placing traction sutures at each end of the proposed incisions before they are made, using these sutures for closure after creation of the atrial septal defect (see Figure 17–1).

Although considered a routine and safe operation, division and suture of a patent ductus arteriosus is associated with many pitfalls in the hands of the uninitiated. The ductus may be an extremely friable structure, particularly when it is large and associated with pulmonary hypertension. It must be freed by sharp dissection under direct vision, especially posteriorly where attempts at completing dissection bluntly may lead to entry into the ductus or into the left pulmonary artery. Another source of difficulty during this operation is placement of suture bites too close together, especially on the aortic side of the ductus, in an effort to prevent hemorrhage. Such an error may result in tearing along the suture line as with perforated cards made for easy separation. Finally, ductus clamps should be checked prior to application, since occasionally they will have been sprung from misuse. Slippage of the ductus from the clamps, particularly on the higher pressure aortic side, can be further assured against by progressive division of the ductus as it is sutured, rather than completely dividing it prior to suture (see Fig. 17–2, a).

Primary control of hemorrhage from a ductus should be with direct finger pressure until preparation can be made for definitive control. When a tear has occurred in the posterior aspect of the ductus, it is usually possible to pass an umbilical tape indirectly around the ductus (see Fig. 17–3, b,c), which then allows elevation of the ductus followed by application of clamps (see Fig. 17–3, d). Hemorrhage on the aortic side of the ductus usually requires temporary occlusion of the descending thoracic aorta above and below, and some have recommended that tapes routinely be placed around the aorta proximal and distal to the ductus should this become necessary. Regardless of whether or not tapes have been preplaced, hemorrhage should be controlled by finger pressure until the aorta is clamped; then sutures should be placed rapidly and the clamps removed as quickly as possible. Attempts to pass sutures through this friable area of aorta and tie them down individually without prior occlusion often are fraught with progressively increasing hemorrhage and even death. We have found it extremely useful to utilize drugs to drop the systemic and pulmonary artery pressures during the time of clamping the ductus. Nipride can be used to reduce the systolic ejection pressure, Arfonad to reduce afterload and decrease

resistance, or the halogen agents in increased amounts to drop the pressure in a high-pressure ductus. If a patient, particularly an adult, has balanced pressures in systemic and pulmonary circuits, it is wise to use the Gott shunt in the arch of the aorta to the descending aorta to facilitate clamping of the aorta above and below the ductus and to provide safe circulation to the distal aorta during the clamp time.

Operative hemorrhage associated with various systemic-pulmonary artery anastomoses can usually be prevented by careful attention to detail and avoidance of hasty or rough maneuvers. Bleeding, however, becomes a more formidable problem in these patients at the time of definitive operation when the shunt must be controlled during bypass and finally obliterated. Adhesions from the original operation may further complicate these maneuvers, both by making control of the anastomosis difficult and by the production of raw surfaces with resultant hemorrhage following operation. For this reason an anastomosis between the ascending aorta and left pulmonary artery has been suggested and allows for easy closure of the shunt through the ascending aorta at the time of definitive repair of the congenital anomaly (see Fig. 17–2, c).

Operative hemorrhage associated with cardiac surgery often results from imperfection of a suture line. Usually this can be adequately controlled by repair sutures, best placed and tied while pressure within the vessel or chamber is reduced during bypass or by temporary occlusion of the vessel. One type of operative bleeding particularly difficult to control is that associated with weakening of the aortic wall by removal of too much calcium at the commissure between the posterior non-coronary cusp and the left coronary cusp during aortic valve replacement for calcific aortic stenosis. The prosthesis tends to hold this area open, and as bypass is discontinued, blood suddenly wells up from the posterior aspect of the aortic annulus. Attempts to control this hemorrhage by rotating the ascending aorta and base of the heart while passing and tying individual sutures often result in further tearing of the aortic wall or in ventricular fibrillation. Again, primary control of this type of hemorrhage is with finger pressure. Cardiopulmonary bypass is then reinstituted, even if recannulation is required. Once pressure on this area is relieved by bypass and reapplication of a clamp to the distal ascending aorta, the ascending aorta and base of the heart are rotated and all necessary repair sutures are placed and tied, often incorporating the sewing ring of the prosthesis as a buttress. Once all sutures are tied, the clamp is removed from the ascending aorta, and bypass again is discontinued.

Operative hemorrhage has become a major concern in the large number of mitral valve replacement operations being done. At the mitral valve, the left atrial and left ventricular junction on the posterior wall may be extremely thin. This is particularly likely to be true in elderly females with long-standing mitral stenosis. Too vigorous an attempt to remove calcium from the posterior leaflet may result in thinning of the posterior wall immediately below the annulus of the mitral valve. Another possible cause of hemorrhage is passage of sutures too deep into the annulus or down into the thin musculature immediately below the annulus (Fig. 17–13). The sutures pulling the valve down into place cut

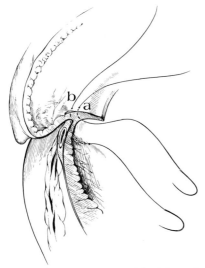

Figure 17–13 A cross section of the left atrial and left ventricular junction showing the proper and improper methods of suture. In a, the suture passes only through the remaining annulus, which is fibrous tissue. In b, however, the suture passes through thinned-out musculature so that with restoration of pressure in the left ventricle, dissection of the muscle might occur. Sutures should not pass through muscle at any point in this back wall. Note also the proximity of the circumflex coronary artery in this area which can easily be snared with a suture placed too deep.

through the musculature as they are tied down. As a result, a layer of only a few cells' thickness may remain in the posterior wall of the left ventricle, and when pressure is returned at the completion of bypass, sudden massive bleeding may occur. Examination by lifting up the heart reveals bleeding points just below the annulus of the mitral valve and the source of hemorrhage can be seen to be the left ventricle. There is no choice in this situation but to go back on complete cardiopulmonary bypass, empty the ventricle by vent, and repair the disrupted myocardium with interrupted buttressed sutures. Attempts to suture this area without bypass will only result in further tearing and probably loss of the patient. The source of this dissection, of course, is almost always immediately beneath the annulus, but the dissection may traverse the left ventricular musculature diagonally and exit near the apex. On finding this dread complication, the diagnosis can be made by simply placing a finger immediately below the artificial valve and observing cessation of bleeding. This will indicate exactly where the sutures should be placed to get at the origin of the dissection. This should be done prior to bypassing and emptying the heart. Prevention of this complication, of course, is by very careful dissection of the posterior leaflet; often some of it should be left in place if possible. If the chordae are massively shortened, the posterior leaflets will provide additional substance in which sutures can be placed. Sutures in this area should be placed only through the annulus itself and not into the muscularis of the left ventricle.

Another complication of mitral valve replacement is suture occlusion of the circumflex artery. Figure 17–13 shows the proximity of this important structure to the annulus of the mitral valve. Deep sutures in this area might result in this catastrophic complication. Also, the proximity of the aortic and mitral annuli at the posterior medial commissure must be kept in mind so that injury to the aortic valve is avoided. Another common problem of aortic valve replacement is the small annulus and obliteration of the left or right coronary orifice by a prosthesis that is too large. Figure 17–14 shows the method that we use of always tying down the sutures encompassing the left and right coronary orifices, and

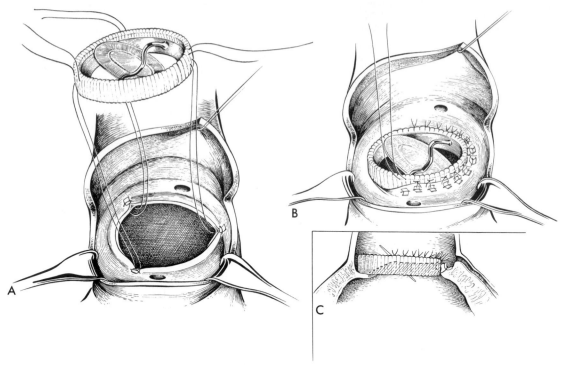

Figure 17–14   Technique of valve suturing to avoid impingement on coronary orifices.

the sutures involving the non-coronary cusps are tied down last. Thus, if there is protrusion of the prosthesis beyond the circumference of the ring, it will be in the non-coronary orifice and adequate openings to the left and right coronary orifices will be assured.

Both operative and postoperative hemorrhage may be associated with defects in the coagulation mechanism, but an extensive discussion of these problems is not within the scope of this presentation. Such problems most frequently arise in patients with cyanotic congenital heart disease and appear related to deficiencies in various plasma clotting factors. Use of fresh whole blood is often helpful in this sort of case, as well as in almost any patient with a generalized bleeding tendency. Use of heparin for extracorporeal circulation requires neutralization with a heparin antagonist such as protamine sulfate, and one should be careful not to give an excessive amount of protamine, which may result in a defect in coagulation referred to as "protamine rebound." This can usually be prevented by giving the calculated amount of protamine in divided doses, erring on the side of using too little rather than too much. The use of

partial thromboplastin time repeatedly during perfusion and immediately after heart-lung bypass has proven to be a good adjunct to coagulation management. Cardiopulmonary bypass, particularly if prolonged, occasionally may be associated with abnormal fibrinolytic activity resulting in a bleeding tendency. Usually this can be managed by the administration of fibrinogen in doses of 2 to 6 gm., but in more severe cases action of plasminogen activator must be neutralized with epsilon-aminocaproic acid. This may be given intravenously, using 5.0 gm. as a priming dose followed by 1.0 gm. per hour until hemorrhage is controlled.

Most often, however, hemorrhage following operations on the heart is associated with technical errors that occur at the time of operation. This fact alone tends to produce a psychologic block in the mind of the surgeon, who must accept his error and reexplore the patient in order to control hemorrhage. No set rules can be followed in terms of how much blood loss following surgery indicates the need for reoperation, since this must be individualized. Nevertheless, in the presence of cardiac tamponade with decreased cardiac output, early evacuation is mandatory. Although a widely open pericardium aids in the prevention of tamponade, it cannot assure against such a development. Clot may seal the pericardial opening with continued hemorrhage beneath this clot producing tamponade, and most cardiac surgeons have been through the unfortunate experience of having tamponade develop in a patient in whom the pericardium had been left completely open. Diagnosis may be difficult to make in the immediate postoperative period, since this type of tamponade is frequently unassociated with classic signs such as increased venous pressure, paradoxical pulse, and distant heart sounds. This is particularly true when circulating blood volume may be diminished, and one must decide whether more blood is indicated or whether tamponade is present and should be evacuated. Central venous pressure often is helpful under these circumstances, lowered central venous pressure in the presence of systemic hypotension suggesting need for further transfusion. The echocardiogram is probably the most helpful diagnostic tool when tamponade is suspected.

It has been our practice to manage pericardial tamponade at the bedside. Often, all the criteria for tamponade are not found. In fact, we have found that paradoxical pulse and rising central venous pressure have occurred in no more than two-thirds of the cases. Figure 17–15 demonstrates our method. Closure of the medial sternotomy is carried out with interrupted sutures in the area below the xiphoid in fascia, subcutaneous tissue, and skin. With this method it is a simple matter, when tamponade is suspected, to drape the patient, remove the sutures, and place a finger into the pericardium, which is left open in its lower portion. If tamponade is present, blood can be released from this space for the patient's immediate improvement. A flexible sucker can be passed completely around the heart to be sure all clots have been removed. A tube is then placed into the anterior mediastinum and retrosternal space and the wound is closed tightly about it. When possible, a tube should be placed in the infracardiac space over the diaphragm. This may be contraindicated, however, in the presence of multiple vein grafts in this area. This bedside procedure has produced no mortality or morbidity and often has been a great help in determining whether pump failure or tamponade is present. The method also permits appropriate treatment when tamponade has been ruled out and the diagnosis of pump failure has been made. We have found that needle aspiration of the pericardium in the postoperative state is not fruitful in most cases. Clot is usually present in the pericardium and the surgeon can be misled.

Hemorrhage following operation on the heart usually occurs from certain areas, all of which should be visualized at the time of reoperation for bleeding. A more fruitful approach is to reinspect each of these areas before closing the wound in an effort to reduce the incidence of postoperative hemorrhage. When the sternal-splitting incision is used, extreme care must be taken in passing the wires about the sternum since

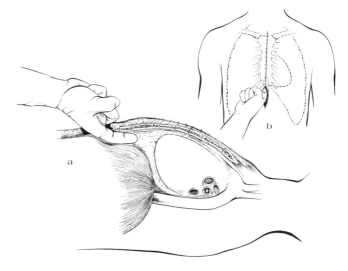

Figure 17–15 This illustration depicts the method of relieving tamponade at bedside. After sterile preparation of the area below the xiphoid and draping of the lower portion of the sternum and epigastrium, sutures are removed below the xiphoid in the skin, subcutaneous tissue, and fascia, so that a finger can be passed into the pericardium. A sucker can then be passed up around the heart to remove all clots, and a tube is placed to drain the retrosternal space.

the internal mammary artery may have a course that does not conform with that usually described anatomically. It may be extremely close to the sternum or even under the extreme margin of the sternum on either side. If wire sutures are to be passed about the sternum, they should ride the periosteal surface of the sternum at all times. Careful inspection for bleeding points should always be made after all wires have been placed. Failure to appreciate this is one of the more common causes of bleeding in cardiac surgery carried out through a sternal-splitting incision.

Each cardiotomy, whether for intracardiac repair or for cannulation, should be inspected carefully prior to closure, as should suture lines in the aorta or pulmonary artery. Small branches of the coronary arteries that may have been divided during ventriculotomy or left atriotomy should be ligated individually to ensure against bleeding from this source. All arterial vessels should be suture-ligated. Pericardial vessels of any magnitude require ligation, particularly if a transverse incision or extension is used in the pericardium. And, in spite of the utmost care in prevention, one must accept an occasional case of postoperative hemorrhage and the necessity for reoperation before massive quantities of blood have been given and a stage of irreversibility is reached. The method for reexploration should be packing off all suture lines except one and investigating them individually. "Wiping" and "suckers" should be avoided. Dabbing with sponges is the procedure of choice.

Heart Block

Like hemorrhage, operative heart block is far easier to prevent than to manage. Precise knowledge of the location of the conduction mechanism of the heart and avoidance of these areas are the best method of prevention, but in spite of such precautions complete heart block will occur occasionally. Although all cardiac surgeons are familiar with techniques aimed at preventing heart block during repair of ventricular septal defects and primum-type atrial septal defects, only recently has the danger of heart block in association with prosthetic replacement of the mitral or aortic valve been fully appreciated. Sutures for fixation of mitral valve prostheses and either sutures or pin fixation mechanisms for attachment of aortic valve prostheses may impinge upon or incorporate the atrioventricular bundle. More frequently, complete heart block follows aortic valve replacement for calcific aortic stenosis in which too vigorous attempts are made to remove calcium as it extends from the aortic annulus onto the interventricular septum just over the location of the bundle. We routinely leave temporary leads attached to the heart in all patients who have undergone valve surgery, because of the significant number of arrhythmias encountered in the postoperative period. As stated before, we now leave permanent leads in the older patient with valvular disease or calcified valves, and in all valvular patients who have preoperative arrhythmias.

When complete heart block occurs under these circumstances, an intravenous drip of isoproterenol hydrochloride is usually helpful in temporary management. Should block persist, however, myocardial leads should be attached and brought out through the chest wall for temporary connection to a battery-powered pacemaker. An implantable pacemaker should not be used at this time, since complete heart block may be only transient and may revert during the postoperative period. If, however, complete heart block persists for 3 to 4 weeks, an implantable pacemaker should be inserted prior to discharge from the hospital. Even though such a patient might be weaned from the temporary pacemaker, Lillehei and associates demonstrated that an unacceptably high long-term mortality rate is associated with Stokes-Adams attacks unless this is done. Later, studies in our patients demonstrated that a new method of insertion of temporary pacemaker wires results in reduced threshold after 10 days (Aris, A., Shebairo, R. A., and Lepley, D., Jr.: Increasing myocardial thresholds to pacing in postoperative cardiac surgical patients. *In* Surgical Forum XXIV, 1973).

Wire breakage may lead to pacemaker failure, either early or late. Several methods are available for differentiating between this and component or battery failure, but exteriorization of the battery and component package usually is necessary. If only one lead has broken, it is usually possible to convert that lead into an indifferent electrode rather than to replace the entire unit and both leads. If the difficulty is found to be component or battery failure, then all that may be required is replacement of the component and battery package. Techniques for such replacement vary with the type of pacemaker used, and reference should be made to literature furnished by the manufacturer.

We have found the arrhythmias encountered in valvular surgery to be so numerous that we routinely leave a temporary right atrial wire and a left ventricular wire in place and bring them out in the epigastrium for use if necessary. Bradycardias — either sinus, nodal, or atrial fibrillation with a very slow ventricular response — are extremely common. They can be managed by using either the ventricular or the atrial pacemaker. The atrial tachycardias may be overridden by an atrial pacemaker wire and this is used quite frequently. The morbidity associated with heart wires is practically nil, and they have saved many lives by permitting use of either a demand or a fixed-rate external pacemaker. In patients with bradycardia, it is our practice to leave the pacemaker attached in the demand mode at a rate slower than the patient's intrinsic rate; if the patient's heart rate falls below the preset level, the pacemaker takes over. The threshold of heart wires placed at the time

of operation should be checked every 8 hours since the rise in threshold to capture is extremely variable. With our recently modified electrode, all the bare wire is buried in the myocardium and all exposed electrode is insulated. This modification has permitted a significant lowering of the threshold at 24 to 48 hours and at 8 days.

Embolism

Peripheral embolization after cardiac surgery may be due to either air or particulate matter and may or may not require or be amenable to specific therapy, depending on its location. Air embolism is usually associated with open operations on the left side of the heart and can be prevented far more easily than it can be treated. Careful attention to evacuation of all air from the heart prior to final closure is far more helpful in this regard than dependence on flooding the operative field with carbon dioxide. Also, at the time the left side of the heart is closed, the head of the table should be lowered to allow any air that possibly has escaped removal to bypass the brachiocephalic vessels and find its way distally into the aorta, where it will do far less harm than in the brain. During the past 2 years, we have routinely inserted a slotted needle into the ascending aorta at the time the clamp is removed from the aorta (Fig. 17–16). This method appears to prevent significant air

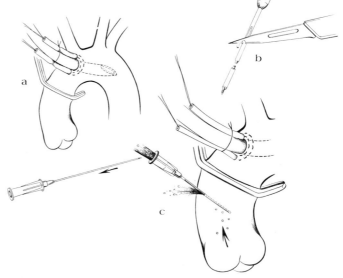

Figure 17–16 This illustration demonstrates the method of removing air from the ascending aorta and a vent that can remain throughout the time that air is being expressed from the heart. In *a* is shown typical aortic cannulation and a clamp placed on the ascending aorta to carry out intracardiac surgery. The method of placing a slot in a common No. 18 Longdwell needle is shown in *b*. The needle then can be inserted as shown in *c* into the ascending aorta with the metal stylet removed. This permits air to regress to the outside from the entire circumference of the aorta rather than just at needle tip. At the conclusion of the procedure, the needle can be simply removed and a single mattress suture used to close the perforation.

embolization to the brain as long as meticulous attention is paid to aspiration of the left ventricular apex, elevation of the heart, invagination of the left atrial appendage at the time air is being removed from the apex, and meticulous aspiration of air at the time of closure of the left atriotomy. Although it is hard to document, it is probably true that most of the problems with left ventricular malfunction at the conclusion of an open-heart procedure are due to air in the coronary arteries. Meticulous attention to removing air from the heart and providing good coronary perfusion throughout the procedure will obviate this problem. A slotted, 14-gauge plastic needle inserted into the elevated apex of the left ventricle has proven very efficient in removing air. Vigorous massage and invagination of the left atrial appendage and the left atrium is carried out while this needle is in place.

Occasionally, however, cerebral *air embolism* will occur. Under these circumstances supportive and symptomatic care is indicated, perhaps aided by an osmotic diuresis with mannitol or urea to reduce cerebral edema. Recent evidence suggests that use of low-molecular-weight dextran may be helpful in such a patient and Decadron 8 mg. every 8 hours should be given immediately and continued for several days when cerebral air embolism is suspected.

Embolism of particulate matter may occur during either open or closed procedures, and again every effort should be made toward prevention. When performing transventricular mitral commissurotomy in a patient with a history of embolism, a purse-string suture should be placed in the base of the atrial appendage without prior occlusion with a clamp, and the atrium should be flushed before inserting the index finger. If thrombus is encountered, no further attempts at a closed procedure should be made, and cardiopulmonary bypass should be instituted, allowing far safer evacuation of clot from the left atrium. When friable calcification is felt on the mitral valve and a closed procedure still appears indicated, it would appear helpful to have the anesthesiologist temporarily occlude the carotid vessels by pressure on the neck during the moment of commissurotomy and for 15 to 30 seconds afterward. In this manner any particulate matter that may break off will probably follow the flow of blood into the right subclavian artery or distally to the lower extremity vessels, from which it can be removed.

Particulate matter may break off during open operations such as valve replacement, and again every effort should be made toward prevention. The tips of the papillary muscles are cut off after the valve is completely free from its wall, and thus the calcium and the valve can be removed in toto. With this method, any particulate pieces of calcium that fall into the ventricle can be readily grasped with a forceps.

In aortic valve replacement, frequently piecemeal resection of calcium must be done. Careful attention is necessary when removing calcium from the area of the junction of the right and non-coronary leaflets because of the position of the conduction system. Removal of mural calcium may result in complete heart block. Copious irrigation of the left ventricle after removal of calcified aortic valve and insertion of a finger into the ventricle to feel for particulate pieces of calcium should be routinely done. To facilitate removal of mural calcium in aortic valve or mitral valve replacement, knife incision of the endocardium and subsequent development of a plane with a Smithwick dissector or a similar spatula-type instrument will often allow removal of the calcium in toto without destruction of the adjacent wall. A plane can usually be established. This instrument is also useful in establishing a plane of dissection in the clotted left atrium so that the clot from the atrial appendage and the mural portion can be removed in toto without the danger of small fragments falling undetected through the mitral valve and subsequently embolizing to the circulation.

During excision of an aneurysm of the left ventricle attention must be paid to removal of all laminated thrombus lest this be allowed to embolize to the peripheral circulation.

The prevention of postoperative emboli associated with valve prostheses is a major problem, since thousands of patients now have artificial valves implanted. Although anticoagulants are usually given, long-term administration has not been entirely effective in reducing the occasional instance of such an untoward occurrence. Perhaps more useful will be recent design changes in the prostheses themselves. Early anticoagulation appears to be of some benefit in preventing thromboembolic phenomena from artificial valves. We have found that after removal of the chest tubes at 24 hours, early heparinization has been advantageous. It would seem that if the patient can be protected with heparin intravenously around the clock over a 7-day period, some pseudointima will form around the sewing ring and knots of the sutures of the valve to prevent thrombus formation in these areas. Heparin administration is continued on a closely controlled basis with frequent measurements of Lee-White clotting time over 7 days. Oral administration of Coumadin is begun as soon as the patient is able to take fluids; at the end of 7 days, the prothrombin time is usually in the 20 to 30 per cent range, which we consider therapeutic. The patient is then given Coumadin alone, and every attempt is made to keep the prothrombin time at the 20 to 30 per cent level.

Once peripheral embolization of particulate matter has occurred, subsequent management is determined by location. If the embolus is in an accessible location, certainly it should be removed. Occasionally, emboli will lodge at a carotid artery bifurcation, and these should be taken out as rapidly as possible. More frequently, however, cerebral embolization occurs to an intracranial location, and only supportive care is possible.

Renal Insufficiency, Acidosis, and Electrolyte Problems

Renal insufficiency and acidosis are more common after open than after closed cardiac procedures. It is our impression that, excluding hemolytic transfusion reactions, the primary cause of both conditions is inadequate perfusion, owing either to poor conduct of bypass or to reduced cardiac output following bypass. Sodium bicarbonate appears far more efficient than sodium lactate in the symptomatic management of acidosis, since lactate must be metabolized before sodium lactate can be effective. Others have suggested use of THAM, and this too would appear symptomatically ef-

fective from reported experience. Definitive therapy, however, must be aimed at correction of the underlying cause, such as reduced cardiac output secondary to tamponade or diminished circulating blood volume.

Renal insufficiency associated with extracorporeal circulation appears to some extent related to use of large quantities of homologous blood to prime various types of pump oxygenators. If oliguria does occur after bypass, use of mannitol has been recommended and may be helpful, but primary attention should be paid to correction of the underlying defect. Close attention to perfusion during open-heart surgery, with adequate flow to produce urine output of 30 to 50 ml. per hour, will usually prevent acute tubular necrosis. Today, furosemide and ethacrynic acid are preferred to mannitol for producing diuresis postoperatively and for keeping the potassium, blood urea nitrogen, and creatinine from rising to dangerous levels in patients with borderline renal failure syndromes.

Once renal shutdown has ensued, administration of diuretic should not be continued. Intravenous fluid intake should be restricted to 500 to 800 ml. per 24 hours plus measured output, and facilities should be at hand for renal dialysis should this prove necessary. In spite of the best of care, however, the mortality rate associated with renal shutdown following open-heart surgery remains high. Patients with renal shutdown after open-heart surgery do not tolerate high levels of potassium; whereas in a patient with chronic renal failure dialysis might be put off until the potassium level reaches 7.0 mEq. per liter, we feel that these surgical patients require immediate renal or peritoneal dialysis when potassium reaches a level of 5.5 to 6.0 mEq. Otherwise cardiac arrest is likely to occur. There is some hope that the pulsatile assist device (PAD), currently popular, may reduce the number of patients with this severe complication.

Electrolyte problems following cardiac surgery most frequently are accelerated manifestations of deficiencies existing before operation. One such problem is the low-salt syndrome, occurring primarily in patients with acquired valvular heart disease on prolonged courses of diuresis before operation. This can usually be managed by the judicious use of electrolyte-containing solutions during and after operation, but on occasion administration of small amounts of hypertonic saline may be required. More of a problem exists in regard to potassium depletion in patients with acquired valvular heart disease who have received thiazide derivatives for long periods without adequate potassium replacement. In such patients serum potassium levels may not adequately reflect true total body deficits, and replacement therapy may be required on an empirical basis. Difficulties arise in this group because the patients are usually receiving cardiac glycosides. Even minor temporary further depression of serum potassium levels associated with open-heart operations (dextrose in distilled water prime and temporary depression of P_{CO_2}) may result in relative digitalis intoxication with severe and occasionally unmanageable arrhythmias. Should such digitalis-induced arrhythmias occur, further potassium replacement as 40 to 100 mEq. per liter of intravenously administered fluids may be required for the first 24 to 36 hours after bypass for control. In addition to adequate potassium replacement during preparation for operation, it is often helpful to omit digitalis for 1 or 2 days before cardiopulmonary bypass in this group. If the patient is taking digitalis leaf, administration should be stopped 5 to 7 days before operation because the leaf extract remains at high levels for a long period of time. It is always possible to give more digitalis, but once given, cardiac glycosides cannot be removed.

Respiratory Complications

In addition to pulmonary complications inherent in all types of thoracic surgery and to be reviewed in a later section of this chapter, certain patients undergoing cardiac surgery have a predilection to respiratory complications secondary to pulmonary vascular damage. Although much of this damage may take place before operation, as in patients with severe pulmonary hypertension from either congenital or acquired heart disease, additional damage may occur during operations requiring cardiopulmonary bypass. Despite inflow occlusion during bypass, coronary sinus return and bron-

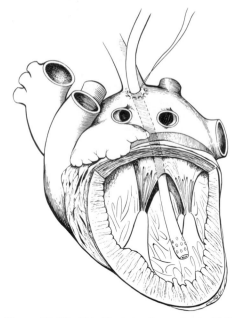

Figure 17–17   This illustrates the method of left heart drainage using the interatrial septum at its junction with the right superior pulmonary vein. A mattress-type suture is placed deep into the atrial septum just at its junction with the right superior pulmonary vein. With a No. 11 blade, a stab wound is made directly through the septum into the left atrium. This is dilated and the cannula is inserted and maneuvered down into the apex of the left ventricle. A purse-string suture with a tourniquet is then tied to the cannula to hold it rigidly in place.

chial artery flow continue to empty into the left atrium through the pulmonary veins. If the left side of the heart is allowed to distend, not only will myocardial damage ensue, but back pressure on the pulmonary vasculature and its attendant complications also will occur. Decompression of the left side of the heart can be accomplished easily by the routine insertion of a small sump into the left atrium and left ventricle. Figure 17–17 shows the method of drainage by this manner. A purse-string suture is placed at the junction of the right superior pulmonary vein and then is brought up through the atrial septum as a mattress suture. A No. 11 blade is used to puncture directly down through the septum; this opening is dilated with a hemostat, and an 18 French catheter is passed into the left atrium. By manipulation with the fingers, the catheter is maneuvered into the apex of the left ventricle. The purse string is pulled down and tied tightly around the cannula to hold it in place. This method avoids violation of the right pulmonary vein, which sometimes is extremely thin, and prevents the complication of left ventricular bleeding in friable ventricles that often attends use of the routine method of sump drainage at the left ventricular apex.

Meticulous tracheobronchial toilet is necessary for the successful postoperative management of patients with preexisting pulmonary vascular damage. This is especially true in those with mitral valve insufficiency who have reached an end stage of decompensation at the time of valve replacement. Intermittent positive-pressure breathing therapy and nebulization with acetylcysteine appear to help these patients in preparation for operation, and one should not hesitate to perform a tracheotomy at the completion of valve replacement if any question exists in regard to its need. Some have suggested that routine tracheotomy and control of respiration for 48 hours or longer are indicated in this group of patients. If such a course of management is followed, however, it is mandatory that adequate humidification be provided, that meticulous cleansing of the tracheobronchial tree be performed frequently, and that physicians knowledgeable in use of the respirator be constantly in attendance. Newer, soft, low-pressure, high-volume endotracheal tube cuffs have diminished the need for early tracheostomy, since the tube can be left in place for many days without danger of erosion of the trachea.

Over the past 4 years, it has been our experience that the use of the Engstrom or other volume respirator has contributed significantly to the reduction in pulmonary complications. When extensive revascularization procedures were first being done, requiring use of the pump oxygenator for up to 4 hours, the adult respiratory distress ("white lung") syndrome was a common complication. With routine use of the volume respirator, addition of cortisone to the regimen, and careful attention to the physiological state of the patient, we have seen these complications dwindle to an extremely small number. The advantage of the volume respirator over the pressure-controlled respirator is that a given volume will be delivered regardless of the pressure. With pressure-regulated respirators, of course,

the resistance climbs and the alveolar ventilation may be markedly reduced without the physician's being aware of it. It has been our practice to leave the endotracheal tube in place until the patient can take over respiratory function well on his own, however long that may be. Blood gases and oxygen and carbon dioxide saturation are measured at 4-hour intervals. Tidal volume is measured periodically with the patient off the respirator. When the patient shows he can maintain a satisfactory Po_2 without the accumulation of carbon dioxide and a satisfactory tidal and minute volume for at least 1 hour off the respirator, the endotracheal tube is removed after thorough tracheobronchial cleansing. Using these methods, we have had to carry out tracheostomy or reintubation in only rare instances.

Infection

Various infections common to any type of thoracic surgery may occur in patients after operations on the heart. Management in general is similar, although the presence of any kind of prosthesis within the heart makes occurrence of infection potentially most hazardous, and every effort should be made to prevent infections in these patients. Studies of Nelson and associates have demonstrated the efficiency of prophylactic antibiotics in this regard, although it is necessary for such therapy to begin well before operation. It also appears helpful to have the patient wash with a hexachlorophene or Betadine soap, including shampooing, for several days before operation.

When mediastinal infection does occur, we use the following method of management. If the sternum seems intact (if a sternotomy approach is used), the inferior pole of the wound is opened below the xiphoid, and a finger is passed up into the retrosternal space. If this space is found to be free of infection, a large 38 French catheter is passed to the superior pole of the wound. For infection that has progressed to the point of sternal destruction, as shown by lateral tomograms, the sternum is completely opened again and as much as possible of the bone involved by osteomyelitis is removed with a rongeur. Figure-of-eight wires are used to reclose the sternum and the catheter is brought out beneath the xiphoid. Subcutaneous tissue is closed, as is the skin if it appears to be clean. More often, the skin has to be left open for drainage. Local irrigation and systemic antibiotics are used until healing is complete. If all precautions are taken — including complete removal of the nidus of infection, meticulous observation of aseptic technique during surgery, and operation of the shortest possible duration — the incidence of serious infections should not exceed 1 per cent.

Changes in the bacterial flora in hospitals in the United States in recent years have influenced the types of infections that follow cardiac surgery. Whereas staphylococci were the most common causative organisms in hospital-acquired infections a few years ago, now gram-negative species and low-grade pathogens or non-pathogens such as *Staphylococcus epidermidis* have become prominent factors in infection of heart valves and in bloodstream infections in general. Prevention requires careful examination of the entire surgical team for the presence of infection, culture of the patient's sputum, and removal of infected teeth and any other potential nidus of infection in the patient before surgery. Identity of bacterial flora must be determined and antibiotic sensitivity studies must be carried out.

In the patient with bacterial endocarditis, either with a valve damaged by rheumatic fever or with a prosthetic valve, adequate medical control of infection must be achieved before removal of the valve or valve prosthesis can be considered. The presence of continued toxemia in spite of adequate antibiotic therapy usually means the infection is disseminated and not localized to the damaged valve or artificial prosthesis. Operation in these instances is usually not successful since the infection cannot be excised.

If a patient continues to be febrile with a high white cell count in spite of an adequate course of antibiotics, it usually means there are microabscesses in the heart and disseminated infection. A new prosthesis or a prosthesis used to replace a damaged valve will also become infected. On the other hand, a patient who becomes afebrile and symptom-free after an adequate course of antibiotics, but then has a recurrence of toxemic symptoms after 5 or 6 days, probably has a localized infection of the valve that was controlled; intensive antibiotic therapy over a 5-day period and then immediate operation to excise the nidus of infection are called for.

Recently, the hemolytic *Staphylococcus aureus* has made a reappearance after being rather uncommon for a few years and has now become a predominating organism. Experience has shown that surgical intervention should be timed according to the organism involved. For instance, the streptococcus family does not invade and destroy but, as seen in the pathology of skin lesions, tends to form a phlegmon rather than to penetrate deeply into the tissues, as does the staphylococcus family. In view of the characteristics of the staphylococcus to invade and destroy tissue, early surgical intervention and replacement after a few days of proper antibiotic therapy appear to be indicated if the patient is to be saved. Delaying surgery in this group of patients only allows for greater destruction of tissue, invasion of the myocardium, and destruction of the aortic or mitral annulus. The principle of the operation is to excise all visible infected tissue regardless of the reconstruction that must be carried out after removal. We use monofilament sutures placed in a mattress fashion over small portions of pericardium as buttresses and soak all sutures and the valvular prosthesis in proper antibiotic solution prior to insertion of the prosthesis as an adjunct to provide a sterile field.

Complications of Prosthetic Valves

Embolic complications of valve prostheses have already been discussed, as have infections and complications occurring during operation. The other major prosthetic valve complication is that of detachment. Synthetic sutures such as Dacron or Dacron coated with Teflon should be used. Using the Teflon pledget reinforced mattress suture method, as depicted in Figures 17–8 and 17–9, we have encountered only eight prosthetic leaks in the past 300 valve replacements. Attention should also be given to removing all calcium since sutures tend to cut through calcium over a long period of time.

Management of prosthetic detachment depends on a variety of factors. Usually only a small portion of the circumference of the prosthesis becomes detached and the occurrence is manifested only by a hemodynamically insignificant murmur. Such a patient should be followed up closely, but unless further detachment occurs, reoperation does not appear indicated. Should leakage around the prosthesis be hemodynamically significant, however, or associated with hemolytic anemia, exploration with correction of detachment or replacement with a new prosthesis should be considered seriously. If progressive detachment is noted, reoperation is mandatory before irreversible myocardial damage occurs, and often must be done as an emergency.

Hemolytic anemias associated with valve prostheses are usually secondary to leakage around aortic prostheses. Cineradiography with supravalvular injection of contrast media may be necessary for diagnosis. Under these circumstances correction of the leakage is indicated if the degree of hemolysis is significant. Rarely, hemolytic anemia occurs in the absence of prosthetic leakage. In these patients complete hematologic studies are indicated. Whenever significant hemolytic anemia develops, whether it is due to a faulty prosthesis or a paraprosthetic leak, the prosthesis must be removed and replaced with some other type. Cloth-covered struts on the more recent ball valves have produced significant anemia, particularly in the smaller sizes. Fracture of the cloth on the strut has also been incriminated. Whatever the cause, anemia that does not respond to iron administration and a significant period of medical management calls for consideration of immediate replacement of the prosthesis.

Postcardiotomy Syndrome

Fever, joint pains, pericardial effusion, pleural effusion, chest pain, and cardiac decompensation occurring in various combinations anywhere from 2 weeks to as long as 3 months after operations on the heart fall into a vague category originally described as the "postcommissurotomy syndrome." Numerous explanations have been suggested for these occurrences, including recurrence of rheumatic activity and low-grade endocarditis. One would be hard pressed, however, to accept recurrent rheumatic activity in patients after operations on the heart for congenital anomalies or trauma. Once these possibilities have been ruled out, no better diagnosis is usually reached than "postcardiotomy syndrome." Perhaps in the same category should be placed patients with similar symptoms following cardiac surgery, but with the addition of leukocytosis and splenomegaly.

In most instances symptomatic therapy, perhaps with the addition of salicylates, is all that is required. On occasion it would appear that the symptoms may be related to some sort of drug reaction, since they clear with discontinuation of all medications, especially antibiotics. Rarely, symptoms persist in spite of stopping all medications except aspirin every 4 hours around the clock, and under these circumstances empirical steroid therapy would appear to be indicated.

THE SECONDARY OPERATION

Increasingly, over the past few years, cardiac surgeons are being faced with the secondary operation to repair the heart on large numbers of individuals. The secondary operation has no relationship to the primary, in that all anatomic planes are obliterated and very tedious and careful dissection must be carried out to expose the heart. In our practice, only those portions of the heart that are to be operated upon are exposed during the secondary operation. Because a large number of valves used in the past have shown a tendency to destruction over the years, and because a significant number of patients undergoing coronary surgery will have either progression of the disease or obliteration of the vein grafts, surgeons will be involved much more in the future with these kinds of operations. If the approach is to the mitral valve, and if the sternal-splitting incision was used before, then that incision is used again; but if the x-rays show that there is obliteration of the retrosternal space to a severe degree, it might be more advisable to use a right anterior thoracotomy incision such as was utilized routinely many years ago for mitral valve replacement. With the thoracotomy incision, only the right atrium and the superior and inferior venae cavae need to be exposed. If the aortic valve is completely competent, it does not need to be isolated for clamping, and incision behind the atrial septum can be facilitated easily. Great care must be taken to avoid injury to the phrenic nerve on the right in either instance. If it is a mitral valve that is to be operated upon, cold solution can be instilled into the left ventricle by pouring it into the pericardial well; or, if one wishes to protect the right ventricle, continuous drip through a 14-gauge plastic needle inserted through the wall of the right ventricle can assist in protection also. If the sternal-splitting incision was utilized, and the aortic valve must be operated upon, only enough of the right ventricle is freed up to eliminate tension on inserting the sternum spreader, which might fracture the anterior wall of the right ventricle. The left ventricle is not isolated. The superior and inferior venae cavae are isolated for cannulation and passing tapes, and the same is done for the aorta, to the extent that a clamp can be placed about the ascending aorta up near the innominate, and an incision can be made above the aortic valve. Venting of the left ventricle can be carried out in the usual manner through the right superior pulmonary vein with a catheter passed down into the apex of the left ventricle (Fig. 17–17). Myocardial protection can be achieved by passing a 14-gauge cannula through the right ventricle, the septum, and into the left ventricle for a continuous drip of 4° C. Ringer's solution. In all of these cases we routinely order fresh frozen plasma and platelets for infusion after the procedure is finished, because of the multitude of bleeding points that cannot be controlled owing to lysis of adhesions. One unique problem that is occurring with greater frequency is the need to approach the circumflex artery in a secondary operation. A left posterior thoracotomy can be used with partial bypass established from the left atrium or femoral vein with return infusion into the femoral artery. The coronary vein bypasses then are sutured from the descending aorta to the circumflex artery, which are in almost absolute proximity at this point.

COMPLICATIONS OF CORONARY BYPASS SURGERY

Many complications are common to all open cardiac surgical procedures. We will deal primarily with those most commonly seen with coronary artery bypass grafting. The list of complications represents a personal experience with more than 3,000 coronary bypass operations spanning 11 years. The complications occur in two general categories, technical and biologic. Technical complications are those involving the vein, the aorta, the coronary anastomosis and the coronary artery, and the heart. Also included in this category are complications of redoing surgery, and postoperative problems such as arrhythmias and pulmonary embolism and neurologic, psychologic, and renal complications. Biologic complications involve vein graft changes over a period of time.

Technical Complications

The Vein

The harvesting of the saphenous vein originally utilized the upper leg. The upper leg saphenous vein usually presents a discrepancy in size between the vein and the coronary artery. This discrepancy led many surgeons to think that a decrease in the velocity of flow in the vein graft predisposed to thrombosis. The major problem with the large leg veins or varicose veins is that they may kink more easily. There is an increased incidence of local wound problems such as hematoma, fat necrosis, or infections when compared to the lower leg. The lower leg saphenous veins are more readily accessible just beneath the surface, more easily removed, and more similar to the coronary artery in size. Frequently, however, the saphenous nerve or lymphatics are damaged or removed. This leads to lower leg complications of paresthesias, numbness, and lymphedema. The lymphedema generally subsides within 2 to 3 months, but occasionally the paresthesias and numbness may be permanent. With meticulous attention paid to the removal of the vein by gentle handling and careful dissection, preservation of the saphenous nerve should be easily accomplished. The side branches of the vein grafts may be sutured; however, careless suturing or suturing by an inexperienced person may lead to kinking of the vein.

For the past seven years, we have used small, metallic "hemoclips" which are placed one millimeter off the main channel of the vein. These carefully applied hemoclips, although subject to being dislodged from the vein if not carefully applied, save time and lead to a smoother vein conduit. Obviously one has to pay attention to the application of the hemoclips. The handling of the veins must be meticulous and gentle. The flushing out of the veins with cold blood will preserve the intimal surface from desquamation. One must be careful not to overdistend the veins in an attempt to enlarge them or to overcome the spasm of smooth muscle, because, over the long term, this may lead to increased biologic problems. One must be careful to reverse the veins. We mark the proximal end of the veins with a suture to be sure that there is no failure to reverse the veins when placed in the aorta. We also utilize the technique of placing the veins on the aorta prior to bypass (Fig. 17–18). After heparinization, we allow the grafts to flow to check for any problems in forward flow. The use of these two techniques has prevented us from placing the vein in backward. If one performs distal anastomosis first, there is a greater chance

of failing to reverse the second or the third or subsequent bypasses and, again, there must be some systematic method for marking the proximal or distal end of the vein grafts so that this cannot occur.

Vein length is measured prior to bypass in our system, since the vein grafts are already attached to the aorta. If one does the distal anastomosis first, the exact length that will be needed can easily be attained in advance by measuring with a heavy, braided silk or some other measuring device from the site of proposed anastomosis to the aorta with the heart full and beating. In general, we make the right grafts always a little longer to allow for cardiac distention. The anterior grafts can be measured quite easily in situ prior to bypass and should not cause any difficulty. If they are too long, veins going to the anterior descending coronary artery may kink when the chest is closed; therefore, tacking down the vein will prevent kinking. However, tacking must also be undertaken carefully, because tacking of a vein graft may lead to a fulcrum point for kinking. The measurement for the circumflex is more difficult. If measuring is done when the heart is filled, it can be accomplished during bypass by clamping the vent and opening any tapes that have been used, letting the heart fill up, and measuring the distance back to the proposed site on the aorta. We have found that kinking of cir-

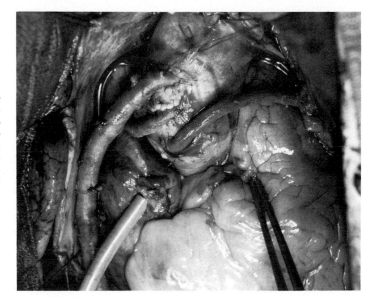

Figure 17–18 Picture shows three vein grafts sutured to aorta *prior* to cardiopulmonary bypass. Upper vein will go to right, middle to circumflex via transverse sinus, and lowermost vein over the pulmonary artery to the anterior descending coronary artery. All vein lengths can be determined prior to bypass with heart full and beating.

cumflex vein grafts can be prevented by using the transverse sinus as the route wherein the vein will lie just like the normal coronary artery.

If forced to attack the main circumflex artery, which is rare, the surgeon has to beware of entering the left atrium or the coronary vein. In this situation we recommend performance of the distal bypass first which will make the technical aspects much easier. If the distal portion of the bypass anastomosis is done first, perfuse the vein with cold blood to be sure that there is flow, eliminating failure of reversal. Locate the valve in the vein and excise the valve immediately, or redo it in the proper direction. If the vein is twisted, this can be determined and corrected and proper orientation marked with an adventitial clip. If at the conclusion of the procedure there is no flow or poor flow, make a transverse slit in the vein and pass a probe through the anastomosis to ascertain patency. The probe may also be passed down the vein and up the vein to be sure that there are no valves obstructing. The handling of the vein grafts is too often left to the most inexperienced member of the team, and he or she is frequently a victim of severe ennui with repeated work on the periphery. One cannot emphasize how important it is that the veins be harvested, handled, and sutured with the most meticulous care and gentleness to prevent later complications.

The Aorta

The handling of the aorta can become the most disastrous part of the operation. Disintegration of the aorta with placement of clamps or multiple placement of clamps can lead to major alterations in the procedure, i.e., replacement of the aorta or dissection. Therefore, prior to placing any cannulas or vein grafts into the aorta, the aorta is palpated carefully by the surgeon so that the graft or the arterial cannula is not placed into an atherosclerotic plaque. This possible complication may be anticipated by observation of a calcified aorta on chest x-ray. This type of aorta may be the source of showers of emboli or the origin of a dissection. If the side-biting clamp is placed too low on the aorta, this may lead to distortion and narrowing of the right coronary orifice and cardiac decompensation. It is our recommendation that the fewest possible side clampings and cross-clampings of the aorta be carried out. Therefore, we have been quite pleased over the last nine years with placing our grafts into the aorta prior to cardiopulmonary bypass and removing as little of the adventitia as possible. We remove the adventitia only in the area planned for suturing the vein bypass grafts on the aorta. After many clampings of the aorta the adventitia may be the saving strength. If the aorta is atherosclerotic, we recommend that one initiate bypass via another route, cool the patient or use cardioplegia, and cross-clamp the aorta to place the proximal anastomosis in soft spots that are more easily palpated when the aorta is cross-clamped. We also recommend the use of the left internal mammary artery in the presence of a poor aorta.

If the aorta is quite thick, we recommend the use of a large caliber, upper leg vein that will not be distorted during the proximal anastomotic suturing. Small veins may well end up being partially occluded by a thick aorta. Also, the innominate or subclavian artery may be used as a source of the proximal vein anastomosis. The surgeon may locate a single, suitable site in the aorta and then use Y grafts off one anastomosis. The use of snake grafts or multiple side-to-side or end-to-side anastomoses will cut down on the number of orifices. We also recommend that the pressure be lowered when one is doing the vein bypass grafts proximally in a poor aorta. A dissection may occur from the site of the vein graft, and this disaster may well lead to the surgeon's instituting all the procedures usually seen with dissection of the aorta to correct the problem. We do recommend that to prevent tension and splaying out of the vein graft the vein used to cover the anastomotic orifice in the aorta be larger than the orifice that is made in the aorta. An aorta punch is commonly used and with small veins this can splay out the vein so that it comes directly off the aorta at right angles, and it may kink as it proceeds to the distal site. We find that the aorta punch is helpful for novices; however, as one gains more experience it is seldom necessary for a proximal anastomosis.

The Coronary Anastomosis

The goal of a coronary distal bypass anastomosis is that one should try to bypass the last plaque in that artery. Certainly, this is desirable and has been shown to have the longest-lasting beneficial effects. However, there is often diffuse non-obstructive wall disease in addition to obstructions that were seen at angiography, and one has to compromise. Exposure for the coronary anastomosis is critical. The surgeon may cross-clamp the aorta, use the occluders described by Mullen et al.,[167] or use cardioplegia. Cardioplegia does have one side hazard of causing coronary artery spasm, which may then cause the surgeon to underestimate the size of a coronary artery as a potential bypass site. The judgment of looking at vessels is quite critical. If the vessel appears too small, one should spray it with papaverine diluted 1:3 with saline and examine it after a cross-clamping of the aorta at a time of maximal dilatation to estimate the size.

A plaque on the back wall of the coronary artery will often be found at the site of intended anastomosis after the artery is opened. Extend the anastomosis 2 to 3 mm above and below the plaque so bidirectional flow can be obtained. If the plaque is extensive, as is often seen in the right coronary artery, then use a bigger vein bypass and sew deeply below the plaque and have the ends of the anastomosis in normal coronary vessel. If the plaque should disintegrate, remove the disintegrated plaque and extend the anastomosis again. Occasionally, the plaque is so bad that as the surgeon places sutures, atherosclerotic material exudes from the artery. At this point we usually stop, carry out an endarterectomy manually, and if we do not obtain what we consider to be good tapered ends of the endarterectomy specimen or if a probe hits an obstruction, we are then forced to go to a point beyond the visible plaque for the coronary anastomosis.

One of the infrequent complications of the coronary anastomosis is cutting through the back wall. Mattress sutures are used to reapproximate the back wall, tying them on the outside. We then extend the anastomosis well beyond the site of the slit in the back of the artery. If fat on the heart prevents visualization of the coronary artery at the site of suitable size or if the artery is intramyocardial, make a distal 1½ mm. slit in the distal coronary vessel, pass the probe up, and dissect down to the probe. The distal arteriotomy can then be closed. The left anterior descending coronary artery (LAD) is usually to the right of the anterior vein in the midportion of the anterior descending artery. Proximally it may be beneath the anterior vein, and distally it can be anywhere. Another method to locate the LAD is to trace a known diagonal vessel back to the anterior descending artery. In the circumflex vessel we usually work on the marginal branches which may be intramyocardial. Look to the junction of the atrioventricular fat and red myocardium when retracting the heart. A red streak may be seen going laterally across the myocardium. The circumflex marginal arteries do not run parallel with veins but run almost perpendicular to them. Another technique that we have used to help us with checking the correctness of our anastomosis is to pass a probe in both directions just to test patency, not to pass it for any distance. This action will determine that there will be an outflow to the vein anastomosis and that no corner stitch has caught a side or back wall.

Protection of the Myocardium During Operation

Anesthesia in the presurgical portion of the operation should be designed to prevent fluctuations in blood pressure and thus, by stabilizing afterload and preload, prevent severe alterations in myocardial oxygen demands. Patients have been kept on propranolol. One gram of steroid is usually given as soon as the patient arrives in the operating room to stabilize the lysosomes of the myocardium to inhibit myocardial necrosis.

Occasionally during operation air enters the coronary arteries. If this occurs after the operation, the surgeon will see sudden left ventricular or right ventricular dilatation and non-contraction. Treatment is to put in the vent again and keep the myocardium decompressed, thus providing better endocardial perfusion. The vent may also remove any residual air. We have vented via the right superior pulmonary veins for the last eight years except in patients who have ventricular aneurysms, in which case we vent through the aneurysm resection. We also place an 18-gauge needle in the aorta with a portion of the needle barrel removed to release any trapped aortic air. Methods have been described using a needle or suction in the aorta. We also vent the bypass veins, and we do not perfuse established vein bypasses with bubbles in the blood solution. If despite this, one finds air in the coronary artery, it is best to resume cardiopulmonary bypass and vent the left ventricle, to create an empty, beating heart for 15 to 20 minutes. This will usually solve the problem. If this procedure is not carried out and the patient is given vasopressors, the situation may worsen and result in an infarction. Perioperative infarction is the most serious short-term complication of coronary bypass surgery. In the operating room it is manifested by low output, serious left ventricular arrhythmias, and occasionally death. The treatment is the intra-aortic balloon pump to decrease afterload. Use of the balloon pump is much preferable to giving vasopressors. The diagnosis of perioperative infarction in the postoperative period is ascertained by the use of CPK-MB fraction, which will peak in 12 to 18 hours. One must check that enzyme at the time rather than at 24 to 36 hours when it usually returns to normal. By combining a check of enzyme levels with EKG and pyrophosphate scans, the surgeon can usually ascertain almost completely whether there has been an infarction, and there can be some estimation of myocardial damage, if any. If any two of the three are positive, it is considered a perioperative infarct. A positive pyrophosphate scan alone is presumptive evidence of an infarction. The CPK-MB alone is highly suggestive if it is definitively elevated. New Q waves on EKG should prompt a full investigation.

The etiology of perioperative infarctions has been much discussed. We still feel that the long pump runs, induced ventricular fibrillation over a long period of time, diffuse disease, technical errors, and kinking of the veins when the chest is reapproximated are some of the major reasons. Prolonged ischemia for any reason without some form of myocardial protection is also an obvious cause. The current term in vogue is "inadequate myocardial protec-

tion." This leads to the question, "Protection from what?" It is obviously protection from ischemia and for this reason cold cardioplegic solutions were introduced to stop the heart in electromechanical dissociation so as to preserve intracellular substrates. Cold solution is quite effective alone if maintained, but potassium or magnesium may be added to this. For periods up to 60 to 80 minutes it is protective, but there is still a perioperative infarction rate associated with coronary bypass no matter what the method used. The cardioplegic solutions are not a panacea; indeed, their optimal composition, osmolarity, and pH are undergoing intensive investigation. Their long-term effects on the intima and methods of getting adequate solution beyond the coronary stenosis or obstruction are still being investigated. The washout of protective solution by noncoronary collateral flow is being compensated for by repeated perfusion of the solution. These solutions do not guarantee protection against sloppy or dilatory surgical technique.

We have been pleased by the control of perioperative infarction with a regimen that includes steroids and mannitol, moderate hypothermia to 28 to 30° C., limited aortic cross-clamping for periods of 15 minutes or less, and intermittent perfusion and defibrillation, venting and beating of the empty, non-working heart. The placing of the grafts onto the aorta prior to cardiopulmonary bypass allows us to establish new flow as soon as the first distal coronary graft is completed. The sequence of bypassing arteries is important in that the most ischemic *yet viable* myocardium receives its new blood supply immediately.

The problem of perioperative infarction may always be with us to some degree, and we must adopt a method to reduce ischemia to the myocardium while we accomplish our stated goal of revascularization. A game plan of attack, expeditiously performed, awareness of any factor leading to ischemia, and a system of protection against ischemia, will keep the perioperative infarction rate at an acceptable level of less than 3 per cent.

A precarious situation in coronary bypass surgery is presented by secondary operations for progression of disease in the native coronaries or in previously performed vein bypass grafts. Besides the pericardial adhesions and obliteration of usual landmarks, the adherence of the right ventricle and vein grafts to the sternum creates potential problems. Reoperation is performed by first exposing the femoral vessels and preparing them for rapid cannulation and partial bypass. The patient is hyperventilated and then as the saw is ready to divide the sternum, all expiratory pressure is removed, allowing the lungs and heart to drop away from the sternum. The oscillating saw or one with a narrow, lower edge is preferable so that the right ventricle will not be injured. The sternum is meticulously sharp-dissected away from the adhesions before any sternal retractor is inserted and opened. The aorta is exposed first, and then the right diaphragmatic surface. The adhesions between the inferior diaphragmatic surface and diaphragm are usually filmy and easily divided. The right atrium is freed next and the left ventricle is usually freed up after cardiopulmonary bypass is established. Adhesions anteriorly and laterally are best lysed by sharp dissection. There is usually a thin filmy adhesion over the entire epicardium that makes coronary vessel identification difficult. This can be wiped away with a sponge to make identification of vessels easier. Also, any previous vein grafts will lead one to the coronary anastomosis and the coronary artery. Some surgeons advocate closure of the pericardium to lessen secondary operative problems. This may lead to kinking of vein grafts, so we have often dissected down the pleura and laid it over the heart. A pericardial incision that allows the right ventricle to be covered is usually all that is necessary. After repeated bypass operations, entrance via the sternum is difficult no matter what was done, and for large circumflex vessels we have gained access to the circumflex coronary artery via a left thoracotomy. The coronary anastomosis is performed first and then the proximal anastomosis to the descending aorta is done. Circumflex marginal branches usually lie within one inch of the aorta. They require very little vein, an additional bonus in this setting. Venting via the left atrium and coronary occluders is helpful in this situation, which is uncommon. This approach provides excellent access to circumflex vessels and some diagonals.

As more coronary bypass procedures are performed and time passes, secondary operations will increase as atherosclerosis progresses in the veins and in the native circulation.

Postoperative Complications

ARRHYTHMIAS

Meticulous attention to blood gases and serum potassium levels will keep ventricular arrhythmias under control. If the patient had arrhythmias prior to operation, they will usually persist. Arrhythmias are seldom due to ischemia. If they can be shown preoperatively to be related to ischemia, they have a good chance of being relieved if ischemia is relieved.

Atrial fibrillation is the most common complication, occurring in 40 per cent of patients. Treatment is digitalis and Inderal, and only if fibrillation is persistent or associated with rapid atrial flutter is countershock necessary. Usually atrial fibrillation is a problem only in the presence of poor left ventricular function where loss of atrial "kick" may make a difference in cardiac output.

Renal insufficiency is more of a problem as the operated population grows older. We have found the pulsatile assist device most helpful for this problem, along with expeditious operation. Mannitol given preoperatively and intraoperatively, as well as early dialysis, if necessary, will tide these patients over.

PULMONARY EMBOLISM

Pulmonary embolism is a rare problem but is most often seen in patients who have had Judkin's-type catheterization and then remain in bed waiting for operation. There is no difference in Judkin's or Sones' technique if a patient is discharged the day following the catheterization and returns for later surgery. Heparin prophylaxis has not been shown to decrease the problem in two groups of about 200 patients. Also, we have noted that complications of heparin are not insignificant. The most unusual of heparin complications is sensitization of platelets to heparin by the catheterization or operation. Then with low-dose heparin,

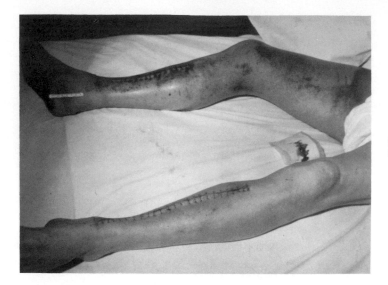

Figure 17–19 Heparin sensitivity led to venous thrombosis in right leg of patient. Normal left leg.

postoperatively, there actually is massive thrombosis due to heparin, detected by a falling platelet count. All patients on heparin or with a heparin flush in a "keep open," capped intermittent IV for drug administration undergo daily or every other day platelet counts. If platelets decrease in the presence of heparin, the tests for sensitization of the platelets are run and all heparin is stopped despite evidence of thrombosis or pulmonary emboli. Dextran and Coumadin are then administered (Fig. 17–19).

NEUROLOGIC COMPLICATIONS

The occurrence of neurologic complications remains the single most severe and devastating complication of coronary bypass surgery. These patients usually have atherosclerosis as a general problem, and it involves the aortic arch, carotids, and small vessels of the brain. These lesions may be occult or asymptomatic but made manifest by cardiopulmonary bypass and altered arterial pressure characteristics. A history of previous strokes or transient ischemic attacks demands preoperative carotid arteriograms; decisions are then made concerning the order of corrective procedures. The incidence of stroke syndrome is about 1 per cent. A review of 900 patients in our series shows that the history of a preoperative stroke was associated with a 5-year survival of only 31 per cent. Indeed, in any patient who has had a previous stroke, the decision for coronary bypass surgery should be made very carefully with full knowledge that there is a markedly lower 5-year survival.

The techniques of perfusion must be meticulous to avoid air or particulate emboli, and then other procedures must be considered when the patient has a calcified or degenerated aorta, which is a notorious source of emboli. Diabetics and patients over 70 years of age present an increased risk for perioperative stroke syndromes.

PSYCHOLOGICAL COMPLICATIONS

There has been a recent conference on the psychological complications following all cardiac surgery and, indeed, they are numerous. The fact that patients undergoing coronary bypass surgery go through a grief response with a period of depression has been well established, and there have been numerous psychological complications, including suicide. The fact that so many young people are undergoing coronary bypass surgery not only offers great hope but also, for the first time, forces the patient to acknowledge his or her mortality. This may wreak havoc with both the patient and his family. A frank preoperative discussion of what the patient may expect of the operation and the concordance of both the patient's expectations and surgeon's expectations will lead to a far more satisfactory postoperative result.

TABLE 17–1

0–6 months	Thrombosis
6 months–1 year	Intimal hyperplasia
1 year–3 years	Stability of vein grafts but with loss of 1–2% per year to occlusion from intimal hyperplasia
>3 years	Atheroma (incidence unknown)

Biologic Changes

In the first 6 postoperative months, vein grafts of autopsied patients reveal thrombosis as the most common pathologic change in vein grafts. In the period up to one year, the vein bypasses all develop intimal hyperplasia to some degree. It is safe to say that after one year, patients do well for about 3 years. At this time those with unusually virulent atherosclerosis will be found to have atherosclerotic plaques in the vein grafts. In the period from 3 to 11 years we have found the most common late vein graft lesion to be an atheroma. This is worst and most virulent in young, Type II hyperlipidemic patients, occurring often within one year of operation. The presence of Type II hyperlipidemia should give pause in consideration for coronary bypass. Table 17–1 contains a summary of the most commonly seen temporal vein graft changes.

There is as yet no proof that diet, exercise, or control of risk factors may diminish the incidence of vein graft sclerosis. There have been many simplistic proposed etiologies such as arterial pressures and distention of veins as the cause, but no one etiologic factor can explain all of the manifestations of this problem. The fact is that radial arteries also develop intimal hyperplasia and occlude when used as coronary bypass grafts. There is no question that meticulous, gentle care in harvesting and preparing the vein grafts is important in prevention of complications, but despite this, the greatest threat to the long-term patency of coronary vein bypass grafts is atherosclerosis.

CONCLUSION

This discussion has attempted to outline some of the complications peculiar to coronary bypass grafting and the methods devised to prevent them. The technical problems may be inherent to the surgical technique used as well as to the vagaries of atherosclerotic disease and its protean manifestations throughout the arterial system. The long-term benefits of vein-coronary bypass surgery will hinge on recognition of the fact that this procedure is palliative in nature and we have much to learn about atherosclerosis. This should not deter us from eliminating every possible complication so that each patient may receive the maximal benefit from the procedure.

"To preserve and renew is almost as noble as to create."

VOLTAIRE

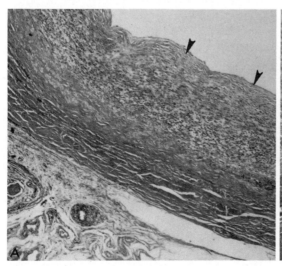 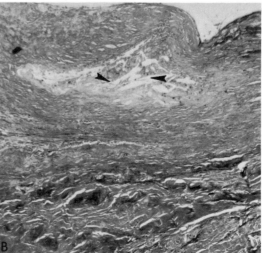

Figure 17–20 *A,* Venous intimal proliferation (arrows) at 18 months (× 160). *B,* Early atherosclerosis in vein with cholesterol clefts (arrows) at 4½ years (× 160).

OVERALL CARE OF THE CARDIOVASCULAR SURGICAL PATIENT

It has been said that once a major complication has become fully developed in an acutely ill patient, such as one undergoing cardiac surgery, the chance of losing the patient is very great. If the complication can be anticipated early, however, before it has become fully developed, there is a good chance of saving the patient. It is for this reason that complete physiological control of the patient must be maintained at all times. This can be done only by complete monitoring during surgery to provide data about the patient's cardiac output, rhythm, urinary output, and homeostasis as revealed by repeated blood gas analyses and oxygen and carbon dioxide saturation determinations during the entire period of anesthesia. These measures all must be continued in the intensive care unit, where nurses who are well grounded in physiology may watch a patient closely and record all data. In addition, they should be alert to indications of rhythm disturbances. Declining ventricular function may well be demonstrated by a falling urinary output and a widening arterial-venous difference. The latter is probably the first sign of declining cardiac output and should be vigorously treated with administration of inotropic agents, that is, increased digitalis or a drip of epinephrine, one ampule of 1:1000 in 250 ml. of fluid. If the decline in output is due to bradycardia, isoproterenol in diluted solutions may be used because of its vasodilatory, chronotropic, and inotropic properties. Any cardiac ventricular dysrhythmias that are potentially life-threatening are treated immediately with intravenous lidocaine.

Potassium levels are watched closely, and assisted ventilation with a volume respirator is instituted immediately after surgery in all patients. The volume respirator is adjusted to provide the tidal volume and minute volume that the patient needs along with the proper concentration of oxygen. The P_{CO_2} is held at a physiologic level by the volume delivered to the patient and the P_{O_2} is also well controlled by changing the concentration of oxygen. The cuffed endotracheal tube is left in place and assisted ventilation with the volume respirator is continued until the patient shows evidence that he can take over complete respiratory function himself without assistance. The endotracheal tube, of course, provides an easy means to cleanse the tracheobronchial tree, and frequent suctioning is carried out while the tube is in place. After the tube is removed, tracheal toilet is carried out by means of a nasotracheal catheter. If these measures are taken, bronchoscopy is usually unnecessary. Constant awareness of the complications of endotracheal tubes is mandatory. Figure 17–27 shows one such complication. In Figure 17–27, insertion of the tube into the right main-stem bronchus has resulted in complete atelectasis of the left lung. Also, the cuff of a tube can be over-inflated to the point of collapse of the tube, resulting in tracheal obstruction.

With these methods and with alertness on the part of the physicians and the nursing personnel, complications can be kept to a minimum or, if they do occur, can be corrected early. The entire approach, then, is maintenance of the patient in a favorable physiological state, with adequate monitoring to detect early changes and correct them immediately, before a full-blown complication occurs.

SURGERY OF THE GREAT VESSELS

Advances in surgery of aneurysms and constrictive lesions of the aorta provided a new area of surgical endeavor that introduced unique anatomic and physiological problems in surgical therapy. Whereas in the past, indirect or palliative measures were usually recommended in surgery of aortic lesions, at present emphasis is placed on a curative approach usually directed at excision of the lesion and restoration of aortic function either by graft replacement or by utilizing some type of bypass procedure. At the turn of the century Carrel demonstrated experimentally that successful resection of the thoracic aorta in animals was possible and that the resulting defects in the aorta could be successfully repaired by vessel grafts. Gross in 1948 first used aortic homografts clinically for replacement of defects in the thoracic aorta, and his results were satisfactory. Indeed, at first aortic homografts were considered to be the most satisfactory replacement material, and many successful operative procedures using either preserved or lyophilized freeze-dried grafts were performed. However, many times these homografts deteriorated rapidly and either developed new aneurysms or ruptured. This led to the development in the late 1950's of synthetic prostheses in the form of knitted or woven tubes of Dacron, Teflon, or other materials. Among the advantages of the synthetic grafts over homografts are ready availability, ease of sterilization, uniformity of strength, and ease of application. Undoubtedly, better materials will become available as more experience accumulates, and ultimately complications related to the graft itself will be eliminated. Although graft materials and other technical details may improve in time, this new surgical concept of a definitive approach toward aortic lesions with emphasis upon restoration of circulatory function will remain firmly established.

Several factors are important in application of this surgical principle to the descending thoracic aorta. The extent to which collateral vessels have formed around the aortic lesion deserves special consideration. Occlusive lesions characteristically produce a much stronger stimulus to development of collateral vessels than do aneurysms, and some occlusive lesions produce more extensive collateral vascular networks than do others. Congenital coarctation, for example, is associated with a rich collateral circulation that begins to develop even before birth. Acquired lesions may also develop collateral vessels, but to a lesser degree than is noted with congenital coarctation. Although in a few massive aneurysms involving the descending thoracic aorta some increase in tolerance to ischemia of tissue located distally may be noted, in general the collateral blood supply is inadequate to prevent damage during a period of temporary aortic occlusion. Blood supply to the spinal cord and central nervous system assumes a vital role in such surgical techniques, and therefore a consideration of normal arterial anatomy is important.

Blood Supply to Spinal Cord and Brain

Studies of the normal blood supply to the spinal cord and brain help to elucidate some of the neurologic complications that may occur after operation. Wide variations are demonstrable in distribution of segmental arterial supply, and the paucity of and small size of the arterial channels is usually striking.

The anterior spinal artery provides the majority of arterial supply to the cord and is located along the anterior midline and sends branches into the substance of the cord. A pair of smaller posterior spinal arteries lies on each side of the cord posteriorly, supplying only a portion of the posterior columns and posterior horn, whereas the more important anterior spinal artery supplies the remaining three-fourths of the cord substance. Various radicular arteries supply these cord vessels along its course through the vertebral spinal canal. In the cervical region the vertebral arteries, posterior inferior cerebellar arteries, and segmental branches contribute to the arterial supply through the spinal vessels. In the thoracic and lumbar regions radicular branches supply the spinal arteries, but since these vessels are scarce, the reserve blood supply is precarious. Fewer than one-fourth of the nerve roots are accompanied by arterial branches, and most of these are in the cervical and upper thoracic regions. Usually six to eight radicular branches supply the vertebral arteries, and three to five of these may be in the cervical and upper thoracic regions. Between C8 and T9 only two unilateral and inconsistently located small branches supply this long segment of cord. Important branches contributing significantly to the anterior spinal artery are usually located between T11 and L3 (usually at L2). Adams has stressed the importance of this arteria radicularis magna in supplying the lumbosacral swelling of the cord and believes that sacrifice of this vessel by aortic resection leads almost inevitably to neurologic sequelae. Another small vessel may enter below this point from L4 or L5. The smaller posterior spinal arteries receive no radicular contributions below the cervical region and are entirely dependent upon the anterior spinal artery. Since the anterior spinal artery is small in the midportion of the cord where few segmental or radicular arteries are located, the lumbosacral cord must receive blood segmentally. Recent studies show that the bronchial arteries may provide a major portion of the blood supply to the anterior spinal artery.

These anatomic studies emphasize the vulnerability of the lower thoracic and upper lumbar portions of the cord to aortic cross-clamping. Moreover, they indicate that no single segmental branch, if preserved, may be relied upon to maintain an adequate supply to the cord either during or after operation. Studies by Dawes et al., however, showed that in dogs prolonged clamp time or division of several intercostals did not consistently cause cord damage. The only significant factor was total heparinization of the animal, which reduced the incidence of cord damage. It should be emphasized, however, that in all human patients clamp time must be kept to a minimum and, if extensive dissection and repair are necessary, a bypass shunt of some kind should be utilized.

Blood supply to peripheral nerves may be compromised during aortic surgery, but for the most part this is an important consideration only in procedures upon the abdominal aorta and peripheral arteries. Such complications are usually associated with embolism and thrombosis of peripheral vessels rather than with the ischemic effects of temporary vascular occlusion by cross-clamping.

In considering the risk of neurologic damage during operations on the descending thoracic aorta, several factors may be enumerated which are important in preservation of the integrity of the central nervous system: (1) duration of aortic or arterial occlusion, (2) level of aortic occlusion, (3) age of the patient, (4) extent and nature of the resected specimen, (5) presence of collateral arterial supply, (6) anatomic variations in blood supply to the spinal cord or brain, (7) adequacy of cardiac output, (8) number of arteries occluded or sacrificed, and (9) measures used to minimize spinal cord or cerebral ischemia.

Experience has revealed that organ systems other than the central nervous system tolerate temporary ischemia from temporary occlusion of the descending thoracic aorta for periods sufficient to permit excision of the lesion without serious effect. Thus ischemia or necrosis of the kidneys, liver, intestines, or other structures is rarely encountered in surgery of the thoracic aorta. Of course, this may not be true if the period of occlusion extends beyond reasonable limits of 1 to 2 hours. All these considerations are important in providing for a successful aortic resection.

TECHNICAL CONSIDERATIONS

Aneurysms

In general, two types of surgical procedures are used for aneurysms of the thoracic aorta; namely, tangential excision with lateral aortorrhaphy and resection of the involved section of aorta with graft replacement. For sacciform aneurysms, tangential excision with lateral aortorrhaphy may be done (Fig. 17–21). A clamp is placed tangentially across the neck of the aneurysm, and the sac distal to the clamp is excised; this permits repair of the aorta without encroachment on its lumen. This is a particularly useful method of dealing with sacciform lesions in the ascending aorta and arch, since it precludes the necessity of temporary arrest of the circulation which, at a high aortic level, could easily produce lethal ischemic damage to the brain as well as left ventricular dilatation and fatal cardiac failure.

Fusiform aneurysms of the thoracic aorta that involve the entire circumference of the vessel present a special problem, since extirpation requires removal of an entire segment of the aorta. Aneurysmectomy for such lesions presents two serious problems: one is concerned with the ischemic effect on tissues distal to the point of aortic occlusion, and the other with bridging the defect created by aortic resection. The latter problem is mostly solved for the present by the use of synthetic graft material. Solution of the former problem, however, remains the critical factor in successful performance of the operative procedure. A number of factors

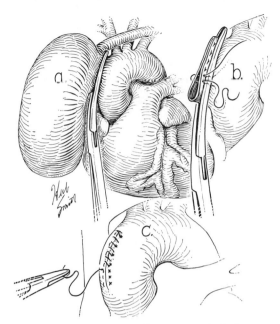

Figure 17–21   Drawings illustrating method of tangential incision and lateral aortorrhaphy for saccular aneurysms of thoracic aorta. *a,* Clamp placed across neck of aneurysmal sac. *b,* Aneurysm excised and sac closed with horizontal mattress sutures distal to the clamp. *c,* Clamp removed and closure reinforced distal to mattress sutures by continuous suture. Since aortic occlusion is unnecessary, ischemic damage to central nervous system does not occur. Care must be taken to prevent dislodgment of fragments of laminated thrombus or cellular debris during dissection or manipulation of aneurysm which may lead to cerebral, mesenteric, or saddle aortic embolism.

influence the degree of ischemic damage occurring during the period of temporary interruption of aortic circulation. The level of occlusion is of particular importance, since even brief periods of occlusion of the ascending aorta or the transverse arch of the aorta are likely to be fatal. In this locality, therefore, resection of aneurysms is accomplished by means of complicated temporary bypass grafts sutured into the vessel or by use of the pump oxygenator for temporary cardiopulmonary bypass. Temporary occlusion of the thoracic aorta distal to the left carotid or left subclavian artery is not as critical and may be tolerated for longer periods of time without producing fatal consequences. The critical period of temporary occlusion of the descending thoracic aorta before serious ischemic damage to the spinal cord occurs is approximately 15 to 20 minutes. Since more time than this is usually necessary to excise such lesions,

provision must be made to protect the spinal cord from ischemic damage.

Use of the simple bypass shown in Figure 17–22 obviates this problem. Over the past couple of years, we have abandoned the use of extracorporeal circulation and femoral-to-femoral or left atrial-to-femoral bypass in surgery for descending aneurysms of the thoracic aorta. Instead, a simple heparin-impregnated cannula, first described by Gott, is placed either in the left subclavian artery in its proximal portion or into the arch of the aorta through purse-string sutures just as is done in cannulating the ascending aorta for total cardiopulmonary bypass (Fig. 17–22). The other end of the cannula is placed into the descending aorta at a point beyond the aneurysm; this provides a shunt that can be placed in a matter of a few minutes and serves satisfactorily while the aneurysm is removed. The greatest advantage in using the Gott shunt is that the patient does not need to be heparinized. The pressure in the ascending aorta and aortic arch and in the brachial cephalic vessels is controlled during the time of pressure with a nitroprusside drip. If the pressure climbs too high, nitroprusside is simply administered to reduce it to a proper level. This simple bypass method avoids the problem of sequestration of blood in the lower or upper parts of the body as was seen with left atrial-to-femoral or femoral-to-femoral bypass in the past. Complications can be reduced significantly with this method.

Several procedures have been advocated and used successfully to minimize the complications of spinal cord ischemia. Induced general body hypothermia was used for a time but has been discarded because of added complications, including ventricular fibrillation, respiratory complications in elderly patients, and postoperative hemorrhage.

Dissecting aneurysms (Type III) of the descending thoracic aorta are usually treated with medication for hypotension unless complications develop. If leakage of blood into the left chest occurs, then these aneurysms may be controlled by the same technique of excision with graft replacement. An effort is made to resect that portion of the aorta containing the greatest fusiform swelling, since this usually represents the point of origin of the lesion. After

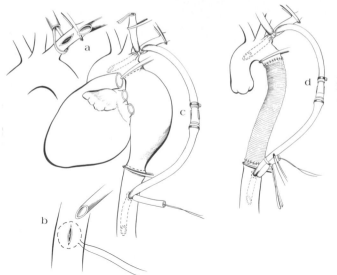

Figure 17–22 An illustration to show the use of a simple bypass for resection of aneurysm of the descending thoracic aorta. In a, an incision is made into the left subclavian artery and the cannula is slipped into place and held by a tourniquet. The other end of the beveled cannula is then placed into the descending thoracic aorta anywhere above the diaphragm, as shown in b. In d, with the completed graft in place, the cannula is simply removed. The opening in the subclavian artery is repaired while it is totally occluded proximally and distally, and a Beck clamp is placed on the descending thoracic aorta to oversew the incision into the aorta at this point.

this area has been resected, the separated layers of the aortic wall located distally may be repaired, after which a graft is used to bridge the aortic defect. The question as to the optimal method of dealing with the false lumen in these cases has not been settled, since certain pathologic features of the lesion may produce an unusually strong tendency to cause ischemic damage to the cord after operation. In some instances the blood supply to the cord is derived from the outer false lumen, and closing off this tract from the aortic flow may lead to ischemia of the cord. Similar complications in the renal arteries may also follow surgical repair of dissecting aneurysm.

Fusiform aneurysms of the ascending aorta and transverse aortic arch present a complicated technical problem, since special consideration must be given to providing cerebral circulation and to relieving left ventricular strain during the period of temporary aortic cross-clamping at this proximal level. Two methods of controlling these factors have been used clinically for such lesions. If the aneurysm extends to a proximal level close to the aortic valve, complete cardiopulmonary bypass must be used with a pump oxygenator. Cardioplegic solution perfused into the coronary arteries for myocardial protection during an anoxic period and carotid perfusion may be necessary, depending upon the extent of the lesion. Occasionally, aortic valve regurgitation associated with extreme dilatation of the valve

annulus requires concomitant replacement of the valve with a prosthesis. For lesions that arise at least 4 cm. above the aortic valve, a system of temporary shunts may be used as a bypass during the period of temporary aortic and carotid occlusion. Although tedious and time-consuming, this latter method appears to be better tolerated in patients from both a cardiac and a cerebral standpoint and should be used when technically feasible.

Dissecting aneurysms arising in the ascending aorta may be limited to the ascending aorta or extend distally as far as the aortic bifurcation or even into the legs. An unusual problem that may occur with chronic dissecting aneurysms is filling of the lumen all the way back to the area of anastomosis. Even though the distal and proximal portions are oversewn so that the false lumen is obliterated, the false lumen from the distal reentry may fill back to the area of anastomosis under pressure. This may cause continued bleeding at the time of operation or the continuation of false aneurysm. It is hoped, of course, that obliteration of the pressure from the proximal source will permit clotting and closure by fibrous tissue reaction of this false channel. The intimal tear from which these aneurysms arise is usually located just above the aortic valve annulus and allows prolapse of the valve with resultant valvular regurgitation. Correction requires use of temporary cardiopulmonary bypass, often on an

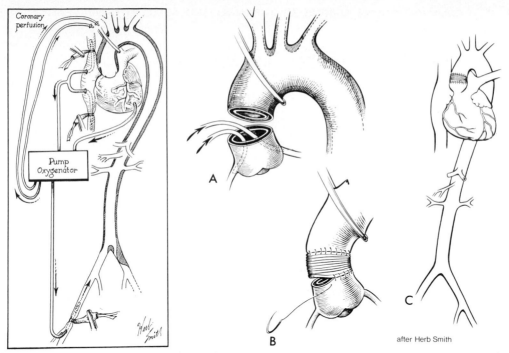

Figure 17–23 Drawings illustrating technique of surgical management of dissecting aneurysm arising just distal to aortic valve annulus and extending through abdominal aorta into left common iliac artery. *Inset,* Extent of aneurysm and connections to pump oxygenator. *A,* Aorta, transected below the clamp, and coronary arteries are perfused with cardioplegic solution. *B,* A piece of woven Dacron graft is interposed and the suture lines usually reinforced with Teflon felt. *C,* With the graft in place and the false lumen obliterated, fibrosis is allowed to obliterate distal extent of dissection.

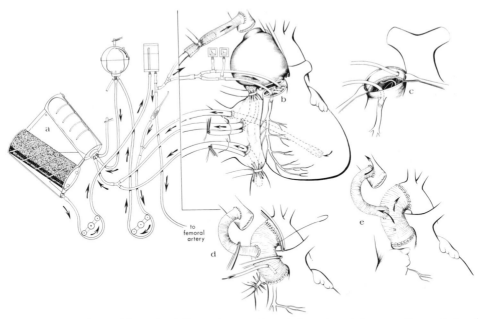

Figure 17–24 A complex problem of calcific aortic stenosis and dissection of the ascending aorta involving the innominate artery. Complete pump-oxygenator bypass is necessary to manage this problem in the circuit, as seen in *a.* The left ventricle is vented and coronary perfusion is carried out in both right and left coronary arteries. A 1-cm. graft is sewn end to side to the innominate artery and the aneurysm is resected. The calcific aortic valve is replaced with a Bjork-Shiley prosthesis with coronary perfusion carried out as seen in *c.* A graft is then used to replace the ascending aorta and a single coronary perfusion cannula is placed just above the coronary ostia and prosthetic aortic valve with the graft clamp. This provides adequate coronary perfusion during the completion of the procedure. The end-to-side graft to the innominate is then sewn end to side to the main ascending aortic graft as seen in *d.* In *e,* the appearance at the end of the procedure is shown.

407

emergency basis. When the dissection extends beyond the limits of the ascending aorta, the area of intimal tear is repaired, with resuspension of the aortic valve, after which the aorta is repaired (Fig. 17–23).

Obliteration of the false lumen is then dependent upon subsequent fibrosis. If the dissecting process is limited to the ascending aorta, the entire area of dissection is excised and replaced with a graft. Concomitant re-

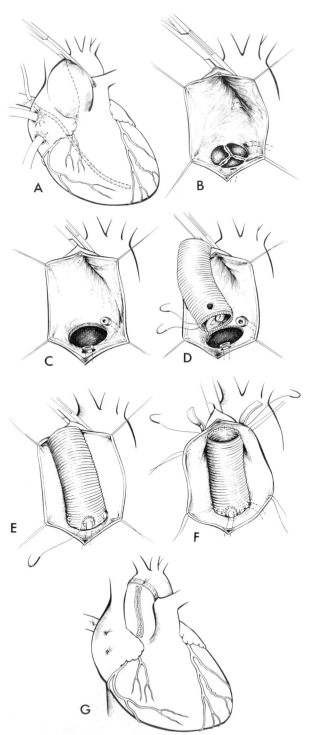

Figure 17–25 Drawing illustrates composite graft replacement of ascending aorta. *A,* Patient cannulated through femoral artery, right atrium and left ventricle cannulated. Line of incision in aorta is seen. *B,* Aorta open and valve and coronaries visualized and infused with cardioplegia. *C,* Aortic valve excised and right and left coronary "buttons" prepared (sometimes it is not necessary to cut out "buttons"). *D,* Valve ring of Bjork-Shiley composite graft sewn in routine fashion. *E,* Left coronary has been sewn in place and right coronary anastomosis being completed. *F,* Both coronary anastomoses complete and distal anastomosis begun. *G,* Completed procedure with aorta sutured together outside the graft for better hemostasis.

placement of an incompetent aortic valve with a valve prosthesis is often indicated in this group. Management of a case of this kind is depicted in Figure 17–24. The patient was a 26-year-old man with congenital aortic stenosis with calcification. Dissection over a large area in the ascending aorta had produced a large fusiform aneurysm that involved the innominate artery. The aortic valve was replaced by a Bjork prosthesis and the ascending aorta and the innominate artery were replaced by grafts as shown in the figure. When the valve had been replaced and the proximal anastomosis of the graft replacing the ascending aorta had been established, a clamp was placed in the midpoint of the graft and coronary perfusion was provided by a single cannula placed into the graft proximal to the clamp. An end-to-side anastomosis was used to perfuse the innominate artery during the clamp time, and ultimately this graft was sewn end-to-side to the ascending aortic graft. For aneurysms extending proximally to the aortic valve, involving both coronary arteries and causing aortic insufficiency, a composite aortic valve Dacron graft prosthesis may be used, with the coronaries being sutured directly into the side of the graft (Fig. 17–25).

Constrictive Lesions

Lesions that produce an obstruction to circulation in the descending aorta may be either congenital or acquired. The usual congenital coarctation occurs in the isthmic region of the aortic arch where it joins the descending thoracic aorta just distal to the origin of the left subclavian artery and the ductus botalli. In typical coarctations only a short segment of aorta is obstructed, and local excision with an end-to-end anastomosis is the procedure of choice (Fig. 17–26, *a*). If the constricted area extends over several centimeters or is associated with local lesions such as aneurysms or atherosclerotic plaques, a longer segment of aorta must be resected with graft replacement (Fig. 17–26, *b*). Aortic anastomosis should not be done under tension, and grafts should be used to prevent unnecessary strain upon the aortic suture line.

Acquired constrictive lesions of the tho-

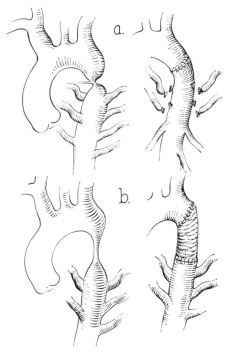

Figure 17–26 Drawings illustrating technique of repair of typical postductal coarctation of aorta. *a*, End-to-end anastomosis performed with division of intercostal vessels. In patients more than 25 years of age this technique may lead to complication from hemorrhage or aneurysm formation if tension on anastomosis is present. Size of anastomosis may be compromised by attempt to pull ends of aorta together. Division and ligation of intercostal vessels also may be tedious, and serious hemorrhage may occur. *b*, Graft used to bridge aortic defect without tension on anastomosis, which is of adequate size. Intercostal vessels not disrupted. This technique is used in avoiding complications following operation for coarctation.

racic aorta are relatively rare and, in general, occur in the descending thoracic aorta or in the supradiaphragmatic region of the thoracic aorta. These lesions may be the result of a localized segmental aortitis of unknown origin that produces a segmental atherosclerosis and obliterative process in the aorta. The length and position of the process vary, but in the majority of cases the involved segment measures several centimeters or more in length and is located in the middle or terminal third of the descending thoracic aorta. Segmental excision of the aortic segment with graft replacement is the optimal method of dealing with these lesions. Often a dense inflammatory reaction is present around the lesion which makes dissection and mobilization of the aorta difficult. A favorable feature of acquired constrictive lesions in contrast to aneurysms is the presence of an adequate collateral network of vessels that provide circulation to the tissues distally. Thus, in these cases if the lesion is producing complete aortic occlusion, there is no need for haste in completing the resection and grafting after the clamps have been applied. Furthermore, there is no necessity for using shunts, hypothermia, or bypasses to protect distal tissues during periods of temporary occlusion. Under these conditions emphasis may be placed upon a complete and precise restoration of a pulsatile distal blood flow.

Aortic Arch Anomalies

Surgical treatment of so-called aortic vascular ring is another development in vascular surgery that deserves brief mention. The most frequent types are the double aortic arch, right aortic arch with left ligamentum arteriosum, anomalous innominate artery, anomalous left common carotid artery, and aberrant subclavian artery. Since the symptoms are usually related to tracheal or esophageal obstruction, operation is directed toward relief of the constriction by division of the least vital arterial element in the ring. Aspiration pneumonia is frequently present in small infants before operation and may lead to complications afterwards. Failure to relieve the tracheal constriction causes respiratory stridor after operation and possibly tracheitis. These complications in infants are managed by oxygen administration and steam inhalations but if the work of breathing is forced, operative intervention is indicated.

COMPLICATIONS

A number of factors contribute to the risk and consequent frequency of postoperative complications in patients with disease involving the thoracic aorta. The critical anatomic location and vital function that the aorta serves impose certain technical obstacles that tend to make recovery complicated. For example, the extensive surgical incisions used in such operations, which often involve both hemithoraces, may be poorly tolerated even in young and other-

wise healthy patients. Many patients with aortic lesions are in the sixth or seventh decade of life, and such patients do not tolerate thoracic operations well. Moreover, other complicating features such as cardiorespiratory disease, generalized arteriosclerosis, renal insufficiency, arterial hypertension, and so on, are frequently present in elderly patients. Although these complicating features are frequent in patients with aneurysm, they are less important in patients with occlusive lesions, who tend to be younger and better surgical risks.

Complications following operations on the thoracic aorta are therefore relatively frequent, and in many instances more than one complication occurs in one patient. Under these circumstances one complication usually aggravates another. Early recognition and diagnosis of complications are of great importance to successful outcome of the operation itself.

Neurologic Complications

Since the central nervous tissue is vulnerable to ischemic damage, neurologic sequelae assume great importance in surgery of the thoracic aorta. For the most part the lesions are produced by anoxia or ischemia during operation, but may also be due to embolic or thrombotic phenomena or to focal hemorrhage occurring after operation has been completed.

BRAIN INJURY. Evidence of brain damage after operation is manifested by confusion, coma, or the presence of a completely decerebrate state. Hemiparesis or hemiplegia suggests ischemic damage to one hemisphere, usually from interference with carotid circulation. Cerebral embolism produces similar manifestations, however, and the source of the emboli is usually discovered in the aortic lesion. Fragments of intraluminal thrombi in an aneurysm are sometimes dislodged during the aortic dissection, clamping, and other manipulations and enter the orifices of major arterial branches. Air may be introduced into a system of extracorporeal shunts and cause cerebral damage from air embolism. In elderly patients with vascular occlusive lesions of an arteriosclerotic nature in the brain, circulatory stasis from whatever cause may lead to cerebral thrombosis during or after operation. Temporary postoperative psychosis of several days' duration is relatively common after operation in such patients, and the cause is often attributable to presence of cerebral hypoxia during or after operation. In patients with aneurysm or coarctation of the aorta, carotid arterial pressure may become extremely elevated during the aortic cross-clamping. Under these circumstances focal or widespread hemorrhage may result in serious cerebral damage.

SPINAL CORD INJURY. Varying degrees of neurologic damage may follow temporary interruption of circulation through the descending thoracic aorta. In some instances vital segmental arteries are resected along with the specimen, making neurologic recovery impossible. Usually the damage is inflicted upon the lumbosacral area of the spinal cord, producing weakness or paralysis in the lower extremities and thighs. Occasionally, in the more severe cases, the cord damage extends as high as the proximal dorsal or the distal cervical segments, but fortunately this is uncommon. Neurologic sequelae may appear as a delayed phenomenon 48 or 72 hours after operation. This suggests a delayed thrombosis of spinal vessels possibly precipitated by sacrifice of smaller segmental vessels. Such delayed paralysis has followed operation for acute dissecting aneurysm. In severe or extensive spinal cord damage death from spinal shock may ensue within a relatively brief period after operation. In these cases peripheral vascular collapse is common and may or may not respond to vasopressor substances. Atony of the urinary bladder and paralytic ileus frequently accompany the motor and sensory loss.

MANAGEMENT. Management of neurologic complications is usually difficult, since specific therapeutic measures are not very effective once the neurologic damage has occurred. General supportive measures should be used in an effort to assist the patient through the early postoperative period. A complete neurologic examination should be made and recorded in the patient's chart for medical and possibly legal reasons. Brain damage usually manifests itself immediately after operation. Soon after recognition of the complication a careful survey should be made of carotid artery

circulation to determine the presence of pulsation in all vessels. An obstruction in the cervical portion of the carotid artery should be recognized early and, if discovered, should be removed as promptly as possible under local anesthesia, since delay usually leads to permanent damage. If labored or inadequate pulmonary ventilation appears as a result of neurologic damage, respiratory assistance is needed and should be provided by an appropriate respiratory assister or tank respirator. Tracheostomy usually facilitates care of the seriously incapacitated patient in providing a reliable airway permitting effective removal of secretions by aspiration.

Since neurologic damage is often associated with vascular collapse and hypotension, vasopressor agents such as Neo-Synephrine or norepinephrine should be used to maintain a relatively normotensive state. Adequate but not excessive blood and fluid replacement is also important. Convulsions are controlled by intravenous administration of pentobarbital as a slow intravenous drip of 0.5 per cent solution. This therapy may be supplemented later by other anticonvulsants such as phenobarbital or phenytoin (Dilantin). If cerebral edema appears, evidenced by papilledema, an attempt may be made to reduce the fluid content of the brain. The most effective method used for this purpose seems to be a mannitol-induced osmotic diuresis, or ethacrynic acid and furosemide may be used. Diuretics and restriction of salt intake are also used for control of cerebral edema as soon as any cerebral ischemia is suspected. Dexamethasone sodium phosphate, 8 mg. every 8 hours, is given intravenously. We have also found that in suspected cerebral hypoxia or air embolus, immediate treatment in the hyperbaric chamber in some instances has significantly reduced the permanent residuals of such catastrophes.

Spinal cord injury is usually first suspected when the patient is unable to move his legs after operation. Deep tendon reflexes are usually absent or sharply reduced during the early phase, but may become hyperactive later if some recovery occurs. Weakness of abdominal muscles is noted in more extensive cord lesions, and the paraplegia may extend into intercostal muscles. In these instances respiratory support with an artificial or mechanical respirator becomes necessary. Sensory loss may also occur. Discrimination of pain and temperature depends upon integrity of the anterior portion of the spinal cord supplied by the anterior spinal artery. Deep sensation and position sense are supplied by portions of the cord nourished by the posterior spinal artery, and these functions may be present or absent at different levels of the cord. Accurate appraisal of these findings by careful neurologic examination is important in determination of the extent of damage and in observation of the progress of recovery.

Patients with extreme neurologic damage usually require an extensive supportive program, including gastric and intestinal decompression, urinary bladder drainage by indwelling catheter, removal of tracheobronchial secretions, prevention of cutaneous compression ulcers, and so forth. Paralyzed muscles should be supported during the acute stages to prevent overstretching, and joints should be manipulated to prevent stiffness. At the first sign of recovery, attention should be directed at rehabilitation through an active physical therapy program. Often patients who appear to have severe neurologic damage immediately after operation may make a striking recovery with little if any neurologic residual.

Renal Complications

Renal complications from ischemia are uncommon after operation for lesions of the thoracic aorta, since temporary occlusion of the thoracic aorta is usually well tolerated by the kidneys for periods of 1 hour or more even without the use of a pump bypass. If the pump bypass is used, measurable aortic pressure between 10 and 30 mm. Hg may be provided by collateral vessels which is apparently sufficient to provide minimal renal function during the period of aortic occlusion. Morris has demonstrated clinically that if a minimal pressure of 30 mm. is maintained in the distal segment, a measurable glomerular function and urinary output may continue during the period of bypass. Severe oliguria or anuria following operation usually implies the presence of some factors other than ischemia as their cause. Among factors to be considered are the presence of nephrosclerosis or arteriosclerotic vascular changes ex-

isting before operation, particularly in elderly patients. Furthermore, in operations of this type large blood transfusions are frequently used, and the possibility of a hemolytic reaction or incompatibility of a blood transfusion must be considered.

Management of renal complications is frequently successful unless the renal damage is severe. It is well known that urinary output is suppressed after extensive operations of any type, and this fact is not unique to aortic surgery. Normal function usually returns after 24 to 72 hours. In aortic operations an indwelling catheter should be used to observe the renal function from hour to hour. Repeated serum electrolyte determinations should be obtained, since in some instances adjustment of electrolyte content of the patient's plasma may cause a dramatic return of renal function. If severe oliguria or anuria occurs, an effort should be made to control the total volume of fluid intake to prevent formation of edema from fluid retention. In the presence of mounting creatinine and serum potassium levels peritoneal and gastric lavage with appropriate rinsing solutions may be considered. In advanced cases the artificial kidney may be used to dialyze the patient's blood.

Vascular Complications

Thromboembolic phenomena may occur, particularly in patients undergoing operation for arteriosclerotic or large syphilitic aneurysm of the thoracic aorta. Thrombi and atherosclerotic debris may be dislodged during the surgical manipulation and may lodge in major vessels distal to the area of aortic repair. Embolism of the carotid vessels produces serious brain damage leading to hemiplegia, total paralysis, or even death in the more severe cases. Mesenteric embolism may lead to intestinal gangrene. Large emboli may lodge at the aortic bifurcation, producing a saddle embolus and extensive aortic thrombosis. Smaller emboli may enter the iliac, femoral, popliteal, or tibial vessels, producing ischemic damage to the lower extremities. Occasionally thrombosis may occur distal to the point of occlusion, being aggravated by stasis and lowered blood pressure during the period of occlusion. These complications are not frequent, and in general, successful management depends upon prompt recognition of the problem with surgical removal of the embolus or thrombus if possible. The introduction of the Fogarty catheter has simplified this procedure, which can be done under local anesthesia in a critically ill patient.

Arteritis following correction of coarctation of the aorta, or the so-called postcoarctation syndrome, is an unusual and striking complication of successful correction of this malformation. The cause of this complication, which is being recognized with greater frequency, has been variously described, but most observers believe that it is a consequence of sudden alteration in pressure relations in the relatively unsupported mesenteric arterial system. The arterial lesions are usually limited to vessels that arise from the aorta distal to the level of coarctation. The pathogenesis of arterial necrosis following aortic resection for coarctation has been well described by Benson and Sealy. Increased pulse pressure results in greater distention of the arteries, which results in intimal and periarterial damage. The lesions that finally result are often indistinguishable from those of periarteritis nodosa. Other factors have been implicated besides hypertension, including hypersensitivity or allergic reaction, increased salt retention, and certain congenital alterations in vascular structure in these vessels, but none of these factors is as important as the hemodynamic factors resulting from the increased head of pressure.

In the typical patient with arteritis after correction of coarctation of the aorta, abdominal pain occurs 2 to 4 days after operation. At first the pain is colicky, but later becomes more constant as paralytic ileus and abdominal distention occur. Vomiting and obstipation ensue, and in the more advanced cases melena and hematemesis occur. Ascites has been reported as a late complication associated with diarrhea and vomiting. Evidence of peritoneal irritation may occur 9 to 14 days after resection of the coarctation. Leukocytosis with 20,000 to 40,000 cells per cubic millimeter is noted, and the differential count shows a strong predominance of polymorphonuclear leukocytes. Intestinal infarction may occur, and laparotomy with resection of the involved segment sometimes becomes a necessity. Nutritional deficiency may become extreme if the disturbance in bowel function persists over several weeks.

Arteritis of the vessels supplying the spinal cord has been described by Singleton and associates, who reported a patient who became paraplegic 3 months after operation for coarctation. This unusual complication occurred explosively in a 35-year-old patient with a preoperative blood pressure of 240/140 mm. Hg. In addition, the patient had necrotizing arteritis of most of the small arteries of the mesentery and small intestines as well as in other abdominal viscera.

The incidence of this complication is not known, but some degree of so-called postcoarctation syndrome appears in as many as 10 per cent of patients operated upon. Severe forms of this complication occur in only 1 to 2 per cent. Although fatal termination is rare, it has been reported in less than 1 per cent of patients undergoing operation.

Antihypertensive agents may have some usefulness if used soon after the complication has been recognized, since control of blood pressure may eliminate the tendency for further arteriolar damage to occur. Cortisone has also been recommended for instances in which adrenal insufficiency may be present. If localized gangrene of bowel occurs, perforation and peritonitis may result, necessitating laparotomy and intestinal resection. In most instances the complication is self-limited and subsides within a few days. Therefore exploratory laparotomy should be delayed until strongly suggestive signs of an intra-abdominal catastrophe appear. It has been our policy over the past 10 years, in more than 100 patients operated on for correction of coarctation of the aorta, to treat postoperative hypertension if the blood pressure rises to the preoperative level or above. Nitroprusside is given immediately as an intravenous drip, and both systolic and diastolic pressures are brought down to near-normal levels. As soon as oral intake is begun, the patient is given propranolol and this is continued until the patient leaves the hospital and often for weeks into the follow-up period. With these methods, our patients have had abdominal pain, ileus, and occasionally melena, but not arteritis producing bowel necrosis.

Pulmonary Complications

Among the pulmonary complications that may follow surgical procedures on the thoracic aorta are atelectasis, hemothorax, pneumothorax, and chylothorax. Since aneurysms of the descending thoracic aorta are frequently extensive and encroach upon the adjacent lung, wide dissection of the lung may be necessary. Partial excision of the lung along with the lesion may produce areas of lung surface in which the blood vessels and bronchi are exposed. Such factors contribute to the postoperative development of pneumothorax and hemothorax. Prolonged compression of the bronchi or tracheal bifurcation by extensive aneurysms may predispose to collapse of these structures during the postoperative period, with resulting respiratory obstruction and atelectasis. Extensive thoracotomy incisions also predispose to development of pulmonary complications because of interference with respiratory exchange. The use of a Carling's endotracheal tube allows selective collapse of the left lung, thereby eliminating trauma to the lung, and will prevent most of the postoperative pulmonary complications.

Pneumothorax is usually controlled by indwelling thoracostomy tubes with subaqueous drainage and light suction. Bilateral pneumothorax may follow operations on the descending thoracic aorta if the right pleural space is entered. Bilateral thoracotomy usually necessitates the use of bilateral tube drainage. Atelectasis due to bronchial obstruction should be relieved as quickly as possible (Fig. 17–27). If the patient is unable to cough vigorously, owing to weakness or pain, aspiration of the tracheobronchial tree should be attempted. Bronchoscopy may be necessary and should be used early if other measures fail. Preferably, bronchoscopy should be performed in the patient's own bed with the head of the bed elevated 45 degrees. Light topical anesthesia is used, and the patient is encouraged to cough. If such complications recur, then tracheotomy should be strongly considered.

Chylothorax may result after operations for aneurysm or coarctation, since the thoracic duct lies in close proximity to the descending thoracic aorta. Usually a chylous fistula closes spontaneously without surgical intervention, but repeated aspirations of chyle are often necessary until the fistula ceases to flow. Chylothorax following operation for ductus arteriosus or coarctation may, however, result in a serious situation.

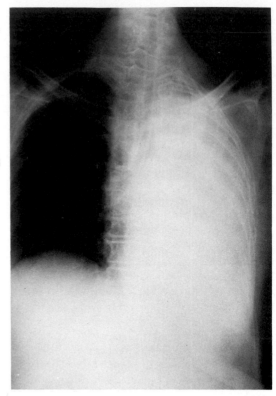

Figure 17–27   Chest roentgenogram showing endotracheal tube in a right mainstem bronchus with resultant atelectasis of the left lung.

In this case, a tube must be placed and the chylothorax drained. If the tube is left in place for several days, sometimes up to 2 weeks, the chylothorax will usually subside and the duct will close. Surgical intervention by thoracotomy is not indicated in most cases. Proper fluid replacement to compensate for the chyle lost through drainage is mandatory for the survival of the patient.

Postoperative Hemorrhage

Bleeding after an extensive operative procedure on the thoracic aorta may be due to several factors. In instances in which an extensive aneurysm is removed, leaving a widespread raw surface in the mediastinum, bleeding may occur postoperatively from multiple vessels that did not bleed while the incision was open. Persistent bleeding from eroded vertebral bodies occasionally complicates operation for extensive aneurysms of the thoracic aorta. The aortic suture line may also bleed, even from small suture holes, particularly if diseased aortic tissue remains after the aneurysm has been removed. Hemolytic blood reactions and defibrination of blood may occur, leading to postoperative hemorrhagic complications. Heparinization of the patient during the procedure may contribute to postoperative hemorrhage. Neutralization of the heparin by means of protamine usually controls this complication. Occasionally, use of epsilon-aminocaproic acid may be indicated if a clotting defect or a euglobulin clot lysis of under 2 hours is found.

In the past, failure of the graft with early rupture and hemorrhage after operation occurred in some patients when homografts were used as the replacement material. Preservation of homografts presented a special problem that was never completely solved even though many techniques were tried. Moreover, suitable graft material was difficult to obtain, and grafts of somewhat marginal quality were sometimes used. Bleeding occasionally occurred from the ligated segmental branches on the graft. Disruption of the graft during the first 24 to 48 hours was usually related to a defective graft, and hemorrhage occurring several days to a month after operation was often related to secondary infection of the graft. Experimental studies by Foster and Scott reveal that homografts do not withstand bacterial infection, since early proteolytic digestion of the graft occurs with resulting hemorrhage. Synthetic grafts, on the other hand, tolerate low-grade infection better than homografts and for these and other reasons previously mentioned are more desirable as a graft replacement. An unfavorable feature of the synthetic grafts has been a tendency of the more porous weaves of cloth to have persistent oozing, particularly in the presence of heparin. Therefore a woven graft should be used whenever heparinization is required. Fortunately wound infection or septicemia is rare in surgery of the thoracic aorta when careful asepsis and prophylactic antibiotics are used in conjunction with operation. Yet once an uncontrolled bacteremia or septicemia occurs, a serious train of events may be expected with secondary hemorrhage often culminating in death. Replacement of the graft with another graft under these circumstances is usually

of no avail, since the second graft placed in the infected site will be subject to the same complications. As more potent antibiotics are being developed, fatal complications produced by septicemia may be completely eliminated.

At times a segment of coarctation may be so long that it would be impossible to approximate the two ends. In a child or teenager, we believe it is preferable to bring down the subclavian artery to bridge the gap between the proximal and distal portions. This artery in children over the age of 7 years is large enough to supply a flow to the distal part of the aorta beyond the coarctation in such a manner that no gradient will remain. It is an uncommon situation, but it is probably better than inserting grafts in children.

Regardless of how meticulous the surgeon may be in an effort to control bleeding at the time of thoracotomy, postoperative hemorrhage with hemothorax will occasionally follow operation for aortic lesions. Although control of shock by blood replacement is obviously important, early surgical reexploration of the thoracotomy wound is of vital importance. Reluctance of the surgeon to accept this fact may lead to a fatal outcome in a patient who could be salvaged by control of a small bleeding point. Under general anesthesia the thoracotomy incision is opened rapidly, and evacuation of the hemothorax relieves respiratory embarrassment. Control of the bleeding points is usually accomplished with suture ligaments. If a diffuse capillary ooze is present, all known hemostatic agents and other adjuncts to control of hemorrhage may be used, including vitamin K, calcium, intravenous administration of fibrinogen or platelet suspension, fresh blood transfusion, topical thrombin, gelatin sponge, and possibly others. One must remember that deaths from postoperative hemorrhage are not usually the result of inability to control the hemorrhage at the time of the second exploration. Failure to recognize serious hemorrhage, the use of insufficient blood replacement, and delay in reexploring the thoracotomy are the usual causes of death from postoperative hemorrhage. Again, the suspicion of tamponade should be indication for bedside examination as previously described (Fig. 17–15).

Bibliography

SURGERY OF THE HEART

1. Bailey, C. P.: The surgical treatment of mitral stenosis (mitral commissurotomy). Dis. Chest. 15:377, 1949.
2. Baker, C., Brock, R. C., and Campbell, M.: Valvulotomy for mitral stenosis. Br. Med. J. 1:1283, 1950.
3. Blalock, A., and Taussig, H. B.: The surgical treatment of malformations of the heart in which there is pulmonary stenosis or pulmonary atresia. J.A.M.A. 128:189, 1945.
4. Gibbon, J. H., Jr.: Application of a mechanical heart and lung apparatus to cardiac surgery. Minnesota Med., 37:171, 1954.
5. Gross, R. E., and Hubbard, J. P.: Surgical ligation of patent ductus arteriosus. Report of first successful case. J.A.M.A., 112:729, 1939.
6. Harken, D. E., Ellis, L. B., Ware, P. F., and Normal, L. R.: The surgical treatment of mitral stenosis. I. Valvuloplasty. N. Engl. J. Med. 29:801, 1948.
7. Rehn, L.: Ueber penetrirende Herzwunder und Herznaht. Arch. klin. Chir., 55:315, 1897.
8. Rehn, L.: Ueber perikardiale Verwachsungen. Med. klin., 16:999, 1920.
9. Souttar, H. S.: The surgical treatment of mitral stenosis. Br. Med. J., 2:603, 1925.

Technical Considerations

10. Andersen, N. B., and Ghia, J.: Pulmonary function, cardiac status, and postoperative course in relation to cardiopulmonary bypass. J. Thorac. Cardiovasc. Surg. 59:474, 1970.
11. Arens, J. F., Ochsner, J. L., and Gee, G.: Volume-limited intermittent cuff inflation for long-term respiratory assistance. J. Thorac. Cardiovasc. Surg., 58:837, 1969.
12. Barboriak, J. J., Rimm, A., Tristani, F. E., Walker, J. A., and Lepley, D.: Risk factors in patients undergoing aorto-coronary bypass surgery. J. Thorac. Cardiovasc. Surg. 64:92, 1972.
13. Barratt-Boyes, B. G., Simpson, M., and Neutze, J. M.: Intracardiac surgery in neonates and infants using deep hypothermia with surface cooling and limited cardiopulmonary bypass. Circulation, Suppl. I, 1971.
14. Beall, A. C., Jr., Cooley, D. A., and De Bakey, M. E.: Surgical management of pulmonary embolism. Experimental and clinical considerations. Dis. Chest, 47:382, 1965.
15. Chardack, W. M., Gage, A. A., and Greatbatch, W.: Correction of complete heart block by a self-contained and subcutaneously implanted pacemaker. J. Thorac. Cardiovasc. Surg. 42:814, 1961.
16. Cooley, D. A., Beall, A. C., Jr., and Alexander, J. K.: Acute massive pulmonary embolism: Successful surgical treatment using temporary cardiopulmonary bypass. J.A.M.A., 177:283, 1961.
17. Cooley, D. A., and Hallman, G. L.: Intrapericardial aorto–right pulmonary artery anastomosis. Surg. Gynecol. Obstet. 122:1084, 1966.
18. Cooley, D. A., and Ochsner, A., Jr.: Correction of total anomalous pulmonary venous drainage: Technical considerations. Surgery 42:1014, 1957.
18a. Cooley, D. A., and Stoneburner, J. M.: Transventricular mitral valvotomy. Surgery 46:414, 1959.
19. Flemma, R. J., Johnson, W. D., Auer, J. E., Tector, A. J., and Lepley, D.: Simultaneous valvular replacement and aorto–coronary saphenous vein bypass. Ann. Thorac. Surg. 12:163, 1971.
20. Flemma, R. J., Johnson, W. D., Lepley, D., Techtor, A. J., Walker, J. A., Gale, H., Beddingfield, G. W., and Manley, J. C.: Late results of saphenous vein bypass grafting for myocardial revascularization. Ann. Thorac. Surg. 14:232, 1972.
21. Flemma, R. J., Johnson, W. D., Tector, A. J., Lepley, D., and Blitz, J.: Surgical treatment of preinfarction angina. Arch. Int. Med. 129:828, 1972.
22. Friesen, W. G., Woodson, R. D., Ames, A. W., Herr, R. H., Starr, A., and Kassebaum, D. G.: A hemodynamic comparison of atrial and ventricular pacing in postoperative cardiac surgical patients. J. Thorac. Cardiovasc. Surg. 55:271, 1968.
23. Garzon, A. A., Seltzer, B., and Karlson, K. E.: Respiratory mechanics following open-heart surgery for acquired valvular disease. Circulation, Suppl. I, 1966.
24. Gazzaniga, A. B., Byrd, C. L., Stewart, D. R., and O'Connor, N. E.: Evaluation of central venous pressure as a guide to volume replacement in children following cardiopulmonary bypass. Ann. Thorac. Surg. 13:148, 1972.
25. Hallman, G. L., and Cooley, D. A.: Surgical treatment of tetralogy of Fallot: Experience with indirect and direct techniques. J. Thorac. Cardiovasc. Surg. 46:419, 1963.
26. Hallman, G. L., Cooley, D. A., Wolfe, R. R., and McNamara, D.: Surgical treatment of ventricular septal defect associated with pulmonary hypertension. J. Thorac. Cardiovasc. Surg. 48:588, 1964.
27. Harding, H. W., Johnson, W. D., Flemma, R. J., and Lepley, D.: Intra-operative physiologic changes incident to improved myocardial perfusion. Surg. Forum 21:160, 1970.
28. Hasbrouck, K. D.: Morphine anesthesia for open-heart surgery. Ann. Thorac. Surg. 10:364, 1970.
29. Herr, R. H., Starr, A., Pierie, W. R., Wood, J. A., and Bigelow, J. C.: Aortic valve replacement: A review of six years' experience with the ball valve prosthesis. Ann. Thorac. Surg. 6:199, 1968.
30. Hodam, R. P., and Starr, A.: Temporary postoperative epicardial pacing electrodes: Their value and management after open heart surgery. Ann. Thorac. Surg. 8:506, 1969.
31. Hodam, R., Starr, A., Herr, R., and Pierie, W.: Early clinical experience with cloth-covered valvular prostheses. Ann. Surg. 170:471, 1969.
32. Hodam, R., Starr, A., Raible, D., and Griswold, H.: Totally cloth-covered prostheses: A re-

view of two years' clinical experience. Circulation Suppl. II, 1970.

33. Johnson, W. D., Dawes, R., Walker, J. A., Leagus, C., and Lepley, D.: Congenital heart disease in adults. Am. J. Surg., *111*:830, 1966.

34. Johnson, W. D., Flemma, R. J., and Lepley, D.: The physiologic parameters of ventricular function as affected by direct coronary surgery. J. Thorac. Cardiovasc. Surg. *60*:483, 1970.

35. Johnson, W. D., Flemma, R. J., Lepley, D. and Ellison, E. H.: Extended treatment of severe coronary artery disease: A total surgical approach. Ann. Surg. *170*:460, 1969.

36. Johnson, W. D., Flemma, R. J., Manley, J. C., and Lepley, D.: Direct coronary surgery utilizing multiple vein bypass grafts. Ann. Thorac. Surg., *9*:436, 1970.

37. Johnson, W. D., Harding, H. W., and Lepley, D.: The aggressive surgical approach to coronary disease. J. Thorac. Cardiovasc. Surg. *59*:128, 1970.

38. Johnson, W. D., Hoffman, J. F., Flemma, R. J., and Tector, A. J.: Secondary surgical procedure for myocardial revascularization. J. Thorac. Cardiovasc. Surg. *64*:523, 1972.

39. Kloster, F. E., Farrehi, C., Mourdjinis, A., Hodam, R. P., Starr, A., and Griswold, H. E.: Hemodynamic studies in patients with cloth-covered composite seat Starr-Edwards valve prostheses. J. Thorac. Cardiovasc. Surg. *60*:879, 1970.

40. Lepley, D., Reuben, C. F., Walker, J. A., Huston, J. H., Gelfand, E. T., and Flemma, R. J.: Experience with the Bjork-Shiley prosthetic valve. Circulation, Suppl. 3:51–55, 1973.

41. Litwak, R. S., Kuhn, L. A., Gadboys, H. A., Lukban, S. B., and Sakurai, H.: Support of myocardial performance after open cardiac operations by rate augmentation. J. Thorac. Cardiovasc. Surg. *56*:484, 1968.

42. Miller, S. E. P., Johnson, W. D., Tector, A. J., Manley, J. C., and Gale, H. H.: The effect of myocardial revascularization on anginal symptoms, ventricular function and exercise performance. Circulation Suppl., to be published.

43. Molokhia, F. A., Beller, G. A., Smith, T. W., Asimacopoulos, P. J., Hood, W. B., and Norman, J. C.: Constancy of myocardial digoxin concentration during experimental cardiopulmonary bypass. Ann. Thorac. Surg., *11*:222, 1971.

44. Morrison, J. D., Moffitt, E. A., Danielson, G. K., and Pluth, J. R.: Circulatory effects of morphine early after open-heart surgery. J. Thorac. Cardiovasc. Surg. *63*:890, 1972.

45. Mundth, E. D., and Austen, W. G.: Postoperative intensive care in the cardiac surgical patient. Progr. Cardiovasc. Dis. *11*:229, 1968.

46. Nathan, D. A., Center, S., Wu, C. K., and Keller, W.: An implantable synchronous pacemaker for the long-term correction of complete heart block. Am. J. Cardiol. *11*:362, 1963.

47. Smith, R., Grossman, W., Johnson, L., Segal, H., Collins, J., and Dalen, J.: Arrhythmias following cardiac valve replacement. Circulation *45*:1018, 1972.

48. Subramanian, S., Wagner, H., Vlad, P., and Lambert, E.:Surface-induced deep hypothermia in cardiac surgery. J. Pediatr. Surg., *6*:612, 1971.

49. Trendelenburg, F.: Ueber die operative Behandlung der Emboli der Lungen Arterie. Arch. klin. Chir., *86*:686, 1908.

50. Trusler, G. A., Bull, R. C., Hoeksema, T., and Mustard, W. T.: The effects on cardiac output of a reduction in atrial volume. J. Thorac. Cardiovasc. Surg. *46*:109, 1963.

51. Vineberg, A. M., and Walker, J. H.: Six months' to six years' experience with coronary artery insufficiency treated by internal mammary artery implantation. Am. Heart J., *54*:851, 1957.

52. Walsh, J. R., Starr, A., and Ritzmann, L. W.: Intravascular hemolysis in patients with prosthetic valves and valvular heart disease. Circulation Suppl. I, 1969.

53. Zeft, H. J., Manley, J. C., Hutson, J. H., Tector, A. J., Auer, J. E., and Johnson, W. D.: Left main coronary artery stenosis: Results of coronary bypass surgery. Circulation *49*:1, 1974.

54. Zoll, P. M., Frank, H. A., Zarsky, L. N., Linenthal, A. J., and Belgard, A. H.: Long-term electric stimulation of the heart for Stokes-Adams disease. Ann. Surg., *154*:330, 1961.

Complications

55. Abbott, O. A., Exarhos, N., and Aydin, K.: Immediate correction of surgical air embolism by regional perfusion with dextran: Experimental and clinical observations. To be published.

56. Andersen, M. N., and Kuchiba, K.: Depression of cardiac output with mechanical ventilation. J. Thorac. Cardiovasc. Surg. *54*:182, 1967.

57. Ashbaugh, D.: The injured lung — CPPB and the concept of total care (Editorial). Ann. Thorac. Surg. *13*:513, 1972.

58. Ashbaugh, D. G., Petty, T. L., Bigelow, D. B., and Harris, T. M.: Continuous positive pressure breathing (CPPB) in adult respiratory distress syndrome. J. Thorac. Cardiovasc. Surg. *57*:31, 1969.

59. Balis, J. U., Cox, W. D., Pifarre, R., Lynch, R., and Neville, W. E.: The role of pulmonary hypoperfusion and hypoxia in the postperfusion lung syndrome. Ann. Thorac. Surg. *8*:263, 1969.

60. Beall, A. C., Jr., and Cooley, D. A.: Renal hemodynamic effect of total cardiopulmonary bypass eliminating heparinized blood. Circulation *27*:858, 1963.

61. Beall, A. C., Jr., Johnson, P. C., Shirkey, A. L., Crosthwait, R. W., Cooley, D. A., and De Bakey, M. E.: Effect of temporary cardiopulmonary bypass on extracellular fluid volume and total body water in man. Circulation *29*:59, 1964.

62. Brown, H. S., Turk, L. N., and Hopkins, W. A.: Management of the white lung syndrome. Ann. Thorac. Surg. *13*:411, 1972.

63. Buckberg, G. D., Towers, B., Paglia, D. E.,

Mulder, D. G., and Maloney, J. V.: Subendo-cardial ischemia after cardiopulmonary by-pass. J. Thorac. Cardiovasc. Surg. *64*:669, 1972.

64. Ching, N. P., Ayres, S. M., Paegle, R. P., Lin-den, J. M., and Nealon, T. F.: The contribu-tion of cuff volume and pressure in tracheos-tomy tube damage. J. Thorac. Cardiovasc. Surg. *62*:402, 1971.

65. Clarke, A. D., and Jackson, P. W.: Postoperative care of patients undergoing cardiopulmonary bypass. Br. J. Anaesth. *43*:248, 1971.

66. Cooperman, L. H., and Mann, P. E. G.: Postop-erative respiratory care: A review of 65 con-secutive cases of open heart surgery on mitral valve. J. Thorac. Cardiovasc. Surg. *53*:504, 1967.

67. Dawes, R. B., Lepley, D., Carey, L., and Ellison, E. H.: Heparin and low molecular weight dextran in thoracic aorta occlusion. Arch. Surg. *88*:699, 1964.

68. Diethrich, E. B., Liddicoat, J. E. Alessi, F. J., Kinard, S. A., and DeBakey, M. E.: Serum enzyme and electrocardiographic changes im-mediately following myocardial revasculariza-tion. Ann. Thorac. Surg. *5*:195, 1968.

69. Dietzman, R. H., Ersek, R. A., Lillehei, C. W., Castaneda, A. R., and Lillehei, R. C.: Low output syndrome. J. Thorac. Cardiovasc. Surg. *57*:138, 1969.

70. Elliott, D., and Roe, B. B.: Aortic dissection during cardiopulmonary bypass. J. Thorac. Cardiovasc. Surg. *50*:357, 1965.

71. Firor, W. B.: Infection following open-heart surgery, with special reference to the role of prophylactic antibiotics. J. Thorac. Cardio-vasc. Surg. *53*:371, 1967.

72. Flemma, R. J., Thurer, R. J., and Reuben, C. F.: Pulmonary complications of non-thoracic trau-ma including burns. *In* Thoracic Trauma. Bos-ton, Little, Brown and Co., 1980.

73. Fogarty, T. J., Cranley, J. J., Krause, R. J., Strasser, E. S.,and Hafner, C. D.: A method for extraction of arterial emboli and thrombi. Surg. Gynecol. Obstet. *116*:241, 1963.

74. Frater, R. W. M.: Intrapericardial pressure and pericardial tamponade in cardiac surgery. Ann. Thorac. Surg. *10*:563, 1970.

75. Friedberg, H. D.: Syncope during standby car-diac pacing. Br. Heart J. *31*:281, 1969.

76. Friedberg, H. D.: Adhesion of pacing catheters to the tricuspid valve: Adhesive endocarditis. Thorax *24*:498, 1969.

77. Gadboys, H. L., and Litwak, R. S.: The postper-fusion hematocrit. J. Thorac. Cardiovasc. Surg. *46*:772, 1963.

78. Gadboys, H. L., Slonin, R., and Litwak, R. S.: Homologous blood syndrome. I. Preliminary observations on its relationship to clinical car-diopulmonary bypass. Ann. Surg. *156*:793, 1962.

79. Gans, H., and Krivit, W.: Problems in hemosta-sis during and after open-heart surgery. Ann. Surg. *155*:268, 1962.

80. Glover, J. L.: Metabolic acidosis in extracor-poreal circulation: Its prevention and treat-ment with THAM. Ann. Surg. *155*:360, 1962.

81. Gomes, M. M. R., and McGoon, D. C.: Bleeding

patterns after open-heart surgery. J. Thorac. Cardiovasc. Surg. *60*:87, 1970.

82. Grillo, H. C., Cooper, J. D., Geffin, B., and Pontoppidan, H.: A low-pressure cuff for tra-cheostomy tubes to minimize tracheal injury. J. Thorac. Cardiovasc. Surg. *62*:898, 1971.

83. Guest, J. L., Sekulic, S. M., Yeh, T. J., Ellison, L. T., and Ellison, R. G.: Role of atelectasis in surfactant abnormalities following extracor-poreal circulation. Circulation Suppl. I, 1966.

84. Hoffman, J. F., Flemma, R. J., Tector, A. J., and Lepley, D.: Cardiac tamponade after open-heart surgery: Description of a rapid safe technique for correction and presenta-tion of six cases. Chest *63*:909, 1973.

85. Hurt, R., Perkins, H. A., Osborn, J. J., and Ger-bode, F.: The neutralization of heparin by protamine in extracorporeal circulation. J. Thorac. Surg. *32*:612, 1956.

86. Javid, H., Tufo, H. M., Najafi, H., Dye, W. S., Hunter, J. A., and Julian, O. C.: Neurological abnormalities following open heart surgery. J. Thorac. Cardiovasc. Surg. *58*:502, 1969.

87. Johnson, W. D., Lepley, D., Lange, R., and Bot-ticelli, J.: A simple method to differentiate postoperative pericardial fluid from cardiac enlargement. Ann. Thorac. Surg. *3*:68, 1967.

88. Kaplan, S. L., Sullivan, S. F., Malm, J. R., Bow-man, F. O., and Papper, E. M.: Effect of car-diac bypass on pulmonary diffusing capacity. J. Thorac. Cardiovasc. Surg. *57*:738, 1969.

89. Krohn, B. G., Urquhart, R. R., Magidson, O., Tsuji, H. K., Redington, J. V., and Kay, J. H.: Metabolic alkalosis following heart surgery. J. Thorac. Cardiovasc. Surg. *56*:732, 1968.

90. Lea, R. E., Tector, A. J., Flemma, R. J., John-son, W. D., Beddingfield, G. W., and Lepley, D.: Prognostic significance of a reduced left ventricular ejection fraction in coronary ar-tery surgery. To be published.

91. Lepley, D., Weisel, W., and Gorman, W. C.: Massive gastrointestinal bleeding as a compli-cation of open surgery in children. Dis. Chest *42*:446, 1962.

92. Lepley, D., Weisfeldt, M., Close, S., Schmidt, R., Bowler, J., Kory, R., and Ellison, E. H.: Effect of low molecular weight dextran on hemor-rhagic shock. Surgery *54*:93, 1963.

93. Mandal, A. K., Callaghan, J. C., Dolan, A. M., and Sterns, L. P.: Potassium and cardiac sur-gery. Ann. Thorac. Surg. *7*:428, 1969.

94. McMullan, M. H.: Low cardiac output and cardiac arrhythmias after open heart surgery. *In* Hardy, J. D. (Ed.): Critical Surgical Illness. Philadelphia, W. B. Saunders Company, 1980.

95. Mundth, E. D., Keller, A. R., and Austen, W. G.: Progressive hepatic and renal failure asso-ciated with low cardiac output following open-heart surgery. J. Thorac. Cardiovasc. Surg. *53*:275, 1967.

96. Nelson, R. M., Jenson, C. B., Peterson, C. A., and Sanders, B. C.: Effective use of prophy-lactic antibiotics in open heart surgery. Arch. Surg. *90*:731, 1965.

97. Nelson, R. M., Jenson, C. B., and Smoot, W. M.: Pericardial tamponade following open-heart surgery. J. Thorac. Cardiovasc. Surg. *58*:510, 1969.

98. Osborn, J. J., et al.: Hemolysis during perfusion. Sources and means of reduction. J. Thorac. Cardiovasc. Surg. *43*:459, 1962.

99. Peters, R. M., Wellons, H. A., and Howe, T. M.: Total compliance and work of breathing after thoracotomy. J. Thorac. Cardiovasc. Surg. *57*:348, 1969.

100. Pillsbury, R. C., Dong, E., Lower, R. R., Hurley, E. J., and Shumway, N. E.: Emergency reoperation following open heart surgery. Ann. Thorac. Surg. *1*:50, 1965.

101. Pontoppidan, H., Laver, M. B., and Geffin, B.: Acute respiratory failure in the surgical patient. Advances Surg. *4*:163, 1970.

102. Porter, J. M., and Silver, D.: Alterations in fibrinolysis and coagulation associated with cardiopulmonary bypass. J. Thorac. Cardiovasc. Surg. *56*:869, 1968.

103. Shelly, W. M., Dawson, R. B., and May, I. A.: Cuffed tubes as a cause of tracheal stenosis. J. Thorac. Cardiovasc. Surg. *57*:623, 1969.

104. Signori, E. E., Penner, J. A., and Kahn, D. R.: Coagulation defects and bleeding in open-heart surgery. Ann. Thorac. Surg. *8*:521, 1969.

105. Thomas, T. V.: Emergency evacuation of acute pericardial tamponade. Ann. Thorac. Surg. *10*:566, 1970.

106. Ulin, A. W., and Gollub, S. S.: Surgical Bleeding. Handbook for Surgery and Specialities. New York, McGraw-Hill Book Company, 1966.

SURGERY OF THE GREAT VESSELS

107. Adams, H. D., and van Geertruyden, H. H.: Neurologic complications of aortic surgery. Ann. Surg. *144*:574, 1956.

108. Alpers, B. J.: Clinical Neurology. Philadephia, F. A. Davis Company, 1954, p. 235.

109. Bering, E. A., Jr., Taren, J. A., McMurrey, J. D., and Bernhard, W. F.: Studies on hypothermia in monkeys and the effect of hypothermia on the general physiology and cerebral metabolism of monkeys. Surg. Gynecol. Obstet. *102*:134, 1956.

110. Bolton, B.: The blood supply of the human spinal cord. J. Neurol. Psychiatry. *2*:137, 1939.

111. Callaghan, J. C., McOwens, D. A., Scott, J. W., and Bigelow, W. G.: Cerebral effects of experimental hypothermia. Arch. Surg. *68*:208, 1954.

112. Eiseman, B., and Summers, W. B.: Factors affecting spinal cord ischemia during aortic occlusion. Surgery *38*:1063, 1955.

113. Laugheed, W., and Kahan, M.: Circumvention of anoxia during arrest of cerebral circulation in cases of intracranial surgery. J. Neurosurg. *12*:226, 1955.

114. McMurrey, J. D., Bernhard, W. F., Taren, J. A., and Bering, E. A., Jr.: Studies on hypothermia in monkeys. I. The effect of hypothermia on prolongation of permissible time of total occlusion of the afferent circulation of the brain. Surg. Gynecol. Obstet. *102*:75, 1956.

115. Moersch, F. P., and Sayre, G. P.: Neurologic manifestations associated with dissecting aneurysms of the aorta. J.A.M.A. *144*:1141, 1950.

116. Owens, J. C., Prevedel, A., and Swan, H.: Prolonged experimental occlusion of thoracic aorta during hypothermia. Arch Surg. *70*:95, 1955.

117. Pontius, R. G., Bloodwell, R. D., Cooley, D. A., and DeBakey, M. E.: The use of hypothermia in prevention of brain damage following temporary arrest of cerebral circulation: Experimental observations. Surg. Forum *5*:224, 1955.

118. Pontius, R. G., Brockman, H. L., Hardy, E. G., Cooley, D. A., and DeBakey, M. E.: The use of hypothermia in the prevention of paraplegia following temporary aortic occlusion: Experimental observations. Surgery *36*:33, 1954.

119. Suh, T. H., and Alexander, L.: Vascular system of the human spinal cord. Arch. Neurol. Psychiatry *41*:659, 1939.

Technical Considerations

120. Bahnson, H. T.: Definitive treatment of saccular aneurysms of the aorta with excision of sac and aortic suture. Surg. Gynecol. Obstet. *96*:383, 1951.

121. Carrel, A.: On the experimental surgery of the thoracic aorta and heart. Ann. Surg. *52*:83, 1910.

122. Cooley, D. A., and DeBakey, M. E.: Surgical considerations of intrathoracic aneurysm of aorta and great vessels. Ann. Surg. *135*:660, 1952.

123. Cooley, D. A., and DeBakey, M. E.: Resection of thoracic aorta with replacement by homograft for aneurysm and constrictive lesions. J. Thorac. Surg. *29*:66, 1955.

124. Cooley, D. A., and DeBakey, M. E.: Resection of entire ascending aorta for fusiform aneurysm using temporary cardiac bypass. J.A.M.A. *162*:1158, 1956.

125. Cooley, D. A., DeBakey, M. E., and Morris, G. C., Jr.: Controlled extracorporeal circulation in surgical treatment of aortic aneurysm. Ann. Surg. *146*:473, 1957.

126. Cooley, D. A., Mahaffey, D. E., and DeBakey, M. E.: Total excision of the aortic arch for aneurysm. Surg. Gynecol. Obstet. *101*:667, 1955.

127. DeBakey, M. E., Cooley, D. A., Crawford, E. S., and Morris, G. C., Jr.: Aneursyms of the thoracic aorta. Analysis of 179 patients treated by resection. J. Thorac. Surg. *36*:393, 1958.

128. DeBakey, M. E., Henly, W. S., Cooley, D. A., Crawford, E. S. Morris, G. C., Jr., and Beall, A. C.: Jr.: Aneurysms of the aortic arch. Factors influencing operative risk. Surg. Clin. North Am. *42*:1543, 1962.

129. DeBakey, M. E., Henly, W. S., Cooley, D. A., Morris, G. C., Jr., Crawford, E. S., and Beall, A. C., Jr.: Surgical management of dissecting aneurysm involving the ascending aorta. J. Cardiovasc. Surg. *5*:200, 1964.

130. DeBakey, M. E., Henly, W. S., Cooley, D. A., Morris, G. C., Jr., Crawford, E. S., and Beall, A. C., Jr.: Surgical management of dissecting

aneurysm of the aorta. J. Thorac. Cardiovasc. Surg. *49*:130, 1965.

131. Edwards, J. E., Chistersen, N. A., Clagett, O. T., and McDonald, J. R.: Pathologic considerations in coarctation of the aorta. Proc. Staff Meet. Mayo Clin. *23*:324, 1948.

132. Ellis, P. R., Jr., Cooley, D. A., and DeBakey, M. E.: Clinical considerations and surgical treatment of annulo-aortic ectasia. J. Thorac. Cardiovasc. Surg. *42*:363, 1961.

133. Gerbode, F., Braimbridge. M., Osborn, J. J., Hood, M., and French, S.: Traumatic thoracic aneurysm. Treatment by resection and grafting with the use of an extracorporeal bypass. Surgery, *42*:975, 1957.

134. Glenn, F., Keefer, E. B. C., Speer, D. S., and Dotter, C. T.: Coarctation of the lower thoracic and abdominal aorta immediately proximal to celiac axis. Surg. Gynecol. Obstet. *94*:561, 1952.

135. Gross, R. E.: Coarctation of the aorta. Circulation *7*:757, 1953.

136. Gross, R. E.: The Surgery of Infancy and Childhood. Philadelphia, W. B. Saunders Company, 1953.

137. Hallman, G. L., and Cooley, D. A.: Congenital aortic vascular ring: Surgical considerations. Arch. Surg. *88*:666, 1964.

138. Morris, G. C., Jr., DeBakey, M. E., Cooley, D. A., and Crawford, E. S.: Subisthmic aortic stenosis and occlusive disease. Arch. Surg. *80*:87, 1960.

139. Section on Cardiovascular Surgery, American College of Chest Physicians: Surgical treatment of coarctation of the aorta. Dis. Chest *31*:468, 1957.

140. Stranahan, A., Ally, R. D., Sewell, W. H., and Krausel, H. W.: Aortic arch resection and grafting for aneurysm employing an external shunt. J. Thorac. Surg., *29*:54, 1955.

141. Warren, W. D., Beckwith, J., and Muller, W. H., Jr.: Problems in surgical management of acute dissecting aneurysm of aorta. Ann. Surg. *144*:530, 1956.

Complications

142. Beall, A. C., Jr., Cooley, D. A., Morris, G. C., Jr., and Moyer, J. H.: Effect of total cardiac bypass on renal hemodynamics and water and electrolyte excretion in man. Ann. Surg. *146*:190, 1957.

143. Beall, A. C., Jr., Morris, G. C., Jr., DeBakey, M. E., and Moyer, J. H.: The various effects of anesthesia, hypothermia and ischemia on the kidney in patients having excisional therapy of thoracic aneurysms. Surg. Forum *7*:323, 1957.

144. Benson, W. R., and Sealy, W. C.: Arterial necrosis following resection of coarctation of aorta. Lab. Invest. *5*:359, 1956.

145. Creech, O., Jr.: Effects of infection and exposure on synthetic arterial prosthesis. Arch. Surg. *78*:271, 1959.

146. Creech, O., Jr., DeBakey, M. E., and Mahaffey, D. E.: Total resection of the aortic arch. Surgery *40*:817, 1956.

147. Foster, J. H., Berzins, T., and Scott, H. W., Jr.: An experimental study of arterial replacement in the presence of bacterial infection. Surg. Gynecol. Obstet. *108*:141, 1959.

148. Lober, P. H., and Lillehei, C. W.: Necrotizing panarteritis following repair of coarctation of aorta. Surgery *35*:950, 1954.

149. Morris, C. G., Jr., and Moyer, J. H.: Artificial dialysis and the treatment of renal failure. GP *15*:102, 1957.

150. Morris, G. C., Jr., Moyer, J. H., Cooley, D. A., and Brockman, H. L.: The renal hemodynamic response to hypothermia and to clamping of the thoracic aorta with and without hypothermia. Surg. Forum *5*:219, 1954.

151. Morris, G. C., Jr., Witt, R. R., Cooley, D. A., Moyer, J. H., and DeBakey, M. E.: Alterations in renal hemodynamics during controlled extracorporeal circulation in the surgical treatment of aortic aneurysms. J. Thorac. Surg. *34*:590, 1957.

152. Moyer, J. H., Heider, C., Morris, G. C., Jr., and Handley, C. A.: Renal failure. I. The effect of complete renal artery occlusion for variable periods of time as compared to exposure to subfiltration arterial pressures below 30 mm. Hg for similar periods. Ann. Surg. *145*:41, 1957.

153. Moyer, J. H., Heider, C., Morris, G. C., Jr., and Handley, C. A.: Hypothermia. III. The effect of hypothermia on renal damage resulting from ischemia. Ann. Surg. *146*:152, 1957.

154. Reid, H. C., and Dallechy, R.: Infarction of ileus following resection of coarctation of aorta. Br. J. Surg. *45*:625, 1958.

155. Ring, D. M., and Lewis, F. J.: Abdominal pain following surgical correction of coarctation of the aorta: A syndrome. J. Thorac. Surg. *31*:718, 1956.

156. Singleton, A. O., Jr., McGinnis, L. M. S., and Eason, H. R.: Arteritis following correction of coarctation of the aorta. Surgery *45*:665, 1959.

157. Williams, G. R., and Spencer, F. C.: The clinical use of hypothermia following cardiac arrest. Ann. Surg. *148*:462, 1958.

158. Wilson, C., and Byrom, F. B.: Renal changes in malignant hypertension: Experimental evidence. Lancet *2*:136, 1939.

ADDITIONAL CURRENT REFERENCES

159. Barboriak, J. J., Barboriak, D. P., Anderson, A. J., Rimm, A. A., Tristani, F. E., and Flemma, R. J.: Risk factors in patients undergoing a second aorta-coronary bypass procedure. J. Thorac. Cardiovasc. Surg. *76*:111, 1978.

160. Barboriak, J. J., Rimm, A. A., Anderson, A. J., Tristani, F. E., and Flemma, R. J.: Risk factors and mortality in patients with aorto-coronary vein bypass operation. Cardiology *63*:237, 1978.

161. Bryant, L. R., Spencer, F. C., and Trinkle, J. K.: Treatment of median sternotomy infection by mediastinal irrigation with an antibiotic solution. Ann. Surg. *169*:914, 1969.

162. Flemma, R. J., Mullen, D. C., Lepley, D., Jr.,

and Assa, J.: A comparative synchronous coronary surgery survival study. Ann. Thorac. Surg. *28*:423, 1979.

163. Flemma, R. J., Singh, H. M., and Tector, A. J.: A method for revascularization of circumflex marginal coronary arteries. Ann. Thorac. Surg., *20*:706, 1975.

164. Galland, R. B., Shama, D. M., Prenger, K. B., and Darrell, J. H.: Preoperative antibiotics in the prevention of chest infection following cardiac operations. Br. J. Surg. *67*:97, 1980.

165. Hoffman, R. G., Blumlein, S. L., Anderson, A. J., Barboriak, J. J., Walker, J. A., and Rimm, A. A.: The probability of surviving coronary bypass surgery — 5-year results from 1718 patients. J.A.M.A. *243*:1341, 1980.

166. Middleton, J., Chmel, H., Tecson, F., Sarkaria, J. S., and Neville, W. E.: Aortotomy site infections: Case presentation and review of the literature. Am. J. Med. Sci. *279*:105, 1980.

167. Mullen, D. C., Lepley, D., Jr., and Flemma, R. J.: Coronary artery surgery without global ischemia. Ann. Thorac. Surg. *24*:90, 1977.

168. Murphy, E. S., and Kloster, F. E.: Late results of valve replacement surgery. II. Complications of prosthetic heart valves. Mod. Concepts Cardiovasc. Dis. *48*:59, 1979.

169. Napier, J. A., Cavill, I., and Ricketts, C.: Measurements of haemolysis in patients with prosthetic heart valves. Cardiovasc. Res. *13*:663, 1979.

170. Read, R. C., Murphy, M. L., and Hultgren, H. N.: Survival of men treated for chronic stable angina pectoris: A cooperative randomized study. J. Thorac. Cardiovasc. Surg. *75*:1, 1978.

171. Reed, G. E., Pooley, R. W., and Moggio, R. A.: Durability of measured mitral annuloplasty. J. Thorac. Cardiovasc. Surg. *79*:321, 1980.

172. Santinga, J. T., Kirsh, M. M., Flora, J. D., Jr., and Brymer, J. F.: Factors relating to late sudden death in patients having aortic valve replacement. Ann. Thorac. Surg. *29*:249, 1980.

173. Watanakunakorn, C.: Prosthetic valve infection endocarditis. Prog. Cardiovasc. Dis., *2*:181, 1979.

18

COMPLICATIONS OF SURGERY OF THE ABDOMINAL AORTA AND OF AORTIC BRANCHES*

Norman M. Rich

In 1759, Hallowell closed an arterial wound by placing a pin through the edges and wrapping a thread around the pin to coapt the edges. He excluded the intima from the pin. In 1899, Dörfler published his results with the technique that is commonly practiced today. He used fine needles and thread and a continuous suture through all layers of the vessel.

Modern arterial surgery began about 25 years ago and has developed rapidly. As surgeons have undertaken repair of arterial injuries and resection of arterial aneurysms, as well as replacement or bypassing of arteriosclerotic segments, numerous complications have been reported. Arterial surgery has become commonplace, and possible complications arising from this surgery are now clearly defined. It is the purpose of this chapter to discuss these complications and their management.

---

*This chapter was contributed by John H. Davis and David B. Pilcher in the previous edition.

PREOPERATIVE COMPLICATIONS

A most serious preoperative complication in patients with acute occlusion of an artery is delay in undertaking correction of the problem; about 6 hours is generally stated to be the maximum permissible delay. The sooner the diagnosis is made and corrective action undertaken, the greater the chance for success. There is no absolute time limit, and successful correction of severe ischemia may be accomplished as late as 48 to 72 hours after onset. In these latter cases, although the ischemia is severe, with intense pain and a cold white extremity, there must be enough circulation through the collateral system to maintain viability. The slight differences in collateral flow that maintain viability can be measured by a variety of relatively new approaches, including Doppler ultrasound, extremity pressures, and radioisotope methods.

Prior to the days of successful arterial surgery, an acute arterial occlusion was often treated by vasodilation accomplished

---

Norman M. Rich was born in Arizona and graduated from Stanford University and Stanford University Medical School. He took his internship at Tripler General Hospital and his residency in General Surgery at Letterman General Hospital, following which he served a fellowship in vascular surgery at Walter Reed General Hospital. Dr. Rich then developed an outstanding career in the United States Army, holding many important positions and assignments. He has built an international reputation in the field of vascular surgery, with many publications in this field. Colonel Rich is Chairman of the Department of Surgery at the Uniformed Services University of the Health Sciences, Associate Chief of the Department of Surgery at the Walter Reed Army Medical Center, and Senior Vascular Surgeon on the Peripheral Vascular Surgery Service at the Walter Reed Medical Center.

by sympathetic blockade. In some instances spasm played a role in ischemia and release provided by sympathetic blockade permitted enough additional circulation to convert a completely ischemic limb into one that would survive. However, limb survival is not the sole desirable goal. Patients treated expectantly for ischemia can have a surviving limb almost functionally useless. All physicians must be aware that once acute ischemia occurs, there is a limited amount of time to carry out necessary diagnostic studies and to correct a lesion by surgical intervention.

ARTERIOGRAPHY

While diagnosis of many arterial lesions is made by careful clinical examination, arteriography is a major adjunct. The arteriogram may provide the diagnosis in some instances such as in renovascular hypertension, or it may substantiate a clinical diagnosis such as transient ischemic attacks with narrowing of the carotid arteries. A most important role of the arteriogram is in providing the vascular surgeon with a clear picture of the arterial tree upon which he must operate. It gives valuable information as to the extent of the lesion and, most importantly, the arterial runoff beyond the point of occlusion or stenosis. Correction of a stenotic arterial lesion or a complete occlusion of an artery is useless unless there is some place for the blood to flow distal to that point.

Arteriography is carried out by injecting a radiopaque dye into the vessel before roentgenograms are taken. The arterial system is usually invaded by means of a percutaneous needle or occasionally by direct cutdown into the vessel. Radiopaque material is injected into the vessel by way of either a needle or a catheter, such as the Seldinger catheter. The contrast may be injected by hand or with an automatic injector under pressure. After roentgenograms have been taken, the needle or catheter is withdrawn and pressure is applied to the puncture site to control hemorrhage. If direct cutdown has been used, the arteriotomy is repaired. Numerous complications can attend arteriography.

Sensitivity to the dye is infrequent but does occur and may result in a severe allergic reaction. Arteriography should never be carried out unless there are supportive measures available for the patient who experiences an allergic response.

Although arteriography is now more commonly carried out through an indwelling arterial catheter, the possibility of infection at the puncture site and in the vascular lumen is present. These procedures require meticulous aseptic technique of the same quality as one would use for any surgical procedure. Contamination of either the catheter or the puncture site resulting from sloppy technique in arteriography is inexcusable.

As the needle or catheter penetrates the wall of the artery, a tear in the intima may occur, and this may be the site of subsequent thrombosis of the vessel (Fig. 18–1). Since most arteriograms are done through abnormal vessels, an atherosclerotic plaque may be torn when the needle or catheter is inserted, with resulting dissection down the medial layer of the vessel and arterial occlusion, or the flap of intima may simply bend into the lumen of the vessel, causing obstruction (Fig. 18–2). Thrombosis may be

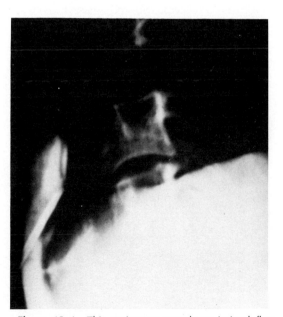

Figure 18–1 This angiogram reveals an intimal flap caused by the tip of a needle during a percutaneous carotid artery puncture. Developing cerebral symptomatology necessitated an emergency carotid thromboendarterectomy. (Rich, N. M., Hobson, R. W., II, and Fedde, C. W.: Vascular trauma secondary to diagnostic and therapeutic procedures. Am. J. Surg. *128*:715, 1974.)

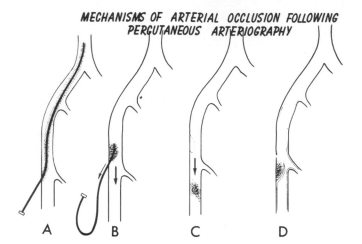

MECHANISMS OF ARTERIAL OCCLUSION FOLLOWING
PERCUTANEOUS ARTERIOGRAPHY

A   B   C   D

Figure 18–2 The mechanisms of arterial occlusion following percutaneous angiography: (*A*) Thrombus forming on outer wall of intra-arterial catheter, (*B*) Catheter withdrawn, thrombus stripped off, adhering to puncture site and occluding the arterial lumen. (*C*) Dislodgement and distal embolization of thrombus. (*D*) Intimal injury at puncture site with plaque elevation at subintimal dissection. (Yellin, A. E., and Shore, E. H.: Surgical management of femoral arterial occlusion following percutaneous femoral angiography. Surgery *73*:772, 1973.)

secondary to prolonged catheterization of the artery for diagnostic arteriography. A small clot forms about the catheter. As the catheter is withdrawn, the clot is wiped free and remains in the lumen where it promotes thrombosis or, if large enough, actually occludes the vessel immediately (Fig. 18–3). It is imperative that the area distal to the arterial puncture site be carefully evaluated before and after arteriography to make sure that ischemia has not occurred. If it has, operative intervention and correction of the localized arterial lesion may be required. Absence of a previously palpable pulse distal to arterial puncture should make one consider surgical correction, but decision about such intervention should be individu-

alized, on the basis of functional expectations.

An additional problem of penetrating a diseased artery is the possibility of fracture of an atherosclerotic plaque, with dislodgement of a portion of it as a peripheral embolus. One must be careful to have a good clinical picture of the area distal to arterial puncture. If embolism of a plaque occurs and ischemia ensues, it will be quickly noted and operative intervention can be promptly undertaken.

Leaking of blood from any arterial puncture is always a potential complication, and it is particularly true when large-bore needles or catheters used for arteriography are inserted. Some hematoma develops in all

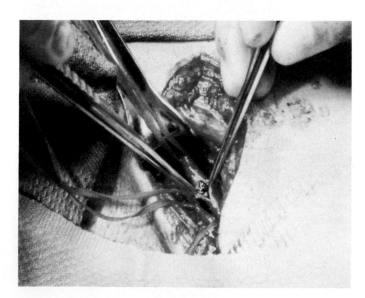

Figure 18–3 Thrombosis is a complication of angiography. There has been an associated increase of brachial artery thrombosis secondary to the increasing use of cardiovascular diagnostic procedures, including angiographic and cardiac catheterization. This photograph taken during surgery demonstrates thrombus in the proximal brachial artery. (Rich, N. M., Hobson, R. W., II, and Fedde, C. W.: Vascular trauma secondary to diagnostic and therapeutic procedures. Am. J. Surg. *128*:715, 1974.)

patients although in most it is not clinically evident. There will usually be some discoloration of tissues about the puncture site within a few days after arteriography. This small hematoma is of little concern. However, the possibility of a false aneurysm must be kept in mind. False aneurysms have been reported in a fraction of 1 per cent of patients in large series in which catheter technique was used for aortography. It may necessitate surgical intervention for correction.

Use of the Seldinger technique has added an additional complication not usually seen with direct needle puncture. This is perforation by either the catheter or the guidewire of a vessel, usually the aorta, at a site distal to the insertion of the catheter. Since the catheter and guidewire are usually inserted into either the femoral artery or the brachial artery, perforation is particularly likely to occur where the catheter is forced around a corner such as in the arch of the aorta or in an area of the aorta that is particularly soft as a result of arteriosclerotic disease. Major hemorrhage may occur and is usually quickly noted because hypotension and all the manifestations of clinical shock develop. This complication occurs in a fraction of 1 per cent of all cases. It is something that the experienced arteriographer is constantly aware of and prepared to combat with help of the surgeon should it occur.

In a review of 13,207 abdominal aortograms, McAfee reported 37 deaths, or an incidence of 0.28 per cent, and 98 additional serious non-fatal complications, an incidence of 0.74 per cent.

In a study of 11,402 Seldinger procedures, the fatal complication rate was 0.06 per cent, the serious non-fatal complication rate 0.7 per cent, and the minor complication rate 3 per cent.

Arteriography has become a standard diagnostic technique in most large hospitals and provides valuable information for the vascular surgeon and the patient. While the incidence of complications is low and the technique of arteriography quite safe, complications do occur and must be considered. The procedure should not be carried out in a cavalier manner, and risk to the patient should be weighed against potential benefit.

COMPLICATIONS OF SURGERY FOR ABDOMINAL AORTIC ANEURYSM

INJURY TO THE SMALL INTESTINE

After brief exploration for other lesions, the small intestine is packed into the right side of the abdomen and covered with moist lap pads. In some patients there is inadequate room for the bowel within the right side of the abdomen. When this is the case the bowel is eviscerated and covered with moist tapes or placed in a polyethylene bag. One should be careful not to place excessive tension on the mesentery that might result in venous obstruction with subsequent engorgement and edema of the bowel. It is important also to keep the bowel moist.

The aorta is exposed by incising the posterior peritoneum in the midline overlying the vessel. It is necessary to gain control of the aorta at the level of the renal arteries. The duodenum is adjacent to the aorta at this point and it must be mobilized with care. The proximal jejunum, as it leaves the ligament of Treitz, is also often adherent to the posterior peritoneum close to the aorta. It is important to keep the incision of the posterior peritoneum slightly away from the bowel wall. When the posterior peritoneum is closed, tissue will hold the sutures adequately. If the posterior peritoneum is incised too near the bowel wall, sutures placed in closing the posterior peritoneum may penetrate the small bowel. This may cause contamination of the surgical area and permit infection of the graft; or, if the sutures attach the bowel firmly against the suture line of the aorta, an aortoduodenal fistula may result. Although this is probably not the most common cause of aortoduodenal fistula, it is one that can be avoided if one leaves a good flap of posterior peritoneum at the time the initial posterior peritoneal incision is made.

Proper peritoneal incision can be particularly difficult when there is a large aneurysm that has elevated a portion of the jejunum, flattened it out against the aneurysm, and smoothed out the posterior peritoneum to a less definable structure. If the incision in the posterior peritoneum is made in the lower third of the aneurysm and carried upward, a plane can usually be found between the posterior peritoneum and the aneurysm wall that provides an adequate layer of posterior peritoneum for subsequent closure. Alternatively, the jejunum may be left attached to the aneurysm, with the latter being opened to the left of the intestine.

INJURY TO THE INFERIOR VENA CAVA AND ILIAC VEINS

The inferior vena cava is usually quite adherent to the normal aorta below the level of the renal arteries. At the aortic bifurcation, the inferior vena cava also bifurcates, with the veins running beneath the two common iliac arteries. Attempts to dissect the cava from the aorta must be carried out with great care. It is quite easy to tear or perforate it with a clamp in the attempt to encircle the aorta in the usual manner. The proper plane should be kept close to the arterial wall. The tip of the dissecting clamp should never be pushed through until a plane has been developed.

With an aneurysm, the inferior vena cava is usually hidden behind the bulge of the aneurysm. Since the first step in managing diseases of the abdominal aorta is usually to encircle the aorta at the level of the renal arteries with a tape to gain proximal control, dissection in this area is usually undertaken first. At the level of the renal arteries, the aorta and vena cava may already be separating. If in dissection one follows the aorta very closely, it is usually quite easy to slip between the vena cava and the aortic wall and to pass an instrument between the two vessels, permitting an umbilical tape to be passed around the aorta for proximal control. Finger dissection is of value, but care must be taken to avoid avulsion of the lumbar arteries.

Dissection of the aortic bifurcation or the iliac arteries, depending upon which is necessary for the procedure being carried out, is perhaps the most difficult dissection in surgery of the abdominal aorta. The iliac veins adhere tightly to the under side of the iliac arteries as well as the bifurcation of the aorta and the plane must be carefully chosen in order to prevent damage to the veins. The artery can be picked up by applying a clamp to its adventitia and elevating it to provide better visualization of the delicate plane between the vein and artery. Dissection at this level must be done extremely carefully under direct vision, or serious injury and massive bleeding may occur. The secret of successful dissection is to stay as close to the arterial wall as possible; in fact, a portion of the adventitia is often stripped in the maneuver of dissecting the vein away from the terminal aorta or either iliac artery.

If either the inferior vena cava or the iliac veins are injured during the dissection procedure, it is important to use digital control or apply an exclusion clamp and to repair the vein with a running fine suture. Far more serious hemorrhage may occur from injury to the vena cava or to the iliac veins than from injury to the aorta or the iliac arteries. Because the hidden veins have inelastic walls with almost no ability to contract around a laceration, and because they adhere tightly to the arteries so that any laceration is actually held open, bleeding may be massive. Pressure on the bleeding area with the finger, a sponge stick, or a lap pad will usually manage it momentarily while dissection is followed by repair of the vein under direct vision. Blood loss occurring from this low pressure system can be severe, and shock or cardiac arrest may result. This complication is more easily avoided than corrected.

In the early days of vascular surgery the aneurysm was dissected free of its surrounding structures and removed in toto. The simpler maneuver of freeing up a cuff of proximal aorta and dissecting either the aortic bifurcation or the iliac arteries, depending upon whether one is going to use a tube or bifurcation graft, permits avoidance of many complications. Once these areas are dissected free and clamps are applied, the aneurysmal sac is opened in its midline. Bleeding from lumbar arteries is controlled by direct suture from inside the sac, and a portion of the sac wall is cut away. This leaves the posterior wall of the aorta and its attachment to the surrounding veins. Thus, complete dissection of the vena cava or the iliac veins from the aneurysmal sac is not only unnecessary but also dangerous.

If cultures of the laminated thrombus with the aneurysmal sac are taken, an occasional one will be positive. For this reason some surgeons have insisted on total extirpation of the sac, because of the fear of infecting the graft. It has been shown, however, that leaving the posterior wall is not associated with an increase in the rate of graft infection. Many surgeons suture a portion of the residual aneurysmal sac around the fabric graft.

URETERAL INJURY

Injury to the ureter during surgery of the abdominal aorta and iliac vessels is uncommon. With abdominal aortic aneurysms, occasionally a ureter will be caught partially upon the wall of the aneurysm and may be inadvertently cut when a part of the aneurysmal sac is removed. Usually the ureter is behind the aneurysm, and the technique of leaving part of the aneurysm wall protects the surgeon from inadvertently damaging the ureter.

In dissection of the iliac vessels down to the iliac bifurcation, there is danger of injury to the ureter. The ureter crosses the artery at this point, and it may be damaged if care is not taken in the dissection. If the ureter is accidentally cut, it should be repaired over a small ureteral catheter which is inserted through the cut end into the bladder. Repair is made with fine interrupted sutures, and the catheter is later removed through a cystoscope during the postoperative course. At the completion of graft replacement of the abdominal aorta, the ureter should be carefully identified to ensure that kinking or constriction of it does not occur at the time of reperitonealization. If ureteral injury is suspected postoperatively, cystoscopy with retrograde pyelography should resolve the question.

In difficult cases ureteral catheters inserted before the abdomen is opened will permit rapid identification of the ureters in the dissection and will help the surgeon avoid damaging them.

THROMBOSIS DURING THE OPERATIVE PROCEDURE

Occasionally one will find thrombosis distal to the point at which occluding clamps have been placed in vascular surgery. It is possible to inject heparin into the distal vessels just before applying the occluding clamp. In the case of surgery on the abdominal aorta, 5000 units of heparin are injected into the aorta just before the proximal clamp is closed. One must be aware that this heparin flushes into the general circulation. No reversal of heparin with protamine at the time of removal of the aortic clamps following the completion of the anastomoses may be indicated. If total body heparinization is used, as many surgeons prefer, an equal amount of protamine sulfate may be administered to neutralize the heparin at the time of declamping the vessel. Backflow out of the distal arteries should be checked before the last few sutures are placed. If this is inadequate, Fogarty catheters should be run down the vessels to free up and remove any clots that have formed. If it is necessary to use Fogarty catheters, distal vessels are filled with dilute heparinized saline before reclamping and the tying of the last few sutures.

Postoperative anticoagulants are not indicated as they will not keep open an inadequate anastomosis, a kinked graft, or a narrow, shaggy vessel into which an anastomosis has been made. The danger of continued bleeding from a suture hole at an anastomotic site in the patient given anticoagulants far outweighs any benefits that have been demonstrated for postoperative anticoagulation.

LENGTH OF GRAFT

Synthetic grafts are usually made of a woven or knitted synthetic fiber and are crimped to permit them to make curves without kinking. These grafts can expand vertically as well as horizontally. It is necessary to position the graft properly and cut it to length. All synthetic grafts should be placed with minimal tension on the graft at the time of suture. Removal of the clamps and reestablishment of blood flow will smooth out the crimped graft and create some elongation of it. If the graft is too long, it may kink and cause obstruction to flow through the graft or favor later build-up of clot due to turbulence. When a bifurcation graft is placed in the abdominal aorta, the bifurcation should be placed slightly higher than the bifurcation of the patient's vessels. This also narrows the angle of the bifurcation and relieves the tension on the crotch of the graft. The upper portion should then be cut just short of the point of anastomosis with the graft stretched out. The upper anastomosis is made in the standard fashion with running synthetic over-and-over sutures starting posteriorly and coming around both sides of the graft. They are tied in the mid-anterior position. It is of utmost importance that the most posterior sutures be well placed and watertight. Once the graft is in place, a leak in the most posterior aspect of the suture line can be difficult to correct. The graft will have retracted a great deal by this time, and it is now necessary to pull the bifurcation back down to its correct position corresponding to the original aortic bifurcation. Each limb is then stretched and cut just short of the point of anastomosis to the iliac artery. While the assistant keeps the graft stretched to avoid tension on the suture line, a running suture is again placed in the distal anastomosis. If one attempts to cut the graft short, and then pull it down by means of tying the first suture posteriorly, the suture may tear out of the artery. Thus, the assistant, keeping traction on the graft, reduces tension while the first sutures are placed.

In addition to cutting these grafts to proper lengths, it is important to suture them in direct line with arterial flow when an end-to-end anastomosis is being made. Occasionally, a kink occurs right at that point, causing reduced flow and setting the stage for thrombosis. When an end-to-side anastomosis is being made, it is important that the graft be cut on the bias so that it enters the distal vessel at approximately the same angle as any normal vessel would.

If a graft has been left too long, resulting in marked kinking or bowing, it is imperative that it be corrected immediately. A kinked graft may lead to thrombosis and necessitate a second procedure. The bowed graft often will preclude the possibility of closing tissues about it in a normal fashion. While it is true that within the abdomen a rather large bow can be accommodated, it is often difficult to close the posterior peritoneum over a bowed graft, and there is always the opportunity for herniation of bowel under the bow. It takes but a few moments to excise the excessive length from the middle of the graft.

INTIMAL EMBOLISM

The surgeon who treats arteriosclerotic vascular disease is very familiar with soft, shaggy, plaquelike material lining vessels. Unless atheromatous material above the anastomotic site is firmly adherent, it should be removed when a vessel is being replaced or a bypass graft is being inserted. When the aorta is cross-clamped for suture of an aortic graft, the mouth of the proximal aortic cuff should be carefully scrutinized for any loose material. After completion of the anastomosis the proximal clamp is released for a few heartbeats in order to flush out any material caught in the clamp but free of the intimal wall.

Prior to the completion of the first distal anastomosis in the placement of a bifurcation graft, a clamp is applied to that limb and the proximal clamp is again removed in order to flush out any debris through the unsutured limb of the graft. Upon completion of anastomosis of one limb of the iliac graft, and after flushing as just described, flow through that leg can be reestablished by placing a clamp across the limb that remains unsutured. Before the second limb of the bifurcation graft is connected, the bifurcation clamp is removed and that limb is flushed out as well. This also permits any soft clot that has adhered to the inside of the graft to be flushed free. The distal anastomosis is then completed and all clamps removed to reestablish flow. Usually the distal pulses are checked within the abdomen at the femoral canal after all clamps have been removed. If good pulsations are felt at this level, one can assume that flow through the graft is satisfactory. Before closing the abdomen, however, uncover the feet and check pulses, venous filling and color. If either or both limbs appear ischemic, the graft can be opened in its largest portion and Fogarty catheters slipped down the arteries in order to remove any thrombus or an embolus that may have formed. Once flow has been reestablished, with venous filling of the feet and return of normal color, the incision in the graft itself is closed.

In the case of aortic grafts, any narrowing of the lumen is so minor that there is little or no hazard in this procedure. Although determination of a patent distal arterial tree following insertion of a graft can usually be made on clinical evidence, other techniques that may be more accurate are available. Increasing use is being made of Doppler and plethysmographic techniques in assessing the patency of a graft and the distal flow at the completion of the procedure. In addition, provision should always be made for the possible use of intraoperative or immediately postoperative arteriography in order to demonstrate the patency of the graft and distal arterial tree.

BLEEDING FROM THE GRAFT OR THE ANASTOMOSIS

The development of synthetic materials such as nylon and Dacron has provided us with satisfactory substitutes for human blood vessels. The grafts most commonly used today are of knitted or woven Dacron, crimped to allow for expansion and angling without kinking of the graft material. Originally, it was felt that grafts should be watertight, but subsequent studies have shown that porosity of the graft is important to allow development of a well nourished neointima within the graft. The greater the porosity of the graft, the more satisfactory the healing of the neointima. It is obvious that too much porosity will permit continued leakage from the graft and major hemorrhage.

In the abdominal aorta, the knitted graft is frequently preferred, but the pore size necessitates that preclotting be carried out in order to prevent major blood loss following the removal of the clamps. Remove 50 ml. of blood from the aorta into a small basin just prior to the application of clamps and administration of heparin. The graft is placed in the basin of blood. This provides a good coating. The graft is then cut to length and inserted as already described. In general, this will prevent any major leakage through the graft itself, although on occasion a point or two will bleed rather briskly following removal of the clamps. The clamps may be reapplied for approximately

3 minutes and then again slowly opened in order to permit clotting to occur at the point of leakage. If only one or two small places in the graft are leaking, place a dry pad over them and maintain finger pressure against them until clotting has occurred. This permits continued flow through the graft and eliminates the possibility of intraluminal clotting.

A second point of blood loss following the removal of clamps is at the suture line. Ordinarily, the suture lines consist of running, baseball-type sutures, the stitches being placed approximately 1/16 to 1/8 inch apart, depending upon the size of the graft being sutured. This closure is watertight for the most part and no reinforcing of sutures is required. Occasionally a point will be found on the circumference of the suture line that is bleeding briskly. Some judgment is needed in controlling hemorrhage at the suture line. If the hemorrhage is no greater than that occurring through the graft, it usually will respond to the same measures, that is, the application of a dry pad held in place over the bleeding point until satisfactory clotting has occurred. The same technique is used for holes in the aorta made by the needle and suture that leak when the clamps are removed. Again, simple occlusive pressure with the finger until a clot has formed in the tract of the suture is adequate management. The hole may be closed by the addition of a simple suture or a mattress suture if the hole is large enough to demand it. One may then detect some heparin effect encouraging bleeding at the suture line. It may be necessary to give protamine to counteract the heparin, if bleeding continues and seems unusually difficult to control.

PARTIAL OCCLUSION OF THE ANASTOMOSIS

Once the clamps have been removed and blood flow is reestablished, it is important to check carefully the areas beyond any anastomotic site for satisfactory flow. At the level of the abdominal aorta, the anastomosis is so large that overt arterial thrombosis is the only type of occlusion that might occur. The discrepancy in graft size or aorta size at the level of the aortic graft anastomosis is relatively unimportant, and one can easily make up for the difference in size of either graft or aorta by proper suture technique.

When a bifurcation graft is used, however, the distal anastomoses are much smaller, usually ranging from 9 to 15 mm. in diameter. At this level suture technique is much more important than it is in the aortic anastomosis. The sutures should be placed from the graft to the artery and the intima should be tacked down. This prevents partial dissection of the intima when blood flow is reestablished, which could lead to partial or complete occlusion. Matching of circumference between the graft and the artery is also of some importance here. Narrowing of the lumen by differential size between graft and distal artery is to be avoided. Choose a bifurcation graft on the basis of the iliac artery size rather than the size of the proximal abdominal aorta. If the graft matches the iliac arterial size fairly well, the use of a fine suture technique running all the way through the graft, into the intima and out through the adventitia of the artery, will almost always assure a satisfactory anastomosis without reduction in size and without dissection of the distal intima at the time flow is reestablished.

It is important to palpate the iliac arteries carefully after the clamps have been applied and the internal pressure is reduced. This permits selection of a site for anastomosis to the iliac artery where the lumen will be of maximal size, By careful palpation. one can find and thus avoid those spots where the iliac wall is particularly thick. This prevents two complications. The first is that an artery cut at this point is already narrowed by the thick wall and the graft is therefore disproportional to the lumen size. The second complication results from suturing through the thickened wall which is often quite cheesy in consistency and may allow the sutures to partially tear out, leaving ragged pieces of intima which may dissect when blood flow is reestablished. If significant stenosis of an anastomosis is seen after its completion, it should generally be resutured unless the patient's condition demands a compromise. The graft should be milked empty and vascular clamps reapplied, if reanastomosis is required, to prevent extensive clotting within the graft.

Paraplegia may be a complication associated with abdominal aortic aneurysmorrhaphy. This may be caused by interruption of limited blood supply to the spinal cord. Ischemia of the left colon can also occur. Fortunately, these are unusual complications.

COMPLICATIONS OF REPLACEMENT OF THE UPPER ABDOMINAL AORTA

When the upper abdominal aorta is involved by either aneurysm or occlusive disease, the magnitude of surgical risk to the patient is greatly increased. The major problem is the duration of ischemia of the celiac, superior mesenteric, and renal arteries.

Involvement of the upper aorta may be an extension of an aneurysm of the abdominal aorta to include the origin of the renal arteries. The caliber of the aorta at the level of the celiac and superior mesenteric arteries is usually normal; the aneurysm begins to flare just below these arteries and involves the renal arteries. Careful inspection and palpation of the aorta at this level should reveal its consistency and show whether or not there are any "thin" spots in the vessel. If there are thin spots, it is easiest to dissect the aorta free above the renal arteries and apply a clamp at this level. The clamp is not closed until all other dissection has been accomplished, as in the technique used in resecting an infrarenal abdominal aortic aneurysm. A clamp is also applied just below the renal arteries with a margin of cuff left beyond it to permit suture of the aortic graft. The clamp above the renal artery is applied momentarily, and a dart is removed from the anterior wall of the aorta with its apex just above the renal arteries at a point at which the aortic size is normal. A running suture is started at the apex and brought down below the renal arteries to the cut end of the aorta. This procedure narrows the aorta to its normal diameter and will serve perfectly satisfactorily if the wall of the aorta is of good quality. The clamp above the renal arteries is removed after the clamp below the renals on the aortic cuff has been applied. This limits cross-clamping of the aorta above the renal arteries to less than 3 or 4 minutes and rarely will cause any damage to the kidneys. The distal aortic graft is sutured in place and the procedure is carried out as described previously for infrarenal aortic aneurysms.

When an aneurysm involves the celiac, superior mesenteric, and renal arteries, it is obvious that the ischemia time must be minimized in order to prevent damage to the liver, intestine, and kidneys. One can reduce the complications by extending the abdominal incision into the chest and gaining control of the descending thoracic aorta just above the diaphragm. With use of a partial occlusion clamp, a tube graft may be sutured in standard fashion end to side to the descending thoracic aorta. The graft is brought through the diaphragm and sutured end to side to the terminal aorta beyond the level of the aneurysm. If the aneurysm involves the bifurcation, it is sometimes necessary to suture a bifurcation graft onto the end of the tube graft in order to provide two limbs for anastomosis to the iliac arteries. These are again sutured end to side into the iliac arteries. Throughout this time blood flow is maintained through the aneurysm and the celiac, superior mesenteric, and renal arteries. There are at least three methods by which anastomosis of the various branches of the aorta can be made. One is simply to cut the celiac axis flush at the aorta and connect it directly to the tube graft end to side. The same procedure can be followed for the superior mesenteric and both renal arteries. Frequently stumps of these arteries will not be long enough to reach the tube graft. In these cases, another method must be used: A partial occlusion clamp is applied to the tube graft and stubs of knitted Dacron equal in diameter to the vessels to which they are to be attached are first sutured to the tube graft. As soon as this has been accomplished, the end of these stubs can be connected end to end to the celiac, superior mesenteric, and renal arteries. Further reduction in ischemia time can be accomplished by suturing these stubs end to side to the celiac, superior mesenteric, and renal arteries. An internal shunt may be of value in such a procedure to maintain blood flow while most of the anastomosis is being completed. The last few sutures are placed but not tied and the shunt is removed. The last sutures are then tied to make a watertight closure. When all flow to the peripheral organs has been reestab-

lished, the aortic aneurysm can be cross-clamped and excised or it may be opened, and the lumbar vessels controlled by direct suture within the aneurysmal sac. The residual sac may be closed around the tube graft if one prefers this approach. In the most recent experience, Crawford has provided a replacement technique of suturing part of the wall of the aorta containing branches to a long window in the bypass prosthesis.

COMPLICATIONS OF CELIAC AND MESENTERIC ARTERY SURGERY

In recent years newer concepts of chronic ischemia due to occlusive disease of the celiac and superior and inferior mesenteric arteries have been put forth. With the advent of aortography and successful vascular surgery in other areas of the body, it was natural to begin to look at the celiac and superior and inferior mesenteric arteries. The entity of abdominal angina has been accepted, and too often patients are subjected to surgical exploration for vague digestive symptoms on the assumption that they have abdominal angina, only to find that the symptoms continue after operation. Szilagyi has studied this problem and found that between 12 and 49 per cent of his patients undergoing arteriography demonstrated a narrowing of the celiac axis. Almost all these patients were asymptomatic, although some had mild digestive symptoms. They usually had additional vascular disease as well. Chronic ischemia of the bowel may improve with time, may cause stricture formation within the gut, or may produce gangrene.

The diagnosis can usually be reasonably established if the patient has these symptoms: (1) need for small meal ingestion; (2) postprandial pain; (3) weight loss; and (4) an arteriogram that shows marked stenosis or occlusion of at least two of the three vessels of the intestine: the celiac, superior mesenteric, and inferior mesenteric arteries. When this group of findings occurs, revascularization of one or more of these narrowed arteries can be expected to produce reasonable improvement in the patient. It is usually unnecessary to improve the circulation through all of them, since it is doubtful that major symptoms occur unless two of the three have major degrees of stenosis.

The only intraoperative complication that is different from the complications of arterial surgery elsewhere results from the fact that the celiac artery tends to be somewhat thin walled and can easily be torn. It does not seem to have the same strength in the portion coming off the aorta that the other major vessels within the abdomen have, and careful dissecting is necessary in freeing it. The easiest method of avoiding this hazard is to place a bypass graft between the aorta and the celiac artery, with the graft sutured to the celiac artery at a convenient point distal to the origin.

Acute intestinal ischemia usually results from arterial thrombosis or embolism in the superior mesenteric artery and is somewhat more easily diagnosed than is chronic ischemia. It is a rapidly fatal disease unless treated by prompt surgical intervention. Its onset is usually heralded by severe abdominal pain and hyperperistalsis. This may lead to ileus and a very quiet, undistended abdomen. Distention is less common with arterial occlusion than with venous occlusion. In the patient with known cardiac disease, either an arrhythmia or a previous myocardial infarction, sudden onset of severe abdominal pain should arouse one's suspicion of acute intestinal ischemia. Immediate arteriography may be helpful, but if there is to be any delay in obtaining an arteriogram, immediate abdominal exploration is indicated. The standard abdominal approach is used and the superior mesenteric artery is reached through either the base of the transverse mesocolon or the gastrohepatic ligament. Since the clot usually is lodged distal to the branching point of the superior mesenteric artery, an arteriotomy is made at a convenient point and the thrombus or embolus is extracted in the usual fashion by means of Fogarty catheters. The arteriotomy is then closed. Occasionally an aorto-superior mesenteric bypass will be necessary. The postoperative complications are the same as those in all other arterial surgical procedures. The great difficulty in superior mesenteric artery reconstruction is to know whether or not the vessel has remained open following the operative procedure. Some surgeons have recommended a second look within 6 to 8 hours and others

advocated waiting 24 to 48 hours. It seems wise, if a second look is to be taken, that it be done within 8 hours, since reocclusion will usually have caused gangrene by 24 to 48 hours. Another approach has been to abandon the second-look procedure and to repeat arteriography 8 to 12 hours after surgery if there is any doubt about the success of the reconstruction.

Antibiotic therapy should be started whenever mesenteric vascular occlusion is suspected and should be well established before the abdomen is opened. Because the integrity of the gut membrane may be damaged by ischemia, it would be dangerous to wait until the gut has been exposed before administering antibiotics.

Management of acute arterial lesions in the superior mesenteric artery is very unsatisfactory, because diagnostic techniques are poor, index of suspicion is low, and the time factor works against the patient. The mortality rate remains frightfully high. Many patients have had symptoms from 8 to 48 hours before they seek medical attention, or at least before they are seen by a surgeon. All too often when the abdomen is entered gangrenous bowel, frank peritonitis, and too short a segment of viable intestine to permit survival are found.

If there has been delay in relieving an embolic occlusion or if revascularization is not feasible, there may be justification for a second exploration when the entire small bowel seems non-viable. There have been reports of management by prolonged hyperalimentation following virtually total small bowel resection.

COMPLICATIONS OF SURGERY FOR RENOVASCULAR HYPERTENSION

Although no one knows with any certainty how many hypertensive people there are in this country, hypertension continues to be a major problem. It is known that there are a variety of etiologies for hypertension, and it is estimated that between 5 and 15 per cent of the hypertensive population have renovascular hypertension. The questions of what screening tests to use and of whom to test are debated. Some centers screen all people who have onset of hypertension at an early age: before 40 years. Also included are all patients who seem to have essential hypertension that shifts suddenly to a malignant type of hypertension. Rapid-sequence intravenous pyelography serves as the most satisfactory screening test, even though false-negative results may be found in as many as 30 per cent of studies. Split renal function tests are of value, but they do not appear to be as satisfactory a method of screening. Split renal function tests of either the Stamey or Howard variety can be helpful. The complication rate varies from 3 to 30 per cent and the complications are those one would expect from placement of ureteral catheters. Most common are urinary tract infection and bacteremia secondary to it. Ureteral edema or obstruction may follow ureteral catheterization and in extremely rare cases may proceed to azotemia and uremia. [This test is now rarely used. Ed.]

Renal vein renin assay should be carried out if possible because it can be of great help. Selective catheterization of the renal veins is now a relatively safe and easily carried out procedure; the blood samples drawn are submitted for renin assay. A positive renal vein renin assay is one in which the ratio of renin activity from the involved to the uninvolved kidney is 1.5 or greater in most centers. The only serious complication of this diagnostic test is the possibility of thrombosis in either the renal veins or the vein in which the catheter is inserted, usually one of the veins of the groin.

The rapid-sequence intravenous pyelogram is diagnostic if there is: (1) a unilateral delay in calyceal appearance time; (2) a difference in the renal length of 1.5 cm. or greater; (3) hyperconcentration of contrast media on the late films; (4) ureteral notching secondary to tortuous dilation of ureteral arteries; and (5) a renal silhouette suggestive of segmental infarction. The only important complication of the procedure is allergic reaction to the dye. Serious reactions have been shown to occur in about one in every 100,000 injections. If the rapid-sequence intravenous pyelogram is positive, aortography may be indicated to examine the renal arteries.

The complications of aortography also are minimal, although greater than those of rapid-sequence intravenous pyelography.

The complication rate for aortography has been about 0.7 per cent in a number of studies that have been reported. Obtain a blood urea nitrogen value both before aortography and on the day after to check for the possibility of renal toxicity.

If surgical intervention for renovascular hypertension is to be carried out and there is any evidence of carotid artery disease, this should be corrected first. Blood flow to the brain may well be dependent on the hypertension that exists in the face of a stenotic carotid artery, and correction of renovascular hypertension with subsequent lowering of the blood pressure may produce cerebral symptoms.

Preoperative antihypertensive drugs such as reserpine and guanethidine should be stopped at least 2 weeks before the operation. Hypovolemia if present should be corrected to prevent thrombosis following surgery. Systemic heparin is given routinely during the procedure, and mannitol is infused before the renal artery is clamped and immediately afterward. These precautions are taken to prevent intraoperative and postoperative complications that may occur with this type of surgery.

When the renal arteries as well as the aorta are exposed, before the bypass graft is placed, attention to several seemingly small technical points may prevent rather major complications. The renal arteries are small and often quite spastic by the time they have been manipulated and dissected free of the surrounding tissues. It is extremely important that the point of the knife used to create the arteriotomy be inserted perpendicular to the artery so that the lumen is entered. Make a small stab wound with the point of a No. 11 blade, and then use angled scissors, feeling the inside of the lumen with the inserted blade. This technique ensures that one does not miss the lumen of the renal artery and damage the artery quite severely before the error is discovered.

Another technical point that must be considered is the angle at which the two ends of the graft are sutured. If the angle exceeds 90 degrees, severe turbulence may develop about the anastomosis. It probably would be ideal to make the aortic anastomosis above the renal arteries, but since this would increase the hazards of the surgery, the graft is usually connected to the aorta below the renal arteries. While this angle does exceed 90 degrees and turbulence probably does occur, thrombosis at the aortic anastomosis rarely results. The flow in the aorta, coupled with the size of the graft (usually at least 8 mm. in diameter), may explain why thrombosis does not occur at this point. The distal anastomosis into the renal artery is usually much smaller, and turbulence becomes a more important factor. The graft should make a gentle curve upward and be connected to the renal artery at as acute an angle as possible. An end-to-end anastomosis is probably more desirable from the point of view of avoiding turbulence, but many times a more satisfactory anastomosis can be made with the end-to-side technique. Great care must be taken in the placement of aortorenal bypass grafts to prevent kinking and twisting of the graft. When a vein graft is used, inadequate tension may cause the graft to elongate when arterial pressure is permitted through it, and a kink may be created. If a kink occurs, one should not attempt to correct it by suturing it or burying it behind tissue since thrombosis almost always will result. One way of handling the problem is to take down one of the anastomoses, shorten the vein graft, and reconstruct the anastomosis. Alternatively, a segment can be excised from the middle of the graft. Use of the synthetic graft leaves available a saphenous vein in the leg which may well be needed for other arterial anastomoses, particularly of the coronary arteries, at a later time.

As with all small vessel anastomoses, there are several technical points that must be meticulously observed to prevent complications. When a small vein graft is used, there is a tendency to cause stenosis of the orifice by drawing the running arterial suture too tight. It is probably better under these circumstances to use interrupted sutures to prevent the stenotic effect of a purse-string.

In the postoperative state a number of complications may occur. Damage to the kidney on the operative side is more common than was suspected in the past. The studies by Foster suggest that in many cases an acute tubular necrosis has occurred, lasting from 1 to 3 weeks before recovery. Foster's group studied a number of their own cases with the triple-isotope renal scan and were surprised at the amount of renal damage that had occurred. They have advocated the technique of washing out the kidney with iced saline, usually with infusion of about 500 ml. of saline at 1° to 2°C. This will lower the core temperature of the kidney to about 15°C. and permit a longer operating time with minimal damage. Foster and his group contend that with routine use of this technique they have found no evidence of renal damage in their patients.

In the postoperative period, once the patient has recovered sufficiently to be up and around, rapid-sequence intravenous pyelography is repeated. If it was positive preoperatively and is now negative, a successful result can be assumed. If it is still positive in the postoperative period, then a repeat arteriogram is obtained.

Another complication in the postoperative period may be hypertension. There are several causes for this, and they should be investigated. In the immediate postoperative period the body temperature should be checked, because if it has fallen during the operative procedure, peripheral vasoconstriction may occur and hypertension may result. A second cause that must be excluded is the possibility that fluid overload has occurred during the operative period. The modern use of vasodilating agents such as halothane for general anesthesia often requires a rather large fluid load in order to maintain a satisfactory blood pressure. At times overzealousness on the part of the anesthesiologist may permit a rather large fluid load to be accumulated during the operative procedure, with hypertension resulting in the postoperative period. Finally, it must be remembered that hypertension often is not immediately corrected by the operative procedure, even though a good result will be obtained eventually. If the possibility of low body temperature and vasoconstriction or fluid overload has been eliminated, one must assume that the hypertension will be best managed in the interim by the use of antihypertensive agents. One choice is alpha-methyldopa, for days to weeks, with the dose gradually diminished as the pressure comes down.

The late complications of renovascular hypertension surgery are graft thrombosis, suture line stenosis, and graft dilation. Thrombosis of the graft occurs in about 5 per cent of patients, usually in the early postoperative period. The rate of thrombosis after a successful graft procedure and reduction of hypertension is unknown, since most patients who have had a satisfactory outcome are not routinely reevaluated by arteriography. If hypertension returns sometime after the successful correction of the problem, repeat studies, including aortography, should be carried out to determine whether thrombosis has occurred.

Suture line stenosis may occur as the anastomosis heals and scarring takes place about it. The incidence of this complication is unknown, but it has been demonstrated at reoperation that a marked stenosis of the suture line is secondary to scarring and not due to additional atherosclerotic disease. If stenosis occurs, reoperation and correction of the stenosis is the only successful way to again reduce the hypertension.

In general, the surgery of renovascular hypertension, when patients are carefully selected and meticulous technique is used during the operative procedure, is most satisfactory. A successful result usually remains so and the incidence of recurrence of hypertension following successful correction is small. One must be aware, however, that the atherosclerotic process is generalized and may well continue and eventually involve the other kidney. If hypertension does occur at some subsequent date, reinvestigation is necessary and one must be prepared for the possible necessity of operation on the opposite kidney.

COMPLICATIONS OF SURGERY FOR OCCLUSIVE DISEASE OF THE TERMINAL AORTA AND ILIAC ARTERIES

The patient with thigh and hip claudication and absence or diminution of femoral pulses can be assumed to have occlusive disease of the terminal aorta or iliac arteries or both. In the male this is frequently accompanied by impotence. Correction of this disease process can be undertaken by means of either aortoiliac thomboendarterectomy or a bypass graft.

When the aortogram reveals a relatively short segment of occlusive disease (a common finding in the terminal aorta and first portion of the bifurcation, often extending over no more than 2 to 6 cm.), thromboendarterectomy can be the treatment of choice. The technique consists of an incision in the terminal aorta in the midline after proximal control has been obtained and extension of the incision down one iliac limb. To prevent undue blood loss, the lumbar arteries should be isolated and controlled before the aorta is entered. A short incision is then made in the opposite iliac artery distal to the bifurcation, and the thrombosis and arteriosclerotic plaque are removed under direct vision. It is important to remove all of the intima and media out to the adventitial wall. This is sometimes disturbing to the surgeon because it appears to leave a very thin vessel wall.

Two planes of cleavage will be noticed when one attempts a thromboendarterectomy, the innermost plane with a yellowish appearance and the outer plane whose removal leaves only a bluish, thin-looking adventitial wall. Endarterectomy must be carried out through the outer plane even though it might appear that the remaining adventitia will not be strong enough to withstand arterial pulsation without aneurysm formation. Actually, aneurysm formation is an extremely rare complication of thromboendarterectomy, and for practical purposes can be ignored. If the surgeon mistakenly uses the innermost plane as the plane of dissection, it is likely that atherosclerotic plaques and shaggy material hanging onto the arterial wall will form again and that thrombosis will recur.

If at the distal termination of an endarterectomy a thickened or loosely adherent intima is left, it probably means that the dissection has not been carried far enough. A good indication that an adequate endarterectomy has been accomplished is a tightly adherent, thin intima or smooth tapering of the distal plaque. When it is difficult to carry the endarterectomy to a point at which the intima is tightly adherent, it is important that the distal intima be sutured to the arterial wall to prevent dissection when blood flow is reestablished. The distal atheromatous intima one encounters may be loosened by the surgical dissection itself. When this occurs, the intima may be dissected away from the adventitia when blood flow is reestablished, with the result that a flap of intima drops into the lumen of the artery and causes acute occlusion. Suture the intima with three or four mattress sutures on the four quadrants of the vessel using fine Dacron of 6–0 or 7–0 size. This procedure leaves a small portion of the suture within the lumen of the artery, but the risk of thrombosis from this foreign body is less than that from dissection of an intimal flap.

Closure of the thromboendarterectomy is done with a standard running baseball stitch of 3–0 to 5–0 Dacron depending upon the size of the vessel. Because of the thinness of the adventitia that remains after endarterectomy, bleeding from the suture holes is common. This is easily controlled by the application of a dry pad held in place for 2 or 3 minutes as already described.

Other factors besides loose distal intima that favor early thrombosis following aortoiliac endarterectomy are poor outflow situations and postoperative hypotension from such factors as hypovolemia or myocardial infarction. Careful preoperative evaluation seems the best means of preventing these complications. Improving outflow by distal bypass grafting or by a more appropriate manner of completion of the endarterectomy may at times change the course of early thrombosis.

When the occlusive disease extends over a longer length of aortoiliac segment, such as from the renal arteries to the iliac bifurcation, a Dacron bypass graft is preferred. The proximal suture line can be either an end-to-end anastomosis of aorta to a bifurcation graft or an end-to-side anastomosis. The latter is accomplished by obtaining proximal and distal control of aorta, applying a partially occluding clamp, and incising a window in the anterior aortic wall. The angled Dacron graft is then sutured with running 3–0 vascular sutures. Next, the distal limbs of the graft are trimmed and sutured as described earlier for resection of an aortic aneurysm. The distal anastomosis may be end-to-side, probably the most commonly used anastomosis, or end-to-end. If no retrograde flow up the iliac arteries is anticipated because of solid occlusion of the vessels, it may be preferable to transect the artery and do an end-to-end anastomosis. Since many patients have some proximal channel of flow, many prefer an end-to-side anastomosis like that just described for

connection of the graft to the aorta. Before the iliac arteries are cross-clamped, heparin solution should be injected distally or given systemically even though the iliac arteries are totally occluded. It is almost impossible to work on the iliac vessels without either dividing or partially occluding some of the collateral channels with the abdominal packs and retractors necessary to gain proper exposure. Therefore, the already sluggish flow in the distal extremity may be further compromised during the operative procedure. It is most disheartening to carry out a rather extensive procedure, remove the clamps, and discover distal occlusion due to the period of low flow in the distal extremity. Open the distal clamp just before completing the anastomosis to allow backflow to flush out any clots that may have formed. If the backflow is not good, Fogarty catheters are used to remove clots from the distal arterial tree. The distal arterial tree is then filled with dilute heparin solution and the anastomosis is rapidly completed. If good pulses are not obtained distal to the graft, the graft or the artery must be opened and all clots must be removed by means of Fogarty balloon catheters. If the patient's feet have not been left exposed during the operative procedure, the drapes should be applied so that they can be turned back for inspection of the feet before the procedure is completed and the incisions are closed. [The aorta must be cleared of intraluminal thrombus at the level of the aortic anastomosis, and systemic heparinization is often preferred. Ed.]

A bifurcation graft from the aorta is tunneled through the retroperitoneal space along the course of the patient's own vessels into the femoral canal in order to provide an aortofemoral bypass. The proximal aortic anastomosis is made through a standard abdominal incision as discussed earlier. Bilateral groin incisions are then made and carried above the inguinal ligament, which is divided when necessary to gain proper exposure of the common femoral, profunda femoral, and superficial femoral arteries. Division of the inguinal ligament for adequate exposure is sometimes necessary in the obese patient.

Once the femoral arteries have been exposed, blunt finger dissection is carried out along the course of the femoral artery up into the abdomen and from the abdominal side down into the groin so that a tunnel is made. The graft must be carefully placed through the tunnel so that it will not twist, and adequate tension must be applied to prevent kinking when blood flow is reestablished.

Groin incisions are especially susceptible to infection, and insertion and suture of a graft here must be done carefully. The preoperative skin preparation is important, as is avoidance of contamination of the operative field during the procedure. Infection rarely occurs when the grafting procedure is carred out quickly and efficiently with minimal exposure of the groin wounds. When infection does occur, it almost always necessitates removal of the graft; otherwise disruption of the suture line will occur.

Administer antibiotics to the patient in whom a synthetic prosthesis has been inserted through a groin incision because this is one area in which prophylactic antibiotic therapy may be of value. Whether or not this therapy is of value is questionable; it is used on an empiric basis rather than because of any conclusive proof of its effectiveness. [Pre- and transoperative antibiotics are indicated. Ed.]

Hemorrhage is an ever-present complication of aortoiliac thromboendarterectomy or bypass grafting. The surgeon must be satisfied that the suture lines are watertight at the time of closure and that no open vessels remain. Whenever hemorrhage is suspected postoperatively, the patient must be returned to the operating room for reexploration and correction of the cause of the bleeding. No surgeon enjoys returning the patient to the operating room, particularly after a long and difficult procedure, but the willingness of the surgeon to do so as often as necessary in order to achieve a satisfactory outcome is one of the major factors in successful vascular surgery. Surgeons who are reluctant to accept the fact that the patient is bleeding, and who attempt to control bleeding from a graft site or arterial suture line by means of multiple blood transfusions rarely succeed.

A rare complication is ureteral obstruction secondary to adherence of the ureter to the synthetic graft. Ordinarily, the ureter is moved out of the way at the time of surgery and remains free of the synthetic prosthesis, but occasionally it drifts into contact with the prosthesis so that as healing and contracture of the tissues occur ureteral obstruction results. The management of this complication is reexploration following diagnosis by means of contrast studies through the ureters. The ureter is dissected free of the graft and tissue is interposed between the two structures. This procedure usually will correct the obstruction satisfactorily.

Aneurysm at the suture line, either proximal or distal, is rare when the anastomosis is carefully done. This was more common when silk sutures were used with synthetic graft materials; the almost universal use of synthetic sutures today has greatly reduced this complication. Occasionally, a suture pulls free sometime after the procedure is completed, with resulting development of hemorrhage and a small false aneurysm. Infection in the suture line eventually softens the vessel wall and allows the sutures to pull free; this may permit hemorrhage or aneurysm formation to take place.

Thrombosis at the endarterectomy site or in the synthetic prosthesis is always a threat in vascular surgery. It would seem natural to use anticoagulant therapy in patients undergoing these procedures, but the hazards of anticoagulants seem to outweigh the benefits that have been proven to date. Most surgeons believe that if a graft is properly placed and anastomoses are satisfactory technically, clotting will not occur and anticoagulant therapy is not necessary.

COMPLICATIONS OF FEMOROPOPLITEAL RECONSTRUCTION

One of the most common sites of atherosclerotic occlusion of peripheral vessels is the superficial femoral artery, where the occlusion produces the symptoms of intermittent claudication of the calf. The occlusion most often occurs at the site where the superficial femoral artery passes beneath the adductor magnus tendon to become the popliteal artery. Another fairly common site is the origin of the superficial femoral artery. In general, the indications for surgical intervention in occlusive disease of the femoropopliteal system are pain at rest and gangrene. Calf claudication alone resulting from superficial femoral artery occlusion may improve as collateral circulation develops. Many patients seek medical advice for non-disabling calf claudication and an explanation of their symptoms may be all that is required. In many patients superficial femoral artery occlusion is well tolerated and the fact that such occlusion exists is not sufficient reason to undertake surgical correction on the basis that gangrene will inevitably result.

Once the decision has been made that surgical intervention is necessary, arteriography is mandatory in order to properly localize the occlusive area within the superficial femoral artery and, of more importance, to visualize the distal runoff of the popliteal artery. The popliteal artery divides into three branches, and the runoff is considered good if all three, or two of the three, are patent. If only one vessel is patent or if the outflow vessels have distal blocks, the runoff is poor and the chances of success of a surgical procedure are markedly diminished.

At the time of operation the skin of the entire leg should be meticulously prepared and draped, in recognition of the higher incidence of infection in femoropopliteal grafts. The value of routine prophylactic antibiotic therapy in these surgical procedures has not been documented, but many prefer to start administration of antibiotics before surgery and continue it throughout the operative period and into the postoperative period in order to minimize infection. Experimental studies in which dogs with synthetic grafts were subjected to deliberate injection of a culture of staphylococci into the bloodstream have shown a protective effect of antibiotics under these conditions. Because the groin tends to be moist and to have a naturally high level of surface contamination, the chances of wound contamination are probably increased. In addition, fluid accumulations from lymphatic interruption and hematoma may be contributing factors.

When the saphenous vein is used as a bypass, large skin flaps may be made, with attendant increased risk of ischemia of the margins of the wound; subsequent breakdown and the invasion of the wound by surface bacteria may produce infection.

When synthetic grafts are used, the presence of a foreign body, if contaminated, again increases the incidence of infection. Since an infected graft can rarely be salvaged, protection against infection has high priority in the operative treatment of atherosclerotic occlusion of the femoral artery.

The superficial femoral artery and the popliteal artery are exposed through medial incisions which may or may not be connected, depending upon the surgeon's choice of procedure. If the occlusive process is quite localized, a small incision and a local endarterectomy may be chosen as the preferred method of managing the problem. Generally speaking, however, the atherosclerotic process, while it may be occlusive only at the level of the adductor magnus tendon, usually extends throughout the femoral vessel and necessitates a long bypass. A "well localized lesion" demonstrated by arteriography almost always proves to be a more extensive lesion on direct inspection. More graft failures are attributable to bypasses that fail to bypass all obstructive areas than to those that extend too far.

In placing the graft or isolating the saphenous vein, the dissection of flaps should be kept minimal; multiple non-connecting incisions often are useful in maintaining viable skin bridges and improving the vascularity of the wound margins. The femoral artery is then dissected free of its surrounding structures and encircled with a tape, as are the profunda femoris artery and the superficial femoral artery. The popliteal artery is isolated similarly and traction tapes are placed about it. Care must be taken in isolating the popliteal artery because the popliteal vein and one or two large tributaries are usually closely attached to it. Gentleness in dissection will prevent tearing of the popliteal vein, which might necessitate its ligation and thus result in impeded peripheral venous outflow. Once these vessels have been isolated, the graft — either a reversed saphenous vein or a synthetic graft — is sutured into the superficial femoral artery and into the popliteal artery. Standard techniques as mentioned elsewhere are utilized: the graft is sutured into each artery by the end-to-side technique. Occasionally, an end-to-end technique is used.

Care in the dissection will minimize the possibility of breaking off pieces of atheromatous material that might result in peripheral embolization. The vascular clamps used in the femoropopliteal reconstruction should be inspected to be sure they are non-crushing. Thrombosis secondary to damage by vascular clamps is probably more common than is realized. It is our practice to close the ratchet on the clamp only far enough to stop blood flow; this is generally at the first notch. Careless use and tightening of the clamp may provide just enough pressure to crack the intima and provide the proper conditions for thrombosis when the clamp is released.

When atherosclerotic plaques are found at the proposed level of graft attachment, there is a temptation to perform a localized endarterectomy. However, in situations in which graft flow is marginal, one advantage of saphenous vein grafts is that they provide a less thrombogenic surface immediately after operation. An intima-to-intima approximation in a non-endarterectomized artery is therefore preferred, as the endarterectomized arterial wall is more thrombogenic. When localized endarterectomy is attempted in the popliteal artery, no reasonably normal vessel wall may be found, and there is a risk of elevating a flap or producing turbulence at the termination of the endarterectomy. If a localized endarterectomy seems necessary at the site selected for distal anastomosis, one might question whether the site is appropriate for an anastomosis.

When a bypass is being constructed around a long stenotic area or into a popliteal artery with stenosis of some outflow vessels, the temptation to improve inflow or outflow by dilatation with a Fogarty catheter should be resisted because such a procedure will often produce complications. Distal embolization or loosening of plaques may result. A well conceived and executed bypass-graft procedure is usually preferable to an attempt at thrombectomy with a Fogarty catheter in management of atherosclerotic occlusion of these vessels. The most recent experience with the Grüntzig catheter has demonstrated a more favorable combined approach.

If the graft is to be tunneled under intact skin or bridges of skin, great care must be taken not to twist the graft, because twisting will result in obstruction when the clamps are released. As in all other arterial reconstructive procedures, the graft should be placed with slight tension so that kinking does not occur when blood flow is reestablished. The surgeon should always be prepared to carry out intraoperative angiography in femoropopliteal reconstructive procedures. If blood flow is not good when the clamps are released, an angiogram should be taken before the wound is closed. The technical skill required for successful reconstruction of the femoropopliteal arterial tree is much more than that necessary in reconstructive procedures on the aorta and iliac arteries, because the large size of the latter vessels and the higher flow rate allow a wider margin of error.

The most common postoperative complication is thrombosis of the graft, and in most instances this is secondary to poor distal runoff. Unfortunately, reconstructive surgery is often mandatory in the very patient in whom the runoff is the poorest. Sound surgical judgment is very important in these patients, because with some experience one can recognize those cases in which attempt at reconstruction is futile. When there appears to be at least a chance of success, even though the runoff is less than one would like, the result often is satisfactory for a matter of a few hours to a few days and then thrombosis occurs.

If thrombosis of the graft occurs in the early postoperative period, particularly in patients in whom outflow is poor, the condition of the limb may be made significantly worse than it was properatively. This should cause hesitancy in recommending an attempt at reconstruction with poor outflow unless the alternative is impending amputation. Late thrombosis of a graft may find sufficient development of collaterals that the limb remains in better condition than before the original graft placement. Late graft failure is more frequent with synthetic grafts than with vein grafts in this area, especially when the graft crosses the knee joint. Avoidance of the complication of late graft failure is best achieved by using vein grafts when a suitable vein is present.

If the limb is in jeopardy after early occlusion, and if a successful outcome is possible, reexplore despite the realization that chances of success are much less than in the initial procedure. Angiography at the time the graft is occluded serves only to confirm occlusion. If technical errors were identified by intraoperative angiograms at the completion of the initial procedure, reoperation may initially correct these problems. Otherwise, intraoperative angiography after graft thrombectomy may demonstrate correctible technical problems or may reveal that a different site of anastomosis seems more appropriate. In all these cases intraoperative arteriography at the completion of the second operation should confirm technical perfection. If reoperation is required by thrombosis of the graft, anticoagulants are routinely used in order to try to maintain patency of the graft, although their value remains in question. If the extremity has been reopened for a second look and thrombectomy or revision of a previously placed graft has been carried out, antibiotics are routinely used, beginning preoperatively and continuing through the postoperative period.

A lesser complication is hemorrhage occurring from the suture line. This usually occurs because a suture placed through a severely diseased artery has pulled through and allowed a bleeding point to develop. When this occurs, control by external means is usually not successful; the wound should be reopened and the bleeding area controlled by direct suture.

Edema of the leg is not uncommon after a successful reconstructive procedure, particularly if the period of ischemia before reconstruction was prolonged. The leg is pink and warm, with a reactive hyperemia; often rather marked peripheral edema follows. Although this state usually is self-limited and clears completely within 3 months, it may be disturbing when first seen. The edema may actually increase with ambulation rather than decrease, as one might expect with venous outflow obstruction. Lymphatic interruption during groin dissection has been implicated as a cause of this edema, and meticulous and accurate groin dissection, instead of needless lymphatic division, may help prevent it. Increased transcapillary escape of fluid has also been noted.

Infection occurring at the anastomotic site or along the course of the graft is perhaps the most serious complication that occurs. It may lead to false aneurysm formation or disruption of the graft with hemorrhage or both. When infection in the wound occurs, a program of aggressive débridement, use of topical and systemic antibiotics, and careful monitoring of the patient permits salvage of the graft in a few cases. Unfortunately, more grafts are lost than saved, and usually it is necessary to remove the graft and replace it. Replacement may be done through another route if it must be done immediately; otherwise, if the leg is viable, the wounds may be allowed to heal and another graft may be considered at a later date.

Occasionally, lymphorrhea will be seen after a femoropopliteal reconstruction; it usually is an exudation from the femoral wound. Treatment consists of bed rest and elevation of the leg for a few days to as long as a week. Spontaneous remission is usual; the condition almost never becomes a serious problem if it is properly managed and secondary infection is avoided. Careful application of the principles of sterile technique in handling the wound to avoid contamination from without is the major treatment.

False aneurysm may occur either in the immediate postoperative period or quite late after the reconstruction. It has been reported in as many as 23 per cent of femoral anastomoses in one series, but in an average of less than 5 per cent from a general survey of the literature. Anastomoses between synthetic graft and artery require continued integrity of the suture material for anastomotic security. The incidence of false aneurysm appears to have markedly decreased with the introduction of synthetic suture materials that maintain their strength indefinitely, unlike silk, which deteriorates and loses strength after many months. When false aneurysm occurs, it is usually necessary to correct the process surgically as soon as feasible. The dissection must be done carefully in order to prevent major hemorrhage, and proximal and distal control of the vessels as well as of the graft must be obtained before the false aneurysm is dissected out. Occasionally the mouth of the aneurysm when isolated is small and requires only closure with a simple suture. At other times disruption of a large area of suture line is found and a more extensive repair or anastomosis at a different level is required.

True aneurysm formation may also

occur. Usually it occurs in the artery above or below the graft. If these aneurysms are small, nothing need be done about them; but if they enlarge or if peripheral embolization occurs, they must be surgically resected.

An interesting complication that is being seen with the passage of time is the occurrence of atherosclerosis in vein bypass grafts. The same complication may be seen after thromboendarterectomy has been carried out. Fortunately, in most cases the patient has had a period of relief from symptoms after the surgical reconstructive procedure, since the atherosclerosis usually occurs only several years after the initial procedure. Prevention of this complication may depend on care in initial handling of the vein and avoidance of trauma to it.

Grafts in the femoropopliteal system are susceptible to progressive thrombosis, and in some carefully evaluated series of patients with vein bypass grafts the rate of thrombosis formation appears to be about 3 per cent per year. The rate is clearly somewhat higher with synthetic grafts but in both synthetic and vein grafts there is relentless progression of the disease.

Reconstruction of the femoropopliteal vessels is most satisfactory, from the patient's point of view, when disabling symptoms are relieved or limb salvage is achieved.

COMPLICATIONS OF SURGERY FOR PERIPHERAL ANEURYSMS

While aneurysmal formation can occur in any vessel of the body, the two most common sites, after the aorta, are the femoral and popliteal arteries. Popliteal aneurysms are far more common than are femoral aneurysms, and their complications may be quite severe. The main complication is thrombosis of the aneurysm with sudden ischemia of the distal extremity and loss of the limb if repair is not undertaken as an emergency procedure. In addition, distal embolization from clots within the aneurysm or rupture of the aneurysm with severe hemorrhage may occur.

Hemorrhage from a ruptured popliteal aneurysm rarely threatens life, since the bleeding is into a confined space and, there-fore, not so massive as that seen with ruptured aortic aneurysm. At the same time, the hemorrhage occurring within a confined space puts additional pressure on nerves and veins as well as muscle and may cause ischemic necrosis. Once hemorrhage has occurred, dissection becomes more difficult because the anatomic structures are not clearly defined and the chance of injuring adjacent veins and nerves makes the procedures more hazardous. It is unwise to wait for complications to arise from these aneurysms before advising operation, and with the present state of the art of vascular surgery, surgical correction of the aneurysm should be undertaken whenever the diagnosis is made. Arteriography may help delineate the outflow tract and give a better picture of what type of reconstruction may be necessary and what kind of a success rate may be anticipated.

Popliteal aneurysms may be approached through either a medial incision or a posterior incision that crosses the knee from one side to the other. Once the skin incision has been made, proximal and distal control must be obtained. If the aneurysm is inadvertently entered before adequate proximal and distal control have been achieved, control by means of finger pressure on the narrow opening from within is preferable to blind clamping, which risks venous damage. If the aneurysm is large, it is often necessary to divide the medial gastrocnemius origin and semimembranosus tendon, and reapproximate them at the completion of the procedure. The popliteal vein is always tightly adherent to the aneurysm and often stretched at that point. If the vein is in danger of being lacerated or divided as it is dissected free of the aneurysm, it is often wiser to clamp the artery proximally and distally, decompress the aneurysmal sac by opening it, and leave a portion of the sac attached to the vein. Damage to the popliteal vein with subsequent thrombosis may jeopardize the successful arterial reconstruction by setting the stage for thrombosis within the graft or by causing severe edema of the lower extremity postoperatively.

The tibial nerve is frequently stretched over the presenting surface of the aneurysm and thinned out because of the expansile mass. The nerve must be carefully dissected free of the aneurysm, and it usually is long enough to be gently retracted to the medial or lateral side to allow an approach to the aneurysm. [The medial approach avoids nerves. Ed.]

Before the aneurysm is dissected free from the surrounding structures and a great deal of retraction is placed on the aneurysmal sac, a distal clamp should be applied in order to prevent the loosening of clots within the aneurysm and subsequent embolization to the distal arterial tree. This is a significant threat in popliteal aneurysms, much more so than in aortic aneurysms.

Extensive aneurysms may originate above the knee, often as high as the middle of the thigh. If there is any question that adjacent structures may be damaged with resection of the sac, it may be preferable to ligate the proximal and distal ends of the aneurysm and bypass it with a vein or synthetic graft. Autologous vein grafts are probably preferable in this situation, but synthetic grafts work quite well in this area. They probably are more satisfactory here than they are in the femoropopliteal area because the artery is somewhat dilated and a graft with a fairly large diameter can be used. In addition, usually no more than 2 or 3 inches of synthetic material is required to bridge the gap. Aneurysmal change in the popliteal artery is usually associated with considerable elongation. The defect left after aneurysm excision is much shorter than it appears initially. Success rates with synthetic grafts for popliteal aneurysm reconstruction are quite high. If the graft crosses the joint, use saphenous vein if at all possible, because a synthetic graft crossing the joint space is less likely to be successful.

Complications occurring in grafts in the popliteal area are the same as those seen in other grafts.

Femoral artery aneurysms are less common than popliteal aneurysms, but the complications are similar. Distal embolization may occur as well as thrombosis or rupture. All three complications usually require immediate surgical intervention.

When extensive or limb-threatening distal embolization occurs, immediate resection is undertaken. After the artery has been controlled proximally and distally, the sac is opened and carefully cleaned of clots. Fogarty catheters are then used to clear the distal arterial tree. Once this has been accomplished, heparin solution is instilled and the distal artery clamped. The aneurysm is then resected and replaced by a graft of either autologous vein or synthetic material. [The graft can also be placed inside the aneurysm. Ed.]

The profunda femoris artery frequently is involved in the aneurysm, and care should be taken to preserve as much of its length as possible. Replant this vessel into either the side of the graft or the adjacent normal artery, to preserve flow as a protection against later atherosclerotic occlusive disease which may occur. At times the use of a bifurcation graft is appropriate.

Thrombosis of the aneurysm will produce serious ischemia of the leg in most instances. Immediate resection and grafting should be carried out. This may be accomplished in even the most debilitated patient with use of local anesthesia.

Rupture of a femoral artery aneurysm is similar to rupture of a popliteal aneurysm in that hemorrhage is usually into a confined space with pressure on surrounding structures. On occasion, these aneurysms are not seen until they have eroded through the skin, become infected, and ruptured onto the surface of the skin. Here the hemorrhage is massive and may be life-threatening. This problem is very difficult to manage because the infection makes grafting a hazardous procedure. Success can be obtained by débridement of the necrotic skin, use of a vein graft, and immediate coverage, using flaps of skin where possible and a split-thickness graft if the development of flaps is not possible. Antibiotic administration is mandatory and should be prolonged for an arbitrary 10 days to 3 weeks in these patients. [An extra-anatomic bypass graft through clean tissue planes may be required. Ed.]

If the rupture has occurred beneath intact, non-infected skin, the technique of resection is similar to that for any other aneurysm. The profunda femoris artery should be replanted into the graft where possible, and a cuff of common femoral artery wall is left on the profunda to provide easier suture with a smoother anastomosis. This is usually possible even if the portion of femoral vessel attached to the profunda orifice is part of the aneurysm wall.

In general, all femoral aneurysms should be resected once they are discovered because of the hazard of thrombosis or hemorrhage.

COMPLICATIONS OF CAROTID ARTERY SURGERY

The surgery of occlusive disease of the extracranial cerebral circulation has proven to be of great benefit for patients with transient ischemic attacks. Most of the patients are initially seen by the family physician or a neurologist before being referred for surgical care, but some are referred directly to a vascular surgeon for correction. Selection of patients is of extreme importance in reducing the complications of this procedure. All patients in whom transient ischemic attacks are suspected, those who have had a mild stroke from which they have fully recovered, and some who have had a completed stroke should be considered for possible surgical intervention.

In addition to the neurologic examination and general evaluation of the patient's condition, four-vessel angiography is valuable. If patients are operated upon on the basis of their symptoms, and perhaps the finding of a bruit or a thrill over the carotid artery, but without the benefit of arteriography, serious mistakes will be made and major complications will occur. Four-vessel angiography usually is accomplished by means of placement of a catheter in the aortic arch and will give satisfactory roentgenograms of the two carotid arteries as well as of the two vertebral arteries and intracranial views. Both direct and oblique views should be obtained. This not only helps to localize the lesion but in many instances is the determining factor in the decision about which lesion should be approached first. For example, marked stenosis of a vertebral artery, even with vertebral basilar symptoms, may well reflect a stenotic lesion in a carotid artery. The stenotic lesion in the carotid artery should be corrected initially and in many instances there will be no need for further surgical intervention. If the vertebral artery is treated first, and the carotid artery is stenotic, the result may be disaster. Four-vessel angiography reveals multiple lesions in approximately two-thirds of the patients.

An interval should be left between the time a completed stroke occurs and surgical intervention. Wait about 6 weeks after a completed stroke before attempting to relieve a stenotic lesion or an ulcerated plaque in the extracranial cerebral vessels, or until a normal brain scan is obtained.

Patients with an elongated tortuous or kinked carotid artery also are referred for evaluation, although this condition is rarely a cause of symptoms. A number of these patients are identified because a bulging pulsating supraclavicular mass is thought by the initial examining physician to be an aneurysm. In the great majority of cases the mass turns out to be a tortuous, kinked carotid artery; aneurysm formation in this area is extremely rare. There is little evidence that correction of the elongated tortuous carotid artery need be undertaken except in those few patients in whom definite symptoms are produced by positional change and in whom there is arteriographic evidence of partial occlusion of the carotid by kinking at this point.

During carotid artery surgery, it is important that the blood pressure be maintained, even if it requires the use of vasopressors. The anesthesiologist should have an appropriate vasopressor mixed and attached to an intravenous line ready to infuse at any time the blood pressure falls. While flow and pressure appear not to be related in most of the peripheral circulation, this is not true of the cerebral circulation and the maintenance of blood pressure during the operative procedure is extremely important. General anesthesia permits improved cerebral circulation. There is still a place for local anesthesia if the patient's condition is such that general anesthesia is thought not to be advisable.

Carotid endarterectomy is undertaken through an incision crossing the carotid bifurcation, usually along the border of the sternocleidomastoid muscle. As soon as the vascular sheath in the neck is entered, gentle dissection around the common carotid artery is carried out and proximal control is thus obtained. The dissection necessary to expose the carotid artery bifurcation will usually necessitate exposure of the hypoglossal nerve. It should be handled gently. Rough handling of the nerve may cause a postoperative paralysis of the tongue, and although it usually is only temporary, it may be troublesome. One must stress that in carotid artery surgery very gentle isolation of the arteries is necessary to avoid the risk of dislodging small pieces of ulcerated plaque as the vessels are manipulated. Generally the twisting and pushing that occurs when vascular structures are rapidly encircled for peripheral arterial reconstruction is of no significance; however, in carotid artery surgery there is danger of releasing emboli if the vessels are not manipulated gently.

Before the internal and external carotid arteries are isolated, the carotid body and carotid sinus nerve area may be injected with lidocaine (Xylocaine) in order to prevent bradycardia and possible hypotension. Some surgeons resect the nerve in this area.

The patient is given aqueous heparin systemically before the vessels are cross-clamped. The question of the use of an internal shunt remains. One may open the clamp on the internal carotid artery and check to see whether the blood flowing back out of it is well oxygenated; if it is, no internal shunt is used. If there is poor flow out of the internal carotid artery or if the blood appears to be somewhat deoxygenated, then an internal shunt is inserted, tapes are secured about it, and the procedure is continued. Others measure carotid artery backpressure to determine whether an internal shunt should be used. Some use routine shunts. When an internal shunt is used, it must be inserted rapidly, but care must be taken during insertion not to elevate the distal intima and produce an embolus or intimal flap.

It is extremely important that all the plaque be removed so that the normal intima of the internal carotid artery is tightly attached to the media in the upper line of resection of the plaque. If any is left, the danger of thrombosis or dissection of the plaquelike material off the wall of the vessel is great and a major complication may well occur. If there is any suspicion that the distal intima in the internal carotid artery is loose, it must be sutured down with very fine mattress sutures, our choice being 6–0 or 7–0 monofilament synthetic suture. Once the endarterectomy has been completed it is essential that the arteriotomy be flushed thoroughly with saline to remove even minute pieces of debris that may remain. Even the smallest amount of debris allowed to

flush up into the brain when the clamps are removed may cause serious cerebral impairment. The clamp on the internal carotid artery also is released for a moment to flush out any loose material that may be wedged in the clamp line; it is then reapplied. The external carotid is unclamped and backflow is allowed to wash out any collected debris. The common carotid clamp is released, so that any remaining debris or air bubbles are flushed up the external carotid artery, and the brain is thus protected. The clamp on the internal carotid artery is then released and flow to the brain is reestablished. The arteriotomy is closed with a single running suture of 5–0 monofilament synthetic suture material. If the vessel is small and it appears that it may be constricted somewhat by the suture line, a venous or Dacron patch is applied. This is not often necessary, but it should be kept in mind if there is any question that the suture line might create stenosis. In general, systemic heparinization will not cause major bleeding at the suture line and a dry sponge held on the suture line for a few moments until all oozing stops is adequate. The wound is closed in layers. Protamine sulfate can be used to reverse the systemic heparinization. If no patch has been used, a drain will prevent the small hematoma collection that often occurs in the neck in the first 24 hours after surgery.

The major complication in the postoperative period is diminution in cerebral function. The most common cause of this is small emboli that were retained in the endarterectomy area or have formed on the suture line and are released. It is of help to have palpated the temporal artery preoperatively and postoperatively because if thrombosis has occurred, it may well involve the external carotid artery and be reflected by a failure of pulsation in the temporal artery. Unfortunately, this is not a completely reliable test because the internal carotid artery can become occluded and the external carotid maintain its flow or vice versa. However, if the temporal artery has lost its pulsation in a patient in whom cerebral function has worsened, it is a good sign that the neck should be reexplored.

If there is no evidence of thrombosis by supra-orbital Doppler exam and/or oculoplethysmography and if the clinical condition has not worsened to suggest a stroke in progress, clinical dextran can be started and a unit is given for its volume expansion effect, its coating effect, and its mild anticoagulant effect.

If a major wound hematoma does occur, it usually means there is a leak at the arterial suture line or the divided facial vein has leaked. The venous system is ordinarily a low-pressure system, but with the coughing that often occurs postoperatively as the patient clears his lungs, high pressure may develop in the facial vein, which is almost always divided during the surgical procedure. If the tie comes off the facial vein, bleeding can be rather extensive and a large hematoma can occur. A leak from the arterial suture line is rare, but occasionally a stitch will pull loose, particularly one in a very friable artery, and may allow hemorrhage to occur. This is usually detected by hematoma formation or by blood coming out the drain left in the operative site; if the bleeding is extensive, reexploration is necessary.

A false aneurysm may occur at the suture line, and is probably slightly more common when vein and Dacron patch grafts have been used. If it should occur, it may require reexploration of the area and correction of the aneurysm at a later date.

Another complication that is seen in the postoperative period is a rather severe hypertension. About 10 per cent of patients become hypertensive in the recovery room, the blood pressure often going as high as 300 mm. Hg. There is no explanation for this phenomenon except to say that it does not appear to be harmful. Some surgeons have treated a number of patients with trimethaphan (Arfonad) in order to bring blood pressure down to a more acceptable range. Actually, there is no evidence that this transient hypertension is serious and no patients suffer cerebral dysfunction because of it. If hypotensive agents are used, one must be very careful in bringing the blood pressure down from these high levels not to allow it to fall below normal.

An occasional patient will have difficulty in maintaining a satisfactory blood pressure and may require the use of vasopressor therapy. Once hypovolemia has been ruled out, a hypersensitive carotid sinus should be considered as a possible cause. This phenomenon is not permanent but has occasionally persisted for several days without other apparent explanation.

Wound infection or infection at the site of the arteriotomy is very rare in carotid artery surgery. Treatment is similar to that for infection at other sites.

COMPLICATIONS OF VERTEBRAL AND SUBCLAVIAN ARTERY SURGERY

As mentioned in the previous section, when stenosis of the vertebral artery occurs, the main lesion should be looked for in the carotid artery and this should be repaired initially. The stenotic lesion of the vertebral artery is corrected subsequently only if symptoms persist; this occurs in less than 10 per cent of patients. Stenosis of the vertebral artery may be caused by a plaque within the vessel, by a fascial band in the neck, or by osseous spurs along the bony canal through which the vertebral artery passes.

One approach is through a supraclavicular incision, dividing the attachment of the sternocleidomastoid muscle and exposing the vertebral takeoff from the subclavian artery. One must be very careful in dissecting out the vessels at this level because if major hemorrhage occurs the proximal artery is difficult to control. A rapid median sternotomy may be required. One should be careful to avoid the recurrent laryngeal nerve as it crosses the right subclavian artery and the thoracic duct on the left side. Both these structures as well as the phrenic nerve may be damaged if dissection is not done with care. If the stenosis is in the takeoff of the vertebral artery, an incision is made in the subclavian vessel up onto the vertebral artery, endarterectomy is carried out, and a vein patch is applied to open the mouth of the vertebral artery.

During the operative procedure the pleural space may be entered and for this reason a postoperative chest film should be obtained and aspiration of tube thoracostomy should be carried out if a pneumothorax has occurred.

The subclavian steal syndromes have evoked increased interest in recent years, having been described by a number of authors. Symptoms of vertebral basilar insufficiency consisting of vertigo, transient blindness, and syncopal attacks, together with a blood pressure differential of more than 20 mm. Hg between the two arms, suggest a subclavian steal syndrome. If retrograde flow down the vertebral into the subclavian can be seen, with a proximal occlusion of the subclavian artery by angiography, the diagnosis of a steal syndrome may be made.

On the right side a subclavian endarterectomy is usually relatively easily carried out through a supraclavicular approach. On the left side, because of the difficulty of identifying the proximal subclavian as it comes off the aortic arch, one can approach it only through a formal thoracotomy. On this side, therefore, many prefer to insert a bypass graft from the left common carotid artery to the subclavian artery distal to the occlusion. The carotid-subclavian bypass should not rob the cerebral circulation, although the arteriograms of the left common carotid artery must be carefully evaluated to ensure that there is no stenotic lesion proximal to the takeoff of the bypass graft.

Ligation of the vertebral artery has been carried out by some authors to prevent the retrograde flow. Subclavian-subclavian bypass graft procedures have also been reported. Complications of running a vein graft across the neck are not great, but these grafts will probably prove to be subject to a higher occlusion rate because of their length. There may be patients in whom technical difficulties preclude the carotid-subclavian bypass and perhaps these situations may provide the rare indication for a subclavian-subclavian bypass or axillo-axillary bypass.

In general, the surgical approach to treatment of stenosis of the extracranial cerebral circulation is very satisfactory when done very carefully. Because many of these patients are relatively asymptomatic, having had only transient ischemic attacks, the surgery must carry a very low morbidity and mortality in order to be justified. It should be carried out only by surgeons with experience in the field, with meticulous technique and a thorough understanding of the changing neurologic picture that may occur with these lesions, and with the ability to do the procedure quickly. The shorter the period of clamping, particularly of the carotid arteries, the better the results will be and the fewer the complications. While the use of an internal shunt may be helpful, it does not carry normal flow and therefore does not give the surgeon time to be inefficient in the operation.

COMPLICATIONS OF SURGERY FOR THORACIC OUTLET SYNDROME

Complications following surgical management of a thoracic outlet syndrome are relatively uncommon. They may be due to improper diagnosis initially or may be secondary to the actual operative procedure.

The thoracic outlet syndrome may be manifested by either neurologic or vascular symptoms, or both. It is included in a section on the complications of vascular surgery because symptoms may involve the vascular system initially and because the operative intervention, even if it is done for purely neurologic difficulties, may well compromise the vascular system.

The selection of the patient for operation is most important in this syndrome because the differential diagnosis of a true thoracic outlet syndrome from other neurologic problems is most important. A complete neurologic examination is necessary in all patients, and consultation with a neurologist is frequently of much help in differentiating the source of difficulty. In addition to careful neurologic and vascular examinations of the extremity involved, films of the cervical spine as well as routine chest films should be obtained. These will help rule out problems such as a Pancoast tumor affecting the brachial plexus or cervical osteoarthritis involving the brachial plexus.

Arteriography is not always necessary and is limited by many to patients with complete occlusion of the axillary artery manifested by absence of peripheral pulses, or patients with a loud bruit.

Studies of conduction time may also be helpful diagnostically in certain circumstances. A nerve conduction velocity of less than 60 meters per second with one electrode in the supraclavicular space and another over an appropriate nerve in the upper arm appears to be of value in suggesting compression between the two electrodes.

Phlebography may also be of help when there is evidence of venous obstruction.

Many of these patients have dilated veins across the chest wall or in the affected arm, and a phlebogram, which is much simpler to carry out than an arteriogram, may give valuable information. Demonstration of a constriction of the vein as it passes through the thoracic outlet is helpful diagnostic evidence of compression.

The thoracic outlet syndrome may be due to a long cervical rib that comes around and attaches to the first rib. In those patients in whom a true cervical rib is identified, resection of this rib through a supraclavicular approach should be the first step in alleviating the compression syndrome. Some authors prefer to attempt to remove the cervical rib through the transaxillary approach at the same time as they remove the first rib. The supraclavicular approach with a small incision made just above the clavicle offers an easy exposure of the cervical rib, and gentle dissection around the brachial plexus allows it to be elevated and the rib to be removed from its origin behind the plexus and its insertion on the first rib. Major complications may occur with this approach if one proceeds without a clear view of the anatomy and without caution. Gentle dissection in the area of the root of the neck will usually allow a favorable outcome with minimal complications. A thorough understanding of the anatomy is mandatory if the surgeon is to avoid trouble.

In the vast majority of patients, a cervical rib is not present, and the thoracic outlet syndrome is secondary to compression caused by scissoring of the clavicle or scalenus muscles against the first rib. Resection of the first rib opens the thoracic outlet and is the treatment of choice in all patients without cervical rib regardless of the original cause of the compression. A transaxillary approach is used. Once the skin and subcutaneous tissues have been incised, the muscles are retracted by gentle blunt dissection. It is important that the retractors not have too deep a blade so that they do not compress the brachial plexus and the vessels. Once the ribs are visualized, one can simply proceed up the chest wall until the first rib is reached. The patient's arm, which has been prepared and draped so that it is free, is held by an assistant and gentle traction is applied at the time of dissection in the region of the first rib. This traction allows the space between the first rib and the clavicle to be opened up so that the dissection is more easily carried out. Too much traction applied by the assistant who is elevating the arm may overstretch the brachial plexus and cause injury. Traction is usually applied with the elbow at a 90-degree angle, and, again, too much traction may damage the ulnar nerve as it runs through its groove at the elbow.

Gentle dissection of the first rib, incision of the periosteum, and removal of the rib with its periosteum are carried out in standard fashion. One complication that may occur at this point in the procedure is damage to the vessels or brachial plexus by the heavy instruments necessary to cut the rib. The working space is quite confined, and one must be very careful upon the insertion of bone-cutting instruments that the brachial plexus and the vessels are clear of the cutting instrument. Although some direct vision is possible in this portion of the procedure, it too demands a thorough knowledge of the anatomy and control with a finger placed ahead of the cutting instrument to protect all soft tissue such as the brachial plexus and vessels. It is equally important, after the rib has been cut and removed, that the remaining ends of the rib be carefully palpated and all bone spicules removed. Both the plexus and the vessels will run over the end of the cut surfaces of the rib, and bone spicules may damage these structures.

It is quite easy to enter the pleural cavity during the procedure because the pleura is occasionally so tightly adherent to the ribs that it cannot be gently pushed away from the rib. At the termination of the procedure the axilla is filled with saline and the anesthetist inflates the lung and an air leak is looked for. If there is no air leak, the axilla is closed in layers in standard fashion. The presence of an air leak demands either the introduction of a thoracostomy tube or the use of one or more aspirations until the lung has reexpanded.

A routine chest film is mandatory at the termination of the procedure, because a saline irrigation of the axilla will not always reveal a defect in the pleura. If there is any pneumothorax, aspiration or tube thoracostomy is the definitive step for managing the air leak. Some hematoma undoubtedly occurs in this wound, as in any other, but it apparently dissects down the chest wall, leaving the axilla flat, so that no drainage is necessary. The avoidance of a drain and the use of a subcuticular closure in the moist axillary region appear to decrease maceration and irritation about the suture line and may be of value in preventing wound infection.

Early active shoulder motion will avoid prolonged disability. The patient is instructed not to abduct beyond 45 degrees at the shoulder for the first 2 weeks in order to prevent wound tension and dehiscence.

COMPLICATIONS OF SYMPATHECTOMY

Although sympathectomy has long been a part of the vascular surgeon's armamentarium, enthusiasm for the procedure has waxed and waned over the past 40 years. Five indications for sympathectomy are now reasonably well documented: (1) to relieve vasospasm, (2) to aid the development of collateral circulation, (3) to relieve causalgia, (4) to relieve hyperhidrosis, and (5) to attempt to increase blood flow to skin with non-healing cutaneous lesions when arterial reconstruction is not feasible.

There is no place for sympathectomy in the treatment of intermittent claudication. The arterioles that supply the muscle are not under sympathetic control — there are no sympathetic fibers controlling these vessels. Thus, sympathectomy has no effect on blood flow into the muscle mass. It does have a role to play in ischemic vascular disease in which the skin is involved. There is ample sympathetic supply to the arterioles of the skin. When one is dealing with ischemic ulcers of the skin, sympathectomy may be indicated to reduce the spasm in these vessels and to aid in the development of collateral circulation and, thus, the healing of a skin ulcer.

The most common role of sympathectomy today is in the treatment of vasospastic disease. In these cases, arteriography is often indicated and it must be remembered that the contrast medium may produce additional spasm in the affected vessels, with subsequent thrombosis. Whenever arteriography is to be carried out in a patient with vasospastic disease, a vasodilator should be used with the contrast medium or should at least be available for immediate injection if necessary. The injection of 0.1 mg. of reserpine intra-arterially may relieve spasm and at times provides long-term relief.

It is sometimes possible to predetermine the effect of sympathectomy by carrying out a sympathetic block with various local anesthetic agents and monitoring the response as manifested by skin temperature and plethysmographic changes. In addition to the complications that may arise from introduction of a needle anywhere in the body, there are some additional complications of sympathetic block. Hypotension may develop, because between 500 and 1000 ml. of blood may be redistributed after sympathetic blockade. This may lead to cerebral or coronary insufficiency, or may cause spontaneous thrombosis elsewhere in the body as blood is redistributed. If hypotension develops at the time of sympathetic blockade, immediate anticoagulation should be undertaken to prevent thrombosis until blood flow is restored.

Realizing the difficulty of predicting the sympathetic block response in the lower extremities, others have used galvanic skin resistance and resting ankle pressure as predictors. To date there is no proven definitive test that accurately predicts response to sympathectomy.

COMPLICATIONS OF DORSAL SYMPATHECTOMY

Dorsal sympathectomy is most often carried out for patients who are suffering from Raynaud's phenomenon or Raynaud's disease. It is rarely effective for any length of time in patients who are suffering from Raynaud's phenomenon secondary to a collagen disease such as scleroderma.

There is an extremely high rate of recurrence of sympathetic activity in the arm, usually within 1 to 2 years after the procedure has been carried out. This high rate of failure to maintain the effects of sympathectomy in a limb is not well understood but it may be due to regeneration of sympathetic fibers or to heightened sensitivity to catecholamines following sympathectomy.

Dorsal sympathectomy may be accomplished through a supraclavicular approach, a transaxillary approach, or the extrapleural posterior approach with or without removal of a section of the third or fourth ribs.

There are two complications that may arise from use of the supraclavicular approach: production of a pneumothorax from an opening in the apex of the pleura and damage to the brachial plexus by retraction or by dissection of the region. The supraclavicular approach has the advantage of allowing more extensive dissection of the sympathetic chain in the cephalad direction, particularly the stellate ganglion. The development of a pneumothorax is not a serious complication as long as the surgeon is aware of its possibility and obtains an x-ray of the chest immediately after operation. If pneumothorax has occurred, insertion of a tube thoracostomy with water-seal drainage will allow reexpansion of the lung and closure of the hole in the pleura. Damage to the brachial plexus and vessels in the supraclavicular region can be prevented only by a thorough knowledge of the anatomy, careful anatomic dissection, and care in the placement and use of retractors.

The complications of a transaxillary transpleural approach include pneumothorax and damage to the vascular structures and brachial plexus. In the transaxillary approach the pleura is opened and the sympathetic fibers are approached through it. A pneumothorax is thus intentionally created. Although it is a part of the operative procedure, it is also a complication of the operation and must be managed as already described. With the transaxillary approach the surgeon works in a deep hole that may be poorly illuminated, and very careful dissection is required to prevent injury to the brachial plexus and axillary vessels secondary to the pull of the retractors necessary to open the space properly. Another complication of this approach may also occur: too much tension on the arm as the assistant lifts it to open the axilla may cause overstretching of the nerves of the brachial plexus and subsequent damage. Complications may be avoided by careful dissection, working in a bloodless field, care in placement and use of retractors, and minimizing tension on the abducted arm.

Pneumothorax may be a complication of the posterior extrapleural approach, too, if the pleura is inadvertently opened. Again, no great harm is done if the condition is recognized and proper treatment instituted. An additional complication results from the fact that the area in which the surgeon must work is extremely limited, and upward and downward dissection for access to more of the sympathetic chain is very difficult. To attempt to remove more of the sympathetic chain that can be easily visualized under direct operative control is hazardous, and major damage and hemorrhage may occur if great care is not taken in the dissection.

If the stellate ganglion is totally resected, the patient will suffer permanently from Horner's syndrome, which consists of ptosis of the eyelid, constriction of the pupil, usually enophthalmos, and absence of sweating on the affected side of the head and face. Resection of only the lower half of the stellate ganglion should produce equivalent sympathectomy while avoiding Horner's syndrome, but it should be carefully explained to the patient prior to surgery that this result may occur. Most patients who need a sympathectomy accept this with minimal complaint.

PARAVERTEBRAL BLOCK AND LUMBAR SYMPATHECTOMY

When the surgeon is dealing with the lower extremity, lumbar sympathectomy is sometimes preceded by a paravertebral block, which provides a temporary sympathectomy and may permit the surgeon to estimate the effect that surgical sympathectomy will have on blood flow in the lower extremity. It is especially valuable when one is trying to separate out any questionable vasospastic element in the patient who has had arteriosclerotic occlusion of the vessels in the leg.

Paravertebral block is usually done with the patient in the prone position, and the needle is inserted through the back to the paravertebral space. This should always be carried out before anticoagulant therapy for occlusive disease in the legs is begun. If anticoagulants have already been given, the paravertebral block should not be attempted until the anticoagulation effect has been reversed or adequate time has been allowed for the anticoagulant to dissipate. Otherwise, needle puncture of an artery or vein in the paravertebral region may produce serious hemorrhage.

A successful paravertebral block with a marked increase in skin temperature secondary to increased blood flow to the skin is an indication that surgical sympathectomy will be successful, but if the paravertebral block fails to provide increased blood flow to the skin, this does not mean that surgical sympathectomy will be of no value. In this case, the decision to operate may have to be made on a clinical basis with full recognition that it may fail. If there is reasonably good evidence of a vasospastic element in the disease, even though large vessels may be occluded in conditions such as Buerger's disease, surgical sympathectomy may be indicated, particularly when there are ischemic ulcers of the skin associated with large vessel occlusion.

If lumbar sympathectomy is planned, there are several complications that must be considered. There seems to be little or no effect of lumbar sympathectomy on sexual function in the female, but a marked decrease in function may be observed in the male. It is wise to leave the ganglion of the first lumbar vertebra intact on one side when bilateral lumbar sympathectomy is carried out in the male. This will help maintain sexual function at whatever degree was present prior to the operation.

Sympathectomy decreases the ability of the skin to sweat, and dry cracked skin is sometimes a significant complication. When cracking occurs because of dryness, the extremity should be carefully protected from external trauma and a good hand lotion containing lanolin should be applied at least twice a day. This will keep the skin oily and soft and prevent the cracking that may lead to infection.

One of the most significant complications is postsympathectomy neuralgia, which occurs in 20 to 30 per cent of patients undergoing a lumbar sympathectomy. The patient has usually almost completely recovered from the operative procedure when sometime between the fifth and twentieth day (usually about the tenth), and often after the patient has gone home, severe pain or hyperesthesia develops along the anteromedial aspect of the thigh or occasionally in the sacroiliac area. Although this pain is usually self-limited and will disappear within 2 to 3 months, it may be so severe as

to necessitate opiates for its control. The dose of the drug should be kept as low as possible and the patient should be encouraged to continue normal activities. The cause of this complication is unknown and there is no effective way to prevent it, although some have felt that preserving the first lumbar ganglion bilaterally lowers its incidence. [We have not observed this incidence or severity. Ed.]

During the operative procedure, the lumbar veins, which may cross in front of or behind the sympathetic chain, must be identified and carefully dissected free to prevent their being avulsed from the vena cava or torn at the time the chain is removed. Control of these bleeding vessels by direct clamping and ligature may be difficult. Use of metal clips has proven to be of significant benefit in managing these small vessels. Control may also be obtained by placing a lap pad in the wound and applying pressure for a few moments. This will stop the hemorrhage in most cases or at least clear the field so that better visualization of the bleeding point is obtained. It is much easier to prevent damage to these vessels than to treat it. Careful dissection should be the goal.

Although the peritoneum is not entered during sympathectomy, paralytic ileus may accompany the retroperitoneal dissection. This possibility should be anticipated and preventive measures should be taken, including insertion of a nasogastric tube and the stopping of all oral intake until bowel activity returns.

COMPLICATIONS OF ARTERIAL INJURY

In various conflicts since World War II significant advances in the management of acute arterial injuries, even under battle conditions, have led to vast improvement in management of civilian arterial injuries. During World War II ligation of an injured artery was the primary method of treatment, and the overall amputation rate was 49 per cent. Direct arterial repair was introduced during the Korean Conflict and reduced the amputation rate to 13 per cent. The same amputation rate prevailed during the war in Vietnam, although isolated late reports from that conflict suggest that an

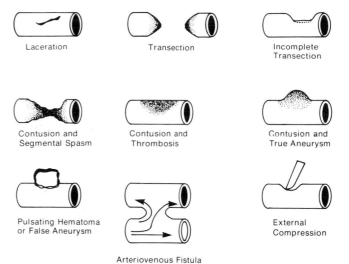

Figure 18–4 Common types of arterial trauma. Lacerations and transections account for the vast majority of arterial injuries. Transections may be associated with avulsions with missing segments of artery. External compression can be caused by displaced bone from comminuted fractures. (Rich, N. M., and Spencer, F. C.: Vascular Trauma. Philadelphia, W. B. Saunders Company, 1978.)

amputation rate as low as 6.5 per cent was obtained.

The development of high-velocity missiles has led to a cavitation type of arterial injury that is somewhat different from the direct injury to the artery by shell fragment and bullet that was commonplace before World War II. As the high-velocity missile penetrates tissue, it creates within the tissue a cavity whose rapid expansion may severely damage a vessel that the missile never touched. Thus, the possibility of arterial injury must be kept in mind, even if the point of entry of the missile is not in the immediate vicinity of the major vessels.

Blood vessels, particularly the arteries, demonstrate some unique responses to injury (Fig. 18–4). They tend to retract when complete transection has occurred. Thrombosis also occurs and blood loss is thus diminished. The partially transected or lacerated vessel does not have this unique ability to contract and tends to continue to bleed, causing a major hemorrhage and sometimes death.

An additional type of injury secondary to blunt trauma has been described in recent years. What often was thought probably to be arterial spasm after blunt trauma is now known to be obstruction to the flow of blood caused by an intimal flap produced by a tear in the intima. The flap may fall into the lumen of the vessel, causing complete obstruction to flow, or dissection may extend behind the flap and push more intima into

the lumen to cause further obstruction. Perivascular hematoma may cause compression of the vessel with subsequent thrombosis.

Concomitant venous injury frequently occurs with arterial injury and may be present in as many as 40 per cent of arterial injuries. Concomitant nerve involvement occurs in about 20 per cent of arterial injuries. Thus, in any patient suspected of having an arterial injury, careful search and evaluation for accompanying venous and nerve injury must be made.

It is important to maintain close observation of an extremity that has been placed in a plaster cast. If typical signs of ischemia appear — namely, a cold, white, pulseless extremity distal to the cast — the cast must be opened immediately and the extremity carefully observed for the return of circulation. If the circulation does not appear to be normal within a few minutes, arteriography is indicated.

The diagnosis of acute arterial injury is not always easy since approximately 50 per cent of the patients are in serious shock, that is, with a systolic blood pressure of less than 80 mm. Hg. Under these conditions the skin tends to be pale and cool, and distal pulses may be difficult to palpate. One can usually detect a difference between the truly ischemic limb and one that simply reflects a low-flow state secondary to hypovolemia. An ischemic limb often is painful if the patient is conscious, there may be difficulty in moving the extremity, and venous filling is minimal to absent. There is also a slightly different color to the truly ischemic limb, in that it may be slightly mottled rather than pale as is the limb of the patient in shock. If the question cannot be answered by direct inspection, arteriography should be carried out immediately. In the patient in shock resuscitation and correction of other, more life-threatening injuries have higher priority than management of the ischemic limb. Once successful resuscitation has been accomplished and the normal limb has begun to regain color, vascular tone, and pulses, the ischemic extremity can be investigated and proper therapy carried out.

In as many as 25 per cent of patients with acute arterial injury pulses are palpable below the injured segment of the vessel. The presence of palpable pulses does not exclude arterial injury. Careful assessment of the type of injury, determination of the course of the missile or knife in penetrating injury, and awareness of possibility of arterial injury in blunt trauma are necessary to prevent serious complications. The routine use of a stethoscope in a suspected area may document an arterial injury by revealing a bruit suggesting partial occlusion of a vessel or a continuous bruit suggesting an arteriovenous fistula. This is more common than is usually appreciated in cases of penetrating injury.

Certain complications can be avoided if a few simple rules are kept in mind when the patient enters the emergency department. Under no circumstances should blind clamping of vessels be attempted for control of hemorrhage in a wound that is bleeding profusely. This is dangerous because serious damage can be done to adjacent structures such as nerves and veins or to the artery if it is clamped at a point where it is not actually bleeding. When uncontrollable bleeding occurs in an extremity, pressure should be applied directly to the wound and satisfactory control achieved.

Since acute arterial injuries often require direct surgical correction with the addition of foreign bodies such as sutures and occasionally synthetic grafts, antibiotic administration should be started as soon as the patient is seen in the emergency department.

In the operating room, complications can be avoided by using an elective incision that will give the best exposure of the vessel. Too often the surgeon attempts to use the incision that has been created by the trauma, merely extending it in one direction or another, and still has difficulty in gaining control of and repairing the vessel. This situation may force the surgeon to resort to dissection of flaps and destruction of viable tissue in order to obtain adequate exposure of the vessel. High-velocity missiles frequently create such large wounds that exposure of the vessel is easily accomplished by simply extending the wound through longitudinal incisions. This type of wound does not require development of flaps for exposure of the vessel. Most wounds in the civil population are of far less destructive force and the ideal approach to the vessel is through a separate incision directly over the course of the vessel.

After satisfactory proximal and distal control has been obtained and the arterial injury identified, the best method of managing the arterial injury is determined. Adequate débridement of the injured artery is important.

If a graft must be used to bridge a gap in the vessel because of loss of tissue, a vein graft is preferred in a patient with an open injury. Danger of infection with use of synthetic grafts in compound injuries is great. If a synthetic graft must be used, antibiotic therapy should be continued for a long period of time. The graft must also be covered with viable soft tissue if infection is to be prevented. If a large skin defect exists, the arterial repair may be covered by the movement of a flap of muscle over the damaged artery or, if this is impossible, a split-thickness skin graft can be applied directly over the arterial repair. Closure of the skin may be carried out in a more satisfactory manner at a later date. In addition to these specific complications, all complications of arterial suture and repair that have been mentioned previously apply to vessels that have undergone severe trauma.

Serious arterial injury may be encountered when the abdomen is explored after penetrating injury or blunt trauma. If the abdomen is contaminated by perforation of a hollow viscus, this should be repaired first, after the hemorrhage has been controlled by the application of appropriate vascular clamps. Once the viscera have been repaired, thorough irrigation of the abdominal cavity with antibiotic solutions is mandatory before correction of the vascular defect is undertaken. The arterial injuries occurring within the abdomen are usually to large vessels, and vein graft repair is totally inadequate. The surgeon is forced to use a synthetic graft. The ingenuity of the surgeon is tested because it is important that a graft for replacement of an injured artery be placed in such a way as to bypass the contaminated peritoneal cavity if possible. This may necessitate tunneling a graft through the retroperitoneal space or moving it anterior beneath the anterior peritoneum of the abdominal wall. If for some reason the graft must run through the peritoneal cavity and contamination has occurred, it is probably worthwhile to wrap the graft with omentum because of its unique ability to collect scavenger cells as well as bacteria, and to satisfactorily manage these particles. The abdomen must subsequently be closed so that the graft is satisfactorily buried. Drainage is unwise because it may permit the ingress of bacteria.

A major complication of arterial injury is obstruction distal to the point of injury and repair. If after satisfactory repair of an arterial injury the distal flow is not adequate, intraoperative arteriograms must be obtained. Because these patients often have multiple injuries, there may be a delay in getting the patient to the operating room, and because a low-flow state distal to the injury may have existed for some time, distal arterial obstruction frequently occurs. Whether the obstruction is due to a clot that has formed in situ, or to a piece of intima or arteriosclerotic plaque that has broken off from the point of injury and slipped on down the artery, or whether an intimal flap has developed with distal thrombosis is unimportant. Arteriography following repair will demonstrate the arterial occlusion, and cleanout of the distal vessel with the Fogarty catheter is mandatory. The patient should not be allowed to leave the operating room in the vain hope that the circulation will improve with time, when under direct vision the arterial outflow appears inadequate. Only by investigating the problem immediately can the patient be assured of the fullest possible recovery.

If the adjacent vein has been injured with a major artery, venous repair should be undertaken. The resultant improvement in venous return decreases the peripheral resistance, thus improving the flow through the arterial repair and reducing the chance of thrombosis. Most veins can be repaired by direct or lateral suture, depending upon the type of injury. Should a defect be present in the vein, a length of vein graft similar to that used in the artery may be used to bridge it. If the ipsilateral vein was partially destroyed by the injury, pieces of it may be used for grafting. If it is intact, a graft should be removed from the opposite leg in order to protect the venous return through the saphenous on the injured side. Should repair or grafting of the deep venous system fail, the saphenous may be the major collateral vessel available for venous return. A thrombosed deep venous system may recanalize but the saphenous will help carry the load in the interim. Synthetic grafts are rarely satisfactory in vein repair, have a very high rate of thrombosis, and probably should not be used.

Whenever an injury occurs in an extremity, swelling within tight fascial compartments may occur. Even in the absence of arterial or venous injury, major compression of arteries, nerves, and veins may occur. The most frequent site of this complication is the anterior compartment of the lower leg, but it may occur in any of the fascial compartments of the extremities. Diagnosis should be suspected if there is swelling of the extremity or if there has been a significant delay from the time of injury to the time of repair or when arterial and venous injury along with massive soft tissue crushing has occurred. When such a situation exists, immediate fasciotomy, opening the entire length of the fascial compartment, must be carried out as an urgent procedure. To be of significant clinical benefit fasciotomy must be performed early. When in doubt, the conservative approach is to perform the fasciotomy. This procedure carries a risk of some complications, although it is relatively simple to perform. In the lower extremity, care must be taken to avoid the peroneal nerve so that a foot drop is not precipitated by the fasciotomy. Large tissue planes are opened to the outside and secondary infection may occur unless meticulous aseptic technique is employed.

Arterial injury can occur in the presence of a major fracture. When this situation exists, the fracture should be immobilized. Internal or external fixation may be necessary. Once the bony parts have been immobilized, the vascular surgeon may repair the artery and expect it to remain intact. A properly performed arterial repair without undue tension will withstand the usual forces that result from traction.

There is a place for the ligation of a major artery, although it may be a difficult decision from an emotional point of view. Primary amputation may also be indicated. In this day of vascular surgery, it is not uncommon to see an arterial injury repaired in an extremity that has an inadequate muscle mass or bone structure and no sensation or movement. Under these circumstances, even though viability may be maintained by repair of the artery, the extremity itself is useless and will create serious problems for the patient.

A major complication of arterial injury is the development of an arteriovenous fistula or a false aneurysm. The latter occurs when a laceration is made into an artery and blood flows out of the artery into the surrounding tissue spaces. Instead of clotting completely, the blood is forced out in a steady stream by arterial pressure and begins to pulsate against the soft tissues. A capsule may form around this blood, creating a hollow cavity with arterial flow out into it and back into the artery. The term false aneurysm is used for this expanding mass. It has no true intimal lining since there is a hole in the entire thickness of the arterial wall.

Arteriovenous fistula may occur when an artery and vein in close proximity to each other are injured. When such an injury is suspected, it can often be diagnosed by the to and fro continuous bruit heard over the fistula. Conversely, a false aneurysm will usually produce only a systolic bruit with no diastolic component. There may also be a thrill over the arteriovenous fistula.

Rapid expansion of a false aneurysm may occur, causing severe neurologic and venous defects secondary to pressure. Continued pulsation of the false aneurysm against a nerve, even without compression, may produce serious damage.

These lesions are susceptible to infection. Many of them occur in the extremities and, as expansion of the aneurysm continues, erosion of the skin may follow. Direct ingress of bacteria from the skin into the area of the aneurysm results in serious infection.

Repair of these lesions should be undertaken when they are diagnosed. Some of the older reports in the literature suggest waiting up to 6 months before attempting repair, to permit adequate development of collateral circulation. There is now ample evidence that collateral circulation develops earlier. Delay in repair may be justified while adjacent infected tissue is allowed to resolve in order to provide a clean field for operative intervention. Proximal and distal control of the vessels is necessary for prevention of major hemorrhage when the fistula is dissected free or the false aneurysm is damaged during the dissection process.

An acute arterial injury may result from penetrating or blunt trauma, it may be extremely difficult to diagnose, it requires a high index of suspicion, and arteriography may be needed to prove the injury. Once diagnosis has been satisfactorily made by clinical findings coupled with arteriographic evidence, direct arterial repair should be undertaken. Injuries should be considered contaminated, and direct repair without a graft is the treatment of choice. If there is loss of vessel substance, a vein graft may be used to bridge the defect. In those rare occasions in which a limb-threatening or life-threatening situation exists and a vein graft is not available, the use of a synthetic prosthesis is required. Careful attention to technique, preoperative administration of antibiotics, and the prolonged use of antibiotics in the postoperative period may reduce the rate of infection and increase the rate of healing in these lesions.

GENERAL POSTOPERATIVE COMPLICATIONS OF VASCULAR SURGERY

In dealing with the problems of occlusive arterial disease, one must work under the assumption that the arteriosclerotic process seen in one vessel probably exists to a varying degree in all vessels. Therefore, the patient who needs a carotid endarterectomy, resection of an abdominal aortic aneurysm, or repair of an occluded femoral artery probably has arteriosclerosis of the coronary arteries as well as of other major arteries.

PREVENTION OF HYPOTENSION

Since vascular surgical procedures may be extensive and can be lengthy, and since sudden blood loss is always a possibility, protection of coronary arterial flow must be constantly in the mind of the surgeon and anesthesiologist. If good exposure of the diseased vessels has been obtained and proximal and distal control secured before the vascular procedure is attempted, blood loss should be minimal. It is important that the patient be adequately hydrated when the incision is made and that the surgeon alert the anesthesiologist when rapid blood loss may be anticipated. The weighed-sponge technique, along with measurement of blood in the suction bottle, to estimate blood loss and serve as a guide to replacement can help insure that adequate blood volume is maintained at all times. Vasopressors are not recommended. Urinary output is used as a measure of normal body perfusion.

One must also be prepared for a drop in blood pressure when the clamps are removed after resection of the aorta. Flow into the legs has been stagnant for some time, and the washout effect may cause a sudden drop in pressure due to peripheral vasodilatation and to release of lactic acid from ischemic cells. Prior to releasing the clamps, adequate blood volume must be present. If the blood pressure falls, the clamps are reapplied, additional fluid is given, and the clamps are again slowly removed. If the declamping process is carried out smoothly and not too quickly, no sudden drop in blood pressure will occur. Metabolic acidosis may require the use of sodium bicarbonate solution. [Many anesthesiologists and surgeons give sodium bicarbonate routinely. Ed.]

RESPIRATORY COMPLICATIONS

Many patients undergoing major vascular surgery have chronic lung disease and many of them are smokers. Delay of the operation 3 to 4 extra days during which the patient undergoes chest physiotherapy in the hospital and is not allowed to smoke, will place the respiratory tract in the best possible condition for anesthesia and surgery. If the patient is intubated for the procedure the tube is usually left in place during the postoperative period for a few hours to several days, depending upon his ability to maintain effective ventilation. Tracheostomy is resorted to early only in those patients in whom severe complications occur, and in whom the endotracheal tube may be necessary for 10 days to 2 weeks.

TUBE GASTROSTOMY VS. NASOGASTRIC TUBE

Some surgeons prefer to use a tube gastrostomy in patients who are undergoing major abdominal surgery rather than an inlying nasogastric tube such as a Levin tube. Others rarely perform a gastrostomy, feeling that the chance of contamination, while not great, is an unnecessary hazard. The evidence that an inlying nasogastric tube actually increases the morbidity rate, particularly in patients using a respirator, is insufficient to justify an additional operation (gastrostomy) with its attendant complications.

PROTECTION OF BOWEL

In an operation in the abdomen, many nearby organs could conceivably be damaged by the dissection process or by the retraction necessary to gain exposure. It is important to handle the bowel in a gentle manner and to prevent it from drying out if it is eviscerated from the abdomen as previously outlined.

Continued untreated distention of the bowel is one of the causes of wound dehiscence, and this in the presence of an aortic graft may be a very serious complication. The mortality rate associated with wound dehiscence remains substantial. The value of retention sutures is a subject of controversy. Evisceration may be prevented by retention sutures.

PREVENTION OF URINARY TRACT INFECTION

Urinary tract infection may occur with use of an inlying urethral catheter during the operative procedure to monitor urine flow. Since most general anesthetics used today are vasodilators that reduce the mean arterial pressure below normal, adequate tissue perfusion may be assured by a good urine flow. Indwelling urethral catheters carry the hazard of contamination of the bladder and subsequent infection. Protect the bladder by care in inserting the urethral catheter and removing it as soon as is feasible after operation. In most instances, the catheter remains in place for 2 to 5 days or until the patient is making a satisfactory recovery and can void satisfactorily. Postoperative urinary tract infection is more often due to unnecessarily prolonged use of the Foley catheter than to its use during operation and immediately afterward.

AORTODUODENAL FISTULA

Aortoduodenal fistula occurring between the duodenum and an aortic graft, although not common, is being reported with increasing frequency. This fistula formation is thought to be secondary to pressure from the sharp edge of the graft against the duodenum, to erosion of uninjured duodenum by persistent infection around the graft, or to involvement of the adjacent graft by a focus of infection produced by duodenal injury.

Prevention of this complication requires avoidance of injury to the duodenum by careful dissection of the posterior peritoneum away from it so that, with closure, reperitonealization does not injure it. If this is not possible, and the duodenum is drawn tightly against the graft when closure is attempted, a piece of omentum should be interposed between the duodenum and the graft. Another approach is to wrap the upper aortic anastomosis with a second piece of graft material to provide a smooth surface for the duodenum to lie against. Neither of these preventive measures has been proven to be effective.

Recognition of this complication requires a high index of suspicion when there is evidence of sepsis or gastrointestinal bleeding after placement of an aortic graft. Aortography may demonstrate a false aneurysm or graft irregularity. Demonstration of an aortic leak by arteriography is not usually practical because the leak has either momentarily stopped or the patient is bleeding so profusely that there is no time for arteriography. If there is time and the patient's condition is stable, an upper gastrointestinal series may show a deformity of the distal duodenum, as may endoscopy.

The method of treatment depends on the location of the fistula. If the proximal or distal suture line is not involved, antibiotic therapy and closure of the hole in the duodenum with interposition of omentum may be successful. However, most of these fistulas involve the proximal suture line. The graft must be removed and the proximal aorta ligated. Then a bypass graft, either axillofemoral or intra-abdominal, attached to the aorta above the fistula, is tunneled behind the peritoneum and anastomosed to the distal aorta or iliac vessels to reestablish blood flow. The hole in the duodenum is repaired simultaneously and an antibiotic is given in massive doses. Repair of the duodenum may be difficult and may require a duodenojejunostomy, proximal gastroenterostomy, or the use of a serosal patch from an adjacent loop of jejunum.

Duodenal repair and suture of the proximal suture line of the graft might seem a very attractive solution in these sick patients, but it is unwise and can lead to a fatal outcome.

Plastic irrigating catheters may be left in the graft bed with continuous antibiotic irrigation of the area for several days. The value of this technique is not proven. [Unfortunately, the mortality rate is high. Ed.]

GRAFT INFECTION

Infection of a synthetic graft requires that the surgeon follow the same principles as those outlined for aortoduodenal fistula. The risk of life-threatening hemorrhage occurring suddenly and without warning is so great that an infection adjacent to a graft suture line is an indication for removal of the graft.

A superficial wound infection over a graft suture line does not always involve the graft initially, but may extend to the graft if not treated vigorously.

If an infection extends to or exposes a synthetic graft not at the suture line, early débridement, the use of systemic and topical antibiotics, and delayed wound closure may permit salvage of some grafts.

Initial apparent success in clearing an infection adjacent to a graft may be misleading, as shown by subsequent late sinus formation, development of a false aneurysm, or thrombosis of the graft.

It should be remembered that an infected graft is not the same as a graft placed in a contaminated field. Experimentally and clinically, when no reasonable alternative exists, placement of a synthetic graft in a contaminated field may be successful, with the aid of vigorous preoperative and postoperative antibiotic therapy, but the use of autogenous graft material or the routing of synthetic grafts in such a way as to bypass the contaminated area is a preferable preventive measure.

VENOUS THROMBOSIS

Venous thrombosis may occur in any patient undergoing a surgical procedure but is probably somewhat more common in patients who have had surgery of the peripheral aorta or the peripheral arteries, because of stagnation of blood in the veins during cross-clamping of the arterial inflow, as well as the trauma imposed by the length of time the patient is on the operating table. Some surgeons feel that they can minimize this complication by elevation of the foot of the operating table about 10 to 15 degrees and wrapping the lower extremity with an elastic bandage prior to the operation. Adequate intraoperative hydration is an important factor in avoiding thrombosis.

The prevention and management of venous thromboembolic phenomena as discussed elsewhere in this text apply equally when thromboembolism is associated with arterial problems.

It is important to recognize that swelling of an extremity after arterial reconstruction is not uncommon even when no venous thrombosis is present. A patient with chronic occlusive arterial disease and arterial hypotension distal to a chronic obstruction often has reduced vasomotor tone. Following a successful arterial reconstruction and the return of a normal blood flow into the extremity, arteriolar dilatation occurs, with

engorgement of the peripheral vessels and the development of edema. Lymphatic interruption incident to groin dissection has also been implicated in the development of postoperative leg edema. The leg is usually warm, edematous, and hyperemic in appearance. This should not be misjudged as deep venous thrombosis but should be accepted as a reaction to be expected after arterial reconstruction and one that subsides spontaneously with time. Elevate the foot of the bed 15 degrees while the patient is at rest and insist on elastic support to the legs when he begins ambulation. This type of edema usually disappears completely within 2 to 3 weeks after operation.

Bibliography

Preoperative Complications

1. Adams, D. F., Olin, T. B., and Kosek, J.: Cotton fiber embolization during angiography. Radiology 84:678, 1965.
2. Allen, J. H., Perara, C., and Potts, D. G.: The relation of arterial trauma to complications of cerebral angiography. Am. J. Roentgenol. 95:845, 1965.
3. Ansell, G.: National survey of radiological complications: Interim report. Clin. Radiol. 19:175, 1968.
4. Bergan, J. J., and Yao, J. S. T.: Invited overview: Role of the vascular laboratory. Surgery 88:9, 1980.
5. Candy, J., Grainger, K., and Guyer, P. B.: Aortoduodenal fistula complicating translumbar aortography. Brit. J. Surg. 52:312, 1965.
6. Coran, A. G., and Tyler, H. B.: Aortic dissection. A complication of translumbar aortography. Am. J. Surg. 115:709, 1968.
7. Gudbjerg, C. E., and Christensen, J.: Dissection of the aortic wall in retrograde lumbar aortography. Acta Radiol. 55:364, 1961.
8. Halpern, M.: Percutaneous transfemoral arteriography: An analysis of the complications in 1000 consecutive cases. Am. J. Roentgenol. 92:918, 1964.
9. Killen, D. A.: Angiographic contrast media: A historical resume. Surgery 73:33, 1973.
10. Lang, E. K.: A survey of the complications of percutaneous retrograde arteriography: Seldinger technique. Radiology 81:257, 1963.
11. Lavenson, G. S., Jr., Rich, N. M., and Strandness, D. E., Jr.: Ultrasonic flow detector value in the management of combat incurred vascular injuries. Arch. Surg. 103:644, 1971.
12. McAfee, J. G.: A survey of complications of abdominal aortography. Radiology 68:825, 1957.
13. Rich, N. M., Hobson, R. W., II, and Fedde, C. W.: Vascular trauma secondary to diagnostic

and therapeutic procedures. Am. J. Surg. *128*:715, 1974.

14. Seidenberg, B., and Hurwitt, E. S.: Retrograde femoral (Seldinger) aortography: Surgical complications in 26 cases. Ann. Surg. *163*:221, 1966.

15. Sewell, R. A., Killen, D. A., and Foster, J. H.: Small bowel injury by angiographic contrast medium. Surgery *64*:459, 1968.

Complications of Surgery for Abdominal Aortic Aneurysm

16. Bernstein, E. F., Fisher, J. C., and Varco, R. L.: Is excision the optimum treatment for all abdominal aortic aneurysms? Surgery *61*:83, 1967.

17. Dickson, A. H., Strandness, D. E., Jr., and Bell, J. W.: The detection and sequelae of operative accidents complicating reconstructive arterial surgery. Am. J. Surg. *109*:143, 1965.

18. Golden, G. T., Sears, H. F., Wellons, H. A., Jr., and Muller, W. H., Jr.: Paraplegia complicating resection of aneurysms of the infrarenal abdominal aorta. Surgery *73*:91, 1973.

19. Johnson, G., Jr., McDevitt, N. B., Proctor, H. J., Mandel, S. R., and Peacock, J. B.: Emergent or elective operation for symptomatic abdominal aortic aneurysm. Arch. Surg. *115*:51, 1980.

20. Moore, W. S., Rosson, C. T., and Hall, A. D.: Effect of prophylactic antibiotics in preventing bacteremic infection of vascular prostheses. Surgery *69*:825, 1971.

21. Perry, M. O.: The hemodynamics of temporary abdominal aortic occlusion. Ann. Surg. *168*:193, 1968.

22. Szilagyi, D. E., Elliott, J. P., and Smith, R. F.: Clinical fate of the patient with asymptomatic abdominal aortic aneurysm and unfit for surgical treatment. Arch. Surg. *104*:600, 1972.

23. Wagern, R. B., and Martin, A. S.: Peripheral atheroembolism: Confirmation of a clinical concept with a case report and review of the literature. Surgery *73*:353, 1973.

24. Zuber, W. F., Gaspar, M. R., and Rothschild, P. D.: The anterior spinal artery syndrome — a complication of abdominal aortic surgery: Report of five cases and review of the literature. Ann. Surg. *172*:909, 1970.

Complications of Replacement of the Upper Abdominal Aorta

25. Crawford, E. S., Snyder, D. M., Cho, G. C., and Roehm, J. O. F., Jr.: Progress in treatment of thoracoabdominal and abdominal aortic aneurysms involving celiac, superior mesenteric and renal arteries. Ann. Surg. *188*:404, 1978.

26. Davis, J. H., Benson, J. W., and Miller, R. C.: Thoracoabdominal aneurysm involving celiac, superior mesenteric and renal arteries. Arch. Surg. *75*:871, 1957.

27. DeBakey, M. E., Crawford, E. S., Garrett, H. E., Beall, A. C., Jr., and Howell, J. F.: Surgical considerations in the treatment of aneurysms of the thoracoabdominal aorta. Ann. Surg. *162*:650, 1965.

28. Elkins, R. C., DeMeester, T. R., and Browley, R. K.: Surgical exposure of the upper abdominal aorta and its branches. Surgery *70*:622, 1971.

Complications of Surgery for Celiac and Superior Mesenteric Vascular Disease

29. Bergen, J. J., Dry, L., Conn, J., and Trippel, O. H.: Intestinal ischemic syndromes. Ann. Surg. *169*:120, 1969.

30. Bergen, J. J., Haid, S. P., and Conn, J.: Systemic effects of intestinal revascularization. Am. J. Surg. *117*:235, 1969.

31. Glueck lich, B., Deterling, R. A., Jr., Matsumoto, G. H., and Callow, A. D.: Chronic mesenteric ischemia masquerading as cancer. Surg. Gynecol. Obstet. *148*:49, 1980.

32. Hertzer, N. R., and Mullally, P. H.: Celiac artery aneurysmectomy with hepatic artery ligation. Arch. Surg. *104*:337, 1972.

33. Ottinger, T. W., and Austen, W. G.: A study of 136 patients with mesenteric infarction. Surg. Gynecol. Obstet. *124*:251, 1967.

34. Rob, C.: Surgical diseases of the celiac and mesenteric arteries. Arch. Surg. *93*:21, 1966.

35. Szilagyi, D. E., Rian, R. L., Elliott, J. P., and Smith, R. F.: The celiac artery compression syndrome: Does it exist? Surgery *72*:849, 1972.

36. Williams, T. F.: Progress in gastroenterology: Vascular insufficiency of the intestines. Gastroenterology *61*:757, 1971.

Complications of Surgery for Renovascular Hypertension

37. Barney, J. D., and Mintz, E. R.: Infarcts of the kidney. J.A.M.A. *100*:1, 1933.

38. Dahl, D. S., O'Connor, V. J., Jr., Walker, C. D., and Simon, N. M.: The morbidity of differential renal function studies: Analysis of 271 studies. J.A.M.A. *202*:857, 1967.

39. Foster, J. H., Dean, R. H., Pinkerton, J. A., and Rhomy, R. K.: Ten years' experience with the surgical management of renovascular hypertension. Ann. Surg. *177*:755, 1973.

40. Lawrie, G. M., Morris, G. C., Jr., Soussou, I. D., Starr, D. S., Silvers, A., Glaeser, D. H., and DeBakey, M. E.: Late results of reconstructive surgery for renovascular disease. Ann. Surg. *191*:528, 1980.

41. Sykes, B. J., Hoie, J., and Schenk, W. G., Jr.: An experimental study into the validity of clearance methods of measuring renal blood flow. Surg. Gynecol. Obstet. *135*:877, 1972.

Complications of Surgery for Occlusive Disease of the Terminal Aorta and Iliac Arteries

42. Buckberg, G. D., Henneg, R. P., and Cannon, J. A.: Postoperative complications of aortoiliac endarterectomy: Incidence, cause and prevention. Surgery *63*:121, 1968.

43. Danto, L. A., Fry, W. J., and Kraft, R. O.: Acute aortic thrombosis. Arch. Surg. *104*:569, 1972.

44. Imparato, A. M., Berman, I. R., Bracco, A., Kim, G. E., and Beaudet, R.: Avoidance of

shock and peripheral embolism during surgery of the abdominal aorta. Surgery 73:78, 1973.

45. Kwaan, J. H., and Connolly, J. E.: Renal failure complicating aortoiliofemoral reconstructive procedure. Am. Surg 46:295, 1980.

46. Moore, W. S., and Hall, A. D.: Late suture failure in the pathogenesis of anastomotic false aneurysms. Ann. Surg. 172:1064, 1970.

47. Mozersky, D. J., Sumner, D. S., and Strandness, D. E.: Long-term results of reconstructive aortoiliac surgery. Am. J. Surg. 123:503, 1972.

48. Pilcher, D. B., Barker, W. F., and Cannon, J. A.: An aortoiliac endarterectomy case series followed 10 years or more. Surgery 67:5, 1970.

49. Thomford, N. R., and Dorfman, L. F.: Ureteral obstruction caused by an aortofemoral bypass prosthesis. Am. J. Surg. 115:394, 1968.

Complications of Femoropopliteal Reconstruction

50. Barner, H. B., Judd, D. R., Kaiser, G. C., Willman, V. L., and Hanlon, C. R.: Late failure of arterialized in situ saphenous vein. Arch. Surg. 99:781, 1969.

51. Caldwell, R. L., DeWeese, J. A., and Rob, C. G.: Femoropopliteal bypass grafts utilizing autogenous veins. Circulation 37:37, 1967.

52. Conn, J. H., Hardy, J. D., Chavez, C. M., and Fain, W. R.: Infected arterial grafts: Experience in 22 cases with emphasis on unusual bacteria and techniques. Ann. Surg. 171:704, 1970.

53. Connolly, J. E., and Stemmer, E. A.: The nonreversed saphenous vein bypass for femoral-popliteal occlusive disease. Surgery 68:602, 1970.

54. Couch, N. P., Wheeler, H. B., Hyatt, D. F., Crane, C., Edwards, E. A., and Warren, R.: Factors influencing limb survival after femoropopliteal reconstruction. Arch. Surg. 95:163, 1967.

55. Darling, R. C., and Linton, R. R.: Management of the late failure of arterial reconstruction of the lower extremities. N. Engl. J. Med. 270:609, 1964.

56. Darling, R. C., Linton, R. R., and Razzuk, M. A.: Saphenous vein bypass grafts for femoropopliteal occlusive disease: A reappraisal. Surgery 61:31, 1967.

57. DeWeese, J. A., Barner, H. B., Mahoney, E. B., and Rob, C. G.: Autogenous venous bypass grafts and thromboendarterectomies for atherosclerotic lesions of the femoropopliteal arteries. Ann. Surg. 163:205, 1966.

58. DeWeese, J. A., and Rob, C. G.: Autogenous venous bypass grafts five years later. Ann. Surg. 174:346, 1971.

59. Foster, J. H., Killen, D. A., Jolly, P. C., and Kirtley, J. H.: Low molecular weight dextran in vascular surgery: Prevention of early thrombosis following arterial reconstruction in 85 cases. Ann. Surg. 163:764, 1966.

60. Kaminski, D. L., Barner, H. B., Dorighi, J. A., Kaiser, G. C., and Willman, V. L.: Femoro-

popliteal bypass with reversed autogenous vein. Surgery 177:232, 1973.

61. Koontz, T. J., and Stansel, H. C., Jr.: Factors influencing patency of the autogenous vein femoropopliteal bypass grafts: An analysis of 74 cases. Surgery 71:753, 1972.

62. Mannick, J. A., and Jackson, B. T.: Hemodynamics of arterial surgery in atherosclerotic limbs. Surgery 59:713, 1966.

63. Morton, D. L., Ehrenfeld, W. K., and Wylie, E. J.: Significance of outflow obstruction after femoropopliteal endarterectomy. Arch. Surg. 94:592, 1967.

64. Mulherin, J. L., Jr., and Edwards, W. H.: The current status of femoropopliteal bypass grafting. Am. Surg. 46:273, 1980.

65. Patman, R. D., and Thompson, J. E.: Fasciotomy in peripheral vascular surgery. Arch. Surg. 101:663, 1970.

66. Richardson, R. L., Jr., Pate, J. W., Wolf, A. Y., Ledes, C., and Hopson, W. B., Jr.: The outcome of antibiotic-soaked arterial grafts in guinea pig wounds contaminated with E. coli or S. aureus. J. Thorac. Cardiovasc. Surg. 59:635, 1970.

67. Shaw, R. S., and Baue, A. E.: Management of sepsis complicating arterial reconstructive surgery. Surgery 53:75, 1963.

68. Szilagyi, D. E., Smith, R. F., Elliott, J. P., and Vrendecid, M. P.: Infection in arterial reconstruction with synthetic grafts. Ann. Surg. 176:321, 1972.

69. Turcotte, J. G., Dent, T. L., and Fry, W. J.: Preparation for femoropopliteal bypass. Arch. Surg. 100:627, 1970.

70. Vaughan, B. F., Slavotinek, A. H., and Jepson, R. P.: Edema of the lower limb after vascular operations. Surg. Gynecol. Obstet. 131:282, 1970.

Complications of Peripheral Aneurysms

71. Baird, R. J., Sivisanker, R., Hayward, R., and Wilson, D.: Popliteal aneurysms. A review and analysis of 61 cases. Surgery 59:911, 1966.

72. Edwards, W. S.: Exclusion and saphenous vein bypass of popliteal aneurysms. Surg. Gynecol. Obstet. 128:829, 1969.

73. Gifford, R. W., Jr., Hines, E. A., Jr., and Janes, J. M.: Analysis and follow-up study of 100 popliteal aneurysms. Surgery 33:284, 1953.

74. Graham, L. M., Zelenock, G. B., Whitehouse, W. M., Jr., Erlandson, E. E., Dent, T. L., Lindenauer, M., and Stanley, J. C.: Clinical significance of arteriosclerotic femoral artery aneurysms. Arch. Surg. 115:502, 1980.

75. Pappas, G., et al.: Femoral aneurysms. J.A.M.A. 190:489, 1964.

Complications of Surgery for Carotid, Vertebral, and Subclavian Artery Disease

76. Ehrenfeld, W. K., and Hays, R. J.: False aneurysm after carotid endarterectomy. Arch. Surg. 104:288, 1972.

77. Hays, R. J., Levinson, S. A., and Wylie, E. J.:

Intraoperative measurement of carotid back pressure as a guide to operative management for carotid endarterectomy. Surgery 72:953, 1972.

78. Hertzer, N. R., and Beven, E. G.: A retrospective comparison of the use of shunts during carotid endarterectomy. Surg. Gynecol. Obstet. 151:81, 1980.

79. Jacobson, J. H., II, Mozersky, D. J., Mitty, H. A., and Brothers, M. J.: Axillary-axillary bypass for the "subclavian steal" syndrome. Arch. Surg. 106:24, 1973.

80. Kaupp, H. A., Haid, S. P., Jurayj, M. N., Jergan, J. J., and Trippel, O. H.: Aneurysms of the extracranial carotid artery. Surgery 72:946, 1972.

81. Max, T. C., Muyshondt, E., Schwartz, S. I., and Rob, C. G.: Studies of carotid blood flow in unilateral occlusion. Arch. Surg. 86:65, 1963.

82. McMullan, M. H., and Hardy, J. D.: Lesions of the subclavian artery: Survey of 38 cases with emphasis on steal syndromes. Ann. Surg. 178:80, 1973.

83. Mozersky, D. J., Sumner, D. S., Barnes, R. W., and Strandness, D. E.: Subclavian revascularization by means of a subcutaneous axillary-axillary graft. Arch. Surg. 106:20, 1973.

84. Mozersky, D. J., Sumner, D. S., Barnes, R. W., Callaway, G. P., and Strandness, D. E., Jr.: The hemodynamics of the axillary-axillary bypass. Surg. Gynecol. Obstet. 135:925, 1972.

85. Thompson, J. E.: Prevention of complications of cerebral arteriography and surgery. In Dale, W. A. (Ed.): Management of Arterial Occlusive Disease. Chicago, Year Book Medical Publishers, 1971, p. 353.

86. Thompson, J. E., Austin, D. J., and Patman, R. D.: Carotid endarterectomy for cerebrovascular insufficiency. Ann. Surg. 172:663, 1970.

87. Towne, J. B., and Bernhard, V. M.: The relationship of postoperative hypertension to complications following carotid endarterectomy. Surgery 88:575, 1980.

88. Yao, S. T., Gourmos, C., Papathanasiou, K., and Irvine, W. T.: A method for assessing ischemia of the hand and fingers. Surg. Gynecol. Obstet. 135:373, 1972.

Complications of Surgery for Thoracic Outlet Syndrome

89. Hurlbut, H. J., Snyder, H. E., Vontz, F. K., and Sumner, W. C.: Thoracic outlet compression syndrome. Am. Surgeon 38:443, 1972.

90. Judy, K. L., and Heymann, R. L.: Vascular complications of thoracic outlet syndrome. Am. J. Surg. 123:521, 1972.

91. Polumbo, L. T.: Anterior transthoracic approach for upper thoracic sympathectomy. Arch. Surg. 72:659, 1956.

92. Rob, C. G., and Standeven, A.: Arterial occlusion complicating thoracic outlet compression syndrome. Br. Med. J. 2:709, 1958.

93. Roeder, D. K., Mills, M., McHale, J. J., Shepard, B. M., and Ashworth, H. E.: First rib resection in the treatment of thoracic outlet syndrome: Transaxillary and posterior thoracoplasty approaches. Ann. Surg. 178:49, 1973.

94. Roos, D. B., and Owens, J. C.: Thoracic outlet syndrome. Arch. Surg. 93:71, 1966.

Complications of Sympathectomy

95. Atlas, L. N.: Lumbar sympathectomy in the treatment of elected cases of peripheral arteriosclerotic disease. II. Gangrene following operation in improperly selected cases. Am. Heart J. 23:493, 1942.

96. Bergan, J. J., and Trippell, O. H.: Arteriograms in ischemic limbs worsened after lumbar sympathectomy. Arch. Surg. 85:135, 1962.

97. Cooley, D. A., and Herman, B. E.: Simple means for prevention of postsympathectomy neuralgia. Surgery 53:587, 1963.

98. deTakats, G., and Fowler, E. F.: The neurogenic factor in Raynaud's phenomenon. Surgery 51:9, 1962.

99. Fowler, E. F., and deTakats, G.: Side effects and complications of sympathectomy for hypertension. Arch. Surg. 59:1213, 1949.

100. Fulton, R. L., and Blakely, W. R.: Lumbar sympathectomy: A procedure of questionable value in the treatment of arteriosclerosis obliterans of the legs. Am. J. Surg. 116:735, 1968.

101. Haxton, H. A.: Gustatory sweating. Brain 71:16, 1948.

102. Litwin, M. S.: Postsympathectomy neuralgia. Arch. Surg. 84:121, 1962.

103. Owens, J. C.: Postsympathectomy pain syndromes. Bull. Soc. Int. Chir. 23:500, 1964.

104. Owens, J. C.: Causalgia. Am. Surgeon 23:636, 1957.

105. Plecha, F. R., Bomberger, R. A., Hoffman, M., and MacPherson, K.: A new criterion for predicting response to lumbar sympathectomy in patients with severe arteriosclerotic occlusive disease. Surgery 88:375, 1980.

106. Shaw, R. S., Austen, W. G., and Stipa, S.: A ten year study of the effect of lumbar sympathectomy on the peripheral circulation of patients with arteriosclerotic occlusive disease. Surg. Gynecol. Obstet. 119:486, 1964.

107. Shumacker, H. B.: Sympathetic denervation of the extremities: Operative technique, morbidity and mortality. Surgery 24:304, 1948.

108. Whitelaw, G. P., and Smithwick, R. H.: Some secondary effects of sympathectomy with particular reference to disturbance of sexual function. N. Engl. J. Med. 245:221, 1951.

Complications of Arterial Injury

109. Amato, J. J., Billy, L. J., Gruber, R. P., Lawson, N. S., and Rich, N. M.: Vascular injuries: An experimental study of high and low velocity missile wounds. Arch. Surg. 101:167, 1970.

110. Collins, H. A., and Jacobs, J. K.: Acute arterial injuries due to blunt trauma. J. Bone Joint Surg. 43A:193, 1961.

111. Drapanas, T., Hewitt, R. L., Werchert, R. L., and Smith, A. D.: Civilian vascular injuries: A critical appraisal of three decades of management. Am. Surgeon 172:351, 1970.

112. Fomon, J. J., and Warren, W. D.: Late compli-

cations of peripheral arterial injuries. Arch. Surg. *91*:610, 1965.

113. Foster, J. H., Carter, J. W., Graham, C. P., Jr., and Edwards, W. H.: Arterial injuries secondary to the use of the Fogarty catheter. Ann. Surg. *171*:971, 1970.

114. Hardy, J. D., Raju, S., Neely, W. A., and Berry, D. W.: Aortic and other arterial injuries. Ann. Surg. *181*:640, 1975.

115. Morton, J. R., and Crawford, E. S.: Bilateral traumatic renal artery thrombosis. Ann. Surg. *176*:62, 1972.

116. Perry, M. O., Thal, E. R., and Shires, F. T.: Management of arterial injuries. Ann. Surg. *173*:403, 1971.

117. Rich, N. M., Baugh, J. H., and Hughes, C. W.: Acute arterial injuries in Vietnam: 1000 cases. J. Trauma *10*:359, 1970.

118. Rich, N. M., Baugh, J. H., and Hughes, C. W.: Significance of complications associated with vascular repairs in Vietnam. Arch. Surg. *100*:646, 1970.

119. Rich, N. M., and Spencer, F. C.: Vascular Trauma. Philadelphia, W. B. Saunders Company, 1978.

120. Wilson, R. F., Arbulu, A., Bassett, J. S., and Walt, A. J.: Acute mediastinal widening following blunt chest trauma: Critical decisions. Arch. Surg. *104*:551, 1972.

General Complications of Vascular Surgery

121. Carter, S. C., Cohen, A., and Whelan, T. J.: Clinical experience with management of the infected Dacron graft. Ann. Surg. *158*:249, 1963.

122. Dass, R.: Small bowel erosion after aortic replacement by synthetic graft. Am. J. Surg. *116*:460, 1968.

123. Donovan, T. J., and Buckman, C. A.: Aortoenteric fistula. Arch. Surg. *95*:810, 1967.

124. Ehrenfeld, W. K., Lord, R. S. A., Stoney, R. J., and Wylie, E. J.: Subcutaneous arterial bypass grafts in the management of fistulae between the bowel and plastic arterial prostheses. Ann. Surg. *168*:29, 1968.

125. Hertzer, N. R., Young, J. R., Kramer, J. R., Phillips, D. F., deWolfe, V. G., Ruschhaupt, W. F., III, and Beven, E. G.: Routine coronary angiography prior to elective aortic reconstruction. Arch. Surg. *114*:1336, 1979.

126. Kluge, T. H., Ro, J. S., Fretheim, B., and Stormorken, H.: Thrombosis prophylaxis with dextran and warfarin in vascular operations. Surg. Gynecol. Obstet. *135*:941, 1972.

127. Moore, W. S., and Hall, A. D.: Late suture failure in the pathogenesis of anastomotic false aneurysms. Ann. Surg. *1064*:172, 1970.

128. Perdue, G. D., Jr., Smith, R. B., III, Ansley, J. D., and Constantio M. J.: Impending aortoenteric hemorrhage. Ann. Surg. *192*:237, 1980.

129. Popovsky, J., and Singer, S.: Infected prosthetic grafts. Arch. Surg. *115*:203, 1980.

130. Sheil, G. R., Reeve, T. S., Little, J. M., Coupland, G. A., and Lowenthal, J.: Aortointestinal fistulas following operations on the abdominal aorta and iliac arteries. Br. J. Surg. *56*:840, 1969.

131. Thomas, J. M., and Silva, J. R.: Dextran 40 in peripheral vascular diseases. Arch. Surg. *106*:138, 1973.

132. Vaughan, B. F., Slavotinek, A. H., and Jepson, R. P.: Edema of the lower limb after vascular operations. Surg. Gynecol. Obstet. *131*:282, 1970.

19

COMPLICATIONS OF GASTRIC SURGERY

Distal Subtotal Gastrectomy, Esophagogastrectomy and Total Gastrectomy, Vagotomy, Pyloroplasty, and Gastrostomy

James D. Hardy

Postoperative complications account for large segments of both the morbidity and the mortality that follow gastric surgery.[67, 69, 78, 79, 95] It is the purpose of this chapter to present a comprehensive but concise review of the complications of gastric operations. Implicit throughout the discussion is the fact that meticulous preoperative and transoperative management reduces the incidence of disturbed convalescence. The complications to be considered are primarily those that may follow distal subtotal gastrectomy or vagotomy accompanied by an emptying procedure. However, problems that follow esophagogastrectomy, total gastrectomy, and gastrostomy will also be touched upon. Illustrative data are presented in Table 19–1. The relative incidence of each of the complications listed would be different at the present time, when the peptic ulcer diathesis is now controlled far more often with vagotomy-pyloroplasty than with distal subtotal gastrectomy of either the Billroth I or Billroth II type.

HEMORRHAGE (EARLY)

Intraluminal Bleeding

The grossly bloody fluid aspirated through the nasogastric tube immediately following subtotal gastrectomy usually changes to a serosanguineous material in a few hours. In the occasional patient, however, bleeding into the stomach continues indefinitely, and under these circumstances a decision regarding reoperation must be made.

The anastomosis is the most common site of hemorrhage in the patient who was not bleeding preoperatively. Pearce, Jordan, and DeBakey[82] reported such postoperative bleeding in 14 of 406 cases (3.4 per cent). In 10 patients the hemorrhage was believed to be due to technical failure to control vessels along the anastomosis at operation, in 3 to a bleeding diathesis, and in 1 to cortisone therapy. The date of onset varied, but it was on the day of operation in 6 patients. Ten were managed conservatively and 4 by operation; in 2 of those operated upon the cause of bleeding was found to be a bleeding diathesis. One death, due to renal failure, occurred.

In addition to bleeding from the suture line or hemorrhagic diathesis, other important sources of early postoperative blood loss are an overlooked ulcer in the unresected portion of the stomach[86] or an unresected duodenal ulcer. When there is a history of recent upper gastrointestinal bleeding and no ulcer is seen or palpated in the lower portion of the stomach or duodenum *at the*

TABLE 19–1 POSTOPERATIVE COMPLICATIONS IN 604 CASES FOLLOWING GASTRIC SURGERY*

Deaths	37
Hemorrhage	29
Continuing (11)	
Anastomotic (9)	
Intermediate (2-20 POD) (9)	
Gastric retention	14
Proximal loop syndrome	21
Duodenal stump dehiscence (15)	
Subacute and chronic (6)	
Anastomotic leakage	7
Marked dumping and/or diarrhea	29
Malnutrition (severe)	28
Intraperitoneal infection (including abscess)	14
Wound complications	76
Infection and abscess (55)	
Evisceration (21)	
Jaundice	18
Hemolytic and absorptive (14)	
Operative (4)	
Common bile duct injury	2
Marginal ulceration	15
Fistulas (other than duodenal)	10
Jejunal (1)	
Pancreatic (2)	
Gastrocutaneous (5)	
Gastrocolic (2)	
Internal hernia	1
Intussusception	1
Pancreatitis	6
Pulmonary complications	54
Total	362

*Elective operations, 82 per cent; emergency operations, 18 per cent. (From Hardy, J. D.: Problems associated with gastric surgery: A review of 604 consecutive patients with annotation. Am. J. Surg. *108*:699, 1964.)

initial operation, the fundus and cardia should be examined with great care. The source of hemorrhage may be a shallow ulcer (or ulcers) that cannot be palpated and must be visualized. Exposure is best achieved by first thoroughly cleansing the stomach with saline and then gently inserting Deaver retractors to permit direct inspection of all areas of the fundus. Naturally all precautions are taken to minimize peritoneal contamination, as in any other intra-abdominal operation. If an ulcer is found the excision of which would require virtually total gastric resection, the surgeon may choose to biopsy the lesion and then simply to oversew it if it is benign. Vagotomy-pyloroplasty should then be performed. In other circumstances the ulcer may be resected by wedge excision. But in any event the bleeding must be controlled.

When gastric surgery is being performed for recent (within 72 hours) or continuing hemorrhage due to a duodenal ulcer, every effort should be made to excise the lesion or surely to control the bleeding. Second operations for bleeding not controlled at recent first operations are associated with a substantial mortality rate, especially in elderly patients.

REOPERATION

Conservative management, consisting largely of adequate blood replacement, suffices in most patients with postgastrectomy hemorrhage. Gastric cooling with iced saline solution, introduced and withdrawn through the inlying nasogastric tube, may be helpful. It not only reduces distention of the stomach by removing liquid blood and clots; it also reduces the gastric temperature below the optimal temperature for maximal digestive activity of pepsin, tending to permit ulcer healing. Antacids may also be injected through the nasogastric tube, and cimetidine may be given parenterally. The use of intravenously administered Pitressin is of questionable value in this situation. But if brisk postoperative bleeding has continued, requiring numerous transfusions to support the blood pressure and urinary output; if the blood clots on standing; and if the platelet count is within normal limits, indicating a grossly normal coagulation mechanism—then reoperation is elected.

Exposure of the suture line and the inside of the gastric pouch is best accomplished by making a new incision in the gastric pouch, thus exposing the anastomosis from above without the necessity of taking it down.[96] Access to the fundus is also afforded by the new gastrotomy incision, should the hemorrhage not be arising along the suture line. The bleeding vessel is securely oversewn with permanent suture material. If diffuse mucosal oozing is found, perhaps from multiple shallow ulcers, bilateral truncal vagotomy should usually be performed if not done previously. If vagotomy was performed and there is diffuse mucosal hemorrhage, the alternative of radical resection of residual stomach should be considered. Finally, one should be certain that continuing hemorrhage does not arise from esophageal varices.

Extraluminal Bleeding

Hemorrhage into the peritoneal cavity may of course occur in association with many operations, but certain features of gastric resection render intraperitoneal blood loss fairly common. The splenic capsule, for example, is often torn by retraction or by dissection along the greater curvature of the stomach. Unaware of this mishap, the surgeon may find a considerable volume of blood in the left upper quadrant at the time of closure — unless hypotension has prompted a search for bleeding earlier. A tear in the splenic capsule was once an indication for splenectomy, but the modern position is that a serious attempt should be made to save the spleen by the application of Gelfoam, Avertin, or judicious suture. Should a splenic injury escape notice, a second operation for control of hemorrhage will often be required. Some surgeons now warn the pateint preoperatively that incidental splenectomy may become necessary.

Another important source of bleeding is the divided omentum. If a large mass of omentum is ligated with a single ligature, the artery may retract out of the mass and produce either a large hematoma or free bleeding.

Bleeding may also derive from the left or right gastric arteries, or from the superior pancreaticoduodenal artery. The vasa brevia may be injured by excessive retraction either during vagotomy or in the course of incidental splenectomy. The liver may also be injured. In efforts to control bleeding from the lacerated pancreas one can injure the common bile duct or the pancreatic ducts, incurring risk of serious postoperative pancreatitis. Thus dissection around the duodenum should be performed carefully so that vessels are identified and ligated before they can retract into the pancreas.

The *diagnosis* of extraluminal hemorrhage postoperatively can be difficult. Whereas intrathoracic hemorrhage can usually be detected on chest x-ray, intra-abdominal hemorrhage is not readily demonstrated by routine films of the abdomen and at times must be diagnosed on the basis of limited physical findings and the monitoring of the vital signs, the patient's appearance, urine output, and central venous pressure.

HICCUPS (SINGULTUS)

Hiccups do not constitute a serious complication of gastric resection, but the condition does deserve mention. These spasmodic contractions of the diaphragm can be distressing and even disabling.

The cause of hiccups is not always clear, but several possibilities should be kept in mind. The stimulus mediated over the phrenic nerve to one hemidiaphragm or the other, or both, may be due to distention of the residual gastric pouch. Thus if a nasogastric tube has not already been introduced, it should be inserted promptly and the gastric contents aspirated. If a nasogastric tube has been in place, it may be obstructed or the suction source may not be supplying adequate negative pressure to empty the stomach. Large volumes of fluid may have produced tremendous distention of the small gastric pouch with outlet obstruction (3 liters in one patient we saw). Extreme gastric distention entails the serious hazard of leakage at the anastomosis, not to mention the risk of "acute gastric dilatation." Severe distention of the stomach may produce shock owing to fluid and electrolyte loss into the organ itself, and to compression of the inferior vena cava and, at times, the portal vein.

Patients with electrolyte and acid-base derangements often suffer hiccups. If ionic imbalance is reflected in the blood chemistry values, the abnormalities should be corrected promptly.

Hiccups may also be due to irritation of the diaphragm and may reflect the development of a subphrenic abscess. However, many instances of hiccups can be attributed to no definite finding, and a central nervous system factor is to be considered. Certainly some of these patients are lethargic and disoriented.

MANAGEMENT

Fluoroscopic determination of unilateral diaphragmatic spasm and blockage of the phrenic nerve on that side may occasionally be indicated. But with the advent of meprobamate and other tranquilizing agents the hiccups can be controlled promptly in most patients, once gastric retention has been excluded and subdiaphragmatic abscess has been ruled out as far as possible. When lesser measures have failed, a plastic catheter may be inserted percutaneously in the neck and anesthetization of the involved phrenic nerve maintained indefinitely by a slow drip of 0.5 per cent lidocaine (Xylocaine).

POSTOPERATIVE PANCREATITIS

PATHOPHYSIOLOGY

Pancreatic injury with resulting severe inflammation is reported to account for possibly 1 to 2 per cent of the mortality that follows gastric resection. In fact, when this complication does occur, it is said to prove fatal in almost 50 per cent of cases.[12] Its precise incidence, however, is difficult to establish, for unless one searches for it carefully with serum amylase determinations, many mild cases will be missed.[65] The writer has encountered the problem but rarely.

There appears to be general agreement that the "pancreatitis" reflects an injury to the head, body, or tail of the pancreas in most instances — whether in mobilizing the duodenum (Fig. 19–1) or in removing the stomach from a large ulcer crater in the body of the pancreas, or from dissecting along the greater curvature in the region of the tail of the pancreas.[12, 13, 90, 127, 128] Burnett and his associates[12] called attention to

ANATOMY OF THE AMPULLARY REGION

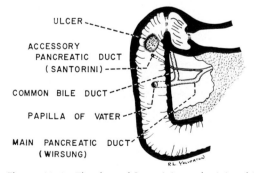

ULCER
ACCESSORY PANCREATIC DUCT (SANTORINI)
COMMON BILE DUCT
PAPILLA OF VATER
MAIN PANCREATIC DUCT (WIRSUNG)

Figure 19–1 The duct of Santorini may be injured in the course of excising a postbulbar duodenal ulcer. In the occasional patient it is the only pancreatic duct entering the duodenum. Postgastrectomy pancreatitis is usually due to pancreatic trauma.

the fact that this "postgastrectomy pancreatitis" need not represent actual pancreatitis in the sense that the organ becomes hemorrhagic and necrotic. Rather, the syndrome may be due to injury to one of the pancreatic ducts, resulting in a flow of pancreatic juice into the peritoneal cavity; this produces a marked inflammatory process that primarily involves the peritoneal surfaces and not the pancreas itself. Even so, some cases of pancreatitis following gastric resection have every feature of the usual hemorrhagic or necrotizing pancreatitis. Thal and Perry[121] pointed out that obstruction of the afferent loop may, presumably by back pressure, cause elevation of the serum amylase level and falsely indicate the presence of pancreatitis, thus adding to the difficulties in establishing an accurate diagnosis.

All agree that the pancreas should be dealt with most carefully in all dissections, for the organ may be injured in a variety of ways. First, dissection around the duodenal bulb or just distal to this point may result in injury to the duct of Santorini. This duct usually has communications with the duct of Wirsung, but occasionally has no communication with the main duct and, in fact, at times may be the only pancreatic duct entering the duodenum. It usually enters separately from the ampulla of Vater, ranging from 1 to 3 cm. proximal to this point (Fig. 19–1). Warren[127] emphasized that the duct of Santorini is the most vulnerable portion of the pancreas in gastric resection, and this fact has been further confirmed by the anatomic studies of Millbourn.[74] The latter concluded that there is serious danger of injury to the duct of Santorini in perhaps 50 per cent of cases, and that such injury may have serious consequences in the 10 per cent of cases in which the duct functions as the chief or sole excretory channel of the pancreas. In collecting from the literature 16 cases of injury to the common bile duct or pancreatic ducts and adding three new cases, Carpenter and Crandell[17] concluded that injury was due usually to anomalous entry of these ducts either into the duodenum or stomach or into the first portion of the duodenum as a result of scarring and contracture. Nevertheless pancreatitis can occur in the absence of any trauma to the pancreas, and it may even develop in ectopic pancreatic tissue.[60]

CLINICAL PICTURE

The typical attack of postoperative pancreatitis occurs within 24 to 48 hours after operation. The patient has abdominal pain, a rapid pulse, mild to moderate fever, and tenderness, together with a leukocytosis and an elevated serum amylase level. Peristalsis is diminished or absent. Nausea and vomiting may or may not occur. The clinical picture ranges from that reflecting a relatively mild condition to an overwhelming attack that terminates fatally in a day or so. Early onset following operation renders pancreatitis a more likely diagnosis than leakage from the pyloroplasty, duodenal stump, or gastrojejunal anastomosis, which complications would be expected to appear later in the postoperative course. Fluid aspirated from the peritoneal cavity may exhibit a high amylase level.

MANAGEMENT

PROPHYLACTIC MEASURES. Since the majority of cases of postoperative pancreatitis appear to be due to either direct or indirect trauma to the pancreas itself, representing in fact a traumatic pancreatitis, every effort should be made to avoid injury to this organ. First, the surgeon should try to determine at the outset whether there is a serious probability of pancreatic duct injury should an attempt be made to extirpate a duodenal ulcer distal to the bulbar portion. All too often, of course, the surgeon belatedly finds that the duodenum has already been perforated at one point, perhaps because the ulcer forms a portion of its posterior wall. Should it be appreciated that the ulcer is situated at approximately the level of the duct of Santorini or even the duct of Wirsung, a vagotomy-gastroenterostomy or vagotomy-pyloroplasty should be elected. Active or recent hemorrhage can often be managed satisfactorily by oversewing the ulcer, without actual excision of the lesion.

If a defect in the bed of the pancreas exists, it is wise not to cauterize or curet this site. There may be instances in which the pancreatic juice from one of the pancreatic ducts had been draining through the bed of the ulcer and into the alimentary tract; or the ulcer may have exposed the wall of a pancreatic duct that is subsequently injured in the dissection. Finally, as the dissection is carried in the general direction of the spleen, one will be careful not to injure the tail of the pancreas in clamping the gastrocolic omentum or the other blood supply along the greater curvature of the stomach.

There is no convincing evidence that the results that follow excision of a duodenal ulcer are substantially better than those obtained when the ulcer is left in situ, provided all gastric mucosa is excised and recent hemorrhage has not occurred. Burton and his associates[13] reported that pancreatitis more frequently follows mobilization of duodenal ulcers than of gastric ulcers. Lahey[56] advocated passage of a catheter from above through the common bile duct into the duodenum as a means of identifying the common duct in the course of difficult dissections, for not infrequently the common bile duct has been drawn by scar tissue into a position much superior or superficial to its usual course. The writer has found this maneuver invaluable on several occasions. Since some cases of postgastrectomy pancreatitis are suspected to have been produced by serious interference with the blood supply to the head of the pancreas, care should be exercised not to produce pancreatic ischemia.

TREATMENT OF THE ESTABLISHED CONDITION. Postgastrectomy pancreatitis is treated as follows: (1) continuous gastric suction to diminish distention of the stomach and perhaps to reduce pancreatic secretion, (2) control of pain with analgesics and paravertebral sympathetic blocks, (3) blood and fluid administration to maintain blood volume and electrolyte balance, (4) management of acute diabetes and hypocalcemia should these conditions occur, (5) cogent antibiotic therapy, and (6) drainage of collections of necrotic material and abscess when present. To these measures Hinton and his associates[94] suggested the addition of propylthiouracil therapy. This modality has not enjoyed wide acceptance, however, nor has the use of antitrypsin agents. Burnett et al.[12] advised immediate peritoneal drainage and irrigations. Anticholinergic drugs such as methantheline bromide (Banthine) have been advocated by some authors to suppress pancreatic exocrine secretions, but we have not been impressed with their value in patients we have treated.

As to the drainage of pancreatic abscesses, the left lumbar approach is particularly satisfactory when the tail of the pancreas is involved. Such collections can frequently be detected on physical examination, and at times roentgen studies may also be helpful. Recently, sonograms and CAT scans have markedly improved the localization of such abscesses. Abscesses involving the head of the pancreas are difficult to drain effectively, in our experience, owing to the presence of vital structures whose precise locations are not easily identified amid the necrotic material.

Pancreatic necrotic material and abscesses may require operative drainage several times before the patient is finally rendered afebrile; or regardless of drainage the patient may ultimately succumb to intra-abdominal sepsis or pulmonary complications or both. Late pancreatic pseudocysts are drained into the stomach, or by Roux-en-Y loop of jejunum, or they may be excised if they are in the tail of the pancreas.

If adequate drainage is provided, an external pancreatic fistula through a well sealed-off tract may be established eventually, provided the injured duct does not close spontaneously. Should the fistulous tract fail to close after many months, it can be implanted into a loop of bowel if partial pancreatectomy is not feasible. The implanted tract may later become occluded, however, and if this results in pancreatic duct obstruction, pancreatitis and sepsis may result. We prefer to excise the involved portion of the pancreas whenever possible. Finally, adequate surgical drainage of the peritoneal cavity should be provided until the fistula has closed.

JAUNDICE

When the surgeon is already apprehensive about the status of the common bile duct after a difficult dissection in the region of the head of the pancreas (Fig. 19–1), he or she is especially dismayed when the patient exhibits jaundice postoperatively. Jaundice is not particularly rare after a gastric resection, although such jaundice is usually mild. Among the possible causes of postoperative jaundice are (1) intravascular hemolysis, (2) partial occlusion of the common bile duct owing to edema around the duodenal stump, (3) bile spillage at operation, (4) leakage of the duodenal stump or of the gastrojejunal anastomosis, (5) liver failure, and (6) actual surgical occlusion of the common bile duct.

The writer has observed mild jaundice on numerous occasions, but with the exception of one case of acute liver failure there has been no instance in which the jaundice did not either clear or prove to be due to an alimentary tract fistula. In several cases in which there was an unusually difficult dissection below the duodenal bulb a catheter was passed from above downward to identify the course of the common duct. In one instance it entered the duodenum about 0.5 cm. distal to where the duodenum had been divided just below the ulcer, and very likely the duct of Santorini had already been ligated. The duodenal stump was closed rather unsatisfactorily, the catheter in the common bile duct being left in place meanwhile, and the nasogastric tube was placed far into the proximal loop and left there for several days of continuous suction decompression. In addition, extensive drainage was afforded in the right upper quadrant in the region of the duodenal stump. This patient exhibited mild jaundice for several days postoperatively, but it then subsided and did not return. There was no leakage at the duodenal stump, and the tube in the proximal loop was withdrawn at the end of several days without event. In this instance, of course, had it been realized initially that the ulcer was situated so close to the papilla of Vater, a vagotomy-gastroenterostomy would have been elected instead of excision of the duodenal ulcer and distal subtotal gastric resection.

Again, jaundice developing several days after operation may be due to leakage at the duodenal stump or at the gastrojejunal anastomosis. Such jaundice is usually associated with the other clinical evidence of intraperitoneal soiling.

INTRAPERITONEAL INFECTION

ETIOLOGY

One of the most serious complications of gastric resection is intraperitoneal sepsis.

This may be due to several causes: (1) contamination from the outside at operation, (2) the harboring of organisms in the nasopharynx that later find their way to the operative field, (3) spillage from the duodenum, the stomach, or the jejunum during the operation itself, and (4) leakage from the duodenal stump, a pyloroplasty, or a gastrojejunal anastomosis during the postoperative period.

Peritonitis with subsequent abscess formation is an extremely serious development. The onset may be obscured by the fact that antibiotic therapy causes the patient not to have the usual evidence of reaction to an intraperitoneal infection. This is particularly true when the infection begins with contamination at the time of operation but develops gradually. It is much less true when the infection starts abruptly because of leakage from the duodenal stump or the gastrojejunal anastomosis some days after a previously uneventful convalescence. Such collections may occur in the midst of the small bowel loops, in the pelvis, or, more commonly, in the left or right upper quadrant. Thus gastric resection may be followed by subphrenic abscess. We drained one such abscess that had traversed the diaphragm and ruptured into a bronchus. An abscess may form in the abdominal wall, or immediately below the abdominal wall but anterior to the stomach in an antecolic anastomosis.

DIAGNOSIS AND MANAGEMENT

Intraperitoneal sepsis may be particularly difficult to diagnose and even more difficult to act upon. The patient may exhibit a general malaise, does not convalesce as rapidly as he should after operation, and runs a protracted febrile course, and the white cell count is often elevated out of all proportion to the tachycardia and fever, although it may be normal. This picture is especially apt to be observed when the patient has been on antibiotic therapy since operation. Again, such therapy often succeeds in combating excessive fever and in limiting the rise in the pulse rate, but it does not, of course, dissipate the purulent collection. Unless the diagnosis can be made and the abscess drained surgically, the patient may not survive.

We have adopted the policy of exploring when in doubt, rather than allowing the condition of the patient who is not eating and whose alimentary tract is not functioning satisfactorily gradually to deteriorate until almost any operation is out of the question. Vigorous intravenous hyperalimentation can do much to preserve the nutritional reserves in such circumstances. By careful physical examination and radiologic assistance a subphrenic abscess can usually be localized. Fortunately, sonography and the CAT scan have dramatically improved the diagnosis of intra-abdominal fluid collections. The abscess can be drained either transabdominally or posteriorly through the bed of the eleventh or twelfth rib. Drainage tubes should not be removed until injection of radiopaque material demonstrates obliteration of the abscess cavity, leaving only the drainage tract.

Intraperitoneal sepsis may also be due to undiagnosed pancreatitis with pancreatic necrosis, or, indeed, to injury to the colon with a colonic fistula. We know of one instance in which colon necrosis resulted from ligation of a bleeder on the wall of this organ, a portion of the colon wall having been included in the ligature.

PROXIMAL LOOP PROBLEMS

The problems and complications that may involve the proximal or afferent loop constructed in the course of a Billroth II gastric resection are numerous and can be serious (Fig. 19–2).[3, 47, 58, 99, 105, 110] They range from minor postoperative symptomatology, with or without some bleeding from a residual unresected duodenal ulcer, to dehiscence of the duodenal closure or necrosis of the wall of the proximal loop owing to enormous distention of this portion of the bowel. The last is usually caused by either obstruction at the gastrojejunostomy or an adhesive band across the proximal loop.

Residual Symptomatology and Bleeding

The fact that further bleeding may occur from an unresected duodenal ulcer left in situ in the course of gastric resection has been mentioned previously. In addition, various other less serious but definitely pathologic circumstances may be present, as

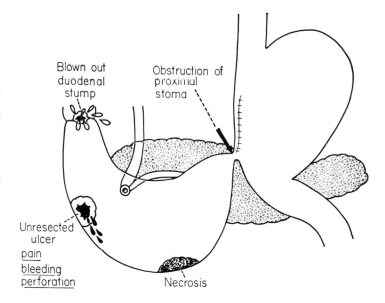

Figure 19–2 The proximal loop syndrome may be acute, subacute, or chronic. Complete obstruction may result in blow-out of the duodenal stump. High-grade partial obstruction may gradually result in enormous distention of the afferent loop, perhaps resulting in gangrene of a portion of its wall with peritoneal soiling. Chronic partial obstruction may be reflected in intermittent vomiting of large amounts of bile-stained material or in a spruelike syndrome because the bile and pancreatic secretions do not overtake the ingested food as it passes along the alimentary tract.

reported by Lorber and Shay.[61] In one patient a "stump ulcer" was demonstrated, in another duodenitis, and in a third a walled-off perforation was observed. Not all patients in whom a lesion was visualized were symptomatic, however. Rarely, such postoperative hemorrhage may be due to conditions such as hemophilia, arteriovenous malformation, or aortojejunal fistula.

Duodenal Stump Leakage

Duodenal stump "blow-out" is unquestionably the most common serious complication and is the main source of mortality in most series of gastric resection with the Billroth II technique. We had 15 instances of duodenal stump leakage in 451 patients (3.3 per cent) who underwent distal subtotal gastrectomy with Billroth II gastrojejunal anastomosis (see Table 19–1). Pearce, Jordan and DeBakey[82] found an incidence of 3.4 per cent in their series of patients in whom gastrointestinal continuity had been reestablished by gastrojejunostomy. All these subjects had been treated for duodenal ulcer.

ETIOLOGY

A number of factors can be important in healing of the duodenal stump. First, the lesion found at operation may be such as to preclude optimal duodenal closure. Second,

it is reasonable to assume that to denude too much of the duodenum distal to the site of actual inversion of the stump may reduce the blood supply and promote poor healing. Third — and perhaps the most important cause of stump leakage — is obstruction of the proximal loop either by adhesions or at the proximal stoma, with distention of the loop by bile, pancreatic juice, and succus entericus. Fourth, infection and a poor general state of nutrition can also be contributing factors. There are other causes of stump leakage, including poor surgical technique, but those mentioned are probably the most important ones.

If there is serious concern as to a safe closure of the duodenal stump — or that the closure, although technically satisfactory, has been achieved with less than optimal tissue with which to work — the abdomen should be drained. We do not drain routinely, but we carefully place drains in every case in which we feel that there is a genuine possibility that duodenal leakage may occur. Some surgeons, perhaps wisely, always drain after gastric resection, and certainly the untoward effects of drainage are few indeed.

CLINICAL PICTURE

Dehiscence of the duodenal closure usually occurs sometime from the third to the fifth postoperative day. The patient, previously convalescing satisfactorily, or possibly with no more than a sense of epigastric fullness and discomfort, may suddenly be seized with severe pain, abdominal rigidity, and fever, and perhaps exhibit a shocklike state. On the other hand, the symptoms may be relatively mild, with only moderate fever and leukocytosis. Jaundice may develop within 48 hours, owing to absorption of bile from the peritoneal cavity.

DIAGNOSIS

If the abdomen was drained, bile-stained fluid may be observed emerging at the drain site. If drains were placed, but no material suggestive of a fistula has appeared, the patient may be given methylene blue by mouth, and this material may be observed to emerge from the drain site. Often bile-stained fluid will extrude from between the skin sutures. The defect may at times be demonstrated with roentgen studies by using a radiopaque medium. A CAT scan may reveal extraluminal fluid or air.

The first and most important step in the diagnosis of duodenal stump leakage is to suspect that it has occurred.

MANAGEMENT

The paramount requirement is to provide prompt and adequate surgical drainage. Successful secondary suture of the duodenal leak has occasionally been achieved, but it usually is not feasible. Nasogastric suction should be instituted and intravenous fluid and nutritional maintenance begun. Within a few days, however, once adequate and walled-off drainage to the outside has been established through a drainage tract, the patient can often be fed by mouth and the nutritional status maintained in this way while the fistula is allowed to close in due course. Thus this "end" type of duodenal fistula is not usually a serious problem, so long as intraperitoneal sepsis is avoided by immediate drainage; this is in contrast to the "side" type of duodenal fistula, which is much more difficult to manage. In fact, a chronic duodenal side fistula has at times been managed successfully by performing a distal subtotal gastric resection with gastrojejunostomy, the duodenal stump being closed or drained, or both. However, there

is a real hazard that anastomoses may break down under such circumstances. A substantial period of intravenous hyperalimentation should usually be tried to improve nutrition whenever indicated. In this way reoperation may be avoided and, if not, the patient will be rendered better able to withstand surgery.

Additional therapeutic measures include protection of the skin surrounding the fistula by catheter aspiration of the fistulous drainage, and by the application of aluminum paste, karaya powder, or an adherent film spray. A heat lamp may be useful in keeping the skin dry, thus reducing skin maceration and promoting healing. It is often possible to seal a disposable ileostomy bag over the drainage tract and thus both protect the skin and measure fluid loss. Antibiotic therapy and general supportive measures are used as indicated. While the patient is on intravenous fluid maintenance the serum chemistry values should be checked every second day. A carefully kept intake-output record is essential. If bed scales are available, it is helpful to weigh the patient daily to determine whether dehydration or overhydration is developing.

In contrast to the stump or end fistula, the duodenal side fistula, of the approximate type that may follow pyloroplasty or a Billroth I gastroduodenal anastomosis, may be much more difficult to manage successfully. In addition to adequate surgical drainage of the right upper quadrant of the abdomen, it is helpful if a nasogastric feeding tube can be passed far into the duodenum and preferably beyond the ligament of Treitz. This permits nutritional maintenance while the associated infection subsides and the fistula gradually closes. Alternatively or as supplementation, intravenous hyperalimentation may be employed. If after six weeks the fistula shows little evidence of closing, a distal subtotal resection of the stomach with Billroth II anastomosis may be considered.

PROGNOSIS

Duodenal end fistulas have a favorable prognosis if prompt diagnosis leads to early and adequate surgical drainage. The major hazard here is sepsis. Duodenal side fistulas carry a less favorable prognosis, because of both sepsis and inanition from lack of oral feeding, but these lesions can usually be managed successfully by vigorous supportive therapy.

Distention and Necrosis of the Wall of the Proximal (Afferent) Loop

Obstruction of the afferent loop is perhaps the most common cause of leakage of an otherwise satisfactorily closed duodenal stump, but closure may be so secure that gradual and continued enlargement of the proximal loop may reach relatively enormous proportions without dehiscence of the stump (Fig. 19–2). When this occurs, the patient notes increasing discomfort and pain in the right upper quadrant, and a mass may become palpable. In fact, in one of the two such cases that we have encountered the firmness of the mass suggested a possible tumor when the patient was admitted some 2 months after the gastric resection. The other patient likewise exhibited a firm mass in the right upper quadrant extending downward almost to the umbilicus. In each instance extreme distention of the proximal loop was found at operation. Such obstruction can result in extensive necrosis and perforation of the bowel wall. The technique of operative management will depend upon the anatomic defect found at exploratory laparotomy.

Proximal Loop Syndrome (Chronic)

When obstruction of the proximal loop is incomplete, the contained bile and other juices may be periodically disgorged in large amounts, with relief of symptoms and reduction in size of the mass if such was previously palpable.

Stasis of pancreatic juice and bile in the proximal loop until the ingested food has passed down the intestine may result in poor digestion and a spruelike picture. Such patients may also be suspected of having pain of pancreatic origin.[73, 121]

Management of Proximal Loop Dysfunction

To prevent distention of the proximal loop, some surgeons routinely pass the tip

PROXIMAL LOOP SYNDROME
ENTERO-ENTEROSTOMY IN MANAGEMENT

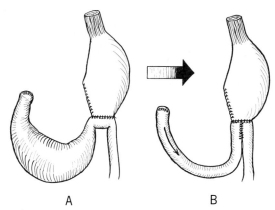

A   B

Figure 19–3 Obstruction of the proximal or afferent loop *(A)* at the gastrojejunostomy anastomosis is a serious matter. By performing a jejunojejunostomy adjacent to the stomach *(B)*, the alkaline fluids draining through the proximal loop continue to exert protection against marginal ulceration at the gastrojejunostomy.

of the nasogastric suction tube into the proximal loop at the close of the gastric resection, leaving it in place for several days. This, however, does not prevent distention after the tube has been withdrawn. Such complications are more effectively avoided by using a short afferent loop and by taking extreme care to reduce the possibility of obstruction at the proximal stoma. Once proximal loop distention is suspected, it can be confirmed by appropriate radiologic studies, including sonography and CAT scan. If the obstruction is not great, alert, conservative management may be used temporarily, but if adequate relief is not achieved, surgical intervention is essential.

The technical procedure to be used at operation will depend upon the anatomic defect found. In one instance the patient was so ill that we merely anastomosed the distended proximal loop to a distal loop of jejunum, with satisfactory results. An alternative procedure is a Finney pyloroplasty on the jejunal loops just at the anastomosis (Fig. 19–3). If obstruction of the proximal stoma is present, revision of the anastomosis may be preferable. Adhesions involving the proximal loop should be divided, but it is hazardous to assume that relatively insignificant adhesions are producing all the obstruction. We know of such an instance in which the obstruction was not relieved and the patient died of extensive duodenal necrosis with peritonitis.

LEAKAGE FROM THE STOMACH OR THE GASTROJEJUNAL ANASTOMOSIS

Ischemic Necrosis of the Gastric Remnant

The rich blood supply of the stomach[11] is shown in Figure 19–4. Although ischemic necrosis of the gastric remnant is a rare complication following gastric surgery, it does occur.[20, 22, 36, 45, 102, 115] In reviewing this problem Fell, Seidenberg and Hurwitt[31] reported two cases and emphasized certain precautions. Inadequate vascularization of the remaining stomach is most likely when the left gastric artery is ligated at its origin and splenectomy is performed. This leaves the gastric pouch precariously vascularized by the phrenic arterial branches, the left gastroepiploic artery and the vasa brevia having been sacrificed in the course of splenectomy (Fig. 19–4). Should the left inferior phrenic artery have arisen from the divided left gastric artery, ischemic necrosis of the gastric remnant is highly likely.[31, 36, 45] Thus one should critically evaluate the blood supply before performing a high gastric resection. In the usual moderately extensive distal gastric resection the phrenic branches, the superior portion of the left gastric artery, the short gastric branches, and the left gastroepiploic artery are all left to supply the remaining gastric pouch. Kilgore and Hardy[54] demonstrated a progressive decline in radiosodium clearance from the gastric wall as the various arteries to the stomach were successively ligated in dogs.

Management of early massive necrosis consists in reoperation and excision of the devitalized tissue, with reestablishment of alimentary continuity and extensive drainage. Unfortunately, this is usually unsuccessful. Spencer[115] was able to save one patient at reoperation by total resection of the ischemic gastric remnant and anastomosis of a jejunal loop to the esophagus.

Dehiscence of the Gastroenteric Anastomosis

Peritonitis due to leakage from the gastrojejunal anastomosis is not as common as that due to blow-out of the duodenal stump following the Billroth II operation, but anastomotic disruption does occur. Of course, the leak is only at the anastomosis when a Billroth I operation, a total gastrectomy, or a gastroenterostomy has been performed, since there is no duodenal stump after these

ARTERIAL SUPPLY OF THE STOMACH

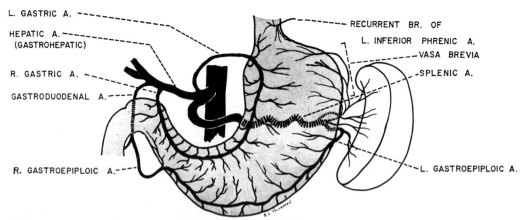

Figure 19–4 High gastric resection, with splenectomy and ligation of the left gastric artery at its origin, may leave the remaining gastric pouch precariously supplied by the recurrent branch of the left inferior phrenic artery. Nevertheless cross-circulation between the several arteries is so extensive that serious ischemia of the remaining gastric pouch following subtotal gastrectomy is rare.

procedures. Peritonitis may be due to technical imperfections, ischemia, poor general health with hypoproteinemia, gastric distention, and other factors. This complication is listed separately from leakage at the duodenal stump because the management of the two conditions is somewhat different. Initially, however, the clinical picture of the one is indistinguishable from that of the other. In both instances evidence of peritoneal contamination develops after the third postoperative day. The signs of leakage are abdominal pain, rigidity, leukocytosis, and tachycardia. If the peritoneal soilage is abrupt and sufficiently massive, a shocklike picture is produced. Should the patient have an initial widespread peritoneal contamination, he may exhibit jaundice during the next 24 to 48 hours resulting from absorption of bile-stained material from the peritoneal cavity. In addition, bile-stained fluid may seep through a drainage site or from between the sutures in the abdominal wound. Administration of indigo carmine or methylene blue by mouth may disclose a fistulous tract by virtue of the appearance of the ingested material on the surface of the abdominal wall. As a rule, the radiologist is able with radiopaque medium to demonstrate leakage at the gastroenteric anastomosis.

MANAGEMENT

The immediate requirement is to establish surgical drainage, with or without an attempt at surgical closure of the defect. After adequate drainage has been established, producing in effect an external fistula if the gastric defect has not been closed along with the placement of drains, therapy is continued in the form of intravenous administration of blood and fluids, nasogastric suction, maintenance of a careful intake-output record, antibiotic therapy, and sedation if indicated. Here again, intravenous hyperalimentation can be very helpful.

Once the patient's condition has become somewhat stabilized and intestinal activity has returned, a long tube may be passed through the stomach and into the distal loop and the patient thus fed. We have seen this maneuver performed in several patients in whom a defect occurred at the anastomosis; after several weeks of such maintenance the fistula closed, and the patients made uneventful recoveries. Intravenous hyperalimentation offers an alternative route for supportive nutrition if a tube cannot be passed into the jejunum distal to the fistula. However, if closure of the fistula is slow and a protracted illness develops, it may be useful to witzel a tube into a loop of jejunum as a feeding jejunostomy.

Should the fistula not close after a reasonable period of conservative management, a secondary operation should be performed after the peritoneal cavity has become generally cleared of contamination and a well-isolated drainage tract has been established. As with duodenal stump leakage, however, a serious sequela of the peritoneal contamination is the not infrequent occurrence of intraperitoneal suppuration with the hazards attendant upon it. Sizable purulent collections must be drained surgically.

The skin surrounding the fistula is protected as outlined under the discussion of duodenal stump leakage. (See also Small Bowel Fistula, p. 505.)

GASTRIC RETENTION

Although rarely fatal and not often seriously disturbing ultimately, failure of the gastric remnant to empty satisfactorily[116, 117, 129] is certainly one of the most common annoyances that follow gastric surgery. Such retention may reach relatively enormous volumes: 3 liters of fluid were present in the stomach of one patient who had had a 75 per cent resection. A special hazard is that of nocturnal aspiration of gastric contents into the lungs, with pneumonitis. There are many causes of this gastric retention, and certain of these will now be examined.

Obstruction of the Distal Stoma

Obstruction of the distal stoma — or, indeed, any obstruction that prevents satisfactory emptying of the stomach and upper small bowel — will result in gastric distention, vomiting, or the recovery of excessive volumes of fluid through an indwelling na-

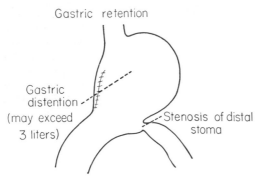

Figure 19–5 There are numerous causes of gastric retention following subtotal gastric resection (see text.)

sogastric tube. Since the distal stoma (Fig. 19–5) has usually been examined by the surgeon after completion of the gastrojejunal anastomosis at the time of operation, it is relatively rare that a lumen of inadequate size was constructed at operation. Therefore edematous swelling is probably the most common cause of early postoperative stenosis of the distal stoma. This is even more credible if one recalls the tremendous edematous swelling that may be observed occasionally in a transverse loop colostomy. Such colostomies may readily become obstructed because of edematous swelling, which usually subsides in a few days. Unquestionably a similar process can develop at the gastrojejunal stoma.

When edema does produce such temporary stenosis of the anastomosis, intravenous supportive therapy and nasogastric suction are continued until the obstruction has been relieved. One can determine this by clamping the tube during the waking hours and leaving it unclamped overnight. If no serious degree of gastric retention occurs, the tube can be clamped for 12 to 24 hours; and if excessive gastric retention still does not occur, the tube is then removed. When nasogastric suction and intravenous fluid maintenance are necessary, however, the plasma chemistry values should be checked every second day and a strict intake-output record maintained.

Operative intervention is not often required, and certainly conservative management should be tried for at least 2 to 3 weeks. In fact, a form of gastric atony may exist, and at a premature reexploration no anatomic distortion may be found. Gastro-

scopy in conjunction with appropriate radiologic studies can be useful in identifying patency of the proximal and distal stomas. If it should become necessary to operate to correct obstruction of the stoma of the distal loop, it may prove expedient to leave the existing anastomosis in place and to bring up another loop of jejunum and perform a second gastrojejunostomy higher up on the stomach.

Infection with Ileus and Anatomic Distortion

That anatomic distortion of the anastomosis and the distal loop may occur because of pancreatitis (Fig. 19–6) or sepsis has been mentioned previously. Postoperative ileus may be inordinately prolonged, or until an abscess is drained. Stomal or proximal jejunal obstruction can be produced by a very small adjacent abscess that has stimulated adverse inflammatory reaction.

Neurogenic Syndrome of the Distal Loop

In some patients the gastric remnant does not empty satisfactorily, but no definite obstruction can be demonstrated by roentgen study with barium. Such patients have often been reoperated upon, but still no definite cause for failure of the gastric pouch to empty was found. Golden[35] reviewed the evidence for functional obstruction of the efferent loop in a number of such patients. The symptoms were epigastric fullness, nausea, and vomiting, beginning during the

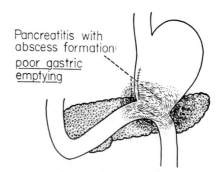

Figure 19–6 Pancreatitis may be a cause of poor alimentary tract function.

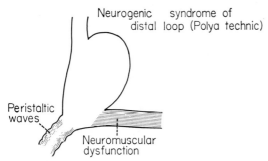

Figure 19–7 The "neurogenic syndrome" of the distal loop appears to be somewhat more common after the Polya than after the Hofmeister modification of the Billroth II type of gastric resection.

latter part of the first or the beginning of the second postoperative week in the majority of cases. These findings usually disappeared spontaneously in a few days, but occasionally they persisted for several weeks. Roentgen studies with barium disclosed a spasm of the efferent loop of the jejunum when the symptoms were present, with delay in emptying of the gastric pouch (Fig. 19–7). It appeared that the disorder occurred less frequently in association with the shorter jejunal incision used with the Hofmeister operation than with the longer incision used with the Polya procedure. Despite these findings by Golden, other workers feel that jejunal adhesions not visualized on roentgenography may well account for a considerable number of these cases of "neurogenic syndrome" of the distal loop. Of course, bilateral vagotomy does produce reduced gastric tone for a variable period of time, and a prolonged period of postoperative nasogastric suction is sometimes required in patients having this procedure. In the absence of vagotomy, gastric atony is rare. (See also Complications of Vagotomy, Pyloroplasty, and Gastrostomy, p. 486.)

MANAGEMENT

A conservative approach with gastric decompression and intravenous fluid therapy is to be preferred. Operative intervention is avoided for at least 3 to 4 weeks, since even at operation no definite organic, pathologic cause may be discovered. Actually, true "neurogenic dysfunction" is rare, the dysfunction usually being due to postoperative adhesions. Gastric atony responds irregularly to drug therapy. (See Complications of Vagotomy, Pyloroplasty, and Gastrostomy, p. 486.)

Transverse Mesocolon Sutured to the Jejunal Loop Instead of to the Stomach in a Posterior Anastomosis

When the anastomosis of the jejunum to the stomach in the Billroth II operation is performed posterior instead of anterior to the colon, the transverse mesocolon should be sutured to the more rigid wall of the stomach and not to the loop of jejunum. The reason for this is that mild compression by the mesocolon will not obstruct the loop of jejunum (Fig. 19–8). Even when the operation has been done correctly, the sutures between the stomach and the mesocolon will ocassionally pull through and allow the stomach to retract upward, dragging the jejunal loop with it and producing obstruction in some patients.

DIAGNOSIS

This condition can be particularly difficult to identify. The usual symptoms are that the patient retains some food and fluid but complains of epigastric fullness, distention, and intermittent vomiting. In effect, the symptoms are those of a high, partial small bowel obstruction. But on barium study it may be observed that the material

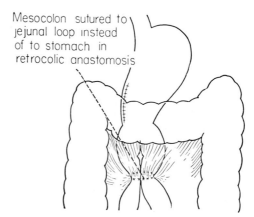

Figure 19–8 Partial obstruction of the jejunal loop by the mesocolon may be difficult to diagnose radiologically.

does leave the stomach. The mild to moderate difficulty that the roentgenologist experiences in massaging the barium out of the stomach at fluoroscopy is perhaps no greater than that associated with the small distal stoma that some surgeons construct deliberately. Therefore in some cases one simply must have a high index of suspicion that this defect exists.

The author had occasion to treat such a patient who had been operated upon elsewhere and who was admitted with an abscess in the lower portion of the abdomen. This collection was drained through a right lower quadrant muscle-splitting incision, but thereafter the patient still did not improve satisfactorily and continued to exhibit evidence of partial obstruction of the upper jejunum. A barium study of the upper gastrointestinal tract revealed no definite evidence of obstruction. When it was learned that a posterior anastomosis had been performed at the original gastric resection, the possibility that the mesocolon had been sutured to the jejunum instead of to the stomach was considered. The patient was operated upon again, and this was found to be the case. All that was required was for the mesocolon to be dissected free from the jejunal loop and sutured to the more rigid wall of the stomach. Thereafter the man rapidly gained almost 20 pounds in weight over the next few weeks. Incidentally, at the second operation for correction of the compression of the jejunal loop it was noted that the site of the huge abscess that had been drained in the lower portion of the abdomen was hardly discernible, so completely had the body defenses cleansed the peritoneal cavity of the products of inflammation and infection.

Adhesions of the Distal Loop

Adhesions of the upper jejunum are a definite cause of poor gastric emptying in some patients (Fig. 19–9). Although various authors disagree as to the incidence with which this occurs, some feeling that it is a rare circumstance, Stammers[116] and Berkas and Ferguson[7] believe that such adhesions constitute an important source of morbidity following gastric resection. The present author has encountered obstruction of the distal loop and of the proximal loop by adhesions on a number of occasions. In one patient, indeed, a tight adhesive band had caused dilatation of the proximal loop associated with leakage of the duodenal stump. The distal loop may be tented upward or

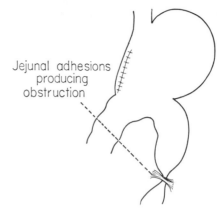

Figure 19–9 Fibrinous adhesions constitute an important cause of early postoperative alimentary dysfunction.

kinked in various directions, depending of course upon the site of these adhesions. Adhesions near the hilus of the spleen will pull the jejunal loop in that direction, while adhesions in the hilus of the liver may cause the efferent loop to be drawn across the anastomosis.

MANAGEMENT

The clinical picture of small bowel adhesions is, again, that of upper small bowel obstruction with epigastric fullness, nausea, and vomiting with or without pain. The diagnosis rests chiefly upon roentgenographic studies, by which distortion of the distal loop can be demonstrated in most instances. Gastroscopy will usually exclude obstruction of the distal stoma itself. Conservative treatment with nasogastric suction and intravenous fluid maintenance usually suffices, particularly if the obstruction is due to the fibrinous adhesions that form shortly after operation. On the other hand, if the obstruction develops after several weeks, being then due to organizing fibrous adhesions, operative intervention may be required. Even so, since in most instances postoperative obstruction owing to fibrinous adhesions will subside on conservative management during the first few weeks after operation, nonoperative measures should be used initially. This is particularly true with high jejunal obstruction, since the ability of the jejunum to decompress itself readily into the stomach minimizes the possibility of ischemic necrosis of the bowel owing to prolonged and severe distention unless closed-loop obstruction exists. Unless nasogastric suction is employed while the gut is returning to normal, acute gastric dilatation and vomiting and pulmonary aspiration remain significant hazards.

Intussusception of the Jejunum

There are numerous reports of intussusception of the upper small bowel either upon itself (Fig. 19–10) or retrograde into the stomach (jejunogastric), or forward intussusception of the proximal loop into the stomach.[43, 111] In one case treated by the author the intussusception was just distal to the stoma and was both forward and retrograde and may have been due to withdrawal of a tube that had been allowed to progress into the upper small bowel. In any event, the intussusception was reduced, and no further difficulty occurred.

Actually, jejunal intussusception, whether into the stomach or not, is a rare complication that may occur years after operation. The symptoms may be acute or chronic, consisting of colicky epigastric pain and vomiting with or without hematemesis, associated with tenderness in the epigastrium. The examiner may feel an epigastric mass,

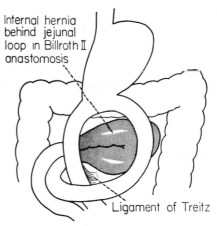

Figure 19–11 Internal herniation of jejunal loop. This has been rare in our experience.

but this will not be palpated if the stoma has retracted beneath the costal margin. The management is surgical, and it may suffice to reduce the intussusception. Gangrenous bowel, however, will obviously need to be resected, and depending upon the judgment of the surgeon at the time, it may be in order to resect the anastomosis and to establish a new one, when the intussusception is into the stomach. Roentgenologic study with barium may permit an accurate diagnosis preoperatively.

Internal Herniation of the Jejunal Loop

The small bowel may herniate behind the jejunal loop used for the anastomosis (Fig. 19–11).[15, 85] This complication has been reported to follow an antecolic anastomosis more often than a retrocolic anastomosis. It may occur soon after the operation or not until years later. Most surgeons reporting such a case have advocated closure of the hiatus formed by the jejunal loop used for the anastomosis, to prevent subsequent herniation of the small bowel behind it. This is the same sort of problem that occasionally follows left colostomy or ileostomy. The pathophysiology may range from that due to a mild degree of obstruction, with some circulatory embarrassment, to actual strangulation and gangrene of a loop of bowel or the omentum. Stammers,[116] who reviewed this problem in some detail, stated that the most common time of onset is between the

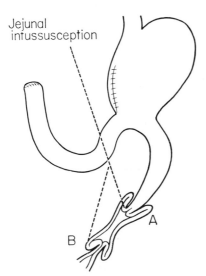

Figure 19–10 Jejunal intussusception may also involve the afferent loop with forward intussusception into the stomach, or the distal loop with retrograde intussusception into the stomach.

third and sixth postoperative days. The patient usually complains of an unpleasant epigastric fullness and feels vaguely less well or actually ill. Vomiting may or may not be present. Radiologic studies, sonography, or CAT scan may be helpful in establishing an accurate diagnosis.

It is felt that a long afferent loop particularly predisposes to herniation, which may be intermittent. Such episodes may explain certain sporadic attacks of nausea and colicky pain lasting from a few hours to a day or so.

MANAGEMENT

Should herniation be found at reoperation, the involved bowel should be reduced and any gangrenous portion resected. After this the defect through which the bowel had previously passed should be closed. If the afferent loop is of excessive length, one may elect to resect a portion of it, with or without construction of a new anastomosis. In one patient we treated it was not possible to reduce the markedly adherent and distended loop until the gastrojejunal anastomosis had been taken down.

Postoperative Filling Defect in the Stomach

Although not necessarily a cause of poor gastric emptying, a filling defect along the lesser curvature may be noted on postoperative follow-up barium study of the stomach. In one such patient the radiologist was sufficiently apprehensive about the possible

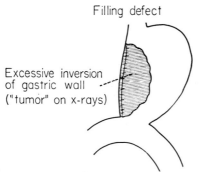

Fugure 19–12 Inversion of an excessive amount of stomach along the lesser curvature may cause a filling defect on postoperative follow-up gastrointestinal series.

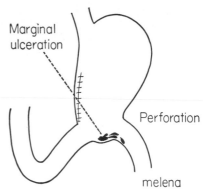

Figure 19–13 Marginal ulceration may occur precisely at the level of the stoma, but more often it develops slightly distal to this point.

presence of an overlooked tumor that the abdomen was reexplored. This was done because the surgeon had not deliberately examined the stomach in this region during the course of the gastric resection. When the stomach was opened above the anastomosis, it was found that the filling defect that the radiologist had believed might well represent an overlooked gastric neoplasm was, in fact, due to inversion of an excessive amount of stomach (Fig. 19–12). Such a negative exploratory laparotomy would now be avoided by gastroscopic evaluation of the lesion.

Marginal Ulceration — Pain, Bleeding, Perforation

The so-called marginal or jejunal ulcer, occurring usually in the efferent loop just distal to the stoma, is still another complication of gastric resection (Fig. 19–13). Such ulceration may follow the Billroth I operation, in which the residual remaining portion of the stomach was anastomosed to the duodenum; the Billroth II procedure, in which the stomach was anastomosed to the jejunum; or vagotomy-gastroenterostomy or vagotomy-pyloroplasty. It is due to the digestive activity of the acid-pepsin factor in gastric juice. The conditions that may predispose to ulcer recurrence include gastric stasis, incomplete vagotomy, retained gastric antrum, inadequate resection of the acid-secreting portion of the stomach, a functioning parathyroid adenoma, or a Zollinger-Ellison or Oberhelman secreting tumor of pancreatic islet cell tissue. Becker[6] has recently reviewed disorders of gastrointestinal hormones after surgery, with an emphasis on gastrin. States of hypergastrinemia without increased gastric acid secretion, as well as those with increased acid secretion, were considered.

It is difficult to compare satisfactorily different series of cases from different clinics, especially for assessing the precise incidence of postoperative marginal ulceration.[75, 80, 92, 112, 125] Nevertheless, it would appear that in most series a two-thirds distal gastric resection results in marginal ulceration in less than 5 per cent of cases. The addition of a bilateral truncal or selective vagotomy further reduces this incidence. The Billroth I operation may have a slightly higher incidence of marginal ulceration than the Billroth II. Most observers feel that the vagotomy-gastroenterostomy operation for duodenal ulcer is followed by a somewhat higher incidence of jejunal ulceration than is a two-thirds distal gastric resection, especially if vagotomy is added to the resection. In recent years there has been an increasing tendency to perform bilateral vagotomy with either a 50 to 60 per cent gastric resection or simple antrectomy, in order to retain a larger gastric pouch with the objective of reducing the incidence and severity of the postoperative dumping syndrome and other impediments to nutrition. This operation abolishes both the vagal and the antral phases of gastric secretion. However, the operation most often used to control the peptic ulcer diathesis is, at present, vagotomy with some type of emptying procedure, usually a pyloroplasty. The vagotomy most often performed is the bilateral truncal type, but the selective and superselective types of vagotomy have gained support. We have had good results with a simple one-layer or two-layer Weinberg pyloroplasty, avoiding tissue inversion, but the Finney and Jaboulay types have recently regained popularity.

The *symptoms* of marginal ulceration are similar to those associated with peptic ulceration elsewhere. The pain may arise slightly to the left of the midline, and point tenderness may be present over the region of the anastomosis in some patients. Occasionally the pain may radiate to the back. The jejunal ulceration may be demonstrated on gastrointestinal series, but often it is not. Gastroscopy may be helpful.

The *complications that may follow marginal ulceration* are obstruction, hemorrhage, and perforation, with or without formation of a gastrojejunocolic fistula. In other words, the complications of marginal ulceration are similar to those of peptic ulceration in the duodenum or esophagus, except that the inflammatory process may erode the wall of the colon and produce a fistula from the stomach, through the jejunum, and thence to the colon — gastrojejunocolic fistula (see Fig. 19–14).

MANAGEMENT

The management of marginal ulceration, in the absence of gastrojejunocolic fistula, is either nonoperative or operative.[34, 68, 91, 124] If the ulceration is mild, the patient may be managed successfully with a strict ulcer regimen. Repeated bleeding, persistent pain, or evidence of penetration or impending perforation, however, may prompt surgical intervention. Many surgeons would next perform a supradiaphragmatic bilateral vagotomy from the thoracic approach, assuming that vagotomy had not been performed at the original operation or that acid secretion tests indicated that the vagotomy had been incomplete. Should this prove insufficient to control the ulcer diathesis, one would usually resect additional stomach with the creation of a new gastroenterostomy. The writer, however, usually prefers to perform the vagotomy through the abdomen, so that the marginal ulcer can be properly examined and assessed. It may prove advisable not only to perform vagotomy, but also to resect the anastomosis and additional stomach. The technical problems attendant upon resection of additional stomach with the creation of a new gastrojejunostomy are usually not difficult. The possibility of a Zollinger-Ellison tumor of the pancreas associated with a particularly intractable ulcer diathesis should be borne in mind.[136]

Gastrojejunocolic Fistula

This complication of gastrojejunostomy, which occurs somewhat more frequently in

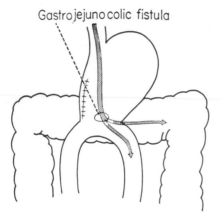

Figure 19–14   Gastrojejunocolic fistulas are less common than they formerly were.

the presence of posterior anastomoses, can be a difficult surgical problem (Fig. 19–14). It is usually a sequel of marginal ulceration following a previous gastric resection and gastrojejunostomy. The writer has also encountered it in connection with a tumor that had allowed passage of material directly from the stomach to the colon (actually a gastrocolic fistula). As with marginal ulceration, the gastrojejunocolic fistula secondary to such ulceration may develop months or even years after the initial operation. In contrast, in one child we treated who had an extremely virulent ulcer diathesis, a gastrojejunocolic fistula had nearly developed within 2 weeks after vagotomy-gastroenterostomy. This 8-year-old boy proved to have a Zollinger-Ellison tumor with small hepatic metastases. His ulcer diathesis was controlled by an almost total gastrectomy, but he died later of metastases.

The usual clinical findings are diarrhea and weight loss, often associated with foul eructations and perhaps fecal vomiting. A spruelike syndrome may be observed. The diarrhea is due less to short-circuiting of the food directly into the colon than to the irritating effect of colonic bacterial flora upon the stomach and the small bowel. The diagnosis is usually established by the use of both an upper gastrointestinal series and a barium enema.

The gastrojejunocolic fistula is best managed by preparing the patient as well as possible, particularly with adequate preoperative blood transfusion, and perhaps with intravenous hyperalimentation, and then

resecting the entire fistula with reconstruction of gastrojejunal and colon continuity at one operation. It is advisable to resect additional amounts of stomach and perhaps to perform vagotomy at the time the gastrojejunocolic fistula is resected, to prevent subsequent recurrence of marginal ulceration. Needless to say, many of these patients are in a poor state of general health preoperatively, and scrupulous attention to postoperative supportive management is essential.

NUTRITIONAL PROBLEMS

The Dumping Syndrome

The incidence of the various groups of signs and symptoms collectively referred to as the dumping syndrome (Fig. 19–15) following gastric resection varies from 10 to 40 per cent, depending upon the extent of the gastric resection performed and upon the clinic reporting its results. It appears to be generally agreed that the incidence of the dumping syndrome is not greatly different after the Billroth I, Billroth II, and vagotomy-gastroenterostomy operations for duodenal ulcer. However, the greater the amount of stomach resected, the more likely is the patient to have serious nutritional disturbances.

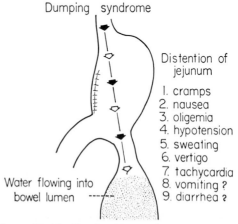

Figure 19–15   The dumping syndrome appears to be due largely to rapid entrance of ingested food into the small bowel. Water flows in from the bowel wall, producing both intestinal distention and a reduction in plasma volume. Generalized vasodilatation may be a factor.

SYMPTOMS AND
PATHOPHYSIOLOGY[16, 25, 33, 52, 130, 131]

SYMPTOMS. The dumping syndrome[86] is actually a rather complex physiologic response to the presence in the small bowel of food of high osmolar concentration.[41, 62] After a meal the susceptible person experiences a prompt onset of varying degrees or combinations of weakness, nausea, epigastric distress, tachycardia, belching, perspiration, and flushing or a sense of warmth; he may exhibit vomiting or diarrhea, or neither. We knew a patient who had severe dumping symptoms without diarrhea for a number of months, after which the symptoms of dumping disappeared but were replaced by diarrhea that occurred shortly after eating. This diarrhea continued for the 2 years' time that he was under observation.

PATHOPHYSIOLOGY. The dumping syndrome was particularly well described by Machella[62] in 1949. In essence, he was able to produce the typical dumping syndrome, even in normal persons, by intrajejunal instillation of hypertonic solutions of glucose, protein hydrolysate, or sodium sulfate — and even at times by distention of the jejunum with an inflated balloon. He pointed out that such symptoms had also been observed after the introduction of 33 per cent magnesium sulfate into the duodenum for the purpose of evacuating the gallbladder. Subsequently Roberts and associates[98] and others[41, 83] showed that the dumping syndrome was associated with a sharp reduction in the circulating blood volume. The reduction in plasma volume appears to be part of a general reduction in extracellular fluid volume.

All in all, the present writer feels that the symptomatology of the dumping syndrome is produced by rapid entrance of hypertonic food products into the jejunum, with a consequent flow of extracellular fluid into the jejunum and a reduction in plasma volume. It is agreed that the dumping syndrome is more common in patients who have a certain psychologic make-up; those who are emotionally unstable are likely to prove to be the ones who are bothered most by the symptoms of the dumping syndrome. In addition to blood volume and psychologic factors, there may be hypoglycemia, ad-

renal stimulation,[89] a fall in the serum potassium level,[100, 114, 134] and an alteration in the digestion of fats. Generalized vasodilatation may be a factor in the hemodynamic changes frequently encountered. The liberation of vasoactive substances from the wall of the intestine may contribute to these changes.

MANAGEMENT

CONSERVATIVE MEASURES. First, the dumping syndrome can be adequately managed in most patients by dietary measures.[37, 48, 53, 87, 101] The patient is put on a diet high in protein and fat, but low in carbohydrate, since carbohydrate is rapidly hydrolyzed and enters the jejunum to increase the osmolar concentration and thus to draw in water. In addition, he is instructed to avoid ingestion of water or other liquid in significant amounts with his meals. Adequate amounts of fluids are taken between meals. Thus proteins are tolerated better than carbohydrates and fairly dry solid foods better than liquids. The patient is advised to avoid foods that he has found aggravate the dumping symptoms. Frequent small feedings, six or more a day, are necessary, especially when the remaining gastric pouch is small and the patient tends to lose weight. With such measures, plus continuous reassurance that the symptoms will gradually recede, most patients gradually recover their normal eating habits without residual symptomatology.

Second, patients who are not sufficiently relieved by dietary measures alone should be instructed to lie down for 20 to 30 minutes after each meal. Gastric emptying is slower when the patient is in a recumbent position, and this appears to be a primary beneficial effect of the supine position.

Third, the use of antispasmodics[93] may be helpful. Various drugs have different effects after meals, as compared with the fasting state. Moreover, certain antispasmodic drugs have a more pronounced beneficial effect in some patients than in others. In each person the method of trial and error must be used to determine which of the various drugs available is the most helpful. It is unusual, however, that adequate relief from symptoms is not obtained by a combination of diet, antispasmodics, and postprandial recumbency. Antiserotonin drugs have been prescribed with various degrees of success.

Fourth, patients with a chronically low blood volume have been assisted by transfusion,[51] but this recourse introduces the hazards of homologous blood and is now rarely used.

Fifth, psychotherapy may be helpful in some patients, and hypnosis has been reported to afford relief in certain patients with severe symptoms.[59, 100]

Fortunately, the symptoms tend to diminish with time, and the patient becomes better able to tolerate them as well.

SURGICAL PROCEDURES FOR RELIEF OF THE DUMPING SYNDROME. Conversion of a Billroth II anastomosis to a Billroth I anastomosis was effected by Perman[84] to ameliorate the symptomatic and the nutritional disturbances associated with the dumping syndrome. Most workers feel that the size of the remaining gastric pouch is the important factor in reducing the incidence and severity of dumping; the larger the portion of the stomach remaining, the less severe will be the dumping symptoms and other untoward circumstances that produce malnutrition following gastric resection. Others have interposed a jejunal segment between the gastric remnant and the duodenum, or constructed a jejunal pouch to enlarge the gastric reservoir. One alternative[39, 49, 50] is shown in Figure 19–16.

Alkaline Reflux Gastritis

The condition termed postoperative alkaline reflux gastritis or bile gastritis[2, 8, 38, 97, 106] has been regularly diagnosed only since the advent of the flexible gastroscope.[104] Before that time it was probably confused with proximal loop problems. The precise incidence is still debatable, for indeed most patients with a distal subtotal gastrectomy and a Billroth II gastrojejunal anastomosis will often exhibit bile in the stomach. In fact, some authors[132] doubt that bile per se is in fact the cause of the gastritis, and still other questions remain.

The clinical picture is that of burning epigastric pain coming on weeks or even years after the gastrectomy. The pain is often aggravated by food intake. Vomiting of bile-stained material is frequent but does not bring relief of pain. Bleeding and anemia are common findings. Weight loss averaging 10 kg. occurred in two-thirds of Sawyers' patients.[104]

The diagnosis is documented by gastroscopy and biopsy of the gastric mucosa. The endoscopic findings are laking or pooling of bile, with a diffuse superficial gastritis that may involve the entire gastric remnant.

Treatment consists of symptomatic medical therapy, although antacids, cimetidine, anticholinergic drugs, and cholestyramine have generally been ineffective. Current surgical treatment consists of the construction of a Roux-en-Y loop to the gastric pouch, so that the alkaline bile and pancreatic juice enter the jejunum about 45 cm. distal to the gastric pouch. In these patients a vagotomy should be performed to protect against anastomotic or pouch ulceration. Herrington, Sawyers, and Whitehead[40] had a 90 per cent success rate with this procedure in patients with chronic alkaline reflux gastritis.

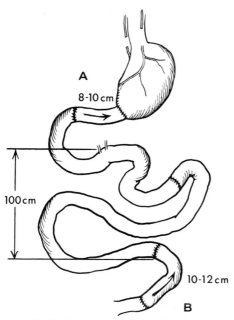

Figure 19–16 The interposition of a reversed jejunal loop (A) between the stomach and the duodenum has been employed in the management of the postgastrectomy dumping syndrome. A similar reversed loop placed 100 cm. distal to the ligament of Treitz (B) has been used in the control of postvagotomy diarrhea. (From Herrington, J. L., and Sawyers, J. L.: A new operation for the dumping syndrome and post-vagotomy diarrhea. *Ann. Surg.*, 175:790, 1972.)

Full-Stomach Discomfort, Bezoar, Dysphagia, and Chronic Diarrhea

Certain patients complain of discomfort in the epigastrium following meals. This is not necessarily combined with the other symptoms usually associated with the dumping syndrome, and it would appear that this "full-stomach discomfort" is actually due to overdistention of the small remaining gastric pouch. These persons usually obtain relief when they follow instructions to take six to eight small feedings daily rather than to consume the customary three meals a day.

Very occasionally, bezoars may form in the stomach of a patient after gastrectomy or vagotomy. These phytobezoars, consisting of undigested food particles, can usually be broken up and removed, or they can be made to progress down the alimentary tract by using a large tube with repeated gastric lavage, turning the patient in different positions, and perhaps instilling the enzyme cellulase.[135] Less often, food bezoars may obstruct the small intestine. Rarely, operation may be required for removal of the bezoar.

At times a patient complains of postoperative dysphagia. This may be due to esophagitis with associated esophagospasm. Hiatal hernia has been described following vagotomy or partial gastric resection, and if present, such symptoms may of course be due to the herniation itself.

Chronic diarrhea, or at least loose stools, may be observed in patients who have had an extensive gastric resection or in those who have undergone vagotomy-pyloroplasty. Mention is again made of a patient whose dumping symptoms of abdominal cramps and sweating subsided, only to be replaced by an intractable diarrhea that occurred shortly after each meal. Apparently the food had previously remained in the jejunum long enough to produce distention and depletion of the extracellular fluid volume, whereas later it simply passed through the intestinal tract so rapidly that there was insufficient time for its increased osmolar effect to draw in fluid and produce the usual dumping symptoms. These loose stools or frank diarrhea can prove exceedingly refractory to all forms of non-operative management. Under these circumstances, the construction of a jejunal loop, as shown in Figure 19–16, has proven helpful in some patients.

Chronic Weight Loss

Most patients lose some weight after an extensive gastric resection. The obese patient may become one of average habitus, the patient of average obesity may become lean, and the lean patient may become even emaciated (Fig. 19–17). For this reason the gastric resection should be less extensive in the thin person than in the obese one if excessive loss of body weight is to be avoided. For example, instead of doing an extensive gastric resection in the already thin patient, one might elect to do hemigastrectomy and vagotomy or vagotomy with pyloroplasty or gastrojejunostomy. Again, there is a rather general trend toward the performance of hemigastrectomy and vagotomy, or especially vagotomy-pyloroplasty, for the surgical management of the peptic ulcer diathesis, to reduce mortality and postoperative nutritional morbidity.

The weight loss following gastric resection, or the inability to regain weight by the person who had become thin postopera-

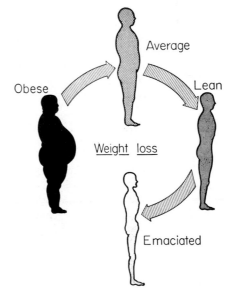

Figure 19–17 *Most patients lose weight after gastric resection. The obese subject may become average size; the average, lean, and the lean, emaciated. Therefore it is wise to avoid an extensive resection for a benign lesion in the lean subject.*

tively, is due to several factors.[4,14,27-30,44,46,64,71,88,109,122,123] First, and often the most important, the patient may ingest less food because food induces unpleasant symptoms. Second, the food may pass through the alimentary canal so rapidly that normal digestion and absorption cannot occur. Third, and perhaps more important than rapid transit, an impairment of fat digestion has been demonstrated by numerous workers. This impairment appears to be somewhat less after the Billroth I operation, which enables the food to pass through the duodenum, than after the Billroth II operation— the measurements being based upon the amount of fat excreted in the stools on a standard diet. The vagotomy-pyloroplasty operation compares favorably with the Billroth I in this respect.

In a study by MacLean and others[64] on the cause of weight loss following subtotal gastrectomy, these findings were noted: (1) Excessive loss of fat in the stools occurred in a number of patients. (2) Excessive stool nitrogen loss was infrequent after subtotal gastrectomy. (3) Thirty-two of 35 patients who were studied had lost weight, the average loss being 20 pounds. (4) Large weight losses were recorded in some patients even when fat and nitrogen excretion in the stool was normal, and such weight losses were found to be closely related to a decreased total food intake despite ingestion of many meals a day. MacLean et al. did not feel that the large weight losses were often closely related to rapid small bowel transit time or to diarrhea. (5) Interestingly, gastroduodenal continuity did not prevent excessive fat loss in the stool. Pancreatic function, as assessed by the secretin test, was found to be normal in most patients after subtotal gastric resection. The possibility was considered that rapid small bowel transit of ingested food separated the food and the enzymes in the presence of normal pancreatic functions. (It will be recalled that a pooling of bile and pancreatic juice in the proximal loop may result in a spruelike syndrome owing to the fact that inadequate amounts of digestive enzymes overtake the food as it progresses down the intestinal tract.) Steatorrhea is present in some degree in many or most patients who have had a total gastrectomy.

Thus, of the factors assessed to explain the weight loss in 35 patients studied after subtotal gastrectomy, MacLean and his associates considered that either a decreased oral intake or a loss of gastric reservoir capacity was of much significance. Some patients admit that they eat less to avoid the relatively mild but nevertheless annoying postgastrectomy symptoms precipitated by food intake. Increased fecal fat excretion was an additional cause of weight loss in some patients. Ellison[27] suggested the use of oral fat preparations to increase the caloric intake in selected patients after partial gastrectomy.

Anemia and Hypoproteinemia

It is not the purpose here to discuss in detail the profound nutritional alterations that may follow a radical subtotal or total gastrectomy. Suffice it to say that great difficulty may be encountered in maintaining even reasonably adequate nutrition in such a patient. For example, iron metabolism is abnormal.[63,118] This is a strong argument against the use of near-total gastrectomy for benign disease and, in fact, for many malignant tumors of the stomach. Weight loss, various avitaminoses, and anemia are encountered. In a study of 27 patients over a decade, Paulson and Harvey[81] found that the following evolutionary sequences occurred: First, an iron deficiency anemia resulted shortly after operation, caused by blood loss from ulcerated areas at the anastomotic site. This was corrected by administration of ferrous salts orally. Next, a macrocytosis of red blood cells occurred within 1 to 2 years after operation; if the patient lived long enough thereafter, this was invariably followed by anemia and, still later, by the development of megaloblasts in the bone marrow. This type of anemia responded to parenteral vitamin B_{12} therapy. A diminished total amount of food was ingested, owing to the reduced pouch capacity.

Bradley and Isaacs[9] consider postresectional anemia to be a preventable complication of total gastrectomy. In their view it is primarily nutritional in origin, although multiple nutritional factors may be involved. During a follow-up period of 32 months, anemia developed in 7 of 10 patients despite parenteral cyanocobalamin. Iron deficiency may also be important.

The nutritional disability of patients having total gastrectomy may be reduced by the construction of a pouch or reservoir from a loop of jejunum. This pouch is interposed between the esophagus and the continuing jejunum below.

Gastroileostomy (Inadvertent)

Gastroileostomy (Fig. 19–18) instead of gastrojejunostomy is occasionally performed inadvertently.[5, 10, 19, 57, 72, 76, 113] This technical error should be suspected when the patient has loose stools in the first few days after operation. Weight loss may occur, and in fact the symptoms may be similar to those present with a gastrocolic fistula, at least to a degree. In reviewing this problem Marshall and O'Donnell[66] found in 6 of 7 patients that there was a complaint of swelling of the abdomen, rumbling, and belching. Three patients stated that the abdomen was visibly distended. The two classic symptoms of diarrhea and weight loss were frequently but not invariably present. It was noted that when diarrhea was present, it had usually begun immediately after the first operation. Three patients had noted that their feces were frothy, contained much gas, and were light tan. The other common feature, weight loss, was particularly noticeable in the patients who had had a subtotal gastrectomy in addition to gastroenterostomy. One patient had lost 50 pounds in 3 years. Actually, however, it was surprising that more of the patients had not lost more weight. Yet it should be recalled that a large

portion of the small bowel can be sacrificed and the patient still manage to maintain a reasonably adequate nutritional status thereafter.

DIAGNOSIS AND MANAGEMENT

The presence of a gastroileal anastomosis is easily demonstrated by means of a gastrointestinal series and barium enema. It is readily corrected by reoperation and formation of a gastrojejunostomy instead of the existing gastroileostomy. It is avoided, of course, by careful identification of the ligament of Treitz at the time of anticipated gastrojejunostomy.

COMPLICATIONS OF TOTAL GASTRECTOMY AND ESOPHAGOGASTRECTOMY

The nutritional complications of these operations have already been touched upon. However, the most serious and life-threatening complications are those associated with a leak at the anastomosis. Total gastrectomy is now most often performed for the Zollinger-Ellison syndrome, usually with a defunctionalized Roux-en-Y loop of jejunum anastomosed to the esophagus. Esophagoenteric or esophagogastric anastomosis always entails some risk of postoperative leakage, which can cause morbidity and not infrequently mortality. Such leakage episodes are minimized by careful operative technique and by maximal preservation of blood supply. If leakage occurs, effective operative drainage, broad spectrum antibiotics, judicious nasogastric tube suction, and prolonged intravenous hyperalimentation will often salvage the situation. Of course, at operation total gastrectomy entails the same risks to surrounding organs as subtotal gastrectomy.

One other serious complication of esophagogastrectomy is postoperative reflux of gastric juice into the esophagus. We recommend simultaneous pyloroplasty, but reflux can produce severe esophagitis and even perforation into the aorta. The reflux of gastric or jejunal contents into the esophagus, especially during sleep, can produce aspiration pneumonitis and respiratory insufficiency.[119]

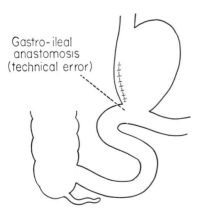

Gastro-ileal
anastomosis
(technical error)

Figure 19–18 A serious but relatively rare technical error is inadvertent anastomosis of the stomach to the terminal ileum.

A late complication of total gastrectomy or esophagogastrectomy is stricture at the anastomosis.[1] This stricture will usually respond to instrumental dilatations, but operative correction may become necessary.

COMPLICATIONS OF VAGOTOMY, PYLOROPLASTY, AND GASTROSTOMY

The widespread use of vagotomy-pyloroplasty requires brief comment upon certain of the complications occasionally met with these operations.[18, 42] These have been reviewed by Santos et al.[103] The principal transoperative complications associated with vagotomy are incomplete division of the vagus nerve trunks at the diaphragm, injury to the spleen or liver, and such disruption of the esophageal hiatus that an esophageal hiatal hernia may develop postoperatively. Since the two vagus nerves may have given off other gastric branches before reaching the diaphragm, not only should the left (anterior) and right (posterior) trunks be divided, but also a careful search for additional branches should be made. Postvagotomy gastric atony and stasis can present a perplexing problem. McClelland and Horton[70] found metoclopramide helpful, in a dosage of 10 mg. 30 minutes before meals. However, Sheiner and Catchpole[108] found bethanechol chloride more successful than metoclopramide in initiating gastric peristalsis. Of course, a mechanical cause of poor gastric emptying must be excluded before resorting to drug therapy.

Late effects of vagotomy include an occasional case of postvagotomy diarrhea[21, 77, 120] and possibly an increased tendency toward gallstone formation.[126] Postvagotomy diarrhea can be protracted and disabling, although it usually improves with time. Duncombe et al.[26] found cholestyramine therapy helpful in the course of a double-blind study. It produced a significant improvement in the urgency and consistency of the stool as well as the frequency of the episodic diarrhea. If after several months the diarrhea persists unabated, a reversed jejunal loop may be constructed as shown in Figure 19–16.

The complications of pyloroplasty are obstruction and leakage. The first is avoided by minimal or no inversion of tissue, and the second by a carefully performed closure.

Gastrostomy is usually performed without event, but leakage has caused peritonitis with sufficient frequency to emphasize the need for careful technique and avoidance of the operation when it is not truly indicated. The writer prefers a simple Stamm gastrostomy, with the stomach surrounding the gastrostomy tube securely sutured to the anterior abdominal wall in the left upper quadrant of the abdomen. The omentum is often wrapped around the gastrostomy site. Feedings are begun on the third or fourth day, though isotonic dextrose or saline solution may be administered as a drip on the first postoperative day.

Bibliography

1. Alexander-Williams, J.: Common problems of gastrectomy and vagotomy. Practitioner 216:649, 1976.
2. Anderson, H. N.: Postoperative alkaline reflux gastritis and esophagitis. Am. Surg. 43:670, 1977.
3. Avola, F. A., and Ellis, D. S.: Leakage of the duodenal or antral stump complicating gastric resection. Surg. Gynecol. Obstet., 99:359, 1954.
4. Babb, L. I., et al.: Evaluation of protein and fat metabolism in postgastrectomy patients. Arch. Surg., 67:462, 1953.
5. Barritt, D. W.: Secondary steatorrhea following gastro-ileal anastomosis. Lancet 2:564, 1952.
6. Becker, H. D.: Disorders of gastrointestinal hormones after surgery. Acta Hepatogastroenterol. 26:516, 1979.
7. Berkas, E. M., and Ferguson, D. J.: Small-bowel obstruction after gastrectomy. Arch. Surg., 76:322, 1958.
8. Boren, C. H., and Way, L. W.: Alkaline reflux gastritis: A reevaluation. Am. J. Surg. 140:40, 1980.
9. Bradley, E. L., III, and Isaacs, J.: Postresectional anemia. A preventable complication of total gastrectomy. Arch. Surg. 111:844, 1976.
10. Brown, C. H., Colvert, J. R., and Brush, B. E.: Gastro-ileostomy, a rare surgical error: Symptoms and x-ray findings. Gastroenterology, 8:71, 1947.
11. Brown, J. R., and Derr, J. W.: Arterial blood supply of human stomach. Arch. Surg. 64:616, 1952.
12. Burnett, W. E., et al.: Studies on so-called postgastrectomy pancreatitis. Ann. Surg. 149:737, 1959.
13. Burton, C. C., Eckman, W. G., Jr., and Haxo, J.: Acute postgastrectomy pancreatitis. Am. J. Surg. 94:70, 1957.
14. Butler, T. J., Capper, W. M., and Naish, J. M.: Ileo-jejunal insufficiency following different types of gastrectomy. Gastroenterologia 81:104, 1954.
15. Cannon, J. A., and Weeks, W. H.: Complications

of the internal hernial ring routinely left unclosed in gastroenterostomy: Report of two cases and method of prevention. Ann. Surg. *138*:772, 1953.

16. Capper, W. M., and Welbourn, R. B.: Early postcibal symptoms following gastrectomy: Aetiological factors, treatment and prevention. Brit. J. Surg. *43*:24, 1955.

17. Carpenter, J. C., and Crandell, W. B.: Common bile duct and major pancreatic duct injuries during operations on the stomach: A report of three cases. Ann. Surg. *148*:66, 1958.

18. Carter, S. L.: Resolution of postvagotomy dysphagia. J.A.M.A. *240*:2656, 1978.

19. Castleton, K. B., and Bailey, F. B.: Syndrome following gastroileostomy. Am. J. Surg. *79*:736, 1950.

20. Cate, W. R., Jr., and Dawson, R. E.: The viability of proximal gastric remnants following radical subtotal gastrectomy and gastroduodenostomy: Experimental study. Surgery *41*:401, 1957.

21. Cerda, J. J., et al.: Postvagotomy diarrhea. Major Probl. Clin. Surg., *20*:144, 1976.

22. Cohen, E. B.: Infarction of the stomach: Report of three cases of total gastric infarction and one case of partial infarction. Am. J. Med. *11*:645, 1951.

23. Dawson-Edwards, P., and Morrissey, D. M.: Acute enterocolitis following partial gastrectomy. Brit. J. Surg. *42*:643, 1955.

24. Dixon, C. F., and Weismann, R. E.: Acute pseudomembranous enteritis or enterocolitis: A complication following intestinal surgery. Surg. Clin. North Am. *28*:999, 1948.

25. Dumping syndrome. (Editorial) J.A.M.A. *168*:1229, 1958.

26. Duncombe, V. M., Bolin, T. D., and Davis, A. E.: Double-blind trial of cholestyramine in postvagotomy diarrhoea. Gut *18*:531, 1977.

27. Ellison, E. H.: Nutritional problems following gastric resection: Fat and protein absorption. Surg. Clin. North Am. *35*:1683, 1955.

28. Everson, T. C.: Experimental comparison of protein and fat assimilation after Billroth II, Billroth I, and segmental types of subtotal gastrectomy. Surgery *36*:525, 1954.

29. Everson, T. C.: Nutrition following total gastrectomy, with particular reference to fat and protein assimilation. Internat. Abstr. Surg., Surg. Gynecol. Obstet. *95*:209, 1952.

30. Farris, J. M., Ransom, H. K., and Collier, F. A.: Total gastrectomy: Effects upon nutrition and hematopoiesis. Surgery *13*:823, 1943.

31. Fell, S. C., Seidenberg, B., and Hurwitt, E. S.: Ischemic necrosis of the gastric remnant: An uncommon complication of radical subtotal gastrectomy. Surgery *43*:490, 1958.

32. Finney, J. R. M.: Gastro-enterostomy for cicatrizing ulcer of the pylorus. Bull. Johns Hopkins Hosp. *4*:53, 1893.

33. Fisher, J. A., Taylor, W., and Cannon, J. A.: The dumping syndrome: Correlations between its experimental production and clinical incidence. Surg. Gynecol. Obstet. *100*:559, 1955.

34. Glenn, F.: Secondary operations for peptic ulcer. Ann. Surg. *132*:702, 1950.

35. **Golden**, R.: Functional obstruction of efferent loop of jejunum following partial gastrectomy. J.A.M.A., *148*:721, 1952.

36. Harkins, H. N.: Discussion of P. P. Jackson: Ischemic necrosis of the proximal gastric remnant following subtotal gastrectomy. Ann. Surg. *150*:1074, 1959.

37. Hayes, M. A.: The dietary control of the postgastrectomy "dumping syndrome." Surgery *37*:785, 1955.

38. Henderson, R. D.: Gastroesophageal reflux following gastric operation. Ann. Thorac. Surg. *26*:563, 1978.

39. Herrington, J. L., and Sawyers, J. L.: A new operation for the dumping syndrome and postvagotomy diarrhea. Ann. Surg. *175*:790, 1972.

40. Herrington, J. L., Jr., Sawyers, J. L., and Whitehead, W. A.: Surgical management of reflux gastritis. Ann. Surg. *180*:526, 1974.

41. Hinshaw, D. B., Joergenson, E. J., Davis, H. A., and Stafford, C. E.: Peripheral blood flow and blood volume studies in the dumping syndrome. Arch. Surg. *74*:686, 1957.

42. Hocking, M. A., and Barth, C. E.: Chylous ascites: A complication of vagotomy. J. R. Coll. Surg. Edinb. *23*:232, 1978.

43. Irons, H. S., Jr., and Lipin, R. J.: Jejuno-gastric intussusception following gastro-enterostomy and vagotomy. Ann. Surg. *141*:541, 1955.

44. Ivy, A. C.: The effects of gastrectomy in animals. Am. J. Dig. Dis. *7*:500, 1940.

45. Jackson, P. P.: Ischemic necrosis of the proximal gastric remnant following subtotal gastrectomy. Ann. Surg. *150*:1071, 1959.

46. Javid, H.: Nutrition in gastric surgery, with particular reference to nitrogen and fat assimilation. Surgery *38*:641, 1955.

47. Jordan, G. L., Jr.: The afferent loop syndrome. Surgery *38*:1027, 1955.

48. Jordan, G. L., Jr.: Treatment of the dumping syndrome. J.A.M.A. *167*:1062, 1958.

49. Jordan, G. L., Jr.: Surgical management of postgastrectomy problems. Arch. Surg. *102*:251, 1971.

50. Jordan, G. L., Jr., Angel, R. T., McIlharey, J. S., Jr., and Willms, R. K.: Treatment of the postgastrectomy dumping syndrome with a reversed jejunal segment interposed between the gastric remnant and the jejunum. Am. J. Surg. *106*:451, 1963.

51. Jordan, G. L., Jr., Overstreet, J. W., and Peddie, G. H.: The use of blood transfusions in the treatment of the postgastrectomy syndrome. Surgery *42*:1055, 1957.

52. Jordan, G. L., Jr., Overton, R. C., and DeBakey, M. E.: The postgastrectomy syndrome: Studies on pathogenesis. Ann. Surg. *145*:471, 1957.

53. Kiefer, E. D.: Progressive dietary care after gastric surgery. Surg. Clin. North Am. *37*:671, 1957.

54. Kilgore, T. L., Turner, M. D., and Hardy, J. D.: Clinical and experimental ischemia of the gastric remnant. Surg. Gynecol. Obstet. *118*:1312, 1964.

55. Krieger, H., Abbott, W. E., Bradshaw, J. S., and Levey, S.: Correlative study of postgastrectomized patients. Arch. Surg. *79*:333, 1959.

56. Lahey, F. H.: The use of an identifying "T" tube in the common bile duct in gastric resection for duodenal ulcer adherent to the bile ducts. Surg. Gynecol. Obstet. 80:197, 1945.

57. Landry, R. M.: Gastroileostomy and gastrocolostomy: Report of three cases. Surgery 30:528, 1951.

58. Larsen, B. B., and Foreman, R. C.: Syndrome of the leaking duodenal stump. Arch. Surg. 63:480, 1951.

59. Leonard, A. S., Papermaster, A. A., and Wangensteen, O. H.: Treatment of postgastrectomy dumping syndrome by hypnotic suggestion: Preliminary report. J.A.M.A. 165:1957, 1957.

60. Longmire, W. P., Jr., and Wallner, M. A.: Pancreatitis occurring in heterotopic pancreatic tissue. Surgery 40:412, 1956.

61. Lorber, S. H., and Shay, H.: Afferent loop studies after subtotal gastric resection. Am. J. Med. Sci. 222:544, 1951.

62. Machella, T. E.: The mechanism of the postgastrectomy "dumping" syndrome. Ann. Surg. 130:145, 1949.

63. MacLean, L. D.: Megaloblastic anemia following total and subtotal gastrectomy. Surg. Gynecol. Obstet. 106:415, 1958.

64. MacLean, L. D., et al.: Nutrition following subtotal gastrectomy of four types (Billroth I and II, segmental, and tubular resections). Surgery 35:705, 1954.

65. Mahaffey, J. H., and Howard, J. M.: The incidence of postoperative pancreatitis: Study of one hundred thirty-one surgical patients, utilizing the serum amylase concentration. Arch. Surg. 70:348, 1955.

66. Marshall, S. F., and O'Donnell, B.: Gastroileostomy — A preventable surgical error. Surg. Clin. North Am. 37:665, 1957.

67. Marshall, S. F., and Reinstine, H. W., Jr.: An analysis of mortality following gastric surgery. Surg. Clin. North Am. 37:637, 1957.

68. Marshall, S. F., and Terrell, G. K.: Postoperative recurrent ulcer. Surg. Clin. North Am. 37:653, 1957.

69. Martin, J. D., Jr., Grady, E. D., and McGarity, W. C.: Complications of partial gastrectomy for peptic ulcer. Am. Surg. 19:593, 1953.

70. McClelland, R. N., and Horton, J. W.: Relief of acute, persistent postvagotomy atony by metoclopramide. Ann. Surg. 188:439, 1978.

71. McCorkle, H. J., and Harper, H. A.: The problem of nutrition following complete gastrectomy. Ann. Surg. 140:467, 1954.

72. McKenzie, A. D., and Robertson, H. R.: Gastroileostomy. Ann. Surg. 138:911, 1953.

73. McMaster, P., and Wijetunge, D. B.: Postgastrectomy afferent loop obstruction due to efferent loop herniation simulating acute pancreatitis. Br. J. Surg. 63:526, 1976.

74. Millbourn, E.: On acute pancreatic affections following gastric resection for ulcer or cancer, and the possibilities of avoiding them. Acta Chir. Scand. 98:1, 1949.

75. Moore, H. G., Schlosser, R. J., Stevenson, J. K., Harkins, H. N., and Olson, H. H.: Clinical analysis of Billroth I and Billroth II subtotal gastric resection. Arch. Surg. 67:4, 1953.

76. Moretz, W. H.: Inadvertent gastro-ileostomy. Ann. Surg. 130:124, 1949.

77. Morris, S. J., and Rogers, A. I.: Diarrhea after gastrectomy and vagotomy. Postgrad. Med. 65:219, 225, 1979.

78. Muller, J. N.: Les complications de la gastrectomie dans la période post-opératoire immédiate. Presse Méd. 64:403, 1956.

79. Nicolaysen, K., and Fretheim, B.: Partial gastrectomy for ulcer and postoperative complications. Surgery 30:597, 1951.

80. Pallette, E. C., and Harrington, R. W.: Long-term results in surgical treatment of peptic ulcer. J.A.M.A. 168:20, 1958.

81. Paulson, M., and Harvey, J. C.: Hematological alterations after total gastrectomy: Evolutionary sequences over a decade. J.A.M.A. 156:1556, 1954.

82. Pearce, C. W., Jordan, G. L., Jr., and De Bakey, M. E.: Intra-abdominal complications following distal subtotal gastrectomy for benign gastroduodenal ulceration. Surgery 42:447, 1957.

83. Peddie, G. H., Jordan, G. L., Jr., and De Bakey, M. E.: Further studies on the pathogenesis of the postgastrectomy syndrome. Ann. Surg. 146:892, 1957.

84. Perman, E.: The so-called dumping syndrome after gastrectomy. Acta Med. Scand. (Suppl. 196) 128:361, 1947.

85. Petersen, W.: Ueber Darmverschlingung nach der Gastro-Enterostomie. Arch f. klin. Chir. 62:94, 1900. (Cited by J. A. Cannon and W. H. Weeks: Ann Surg. 138:772, 1953.)

86. Phillips, R. B., and Childs, W. A.: Postgastrectomy hemorrhage. Am. J. Surg. 95:411, 1958.

87. Pitman, A. C., and Robinson, F. W.: Dumping syndrome — control by diet. J. Am. Diet. Assoc. 34:596, 1958.

88. Polak, M., and Pontes, J. F.: The cause of postgastrectomy steatorrhea. Gastroenterology 30:489, 1956.

89. Pontes, J. F., and Neves, D. P.: Adrenal stimulation in the dumping syndrome. Gastroenterology 23:431, 1953.

90. Priestley, J. T.: Pancreatitis. Surg. Clin. North Am. 37:953, 1957.

91. Priestley, J. T., and Gibson, R. H.: Gastrojejunal ulcer. Clinical features and late results. Arch. Surg. 56:625, 1948.

92. Ransom, H. K.: Treatment of jejunal ulcer, comparative follow-up study. Arch. Surg. 58:684, 1949.

93. Rauch, R. F., and Bieter, R. N.: The treatment of postprandial distress following gastric resection. Gastroenterology 23:347, 1953.

94. Reid, L. C., Paulette, R. E., Challis, T. W., and Hinton, J. W.: The mechanism of the pathogenesis of pancreatic necrosis and the therapeutic effect of propylthiouracil. Surgery 43:538, 1958.

95. Rienhoff, W. F., Jr.: Analysis of results of surgical treatment of 260 consecutive cases of chronic peptic ulcer of the duodenum. Ann. Surg. 121:583, 1945.

96. Robb, H. J., and Nickel, W. O.: Surgery in postgastrectomy bleeding. Surgery 42:474, 1957.

of the gastrointestinal tract may help in differential diagnosis, but laparotomy may be required in some patients for accurate diagnosis.

NEGATIVE X-RAY FINDINGS

The diagnosis of intestinal obstruction can be made in about 90 per cent of cases from roentgenographic examination alone. In a small percentage of cases characteristic x-ray findings are absent when intestinal obstruction exists.[23] When obstructed loops of bowel are filled with fluid and very little gas, the usual roentgenographic changes do not appear. This set of circumstances accounts for negative x-ray findings when obvious obstruction is observed clinically. A realization of this possibility will obviate undue delay in the diagnosis and institution of appropriate management of obstruction.

UNDIAGNOSED STRANGULATION

The preoperative detection of compromised intestinal circulation remains a challenge to those interested in the management of patients with obstruction. The problem lies chiefly in detecting this change early in its course, before irreversible damage has occurred in the bowel. At this time, surgical correction of the obstructing mechanism will avoid the necessity for bowel resection and the hazards of prolonged peritoneal exposure to gangrenous bowel. Findings that strongly suggest strangulation obstruction include the presence of continuous, severe abdominal pain, a palpable abdominal mass, or hypotension that does not respond to intravenous fluid therapy. The presence of fever above 100° F., a pulse rate over 100 per minute, or a leucocyte count above 10,000 per cubic millimeter is found more commonly in patients with strangulation obstruction than in those with "simple" intestinal obstruction.[24, 38] One or more of the findings described above is almost invariably present when established strangulation has occurred.[41] Unfortunately, developing strangulation may be associated with remarkably few findings, especially in the elderly patient. There is, at present, no completely reliable non-operative method

for distinguishing evolving strangulation from "simple" intestinal obstruction. This fact, combined with the observation that delay in diagnosis of strangulated intestine is associated with a significantly increased morbidity rate, indicates that, with rare exceptions, non-operative intestinal decompression should not be relied upon as definitive management of intestinal obstruction. Most patients with complete small intestinal obstruction should undergo early surgical correction.[6, 31, 38]

BOWEL PERFORATION FROM PRESSURE NECROSIS

Adhesions that are responsible for intestinal obstruction may assume many different forms, varying from thin, filmy structures as seen in peritonitis to tough fibrous bands. When the obstructing mechanism consists of the latter type of adhesions, considerable pressure is exerted against a small area of the bowel wall. This interferes with the circulation of the intestinal wall and may lead to necrosis. If operation is performed at this stage, resection of the altered bowel will be necessary. In more advanced cases frank perforation of the intestine will result. Leakage of stagnant content from the obstructed bowel into the peritoneal cavity constitutes a grave and often fatal complication. In spite of immediate operation, irrigation of the peritoneal cavity, and liberal antibiotic administration, these patients may fail to recover. Chiefly responsible for this avoidable complication is undue prolongation of the non-operative treatment of intestinal obstruction. This has come about largely since the introduction of intubation as a definitive method for the management of obstruction. Successful management of bowel perforation from pressure necrosis lies in its prevention rather than in its treatment. Institution of operation before the lapse of long periods of time is the logical prophylactic measure.[5]

COMPROMISE OF BOWEL VIABILITY FROM DISTENTION

The accumulation of solid material, liquids, and especially gas proximal to the site of intestinal obstruction results in gradual and progressive increases in intraluminal bowel pressure. The small arteries and veins that supply the wall of the gut are exposed to this rising pressure, and increasing degrees of circulatory impairment result. Eventually, because of lower pressure, the veins become occluded, while the arteries continue to admit blood. This circulatory congestion proceeds to anoxia and necrosis of the intestinal wall. The close proximity of the duodenal vessels to the mucosal surface renders this segment of bowel even more susceptible to these changes. It is reasonable to conclude, therefore, that intestinal distention must not be allowed to persist or progress indefinitely when obstruction exists. Relief may be obtained through the introduction of a long tube into the gastrointestinal tract.

FAILURE TO CORRECT WATER AND SALT DEFICITS

Fluid loss, which may attain serious proportions, is a prominent clinical feature of intestinal obstruction (Fig. 20–1). The normal process of water ingestion is not available to compensate for the continuous obligatory losses through the skin, kidneys, and lungs. This is further complicated by profuse vomiting in many cases which represents an important route of loss of gastrointestinal secretions. Sequestration of large quantities of fluid in the distended intestine accounts for another avenue of fluid deprivation. Inadequate fluid replacement therapy usually results in oliguria, a rising hematocrit and blood urea nitrogen content, progressive metabolic acidosis, and hypotension. It has been estimated that when early x-ray signs indicative of obstruction appear, the fluid deficit will be approximately 1500 ml. When the obstruction is well established, and there is a history of vomiting, this value will approach 3000 ml. In advanced obstruction when there is a rapid pulse rate or hypotension, 4000 to 6000 ml. of fluid may be necessary to satisfy the losses.[7] The nature and rate of initial intravenous fluid and electrolyte therapy must be guided not only by estimating the patient's preexisting losses but also by monitoring any continuing losses, especially from gastrointestinal tubes, and by consideration of cardiopulmonary and renal status. The adequacy of intravenous volume replacement should be monitored by frequent measurement of pulse rate, arterial blood pressure, and, in the absence of renal disease, hourly urine output. In most patients,

FLUID LOSSES IN SMALL BOWEL OBSTRUCTION

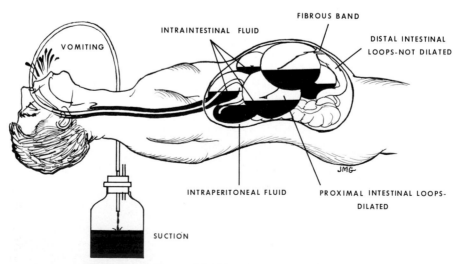

Figure 20–1   Routes of fluid loss during intestinal obstruction.

a central venous catheter should be introduced and central venous pressures monitored. In patients who have significant cardiopulmonary disease or who require rapid infusions of large volumes of fluid, introduction of a Swan-Ganz catheter and measurements of pulmonary arterial wedge pressures increase the safety of fluid volume therapy.

The fluids lost from the body in obstruction of the small intestine are usually approximately isotonic and initial replacement should be by appropriate isotonic sodium solution such as Ringer's lactate. Significant loss of potassium also occurs secondary to vomiting and nasogastric aspiration. Initial serum potassium levels may be normal, but total body potassium is reduced. Potassium should therefore be added to the intravenous infusion as soon as serum potassium levels have been determined and adequate renal function has been established.

In the majority of instances of small bowel obstruction, losses of acid and alkaline ions are approximately equal, so that severe deviations from the normal blood pH are not common. The most frequent acid-base disturbance is a metabolic acidosis related to loss of bicarbonate ions from the bowel, sometimes combined with tissue hypoperfusion. This can be most readily corrected by administration of sodium bicarbonate with close monitoring of mixed venous blood pH and Pco_2. [Arterial blood pH and the carbon dioxide–combining power of plasma may be used instead. Ed.]

OVERCORRECTION OF FLUID AND SALT ABNORMALITIES

Overenthusiastic or inappropriate attempts to correct fluid and electrolyte deficits may result in complications of serious and potentially lethal proportions. Intravenous therapy must, at the very least, replace continuing losses by the patient from the gastrointestinal tract, by urinary output, and by insensible loss. The rate at which preexisting losses should be replaced depends upon their severity, the patient's cardiopulmonary reserve, the adequacy of renal function, and the urgency of possible anesthesia and surgery.

WATER INTOXICATION. This complication is usually the product of infusion of large amounts of glucose in water combined with impaired renal function. These patients usually exhibit a stage of confusion which may be followed by convulsive seizures. Increased intracranial pressure is thought to be responsible for these changes. Restriction of salt-free intravenous infusions and the administration of saline solution promote restoration of normal tonicity to the extracellular fluids, with relief of symptoms.

EXCESS SALT INFUSION. Intravenous infusion of excessive volumes of saline solutions may result in pulmonary insufficiency, weight gain, and peripheral edema. Patients with impaired cardiac or renal function are particularly vulnerable to excessive volume infusions and require close monitoring of central venous or pulmonary arterial pressures. In addition, serial measurements of arterial oxygen tension and periodic chest radiographs may provide early evidence of developing volume overload.

Excessive elevation of serum concentrations of potassium are particularly hazardous because of their effect on the myocardium and the risk of diastolic arrest. This may result from rapid intravenous infusion of potassium chloride before adequate urinary output has been established or by the administration of highly concentrated preparations of this salt. Characteristic electrocardiographic changes, with sharply peaked T-waves, may indicate hyperkalemia. If hyperkalemia occurs, serum potassium must be reduced by the administration of cation exchange resins via retention enemas, by the intravenous administration of glucose and insulin, or by hemo- or peritoneal dialysis. When hyperkalemia is due to impaired kidney function, the treatment is essentially that of renal shutdown.[17]

OVERCORRECTION OF ACID-BASE DEFICITS

The blood pH is maintained close to the normal value of 7.45 largely as a result of the relative concentration of carbonic acid and sodium bicarbonate. The absolute quantities of these substances in the blood are not nearly as important as their relative concentrations. Blood pH values reflect pulmonary and renal function as well as the adequacy of tissue perfusion. In patients with intestinal obstruction, abnormal pH may also result from enteric fluid losses or inappropriate electrolyte therapy. Whatever the cause, variation of blood pH outside the range of 7.35 to 7.50 may be associated with significant cardiac arrhythmias and metabolic impairment. The key to prevention and management of these problems is regular measurement of central venous blood pH and P_{CO_2}.

TUBES

Gastrointestinal suction through nasal tubes has enjoyed widespread usage in the management of small bowel obstruction. In spite of mounting experience and attempts at outlining precautionary measures, the prevalence of complications, some of which assume serious proportions, is becoming more and more apparent.[14]

INABILITY TO INTRODUCE LONG TUBE INTO SMALL BOWEL. The introduction of long intestinal tubes into the upper reaches of the jejunum is a valuable adjunct in the management of small bowel obstruction. Successful introduction of the tube, however, requires considerable attention and effort by nursing and medical staff. Too frequently, a long tube is introduced into the stomach and its further advancement is relegated to chance. Progression of the balloon from the stomach to the duodenum is encouraged by moderate elevation of the head of the bed and turning the patient upon his right side. After a period of 2 to 3 hours, the position of the tube should be determined radiographically. If it has not advanced through the pylorus, an attempt should be made to pass the tip of the tube into the duodenum under fluoroscopic control. Instillation of water or mercury into the balloon facilitates passage from the stomach. In many instances these maneuvers will culminate in successful small bowel intubation. In the presence of advanced distention, however, and especially when there is paralytic ileus, success is often wanting. Those cases that present the greatest need for long tube decompression are often the ones that must be classified as failures. Prolonged attempts at non-operative decompression should not be undertaken.

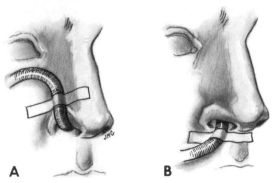

Figure 20–2 *A*, Excessive pressure by the tube on the ala nasi should be avoided. *B*, Satisfactory method for securing the tube.

INJURY TO THE NASOPHARYNGEAL PASSAGES. Improper fixation of the tube to the nostril can result in erosion of the ala nasi if this condition is allowed to persist for extended periods of time. We prefer to maintain the tube in position as shown in Figure 20–2, with overlapping strips of tape applied to the upper lip to avoid continuous pressure against the nasal cartilage. Otitis media in infants and children is an additional troublesome complication. It is seen with greater frequency in the younger age groups, probably because of the less circuitous route pursued by the eustachian tube.

MOUTH-BREATHING. Normal respiration through the nostrils is virtually impossible in the presence of a nasogastric tube. As a result of breathing through the mouth, excessive drying of the mucosa in this area usually occurs. Cracking of the lips which may advance to frank ulceration can occur in neglected cases. Liberal utilization of mouthwashes and gargles is helpful. Frequent application of lubricating materials will effectively minimize complications involving the lips.

LARYNGEAL INJURY. This complication results from pressure necrosis of the upper part of the esophagus opposite its attachment to the cricoid cartilage. A spreading perichondritis of the larynx with edema may progress to complete respiratory obstruction necessitating tracheostomy. Less extensive involvement results in hoarseness or inability to talk above a whisper. Although usually occurring after long periods of intubation, these changes have been observed after intervals as short as 6 days.[14]

ACCIDENTAL INTRODUCTION OF THE TUBE INTO THE TRACHEA. In most instances the cough reflex will effectively warn against inadvertent tracheal intubation. No great harm occurs from this mistake if it is recognized before foreign material is injected into the tube. The error can be avoided by assuming that the tube is in the stomach only after aspiration of obvious gastric content. Additional evidence can be gained by listening with a stethoscope over the stomach while air is injected through the tube. This accident assumes catastrophic proportions usually only in those cases of tube feedings in which huge quantities of foreign material may flood the respiratory passages.

ASPIRATION. Regurgitation and aspiration of gastric contents into the tracheobronchial tree are ever-present hazards. Patients who are elderly or whose neurological function is impaired are particularly at risk. The possibility of massive aspiration in patients with intestinal obstruction may be reduced by maintenance of effective nasogastric decompression and by the introduction of a cuffed endotracheal tube prior to induction of anesthesia. If the occurrence of pulmonary aspiration is recognized, the tracheobronchial tree should be suctioned at once and carefully irrigated with physiologic saline under bronchoscopic control.

INTERFERENCE WITH TRACHEOBRONCHIAL CLEARANCE. Maintenance of a clear airway is distinctly impaired by the presence of a nasogastric tube. Additional effort must be expended by the patient to raise mucus and other foreign material. Increased demands could precipitate impaired efficiency with progressive atelectasis and increasing pulmonary insufficiency. Tracheostomy may be the only effective means by which a clear respiratory passage can be maintained. Pulmonary problems have contributed to the rationale for more widespread use of catheter gastrostomy for postoperative gastrointestinal decompression.

ESOPHAGEAL EROSION AND STRICTURE. Pressure erosion of the lower part of the esophagus is a common complication of prolonged intubation. It probably occurs more frequently than is realized because of spontaneous healing where reversible changes have occurred. Although erosion of the full thickness of the esophageal wall is uncommon, it has been observed in isolated instances. An additional complication is erosion of esophageal varices with bleeding. Esophageal stenosis or complete obstruction may follow healing and contraction of more advanced lesions. Management is then resolved to prolonged dilatations or surgical reconstruction.

LOSS OF FLUIDS AND ELECTROLYTES. The objective of nasogastrointestinal intubation is the reduction of distention by removal of the accumulated gas and fluid. Great benefit can result from prolonged aspiration of gas from the obstructed bowel, since this material serves no useful function. On the other hand, removal of large quantities of liquids over a prolonged period may result in depletion of water and salt stores, with precipitation of dehydration and electrolyte deficits. This material should be measured so that accurate replacement of these elements may be included in the daily fluid and electrolyte quotas. Strict maintenance of no oral intake further reduces the amount of salts that may be washed out of the body.

ACUTE GASTRIC DILATATION. After a long tube has been passed into the lower reaches of the intestinal tract there are instances in which acute gastric dilatation may supervene. This is especially true if an element of paralytic ileus has occurred so that the propulsive power of the gastrointestinal tract is decreased. This course of events necessitates immediate insertion of a Levin tube into the stomach, after which the patient usually experiences immediate relief from upper abdominal discomfort.

OBSTRUCTION OF THE TUBE. The passage of gastric or small bowel contents through nasogastric tubes is usually accomplished without significant difficulty. Occlusion of the tube by either small food particles, mucus, or adjacent bowel mucosa is largely prevented by frequent irrigation with 30 ml. of saline solution. Saline is preferred to distilled water as an irrigation solution because it more effectively promotes conservation of body salts.

At various levels of the gastrointestinal tract, usually in the stomach, tubes may become coiled and subsequently tied in a knot. Further benefit from such a tube is precluded, and a new one must be substituted.

BOWEL PERFORATION. Local bowel wall

ent until frank perforation has occurred, with flooding of the peritoneal cavity by toxic intraluminal material. Earlier utilization of operative treatment should decrease the incidence of this often fatal complication.

GASEOUS DISTENTION OF THE BALLOON. This complication may occur only in those instances in which a closed bag is used, such as those described by Cantor, Kaslow, or Harris. Once the balloon has passed into the intestine, gases tend to migrate into its lumen, with progressive increase in its size. The enlarged balloon may distend the small bowel and precipitate intestinal obstruction. The balloon becomes anchored in the bowel by its distention, and operative removal is frequently needed.[35] Cantor recommends puncture of the mid-portion of the rubber bag with a 21- or 22-gauge needle before passage is attempted. An opening of this size allows accumulated gas to escape without spillage of mercury.

RUPTURE OF THE BAG. This mishap may occur as a result of the use of defective material during manufacture, inadequate

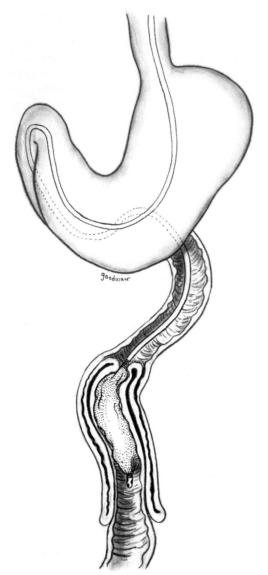

Figure 20–3 Method of creating reverse intussusception during tube removal.

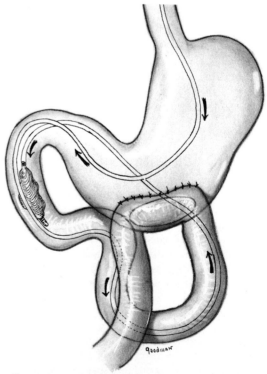

Figure 20–4 Multiple loops through gastroenterostomy complicate tube removal.

changes may occur as a result of continued tamponade from a mercury-filled bag. Eade et al.[12] reported 13 cases of stomach or intestinal perforation as a result of erosion of all layers of the visceral wall. Indirectly, tubes may be responsible for intestinal perforation during unduly prolonged nonoperative treatment of adhesive intestinal obstruction. A false sense of security is gained because of effective decompression of the intestine. The increasing degree of pressure exerted against the bowel wall is not appar-

fixation to the tube, or irrigation of the bag rather than the suction compartment of the tube. When the Miller-Abbott tube is used, the last complication occurs when there is a lack of familiarity with the construction of the tube. It is important to test the tube before it is inserted to make sure that the labels on the metal suction tip have not been reversed. Spillage of mercury into the lumen of the bowel after perforation of the bag is not usually followed by untoward complication.

INABILITY TO REMOVE TUBE. This problem is encountered only in those instances in which long tubes are used. If a Miller-Abbott tube is used, extubation is accomplished in most cases after the balloon has been emptied. If a Cantor tube is used, however, there may be resistance to with-

drawal. Reverse intussusception of the small bowel can occur, as shown in Figure 20–3. Vigorous traction upon nasogastrointestinal tubes must be avoided. When resistance is being encountered, it is much safer to institute further attempts at removal after the lapse of a period of time. Multiple loops through a gastroenterostomy may also complicate tube removal (Fig. 20–4). When prolonged attempts at removal have been unsuccessful, it may be advisable to attempt passage of the tube through the intestinal tract. The posterior pharynx is exposed, and the tube is divided as low as possible. If intestinal obstruction has been relieved, the tube will be passed per rectum in many instances. Operative intervention for removal of the tube may be necessary when all other techniques have failed.

OPERATIVE PERIOD

CONTAMINATION OF PERITONEAL CAVITY

Sepsis is one of the major causes of morbidity and mortality following operations for intestinal obstruction. In the presence of obstruction, gross overgrowth with both aerobic and anaerobic organisms occurs in the small bowel proximal to the obstruction.[42] Opening of the obstructed bowel and spillage of its contents are therefore associated with a marked increase in infectious complications and must be carefully avoided.[41] In addition, preoperative broad spectrum antibiotics should be administered parenterally.[6, 38]

INADVERTENT LACERATION OF THE BOWEL WALL. A sizeable percentage of patients with intestinal obstruction have undergone previous abdominal surgery that has resulted in the firm adherence of small bowel to the anterior abdominal wall, especially in the vicinity of the old scars. The chances for intestinal injury are significantly decreased if the abdominal cavity is entered at a site considerably removed from the area of healed incisions. If a previously healed incision is reused, extension of the incision into a fresh area of abdominal wall and initial peritoneal incision through this extension

often permit entry into the peritoneal cavity in an area that is relatively free of adhesions.

Laceration of the bowel wall may also occur during attempts to release the obstructive agent, as in the division of an adhesion. Avoidance of this technical mishap depends largely upon securing adequate exposure before intra-abdominal structures are divided. Utilization of an abdominal incision of generous proportion is of great importance. A right or left paramedian incision with lateral retraction of the rectus muscle provides good exposure and may be enlarged without irreparable abdominal wall damage.

When intestinal distention is only moderate, the site of obstruction can usually be visualized without great difficulty. When advanced distention exists, it is often advisable to withdraw the greatly enlarged coils of bowel upon the abdominal wall. This maneuver facilitates rapid detection of the site and nature of the obstructing agent. Admittedly, the bowel is subjected to more trauma under these circumstances, but insurance against complications that result from poor exposure as well as shortening of operative time probably outweigh this disadvantage. Gentle manipulation of the bowel along with the application of warm saline packs minimizes the chances of bowel injury.

SPILLAGE OF BOWEL CONTENT DURING ANASTOMOSIS. Open small bowel anastomosis is being performed with increasing frequency after intestinal resection. Greater accuracy in the placement of sutures usually results in a more satisfactory stoma with the use of this method as opposed to the closed technique. The chances for peritoneal contamination are minimized by prior decompression of the proximal intestine and by the placement of packs around the incision as well as the divided ends of the bowel. Leakage from the open bowel may be prevented by application of non-crushing clamps to both the proximal and distal loops 6 to 12 inches from the site of division. Effecting the anastomosis upon the abdominal wall further decreases the chance of peritoneal contamination.

Contamination may be further minimized by creating a limited dirty-field during opening of the bowel and construction of the anastomosis. Instruments used during this period of the operation are confined to this field and are discarded from the operative field together with all contaminated towels and packs after completion of the anastomosis. Gloves should also be changed prior to continuing the operative procedure.

IMPROPER MANAGEMENT OF HERNIA. Contamination of the peritoneal cavity during the operative management of strangulated hernia should never occur if proper precautions are observed. The neck of the hernia sac is usually tightly constricted about the segment of involved bowel, so that leakage of the toxic material into the peritoneal cavity is prevented. The hernia sac should be opened for removal of the material contained therein before the neck of the sac is divided.

DECOMPRESSIVE ENTEROSTOMY. If decompression of the bowel by way of an enterotomy is considered mandatory, this should be carried out in a field isolated by packs and with every precaution to prevent spillage of bowel content. The whole bowel may be decompressed by a catheter introduced through one enterostomy, but advancement of this catheter or of a long tube introduced by the nasogastric route must be careful and gentle. Careless advancement of the tube may result in perforation of the edematous, friable bowel.

MANAGEMENT OF THE CONTAMINATED PERITONEAL CAVITY

The singular introduction of minimal amounts of foreign material into the peritoneal cavity requires little alteration in patient management from that utilized for the uncontaminated case. Generalized peritoneal exposure to normal and abnormal bowel content in large quantities necessitates the use of all therapeutic modalities that hold promise of benefit. Small bowel content incident to intestinal obstruction is usually in a fluid state and may spread extensively over the peritoneal cavity.

Experimental evidence indicates that the longer peritoneal exposure is allowed to exist, the greater is the possibility for irreversible damage. Immediate removal of material can certainly be logically applied to the management of patients. Aspiration with the abdominal suction apparatus should be used as long as success is apparent. Aspiration will certainly remove gross contaminating material, but after this maneuver a layer of the material usually remains over the peritoneal surface. Irrigation of the peritoneal cavity with warm saline solution is beneficial in removal of residual portions of the contaminating material. For the most part, the toxic properties of bowel content are related to the bacterial content of the material. Experimental evidence suggests that intraperitoneal administration of antibiotics may be helpful in the management of the contaminated peritoneum.[4]

FAILURE TO RESECT NON-VIABLE BOWEL

Thorough inspection of the altered bowel is mandatory after the release of intestinal obstruction so that segments showing irreversible changes may be revealed. Particular care must be exerted during the operative management of incarcerated inguinal hernias, since early division of the external oblique fascia that forms the external inguinal ring will allow the bowel to escape into the peritoneal cavity before adequate examination has been made. When this mishap occurs, it is occasionally possible to grasp the questionable segment and withdraw it again through the inguinal opening for observation. This maneuver failing, the operator must make an abdominal incision so that the exact status of the bowel can be established.

The ability of ischemic, traumatized bowel to resume its normal appearance and characteristics is indeed remarkable. After release of the obstructive agent, warm moist packs should be applied to the bowel for at least 10 minutes, after which a decision concerning its viability should be made. Survival of the segment in question is virtually assured if the intestine resumes a pink color, exhibits pulsating vessels in the mesentery, presents a bright glistening surface, shows no evidence of damage to the serosal surface, and demonstrates a capacity to transmit peristaltic waves. On the other hand, the capacity for survival can be seriously challenged when a dark blue or black color persists, the serosal surface is dull and without luster, mesenteric vessels no longer demonstrate pulsation, and there is no evidence of peristalsis.

Unfortunately, the criteria upon which bowel viability is based are not always positive and clear-cut. Inordinately long periods of examination and pondering should be avoided in arriving at a decision concerning the advisability of intestinal resection. If the capacity for survival is still in doubt after 10 to 15 minutes of examination and treatment, then intestinal resection should be performed without further delay. The disastrous consequences that can be expected to follow prolonged peritoneal exposure to gangrenous bowel far outweigh the disadvantages of an intestinal resection performed in the absence of ironclad indications.

UNRELIEVED INTESTINAL DISTENTION

Decompression of distended small bowel has long been recommended in order to improve blood flow to the bowel wall and to hasten the return of peristaltic activity and bowel absorptive capacity.[43] Additional operative trauma to the bowel may, however, increase the period of postoperative ileus and, if enterotomy is required, an additional risk of infection is introduced.[41, 46] The risks and benefits of operative bowel decompression must therefore be weighed in each patient. Relief of proximal intestinal obstruction will usually relieve distention by allowing passage of bowel contents into the distal bowel. When operative decompression of the bowel is required, this may be accomplished by gentle advancement of a tube that was introduced preoperatively into the small intestine by the nasogastric route. When such a tube has not been placed, a Baker tube[3] can usually be introduced either transnasally or by way of a gastrostomy, avoiding the need for enterostomy. If none of these methods is practical, a Baker tube can be introduced through an enterotomy within a purse string suture, with meticulous attention to the avoidance of spillage of bowel contents. The tube may be left in place for postoperative drainage or removed with careful closure of the enterostomy. If the tube is to be left in place, it must be exteriorized through a separate stab incision in the abdominal wall. The bowel wall immediately adjacent to the enterostomy must be carefully sewn to the peritoneum circumferentially around the stab wound.

BOWEL ANASTOMOSIS

After bowel resection, intestinal continuity may be established by either side-to-side or end-to-end anastomosis. Although side-to-side anastomosis may sometimes appear simpler to construct, it can be associated with late complications related to dilatation of the distal portion of the afferent loop and the formation of a blind pouch. With time, this pouch may reach considerable size and give rise to abdominal pain, distention, diarrhea, and anemia. For these reasons, side-to-side anastomosis should be avoided whenever possible. Following small intestinal resection, end-to-end anastomosis is virtually always possible. If very marked discrepancies in bowel lumen are present, end-to-end anastomosis may be facilitated by tailoring the end of the distal bowel using a short incision from its cut end along the antimesenteric border.

INVERT SMALL AMOUNT OF
BOWEL WALL

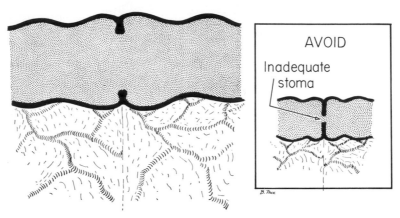

Figure 20–5 Excessive inversion of tissue may cause postoperative obstruction.

DIVIDE INTESTINE AT ANGLE TO INSURE
BLOOD SUPPLY TO ENTIRE BOWEL WALL

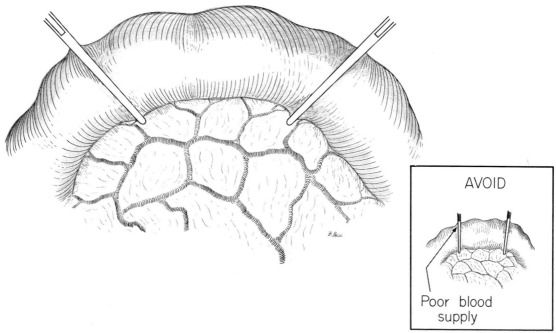

Figure 20–6 Compromise of circulation to the antimesenteric border of the bowel must be avoided.

LEAVE ADEQUATE BLOOD SUPPLY
FROM MESENTERY

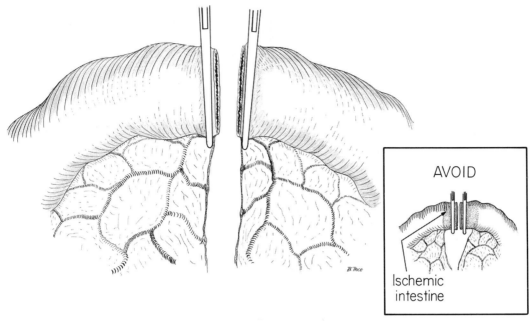

AVOID

Ischemic
intestine

B.Pace

Figure 20–7 Excessive stripping of mesentery from the bowel must be avoided.

We prefer to use the open technique for small bowel anastomosis because of the possibility of undue encroachment upon the lumen, which is probably more likely to occur during the execution of closed methods (Fig. 20–5). In contrast to that of experimental animals such as the dog, human small bowel is not richly endowed with intramural vascular anastomoses. This fact must be remembered during the application of clamps for division of the bowel in preparation for anastomosis. As illustrated in Figure 20–6, the bowel must be divided in an oblique fashion, to eliminate the possibility of infarction of the bowel edges that are to be utilized during the anastomosis. Although it is important that sufficient muscular substance of the bowel wall be available for the placement of sutures in the area of the mesentery, undue "cleaning" of the bowel may impair healing of the anastomosis. Ischemia is certain to result if more than the minimal degree of division and ligation of the mesenteric blood supply is effected (Fig. 20–7). All bleeding vessels should be painstakingly ligated before the anastomosis is begun (Fig. 20–8). Hematoma formation in this area could impair proper healing to the point of leakage at the suture line.

Insurance against anastomotic leakage is also obtained by accurate approximation of the serosa during the placement of the second row of sutures. Under no circumstances should the mucosa be visible in the suture line after completion of the anastomosis (Fig. 20–9). Particular attention must be directed to accurate apposition of the serosal surfaces at the mesenteric angle. Any mesenteric defect must be carefully closed to reduce the risk of postoperative internal herniation. During the construction of the anastomosis, the bowel must be treated with precision and gentleness. Fine suture materials on fine atraumatic needles should be used, and handling of the divided ends of the bowel with forceps should be minimized.

End-to-end anastomosis of distended small intestine frequently involves approximation of two segments of bowel with

CONTROL BLEEDING FROM END OF BOWEL

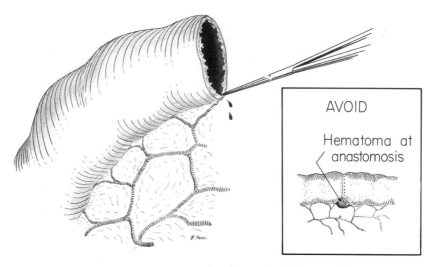

Figure 20–8   Complete hemostasis should be attained.

marked disparity in lumen, requiring appropriate tailoring of the anastomosis. In addition, there is usually considerable edema and thickening of the wall of the proximal intestine. Much of this edema occurs in the subserosal layers and the distance from the serosa to the relatively collagenous submucosa may be 3 to 4 times greater than normal. Therefore, when seromuscular sutures are placed, particular attention must be paid that they are of adequate depth to include the submucosa. Sutures placed to a normal depth in obstructed intestine will frequently include only serosa with edema fluid.

Stapling devices have been used recently in the performance of gastrointestinal anastomoses in some centers. The technique most widely recommended for stapled small bowel anastomosis results in a side-to-side

SEROSA-TO-SEROSA ANASTOMOSIS

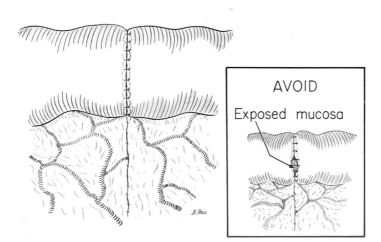

Figure 20–9 Muscosal inversion must be complete.

anastomosis, the ends of the bowel being closed by an everting staple line. The long-term adequacy and relative safety of this technique, in particular with obstructed bowel, have not as yet been established. Recognized complications of staple technique include malfunctioning of the staple equipment, inadequate preparation of the bowel with inclusion of mesentery in the staple line, and inappropriate selection of staple size, resulting either in undue tissue crushing or in poor apposition and excessive bleeding.[13, 44]

POSTOPERATIVE PERIOD

EVISCERATION

For several days, and sometimes longer, after the operative treatment of patients with intestinal obstruction, considerable abdominal distention must be anticipated. During this period severe stress upon the abdominal incision may precipitate wound disruption, with extrusion of the intestine in many instances. This serious complication necessitates immediate return to the operating room for closure of the abdominal wound. This may be accomplished with a large suture (No. 2 nylon) passed through all layers of the abdominal wall.

The incidence of postoperative evisceration can be materially decreased by the routine use of retention sutures in the abdominal wound closure. The presence of these sutures is a source of considerable satisfaction, especially in those instances in which advanced intestinal distention has occurred.

ADYNAMIC ILEUS

Adynamic ileus of a degree commonly follows all abdominal operative procedures. It is particularly likely to occur after surgical relief of bowel obstruction. Rough manipulation of the bowel during the operative procedure is a factor. Advanced stages of intestinal distention resulting from prolonged non-operative treatment of simple obstruction postpone the return of normal bowel activity during the postoperative period. Adynamic ileus also results from inadequate replacement of fluid and potassium deficits. Peritoneal contamination, even of relatively small proportions, usually prolongs and intensifies the period of postoperative adynamic ileus.

Abdominal distention, hypoactive to absent bowel sounds, and obstipation characterize the clinical picture of adynamic ileus. Abdominal tenderness is usually minimal in the absence of peritonitis. In the early postoperative period it is difficult to evaluate the significance of abdominal tenderness. X-ray examination reveals bowel distention along with gas scattered throughout the stomach, small intestine, and colon.

The management of postoperative ileus is simplified if the surgeon has manipulated the bowel with gentleness during release of the obstructing mechanism. This is also true when operative decompression of the dilated bowel has been carried out. Abnormalities of serum potassium, calcium, or magnesium must be corrected. Antibacterial agents must be utilized when peritonitis is a factor. Progression of abdominal distention is prevented by eliminating the oral intake of both solid and liquid materials and maintaining continued nasogastric decompression. This will serve to remove swallowed air, as well as to evacuate such liquids as may be regurgitated into the stomach. The administration of agents designed to stimulate peristalsis, such as neostigmine, has in our experience yielded little benefit during the postoperative management of the patient with obstruction.

RECURRENT OBSTRUCTION

EARLY OBSTRUCTION. The most common cause of early postoperative bowel obstruction is adhesions. Internal hernia such as may occur through a mesenteric defect after bowel anastomosis may account for this complication. Partial separation of the deeper layers of the abdominal wound with entrapment of bowel has also been encountered. Anastomotic obstruction as a result of excessive narrowing of the stoma is a real possibility when one is dealing with the small bowel. Partial volvulus or acute angulation of distended loops of small bowel may also precipitate obstruction. Of chief concern in diagnosis is the differentiation between postoperative bowel obstruction and adynamic ileus. In both conditions there is abdominal distention. The pain that results from obstruction is more likely to be intermittent, colicky, and sharp, whereas adynamic ileus produces continuous abdominal discomfort of less intensity. Bowel sounds are usually loud, indicating intestinal hyperactivity where obstruction exists, whereas they are hypoactive or absent in adynamic ileus. Drainage through the nasogastric tube will be more profuse in obstruction than in adynamic ileus. Films of the abdomen taken with the patient in the erect position reveal air-fluid levels, stepladder appearance of the bowel, and absence of gas in the colon and rectum when small intestinal obstruction exists.

In addition to the elimination of oral intake and the parenteral administration of fluids and electrolytes, nasogastric suction should be instituted. Since obstruction occurring in the first 14 to 30 postoperative days is often related to fibrinous adhesions or angulation of heavy distended bowel, decompression of the intestine by passage of a long tube is frequently successful in providing permanent relief of obstruction. In most patients, therefore, with early, as opposed to late, intestinal obstruction, nonoperative initial therapy by intestinal intubation is justified[32] and may be utilized with considerable expectation of success.

LATE OBSTRUCTION. The abdominal surgeon faces no greater challenge than the patient with obstruction who exhibits multiple abdominal scars and gives a history of numerous previous laparotomies for relief of mechanical ileus. Non-operative attempts at relief through the use of intestinal suction are probably justified for longer periods under these circumstances than is the usual practice. This failing, the only hope for recovery of the patient rests upon the successful execution of laparotomy with lysis of adhesions and complete mobilization of the small bowel. Two maneuvers are available for attempted control of re-formed adhe-

sions in such a manner as not to compromise the lumen of the small bowel. The first is the plication procedure described by Noble[27] in 1939 (Figure 20–10). The essential features of this operation were lysis of all adhesions and suturing adjacent loops of bowel along their mesenteric borders. Angulation of the bowel was minimized by beginning and ending the suture lines 3 centimeters from each turn and the average length of each turn was 6 to 8 inches.[45] Childs and Phillips[10] reported a modified technique for plication of the small bowel (Fig. 20–11). The small bowel is first freed completely from adhesions. The loops are then arranged in segments approximately 8 inches in length. A long straight needle is used to pass a No. 2 silk suture through the mesentery. The suture is tied loosely to prevent bowel obstruction due to kinking or compression. Neither of these operative procedures has gained wide acceptance.

The second procedure involves internal fixation of the bowel with the hope that a semirigid tube will avoid acute angulation of the bowel with preservation of the lumen.[3] The tube may be introduced by either gastrostomy or jejunostomy, gastrostomy being preferred if the patient is operated upon in the obstructed state. Since the tube will remain in place for a prolonged postoperative period, transnasal introduction is not recommended. The Baker tube is advanced until the balloon reaches the cecum. Care is taken

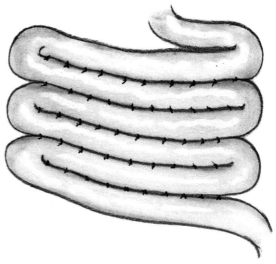

Figure 20–10   Noble plication.

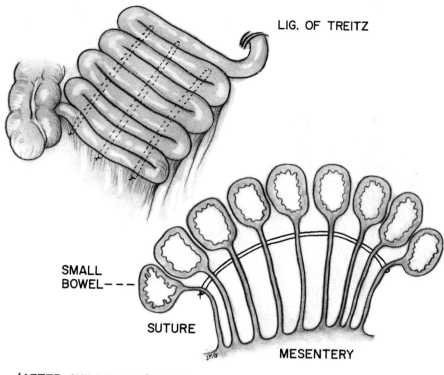

LIG. OF TREITZ

SMALL BOWEL---

SUTURE

MESENTERY

(AFTER CHILDS & PHILLIPS)

Figure 20–11 Method of plication described by Childs and Phillips.

to insure that an adequate length of tube has been introduced so that retraction of the tube into the small bowel will not occur spontaneously. The balloon is then emptied. The tube is left in place for ten days.

Recurrence of small bowel obstruction has been observed to follow the use of both these procedures. We believe that one or the other of these operations should be done when proper indications exist, since the evidence indicates that a significant reduction in recurrence can be expected. Our preference is the splinting procedure with use of a long intraluminal tube.

ANASTOMOTIC DEHISCENCE, PERITONITIS, AND FISTULA

Postoperative extravasation of enteric content with the occurrence of peritonitis or fistula formation is one of the most frequently lethal complications of small intestinal surgery. It may result from anastomotic failure, from unrecognized or inadequately treated injury to the small intestine, or from progression of small intestinal disease.[26, 40] Clearly, meticulous attention to operative technique is of fundamental importance in the prevention of the first two causative categories.

NATURAL HISTORY. Development of a full-thickness defect of the small bowel is often followed by rapid and profuse discharge of enteric content into the peritoneal cavity with resulting generalized peritonitis. This is illustrated as Stage I in Figure 20–12. The insult may be fatal, or in less extensive cases the host may localize the contaminant as depicted in Stage II (Fig. 20–12). Stage III follows drainage of the peritoneal cavity (surgical or spontaneous) with formation of a firm tract from the bowel lumen to the body surface. Stage IV occurs after fibrous obliteration of the tract with healing of the fistula.

DIAGNOSIS. Recognition of enteric leakage into the peritoneal cavity (Stage I) before actual fistula formation to the skin may be extraordinarily difficult and requires careful monitoring of all patients who have undergone intra-abdominal surgery. Fever, tachy-

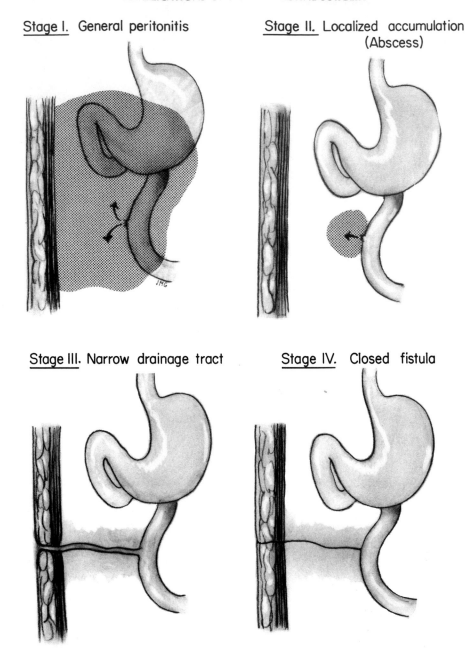

Stage I. General peritonitis

Stage II. Localized accumulation (Abscess)

Stage III. Narrow drainage tract

Stage IV. Closed fistula

Figure 20–12   Usual stages during the course of small bowel fistula.

cardia, and abdominal pain and tenderness are usually present but are frequently attributed to the early postoperative state. Persistent abdominal distention (often associated with remarkably little direct tenderness), fluid retention, prolonged postoperative ileus, developing jaundice, and pulmonary insufficiency all suggest possible postoperative peritonitis. Measurement of central venous and pulmonary arterial pres-

sures may help to distinguish fluid retention or hypotension secondary to cardiac insufficiency from that due to peritonitis. Cardiac output is usually greatly increased in patients with peritonitis, and this finding may help to distinguish postoperative sepsis from other causes of collapse.

When enteric content drains from the abdominal incision or drain sites, the diagnosis of fistula formation is usually clear. Any doubt that may exist can be resolved by enteric administration of charcoal or methylene blue. Effective management of the fistula also requires accurate anatomical diagnosis. Specifically, determination of the presence or absence of associated intra-abdominal abscesses or of distal obstruction requires careful clinical and radiographic evaluation, including contrast studies of the fistula itself and of the gastrointestinal tract.[1, 19]

GENERAL MANAGEMENT. The most frequent complications of enteric leakage fall into *four* major categories: malnutrition, infection, fluid and electrolyte imbalance, and local erosive problems.[40]

The rapid occurrence of malnutrition, related to interference with enteric function and the increased caloric requirements that may be present owing to associated sepsis, is well recognized in patients with gastrointestinal fistulae.[1, 9, 18, 22, 25, 33, 40] Adequate nutritional support is essential to achieve healing of the fistula itself or following surgical treatment of the fistula. This vital feature of the management of patients with gastrointestinal fistulae is discussed in detail in Chapter 12. At least 3000 calories per day are required in most patients. Nutritional support may be provided by intravenous hyperalimentation and by enteric feedings using chemically defined diets.[9, 25, 33] Utilization of enteric feedings must clearly be adjusted to the anatomy of the fistula and usually requires introduction of fine feeding tubes or operative placement of a feeding jejunostomy below the fistula.

Sepsis may be related to undrained intra-abdominal abscesses or to abscesses along the fistulous tract. Management of sepsis includes early surgical drainage together with vigorous antibiotic therapy. Administration of nystatin into the proximal small intestine appears to reduce the risk of eventual monilial overgrowth.

The severity of fluid and electrolyte complications is related to the volume of fistulous drainage and of other losses that may be related to nasogastric or enteric tube suction. All such losses must be carefully measured and appropriate replacement undertaken.

In general, the severity of erosive complications of small intestinal fistulae is inversely related to the distance of the fistulae from the ampulla of Vater, the more severe problems occurring with fistulae of the duodenum or proximal jejunum. The most obvious erosive complication is excoriation and digestion of the skin, which may occur with great rapidity. Prevention of this complication requires meticulous nursing and medical care. Sump suction catheters introduced superficially into the fistula tract help to reduce the volume of spillage. Applications of aluminum and other pastes to the skin surrounding the fistula are of limited effectiveness, and in our experience the best protection has been provided by careful application of karaya sheeting to the skin. The karaya must be carefully tailored and meticulously applied. In addition, when any leakage occurs, the karaya must be changed at once. Disposable collection appliances can usually be affixed readily to the surface of the karaya sheet.

Drainage of enteric content may also be associated with erosion of structures within the abdominal cavity. Damage to blood vessels is most serious and may result in exsanguinating hemorrhage along the fistula tract. Such bleeding may be heralded by a smaller self-limiting bleed, and the possibility of major vascular injury and of imminent massive hemorrhage must be considered when any bleeding occurs from the fistula.

SURGICAL MANAGEMENT. When enteric leakage is recognized early and is associated with spreading or generalized peritonitis, urgent reoperation is indicated. The purpose of such surgery is to evacuate enteric contents from the peritoneal cavity and to prevent continuing spillage. In some cases, this latter goal may be achieved by resection or repair of the source of leakage. In patients with postoperative generalized peritonitis, however, the risk of renewed anastomotic leakage is high. In such patients, resection of the area of leakage and exteriorization by means of an ileostomy or jejunostomy as described by Goligher[15] prevents possible continuing peritoneal contamination. If the area of exteriorization is high in the small intestine, a small soft tube should be introduced into the end of the exteriorized distal intestine prior to closure of the abdominal incision. Subsequent management may be simplified by use of this tube to reinfuse drainage from the proximal bowel and to administer enteric feedings.

When exteriorization is not practical, as in the case of duodenal leakage, repair of the bowel must be attempted. The probability of healing of the duodenal suture line may be increased by constructing a duodenal bypass by gastric resection combined with gastrojejunostomy, together with a tube duodenostomy and local peritoneal drainage. The volume of fluid entering the duodenum may be further reduced by external choledochostomy by means of a T-tube.

In patients with established small intestinal fistulae, surgical intervention may be required to provide drainage of intra-abdominal abscesses and control of sepsis. In addition, early surgical intervention may be required because of the demonstration of unrelieved distal obstruction, retained foreign material, or other factors that may prevent spontaneous closure of the fistula. A fistulous tract less than 2 cm. in length, visible everted mucosa, Crohn's disease, radiation enteritis or associated malignancy are all associated with reduced rates of spontaneous fistula closure.[33, 40] Fistulae that persist for more than 30 days following control of sepsis will frequently require operative closure.[33]

Operative procedures undertaken to achieve fistula closure must include excision or drainage of any residual intra-abdominal abscess and determination that the distal intestine is patent. Simple closure or repair of the fistulous opening is associated with a high probability of failure and should be avoided. Most small intestinal fistulae are best treated by resection of the involved segment and end-to-end anastomosis employing healthy small intestine.

SMALL BOWEL INSUFFICIENCY

Improved methods for management of patients with small bowel gangrene and other lesions necessitating extensive resection have resulted in the survival of an increasing number of these patients who are left with only a small percentage of the normal alimentary tract. The response to such an operation may be variable from one patient to another, depending upon many factors. The length of small bowel among normal persons may vary from 10 to 40 feet.[21] It is thus of great importance, when carrying out extensive resection of the small intestine, to measure not only the length of resected intestine but also the length of residual jejunum and ileum. As much bowel as possible should be preserved and, in particular, the probability for long-term survival is increased if the ileocecal valve and a portion of terminal ileum can be retained. In patients undergoing operation for infarction secondary to vascular occlusion, arterial embolectomy or reconstruction should be undertaken before intestinal resection. Restoration of blood supply may reduce the extent of necessary intestinal resection and may also improve the functional capacity of the residual intestine.[39]

CLINICAL COURSE AND COMPLICATIONS. The initial postoperative period in patients surviving massive intestinal resection is marked by severe diarrhea related to decreased absorptive surface, passage of bile salts into the colon, and possible gastric hypersecretion. During this period, fluid and electrolyte disturbance may be a major threat and significant deficiencies in calcium and magnesium may occur.

The pattern and severity of complications related to malabsorption are related not only to the extent of resection but also to which portion of small intestine has been resected. Resection of the jejunum is relatively well tolerated, since the ileum can adapt to perform most jejunal functions. Resection of the ileum, however, results in a loss of absorption of bile salts and vitamin B_{12} for which the jejunum cannot compensate. Fat malabsorption, steatorrhea, and vitamin B_{12} deficiency may therefore result. Deficiency in fat soluble vitamins, specifically vitamins D and K, may occur, and following resection of the terminal ileum there is an increased risk of cholelithiasis and of urinary oxalate calculi.

MANAGEMENT. Initial management is directed toward monitoring and maintenance of fluid and electrolyte balance. Administration of diphenoxylate hydrochloride or codeine may help to reduce persistent diarrhea. Gastric hypersecretion may be controlled by cimetidine. Initially, nutritional support should be by intravenous hyperalimentation.

Following the initial postoperative period, fat-free oral feedings may slowly be introduced but must be adjusted to the patient's tolerance. Chemically defined dietary supplements are helpful if tolerated. Fats may be tolerated if given as medium chain triglycerides.[11]

As intestinal adaptation progresses, oral intake can be increased, and in most patients a low-fat diet is eventually well tolerated.

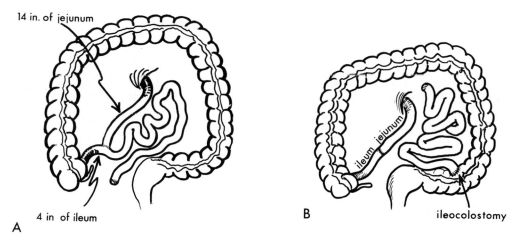

Figure 20–13 *A,* End-to-side jejunoileal reconstruction, *B,* End-to-end jejunoileal reconstruction.

There remain, however, some patients who will require long-term parenteral nutritional supplements.[8, 20, 47]

INTESTINAL SHUNTING FOR OBESITY

Over the past 20 years, there has been considerable interest in the relief of morbid obesity by various small intestinal bypass procedures such as those illustrated in Figure 20–13.[28-30, 36, 37] Recently, an end-to-end small intestinal reconstruction has been preferred, and weight loss has been most satisfactory when 12 inches of jejunum and 6 to 8 inches of ileum were retained in continuity.[37]

Complications associated specifically with small intestinal bypass procedures are similar to those associated with massive small bowel resection and include diarrhea with attendant fluid and electrolyte disturbances, hypocalcemia, and cholelithiasis. In addition, significant hepatic changes have been described following intestinal bypass surgery. In some degree, fatty infiltration of the liver may be related to preexisting obesity. Nonetheless, deterioration in hepatic function and frank hepatic failure have occurred in some patients and may require revision of the bypass.[30]

Some recent studies have suggested that, because of long-term complications of small intestinal bypass operations, gastric bypass or exclusion procedures may be the preferred management of patients requiring surgical treatment for obesity.[2, 16]

THE BLIND-LOOP SYNDROME

Any lesion that predisposes to intestinal stagnation may result in the blind-loop syndrome. Stenosis of the small bowel as a result of tuberculosis or regional enteritis may be responsible. Other etiologic circumstances include side-to-side anastomosis, diverticula, stenosis from adhesions, bypass procedures, and Billroth II type of gastric resection (Fig. 20–14). When the syndrome follows surgery, the patient usually experiences a symptom-free period of variable length, after which the various manifestations of the blind-loop syndrome appear. Among the complaints are abdominal discomfort, diarrhea, abdominal distention, nausea and vomiting, electrolyte disturbance, and steatorrhea. Physical findings may include abdominal fullness, tenderness, and increased peristaltic activity. Late cases are often characterized by progressive weight loss, weakness, glossitis, and icterus. Deficiency of biotin, folic acid, riboflavin, thiamine, and vitamin K is not uncommon. Tetany, osteomalacia, and hypoproteinemia have also been described. An additional finding of considerable interest is the presence of macrocytic anemia in the blind-loop syndrome. The Schilling test (absorption of cobalt-60–labeled vitamin B_{12}) is of value in clarifying the differential diagnosis in the presence of anemia.[34] The normal excretion of labeled vitamin B_{12} is 7 to 25 per cent; this value is 0 to 6 per cent in the blind-loop syndrome. The test is repeated with the additional use of intrinsic factor. The uri-

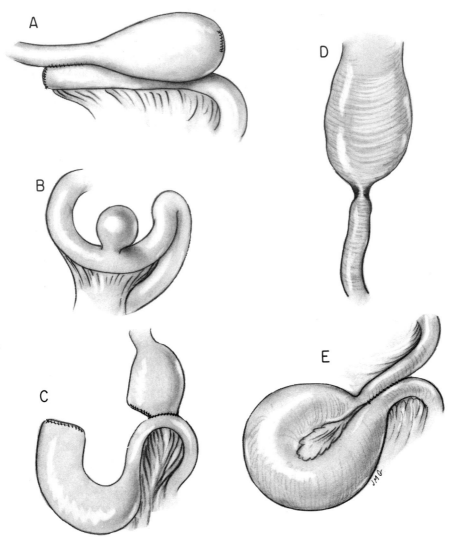

Figure 20–14   Some causes of the blind-loop syndrome. *A,* Side-to-side anastomosis. *B,* Diverticulum. *C,* Billroth II anastomosis. *D,* Stenosis. *E,* Bypassed loop of bowel.

nary excretion of labeled vitamin B$_{12}$ should then rise to normal if the patient has pernicious anemia. Intrinsic factors will not increase excretion of labeled vitamin B$_{12}$ in the blind-loop syndrome. Finally, the patient is given 2 gm. of tetracycline daily for 5 days, and then absorption of labeled vitamin B$_{12}$ is again evaluated. The antibiotic will improve absorption of the vitamin when the blind-loop syndrome exists but will not improve macrocytic anemia due to steatorrhea.

Treatment for the blind-loop syndrome consists of the appropriate surgical procedure that will accomplish adequate drainage of stagnant segments of bowel. This should be preceded by the necessary preoperative

therapy, including the administration of tetracycline, to render the patient an optimal surgical risk.

Bibliography

1. Aguirre, A., Fischer, J. E., and Welch, C. E.: The role of surgery and hyperalimentation in therapy of gastrointestinal-cutaneous fistulae. Ann. Surg. *180*:393, 1974.
2. Alden, J. F.: Gastric and jejunoileal bypass. Arch. Surg. *112*:799, 1977.
3. Baker, J. W.: Stitchless plication for recurring obstruction of the small bowel. Am. J. Surg. *116*:316, 1968.
4. Barnett, W. O.: Experimental strangulated intestinal obstruction — A review. Gastroenterology *39*:34, 1960.

5. Barnett, W. O.: Mechanical small bowel obstruction. Am. Pract. Digest Treat. *11*:389, 1960.
6. Barnett, W. O., Petro, A. B., and Williamson, J. W.: A current appraisal of problems with gangrenous bowel. Ann. Surg. *183*:653, 1976.
7. Berry, R. E. L.: Obstruction of the small and large intestine. Surg. Clin. North Am. *39*:1267, 1959.
8. Broviac, J. W., and Scribner, B. H.: Prolonged parenteral nutrition in the home. Surg. Gynecol. Obstet. *139*:24, 1974.
9. Bury, K. D., Stephens, R. V., and Randall, H. T.: Use of a chemically defined, liquid, elemental diet for nutritional management of fistulas of the alimentary tract. Am. J. Surg. *121*:174, 1971.
10. Childs, W. A., and Phillips, R. B.: Experience with intestinal plication and a proposed modification. Ann. Surg. *152*:258, 1960.
11. Conn, J. H., Chavez, C. M., and Fain, W. R.: The short bowel syndrome. Ann. Surg. *175*:803, 1972.
12. Eade, G. G., Metheny, D., and Lundmark, V. O.: An evaluation of the practice of routine postoperative nasogastric suction. Surg. Gynecol. Obstet. *101*:229, 1955.
13. Edis, A. J.: Pitfalls in gastrointestinal stapling. *In* Maingot, R. (Ed.): Abdominal Operations. Volume II. New York, Appleton-Century-Crofts, 1980, pp. 2210–2220.
14. Farris, J. M., and Smith, G. K.: An evaluation of temporary gastrostomy — A substitute for nasogastric suction. Ann. Surg. *144*:475, 1956.
15. Goligher, J. C.: Resection with exteriorization in the management of faecal fistulas originating in the small intestine. Br. J. Surg. *58*:163, 1971.
16. Griffen, W. O., Jr., Young, V. L., and Stevenson, C. C.: A prospective comparison of gastric and jejunoileal bypass procedures for morbid obesity. Ann. Surg. *186*:500, 1977.
17. Hardy, J. D.: Fluid Therapy. Philadelphia, Lea & Febiger, 1954.
18. Holmes, J. T.: Nutritional support of fistulas. Br. J. Surg. *64*:695, 1977.
19. Irving, M.: Local and surgical management of enterocutaneous fistulas. Br. J. Surg. *64*:690, 1977.
20. Jeejeebhoy, K. N., Langer, B., Tsallas, G., *et al.*: Total parenteral nutrition at home: Studies in patients surviving 4 months to 5 years. Gastroenterology *71*:943, 1976.
21. Kalser, M. H., Roth, J. A., Tumen, H., and Johnson, T. A.: Relation of small bowel resection to nutrition in man. Gastroenterology *38*:605, 1960.
22. Kaminsky, V. M., and Deitel, M.: Nutritional support in the management of external fistulas of the alimentary tract. Br. J. Surg. *62*:100, 1975.
23. Kingsnorth, A. N.: Fluid-filled intestinal obstruction. Br. J. Surg. *63*:289, 1976.
24. Leffall, L. D., and Syphax, B.: Clinical aids in strangulation intestinal obstruction. Am. J. Surg. *120*:756, 1970.
25. MacFadyen, B. V., Dudrick, S. J., and Ruberg, R. L.: Management of gastrointestinal fistulas with parenteral hyperalimentation. Surgery *74*:100, 1973.
26. Monod-Broca, P.: Treatment of intestinal fistulas. Br. J. Surg. *64*:685, 1977.
27. Noble, T. B., Jr.: Plication of the small intestine. Am. J. Surg. *45*:574, 1939.
28. Payne, J. H., and DeWind, L. T.: Surgical treatment of obesity. Arch. Surg. *118*:141, 1969.
29. Payne, J. H., DeWind, L. T., and Commons, R. R.: Metabolic observations in patients with jejunocolic shunts. Am. J. Surg. *106*:273, 1963.
30. Phillips, R. B.: Small intestinal bypass for the treatment of morbid obesity. Surg. Gynecol. Obstet. *146*:455, 1978.
31. Playforth, R. H., Holloway, J. B., and Griffen, W. O., Jr.: Mechanical small bowel obstruction: A plea for earlier surgical intervention. Ann. Surg. *171*:783, 1970.
32. Quatromoni, J. C., Rosoff, L., Halls, J. M., and Yellin, A. E.: Early postoperative small bowel obstruction. Ann. Surg. *191*:72, 1980.
33. Reber, H. A., Roberts, C., Way, L. W., and Dunphy, J. E.: Management of external gastrointestinal fistulas. Ann. Surg. *188*:460, 1978.
34. Reilly, R. W., and Kirsner, J. B.: Blind loop syndrome. Gastroenterology *37*:491, 1959.
35. Rozanski, J., and Kleinfeld, M.: Complication of prolonged intestinal intubation: Gaseous distension of the terminal balloon. Dig. Dis. *20*:1067, 1975.
36. Scott, H. W., Jr., Dean, R., Shull, H. J., *et al.*: New considerations in the use of jejunoileal bypass in patients with morbid obesity. Ann. Surg. *177*:723, 1973.
37. Scott, H. W., Jr., Dean, R. H., Shull, H. J., and Gluck, F.: Results of jejunoileal bypass in two hundred patients with morbid obesity. Surg. Gynecol. Obstet. *145*:661, 1977.
38. Shatila, A. H., Chamberlain, B. E., and Webb, W. R.: Current status of diagnosis and management of strangulation obstruction of the small bowel. Am. J. Surg. *132*:299, 1976.
39. Simons, B. E., and Jordan, G. L., Jr.: Massive bowel resection. Am. J. Surg. *118*:953, 1969.
40. Soeters, P. B., Ebeid, A. M., and Fischer, J. F.: Review of 404 patients with gastrointestinal fistulas. Ann. Surg. *190*:189, 1979.
41. Stewardson, R. H., Bombeck, C. T., and Nyhus, L. M.: Critical operative management of small bowel obstruction. Ann. Surg. *187*:189, 1978.
42. Sykes, P. A., Boulter, K. H., and Schofield, P. F.: The microflora of the obstructed bowel. Br. J. Surg. *63*:721, 1976.
43. Wangensteen, O. H.: Understanding the bowel obstruction problem. Am. J. Surg. *135*:131, 1978.
44. Wassner, J. D., Yohai, E., and Heimlich, H. J.: Complications associated with the use of gastrointestinal stapling devices. Surgery *82*:395, 1977.
45. Weckesser, E. C., Lindsay, J. F., Jr., and Cebul, F. A.: Plication of small intestine for obstruction due to adhesions — Noble procedure. Arch. Surg. *65*:487, 1952.
46. Wickstrom, P., Haglin, J. J., and Hitchcock, C. R.: Intraoperative decompression of the obstructed small bowel. Surgery *73*:212, 1973.
47. Winawer, S. J., Broitman, S. A., Wolochow, D. A., *et al.*: Successful management of massive small-bowel resection based on assessment of absorption defects and nutritional needs. N. Engl. J. Med. *274*:72, 1966.

21

COMPLICATIONS FOLLOWING OPERATIONS UPON THE BILIARY TRACT AND THEIR MANAGEMENT

Frank Glenn and John L. Cameron

Surgery for biliary calculi began to be accepted a century ago. For some time thereafter, however, the medical profession viewed the risk of complications of the operation to be about equal to the risk of the sequelae and complications of the gallstones themselves. In 1934, a review of reports from various clinics throughout the world placed the mortality of surgery at 6.6 per cent.[18] Great progress has been made in the interim with a current overall mortality of 1 to 2 per cent. At this time, biliary tract disease is treated most effectually by surgery. Until we are able to prevent the formation of biliary calculi, the role of calculous disease as a national health problem increases.

The incidence of calculi in the biliary tract as observed by pathologists post mortem ranges from 10 to 30 per cent. A large proportion of these have not had clinical symptoms. Clinicians, internists, and surgeons place the incidence much lower, at 6 to 8 per cent among adults. The life span for those born in 1900 was estimated at 47.3 years, and for those born in 1978 it has been placed at 73.3 years. As the life span has increased so has the proportion of the population 65 years old and older. In 1930, among a population of 122,775,000 there were 6,634,000 people in the category of 65 years old or older, slightly more than 5 per cent. Today, among an estimated population of 220,000,000, it is believed that 11 per cent or 24,400,000 are in the older age category.[30] The health care of the elderly is of increasing importance and requires more and more personnel, facilities, and attention than the care of those who are younger and in the robust period of life.

Frank Glenn is a Midwesterner, born in southern Illinois and educated at Washington University and its medical school. He was trained in surgery at the Peter Bent Brigham Hospital and later became associated with Cornell. A lifetime interest in the physiology and surgery of the liver and biliary system has brought many contributions that are recognized throughout the world. He succeeded Dr. George Heuer in brilliantly occupying the Lewis Atterbury Stimson Chair of Surgery at Cornell University and is now an active Professor Emeritus of Surgery.

John Lemuel Cameron was born in Michigan. After graduating from Harvard University and Johns Hopkins University Medical School, where he was elected to Alpha Omega Alpha, he served his internship and residency at Johns Hopkins Hospital. He joined the Hopkins faculty as Assistant Professor of Surgery in 1971 and was made Professor of Surgery in 1978. Dr. Cameron is a member of the distinguished surgical societies and is widely known for his publications dealing with the biliary tract.

Continual retrospective reviews of patients' records seeking the cause of biliary tract complications does much to reduce the incidence. Most hospitals throughout the United States are well equipped to do this. The avoidable complications may be divided into two main groups. The first group contains the largest number, those complications that may be anticipated. Meticulous and thorough examination followed by indicated preoperative preparation is essential. The second group includes those complications that are difficult to anticipate but that are recognizable, if it is kept in mind that they may occur. Retrospective reviews of large case series in which records are complete attest to the probability of the complications in this category. Continuous and unrelenting observations in the early postoperative period alert those in attendance to early recognition and the immediate utilization of measures to correct them. Morbidity and mortality in surgery are not to be accepted on the basis of past averages. It is the surgeon's responsibility to avoid or reduce the risk by using all possible means, now so much more readily available than in the past.

Anticipation of complications preoperatively and during operation tends to prevent postoperative complications. Precision and accuracy in diagnosis and preoperative preparation, attention to detail and carefulness in surgical technique in performance of the operation, and close observation with well-defined steps in management in the early postoperative period offer an opportunity to reduce complications significantly. To accept an incidence of complications and a rate of mortality that are but average for reported series is to be satisfied with the status quo and to disregard the potential for improvement.

SUBHEPATIC ACCUMULATION

A subhepatic accumulation of material is the most frequent complication following operations upon the biliary tract.[25] This material consists of blood, bile, lymph, and peritoneal fluid. The hemorrhage stems from the blood vessels that have been injured or divided in the course of the operation. The liver is readily lacerated and in-

jured if the capsule to which the gallbladder is adherent is penetrated or torn from the liver.[2, 28] Bile is derived from the extrahepatic ductal system of the liver. The small bile ducts that enter the gallbladder directly from the liver and those that are prominent near the gallbladder site may be inadvertently opened during cholecystectomy. Lymph channels are rarely grossly visible at operation but are luxuriant in the area about the gallbladder. The irritative reaction to blood, lymph, and bile may cause an increase in the permeability of the peritoneum, resulting in an escape of plasma. If bacteria are present in addition, this response may be greater. The effects of all these factors in contributing to the accumulation will vary with the degree to which they are present. If only small amounts of blood, bile, and lymph are present and there is little or no bacterial growth, the peritoneum will absorb and remove them efficiently. If, on the other hand, one or all are present in large quantities and evoke an outpouring of plasma rather than absorption of these substances, then the accumulation increases.

It is a common practice to place a drain of some kind in the subhepatic area and to have it extend through the abdominal wall to facilitate the evacuation of such accumulations. For many reasons these drains not infrequently fail to fulfill their intended function. They may not be properly placed, or they may be dislocated. Sometimes they evoke an increased foreign body reaction on the part of the peritoneum, thus leading to a further sealing off of a localized accumulation. In still other instances, the drain may be removed before the accumulation develops to any significant size. In any event, a subhepatic accumulation frequently occurs. If it persists or increases to an important degree, there is discomfort and pain in the right upper quadrant, an elevation of temperature, and leukocytosis. There is then a localized peritonitis. At any stage in the process, the accumulation may regress or establish escape of its contents externally, or it may extend to involve the subdiaphragmatic area or even spread into the free abdominal cavity.[9] A severe reaction of the tissues near the origin of this accumulation may result in obstruction of the common duct or reflex spasm of the sphincter of

Oddi. If the bacterial content of the bile is high and there is cholangitis, then the systemic manifestations may be heightened.

Some degree of subhepatic accumulation occurs in the majority of patients subjected to operations upon the biliary tract. It is the extent of accumulation that determines whether it becomes clinically significant. Subhepatic accumulation has been the most frequent complication to be diagnosed in the experience at the New York Hospital and the most frequent cause leading to requests to one of us (F.G.) for consultation after biliary tract surgery elsewhere. Its prevention depends upon careful surgical technique and the maintenance of drainage of the subhepatic area for 3 to 4 days or more after operation. Drainage is enhanced and rendered efficient by placing a Penrose drain and a No. 10 or 12 red rubber catheter down to the foramen of Winslow and allowing it to emerge externally through a small incision in the abdominal wall at the level of the eleventh rib (Fig. 21–1). Various closed suction catheter systems can also be used effectively.

CASE REPORT. A 30-year-old housewife underwent a cholecystectomy for chronic cholecystitis with cholelithiasis. Her postoperative course

in the hospital was uneventful, and she was discharged from the hospital on the eighth postoperative day. Five days later she experienced pain in the right upper quadrant radiating through to the back, and this increased on activity. Because of this pain, she was readmitted to the hospital. Physical examination revealed evidence of a subdiaphragmatic accumulation. Reexploration was done, and 4000 ml. of bile-stained ascitic fluid was evacuated. No biliary fistula could be demonstrated. Numerous drains were used to provide for the escape of bile that might accumulate. The patient's postoperative course was uneventful, and she remained well thereafter.

COMMENT. This is an example of gradual accumulation of bile after operation that was so insidious that the patient noted no symptoms until 12 days after operation. At the time of reexploration, the source of this bile was not evident.

HEMORRHAGE

It is an old adage that hemorrhage is one of the important hazards of surgery. Operations upon the biliary tract are no exception to this statement. An analysis of the complications following surgical therapy for biliary tract disease as reported in any sizeable

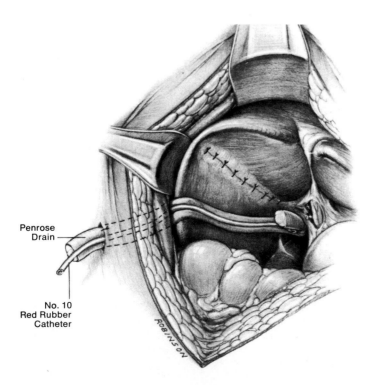

Penrose Drain

No. 10 Red Rubber Catheter

Figure 21–1 Penrose drain and No. 10 red rubber catheter are placed down to foramen of Winslow and emerge externally through a small incision lateral to the initial incision at the level of the tip of the eleventh rib.

clinical series reveals that hemorrhage continues to contribute materially to the morbidity rate. The more common sources of hemorrhage associated with biliary tract surgery include the cystic artery, anomalous branches of the hepatic and right hepatic arteries, the gallbladder bed, the liver, and the vessels of the common duct and of the abdominal wall. An occasional hemorrhage has been reported from injury to the inferior vena cava.

Massive hemorrhage after operations upon the biliary tract is recognized by the same systemic manifestations associated with hemorrhage from any other area.[14] There is an increase in pulse rate and a fall in blood pressure. The patient is often apprehensive and thirsty and may exhibit air hunger. Relief of these manifestations by blood replacement should be a confirmation of the diagnosis whether hemorrhage has been continuous since operation or began later. Bleeding in the immediate postoperative period may result from other sources such as a peptic ulcer or diverticulosis, but this is rare. Hemorrhage sufficient to require blood replacement is an indication for immediate reoperation and search for the source of blood loss. There are two reasons for this approach. First, the hemorrhage may continue or recur, and exsanguination may result in death. Second, blood in such amounts is not readily absorbed by the peritoneum, and if it is mixed with bile that contains organisms, a subhepatic or subphrenic abscess may follow.

This complication may be prevented by carefully identifying all blood vessels before division and then securing them by ligature or transfixing suture. There are so many variations in the blood vessels in the subhepatic area and in their relation to the biliary tract that it is hazardous to divide any structure that is not identified. Furthermore, divided structures should be carefully occluded to prevent escape of the fluid they may contain, be it blood, bile, or lymph.

Although the more frequent sources of hemorrhage are the cystic artery, anomalous branches of the hepatic artery, vessels within the wall of the common bile duct, and aberrant vessels that reach the gallbladder through the bed of the liver, injury to the liver by incision or laceration as the surgeon removes the gallbladder may be the cause of the bleeding. Such bleeding may be noted at operation, and although it usually subsides rather quickly, it may begin again within a matter of hours when bile causes the clot to separate from the liver surface. Massive hemorrhage following surgical procedures upon the biliary tract is an indication for immediate reoperation. The search for the bleeding vessel and proper control of that vessel should not be delayed.

CASE REPORT. A 40-year-old hockey player sustained a severe blow to the upper abdomen. Pain was immediate and persisted. Sixteen hours later, he underwent cholecystectomy. Tube drainage of the common duct was established, and multiple drains were placed in the subhepatic area. He did well for 12 days. Then a massive hemorrhage from the wound led to exploration and evacuation of about 1500 ml. of blood clot. A small laceration on the under surface of the liver noted at the first operation was considered the source of the hemorrhage. Progress was thought to be satisfactory thereafter for 13 days, when bleeding again became profuse. He was transferred to the New York Hospital-Cornell Medical Center. Evaluation, including celiac arteriography, revealed a false aneurysm near the left hepatic artery and a large avascular area within the left lobe of the liver (Fig. 21–2). This was confirmed at operation, and a large clot (500 ml.) unstained by bile was evacuated. Twelve hours later the patient died suddenly of an embolus originating from the left and right hepatic veins and inferior vena cava.

COMMENT. This is an example of the elusiveness of intrahepatic injury caused by external blunt forces, the seriousness of intrahepatic bleeding uncontrolled by ligature of the vessel, and the tendency to thrombosis in hepatic veins when there is an expanding intrahepatic lesion.

HEMORRHAGE DUE TO VITAMIN K DEFICIENCY

Patients with jaundice usually have an increased tendency to hemorrhage. If the degree of icterus is great and of long standing, hemorrhage may be severe. The clotting and bleeding times of these patients are usually normal, but the clot retracts poorly and is fragile. Such clots do not seal the open end of the divided vessels, and there is oozing. Fluctuations of the blood pressure may result in complete dislodgment of the partially occluding clots, and any vessel not

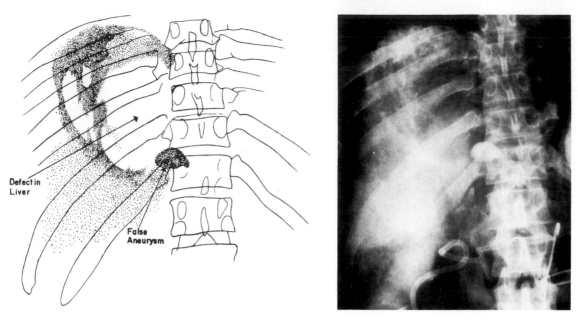

Figure 21–2 A celiac arteriogram demonstrates an intrahepatic hematoma and false aneurysm. This was evacuated. Death occurred 12 hours later and was due to emboli from thrombosis of the hepatic vein.

carefully ligated may bleed actively. That the defect in this clot formation was due to a deficiency of prothrombin in the blood was demonstrated by Dam,[8] Almquist and Stokstad,[1] Quick, Stanley-Brown, and Bancroft,[27] and others in the early 1930's. If the prothrombin content of normal blood is reduced 30 per cent, the bleeding tendency is heightened. This can best be corrected rapidly by the parenteral administration of vitamin K.

Absence of bile from the intestinal tract interferes with the digestion and absorption of fats. Vitamin K is a sterol, soluble in lipids, and requires bile salts to be absorbed by the intestine and carried by the blood stream to the liver, where it is converted into prothrombin. Parenteral administration of vitamin K to jaundiced patients assures control of the tendency to increased bleeding caused by reduced prothrombin, as long as their liver function remains good. Since it was generally accepted in 1936, vitamin K therapy has been so effective in patients with jaundice with a hemorrhagic tendency that the fatalities attributable to this condition have almost completely disappeared. All patients being considered for operation upon the biliary tract should have careful measurements of the prothrombin level,

and if it is lowered, vitamin K should be administered. If the prothrombin level is not satisfactory after vitamin K administration, the operation should be postponed. At present, we recommend that patients with a prothrombin level 50 per cent below normal be given vitamin K parenterally. There should be a rapid response, but if this does not occur, such severe liver disease is probably present that surgery will not be well tolerated.

BILE PERITONITIS

Escape of bile into the peritoneal cavity from the common duct, from the cystic duct remnant, from small radicles extending directly from the liver to the gallbladder, and from breaks in the continuity of liver substance results in peritonitis. If the rate of escape is slow, there is a strong likelihood that the reaction to bile of the omentum and the peritoneal surfaces of the viscera adjacent to the area of operation will prevent its escape into the remainder of the abdomen. Thus, a localized accumulation of bile may occur. The greater the area of peritoneal surface that comes in contact with bile, the greater the effect is likely to be. The local accumulation of bile, by the walling off of an area by the omentum and adjacent viscera, is a response of the body to keep this hazard to a minimum. Free bile in large amounts within the peritoneal cavity may cause a fall in blood pressure, may precipitate the clinical manifestations of shock, and may terminate in death. Although this is the result most to be feared, large quantities of bile escaping into the peritoneal cavity may cause abdominal distention but little evidence of peritoneal irritation and no changes in blood pressure. One of the authors (F.G.) has removed as much as 10 liters of bile-stained fluid from a patient several days after operation.

Clinicians have been perplexed by the fact that these two situations may occur from comparable amounts of bile liberated into the peritoneal cavity. Much study and research have been directed at the solution of this problem. No one explanation seems to account for the various effects that free bile in the peritoneal cavity can produce. In some instances, as bile escapes into the abdomen, the patient appears to become more and more restless and uncomfortable. Pain generalized over the abdomen is frequent. The temperature becomes elevated. The pulse may become rapid or slow, but the blood pressure falls. It is believed that this picture of shock results because bile increases the permeability of the peritoneum, thus permitting rapid escape of plasma with a reduction of the circulating volume. When this continues, death from shock may result. The time lapse between the beginning of liberation of bile into the abdomen and the appearance of shock varies greatly; in some cases, it is a matter of hours, and in others it may extend over 7 to 10 days. It is generally agreed that extending infection, or even the presence of bacteria, may accelerate this course of events. On the other hand, there are instances in which accumulations of bile within the abdomen in amounts of up to 6000 to 8000 ml. appear to be innocuous and produce only those symptoms attributed to abdominal distention by fluid. Analysis of bile removed from the abdominal cavity has not revealed any consistent difference between that removed from the moribund patient and that removed from one with few symptoms. Bile salts, bile acid content, and the bacteria present have been studied with considerable care. While the slow escape of bile into the peritoneal cavity following an operation upon the extrahepatic ductal system may follow a benign course, free flow of bile from the ductal system, such as may occur from an unligated cystic duct or injury to the common duct, usually results in a diffuse bile peritonitis. This may run a rapidly fulminating course to end fatally in a matter of hours.[7, 24]

Treatment of bile peritonitis is dependent upon the reaction that results. Shock is best treated by replacement of reduced circulating volume. At operation it is essential to remove the bile that has accumulated in the abdomen, to irrigate the peritoneal cavity copiously, and to divert the flow of bile to the exterior if it cannot be channeled into the intestinal tract.

EXTERNAL BILIARY FISTULA

When bile escapes from its normal course, it either accumulates near its source and spreads over the peritoneum or reaches the exterior, usually by means of a drain. If the local accumulation persists and increases, it may form a tract to the exterior. When bile is free in the peritoneal cavity, operation may reveal its source and correct the condition by redirecting its flow into the intestine or diverting it to the exterior. In all three instances, however, an external biliary fistula may result. This complication may be burdensome to manage and difficult to correct, but it reduces the seriousness of the situation by replacing a condition associated with a high mortality rate with another with a much lower rate. Complete diversion of bile requires replacement that for many patients is quite burdensome but effectual. In addition, hyperalimentation for those markedly debilitated is mandatory.

An external biliary fistula that develops after an operation upon the biliary tract is the result of an interruption of the flow of bile through its normal path from the liver to the duodenum. This fistula may follow any operation upon the biliary tract, and the cause may be the nature or extent of the biliary tract disease or distortion or injury resulting from the surgical procedure.[31] Fistula after cholecystectomy usually indicates an injury to the external hepatic ductal system or an obstruction distal to the cystic duct, in most instances usually by a stone, ligature, or metallic clip. The diagnosis and exact location of the obstruction can be established by sonography,[15] injection of radiopaque material into a sinus opening, percutaneous or endoscopic cholangiography, and gastrointestinal series. Direct treatment is by stone removal or surgical correction of the ductal injury.

Biliary fistula frequently follows cholecystostomy. In the majority of instances the abdominal wound that is the site of the tube draining the gallbladder closes a few days after the drainage tube has been removed. Within days or weeks the site may reopen, and bile and mucus are discharged. In 50 per cent of patients gallstones re-form within 2 years after the gallbladder has been evacuated of stones and drained by cholecystostomy.[16] It is probable that stones remaining in the gallbladder act as ball valves and obstruct the return flow of bile into the common duct. Cholecystectomy should be done within 6 months after a cholecystostomy to prevent this complication. Cholecystectomy is, of course, indicated when a biliary fistula persists after cholecystostomy.

Cholecystectomy is by far the most frequently performed operation upon the biliary tract. Biliary fistula following this procedure may be the result of obstruction to the flow of bile distal to the cystic duct junction with the common duct. Calculi, neoplasm, and ductal injury within the distal segment may cause obstruction that results in rupture of the occluded cystic duct remnant with escape of bile through a fistula to the exterior. Actually, obstructive jaundice following cholecystectomy may result in a fistula, if the integrity of the wall of the duct is impaired or lost. Thus, obstructive jaundice may precede the formation of a biliary fistula. The amount of bile that escapes from the fistula in the now jaundiced patient is an indication of the degree of obstruction or distortion of the normal path of flow.

When the gallbladder or any significant amount of its mucosal lining is not removed, a fistula that discharges mucus alone or mucus and bile may develop. It is not unusual to operate upon patients who give a history of having had a cholecystectomy for cholecystitis and cholelithiasis and to find a fistulous tract leading from the abdominal wall to a remnant of the gallbladder, usually the ampullary portion, which contains calcareous material. Such patients become symptom free after removal of the remnant of the gallbladder and its cystic duct down to within 3 mm. of its true junction with the common duct.

Establishment of biliary fistula soon after an operation upon the biliary tract is always a cause for grave concern. The greater the amount and proportion of bile that is lost through it, the more serious is its import. It is an indication that an opening has been produced in the ductal system and that there is probably obstruction distal to the defect. The mechanisms by which such injuries are produced will be discussed later in this chapter. Jaundice preceding the discharge of bile usually indicates occlusion and possible interruption of the common duct. If there has been no preceding jaundice, the discharge of bile is more likely to be the result of an unligated cystic duct or a defect in the wall of the common duct due to operative injury. Division of small bile ducts leading from the liver to the ampulla of the gallbladder may give rise to a subhepatic accumulation of bile and then a fistula. The amount of bile ordinarily decreases gradually over a matter of 10 to 20 days, as the fistula closes. Injury to the intrahepatic ducts either in the area of the gallbladder bed by too deep dissection or elsewhere within the operative field by improper retraction may also lead to bile fistula formation. These, too, are usually of short duration and require no surgical intervention other than the maintenance of free drainage until escape of the bile ceases.

After the transduodenal approach for operative procedures upon the ampulla of Vater and the sphincter of Oddi, including the removal of calculi from that part of the common duct that is within the duodenal wall, dehiscence of the duodenostomy wound may occur. A fistula may thus be established that is, strictly speaking, duodenal in origin but that discharges bile as well as other intestinal juices. Fortunately, this complication is less frequent than it was formerly, owing to the more careful closure of the incision in the duodenal wall (Fig. 21–3).

A duodenal fistula is to be suspected when bile and intestinal drainage follows an oper-

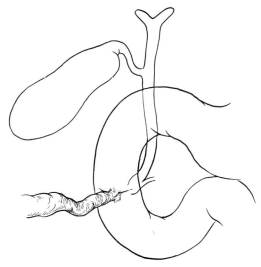

Figure 21–3   Fistula following dehiscence of duodenal incision.

ative procedure upon this segment. Opaque material in the duodenum taken by mouth may demonstrate the fistula. Although these fistulas may close without operation, they are usually slow in doing so. Intravenous hyperalimentation is mandatory in such patients. With careful and appropriate fluid and electrolyte replacement, good wound care, and parenteral nutritional support, many duodenal fistulas will close spontaneously. The remaining patients will require surgical repair, which often includes a serosal patch repair of the duodenal defect.

Nutritional depletion tends to follow complete diversion of the bile from the intestinal tract. Since it escapes from a fistula, bile should be collected and returned to the patient at regular intervals. Many methods have been developed to accomplish this objective, ranging from having the patient drink the bile to introducing it into the stomach through a small tube. The latter measure supplemented by hyperalimentation is usually very effective. An external biliary fistula not involving the duodenum that does not close spontaneously will require surgical correction. In attempting to determine the cause of a biliary fistula, it is important to know what the findings were at the primary operation and exactly what operative procedure was done. Sometimes this information is not available, and the surgeon must rely upon diagnostic measures for guidance. In the absence of jaun-

dice, percutaneous or endoscopic cholangiography and sonography may give much information by revealing calculi, distortion of the ductal system, or abnormalities, sometimes unexpected. Additional information may be gained from a gastrointestinal series focusing on the duodenum. Radiographic visualization of the fistulous tract with radiopaque material is usually the most informative method.

If the cause of the biliary fistula can be determined, the surgeon's problem becomes evident, and an attack may be planned. On the other hand, an attempt at correction of a biliary fistula without obtaining all possible information may result in a frustrating experience to the surgeon and prove of no benefit to the patient. Currently, the treatment of choice, if a patient has a retained calculus following cholecystectomy or common duct exploration, with or without a biliary fistula, is either non-operative extraction through the T-tube tract or endoscopic papillotomy with stone extraction. If these procedures are not successful, then laparotomy and duct exploration should be performed. The other sources of a persistent external biliary fistula following biliary surgery will require operative repair. This will be discussed later.

DISLOCATION, OBSTRUCTION, RETENTION, AND DISINTEGRATION OF DRAINAGE TUBES

Dislocation of Common Duct Tubes

Tubes placed to provide decompression and drainage of the common duct may be displaced or occluded, may disintegrate, or may become difficult to remove. After exploration of the common duct, it is common practice to maintain decompression and afford drainage by means of a T-tube placed through the incision in the duct wall. The tube may be displaced by any one of a number of inadvertent occurrences. It may be caught in the bed clothing or may be attached to some part of the bed so that, as the patient turns, the tube is dislocated. Sometimes the patient may pull upon the tube. There are many methods whereby the tube may be secured so that dislocation will rarely occur. The tube may be anchored to

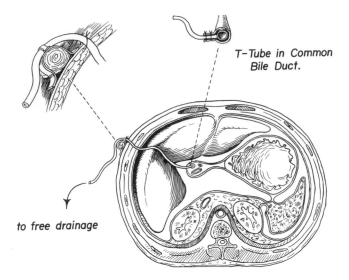

T–Tube in Common
Bile Duct.

to free drainage

Figure 21–4 Location of T-tube from common duct to skin with fixation of adhesive to prevent distortion.

the skin by sutures or fastened to a roll of bandage held to the skin by silk sutures (Fig. 21–4). It is worthwhile to instruct the patient before operation about the function of such a tube.

The shorter the lapse of time from operation until the inadvertent displacement of the tube, the more serious is the accident likely to be. Formation of a tract along the course of such drains tends to allow the bile that escapes from the common duct to pass to the exterior rather than to accumulate in the periductal and subhepatic areas.

When any tube draining the common duct is inadvertently displaced within the first few hours after surgery, bile leakage is to be expected and reexploration for its reinsertion carried out immediately. However, if the tube has been in place for several days, and if there is no obstruction distally, one may expect that little bile will escape. On the other hand, if there is obstruction in the distal part of the common duct, then the amount will be large. The size of the defect in the wall of the choledochus is of less importance than the degree of obstruction. Thus, bile loss depends on the time elapsed since surgery, the patency of the choledocho-duodenal junction, and the presence of calculi in the distal common duct.

The question may arise as to whether tubes that have been displaced from the duct and remain within the abdomen should be left alone or removed. Because

bile may be expected to drain into the subhepatic area, the tube may serve a useful purpose in facilitating escape of bile through the abdominal wall. A further protection is provided by drains that extend from opposite the foramen of Winslow along the bed of the gallbladder to and through the abdominal wall.

Patients who have this unfortunate accident should be observed carefully. If there is no external drainage of bile and there is evidence of diaphragmatic irritation, abdominal distention, or any other sign of the escape of bile into the peritoneal cavity, operation should not be postponed. Many patients will drain bile into the exterior for a few hours and thereafter do well. Others may suffer a bile peritonitis that is general or is localized to the subhepatic area. This readily extends into the subdiaphragmatic area.

Obstruction Caused by Occluded Tubes

In the early postoperative period, tubes may become occluded by blood clot, calcareous gravel, or distortion. The introduction of sterile saline solution under gentle pressure will usually suffice to correct this. The longer a tube remains within the ductal system, the more likely it is to become obstructed by encrusted material. Tubes have been found to remain patent for years, however. Those that become clogged by encrusted material should be removed, because additional layers of encrustations may result in complete occlusion of the common duct. The use of solvent materials other than water and saline is not recommended, since the sludge is not high in cholesterol content and thus not soluble in the currently available biliary solvents.

Retention of Drainage Tubes

Some surgeons seek security from the inadvertent displacement of tubes in the bile duct by suturing them in place. When plain 3-0 catgut is used, the tube usually is readily removed after 10 days. If it cannot be withdrawn readily, it is better to let a few days elapse and then make another attempt. Force should not be applied.

A bile-tight closure about a T-tube is advocated in order that periductal accumulations be kept to a minimum. Since large or stiff T-tubes may be difficult to withdraw, the surgeon should select tubes that are flexible and of suitable size. It is a good practice to cut a small V segment in the T-tube wall opposite the limb that will lead to the exterior. Half of the circumference of the tube within the duct may be cut away before it is placed in order to facilitate later removal. When removal is not readily accomplished, slight traction upon the external limb of the tubing followed by setting a clamp across it and having the patient walk about may initiate its dislocation. Performing the procedure under fluoroscopic control with contrast material in the T-tube and biliary tree may also be helpful.

Disintegration of Tubes

The material used in T-tubes and catheters commonly available in operating rooms of general hospitals is of good quality and, if indicated, the tubes may be left in place for a few weeks. When they are not removed because of a tendency to formation of scar tissue in patients who have had repeated operations for common duct stricture, the tubes become brittle and fragile and readily come apart near the site of exit in the skin. Retained segments of drainage tubes tend to become occluded and may be a nidus of deposition of calcareous material. Their surgical removal is indicated.

JAUNDICE FOLLOWING OPERATIONS UPON THE BILIARY TRACT

The development of jaundice within the first few days or weeks following an operation upon the biliary tract is suggestive of a serious complication. The time of its onset, the degree of jaundice, and the presence of associated systemic manifestations that accompany it provide important information for suspecting its cause and probable course. The jaundice can be secondary to a variety of causes. Perhaps the most serious cause is that of an operative injury to the extrahepatic biliary tree. As with most operative complications, injury to the biliary tree is entirely avoidable, but once it occurs it can be a very difficult and complicated problem with which to deal. Because of the complexity of the problem this topic will be dealt with separately in the next major section of this chapter. Perhaps the most common cause of postoperative jaundice is a retained stone within the biliary tree. Pancreatitis can follow any operative procedure but is more common after biliary tract surgery and can result in partial ampullary obstruction and postoperative jaundice. Halothane hepatitis can also present as jaundice in the postoperative period and is a particularly serious complication with a high mortality rate. A malignant biliary tract tumor that is missed during surgery but subsequently obstructs the biliary tree because of operative manipulation and edema can also present as postoperative jaundice. A wide variety of other entities such as transfusion reactions, sepsis from a non-biliary source, and pulmonary emboli can result in hyperbilirubinemia in the postoperative period.

RETAINED BILIARY CALCULI

The most common cause of postoperative jaundice following cholecystectomy alone or in combination with common duct exploration is a retained calculus within the biliary tree. Following cholecystectomy alone, when there has been no indication for common duct exploration, the incidence is probably in the range of 1 per cent. Following a negative common duct exploration the incidence of a retained stone is in the range of 2 to 3 per cent.[32] Following a common bile duct exploration during which stones are retrieved, retained stones occur in 5 to 10 per cent of patients.[12] Even though these incidences are relatively low, because close to a half million patients in the United States undergo operations upon the biliary tract each year, between 4000 and 6000 patients are left with retained biliary calculi.[34]

There are techniques and procedures currently available that should allow for a significant decrease in the number of patients with retained stones. All patients admitted for elective cholecystectomy, in addition to the appropriate history and physical examination, should have a biochemical profile performed prior to surgery. Obviously, if the patient's bilirubin is elevated, one considers the likelihood of a common duct stone. In addition, if the alkaline phosphatase, SGOT, or SGPT is elevated, this should also alert the clinician to the possibility of common duct calculi. In contrast, if these four preoperative determinations are entirely normal, this does not exclude the possibility of a common duct stone. In many patients who are to undergo cholecystectomy or common duct exploration and who have a high likelihood of common duct stones, the biliary tract anatomy and pathology should be defined prior to surgery. With the aid of endoscopic retrograde or transhepatic cholangiography, the surgeon can be aware of the ductal anatomy, the presence or absence of stones, and the exact number of ductal stones, if present, before surgery. A preoperative cholangiographic work-up may be indicated for a diagnostic problem, in an ill patient in whom operative time should be kept to a minimum, and perhaps in an obese patient in whom operative cholangiography might be difficult. Adequate preoperative cholangiographic information in these situations is exceedingly helpful in avoiding retained stones. In the past, intravenous cholangiography (IVC) has been relied upon to define ductal anatomy prior to surgery. However, the resolution of an IVC is so inferior to transhepatic or endoscopic retrograde cholangiography that its use should be greatly curtailed. More often than not it falsely reassures the surgeon preoperatively, rather than providing helpful information.

During cholecystectomy early control of the cystic duct is important in avoiding retained common duct stones. It is possible for the surgeon to force a stone from the gallbladder into the common duct by manipulation during removal. If at the beginning of the dissection the surgeon identifies the structures in the porta hepatis, loops the cystic duct with a 2-0 silk tie, and places one occluding but not crushing throw, this can be avoided. The cystic duct should not be ligated or divided at this point during the procedure, since anatomic anomalies could result in ductal injury. Only after the gallbladder has been completely mobilized from above downward and the anatomy is clear should the cystic duct actually be ligated and divided. When common duct exploration is carried out, a very careful and thorough duct exploration will decrease the chance of a retained stone. Not only should the usual stone forceps and scoops be used, but also copious irrigation of the biliary tract should be performed to flush out stones and sludge. The routine use of the Fogarty balloon catheter should decrease the likelihood of missing a common duct stone. Ductal injuries in the liver have been reported secondary to overinflation of the balloon, so caution should be used with the Fogarty as with any instrument placed in the biliary tree. Since the incidence of common duct stones increases strikingly with age, the increased use of operative cholangiography and a lower threshold for duct exploration in the elderly should also help decrease the incidence.

Many studies have demonstrated that operative cholangiography with every cholecystectomy will result in uncovering stones that otherwise would have gone unnoticed in as many as 5 per cent of patients. Whereas the controversy continues as to whether or not routine cholangiography should be performed, there is no question that its judicious use in any clinical situation in which biliary tract pathology is a possibility should be encouraged. When one performs operative cholangiography, particular attention should be paid to filling of the left hepatic duct. Because the left hepatic duct is in a non-dependent position, filling is often inadequate. If the patient has a dilated intrahepatic biliary tree, and intrahepatic stones are a possibility, appropriate position changes of the operative table should be carried out and cholangiography repeated until the left hepatic duct is completely visualized. When fluoroscopy becomes widely available in the operating rooms in this country, this will be a further aid in decreasing retained common duct stones.

Some surgeons feel that the incidence of retained stones following biliary tract surgery can be decreased by use of the choledochoscope. Most experience has been with the rigid right angle scope, but more recently, improved flexible fiberoptic instruments have also become available. In a series of 140 patients undergoing operative choledochoscopy with the rigid scope reported by Feliciano et al.,[10] 20 patients were found with the instrument to have stones that had been missed during the routine duct exploration. The authors also felt that the choledochoscope was an aid in removing intrahepatic stones and in clarifying atypical anatomy. They recommended that choledochoscopy be performed during all common duct operations. Keighley and Kappas[21] have also recommended that routine choledochoscopy be performed during common duct exploration. They found that it was not adequate to replace T-tube cholangiography, but it was a helpful adjuvant. When both postexploratory operative cholangiography and choledochoscopy were combined, the authors had a zero incidence of retained common duct stones. Operative biliary tract manometrics have been suggested by some as valuable in decreasing the incidence of retained stones.[35] Currently, very few surgeons in this country perform operative manometric examinations, but it appears that if one becomes familiar with its performance, it can be helpful in identifying stones during biliary tract surgery.

Finally, a more liberal use of biliary drainage procedures at the time of common duct exploration can also be helpful, if not in detecting a retained stone, then at least in eliminating the serious consequences. If the common duct is dilated to 1.5 cm. or greater, a side-to-side choledochoduodenostomy can be safely and quickly performed. This will leave a wide opening between the biliary tree and duodenum and should allow any retained stone to pass easily. If the stone passes distal to the anastomosis and impacts at the ampulla, in most instances this still does not result in symptoms because of the more proximal large anastomosis. The performance of a large sphincteroplasty carried out through a duodenostomy will serve the same purpose. This operation is, in fact, a side-to-side choledochoduodenostomy performed from within the duodenum. This also leaves an enlarged opening between the biliary tree and duodenum so that a retained stone can easily pass. In patients who have multiple stones within the biliary tree or intrahepatic stones, or if it has been demonstrated that a patient recurrently forms stones, one of these biliary drainage procedures should always be performed. In instances in which the surgeon is not certain that all biliary calculi have been completely removed, use of a side-to-side choledochoduodenostomy or a sphincteroplasty should be seriously considered.

Retained Stones Following Cholecystectomy

When a patient develops symptoms of right upper quadrant pain in association with nausea and vomiting, fever, and jaundice following a cholecystectomy, one should be suspicious that a common duct stone was missed. In some instances the episode is not severe, passes quickly, and is only subsequently related to a physician. Under these circumstances the patient might have passed the common duct stone and be free of any biliary pathology. However, in most instances, except the most minor of episodes, cholangiography should be performed to confirm the presence or absence of a retained stone and to rule out the possibility of a ductal injury. In the past, the IVC was used in this situation. However, because of the poor resolution of IVC and the availability of superior techniques, the IVC should no longer be used. Endoscopic retrograde cholangiography can easily confirm the presence of a biliary tract stone. If the patient's jaundice has cleared or is low-grade, this would be the cholangiographic method of choice. If the patient is deeply jaundiced, a transhepatic cholangiogram is more likely to be informative.

A retained stone following cholecystectomy without common duct exploration is

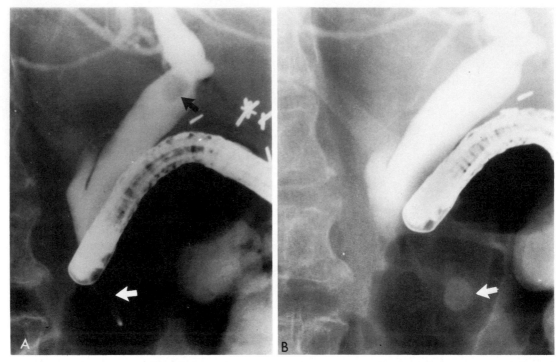

Figure 21-5 *A*, 55-year-old patient who developed cholangitis several months after a cholecystectomy. Endoscopic retrograde cholangiogram demonstrates a large retained common duct stone (*white arrow*). A papillotomy was performed by inserting the papillotome (*black arrow*) into the ampulla and applying an electrical current. *B*, Immediately following the papillotomy, the stone (arrow) spontaneously passed into the duodenum.

apt to be small. In most instances there will have been few signs or symptoms to suggest common duct disease at the time of cholecystectomy, and a stone left under these circumstances will usually be small. Therefore, spontaneous passage may occur, possibly in as many as 20 per cent. If one minor episode of right upper quadrant pain and jaundice has occurred, cholangiography might demonstrate that the stone has passed. However, if a retained stone is demonstrated, treatment will be required. In the past, reoperative biliary surgery with common duct exploration was mandatory. Currently, however, endoscopic papillotomy with stone extraction through the ampulla is the treatment of choice. Through a fiberoptic duodenoscope a wire is passed into the ampulla and an electrical current applied. Most stones less than 1.5 cm. in diameter will spontaneously pass through the enlarged ampulla (Fig. 21-5*A, B*). Those that do not can be extracted through the ampulla with a basket or Fogarty balloon. A collected series of over 1000 papillotomies for common duct stones has been reported with a success rate in excess of 90 per cent.[37] The procedure is not without risk and has a complication rate of 8 per cent and a mortality rate of approximately 1 per cent. However, compared with the risks of reoperative biliary surgery, these figures are acceptable. In addition, in terms of cost and hospital stay, endoscopic papillotomy and stone extraction offer a great advantage. If papillotomy and stone extraction are unsuccessful, then reoperation with common duct exploration will be necessary.

Retained Stones Following Common Duct Exploration

The diagnosis of a retained common duct stone following common duct exploration will be made at one week following surgery when one obtains the postoperative T-tube cholangiogram. In the past, this was a catastrophic situation that every surgeon dreaded. Reoperative biliary tract surgery and a second common duct exploration for a retained stone were not only technically demanding and difficult for the surgeon but also carried a significant chance of postoperative morbidity and mortality. Fortunately, with the improvement in techniques for managing retained common duct stones, very few of these patients currently need to undergo reoperation. There are many options for managing the patient with a retained common duct stone following common duct exploration. It has been estimated that as many as 20 per cent will pass spontaneously.[22] Thus, if the stone is relatively small and is not obstructing the ampulla, and if the patient will tolerate having the T-tube clamped, one option is to discharge the patient from the hospital for a period of several weeks with the hope that the stone will pass. A second option is that of infusing a solvent through the T-tube in an attempt to dissolve or fragment the retained stone. The largest recent experience has been with the solvent sodium cholate. This was first reported by Way et al. in 1972.[33] The technique has the advantage that it can be used as soon as the retained stone has been identified at one week following surgery. A 200 millimole solution of sodium cholate is infused into the T-tube at 30 to 60 ml. per hour, taking care not to elevate the intrabiliary pressure over 20 to 30 cm. of water. This requires the patient to remain at bed rest in the hospital. Dissolution often requires up to 10 days. The success rate is in the range of 60 per cent. Heparin infusion into the T-tube has also been advocated by some, but other investigators have found it to be ineffective. More recently, Capmul (monoctanoin acid) has been shown to work more rapidly than sodium cholate, resulting in dissolution within the first 4 or 5 days. However, the success rate of Capmul is also only in the range of 60 per cent.

Currently, the most effective and preferred technique for removing retained common duct stones following common duct exploration is extraction through the T-tube tract. In the past some surgeons felt a T-tube was unnecessary following common duct exploration, and actually increased the likelihood of a postoperative complication. However, with the development in recent years of the technique of non-operative T-tube tract extraction of re-

tained common duct stones, in no instance should a T-tube not be used. The size of the T-tube is also very important. At least a size 16 French T-tube should be inserted so that the tract leading from the skin to the common duct is large enough to insert instruments for stone removal. When a common duct is small and will not accept a size 16 French, tubes with small T's but large caliber long arms are available so that in no instance does one need to use a T-tube with a long arm less than a 16 French. In addition, the surgeon should pay particular attention to bringing the T-tube out in a relatively straight course without any bends or acute curves. This will allow the radiologist to cannulate the tract and introduce instruments into the biliary tree with less difficulty. Some extraction through the T-tube tract requires waiting a period of 6 weeks following common duct exploration so that the tract leading from the choledochotomy to the skin can mature. A variety of baskets and forceps can be used, and a success rate of greater than 90 per cent can be achieved.[4] This technique often requires the crushing of stones too large to extract through the T-tube tract. In some instances after crushing, the pieces are extracted through the tract; in other instances, they are washed through into the duodenum (Fig. 21–6). In some institutions this procedure is performed on an outpatient basis, but in most instances the patient is admitted to the hospital and placed on antibiotics. If extraction through the T-tube tract is unsuccessful, endoscopic retrograde papillotomy with extraction through the ampulla can be attempted. As mentioned previously, this technique also has a success rate in excess of 90 per cent. Thus, with the combination of T-tube tract extraction, papillotomy and stone extraction, or stone dissolution if the first two are unsuccessful, there should be virtually no failures in managing patients with retained stones. Recently, inserting a flexible fiberoptic choledochoscope through the T-tube tract for retained stone extractions has also been reported. In one small series this technique had a success rate of 100 per cent.[3]

In unusual circumstances, reexploration of a common duct may still be necessary. This should be performed, however, only when all of the non-operative techniques

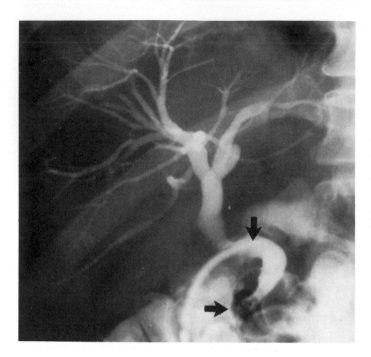

Figure 21–6 A 44-year-old patient who was found to have a retained common duct stone at the ampulla (arrow below) on a T-tube cholangiogram performed one week after common duct exploration. Five weeks later, when the T-tube tract was well established, the T-tube was removed and the Burhenne instrument (arrow above) inserted into the common duct. With the aid of a basket, the stone was grasped and removed through the T-tube tract.

have been used and have failed. In most instances when one reoperates for a retained stone, the surgeon will want to add a side-to-side choledochoduodenostomy or a sphincteroplasty to be certain of not having a repeat performance.

Retained Stones After Cholecystostomy

Even though not frequently used in the United States today, cholecystostomy still has a place in biliary tract surgery. The procedure can be life-saving in the patient who develops acute cholecystitis requiring surgery and who is too severely ill to survive cholecystectomy; in the patient in whom chronic underlying systemic disease makes cholecystectomy too risky; and in the patient in whom technical difficulties arise at the time of surgery, making cholecystectomy technically impossible. When cholecystostomy is performed, the incidence of retained common duct stones is high, in the range of 25 per cent.[29] The procedure is usually performed under local or light general anesthesia, with no attempt being made to examine the common duct. Under these circumstances, the likelihood of leaving a common duct stone behind is high. The diagnosis will be made postoperatively when

the patient is stable and has recovered sufficiently to undergo cholangiography through the cholecystostomy tube. If a common duct stone is identified, its management will depend upon the patient's condition. If the patient is otherwise healthy and is recovering from an acute illness, surgery should be planned. Since the patient's gallbladder is still in place and requires removal, cholecystectomy and common duct exploration should be performed in 6 weeks to 3 months. If the patient is adequately decompressed through the cystic duct and cholecystostomy tube, waiting this interval should be safe. If the patient develops cholangitis and one cannot safely wait 6 weeks to 3 months, or if it is felt that the patient will not recover sufficiently to be able to tolerate cholecystectomy and common duct exploration, endoscopic retrograde papillotomy and stone extraction can be carried out. In most instances instrumentation through the cholecystostomy tract will not be feasible, because the instruments will not pass through the cystic duct. There is little experience with infusing solvents through cholecystostomy tubes to dissolve retained common duct stones, but this approach is possible. In most instances, however, either subsequent surgery with cholecystectomy and common duct exploration or endoscopic retrograde papillotomy will be the treatment of choice.

PANCREATITIS

Pancreatitis can follow any intraabdominal operation but is more frequently seen following procedures on the biliary tree.[20] Its incidence depends upon the degree to which it is looked for. If one routinely obtains amylase determinations following biliary tract surgery, elevations probably representing minor degrees of postoperative pancreatitis will frequently be seen. Occasionally, the attack can be severe, and in some series postoperative pancreatitis carries considerable mortality. Jaundice and partial biliary obstruction may result from periampullary edema and inflammation in the head of the pancreas. Pancreatitis can occur following cholecystectomy alone, as well as following common duct exploration. Heimbach and White[17] have demonstrated that the passage of progressively larger Bakes dilators through the ampulla of Vater will result in a progressively higher incidence of postoperative pancreatitis. An older practice not commonly seen now is that of placing the long arm of a T-tube through the ampulla. This is associated with a significant incidence of postoperative pancreatitis and should never be done unless a wide sphincteroplasty has been performed.

The course of postoperative pancreatitis is quite variable and can range from a minor attack that is only recognized by an amylase elevation to a severe postoperative illness resulting in necrosis of the pancreas and death. The degree of jaundice seen in association with the pancreatitis often is proportional to the severity of the attack. The treatment for postoperative pancreatitis, as well as for pancreatitis that occurs in the absence of surgery, is primarily supportive. Appropriate intravenous fluids and analgesics are the mainstay of therapy. Other specific treatment modalities that are primarily aimed at decreasing pancreatic secretion, such as nasogastric suction, atropine administration, glucagon administration, and cimetidine administration have proven ineffective in controlled clinical trials. In addition, antibiotic administration has been evaluated in prospective studies and has been ineffective in preventing septic complications. In most instances acute pancreatitis is a self-limited disease. The patient will recover and the jaundice will abate without further specific therapy being necessary.

HALOTHANE HEPATITIS

Halothane was introduced clinically as an anesthetic agent in the middle 1950's. Because it is non-explosive, easily controlled, and a clinically safe agent, halothane came into extensive use very rapidly. In the early 1960's, cases of jaundice and hepatic necrosis were reported following its use. Subsequently, the entity halothane hepatitis or halothane-induced hepatic necrosis has become well documented, and by 1976 there were over 900 cases reported in the English language literature.[36] The actual incidence of jaundice resulting from halothane use is very small, probably in the range of one per several thousand exposures. However, this fluorinated hydrocarbon anesthetic agent is used so extensively that a large number of cases have been seen. Halothane hepatitis does not occur with any higher frequency following surgery on the liver or biliary tract than with other operative procedures, but when it occurs in this setting it is often confusing and the diagnosis delayed because of the preceding biliary surgery.

The presentation of halothane hepatitis following biliary tract surgery is particularly perplexing, because it can closely simulate a complication of the surgery itself.[28a] Fever is usually seen from 3 to 6 days following surgery, and jaundice occurs within 6 to 11 days. Nausea and vomiting are also prominent, as is right upper quadrant abdominal pain. These symptoms are often preceded by a latent period of several days during which there is no clinical evidence of a problem. Approximately a quarter of the patients who develop halothane hepatitis have had no prior exposure to the drug. The remaining three quarters have received halothane in the past. The diagnosis can be confirmed as soon as it is suspected by determining the serum transaminase values and performing a liver biopsy. The SGOT and SGPT values are often in the thousands, and a liver biopsy shows a fairly characteristic pattern of central lobular necrosis. The clinical course can vary from a mild subclinical case that is detectable only if transaminase values are drawn to a catastrophic illness leading to death within a few days. If clinical jaundice occurs, the prognosis is grave, with the mortality being in excess of 50 per cent.[36] The shorter the interval between exposure to the anesthetic agent and the development of symptoms, the worse is the prognosis. A history of prior exposure to halothane makes the prognosis even more dire. Treatment is merely supportive. Steroids have been used and are recommended, but their efficacy is uncertain. The disease is thought to be secondary to an idiosyncratic hypersensitivity reaction and not secondary to a general hepatotoxic property of the anesthetic agent itself. Since repeated exposures to halothane increase the chances of developing halothane hepatitis by as much as sevenfold, they should be avoided. If a patient has had prior halothane anesthesia, particularly within the past 3 months, halothane should be avoided.

OCCULT BILIARY TRACT TUMORS

Occasionally, postoperative jaundice may be the result of missing an occult biliary tract tumor at the time of cholecystectomy or common duct exploration. Symptoms of occult biliary tract tumors frequently simulate those of calculous disease and result in an exploratory laparotomy. These tumors are often associated with stones and occasionally are so small that unless one is specifically looking for a malignancy they can easily be missed. Postoperatively, jaundice then appears in the days or weeks that follow, because of edema from operative manipulation or progression of the tumor. The tumor with which this sequence is most frequently associated is the so-called Klatskin tumor, a small adenocarcinoma occurring at the bifurcation of the right and left hepatic ducts. These malignancies are small and slow-growing and slow to metastasize. Even though they originate at the hepatic duct bifurcation, they usually initially obstruct only the right or left hepatic duct. This results in mild non-specific right upper quadrant symptoms and alkaline phosphatase and transaminase elevations. The bilirubin remains normal because one-half of

the liver continues to drain normally. At the time of surgery the extrahepatic biliary tree may look entirely normal. The Klatskin tumor at the bifurcation may be so small that palpation of the porta hepatis will not reveal its presence. The gallbladder, whether or not it contains stones, often is removed because of the liver function abnormalities. An operative cholangiogram will reveal a perfectly normal extrahepatic biliary tree and portions of a normal intrahepatic biliary tree. Because of the general propensity of surgeons to accept less-than-perfect operative cholangiography, often the operation will be terminated at this point. Postoperatively, the patient becomes jaundiced, because the surgical manipulation has produced enough edema to occlude the remaining open duct at the bifurcation. At this point, because of the recent negative biliary exploration, further consideration of a mechanical biliary tract obstruction may be put off for a period of weeks or months until the jaundice has deepened. The patient will eventually come to reoperation for biliary decompression. At reexploration careful dissection of the porta hepatis will allow resection of only 20 to 30 per cent of lesions. In the remainder, it will be necessary to dilate the tumor and stent the malignant stricture, preferably with a transhepatic Silastic biliary stent.[5] This sequence can be avoided if one is aware of the manner in which a Klatskin tumor presents and if one obtains either percutaneous or endoscopic retrograde cholangiography preoperatively when one is suspicious of the lesion (Fig. 21–7). In addition, one must insist upon technically adequate cholangiography visualizing the entire intra- and extrahepatic biliary tree at the time of surgery. If the lesion is missed and the patient becomes jaundiced days or weeks following surgery, at this point transhepatic cholangiography probably will reveal the anatomy most satisfactorily.

Carcinoma of the gallbladder can also result in this sequence of postoperative jaundice developing after a cholecystectomy. Carcinoma of the gallbladder presents as acute cholecystitis in 20 per cent of cases. If the tumor is relatively small and is present in a markedly dilated, thickened, and inflamed gallbladder, the surgeon may not appreciate the primary diagnosis. Tech-

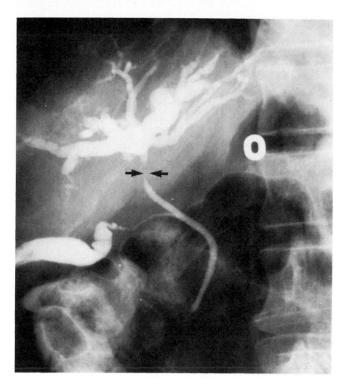

Figure 21–7 A 52-year-old patient with a malignant tumor (arrows) identified just below the hepatic duct bifurcation (Klatskin tumor). These lesions are so small that their identification either grossly or by cholangiography at the time of surgery can be very difficult.

nically, the cholecystectomy may be difficult to perform and a portion of the gallbladder often is left in place. Only postoperatively when the specimen has been examined will the diagnosis be made. This is usually followed in a matter of days or weeks by the development of jaundice from perioperative edema and from progression of the tumor. Carcinoma of the gallbladder is essentially an incurable lesion, except in those instances when a small occult malignancy is removed in its entirety at the time of a cholecystectomy. Rarely, reexploration with the hopes of a curative resection may be indicated. However, in most instances when jaundice develops, the patient will be best treated by non-operative biliary decompression. This can best be accomplished by the percutaneous insertion of a Ring catheter stent.[26] In most instances these catheters can be threaded through the obstructed biliary tree into the duodenum, and internal drainage can be established. If the catheter cannot be passed through the tumor into the duodenum, external decompression is established. This may be combined with radiotherapy and allow adequate palliation for the patient without the need for reoperation. Reexploration in such instances often is unsuccessful in establishing decompression and may not be well tolerated in patients with incurable malignancies.

The presence of a distal bile duct or periampullary carcinoma may also occasionally be missed at the time of cholecystectomy and present in the postoperative period with jaundice. Periampullary tumors early in their course, prior to the development of jaundice, may result in non-specific right upper quadrant symptoms and a distended gallbladder. If the surgeon does not carefully examine the periampullary area at the time of surgery and is not alerted by the minimally dilated biliary tree, an early periampullary tumor responsible for the patient's clinical presentation may be missed. Gallstones are so common in this country that the patient may indeed have gallstones. If the surgeon attributes the patient's signs and symptoms to gallstone disease, the periampullary tumor will be missed. Even a cholangiogram at the time of cholecystectomy, if not technically of excellent quality, may not show the lesion. In such a situation if jaundice develops in the postoperative period, further work-up with either endoscopic retrograde or transhepatic cholangiography will be necessary and should reveal the pathology. Such a patient will require reexploration with the hopes of performing a curative pancreaticoduodenectomy.

OPERATIVE INJURY TO THE BILIARY TREE

There is perhaps no situation in surgery in which a routine operative procedure becomes more complicated, with more potential for tragic long-term results, than when a bile duct injury occurs during a cholecystomy. In all likelihood some of the injuries result during an attempt to control bleeding. In over 30 per cent of the strictures referred to the Johns Hopkins Hospital for repair, hemoclips had been used during the preceding cholecystectomy, and in several instances the clips have been identified across the biliary tree (Fig. 21–8). When one is in the habit of utilizing hemoclips, it is very tempting in the face of bleeding to insert a clip in the base of a pool of blood. It is much safer to control bleeding with pres-

sure and suture ligate with adequate suction visualization than to use hemostats or clips without adequate visualization. If hemoclips are used during cholecystectomy, they should be used with great caution. In most instances, however, bile duct injuries are probably secondary to either inadequate visualization of the junction between the cystic duct and common duct or secondary to an anatomic anomaly.

Iatrogenic biliary tract injuries are all avoidable. If one is exploring a patient with an acutely or subacutely inflamed gallbladder and it is technically impossible to differentiate the structures in the porta hepatis, it is acceptable to perform a cholecystostomy. The patient can be reexplored several months later at a time when the inflammation has subsided. Absolute identification of the anatomy at the time of cholecystectomy is essential. Before ligating and dividing the cystic duct, its junction with the common and common hepatic ducts should be identified clearly. Relying upon size of the tubular biliary tract for identification is inadequate. A normal common bile duct may be as small as 2 to 3 mm. Therefore, small size does not

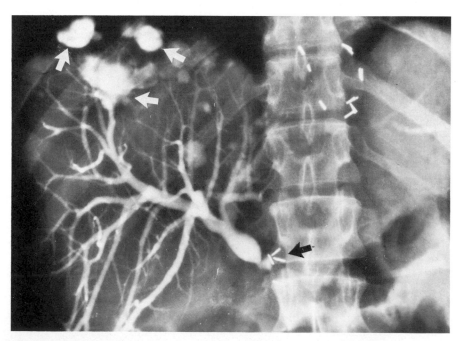

Figure 21–8   Percutaneous transhepatic cholangiogram in a deeply jaundiced patient who had recently undergone a cholecystectomy and pyloroplasty and vagotomy. The cholangiogram demonstrates complete obstruction of the biliary tree at the site of the cystocholedochal junction. At reoperation, a hemoclip was found across the common duct (black arrow). The cholangiogram also demonstrates liver abscesses (white arrow) secondary to cholangitis.

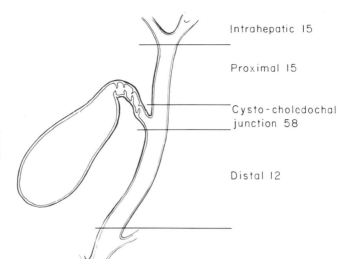

Intrahepatic 15

Proximal 15

Cysto-choledochal junction 58

Distal 12

Figure 21–9 The site of injury in 100 patients with iatrogenic biliary tract injuries with complete obstruction to the flow of bile from the liver to the duodenum. (From Glenn, F.: Iatrogenic injuries to the biliary duct system. Surg. Gynecol. Obstet. *146*:430, 1978.)

identify a duct as the cystic duct and exclude the possibility of it being the common, common hepatic, or right hepatic duct. Anatomic anomalies can present very confusing anatomic patterns. A low confluence of the junction between the right and left hepatic ducts can place the right hepatic duct at risk of ligature, confusing it with the cystic duct. Origin of the cystic duct from the right hepatic duct can also be confusing at the time of cholecystectomy. Possibly one of the more common anatomic anomalies resulting in biliary tract injury is that of a short cystic duct. In this instance if the anatomy of the junction between the cystic and common ducts is not clearly identified, stenting of the common duct at the time of gallbladder removal can result in a tangential injury. In a series of 100 bile strictures reviewed by Glenn,[13] 88 per cent involved the junction of the cystic and common ducts (58 per cent), the common hepatic duct (15 per cent), or one of the hepatic ducts at the bifurcation (15 per cent). In only 12 instances was the injury to the common bile duct (Fig. 21–9). This suggests that inadequate visualization of the anatomy in the porta hepatis in the area of the junction of the cystic duct with the biliary tree was the cause of the majority of injuries. Perhaps the single most important technique that surgeons could adopt in an effort to decrease or eliminate iatrogenic biliary tract injuries is the routine of cholecystectomy described some time ago.[11] This

technique involves identification of the structures of the porta hepatis first, with the looping of the cystic duct and cystic artery with 2-0 black silk. One throw is placed in each suture so as to occlude the presumed cystic duct and cystic artery, without crushing or injuring the structures. The gallbladder is then removed from above downward, maintaining the dissection immediately adjacent to the gallbladder wall. If one is unsure of the anatomy any time during the dissection, the dissection should be interrupted and an operative cholangiogram performed through the already isolated cystic duct. If no confusion arises during the cholecystectomy, then at the point where the gallbladder is completely mobilized and connected only by the cystic duct, an operative cholangiogram should be performed. It is our feeling that routine operative cholangiography is of benefit not only in attempting to detect silent common duct stones, but also, and perhaps even more important, in defining anatomic anomalies that might lead to ductal injury.

Ductal Injury Recognized at the Time of Surgery

If the ductal injury is recognized at the time it occurs, the course of action depends upon what portion of the biliary tract has been injured and the extent of the injury. If a subsegmental duct has been divided that is 2 mm. in diameter or less, any attempt at repair is certain to fail and is unnecessary. If the biliary tree is not infected, as will most frequently be the case, secure ligature of the divided duct with adequate drainage of the stump is the appropriate course of action. As long as the biliary tree does not become infected postoperatively the patient will remain asymptomatic, and that portion of the liver drained by the ligated duct will atrophy. This is also the appropriate course of action when a small segmental branch of the right or left hepatic duct is injured. This will involve most frequently the segmental branch to the right dorsal caudal segment of the liver, which arises from the right hepatic duct. This segmental branch occasionally arises from the right hepatic duct low enough in the porta hepatis to be mistaken for the cystic duct. The outside diameter of this duct may be only 3 mm. The chance of a successful repair with a structure this small is very low. It has been well documented that there is sufficient liver reserve so that one can safely ligate a segmental branch without danger of a clinically significant decrease in hepatic function. Longmire and Tompkins[23] have demonstrated that even in the face of complete lobar obstruction, sufficient hepatic function remains to maintain a normal serum bilirubin. Surgeons should consider an injury to any biliary structure of any size at the time of cholecystectomy as a tragic error and make every effort to avoid its occurrence. Nevertheless, when the structure is small in diameter and segmental or subsegmental in distribution, it is better ligated without attempt at repair.

More frequently, however, the injury will be to the common or common hepatic duct in the area of the junction with the cystic duct. If the injury is small or tangential, such as with a cautery burn, and does not include most of the circumference of the duct, a local repair may be feasible. Also, in rare instances, if the area of injury is small, it may be used as the site for insertion of a T-tube with closure of the defect around the long arm. In most instances, however, local repairs will not be possible. There will be either a circumferential defect in the biliary tree or, in order to obtain uninjured tissue both proximally and distally, a segment of duct will need to be debrided and resected. If the defect remaining is 1 cm. or less in length, the duodenum can generally be mobilized adequately and the ends of the duct brought together without tension for an end-to-end anastomosis (Fig. 21–10). A T-tube should be inserted above the line of repair to decompress the anastomosis. The T-tube should not be brought out the suture line, but one arm should extend through the anastomosis. The T-tube is used not so much as a stent but as a means to decompress the biliary tree and prevent bile leakage through the anastomosis that subsequently could lead to fibrosis, scarring, and stricture formation. If the repair is technically satisfactory, the T-tube should be removed in 6 weeks to 3 months. If more than

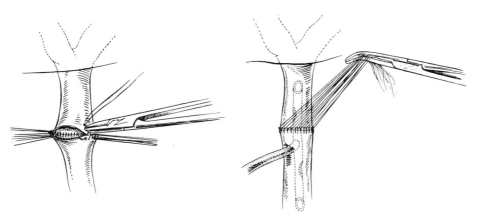

Figure 21–10 An end-to-end anastomosis is performed when an acute biliary tract injury is identified. Fine suture material is used on atraumatic needles, taking care to place the ties on the outside. The T-tube is inserted with one arm of the T extending through the anastomosis.

1 cm. of duct has been injured or removed, and the resulting defect is in excess of 1 cm., an attempt should not be made to perform an end-to-end biliary anastomosis. Tension on the anastomosis will almost certainly result in at least partial dehiscence with subsequent stricture formation. In this instance a defunctionalized Roux-en-Y jejunal loop should be constructed. The end of the Roux-en-Y loop should be closed and an end-to-side choledochojejunostomy performed. This anastomosis should also be decompressed by the placement of a T-tube in the common duct with one arm through the anastomosis into the jejunum. In this instance also the T-tube is placed for decompression rather than for stenting and should probably be removed between 6 weeks and 3 months following the repair, if cholangiography demonstrates adequate healing. A variety of suture materials have been advocated for biliary anastomoses, with no one being clearly superior. The synthetic absorbable sutures would appear to have certain theoretical advantages. Care should be taken to place all knots on the outside of the anastomosis.

One would assume that the primary repair of a bile duct injury recognized at the time of occurrence would be followed by long-term results superior to those obtained from delayed repairs. This is often stated in texts, but there are very few data to support this conclusion. In a review published by Longmire,[22] only one of eight immediate repairs was successful, in comparison with 11 of 16 delayed primary repairs. Perhaps the lack of experience of the initial surgeon results in the biliary tract injury and also is responsible for the less-than-acceptable results with primary repair. Certainly under any circumstances it is recommended that if a bile duct injury occurs, a consultation in the operating room should be obtained with the surgeon in the hospital or community who has the greatest experience in reconstructive biliary tract surgery. Under certain circumstances, such as many hours into an operative procedure with an unstable patient, it might be best merely to ligate the biliary tract, particularly if the common duct is very small and a primary repair exceedingly difficult. This would allow time over the succeeding days or weeks for the biliary tract to dilate and for the surgeon to obtain

consultation and advice from an experienced biliary tract surgeon, or possibly to transfer the patient to a center in which reconstructive biliary tract surgery is performed.

Ductal Injury Recognized Following Surgery

In most instances injury to the biliary tract is not recognized at the time of cholecystectomy. Only subsequently when it is apparent that the patient's postoperative course is not routine will a common duct injury be suspected. The development of jaundice within the first few days of surgery will often be the presenting sign. Copious drainage of bile through the wound or along a drain tract is also a common means of presentation. Sepsis secondary to cholangitis, or less frequently, sepsis secondary to the accumulation of bile in the subhepatic space or throughout the peritoneal cavity is another means by which an iatrogenic bile duct injury can be manifested.

In rare instances evidence of an injury will not become apparent for weeks, months, or even years following surgery. In most instances, however, a significant bile duct injury will be obvious in the immediate postoperative period. If the injury is accompanied by the accumulation of significant quantities of bile in the peritoneal cavity, with or without infection, the initial management may require reexploration, drainage, and the establishment of an external biliary fistula. Most of the time, however, immediate reexploration will be neither necessary nor advisable. The patient will have evidence of increasing jaundice or copious bile flow along the drains and should be placed on antibiotics to prevent biliary tract sepsis. Then, at an appropriate time, perhaps 2 to 3 weeks following surgery, cholangiography should be performed to confirm the diagnosis and to identify the site of injury. With current techniques, the anatomy of the biliary tract and the site of pathology should be identifiable in every instance. If the patient has significant bile flow through the drain site, a sinogram may well identify the site of injury and fill the biliary tree satisfactorily to obtain all necessary information. In those instances in which bile drainage has not occurred and the patient has developed progressive jaundice, a transhepatic cholangiogram will identify the site of injury (see Fig. 21–8). In addition, the catheter can be left in place to establish external biliary drainage to allow for improvement in hepatic function prior to reexploration for repair.

Less frequently, endoscopic retrograde cholangiography will be helpful. Since in many instances there will be a complete division or occlusion of the biliary tree, cholangiography performed retrograde will demonstrate only the distal blind end of the biliary tree and will not provide the needed information concerning the proximal biliary tract. Only if the injury is partial and the hyperbilirubinemia in a low or intermediate range will endoscopic retrograde cholangiography be helpful.

The appropriate management of a bile duct injury recognized several days after cholecystectomy depends upon the clinical status of the patient. As mentioned above, if the patient is septic and has accumulated a significant amount of interperitoneal bile, or if an interperitoneal abscess has developed, reexploration is necessary for drainage. In most instances, however, the biliary tree will be completely occluded with no external drainage, or satisfactory drainage will occur along the drain tract. There often

is a sense of urgency with the surgeon who has performed the cholecystectomy to reoperate upon the patient and carry out an early repair. However, the reexploration of a patient for reconstructive biliary surgery who has undergone a cholecystectomy only 1 or 2 weeks earlier is technically very difficult. If possible, one should wait for at least 3 to 4 weeks before reexploring the patient. If the patient is completely obstructed, one of two courses may be pursued. If the patient is young and healthy and has adequate liver reserve, one may choose to allow the patient to remain obstructed with the plan of reexploration in 3 or 4 weeks, at a time when the biliary tract is maximally dilated. With a markedly dilated biliary tree one has the best opportunity to effect a satisfactory repair. On the other hand, if the patient is elderly or does not have a great deal of hepatic reserve, or if the patient has evidence of cholangitis, percutaneous decompression with a transhepatic catheter can be performed (Fig. 21–11).[26] This procedure can be performed under local anesthesia by radiologists in most hospitals in this country. It is performed by first obtaining a percutaneous cholangiogram. Once the biliary tree is visualized, a guide wire can be inserted and positioned. A drainage catheter can then be placed into the biliary tree

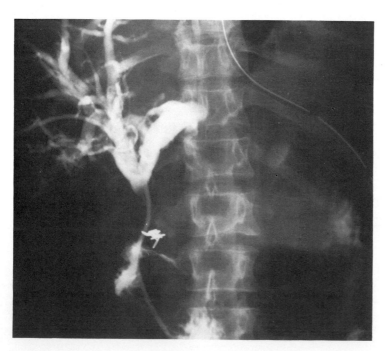

Figure 21–11 Internal decompression by a Ring catheter in a 50-year-old patient with an iatrogenic common duct injury. The patient became septic one week following the duct injury and was not a good risk for re-exploration and stricture repair at that time. A percutaneous cholangiogram was performed, and then using a guide wire, the Ring catheter was inserted through the stricture and into the duodenum. The Ring catheter contains multiple side holes so bile can drain into the catheter above the stricture and then out into the duodenum. This form of decompression can be utilized until the patient is in suitable condition for stricture repair.

over the guide wire. The catheter can be connected to external bile bag drainage, thereby decompressing the liver. This will allow for recovery of hepatic function and control of sepsis by decreasing intrabiliary pressure. Thereafter, the timing of the repair is important. Even though the patient can be left in this situation for weeks or indeed months, the decompressed biliary tract will eventually return to normal size, making the repair more difficult. Therefore, the patient should probably be reoperated upon after allowing approximately 2 weeks to pass to gain control of sepsis and improvement of liver function.

Technique

Over the past several decades biliary tract surgeons have debated two major technical aspects of stricture repair: whether or not to use a long-term biliary stent, and whether to use the distal bile duct, duodenum, or jejunum for the anastomosis to the proximal biliary segment. These questions are now fairly well resolved. For most established strictures when a mucosa-to-mucosa anastomosis cannot be carried out, the majority of surgeons prefer long-term stenting in the range of 6 months to 1 year. In addition, very few surgeons now feel that an end-to-end anastomosis between the dilated proximal biliary segment and the distal small biliary segment offers any benefit. The distal segment is usually difficult to find, often is small, thick-walled, and fibrotic, and technically is difficult to anastomose to the dilated proximal segment. In addition, there is often a gap that greatly exceeds 1 cm., and the repair will be under tension. Therefore, except in the acute situation when the injury is recognized at the time of its occurrence, biliary-to-biliary reconstruction is seldom indicated. Anastomosis of the proximal biliary segment to the duodenum also is not currently favored by most biliary tract surgeons. Although the duodenum can usually be mobilized sufficiently to reach the porta hepatis for an anastomosis, if a leak occurs following repair, one is dealing not only with a biliary-cutaneous fistula but also with a duodenal-cutaneous fistula, which greatly complicates management. Thus, most surgeons feel that an anastomosis to a defunctionalized Roux-en-Y jejunal loop, in combination with long-term stenting, is the preferred method for dealing with an established stricture. Following this repair, if a leak occurs at the anastomosis because the jejunum is defunctionalized, it will not interfere with normal bowel recovery and alimentation. The presence of a long-term stent will allow healing at the anastomosis, even in the face of a leak, and if left in long enough will allow a stable scar to form and contract so that when the stent is removed 6 months to a year later, recurrence of the stricture is less likely.

A technique of repair for benign strictures that has met with a high degree of success has been used at the Johns Hopkins Hospital for the past 10 years.[5, 6] All patients undergo percutaneous cholangiography immediately prior to repair, with the placement of a catheter in the biliary tree at the site of the stricture in the proximal biliary segment. The patient is then taken to the operating room and under general anesthesia is explored through a generous right upper quadrant incision. In a particularly obese patient with a deep chest, we have occasionally teed the incision off into the right chest to achieve adequate exposure. The most difficult and time consuming part of the operation is the identification of the proximal biliary segment. This may take a matter of only 30 or 45 minutes, or it may take the operating surgeon several hours if there is a good deal of edema and fibrosis in the porta hepatis. The prior placement of the catheter by the radiologist aids in the identification of this proximal segment, and when located, reassures the surgeon that he has correctly entered the biliary tree at the point of the stricture. If an adequate proximal segment with good mucosa and little fibrosis is present, an end-to-side hepaticojejunostomy can be carried out with a mucosa-to-mucosa anastomosis. The anastomosis is performed with one of the synthetic absorbable sutures, carefully placing the knots on the outside. A T-tube can be placed in the proximal biliary segment with one arm through the enteric anastomosis to decompress the biliary tract, much as with an acute primary repair. Following a mucosa-to-mucosa repair, it is not necessary to leave the stent in for a long period, and it can be removed in 6 weeks to 3 months.

However, in the great majority of repairs one will not have a normal proximal biliary segment with good normal mucosa. Even though the injury in most instances will have been to the biliary tract near its junction with the cystic duct, the inflammation will extend to the porta hepatis, because of bile leakage and infection. Thus, in many stricture repairs one will be dealing with a short proximal biliary segment high in the hilum of the liver. In this instance a good mucosa-to-mucosa repair will be unlikely. In such a situation the anastomosis should be stented long-term with a Silastic transhepatic biliary stent. This can be inserted by placing stone forceps into the intrahepatic biliary tree through the proximal biliary segment, into either the right or left hepatic duct. The instrument is passed as close to the surface of the liver as possible. This will usually take it within a centimeter of Glisson's capsule. The instrument is then forced through Glisson's capsule, and a Silastic transhepatic biliary stent grasped and pulled back down through the liver parenchyma, through the intrahepatic biliary tree, and out the proximal biliary segment into the porta hepatis. The end that emanates from the superior surface of the liver is brought out through a stab wound in the anterior abdominal wall and is connected to bile bag drainage. The end that exits through the proximal biliary segment is placed into a stab wound in the side of a Roux-en-Y loop. The Roux-en-Y loop is anastomosed or tacked up to the porta hepatis in the vicinity of the proximal biliary segment. Usually part of the proximal biliary segment can be used for the anastomosis. Often, however, it is not intact circumferentially and one has to tack the loop to liver parenchyma, Glisson's capsule, or any other tissue in the vicinity of the porta hepatis (Fig. 21–12). The Silastic transhepatic stent should have an outside diameter of at least 6 mm. It can be made from a 60 cm. length of medical grade Silastic. Side hole perforations are placed in 40 per cent of the length. The stent is positioned so that the portion of the tube within the intrahepatic biliary tree, the anastomosis, and the Roux-en-Y loop contains the side holes. That portion of the stent that emanates from the top of the liver, through the peritoneal cavity, and out through a stab wound in the upper abdomen obviously should contain no holes. The anastomosis is drained, as is the stent exit site on the diaphragmatic surface of the liver. The stent is left to bile bag drainage postoperatively, until cholangiography demonstrates no bile leaks at the anastomosis or at the exit site of the stent through the superior surface of the liver. At that point the tube is clamped. The patient is taught to irrigate the tube twice a day with 50 ml. of saline. The stent is left in place for 1 year. Since the stent is Silastic, it tends to collect sludge very slowly. However, if side holes become occluded with sludge, the stent can easily be changed as an outpatient procedure by first inserting a stylet through the entire length of the stent, then removing the old stent,

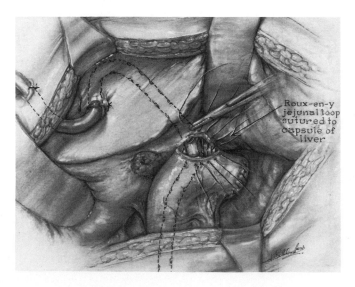

Roux-en-y jejunal loop sutured to capsule of liver

Figure 21–12 After insertion of the transhepatic Silastic biliary stent, the Roux-en-Y jejunal loop is tacked up to the porta hepatis to any available structures. That portion of the stent that resides in the liver, biliary tree, and jejunum contains multiple side holes. That portion of the stent that exits from the liver and is brought out the anterior abdominal wall to be connected to bile bag drainage contains no side holes. (From Cameron, J. L. et al.: The use of Silastic transhepatic stents in benign and malignant biliary strictures. Ann. Surg. *188*:552, 1978.)

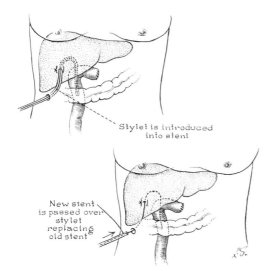

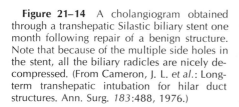

Figure 21–13 The transhepatic Silastic biliary stents can easily be changed by first inserting a guide wire or pliable stylet into the jejunum through the old stent. The old stent is then removed and a new stent inserted over the guide wire. The guide wire is then removed. (From Cameron, J. L. et al.: Long-term transhepatic intubation for hilar hepatic duct strictures. Ann. Surg. *183*:488, 1976.)

leaving the stylet in place, and, finally, threading a new stent over the stylet back into the Roux-en-Y loop (Fig. 21–13). Changing of the stent may be necessary as often as every 3 to 4 months. Use of a Silastic transhepatic stent has several advantages: it can be securely fixed at the skin with wire sutures so that migration cannot occur; it tends to accumulate biliary sludge more slowly than rubber stents; since Silastic is relative non-reactive it allows healing to take place with a minimum of foreign body reaction; serial cholangiograms can be performed (Fig. 21–14); and if left in for an entire 12-month period the scar at the anastomotic site will have matured, contracted, and stabilized so that when the stent is removed, restricture is unlikely. The technique is easy to perform and is followed by a high rate of success.

Bibliography

1. Almquist, H. J., and Stokstad, E. L. R: Hemorrhagic chick disease of dietary origin. J. Biol. Chem. *111*:105, 1935.
2. Altemeir, W. A., Schowengerdt, C. G., and Whitely, D. H.: Abscess of the liver. Surgical considerations. Arch. Surg. *101*:258, 1970.
3. Birkett, D. H., and Williams, L. F.: Choledochoscopic removal of retained stones via a T-tube tract. Am. J. Surg. *139*:531, 1980.
4. Burhenne, H. J.: Complications of nonoperative extraction of retained common duct stones. Am. J. Surg. *131*:260, 1976.
5. Cameron, J. L., Gayler, B. W., and Zuidema, G. D.: The use of Silastic transhepatic stents in benign and malignant biliary strictures. Ann. Surg. *188*:552, 1978.

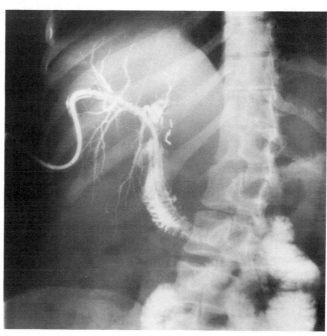

Figure 21–14 A cholangiogram obtained through a transhepatic Silastic biliary stent one month following repair of a benign structure. Note that because of the multiple side holes in the stent, all the biliary radicles are nicely decompressed. (From Cameron, J. L. et al.: Long-term transhepatic intubation for hilar duct structures. Ann. Surg. *183*:488, 1976.)

6. Cameron, J. L., Skinner, D. B., and Zuidema, G. D.: Long-term transhepatic intubation for hilar hepatic duct strictures. Ann. Surg. *183*:488, 1976.
7. Conn, J. H., Chavez, C. M., and Fain, W. R.: Bile peritonitis. Am. Surgeon *36*:219, 1970.
8. Dam, H.: The antihemorrhagic vitamin of the chick: Occurrence and chemical nature. Nature *135*:652, 1935.
9. Dineen, P., and McSherry, C. K.: Subdiaphragmatic abscess. Ann. Surg. *155*:506, 1962.
10. Feliciano, D. V., Mattox, K. L., and Jordan, G. L.: The value of choledochoscopy in exploration of the common bile duct. Ann. Surg. *191*:649, 1980.
11. Glenn, F.: Atlas of Biliary Tract Surgery. New York, MacMillan Company, 1963, p. 28.
12. Glenn, F.: Common Bile Duct Stones. Springfield, Ill., Charles C Thomas, 1975, p. 68.
13. Glenn, F.: Iatrogenic injuries to the biliary ductal system. Surg. Gynecol. Obstet. *146*:430, 1978.
14. Haff, R. C., and Wise, L.: Postoperative hemorrhage and abscess formation following biliary tract surgery. Am. Surg. *38*:295, 1972.
15. Hagen-Ansert, S. L.: Textbook of Diagnostic Ultrasonography. St. Louis, C. V. Mosby, 1978.
16. Hays, D. M., and Glenn, F.: The fate of the cholecystostomy patient. J. Am. Geriatrics Soc. *3*:21, 1955.
17. Heimbach, D. N., and White, T. T.: Immediate and long term effects of instrumental dilation of the sphincter of Oddi. Surg. Gynecol. Obstet. *148*:79, 1979.
18. Heuer, G. J.: The factors leading to death in operations upon the gall bladder and bile ducts. Ann. Surg. *99*:881, 1934.
19. Historical Statistics of the U.S. Colonial Times to 1970. Washington, U.S. Dept. of Commerce, Bureau of the Census, 1975, Part 1, p. 15.
20. Imrie, C. W., McKay, A. J., Benjamin, I. S., and Blumgart, L. H.: Secondary acute pancreatitis: Aetiology, prevention, diagnosis and management. Br. J. Surg. *65*:399, 1980.
21. Keighley, M. R. B., and Kappas, A.: Evaluation of operative choledochoscopy. Surg. Gynecol. Obstet. *150*:357, 1978.
22. Longmire, W. P.: The diverse causes of biliary obstruction and their remedies. Curr. Probl. Surg. *14*(7):1, 1977.
23. Longmire, W. P., and Tompkins, R. K.: Lesions of the segmental and lobar hepatic ducts. Ann. Surg. *182*:478, 1975.
24. Means, R. L.: Bile peritonitis. Am. Surg. *30*:583, 1964.
25. Pilcher, D. B.: Penetrating injuries of the liver in Vietnam. Ann. Surg. *170*:793, 1970.
26. Pollock, T. W., Ring, E. R., Oleaga, J. A., Freiman, D. B., Mullen, J. L., and Rosato, E. F.: Percutaneous decompression of benign and malignant biliary obstruction. Arch. Surg. *114*:148, 1979.
27. Quick, A. G., Stanley-Brown, M., and Bancroft, F. W.: A study of the coagulation defects in hemophilia and in jaundice. Am. J. Med. Sc. *190*:501, 1935.
28. Robson, M. C., Bogart, J. M., and Heggers, J. P.: An endogenous source of wound infections based on quantitative bacteriology of the biliary tract. Surgery *86*:471, 1970.
28a. Sherlock, S.: Halothane hepatitis. *In* Davison, C. S. (Ed.): Problems in Liver Diseases. New York, Stratton International Book Corp., 1979.
29. Skillings, J. C., Kumai, C., and Hinshaw, J. R.: Cholecystostomy: A place in modern biliary surgery? Am. J. Surg. *139*:865, 1980.
30. Statistical Bulletin. Metropolitan Life Ins. Co. *61*: (2) 13, 1980.
31. Stull, J. R., and Thomford, N. R.: Biliary intestinal fistula. Am. J. Surg. *120*:27, 1970.
32. Way, L. W.: Retained common duct stones. Surg. Clin. North Am. *53*:1139, 1973.
33. Way, L. W., Admirand, W. H., and Dunphy, J. E.: Management of choledocholithiasis. Ann. Surg. *176*:347, 1972.
34. Way, L. W., and Motson, R. W.: Dissolution of retained common bile duct stones. Adv. Surg. *10*:99, 1976.
35. White, T. T., and Bordley, J.: One percent incidence of recurrent gallstones six to eight years after manometric cholangiography. Ann. Surg. *188*:562, 1978.
36. Zimmerman, H. J.: Hepatotoxicity: The Adverse Effects of Drugs and Other Chemicals on the Liver. New York, Appleton-Century-Crofts, 1978, p. 376.
37. Zimmon, D. S.: Endoscopic diagnosis and management of biliary and pancreatic disease. Curr. Probl. Surg. *16*(3):1, 1979.

22

COMPLICATIONS OF PANCREATIC AND SPLENIC SURGERY

George L. Jordan, Jr.

COMPLICATIONS OF PANCREATIC SURGERY

Historically, the incidence of complications following pancreatic trauma and surgery, including those ending fatally, was so high that many surgeons avoided operations upon this gland. The complication rate remains relatively high, as compared with that following operation on other organs, but fortunately these complications can usually be treated successfully (Table 22–1).

Some of the problems of pancreatic surgery relate directly to the anatomy of this organ (Fig. 22–1), and certain points deserve emphasis.

The blood supply is unusual in that the arterial supply is from multiple sources. Most of the pancreatic arteries are short branches from a major artery that primarily supplies another viscus. The venous drainage is similar, there being multiple short, friable veins that enter directly into a major vein draining other organs. These major veins — the splenic, superior mesenteric, and portal veins — are often completely surrounded by pancreatic tissue. It is impossible to remove the entire head and uncinate process without removing the duodenum, and the hepatic artery must be dissected carefully. In most instances, removal of the tail is accomplished more easily by removing the spleen as a part of the specimen than by trying to dissect the splenic artery and vein from the pancreas. Furthermore, chronic inflammation or neoplastic lesions may cause adherence to other major vessels, particularly the vena cava and the superior mesenteric artery. In addition to having a common blood supply with the pancreas, the duodenum is firmly attached to the head of the pancreas so that its removal requires dissection of the head of the pancreas, as well as division of the major and minor ducts at their points of entrance into the duodenum. Lastly, the common bile duct runs in a groove on the under surface of the gland, and a part of the duct is completely surrounded by pancreatic tissue. In most instances, the common bile duct joins the duct of Wirsung before entering the duodenum. Consequently, detailed evaluation of disease of the head of the pancreas requires dissection and exploration of the

---

George L. Jordan is a North Carolinian who was elected to Phi Beta Kappa at the University of North Carolina and to Alpha Omega Alpha at Baylor College of Medicine. After interning at Grady Memorial Hospital, he received his surgical training at Tulane University and the Mayo Clinic. In 1952 he joined the faculty at Baylor University and in 1964 was made full Professor. A member of many important national committees and surgical societies covering a wide range of clinical and scientific expertise, Dr. Jordan has been especially interested in the physiology and diseases of the pancreas. His significant contributions in this field are universally recognized.

TABLE 22–1   COMPLICATIONS OF PANCREATIC
SURGERY

  I. Fistula
   A. Pancreatic
   B. Duodenal
   C. Biliary
   D. Gastric
  II. Pancreatitis
 III. Hemorrhage
 IV. Operative injury to adjacent structures
  V. Mesenteric thrombosis
 VI. Infection
   A. Intra-abdominal abscess
   B. Peritonitis
VII. Hepatic failure
VIII. Renal insufficiency
 IX. Stricture of the common bile duct
  X. Marginal ulcer
 XI. Metabolic problems
   A. Diabetes
   B. Deficiency of exocrine secretion

duodenum and the common bile duct as well as of the gland itself.

Another anatomic factor of importance is the retroperitoneal location of the gland. It is not surrounded by a serosal surface, and an extensive dissection of the retroperitoneal area must be accomplished to perform a detailed exploration of the organ. The tensile strength of the normal gland is low, so that sutures easily tear through its substance. Thus, sutures must be placed with precision and tied with care. This problem is less pronounced when surgery is performed for chronic pancreatitis, for this disease process results in dense fibrosis that increases the strength of the tissue. It is not possible, however, to enfold the gland to obtain good approximation of the external surfaces.

The anatomy of the gland is of further importance because it is impossible to place sutures without damage to actively secreting cells, and the potential for leakage of pancreatic juice along a suture tract always exists. Because of the potency of the pancreatic enzymes in digestion of carbohydrates, fats, and proteins, any leakage of pancreatic juice is potentially serious.

PANCREATIC FISTULA

The most common complication of pancreatic surgery is pancreatic fistula. Because of its frequency and because of earlier reports concerning morbidity and mortality, it is one of the most feared complications of pancreatic surgery. The frequency with which pancreatic fistula develops is predicated, to some degree, upon the anatomy and physiology of the gland. As already noted, any injury or incision into the gland necessarily transects cells that normally secrete proteolytic enzymes and pancreatic ducts draining these cells must also be transected. The anatomic factors previously noted make fistula formation a special hazard. The incidence of pancreatic fistula is significantly greater when there has been deep penetration of the head of the gland by external trauma, so that one of the major ducts is injured, in contradistinction to a very superficial laceration or biopsy near the tail where the ducts are small. Furthermore, as noted previously, pancreatic fistula occurs more commonly after surgery on the normal gland than when operation is performed after several attacks of pancreatitis.

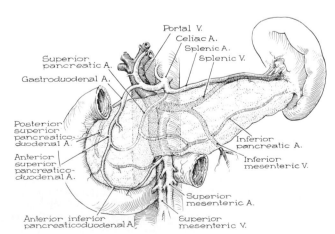

Figure 22–1 An illustration to demonstrate the blood supply and some important anatomic relations of the pancreas. The common bile duct is not shown.

Thus, if sutures are not placed carefully in the normal pancreas, the suture itself may produce some laceration of the gland and a pancreatic fistula may occur from the area of the suture placement rather than from the area of injury or incision into the gland.

Etiologic Factors

TRAUMA. The most common cause of pancreatic fistula in the United States is external trauma. External trauma to the pancreas was considered an uncommon lesion as recently as 10 to 15 years ago, but throughout the United States traumatic lesions of the pancreas are seen with increasing frequency. In the Baylor Affiliated Hospitals, more patients are treated for traumatic lesions of the pancreas than for all other pancreatic lesions combined; and the incidence of pancreatic fistula following external trauma is higher than the incidence of pancreatic fistula following treatment of any other lesion.[40, 44] In many instances, there is actual loss of pancreatic tissue which prevents reapproximation of the gland, and even if the damaged area is resected, closure of the transected end cannot always be performed without development of fistula. This is of particular significance because there is increasing interest in resective management of pancreatic injuries.[3, 6, 43] To date, however, the evidence does not support the concept that resective treatment can be accomplished with a lower mortality rate than simple repair and drainage. It does not decrease significantly the incidence of subsequent pancreatic fistula. In our experience, pancreatic fistula develops in 31 per cent of patients sustaining pancreatic trauma. The incidence of pancreatic fistula is higher after blunt trauma than after penetrating trauma, owing to delay in diagnosis in some patients with blunt trauma and inability to accomplish proper surgical repair of the pancreatic lesion at the time of operation. Thus, with blunt injuries pancreatic fistulas develop in approximately 45 per cent of patients.[34, 44] Wounds of the head of the gland are more commonly associated with development of fistula than those in the tail, because the ducts in the head are larger and because pancreatic juice nor-

mally drains from the tail of the pancreas through the head into the duodenum. If the major pancreatic duct has been injured, the likelihood of fistula is particularly great. Thus, it is important to ascertain whether or not the major pancreatic duct is intact at the time of the exploration of the pancreatic wound, unless other major injuries immediately jeopardize the life of the patient. If the pancreatic duct has been injured, repair of this lesion is important to prevent a pancreatic fistula and to allow healing of the wound.

DRAINAGE OF PSEUDOCYSTS. Until recent years, the treatment of pseudocysts of the pancreas was external drainage by marsupialization or the placement of a catheter into the cyst. Some pseudocysts have a persistent or intermittent communication with the main pancreatic duct, and these fistulas drain 200 to 300 ml. of pure pancreatic juice each day (Fig. 22–2). Currently, the procedure of choice for treatment of pancreatic cyst is internal drainage. Regardless of the technique used, the complication of pancreatic fistula is virtually eliminated. There is

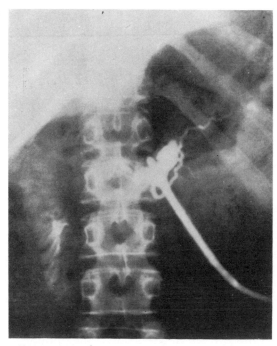

Figure 22–2 A roentgenogram demonstrating communication of a pseudocyst of the pancreas with the distal portion of the pancreatic duct. (From Howard, J. M., and Jordan, G. L., Jr.: Surgical Diseases of the Pancreas. Philadelphia, J. B. Lippincott Co., 1960.)

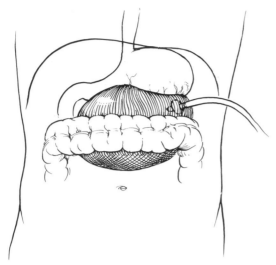

Figure 22–3 Catheter drainage is the preferred method when external drainage of a pseudocyst is necessary. An external pancreatic fistula usually develops when this technique is used.

no possibility of development of an external pancreatic fistula following cystgastrostomy when the pseudocyst is in the lesser sac, for example, and even after formal anastomosis of the fibrous cyst wall to a defunctionalized loop of jejunum for cystjejunostomy, the incidence of leakage and formation of external pancreatic fistula is quite low. There are still indications, however, for external drainage of pancreatic pseudocysts. These include treatment of cysts with poorly developed walls, those in which secondary infection has occurred, and those in which hemorrhage occurred prior to surgery. External drainage may also be performed in the very ill patient when a longer surgical procedure seems contraindicated (Fig. 22–3).

PANCREATIC BIOPSY. There is a great deal of discussion in the surgical literature about the value of pancreatic biopsy. Most of this discussion concerns the biopsy of lesions in the head of the pancreas. In the opinion of the author, biopsy of malignant lesions of the head of the pancreas is fraught with the danger of the creation of a pancreatic fistula unless the lesion is extremely large and gross tumor can be seen on the surface of the gland. If the tumor is small and appears to be resectable, the biopsy, unless taken very deeply, will be misleading to the pathologist because the cancer is surrounded by a zone of pancreatitis and

the malignant lesion is in the center of the mass rather than extending to the periphery of the palpable lesion. These tumors usually arise from the major pancreatic ducts and thus, once an accurate biopsy of a relatively small lesion has been performed, the ductal system may have been entered. Consequently, deep incisional biopsies into the head of the pancreas are best avoided. To obviate this possibility, needle biopsy of lesions of the pancreas has been advocated by some, and this is less likely to produce pancreatic fistula, but this complication does sometimes occur. Recognizing this, there have been those who have advocated needle biopsy transduodenally so that any leakage of pancreatic juice will drain into the duodenum rather than to the exterior. This technique is least likely to produce pancreatic fistula, but it is attended by other complications that will be discussed later. Biopsy of specific lesions of the body and tail of the pancreas is usually not followed by the development of pancreatic fistula, and if a pancreatic fistula does occur, it will be small. Thus, in contradistinction to lesions deep in the head of the pancreas, lesions of the body and tail can usually be biopsied successfully if desired, without fear of a major complication. Under such circumstances, however, the incisional biopsy area should be carefully repaired.

Drains should always be placed when the pancreas has been incised, for it is impossible to be sure that leakage of pancreatic juice will not occur.

PANCREATODUODENECTOMY. After pancreatoduodenectomy several different types of fistula may develop. The most common fistula is pancreatic fistula, and the reported incidence varies from 10 to 20 per cent of patients having this operation.[19, 26, 39] At times, the fistula is a pure pancreatic fistula representing a simple tear of a suture placed into the gland. A pure fistula also may develop when the technique of simple closure of the stump of the pancreas without anastomosis to the tubular gastrointestinal tract is performed. Under these circumstances, however, the fistula represents complete drainage of all of the remaining portion of the gland that is left intact, and consequently is a major fistula. In the early experience with pancreatoduodenectomy, this technique was used by many surgeons. Because of the high incidence of pancreatic fistula, however, ranging from 25 to 50 per cent, the technique was abandoned and the procedure of choice became anastomosis of the gland to the gastrointestinal tract, both to decrease the incidence of pancreatic fistula and to provide a source of drainage of digestive enzymes into the gastrointestinal tract. It is interesting that in recent years, simple closure of the pancreatic stump has again been recommended by some. Those who advocate this, however, are doing so on the basis of a relatively small experience, and in the opinion of the author, it is not the preferred method of performing this operation. Others believe that pancreatic fistula is such a major complication when it occurs that total pancreatectomy should be performed for the treatment of carcinoma of the pancreas to prevent this complication.[10, 31] Total pancreatectomy carries its own additional complications, however, and the experience with this technique does not indicate that the mortality rate for total pancreatectomy is less than for pancreatoduodenectomy, despite the elimination of the complication of pancreatic fistula. Consequently, the ultimate determination concerning the value of total pancreatectomy in treatment of carcinoma will rest more upon considerations of long-term survival than on any technical considerations, particularly the consideration of the development of pancreatic fistula.

When fistula does occur after pancreatoduodenectomy, in which the pancreas has been anastomosed to the jejunum, the fistula usually represents a partial breakdown of the anastomosis, and thus in effect is more comparable to an "end" duodenal fistula than to a pure pancreatic fistula, because the pancreatic anastomosis is usually not far distant from the biliary anastomosis. Consequently, the material draining from the fistula is activated pancreatic juice containing the usual potent digestive enzymes that impair healing of the fistula and result in significant digestion of the skin around the site of the fistula. Furthermore, the volume drainage from the fistula may be large, as it will include a portion of the biliary drainage as well as pancreatic drainage.

ANNULAR PANCREAS. Resection of annular pancreas involves transection of major ducts, and the incidence of pancreatic fistula and the mortality rate following resection are so high that the procedure has been abandoned.

PANCREATITIS. In the United States, the majority of patients with pancreatitis have a relatively mild form of the disease associated with a limited amount of gross destruction of the pancreatic tissue. With severe necrotic pancreatitis, however, and particularly with hemorrhagic pancreatitis and extensive necrosis, loss of significant amounts of pancreatic tissue may occur, as well as loss of tissue of adjacent organs. Consequently, if the patient survives, pancreatic fistula may occur. This is why the author advocates surgical treatment of hemorrhagic pancreatitis, with adequate drainage. If fistula formation occurs, established drainage tracts prevent leakage of pancreatic juice into the peritoneal cavity. Although fistula formation is uncommon in pancreatitis, in our experience it has occurred in 20 per cent of patients treated surgically for hemorrhagic pancreatitis. The number of surviving patients is small, and thus, at the present time, our total experience with fistula resulting from pancreatitis includes only five patients. In each of these, however, the pancreatic fistula was a major one and represented a therapeutic challenge.

MISCELLANEOUS. Pancreatic fistula has also occurred after a variety of other procedures such as gastrectomy for benign ulcer when the ulcer penetrated deeply into the pancreas, erosion of an abscess into the pancreatic tissue, and pancreatojejunostomy for treatment of chronic pancreatitis. These are all uncommon causes of pancreatic fistula, but emphasize the fact that a fistula may occur after any surgical procedure or traumatic wound to the pancreas. Consequently, all wounds of the pancreas, whether due to external trauma or surgical procedures, should be drained.

Clinical Features

Pancreatic fistula is heralded by the development of a clear, colorless fluid draining from the area of the pancreatic wound. If proper drains have been placed at the time of surgery, this will occur without development of any systemic symptoms. The drainage commonly has a "musty" odor that is quite different from the odor of drainage from a duodenal fistula containing activated juices admixed with bile. At times, it may be difficult on gross examination alone to ascertain whether the drainage is pancreatic juice or simply represents weeping of lymph from areas of dissection. Also, in the early postoperative period, there is often a sanguineous component to the drainage from the extensive dissection that may be necessary in the removal of the pancreas, and therefore the typical appearance of the pancreatic juice is not immediately appreciated. Whenever a question is raised concerning the development of pancreatic fistula, however, the diagnosis can be confirmed by demonstrating the presence of amylase or other digestive enzymes within the juice. A common test utilized in the past has been the placement of a drop or two of juice on x-ray film. If the fluid is pancreatic juice, the emulsion of the film will be digested. More accurate determination can be accomplished by making a chemical determination of the amylase concentration. The amylase concentration in drainage from a pancreatic fistula will depend upon the activity of the gland, the amount of associated lymph drainage admixed with pancreatic juice, the status of the gland, and the size of the fistula. One can anticipate amylase values ranging from 10,000 to 50,000 Somogyi units in fistulas draining high concentrations of pancreatic juice.

The volume of pancreatic juice will vary considerably depending upon the location in the gland, whether or not the major ductal system is involved, and whether there is obstruction in the ductal system. Thus, fistulas from the tail of the gland, under circumstances in which the pancreatic duct draining into the duodenum is normally patent, rarely discharge more than 200 to 300 ml. a day; on the other hand, those fistulas involving the major duct in the head of the gland may discharge virtually the entire pancreatic secretion, ranging from 700 to 1000 ml. a day. In an occasional patient, even larger amounts of juice may be discharged through a fistula. The largest volume observed by the author has been 1800 ml. a day.

Spontaneous closure is the natural conclusion of pancreatic fistula, unless complications develop.[20]

Complications

LOSS OF FLUID AND ELECTROLYTES. The presence of a pancreatic fistula in itself implies loss of fluid and electrolytes, and therefore some might not consider this a complication. With a small pancreatic fistula the loss of fluid and electrolytes is minimal and of no great physiologic consequence. If the patient can ingest a normal diet, for example, the ingestion of an extra 200 ml. of fluid plus the quantity of electrolytes that would be lost in pancreatic fistula is not difficult. Thus, the metabolic consequences are no greater than those of the increased losses that may occur from the body during heavy exercise or sweating on a hot day. When losses reach volumes of 1000 to 1500 ml., however, dehydration, hyponatremia, hypokalemia, and hypochloremia may result. Pancreatic juice is alkaline, with a pH of 8.0 to 8.4. Thus, uncorrected loss will lead to metabolic acidosis.[33] Management will be discussed in the section on treatment.

INFECTION. The most serious frequent complication of pancreatic fistula is the development of infection in the cavity that may form around the origin of the pancreatic fistula. Infection almost always implies inadequate drainage, because in the absence of the development of a large pocket that results in stagnation of pancreatic juice and tissue fluid within the body cavity, secondary infection of clinical significance rarely occurs. Bacteria are almost invariably present in a fistulous tract, having entered along the drain tract from the exterior, and therefore a positive culture from pancreatic fistula drainage can usually be obtained. The presence of bacteria, however, does not constitute evidence of active infection any more than does the presence of bacteria upon the skin; infection is diagnosed only when there are clinical findings of infection, such as temperature elevation, or when frank pus drains from the area of the fistula. The most important factors in treatment of infection are adequate drainage and the administration of appropriate antibiotics.

HEMORRHAGE. The most lethal complication of pancreatic fistula is hemorrhage. Hemorrhage from the pancreatic substance rarely occurs, and the author has never observed a fatal hemorrhage from the area of the pancreatic wound in a patient with a well established pancreatic fistula. Severe hemorrhage results from erosion of the fistula into adjacent major vessels and is more likely to occur when a major artery or vein has been transected, with drainage of the fistulous tract across the area of the ligature placed around the vessel. Under these circumstances, either the drainage may digest the transected end of the artery, resulting in hemorrhage, or a low-grade chronic infection from bacteria caught in the interstices of the ligature may develop, with breakdown of the closure of the vessel, and consequent massive hemorrhage. It is unusual for a pure pancreatic fistula to erode through the normal adventitia of a normal vessel and cause hemorrhage. In an experience of more than 100 pancreatic fistulas, the author has never observed a fatality owing to erosion of a normal vessel, whereas death resulting from erosion of a transected end of an artery has been observed on several occasions. Consequently, the conservative surgical procedures for traumatic wounds of the pancreas that can be accomplished without dissection of major vessels remain the treatment of choice.

When major vessels must be transected, in performing major pancreatic resections such as during pancreatoduodenectomy, it is desirable to separate the vessels from the transected end of the pancreas or the pancreatic anastomosis; often this can be accomplished with the omentum. Thus, if a fistula does develop, the omentum may prevent the drainage from coming into contact with the vessel and thereby prevent the development of hemorrhage.

EROSION INTO ADJACENT VISCERA. The pancreatic juice in a pure pancreatic fistula is relatively inactive in its fresh form. However, if there is stagnation, spontaneous activation may occur. Furthermore, those fistulas that also drain bile or succus entericus contain very active digestive juices. Consequently, erosion into an adjacent viscus may occur. Erosion from actual digestion, however, is most likely to occur when there has been dissection or decreased viability of the adjacent viscus. The placement of large hard rubber or hard plastic drains in the management of pancreatic fistula may also contribute to erosion into an adjacent viscus, for these drains may in themselves cause erosion even when a fistula does not exist.

Consequently, although the use of sump drains is advocated by many authors for the initial treatment of pancreatic wounds, we initially drain the pancreas almost routinely with soft Penrose drains. When a sump drain or hard rubber catheter is necessary, it is preferably placed only through the skin and fascia and not into the peritoneal cavity where it may come in contact with the stomach, colon, or small intestine. On occasion, however, it may be desirable to place a rubber catheter for management of a chronic fistula. This should be done only after the fistulous tract is well established so that the walls of adjacent viscera are protected by a thick layer of fibrous tissue (Fig. 22–4).

The true incidence of erosion into adjacent viscera is not known because many who treat these lesions do not routinely perform sinography at regular intervals. It has become apparent that many such complications are not recognized clinically, as they are small and the drainage from the eroded viscus is not appreciated. They may, therefore, be diagnosed only if a sinogram is taken (Fig. 22–5). No special treatment is

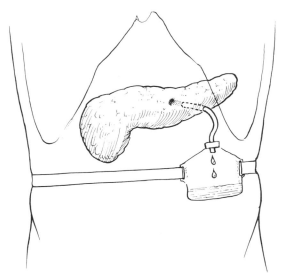

Figure 22–4 A drawing to illustrate management of a chronic pancreatic fistula on an outpatient basis. A catheter is inserted through the abdominal wall to prevent premature closure of the skin or fascia, but it is not passed deep into the abdomen where it might serve as a foreign body and thus prevent healing of the fistula. This catheter can be connected to a bag so that the drainage from the fistulous tract can be conveniently collected without irritation of the skin.

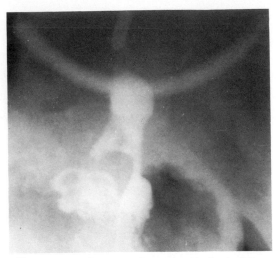

Figure 22–5 Sinogram of a pancreatic fistula following trauma. Erosion into the colon is demonstrated. The colonic fistula had not been suspected before this examination was performed.

required when the communication with the adjacent viscera is small, for it heals as the pancreatic fistula heals. If the communication is large, however, serious problems may arise. Unless there is prompt evidence of healing, surgical exploration should be performed with drainage of the pancreatic fistula into a Roux-en-Y loop of jejunum and surgical closure of the eroded viscus.

NUTRITIONAL DEFICIENCY. In the presence of major pancreatic fistulas, the loss of pancreatic juice from the body results not only in fluid and electrolyte loss, but also in loss of digestive enzymes from the tubular gastrointestinal tract. Thus, adequate digestion of protein and fat may be impaired. The problems of deficiencies of external pancreatic secretion are discussed elsewhere in this chapter.

Treatment

The primary approach to pancreatic fistula should be concerned with its prevention. Careful and meticulous repair of pancreatic wounds should be performed when possible, with the sutures placed so that adequate approximation is obtained and tied carefully so that they will not cut through the pancreatic tissue. A careful and meticulous anastomosis should be constructed when pancreatojejunostomy is accomplished. There are a variety of methods of performing pancreatojejunostomy and there is no agreement concerning the best technique even among surgeons with extensive experience in pancreatic surgery. The author prefers that in which a careful two-layer anastomosis is made end to end with approximately 2 cm. of pancreas invaginated into the jejunum.[42] Unfortunately, the technical details of this procedure are not appreciated by many surgeons, for, performed in its proper manner, it constitutes almost (though not quite) a ductal anastomosis to the jejunal mucosa with the anastomosis protruding well into the jejunum rather than the end of the pancreas lying against the side of the jejunum, as is the usual circumstance when a true duct-to-mucosa anastomosis is accomplished. When a Roux-en-Y loop of jejunum is utilized, careful attention must be given to the management of the loop to prevent obstruction of the afferent loop and thereby prevent rises in pressure that might result in disruption of the anastomosis. Proper placement of a large T-tube can serve to decompress both the biliary tree and the afferent loop of jejunum. Thus, the T-tube is placed into the common bile duct and a long arm is passed through the anastomosis into the afferent loop; multiple openings are cut into the tube to allow egress of jejunal contents, should partial obstruction of the afferent loop occur. In addition, this method allows filling of the afferent loop with contrast material for radiographic examination when development of an afferent loop obstruction is suspected (Fig. 22–6). Howard prefers decompression of the afferent loop by an additional jejunostomy tube placed into the afferent loop for this purpose.[18] Smith recommends an additional tube placed into the pancreatic duct, brought through the anastomosis and out through a jejunotomy wound.[35] It is believed that this will maintain a tract for pancreatic juices to drain directly into the jejunum and thereby help prevent the development of pancreatic fistula, or to aid in proper healing if a fistula should develop. Additional precautions include protection of exposed arteries and veins with omentum or other peritoneum-covered surfaces, as well as separation of areas of repair of adjacent viscera from the region of the pancreatic anastomosis.

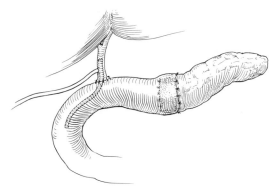

Figure 22–6 A drawing to illustrate pancreatic and biliary anastomoses used for reconstruction of gastrointestinal continuity following pancreatoduodenectomy. An end-to-end pancreatojejunostomy is first performed as a careful two-layer anastomosis, followed by an end-to-side choledochojejunostomy. A T-tube with a long arm is placed through the anastomosis to prevent any biliary obstruction in the immediate postoperative period. The long arm is placed into the jejunal loop to prevent a rise in pressure in the early postoperative period that might endanger the anastomoses.

Because of the possibility of development of pancreatic fistula following any pancreatic surgery, drainage should be instituted. When an incision into the pancreas has been made, it is important to place the drains properly so that they do not come in contact with the area of pancreatic repair, for if there is direct contact with the pancreatic wound, the drains may actually contribute to the formation of a fistula. The drains should be placed in proximity, though, so that if a fistula does occur, egress along the drain tract will be the most direct route for the drainage and thus contamination of the peritoneal cavity will be prevented.

Once diagnosis of pancreatic fistula has been confirmed, the most important initial consideration is adequate drainage. This should have been accomplished at the time of surgery if the drains were properly placed. If not, surgical drainage should be performed promptly. If the fistula is small, a plastic bag that can be cemented to the skin may be used to collect the drainage. In this way, the skin is adequately protected and the collection of drainage into the bag allows proper documentation of the total fluid loss, and thus proper calculations of adequate replacement. If drainage from the tract is large, initial collection is best accomplished through sump suction. The sump catheter should be inserted into the drainage tract

through the fascia but not deep into the peritoneal cavity. This, too, will provide protection of the skin and collection of the discharge to document volume of fluid loss. If this technique is utilized, aluminum paste should be placed to protect the skin immediately around the fistula. The paste should be applied as soon as fistula is suspected, before irritation of the skin has occurred. It will promptly stick to the skin and will serve as permanent protection throughout the period of treatment of the fistula. It should not be removed until the fistula is healed. If some of the paste is accidentally brushed off, the area should be cleaned gently and an additional layer of paste should be applied to cover it. In this way, the skin beneath the aluminum paste stays quite healthy and will be in excellent condition when the paste is removed. It must be emphasized that once aluminum paste is applied, it is never removed — only reinforced — until complete healing has occurred. Thus, the skin may remain completely covered with paste for 1 or 2 months. When removal of the paste is desired, this is best accomplished with use of generous quantities of mineral oil as a solvent.

The drainage from the fistulous tract should be cultured, and initially a broad-spectrum antibiotic should be administered to prevent the development of a clinical infection during the early phase of development of the fistula. If a chronic fistula develops without contamination of the peritoneal cavity, long-term antibiotic therapy is not necessary.

After 2 to 3 weeks of drainage from the fistula, a sinogram should be made to ascertain the development of the fistulous tract and to determine whether or not there are multiple tracts and whether or not a cavity exists within the abdominal cavity. The sinogram will show, in addition, whether perforation of adjacent viscera has occurred and whether or not the fistula communicates directly with the major pancreatic duct. These observations will be of both prognostic and therapeutic value (Fig. 22–7).

In the early postoperative period, particularly in patients with abdominal wounds, other injuries of the gastrointestinal tract may prevent the ingestion of a normal diet. Under these circumstances, the use of intravenous hyperalimentation is indicated.

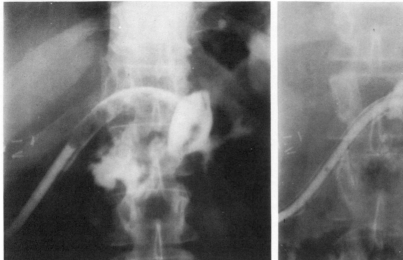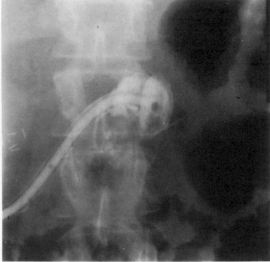

Figure 22–7   *Left,* Roentgenogram following injection of radiopaque material through a catheter after external drainage of a pseudocyst reveals persistence of the cystic cavity. If catheter drainage is discontinued at this time, recurrence of the cyst is likely.

Right, Sinogram performed 4 weeks later. The cavity is completely obliterated and only a persistent tract along the course of the catheter remains. At this point, the catheter can be removed slowly over a period of 2 to 3 weeks to allow firm healing.

The value of this technique, which is described in detail in Chapter 12, will not be reiterated here. It will allow the administration of sufficient calories and protein to provide for healing of the fistulous tract, as well as adequate fluid and electrolytes. Of particular interest in the management of pancreatic fistula is the observation of Hamilton and associates that the administration of hyperalimentation solutions results in significant decreases in the volume of fluid and amylase lost through fistulas of the upper gastrointestinal tract.[16] There may therefore be a tendency to utilize this technique preferentially in the treatment of pancreatic fistula. It should be used only until food can be ingested normally because of the morbidity occasionally associated with it, because of its expense and the requirement of constant nursing supervision in the hospital, and because it does not provide nourishment equal to that obtained from a solid diet ingested orally.

Most pure pancreatic fistulas will close spontaneously without the development of any major complication if adequate drainage is maintained. Once the tract is definitely well established, drains placed at the time of surgery should be gradually removed. If the drains remain in the area of

the pancreas, they themselves may serve as a foreign body, perpetuating the drainage from the fistula. Consequently, drains should be shortened as soon as a thick fibrous tract has developed and then should be totally removed, being replaced with sump drainage if the volume is great. If the volume is small, a small rubber catheter can be used as a long-term drain and connected to a bag, in the same manner as bile is collected from T-tube drainage; or this area may be covered with an adhesive plastic bag. If a rubber catheter is used, it should be inserted well into the tract, but not to the region of the pancreas (see Fig. 22–4).

It is important that an opening in the abdominal wall be maintained until complete healing of the fistula at the site of the pancreatic wound has occurred. A common error in treatment of pancreatic fistula has been failure to maintain an adequate tract through the abdominal wall, particularly at the skin level. Rarely will pocketing occur along the drainage tract within the abdominal cavity. However, the abdominal wall, particularly the skin, has a propensity to close and thus closure at the skin level may occur before healing has occurred deep within the sinus tract. Closure at this level while the fistula is still draining causes accumulation of fluid within the abdominal cavity, with the development of secondary infection and undue complication of the patient's course. Complete healing is best documented by serial sinographic examinations if the fistula remains open for a long time.

Various medications and techniques have been advocated to help decrease secretion from the pancreatic fistula in attempts to promote healing. Since it is known that ingestion of food is one of the most potent stimuli to pancreatic secretion, many surgeons make the erroneous assumption that maintaining the patient on nasogastric suction with no oral intake is a desirable feature in treatment of the fistula. This is not the case. Once proper progression of food through the gastrointestinal tract is assured, the ingestion of a normal diet is one of the most significant factors in healing of a pancreatic fistula, because this will allow adequate provision of calories, protein, vitamins, and minerals, which will not only replace the losses from the fistula but also will create an optimal nutritional state for healing.

The use of anticholinergic agents, recommended by some to aid in decreasing drainage, has not been useful in the treatment of chronic fistula. It can be demonstrated that in the fasting state the administration of an anticholinergic drug will temporarily decrease the secretion from a pancreatic fistula, but experience has shown that regular administration of these agents does not produce a constant and predictable decrease in fluid loss. The side effects from the use of these drugs far outweigh their advantages.

Once a pancreatic fistula is well established and the volume of drainage does not exceed 200 to 400 ml. a day, the patient can be managed on an outpatient basis if he is eating a normal diet and is progressing satisfactorily except for the drainage from the fistula.

The length of conservative therapy will depend upon the course of the fistula. As long as there is a progressive decrease in the amount of drainage, conservative therapy may be continued for relatively long periods. Most pancreatic fistulas close within 4 to 6 weeks, but occasionally one will drain for several months, and we have treated patients for as long as a year with ultimate closure of the fistula when the drainage

amounted to only 25 to 50 ml. a day. Under such circumstances, the drainage is a nuisance but does not impair weight gain and return to usual normal activities. As emphasized earlier, it is mandatory that the tract through the abdominal wall be maintained.

Few surgeons have experience with surgical treatment of fistula, since most fistulas heal spontaneously.[19] Our current experience supports this observation, with surgical closure required in only 5 or 6 per cent of patients.

The primary indication for surgical closure is the continuous drainage of large volumes of secretion with no evidence of improvement for a period of 3 to 4 weeks. Under these circumstances, a prolonged period of morbidity can be anticipated and surgical closure will be the most expeditious method of rehabilitation of the patient.

When surgical treatment is indicated, the technique used will depend upon the location of the fistula and the presence or absence of additional abdominal lesions. In most instances, when the fistula is well established it can be easily identified, and the tract followed surgically to its origin from the pancreas. Older texts describe a technique of dissection of the tract and implantation of it into an appropriate portion of the bowel. This method is no longer used. The repair of a pancreatic fistula should consist of total excision of the fistulous tract, identification of the area of drainage from the pancreas, and accurate construction of an anastomosis between the pancreas and a Roux-en-Y limb of jejunum (Fig. 22–8). On occasion, the anastomosis has been made between the fistula and the stomach or the duodenum, but these techniques are used only under special circumstances, and in most instances anastomosis to the jejunum is satisfactory.[20] The fibrosis surrounding the area of the fistula allows accurate placement of sutures into tissues that have good tensile strength; therefore, leakage from placement of a suture or breakdown of anastomosis has been quite rare. Up to now, none of our patients have died after surgical management of pancreatic fistula with this technique. Repair of fistula has also been accomplished by resection of the portion of the gland containing the fistula, particularly when the fistula is in the tail of the gland,

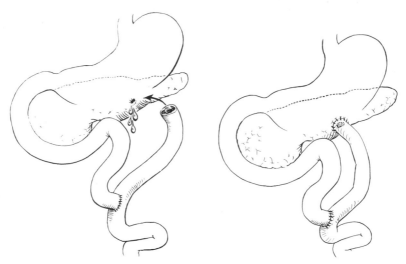

Figure 22–8 A drawing to illustrate the preferred method for surgical treatment of pancreatic fistula. The fistulous tract is excised to the point of the opening in the gland and an anastomosis is made between the pancreas and a Roux-en-Y loop of jejunum to allow drainage of the fistula into the gastrointestinal tract. (From Jordan, G. L., Jr.: Pancreatic fistula. Am. J. Surg. *119*:200, 1970.)

and pancreatoduodenectomy has been advocated for fistula of the head. These are less satisfactory techniques than a Roux-en-Y anastomosis, for a new fistula may develop from the transected end of the gland and the problem will begin again.

Mortality

The mortality rate associated with pure pancreatic fistula is low. In our entire experience, only one patient has died from the effects of malnutrition from a fistula, and this occurred many years ago. Thus, if adequate drainage is maintained and hemorrhage from transected vessels is prevented, one can anticipate an ultimately favorable outcome in most patients, even if surgical intervention is required. Excluding the fistulas that have developed after pancreatoduodenectomy for cancer, which, as noted earlier, are not pure pancreatic fistulas, the over-all mortality rate has been 4 per cent. The fistulas developing after pancreatoduodenectomy are special problems. They are associated with greater fluid losses of juice with potent digestive enzymes, and they occur in patients who are seriously ill at the time of operation. Thus, the mortality rate in this group is 40 per cent, with massive hemorrhage from erosion of the stump of

the gastroduodenal artery being a major problem.

PANCREATITIS

Some degree of inflammation is anticipated following trauma to any part of the body, and the pancreas is no exception. The term "traumatic pancreatitis" commonly occurs in literature. However, in general, the degree of inflammation that follows surgical or external trauma to the pancreas is no greater than that following injury to any other organ. Whereas an elevation of the serum amylase concentration often occurs after pancreatic trauma or surgery, the inflammation is self-limiting and does not have the clinical significance of spontaneously occurring pancreatitis. Thus the term "traumatic pancreatitis" as usually applied is misleading. In the occasional patient, however, trauma to the pancreas or its duct may result in the development of frank, severe pancreatitis with the anticipated clinical course. Of more importance is the fact that when such pancreatitis does occur, it is likely to be of the severe necrotic or hemorrhagic type, and the mortality associated with this complication is quite high. In some patients, it is probable that the disease process is actually an intrapancreatic hematoma, resulting from trauma to a large intrapancreatic artery. Although in rare instances pancreatitis may follow minimal trauma to the gland, it would appear that in most instances acute pancreatitis is the direct result of a major insult, including damage to the major pancreatic duct. Pancreatitis has been observed after simple biopsy of the pancreas, however, and fatal pancreatitis has occurred after needle biopsy. Furthermore, partial ligature of the pancreatic duct and particularly inadvertent ligation of the ampulla of Vater may produce fatal pancreatitis.

The diagnosis of postoperative pancreatitis is based upon the same findings as those in pancreatitis in the patient without previous surgery. Unfortunately, the diagnosis is sometimes missed until the disease has progressed, because of the presumption that the abdominal pain and tenderness are the result of the surgical procedure or trauma. When upper abdominal pain — particularly if it radiates straight through to the back — is of greater severity or lasts longer than one would anticipate after a surgical procedure, postoperative pancreatitis should always be suspected. Leukocytosis and elevation of the serum concentrations of amylase and lipase will be present.

The use of a long T-tube after exploration of the common bile duct and after sphincteroplasty has been advocated by some. A number of cases have been reported in which pancreatitis developed when a long-arm T-tube was used, and many authors believe that the tube may be a factor in causing the pancreatitis by partially occluding the pancreatic duct.[1, 28] The most extensive experience with this technique has been reported by Cattell and associates, and in a review of this subject they found that the incidence of pancreatitis was no greater in their experience when the long-arm T-tube was used than when other techniques were employed.[8] Still, most surgeons use a long-arm T-tube only in special circumstances.

After upper abdominal surgery, pancreatitis must be carefully differentiated from other lesions that may simulate it. Burnett and associates have emphasized the fact that the diagnosis of pancreatitis after gastrectomy must be made with some caution, since leakage from the duodenal stump may mimic pancreatitis, even causing elevation of serum amylase concentration, and thus lead incorrectly to conservative therapy.[7] A second lesion that may follow gastrectomy and be mistaken for pancreatitis is acute obstruction of the afferent loop. Under these circumstances, the pressure in the afferent loop rises so that pancreatic secretion must be accomplished against an elevated pressure. This results in a marked elevation of the serum amylase concentration, even though frank pancreatic inflammation does not develop. This lesion can be diagnosed by the absence of bile in the efferent loop and is discussed in more detail in Chapter 19. Differentiation from pancreatitis is critical because early operation is mandatory to prevent rupture of the afferent loop and leakage therefrom.[29]

Treatment

Mild episodes of pancreatitis occurring in the postoperative period should be treated non-operatively in the same manner as pancreatitis occurring spontaneously without previous surgery. As noted earlier, however, many of these patients have hemorrhagic pancreatitis, and when this develops, the treatment of choice is surgical intervention. Thus, if postoperative pancreatitis of any severity is diagnosed, surgical intervention should be considered for a number of reasons. First, diagnosis may be in error, and if there is obstruction of the afferent loop or leakage of a duodenal stump, operative intervention will permit accurate early diagnosis and indicated surgical treatment. Second, hemorrhagic pancreatitis can best be treated surgically. Surgical intervention allows aspiration of the toxic fluid that accumulates in the peritoneal cavity, and the proper placement of drains prevents the reaccumulation of this material in the peritoneal cavity, allowing it to drain to the exterior. Furthermore, the placement of drains prevents contamination of the peritoneal cavity if a major portion of the pancreas becomes necrotic and sloughs, with creation of a pancreatic fistula. Under these circumstances, it is also well to place a tube in the stomach for gastrostomy drainage, as prolonged gastric drainage may be necessary. A second tube should be placed into the jejunum for jejunal feedings, for many patients are able to tolerate feedings into the small bowel long before the inflammatory process in the pancreas has subsided sufficiently so that the food placed into the stomach or duodenum will be tolerated. There are those who advocate performing a cholecystostomy to drain the biliary tree under these circumstances. The author, however, prefers to reserve this procedure for those patients who have stones in the gallbladder. In these patients, evacuation of the stones and the placement of a tube in the gallbladder seems desirable. Detailed exploration of the common bile duct is usually not indicated because extensive dissection in the region of the porta hepatis may result in further exacerbation of the pancreatic inflammation.

Reports in recent years indicate that the mortality rate for postoperative pancreatitis still remains extremely high.[30] More aggressive treatment of these lesions, including these surgical procedures and the use of intravenous hyperalimentation, has resulted in some decrease in the mortality rate, but in those patients with the hemorrhagic variety, the mortality rate remains around 50 per cent.

In addition to the acute problem that may develop in the early postoperative period, recurrent pancreatitis may develop in the late postoperative period in some patients undergoing surgical treatment for pancreatic trauma. In some cases, the development of recurrent pancreatitis is probably unrelated to the operation that was performed, and thus treatment should not differ from that of pancreatitis occurring in patients who have not had previous operations. Patients who sustain pancreatic trauma, for example, include some who indulge in excessive alcohol ingestion, and may incur spontaneous pancreatitis on this basis. Recurrent pancreatitis definitely may follow external trauma to the pancreas, however, though this complication has been quite rare in our experience. It most likely represents a partial ductal obstruction at the site of the injury, and thus can be treated successfully by resection of the distal portion of the gland or by drainage of the ductal system distal to the area of stenosis.

In all patients with recurring pancreatitis elective exploratory surgery should be done at a time when the disease is quiescent. Careful examination of the gland should be made to locate the area of the pancreatitis, and pancreatography should be performed to delineate ductal lesions. The exact method of treatment will depend upon the pathologic changes found. Pseudocysts should be treated by internal drainage. Lesions limited totally to the tail of the pancreas should be treated by resection, and Roux-en-Y drainage of the pancreatic duct should be accomplished if there is obstruction near the head or neck of the pancreas. When recurrent disease has resulted from stricture of the pancreatic duct due to trauma, good or excellent results will be obtained when the obstructing stenosis is relieved.

HEMORRHAGE

Massive hemorrhage is one of the most common causes of death after major pancreatic resections, particularly after resection of the head of the pancreas.

Intraoperative Hemorrhage

The head and neck of the pancreas are so intimately associated with a large number of major vascular structures that hemorrhage may be encountered whenever a difficult resection is undertaken, and at times even when the resection does not appear difficult. Although massive hemorrhage from the vena cava may be encountered, this is rare because few surgeons attempt resection when there appears to be firm adherence to this structure. One might also encounter massive hemorrhage from the hepatic artery, but this, too, is uncommon for the same reason. Thus, the portal or superior mesenteric vein is the most common source of intraoperative hemorrhage, which is caused by attempts to dissect these structures from the pancreas.

The usual method of the initial dissection of the portal and superior mesenteric veins in pancreatic resection is to establish a plane between the anterior surface of these vessels and the posterior surface of the neck of the pancreas. Dissection proceeds bluntly between the vein and the pancreas with the finger. In most instances, there are no veins entering directly from the anterior side of the portal vein and the neck of the pancreas, and this dissection can be accomplished safely. On the other hand, it must be performed with considerable care because occasionally such veins are present; and if they are torn, massive hemorrhage will occur under circumstances in which direct visibility of the gland is not possible. When difficulty of dissection develops because a vein traverses this area, the dissection should be discontinued and the pancreas transected lateral to the superior mesenteric vessels. The transected end may then be reflected to the right and the vein exposed under direct vision, divided, and ligated. A second problem in dissecting the anterior surface of these veins occurs when carcinomatous invasion of the vein has occurred. When this problem exists, the vein may be extremely friable and easily torn, and the vessel may be inadvertently injured, despite gentle dissection. It is important to make this determination early in the course of dissection and to abandon the operation when carcinomatous invasion is encountered, for direct invasion of the portal or superior mesenteric vein is a contraindication to pancreatic resection for carcinoma. Although it is possible to resect this portion of the vein, the mortality rate after this procedure has been high and there is no evidence that it improves the survival rate. Difficulty may also be encountered in this dissection when resecting the head of the pancreas for chronic pancreatitis. Firm inflammatory adherence between the pancreas and the associated venous structures at times occurs, which may require sharp dissection for removal. Under these circumstances, blunt dissection should be abandoned, the pancreas should be divided distally, and a careful dissection of the vessels should be made after proper exposure has been gained by reflecting the pancreas to the right. Even leaving a small cuff of pancreatic tissue on the vein will not jeopardize the ultimate results of treatment of pancreatitis.

The literature on pancreatoduodenectomy documents a high mortality rate following inadvertent damage to the portal or superior mesenteric vein beneath the neck of the pancreas. The hemorrhage can be successfully controlled, however. Immediate control is obtained by simple manual pressure, with compression of the vein between the thumb and forefinger. One finger

placed behind the uncinate process of the pancreas and one anterior to the area of the hemorrhage will readily give full control of hemorrhage. The pancreas can then be transected rapidly directly over the vein, with a scalpel. The area of bleeding can be identified and the bleeding controlled, again temporarily, with finger pressure. Vascular occluding clamps can then be applied and repair of the vein accomplished under direct vision with use of a running vascular suture. The application of the vascular clamps will depend upon the extent of the tear and degree of damage to the vein. Thus, if hemorrhage occurs from simple transection of an anomalous vein, finger pressure may be all that is necessary and the bleeding may be controlled with a simple figure-of-eight suture around the entrance of the vein. When a longer tear has occurred in the vein, it will be possible to control bleeding from the vein by placing a partially occluding vascular clamp which will allow repair of the vein without total interruption of venous flow for any prolonged period. In the occasional patient with a severe tear, it will be necessary to occlude totally the venous inflow and outflow. This requires placement of vascular clamps upon the portal vein, the superior mesenteric vein, and the splenic vein to occlude these structures temporarily until good visibility of the area of laceration can be obtained and a proper repair made (Fig. 22–9). The author has never encountered a

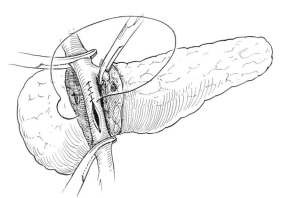

Figure 22–9 A drawing to illustrate the method for control of hemorrhage from a long tear in the anterior surface of the superior mesenteric vein. The pancreas has been transected rapidly with a scalpel and clamps have been placed upon' the superior mesenteric, portal, and splenic veins to control hemorrhage. The tear is repaired with a running vascular suture.

laceration that could not be repaired satisfactorily.

Hemorrhage may also occur from the
portal or superior mesenteric vein as the
dissection proceeds to free the vein on its
right lateral surface and on its posterior
surface where the major venous drainage
normally enters the vein from the head and
uncinate process of the pancreas. These
veins are short and friable and tear very
easily; consequently, dissection should proceed carefully and each vein should be carefully ligated. The author prefers to ligate
these veins without placing a clamp upon
them, having found that many of the small
veins tear when clamped. Thus, ligatures
are placed proximally and distally on the
vein and the vein is cut between. This prevents not only bleeding from the major
vessels but also back-bleeding from the pancreas, which might obscure and complicate
the dissection. In an occasional patient undergoing resection for a malignant lesion,
adherence of the tumor to the posterior side
of the vein will be encountered after dissection has proceeded to the point that removal
of the pancreas must be accomplished.
Some have described the removal of the
pancreas by use of a cautery. A better removal of the tumor can be accomplished,
however, simply by placing a partially occluding vascular clamp on the portal vein
and removing a small wedge of the vein with
the tumor. This allows complete removal of
the tumor; at the same time, this excision of
a small portion of a vein does not significantly increase the complexity of the procedure, and it eliminates the possibility of
major hemorrhage that might result from
an attempt to dissect the tumor away from
this major vessel. After resection, a lateral
repair with a vascular suture can be accomplished. This technique has been utilized a number of times and no major hemorrhage has been encountered in the early
or late postoperative period (Fig. 22–10).

Hemorrhage may also occur from injury
to the superior mesenteric artery. In removing the head of the pancreas, careful identification and dissection of all vascular structures must be accomplished. Hemorrhage
from the superior mesenteric artery should
be treated intraoperatively, as hemorrhage
from any other major vascular structure.
Immediate control is obtained with finger

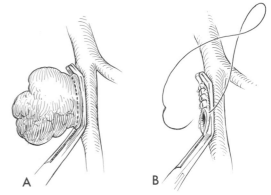

Figure 22–10 Technique of removal of pancreas
when adherence of the uncinate process to the portal vein
is encountered unexpectedly. A partial occluding clamp is
placed and the involved portion of the vein excised *(A)*. The
defect thus created is closed with a running vascular suture
(B).

pressure and suitable exposure is obtained
by satisfactory division of the pancreas. Vascular clamps can then be applied and the
laceration repaired as a wound of any other
artery. When complete division of the superior mesenteric artery has occurred, vascular clamps should be applied proximally and
distally and a careful end-to-end reanastomosis accomplished. If the problem is
promptly recognized, reanastomosis can be
accomplished with sufficient rapidity to prevent irreversible ischemia to the bowel. If
the anastomosis is unduly difficult, the viability of the bowel can be prolonged by
cooling the abdominal contents with iced
saline so that the time available for repair is
significantly lengthened. In an occasional
patient, division of the superior mesenteric
artery may have occurred under circumstances in which removal of a segment prevents direct reanastomosis. Correction of
this technical error can be accomplished by
rapidly dissecting the abdominal aorta and
performing an end-to-side anastomosis between the distal end of the superior mesenteric artery and the aorta, thus reestablishing blood flow to the intestinal tract.

Injury to the superior mesenteric artery
or one of its major branches may also occur
during the dissection of the uncinate process of the pancreas. After the pancreas has
been dissected from the superior mesenteric
and portal veins, the vein can be retracted to
expose the mesentery of the uncinate process. The mesentery of the uncinate process

should be clamped progressively and ligated, preferably with figure-of-eight sutures of silk. In accomplishing this dissection, the inferior pancreatoduodenal artery should be identified and specifically ligated. Since this dissection is performed very close to the superior mesenteric artery, this artery must be kept in view at all times during this portion of the procedure. Should injury occur inadvertently, repair is effected in the manner already described.

Hemorrhage may occur from the splenic vein during dissection of the tail of the pancreas. Normal variation in the course of this vein causes difficulty in dissecting the pancreas from it in some patients. The vein may appear to be almost surrounded by pancreatic tissue, lying in a well defined groove, with some adherence to the gland. When severe pancreatitis has existed, the vein is almost uniformly adherent to the gland. In these cases, it is best to proceed with mobilization of the spleen and reflection of the body and tail of the pancreas to allow placement of clamps on the splenic artery and on the splenic vein proximal to the area of laceration. The artery and vein can then be divided at that point and the pancreas transected in this area, to provide control of hemorrhage. In rare instances, laceration of the vein will occur beyond the point where division of the pancreas is desired. Control of hemorrhage by finger pressure should be accomplished and the laceration repaired with simple suture. Major hemorrhage from the splenic artery is fortunately uncommon. It can be controlled simply by placing a clamp on the artery and performing proper ligation or suture of the vessel.

Patients requiring resective procedures on the pancreas frequently have an obstruction of the common bile duct that may have caused impairment of the clotting mechanism. Consequently, prior to operation the clotting mechanism should be thoroughly evaluated, and if significant abnormalities are found, operation should be postponed until they are corrected. In the usual patient with carcinoma of the head of the pancreas and ductal obstruction, abnormalities in the prothrombin time result from failure of absorption of vitamin K for utilization by the liver in the formation of prothrombin. Thus, parenteral administration of vitamin

K will result in return of the prothrombin time to normal and will allow the safe performance of surgery. Prior to the recognition of this prothrombin abnormality and the availability of vitamin K, death from hemorrhage often occurred in patients with jaundice because of uncontrollable bleeding, even though a major vessel was not transected, for in addition to hemorrhage from specific vessels, considerable weeping may occur from the large denuded raw surface from which the head of the pancreas and uncinate process is removed. Bleeding from this area is rarely a significant problem if the clotting mechanism is normal, for despite the relatively large area of dissection, control of individual vessels results in good hemostasis. When there has been an extensive inflammatory process surrounding a lesion or when the lesion has been unusually large, requiring extensive sharp dissection for its removal, however, multiple small bleeding points may be observed. These may be difficult to control by individual suture ligation. Use of the cautery may be of value in obtaining adequate hemostasis.

Late Hemorrhage Following Pancreatic Resection

In the postoperative period, maintenance of a normal clotting mechanism is mandatory, for even though adequate hemostasis is obtained at the time of surgery, bleeding may occur in the postoperative period if the patient's coagulation mechanism is not maintained at normal levels.

HEMORRHAGE FOLLOWING TREATMENT OF PANCREATIC PSEUDOCYSTS. During the development of a pseudocyst, erosion into major vessels may occur, with hemorrhage into the pseudocyst. It is not uncommon to find some evidence of old blood in a pseudocyst at the time of operation, and on occasion fresh blood will be encountered in the absence of continued hemorrhage. Rarely, massive hemorrhage into the cyst will require emergency operation for control, and direct control of the bleeding point is mandatory.

The problem that has received the greatest attention is the development of hemorrhage in the postoperative period following surgical treatment of pancreatic pseudo-cysts. Hemorrhage has occurred after all methods of therapy but has been reported to be more common after cystgastrostomy. There is some disagreement among authors reporting on this procedure, for some have not encountered this problem at all, while others believe that it is a problem of such proportion that cystgastrostomy should not be performed.[2, 21, 32, 45]

A number of explanations have been offered for hemorrhage that follows cystgas-trostomy,[11] including: (1) Failure of adequate control of the vasculature of the posterior stomach wall through which incision is made for drainage. Most have utilized a running catgut suture placed around the posterior wall for this purpose. There are those who believe that this is not adequate and that the vessels should be ligated individually with non-absorbable sutures. (2) Rigidity of the wall. Zeppa and associates[45] believe that a running suture of chromic catgut produces rigidity of the wall around the incision from the stomach into the cyst and that this rigidity impairs proper emptying of the cyst. Thus, material may be forced out of the stomach and may not be able to return because the rigid wall serves as a flap valve. Under these circumstances, dissolution of the suture may occur before complete healing of the gastric wall has been completed, with resulting hemorrhage. Furthermore, the presence of material in the cyst may result in fermentation, infection, and persistence of the cyst, with erosion into adjacent vessels. (3) An inadequate incision for drainage. This also may allow gastric contents to be forced into the cyst cavity under circumstances in which they will not return into the stomach, even though there is no rigidity of the wall. The gastric contents that enter the cyst cavity, as well as fermentation of material, may result in digestion of the cyst wall, as already noted, with major hemorrhage.

The most common site of hemorrhage found at the time of exploration in patients with massive hemorrhage after treatment for pseudocysts has been the area of the incision through the stomach; thus, care in control of bleeding from this area is mandatory. In other circumstances, however, the area of hemorrhage has been from within the cyst, the result of erosion of one of the major vessels, such as the superior mesenteric vein or the splenic artery. Repair of the defect in the vessel is necessary. As noted, some believe that the propensity for hemorrhage after cystgastrostomy is so great that this particular procedure is contraindicated in the treatment of pancreatic cysts. This opinion is not generally held, however, and the majority of surgeons with experience in the treatment of pancreatic pseudocysts use cystgastrostomy when the cyst is in the lesser sac and drainage into the stomach can be accomplished without requiring a formal anastomosis. If a formal anastomosis between the cyst and one of the intra-abdominal viscera is required, however, a Roux-en-Y cystojejunostomy is preferred.

The appearance of massive hemorrhage after drainage of a pancreatic pseudocyst is an indication for immediate reoperation. Study of the clotting factors should be repeated, blood should be typed and cross-matched for operation, and the abdomen should be opened as rapidly as possible. When bleeding has occurred from the gastric wall, it is easily controlled with interrupted sutures.

If massive hemorrhage from deep inside the cyst is encountered, the cyst must be opened widely to provide detailed inspection.

GASTROINTESTINAL HEMORRHAGE. *Gastrointestinal hemorrhage* may occur in the early or late postoperative period. Early hemorrhage is usually from a suture line or from the transected end of the pancreas. In many patients, spontaneous cessation will occur with conservative therapy. If severe bleeding occurs, however, reoperation with suture ligation of the points of bleeding will be required.

Stress ulceration is infrequent but must be considered in the differential diagnosis.

In the late postoperative period, hemorrhage may occur from a marginal ulcer. This problem is discussed elsewhere in this chapter.

HEMORRHAGE ASSOCIATED WITH PANCREATIC FISTULA FORMATION. Hemorrhage from a major artery or vein is usually associated with *pancreatic fistula formation* and is discussed elsewhere. When the splenic artery or vein has been eroded, ligation should be accomplished. Depending upon the collateral circulation, the spleen may or may not require removal. When the superior mesenteric artery or vein has been eroded, repair of the area of erosion should be accomplished if at all possible. In the rare circumstances when this cannot be done, a bypass arterial procedure may be necessary to reconstitute the superior mesenteric artery. This may be accomplished with a vein graft or a Dacron prosthesis from the aorta to the superior mesenteric artery, using a technique that would be suitable for the reconstruction of the superior mesenteric artery after spontaneous thrombosis.

DISSEMINATED INTRAVASCULAR COAGULATION. In an occasional patient with pancreatic disease *disseminated intravascular coagulation* may develop, with the resulting failure of normal clotting in the remainder of the circulating blood. This is most often associated with cancer. The defect can be determined by appropriate tests for the fibrinogen content of the blood, and fibrinogen has been administered parenterally as a therapeutic measure. The majority opinion at this time, however, is that heparin is the agent of choice for this condition, as the administration of additional fibrinogen may result in a progression of the clotting mechanism and consequently perpetuate, rather than solve, the problem. When both hemorrhage and intravascular clotting are occurring simultaneously, however, the maintenance of a proper balance between suitable coagulability of the blood and prevention of further intravascular thrombosis may be difficult.

INJURY OF ADJACENT STRUCTURES WHEN PERFORMING CYSTODUODENOSTOMY

Drainage of a pancreatic pseudocyst into the stomach or into a Roux-en-Y limb of jejunum can be accomplished without any special danger of injuring adjacent structures in the process. Cystoduodenostomy is occasionally employed for treatment of a cyst in the head of the gland, when approximation to other structures might be difficult. This procedure is fraught with considerable danger of damage to the common bile duct, the superior mesenteric artery, or the superior mesenteric vein, and thus it should be undertaken only by surgeons with

an intimate knowledge of this area and with experience in judging the displacement of the structures due to pancreatic lesions. The inflammatory process surrounding the area of pancreatitis that is usually present and that of the pseudocyst may not only distort the anatomy by displacement of these structures, but also makes identification more difficult because of the surrounding fibrous tissue. If there is any question, therefore, of the relationship of these structures to the cyst, attempted drainage into the duodenum should not be made. There are reports of total transection of each of these structures during the performance of this operation, and in some instances the complications have ended fatally. If transection is immediately recognized, however, repair can be accomplished as noted elsewhere.

INJURY TO THE COMMON BILE DUCT

Purposeful division of the common bile duct is performed routinely in resection of the head of the pancreas, and thus inadvertent injury rarely occurs in this operation. Before the 95 per cent distal pancreatectomy came into use for treatment of chronic pancreatitis, therefore, inadvertent injury to the common bile duct was relatively uncommon in pancreatic surgery, though it had been reported as a rare complication of cystoduodenostomy for treatment of pseudocysts in the region of the head of the pancreas. There is a definite hazard of injuring the common bile duct, however, in performing distal 95 per cent pancreatectomy. In this operation, only a small rim of pancreas is left immediately adjacent to the duodenum to preserve the duodenal blood supply; therefore, careful dissection is required if injury of the bile duct is to be prevented. Placement of a T-tube into the common duct during the period of dissection may aid in the identification of the intrapancreatic portion of the duct, though not all authors believe that this is necessary. Child and associates, who have had the greatest experience with this operation, report a 6 per cent incidence of common duct injury.[9] The injury should be recognized at the time of operation and proper repair accomplished. The type of repair to be used depends upon the injury. A small injury of the lateral wall may be repaired primarily with suture, and, if necessary, a T-tube may be placed in the common duct as a stent to support this repair. Even if the duct is totally transected, a primary end-to-end repair may be accomplished. In other patients, however, repair will best be accomplished by performing choledochojejunostomy with Roux-en-Y anastomosis. Injuries of the biliary tract are discussed in more detail elsewhere.

POSTOPERATIVE STRICTURE OF THE COMMON BILE DUCT

Stricture of the common bile duct at the point of anastomosis to the bowel following resection of the pancreatic head is uncommon, but occurs in approximately 2 per cent of cases. The management of biliary obstruction is discussed in the preceding chapter and will not be repeated here. It is important, however, to recognize this as a possible cause of jaundice after pancreatic resection, and not presume that recurrence of cancer or other pancreatic disease has occurred without proof.[22]

BILIARY FISTULA

A variety of techniques have been described for reconstitution of gastrointestinal continuity after pancreatoduodenectomy. Most of the original techniques utilized the gallbladder for anastomosis between the jejunum and the biliary tract. The common duct was simply ligated or was closed with suture. This closure of the common bile duct was frequently insecure, and breakdown leading to biliary fistula occurred. Biliary fistula may also occur after an anastomosis between the common bile duct and the jejunum, but in our experience this is an uncommon complication, having been recorded in only 1 per cent of our patients. Biliary fistulas also occur as a result of severe pancreatitis in which erosion of the intrapancreatic portion of the common bile duct occurs.

When proper drainage has been accomplished after pancreatoduodenectomy, the first suggestion of a biliary fistula is the appearance of bile on the dressing. This occurs without the development of systemic symptoms or signs if proper drainage has prevented contamination of the general peritoneal cavity. The volume of drainage from the fistula varies, depending upon the volume of output of the liver as well as the extent of the dehiscence of the anastomosis.

Once a fistula is well established, management should proceed in a manner similar to that described for pancreatic fistula. A sinogram should be obtained to delineate the degree of dehiscence of the anastomosis and the exact site of the leakage. If the sinogram demonstrates that the fistula is of small size, conservative therapy is in order — sump suction to collect the drainage and protection of the skin with aluminum paste or an appropriate covering. Adequate drainage should be insured to prevent pocketing of the drainage material within the abdomen, which could lead to infection. Bacterial contamination of the drainage tract occurs uniformly, and thus antibiotics may aid in preventing the development of a clinical infection.

To aid in prevention of this problem and in its management, a T-tube is placed into the common duct and one arm is threaded through the anastomosis into the jejunum at the time of the operation. This will prevent rises in pressure in the jejunal loop that might cause disruption of the anastomosis. It will also serve to decrease the amount of leakage from the anastomosis if a fistula develops and thus decrease the period required for healing. When a fistula develops, the T-tube should be left in place until the fistula is completely healed and the inflammatory process has subsided. Available evidence indicates that when properly treated, a fistula will usually heal with conservative therapy alone, and early stenosis following healing is not common, though it may occur in the late postoperative period.

Large biliary fistulas may create problems in fluid and electrolyte balance. The author has observed one fistula that drained 3000 ml. a day. Under these circumstances, as with pancreatic fistulas, refeeding of the bile that is collected can provide a simple means of eliminating this potentially serious problem. When oral alimentation is impossible, fluid and electrolyte balance can be maintained by appropriate administration of intravenous fluids. Accurate determination of the mineral content of the bile to allow better replacement is desirable. This technique is described in more detail in the preceding chapter.

GASTRIC FISTULA

Following pancreatoduodenectomy, leakage at the gastrojejunal suture line may occur, as it may following gastrectomy for other reasons. The factors contributing to this complication and details of therapy are found in Chapter 19.

DUODENAL FISTULA

A duodenal fistula is one of the most serious complications following surgical incision into this organ and is undoubtedly a factor that limits the number of times exploration of the duodenum is performed. In actuality, the incidence of duodenal fistula following incisions into the normal duodenum has not been high, and duodenotomy should be performed whenever accurate delineation of disease in the region of the ampulla is necessary. The likelihood of fistula formation can be significantly reduced by proper repair of the duodenum. A longitudinal incision and transverse closure of the duodenum have been advocated by many surgeons; however, if the incision is long, the transverse closure tends to place tension on the suture line, since the wall of the duodenum in juxtaposition to the pancreas is not mobile. For this reason, closure in the line of the incision is preferred. A three-layer closure of the duodenum, with the closure made in the same direction as the incision, may be accomplished without causing duodenal obstruction. This is performed with two running layers of 4–0 chromic catgut. In the first layer a baseball stitch is used to control hemorrhage, but the suture should encompass a minimal amount of tissue; the second row is a running row of horizontal mattress sutures — again, with a minimal amount of tissue turned in. Security of this closure is then obtained by the third row of horizontal mattress sutures of 3–0 silk so that the total cuff is not more than 2 to 3 mm. in thickness. The author

has never encountered a problem with duodenal obstruction following a meticulous closure of this type. This closure is reinforced by tying over it a piece of omentum or nearby serosa-covered mesentery. Thus, proper incision and careful closure of the duodenum can be made safely.

Duodenal fistulas are more likely to occur after trauma to the duodenum, particularly in association with trauma to the head of the pancreas. Under these circumstances, and particularly if there is loss of duodenal substance, repair of the duodenal defect may result in compromise of lumen, and development of a pancreatic fistula may endanger the repair. A safe procedure is closure of the pylorus, creation of a gastrojejunostomy, and creation of a gastrostomy for gastric drainage and a jejunostomy for feeding. If a fistula does occur, it will be an "end" rather than a "side" duodenal fistula.

The reported mortality rate in the past for side duodenal fistula has been very high, ranging from 40 to 60 per cent. In recent years, however, it has decreased significantly, owing to a number of significant improvements in the care of patients with this problem. These include the use of intravenous hyperalimentation, the utilization of defunctionalization of the pylorus, and the placement of a feeding jejunostomy, as well as improved techniques for repair of the duodenal defect.

Duodenal closures should always be drained; thus, when a fistula develops, it should develop as a duodenocutaneous fistula without contamination of the peritoneal cavity. Under these circumstances, the problem is that of loss of large quantities of gastrointestinal fluid because gastric contents as well as bile and pancreatic juices are lost. Furthermore, this is the most active digestive juice that may exit onto the skin, and it impairs healing and rapidly produces severe irritation and maceration of skin that is not properly protected. The approach to the treatment of the lateral duodenal fistula, therefore, should be as follows: All oral alimentation should be immediately discontinued and nasogastric suction instituted. Intravenous hyperalimentation should then be instituted to provide adequate fluid, electrolytes, and nutrition during this early phase. Suction should be applied to the fistulous tract to assure proper collection of the material draining in order that this may aid in calculation of fluid and electrolyte needs. The skin around the fistula should be immediately covered with aluminum paste, and this skin protection should be maintained until the fistula has healed completely.

After institution of this treatment, the progress of the fistula may be followed over a short period of time to determine its course. Some will heal spontaneously under this program, and continuation of intravenous hyperalimentation and maintenance of an empty gastrointestinal tract may be all that is neeeded. The addition of an anticholinergic agent may also be helpful to decrease secretions from the gastrointestinal tract as well as to put the gastrointestinal tract at rest so that a minimal amount of material will be presented to the fistula for drainage. If this produces a rapid decrease in volume from the fistula, spontaneous healing may occur and therefore continuation of this program is desirable. Under this program, if a decrease is occurring, and a well established fistulous tract has developed, a sinogram should be taken to determine the size of the fistula, to ascertain whether or not a single, well established fibrous tract exists, and to insure that there is no obstruction distally in the intestine. Once this circumstance has been reached, the fistula may be plugged with chewing gum or other appropriate agents to eliminate totally the loss from the fistula and to obviate the need for further nasogastric suction. This technique may significantly decrease the time of morbidity of the fistula.

Not all fistulas heal with this program, however, and if continued loss of large amounts of gastrointestinal juices occurs despite intravenous hyperalimentation and nasogastric suction, operative intervention should be undertaken because even with intravenous hyperalimentation it is difficult to replace all of the important contents of gastrointestinal fluid if the volume is large. When primary repair of the fistula can be accomplished, the repair should be reinforced by the use of omentum or by use of a patch of jejunum. The technique used will depend somewhat upon the pathologic change found. If the defect is large, primary suture of the defect should not be undertaken. Rather, the defect should be converted to a duodenojejunostomy with a formal two-layer anastomosis, or a serosal patch of the jejunum should be placed over it. This technique has resulted in the development of a duodenal-jejunal fistula in the late postoperative period in some patients. However, if this occurs into the proximal portion of the jejunum, it will cause no particular difficulty and should be not greatly different from the creation of a duodenojejunostomy.

The occasional fistula will be so large that the repair will be tenuous, irrespective of the technique used. Under these circumstances, the author prefers to protect the repair by closure of the pylorus with sutures and performance of a gastrojejunostomy. A gastrostomy tube can be placed to keep the stomach empty in the early postoperative period, and a feeding jejunostomy tube can be placed either by passing it through the stomach into the jejunum, or as a standard jejunostomy using the Witzel technique. Once this has been accomplished, adequate nutrition without prolonged use of intravenous feedings can be assured by feeding through the jejunostomy tube not only nutriment but also any drainage from the stomach or from the fistula. Under these circumstances, if the fistula repair is not immediately successful, one has the problem of an end, rather than a side, duodenal fistula, so that the patient can soon resume feedings by mouth with emptying through the gastrojejunostomy if the inflammatory process in the upper gastrointestinal tract allows oral ingestion of food without nausea. The placement of the jejunostomy tube will serve as a safety valve to allow feeding below the area of inflammation if food ingestion by mouth cannot be resumed promptly. With these techniques, the current success rate in treatment of duodenal fistulas is quite high. Pancreatoduodenectomy has been advocated for treatment of difficult combined duodenal and pancreatic fistulas, but we have never found this necessary.

MESENTERIC THROMBOSIS

Thrombosis of major intra-abdominal arteries or veins secondary to resection of the pancreas may occur. The mesenteric, portal, splenic, or hepatic vessels may be involved. This complication has been observed most often after pancreatoduodenal resection for carcinoma of the pancreas. Its occurrence after other operations on the pancreas is unusual. In some patients, thrombosis of mesenteric vessels is not actually a complication of surgery, but represents involvement of the vessels with malignant disease, for the entire vein or artery at times becomes occluded with malignant cells. One patient was operated upon recently because of gangrene of the bowel resulting from vascular occlusion due to an islet cell tumor of the pancreas. This is the only such patient with which the author is familiar. In other instances, however, the trauma of dissection in addition to injury during the operation results in occlusion in the postoperative period. It is also well known from autopsy studies that carcinoma of the pancreas is associated with a high incidence of vascular occlusive lesions. These may involve vessels not only in the region of the tumor, but also elsewhere in the body. The precise cause for this thrombosis has not been fully delineated, but it is presumed to be directly related to some secretion from the pancreatic tumor or the effect of the circulating pancreatic tumor cells.

The clinical findings in such patients are the same as those after vascular thrombosis from any other cause. The clinical picture after portal vein thrombosis, for example, is that of an acute abdomen typical of intestinal infarction. Immediate operation should be carried out in an attempt to remove the thrombus and reestablish circulation. The author is at present aware of only one report in which this procedure was carried out successfully after pancreatic resection. In other patients, however, a sufficient length of intestine remains to support life, and resection of the infarcted bowel will allow survival.

INTRA-ABDOMINAL ABSCESS

Infection may complicate pancreatic surgery, as it may any other operation upon the gastrointestinal tract.[13] Abscesses occur most frequently in the upper abdomen, with the lesser peritoneal sac being a common location. Left subphrenic abscesses are likely to occur when left pancreatectomy has been performed in association with splenectomy, and right subphrenic abscesses may also occur. Although these abscesses may occur

in the absence of other demonstrable complications, in most instances they are related to pancreatitis or to the development of pancreatic fistula. In our experience with the treatment of pancreatic trauma, a number of intra-abdominal abscesses have occurred, but in a critical review of this problem, the incidence of intra-abdominal abscess directly attributable to the pancreatic wound was only 1.5 per cent. In contradistinction to this, Child and associates note that subphrenic or subdiaphragmatic abscesses occurred in approximately 10 per cent of 51 patients treated for chronic pancreatitis by pancreatic resection.[9]

Subphrenic or subdiaphragmatic abscess associated with pancreatic disease presents no specific diagnostic problems. An abscess localized within the lesser peritoneal sac deserves specific consideration, however.[5] Under these circumstances, one may anticipate upper gastrointestinal symptoms, including pain and anorexia, frequently associated with nausea and vomiting. Vague epigastric tenderness may be observed, but in some patients the degree of tenderness is much less than one would anticipate in association with a frank infection. An elevation of temperature occurs. Roentgenographic studies of the upper gastrointestinal tract may be helpful in demonstrating external pressure on the posterior wall of the stomach, and it is possible to make an incorrect diagnosis of pseudocyst.

An abscess may form in the lesser peritoneal sac after pancreatic surgery, despite placement of drains at the time of operation, if the drainage is inadequate. Consequently, if findings of sepsis develop, even though there appears to be drainage along a drain tract, one must reoperate and provide more definitive drainage. Adequate cultures must be taken, and current experience emphasizes the need to culture properly for anaerobic as well as aerobic organisms in order that appropriate antibiotic therapy may be administered.

PERITONITIS

Generalized peritonitis has been reported as a cause of death after pancreatic surgery in the past, but today it is a rare complication. When it does occur, it usually represents inadequate drainage of the area of pancreatic surgery or rupture of a neglected pancreatic abscess into the peritoneal cavity. The diagnosis should be suspected when in the postoperative period generalized abdominal pain, anorexia, nausea, vomiting, tenderness, and temperature elevation develop. Bowel sounds, which may previously have been active, will become decreased or absent. If necessary, the diagnosis can be confirmed by a peritoneal tap.

Treatment is immediate operative intervention with thorough cleansing of the entire peritoneal cavity. The site of contamination of the peritoneal cavity should be identified and properly drained. During the operative procedure, introduction of an antibiotic solution into the peritoneal cavity may be of benefit. Systemic administration of a wide spectrum antibiotic should be begun preoperatively as soon as the diagnosis is made. More specific antibiotic therapy may be chosen as soon as culture and sensitivity data are available.

HEPATIC FAILURE

Varying degrees of hepatic dysfunction are found in association with many pancreatic lesions. Perhaps the most common is the association of cirrhosis with alcoholic pancreatitis. Impaired hepatic function also occurs as a direct result of long-term obstruction of the biliary tract. In the early stages of obstructive jaundice hepatic function remains relatively normal and operation can be undertaken without a significantly increased risk of postoperative hepatic problems. If obstruction is not relieved, however, damage to hepatic cells generally results and this may progress to biliary cirrhosis. Tests of hepatic function are usually abnormal within 1 month after the onset of jaundice. It is thus desirable to differentiate between intrahepatic jaundice and extrahepatic obstruction as expeditiously as possible, for failure to operate early in the course of obstructive jaundice not only allows progression of the basic disease process, but also results in progressive hepatic damage. The possibility of hepatic failure in the postoperative period was one of the reasons why a two-stage operation was advocated for treatment of pancreatic cancer in years past, and it is of interest that a recent report indicates that a two-stage operation

results in a lower mortality rate even today. This is no doubt true if one considers only the mortality rate following the second operation, but the true mortality rate of a two-stage procedure is the combined rates of the first and second procedures, and our experience indicates that only rarely is a two-stage procedure of possible advantage.

Hepatic insufficiency is best treated by prevention. However, when evidence of hepatic failure is found postoperatively, it should be treated in the same manner as hepatic failure occurring in the absence of surgery. Bed rest is an important factor in treatment, and the usual program of exercise and ambulation prescribed postoperatively must be modified. An adequate diet high in carbohydrates and vitamins must be provided. If the patient has an anemia it should be corrected with blood transfusions. A maximal effort should be made to prevent atelectasis and pneumonia, not only because of the risks of these complications but also to insure adequate oxygenation of the liver. Equipment to supply positive pressure as an aid to respiration should be used if needed, and if the sensorium becomes clouded, tracheostomy may be necessary to maintain a good airway.

The value of steroids in such problems is still debated, but we recommend their use.

The preceding description has dealt with hepatic insufficiency resulting from hepatic disease existing preoperatively. Damage to the liver can also occur as a result of the operation. The most common problem is damage to the blood supply of the liver during dissection of the main trunk of the hepatic artery when freeing the pancreatic head, or to the right hepatic artery during cholecystectomy or a difficult dissection of the porta hepatis. In many patients the right hepatic artery is anomalous and may arise from the superior mesenteric artery or directly from the aorta. In these instances it may course posterior to the pancreas and be mistaken for a pancreatic artery and divided. It may also course on the right side of the common bile duct, so that careful dissection to identify the vasculature of the liver should be performed before any major structures are taken. Should damage to the hepatic artery occur, immediate repair should be accomplished. Damage to one wall, such as may occur if a tie cuts through the base of the gastroduodenal artery, can be readily repaired with one or two sutures of 6–0 arterial suture. If more severe damage occurs, vascular clamps should be applied proximally and distally and an end-to-end anastomosis accomplished. If this cannot be performed rapidly, the liver may be protected by cooling with sterile iced saline.

Lastly, a rare cause of hepatic failure is infarction of the liver in the absence of injury of the hepatic artery. This is a rare lesion and the cause may not be identified. It could, however, be due to inadvertent occlusion of the hepatic artery by retractors during the operation or to embolization of atheromatous plaques dislodged from the hepatic artery during dissection. Therefore, particular care must be taken in the dissection of the hepatic artery in older persons. Infarction of the liver is heralded by the development of high fever and jaundice, and if the infarction involves enough hepatic tissue, death occurs. If the diagnosis is suspected, antibiotics should be administered to prevent secondary infection, and the use of steroids may decrease the inflammatory response in adjacent viable hepatic cells. Experience with treatment of hepatic infarction is so limited that the precise value of any specific therapy is unknown. The diagnosis has often been made only at necropsy.

RENAL INSUFFICIENCY

Renal failure has been a major cause of death after pancreatoduodenal resection for carcinoma of the pancreas. Renal insufficiency may arise from a variety of causes. It is particularly likely to occur in elderly patients who are quite ill and are subjected to a prolonged operation. The development of shock due to surgical trauma or hemorrhage during the procedure may precipitate renal insufficiency, and the administration of transfusions during the operation may result in a transfusion reaction. In these elderly patients there may be some preexisting renal disease that accentuates the severity of the problem. Consideration must be given also to what in the past has been called the "hepatorenal syndrome." There is not general agreement as to whether or not

such a syndrome actually exists, but there are those who believe that precipitation of bilirubin in the renal tubules, particularly in patients with inadequate hydration, may impair renal function and thus increase the risk of renal failure in patients with jaundice. Hori and associates reported that impairment of renal function occurred in the dog after experimental and temporary occlusion of blood flow to the kidney and after crush stimulation of the nerve plexus around the hepatic artery and gastrohepatic ligaments.[17]

Other causes of renal insufficiency include the development of sepsis postoperatively and administration of antibiotics that have a high degree of renal toxicity, particularly the aminoglycosides such as kanamycin and gentamicin. Nephrotoxic drugs should not be used prophylactically in these patients. Their use should be reserved for special problems in which they represent the drug of choice for treatment of an established infection.

Periods of oliguria or even short periods of anuria in the postoperative period after major pancreatic resection are not uncommon if adequate fluid replacement is not maintained. In the past the usual cause was simple inadequacy of fluid administration owing to reluctance to replace fluids in elderly patients. Additional factors may be operative in these patients that are of significance in this regard. Drains are usually placed in the region of the anastomosis during the first few days after pancreatoduodenectomy. Large amounts of fluid may drain from the raw surfaces during the operative dissection. If an accurate estimate of this fluid loss is not made and considered in prescribing replacement, inadequate fluid administration may result. Consequently, in the early postoperative period, fluid loss at the drain site should be estimated with reasonable accuracy. If drainage is unusually excessive it should be collected by sump suction so that an accurate record can be maintained. An accurate record of loss by nasogastric suction also is mandatory. Furthermore, fluid may accumulate in the abdominal cavity, and if the patient does not rapidly begin to have normal bowel activity, a significant amount of fluid may accumulate in the gastrointestinal tract. All of these factors lead to decreased urinary output.

In view of these considerations, it is important that patients undergoing pancreatoduodenectomy be maintained in a good state of hydration. As the average age of these patients is 60 years, other associated diseases such as myocardial insufficiency may also be present that make it important to avoid fluid overload. Thus, as accurate an estimate as possible of the patient's needs must be made at all times and proper fluid replacement must be maintained.

In most instances, the diagnosis of renal insufficiency can be readily made by measurement of urine osmolarity, the ratio of plasma to urinary osmolarity, and the urine sodium excretion. A high urine osmolarity in the presence of diminished or absent excretion of sodium and chloride should lead one to the conclusion that there has been inadequate administration of both fluid and electrolytes. Thus, a trial of rapid administration of 1000 ml. of 5 per cent dextrose in normal saline is justified. This will frequently result in prompt resumption of urinary output. Replacement of the fluid deficit can then be accomplished and accurate estimations of fluid loss and replacement continued at that time. When fluid administration alone does not result in diuresis, a specific diuretic may be administered. In the past, mannitol was the drug most commonly used. This is an osmotically active diuretic, however, and if response is not forthcoming, it may result in a significantly increased intravascular fluid volume; thus, use of large doses of mannitol may increase the strain on cardiac reserve. Consequently, in recent years, furosemide (Lasix) has been more popular. This drug acts directly upon the kidney and is a more potent diuretic than mannitol. It does not have a persistent effect in patients in whom diuresis does not develop, for it is estimated that its length of action does not exceed 4 hours. This drug is initially used in doses of 10 to 40 mg. intravenously, and when given in addition to fluids it usually will produce a prompt diuresis. Larger doses may also be used, and doses as large as 400 mg. intravenously are not uncommon. Such doses may produce an increased volume of urine even in the presence of lower nephron nephrosis, and in some patients an oliguric renal insufficiency may be converted to a high-output renal insufficiency. Thus, when this drug is used, it is mandatory that careful and repeated estimations of the concentrations of blood urea nitrogen, creatinine, and serum electrolytes be made to follow the progress of the patient. The increased volume may lead one to the erroneous conclusion that the problem of renal insufficiency has been overcome, when in actuality there has been a simple change in the form of the renal insufficiency.

When mild degrees of oliguric renal insufficiency develop, treatment is similar to that classically used in the past, namely, careful calculation of the specific fluid requirements of the patient, taking into account insensible loss, urinary output, loss through nasogastric suction, and loss through other areas of drainage. Administration of hypertonic glucose and insulin aids in preventing a rapid rise in the serum potassium concentration, and acidosis is controlled by administration of sodium bicarbonate.

When severe oliguric or anuric renal insufficiency develops, prompt institution of renal dialysis is important. In these patients, the period of anesthesia and surgical trauma produces a catabolic state that results in a rapid rise in serum potassium and accumulation of metabolic acid waste products — a somewhat different metabolic state from that in patients in whom renal insufficiency develops slowly. Furthermore, in such patients the operative procedure and the presence of a highly malignant lesion have already made considerable demand upon basic reserves. Maximal support is needed from the beginning of treatment and this can best be provided by prompt institution of renal dialysis, maintaining the blood pH, blood urea nitrogen, and serum potassium concentration at as near normal levels as possible at all times. In the past, severe oliguric renal failure in patients undergoing major surgery was attended by mortality rates ranging from 60 to 90 per cent. How much this mortality rate can be reduced by the early institution of renal dialysis has not yet been adequately documented, but dialysis is the best method of treatment currently available.

MARGINAL ULCER

A late complication after pancreatoduodenectomy is marginal ulcer. It has been recommended that partial gastrectomy or vagotomy be performed to decrease the likelihood of this complication, and, in fact, in recent years there has been increasing interest in the combination of both vagotomy and partial gastrectomy with pancreatoduodenectomy. The incidence with which marginal ulcer occurs varies considerably among reports by different authors. Waddell and Loughry observed marginal ulcers in the late follow-up period after pancreatoduodenectomy in 2 of 14 patients treated for tumors and for trauma.[36] In one patient the ulcer occurred 8 years after operation. The authors performed gastric acid studies, and the basal acid values were within the low-normal range. Interestingly enough, the two patients in their series with ulcer disease had lower average acid secretions (0.7 mEq. per hour) than those without the development of ulcer (1.0 mEq. per hour). A relatively high incidence of marginal ulcer has also been reported by other authors, and thus today the standard procedure for resection of the head of the pancreas includes removal of a portion of the stomach. We remove the distal portion of the stomach in performing pancreatoduodenectomy, but do not include vagotomy because our experience does not reflect the high incidence of marginal ulcer reported by others. In a review of 100 consecutive patients undergoing pancreatoduodenectomy, there has been only one documented marginal ulcer, which occurred 4 years postoperatively.

There is reason to believe that one of the factors accounting for the differences in the reported incidence of marginal ulcer is the technique of reconstruction of the gastrointestinal tract. More than 30 different techniques have been described; some of these divert all of the bile and pancreatic juice away from the gastroenteric anastomosis, creating, in the human, a physiol gical abnormality similar to that created in the Mann-Williamson operation devised for the experimental production of ulcer in the dog. We prefer, therefore, a technique of reconstruction such as described by Hunt or Waugh in which both the pancreatic and biliary anastomoses are placed into a loop of jejunum which functionally simulates the afferent loop following a Billroth II reconstruction after gastrectomy.[42] Thus, all bile and pancreatic juices drain past the gastrojejunal anastomosis and give protection against the development of marginal ulcer.

In the occasional patient with pancreatitis in whom cicatricial stenosis of the common duct occurs, a choledochojejunostomy with Roux-en-Y anastomosis to drain the biliary tract and a retrograde pancreatojejunostomy to drain the obstructed pancreatic duct may be performed. If these procedures are required, a vagotomy should be performed. In a recently treated patient an ulcer developed despite vagotomy and required a gastric resection for control of hemorrhage.

It is apparent, therefore, that patients who return with symptoms of abdominal pain after pancreatic surgery will, in some instances, have an ulcer of the duodenum or, if the stomach has been resected, a marginal ulcer, and thus, evaluation of this possibility should always be included as a part of the diagnostic procedure. A trial of medical therapy is justified, and in the occasional patient a good response will be obtained. In one of Waddell and Loughry's patients, for example, a marginal ulcer that occurred 8 years postoperatively was treated conservatively, and the patient was alive and well without further difficulty at the time of the report, 16 years after operation. Failure to respond to medical therapy or development of life-endangering hemorrhage, perforation, or obstruction will require operative therapy, however; it should consist of a higher resection of the stomach and the assurance of a complete vagotomy.

DIABETES

Islets of Langerhans are scattered throughout the entire pancreas. Whereas it is commonly stated that the majority are in the body and tail, there is little accurate evidence to indicate that there is a significant difference in the insulin production from various portions of the gland. Most investigators report that 80 per cent of the gland may be removed without producing diabetes, and these data are derived from clinical and experimental studies following removal of the head and body and a portion of the tail, or removal of the tail and body. There is adequate evidence to support this observation, and the present experience with extensive distal subtotal pancreatectomy for the treatment of pancreatitis, as advocated by Child and associates, in which it is estimated that 90 per cent or more of the pancreatic tissue is removed, with only a small rim of the pancreas left adjacent to the duodenum to preserve the duodenal blood supply, supplies documentation that survival of only a very small amount of the head of the pancreas is sufficient to prevent diabetes in some patients. Child et al. report that approximately 10 per cent of the patients having an extensive resection of this type do not incur diabetes, even though the remainder of the gland is presumably involved with severe pancreatitis.[9] Diabetes invariably ensues, however, when total pancreatectomy is performed.[12, 38]

The diabetes created by pancreatic resection differs in several significant respects from spontaneously occurring adult-onset diabetes and is not the same disease.[27] The clinical and laboratory findings are strikingly different. The amount of insulin necessary to control the diabetes following total pancreatectomy is relatively small. In some patients, as little as 10 units per day is satisfactory, and rarely is more than 25 units or 30 units per day necessary. These patients also seem to be unduly sensitive to insulin, for profound hypoglycemic coma may develop with doses as small as 20 units of insulin, which, in many normal patients, may not even produce symptomatic hypoglycemia. In the past this apparent sensitivity to insulin was presumed by some to be due to the fact that many of the patients requiring the operation were malnourished and underweight. At the present time, however, it is generally conceded that this is not the full explanation, although it may be a factor. Another factor is that, unlike spontaneously occurring adult-onset diabetes, this is an insulin-deficient diabetes, so that lower absolute insulin values are found on plasma insulin determination, with no insulin response to glucose feeding, whereas in spontaneously occurring adult-onset diabetes, plasma insulin values are usually within normal range and there is frequently an exaggerated insulin response to carbohydrate ingestion. Total pancreatectomy removes all of the pancreatic islet cells, not only insulin-producing cells, but also glucagon-producing cells. Furthermore, it is possible that the islet cells produce other, as yet unrecognized, hormones that are effective in regulation of carbohydrate metabolism. Total pancreatectomy in a patient with previously established adult-onset diabetes usually results in no significant change in insulin requirements, though in an occasional patient the insulin requirement may be reduced.

For these reasons, in managing a patient in the postoperative period after total pancreatectomy, hypoglycemia is a greater problem than diabetic coma. Insulin should be administered in small doses with careful monitoring of urinary sugar loss and blood glucose concentration. In the immediate postoperative period the initial use of 10 per cent glucose solutions with 5 units of insulin added to each bottle will be sufficient in some patients. When blood sugar concentration and urinary sugar level indicate that this is an insufficient amount, it can be increased to 10 units of insulin per bottle, but rarely will it be necessary to exceed this dosage; it is safer to allow a moderate elevation of the blood sugar concentration and positive urine findings than to try to keep the blood sugar concentration at a normal level and to keep the urine sugar-free by increasing insulin dosage. There have been a number of deaths postoperatively due to hypoglycemia, but diabetic coma has been encountered infrequently.

When the patient is ready to receive a normal diet, a 2500-calorie diabetic diet can be prescribed with the dosage of insulin suited to his individual needs. Most patients do well with one daily dose of NPH or a similar long-acting insulin. Careful instructions in care of their diabetic state must be given before discharge, particularly in view of the fact that these patients have an absorption defect, and the amount of fat and nitrogen absorption may vary from day to day and also may change with time.

The long-term experience with surgically created diabetes in the human is relatively meager, for only a few patients with total pancreatectomy have survived 5 or more years, and an even smaller number have survived into old age. In general, however, those patients who do well in the early postoperative period continue to do well. Diabetic complications have been reported, but the incidence of such complications is not known.[31, 38]

LATE NUTRITIONAL EFFECTS

Chronic pancreatitis may result in great diminution of external pancreatic secretion, to the point of development of clinical manifestations of steatorrhea and weight loss, leading ultimately to varying degrees of emaciation. Increased loss of fat and nitrogen immediately follows total pancreatectomy and may occur after limited resections as well.[4, 19, 24] Fish and associates, in a study of patients who had undergone pancreatoduodenectomy for carcinoma, for example, found, on the basis of chemical studies, that all the patients had increased loss of fat in the stool as compared to normal, and three of six patients studied had been unable to regain their weight.[14] In view of the fact that partial gastric resection was part of the procedure in these patients, it is not possible to determine how much of the problem was due to the gastric resection and how much was due to loss of pancreatic enzymes. The authors further concluded that the pancreatojejunostomy often did not remain functional and that stenosis or complete occlusion of the pancreatic ductal system was the usual circumstance. Warren believes that duct stenosis can be prevented by an accurate anastomosis between duct and jejunal mucosa rather than simple implantation of the pancreas into the jejunum.[39]

The initial symptom of exocrine pancreatic insufficiency is usually diarrhea, which may progress to frank steatorrhea. As already noted, chemical determinations of fecal content will show an increased loss of fat and of protein in some patients with diarrhea, despite the physical appearance of the stool.[23, 41] Weight loss may ensue. Though the most recent patient in our series of those having total pancreatectomy gained 5 pounds during the first 2 weeks after discharge from the hospital, most patients with total pancreatectomy and some with partial pancreatectomy will have difficulty in maintaining their weight without oral supplementation of pancreatic enzymes. Fortunately today there are more potent enzymatic replacement products than were available many years ago. Two of the most potent are Cotazym and Viokase.[15] Cotazym is given in doses of two to four tablets three to four times a day. Longmire

and associates observed that if the patient is on a six-meal-per-day diet or is eating more frequently, more frequent feeding of Viokase is useful in aiding them to digest their food.[25]

Establishment of a pancreatojejunostomy in patients with pancreatic duct obstruction due to pancreatitis may result in significant weight gain and general improvement in nutritional status. It is rational to presume that this desirable result is due to reinstitution of flow of pancreatic juice. This is not well documented, however, and it is possible

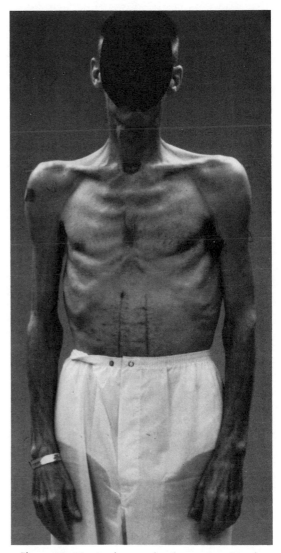

Figure 22–11 A photograph of a patient in whom severe malnutrition secondary to pancreatitis developed despite surgical attempts to relieve his disease.

that cessation of attacks of pancreatitis and increased oral intake of food are more important factors, for in our experience longitudinal pancreatojejunostomy does not result in significant weight gain unless the attacks of pancreatitis are controlled.

Most patients with external pancreatic insufficiency survive this complication despite some weight loss, steatorrhea, and the resulting weakness. In the rare patient, however, malnutrition may be life-endangering (Fig. 22–11).

Treatment of chronic steatorrhea and malnutrition requires good dietary supervision, trial of various drugs and regimens (for there is a definite difference in the response of patients to different programs), and patience on the part of the physician. A diet must be prepared that is attractive to the patient. The fat content should be limited. Frequent small feedings may be tolerated better than three large ones. If diarrhea is the basic problem, the use of diphenox-ylate (Lomotil) or other drugs to decrease speed of transit may be helpful. Dietary supplements are beneficial in some patients. Medium-chain triglycerides as a dietary supplement are useful, but in the author's experience existing products have had poor patient acceptance because of taste. Predigested protein supplements or "elemental diets" may also be helpful.

Patients may have periods when nutritional problems are uncontrollable on an outpatient basis. Hospitalization should be recommended. Nutritional improvement can usually be accomplished with tube feedings of predigested foods plus medication. If this technique is not successful, and particularly if diarrhea is difficult to control, cessation of all oral intake and institution of intravenous hyperalimentation may produce sufficient weight gain and return to satisfactory sense of well-being that the patient can subsequently sustain himself on an oral diet.

COMPLICATIONS OF SPLENECTOMY

The spleen, unlike the pancreas, has no particularly complex anatomic relationships. It has a major blood supply from the splenic artery and splenic vein. The splenic artery gives rise to the left gastroepiploic artery and to short gastric vessels to the stomach, but division of these vessels rarely affects the blood supply to that organ. Of equal significance is the fact that for the most part only one operation is performed on the spleen, as compared to the multiple complex procedures often performed dur-ing surgery for pancreatic lesions. In recent years, however, because of concerns of immunologic deficits in patients subjected to splenectomy, particularly children, there has been an increasing number of reports of salvage of the spleen or of portions of the spleen. Furthermore, elective partial splenectomy has been performed in the treatment of some diseases. The complications of partial splenectomy, however, are the same as those of total splenectomy (Table 22–2).

HEMORRHAGE

A small spleen may be removed from the abdomen with minimal blood loss. However, when the spleen is extremely large, so that exposure of the major splenic vessels is difficult, and when there are multiple vascularized adhesions between the spleen and the surrounding organs and the diaphragm, severe hemorrhage may be encountered during splenectomy. Splenectomy may be particularly difficult in the presence of portal hypertension. Hemorrhage may occur from an inadvertent tear in the splenic capsule or from an extremely vascular adhe-

TABLE 22–2 COMPLICATIONS OF SPLENECTOMY

I. Intra-abdominal
  A. Hemorrhage
  B. Infection
  C. Fistula
    1. Gastric
    2. Pancreatic
  D. Delayed rupture
  E. Splenosis
  F. Stress ulceration
II. General
  A. Thrombosis
  B. Late infection
III. Intrathoracic
  Atelectasis and pneumonia

sion that may retract behind a large spleen and be difficult to expose, or it may be due to inadvertent damage to the major splenic vessels. Thus, when removing a large spleen, it is preferable to have control of the splenic artery and the splenic vein before the spleen is mobilized. When removing a spleen with many vascular adhesions, the adhesions should be carefully divided and ligated sequentially as the dissection proceeds, with care not to tear these vessels.[54]

Because of the vascularity of the spleen and the danger of hemorrhage, blood should be available for transfusion whenever splenectomy is planned. Deaths have occurred during the operations because of uncontrollable hemorrhage from the spleen, but with rapid transfusion and expedient removal of the organ, ultimate control of hemorrhage and replacement of blood volume should be possible even under dire circumstances.

When severe hemorrhage from the spleen occurs, immediate control of the splenic artery and vein is necessary if it has not already been obtained. Control is most easily first accomplished by grasping the tail of the pancreas and compressing the splenic vessels in this area (Fig. 22–12). If exposure is difficult, further control can be obtained by placing a non-crushing vascular clamp across the splenic pedicle, which will immediately control blood flow through these vessels without the serious damage to adjacent tissues that a large crushing clamp could cause. The vessels controlled, the spleen can then be rapidly removed and any

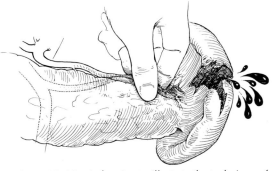

Figure 22–12 A drawing to illustrate the technique of immediate control of hemorrhage due to laceration of the spleen. The lesser sac is rapidly opened and the tail of the pancreas is grasped between the fingers, so that the splenic artery and splenic vein are compressed.

vascular adhesions that have been difficult to expose can be immediately controlled with packing and then definitively controlled by individual clamping and ligation of the bleeding areas. The splenic vessels can be controlled under these circumstances by closing the transected ends with vascular suture, rather than attempting to ligate them individually, if the splenic vessels are very friable and individual dissection seems hazardous.

When the splenic bed has been drained, massive hemorrhage may occur from the splenic vessels as a late complication. The bleeding usually occurs after a firm, fibrous tract has formed around the drains, and under these circumstances, bleeding into the peritoneal cavity does not occur. Massive hemorrhage may suddenly appear while the patient is apparently recovering uneventfully from his surgical procedure, as it may be a complication of infection. When this happens, if drains are still in place, they should be rapidly removed and the bleeding controlled by placing a finger into the drainage tract to occlude it, or by rapidly placing a pack of Surgicel gauze. This will control bleeding immediately and allow replacement of blood volume by appropriate intravenous administration of blood and other fluids. The patient should be taken to the operating room soon and definitive control of hemorrhage accomplished at laparotomy by ligation of the splenic artery and vein at a point proximal to the site of hemorrhage. If bleeding is recognized soon after it begins, prompt control and successful outcome should be anticipated. If bleeding is not recognized promptly, or if immediate control is not obtained, fatal hemorrhage may occur.

The fact that hemorrhage represents the most common cause of death leads to important considerations in the management of patients with splenic injury. On admission to the hospital, rapid evaluation should be accomplished. If splenic injury is suspected but cannot be unequivocally diagnosed, peritoneal tap should be performed, and if hemorrhage is found, the patient should be promptly moved to the operating room without detailed diagnostic roentgenography or other prolonged tests. Furthermore, one should not spend time attempting to "improve the patient's condition" before operation is undertaken. When active hemorrhage from the spleen is occurring, the most important resuscitative measure is control of the hemorrhage. Bleeding from the splenic artery and from the splenic vein can occur more rapidly than replacement therapy can be administered.[50, 53, 59]

When splenic repair is attempted after traumatic rupture or after partial splenectomy is performed, hemorrhage from the raw surface of the spleen is controlled by use of hemostatic agents such as Avitene or Surgicel, plus suture. Suture control of hemorrhage, particularly in children, can be accomplished much more readily than previously believed, and in cases reported both in children and adults, the incidence of rebleeding from the traumatized or transected spleen in the late postoperative period has been low. Rebleeding may occur, however, and for this reason the author recommends drainage of this area so that hemorrhage can be detected, should it occur. If recurrent hemorrhage occurs, it should be treated by splenectomy.

When the spleen is removed as an elective procedure, the type of incision is of little consequence, in the opinion of the author, as long as it gives adequate exposure. Thus, some surgeons prefer a left subcostal incision, some prefer a left paramedian, and some perform the procedure through a midline incision. If the spleen is very large, a thoracoabdominal approach may even be helpful. When massive hemorrhage is the problem, however, the most rapid and expeditious incision possible should be made. This, in the opinion of most surgeons, is a long midline incision, which will give adequate exposure of the splenic fossa and in addition will allow adequate inspection and examination of all other organs to eliminate the possibility of associated injuries and will provide adequate exposure to treat them should any be found.

ABSCESS

There are few data to document accurately any superiority of drainage over nondrainage of the splenic bed after splenectomy. The final decision has usually reflected the experience of the surgeon and, to some degree, his emotional response to the various factors that have been thought to be of importance. It would appear rational to drain the splenic bed when there has been associated injury of the pancreas (and therefore the possibility of development of pancreatic fistula or collection of the pancreatic juice in the splenic bed), when there has been associated injury of the colon and the area has been contaminated, when there is injury to an adjacent portion of the stomach, and when there has been injury to the kidney from which a fistula might arise. Under these circumstances, drainage is established primarily because of the associated organ injury, rather than specifically because the spleen is removed. It is important, however, to remove the spleen carefully, to control hemorrhage from the splenic vessels properly, and to make sure that there is adequate hemostasis in the splenic bed. The divided peritoneal surfaces should be reapproximated with a running catgut suture so that the raw surface created by removal of the spleen is completely covered with peritoneum. In this way, one further assures adequate control of bleeding, the end of the pancreas is covered with peritoneum, and there is no raw area from which drainage directly into the left subphrenic space will occur.

As noted previously, there are strong differences of opinion concerning the value of drainage. Slate and associates believe that postoperative complications are more prevalent if the splenic bed is not drained.[60] Olsen and Beaudoin, on the other hand, concluded that prolonged prophylactic drainage of the left subphrenic space actually increases the incidence of subphrenic abscess and significant drain tract infection without offering any advantages.[56] A careful review of the data available in the literature on this subject, as well as an evaluation of the experience in our own institution, leads us to the conclusion that drainage does not decrease the incidence of subphrenic abscess. We have observed the development of subphrenic abscess in patients who had apparently adequate drainage as well as in those who had none, and thus we do not recommend routine drainage. If the splenic bed is properly closed, if there is no contamination of the subphrenic space, and if careful attention has been paid to division of arteries along the greater curvature of the

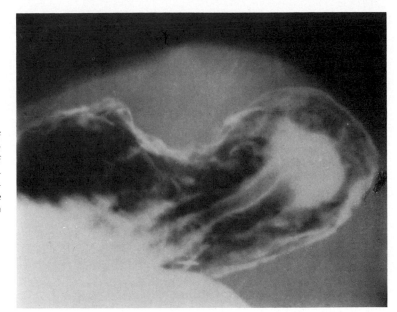

Figure 22–13 Roentgenogram of the upper gastrointestinal tract may be helpful in the diagnosis of subphrenic abscess following splenectomy. This roentgenogram demonstrates external compression of the stomach due to a subphrenic mass in the left upper quadrant.

stomach and dissection of the pancreas away from the spleen, a subphrenic abscess should not occur.

An abscess that develops after removal of the spleen is almost always in the left subphrenic space. Temperature elevation and symptoms of malaise occur, and there may or may not be actual pain in the region of the subphrenic space. The diagnosis should be suspected when there is elevation of the left leaf of the diaphragm as well as tenderness either anteriorly or over the twelfth rib posteriorly. The presence of an air-fluid level in the left upper quadrant that can be proved to be outside the gastrointestinal tract is virtually pathognomonic. In some patients, the diagnosis may be difficult. Examination of the upper gastrointestinal tract radiographically using barium as well as a barium enema may be of aid in demonstrating displacement of these organs from the anticipated position in the left upper quadrant or in revealing an actual pressure defect on the cardiofundus of the stomach (Fig. 22–13).

In recent years, ultrasonography has been the most valuable technique for early diagnosis of abscess. This examination is often positive before other classic roentgenographic findings are present. Computerized axial tomography would also aid in the diagnosis, but in our experience, results

with ultrasound have been as accurate as computerized tomography, and much less expensive.

Once the diagnosis has been made, the treatment is drainage, which may be accomplished posteriorly through the bed of the twelfth rib. This will prevent contamination of the general peritoneal cavity, as well as providing the most dependent drainage. In some patients, on the other hand, the abscess occurs in an anterior position and can best be drained transabdominally. The decision concerning the proper incision must be made on the evidence of the site of localization of the abscess cavity. At the time of drainage, proper culture should be taken and appropriate antibiotic therapy instituted. At present, it is possible to treat most subphrenic abscesses successfully.

After hemorrhage, which is the most common serious complication of splenic rupture, infection, usually in the subphrenic space, leads the list of complications in most series. In our experience, intra-abdominal infection of all types has occurred in approximately 10 per cent of patients undergoing splenectomy for traumatic rupture. In many instances, however, the subphrenic space has been contaminated by injuries to other organs, and consequently this infection rate represents not the infection rate of splenectomy but that of splenectomy performed in the presence of an already contaminated peritoneal cavity. Splenectomy performed as a single intra-abdominal procedure under elective conditions should be attended by a very low incidence of subphrenic abscess; in some series, the incidence has been as low as 1 per cent. Of particular interest is the very low incidence of infection of the subphrenic space after splenectomy performed as a part of renal transplantation studies, in which the patients underwent splenectomy, often associated nephrectomy, as well as concomitant subsequent renal transplantation. These patients were often in a poor state of nutrition and had chronic uremia. Furthermore, they were given immunosuppressive drugs at the time of renal transplantation, and thus had decreased resistance to infection. Under these circumstances, most surgeons have not drained the splenic bed, but the incidence of infection has been quite low, and it has been a rare cause of death in such patients. These data support the contention that drainage of the splenic bed is not necessary in the absence of extenuating circumstances.

LATE INFECTIONS

There is evidence to indicate that the spleen is actively involved in the development of the general immune response in young children. Just how long the spleen plays an important role is not well documented, though most observers support the concept that full immunologic maturation has occurred by the age of 2 years and that, in the absence of other disease, splenectomy does not create any greater degree of hazard in children beyond the age of 2 than in the adult. Current evidence would suggest that some patients undergoing splenectomy before the age of 2 may not develop full immunologic competence and may have decreased resistance to infection. Severe infections may occur and may be fatal. Some pediatric surgeons are so concerned about this problem that they attempt to salvage a part of the spleen even in the management of traumatic rupture in children. Haller and Jones studied this problem in 51 children under the age of 10 treated at Johns Hopkins Hospital, with an average follow-up of

6.2 years.[52] The postoperative mortality rate was 10 per cent, two patients dying of infection. These authors concluded that fear of infection should not interfere with performance of splenectomy when specific indications are present, though consideration of prophylactic antibiotics in children under 1 year of age was suggested.

Further evidence is found in the report of Bilski-Pasquier and Bonnet-Gajdos, who reviewed the progress of 1255 children subjected to prolonged medical observation following splenectomy.[47] One hundred and four (8 per cent) of these child had one or more serious infections, and 43 died of them. The most common infections were purulent meningitis and septicemia, though all types occurred. The pneumococcus and meningococcus were the bacteria most commonly isolated. The interval between operation and the first serious infectious manifestation varied from a few days to several years, but was usually 2 to 3 years. These authors believe that the risk of infection varies with the disease process and that it is particularly high in the Aldrich syndrome. They concluded that in this disease the dangers of splenectomy are far greater than its benefit.

In recent years concern about the possibility of early or late infection, particularly with pneumococcus, has steadily increased. There is now a concern about postsplenectomy infection in adults, as well as in children. Until a few years ago, it was generally believed that the immune system was well developed in the normal adult and that splenectomy might impair immunocompetence only in patients with specific diseases which in themselves impaired immunocompetence. However, there have been reports of fatal pneumococcal infections occurring in adults following splenectomy. In a recent review of this subject, Sherman collected reports of a total of 10 postsplenectomy patients in whom pneumococcal pneumonia occurred, and 6 of these patients expired.[58] Thus, some surgeons are advocating salvage of the spleen even in the adult, and there are ongoing studies to delineate more specifically the indications and safety of this procedure.

Concern about postsplenectomy infections has reached a point at which some clinicians advocate routine immunization of all splenectomized patients against pneumo-coccus, and some advocate prophylactic antibiotic therapy for the remainder of the life of the individual. It is unfortunate that some statements have been made as strongly as they have, for vaccine-type pneumococcal pneumonia has occurred after vaccination in an asplenic patient, and fatal pneumococcal bacteremia has occurred in a splenectomized child despite vaccination.[46, 51] Furthermore, in the opinion of the author, the use of prophylactic antibiotics over a period of 40 to 60 years — which would be the normal life expectancy of most patients undergoing splenectomy for trauma — is highly questionable, since morbidity and mortality rates from the antibiotics may be greater than those from the splenectomy. Thus, in our institution, we are not using long-term prophylactic antibiotics at this time, but rather, we believe that the patient should be advised of the potential problem.

THROMBOSIS

A complication of splenectomy that received a great deal of attention in older standard textbooks is the development of thrombosis. Thrombosis is commonly attributed to the increase in platelet count that may occur after the operation and the resulting increased coagulability of the blood.[49, 54, 55, 62] Some rise in platelet count is anticipated after splenectomy under any circumstances. It may be transient or prolonged. In cases in which splenectomy is necessitated by trauma, when the spleen was normal preoperatively and the patient had no other concurrent disease, platelet count elevations to 500,000 to 700,000 per cu. mm. are often seen, but increases beyond this level are relatively uncommon. In certain diseases, such as congenital hemolytic jaundice and hypersplenic states, however, splenectomy produces marked rises in platelet count. The greatest rise in platelet count observed by the author occurred in a patient with an idiopathic hypersplenism; after splenectomy the platelet count rose to 3 million per cu. mm. and remained at this level throughout the patient's life. No spontaneous thrombosis occurred, however.

Whether or not the patient should be treated with anticoagulants when elevation of the platelet count occurs is a subject on which there is not complete agreement. Approximately 20 years ago, anticoagulant therapy was commonly recommended if the platelet count exceeded 750,000 per cu. mm. It is not clear just why this particular figure was used. Experience showed, however, that despite the elevated platelet count, thrombosis is really not common, and the complications of anticoagulant therapy appear to be as great as the complications of thrombosis resulting from the increased number of circulating platelets. Consequently, it seems at this time that most clinicians reserve anticoagulant treatment for patients in whom clinical findings of thrombosis develop.

When it occurs, thrombosis is more likely to involve veins than arteries, although coronary thrombosis after splenectomy has been reported on a number of occasions. In general, however, the patients have been in the age range in which coronary thrombosis is likely to occur. In our experience, thrombotic complications in young patients remain quite rare despite high platelet counts.

When thrombotic complications occur, they are seen more frequently during the second and third postoperative weeks. In the report by Slate and associates, the only deaths following splenic injury when the spleen was the only organ injured occurred from postoperative thrombosis during the third week.[60]

SPLENOSIS

The spleen of the dog varies considerably from that of man. After trauma, fatal hemorrhage is much less likely to occur in the dog, as the spleen is a very contractile organ, and, unlike the human spleen, the dog's spleen can be biopsied and sutured with very little danger. Consequently, after significant abdominal trauma resulting in rupture of the spleen, many dogs may subsequently be found at autopsy or at surgery to have small implants of the spleen growing throughout the peritoneal cavity. We have observed this on many occasions in our experimental laboratories.

Splenosis in the human, however, is quite

uncommon. In 1971, Widmann and Laubscher were able to find only 70 cases of splenosis reported in the world literature.[61] Undoubtedly many additional cases have been observed but have not been worthy of a specific report. Although the incidence remains quite small, small pieces of spleen may be found growing in the peritoneal cavity after splenic rupture. When present, the splenic implants are usually multiple. They are small and encapsulated, as a rule, though sessile and slightly pedunculated implants may be seen. The size varies from a few millimeters to 2 or 3 cm. in diameter and there is no surrounding inflammatory response or fibrosis. Splenic implants are commonly seen throughout the entire abdominal cavity, including the pelvis, and they have been observed in the chest as well. Whether or not splenosis is a beneficial phenomenon allowing continued splenic function is not documented. On the other hand, neither is it harmful; the author has never observed an intra-abdominal complication that could be attributed to splenosis, and in the review by Widmann and Laubscher, there were only four cases in which the possibility existed, these being patients in whom an obstructing band was directly related to an implant. In these cases, an intra-abdominal adhesion may simply have occurred near the area of implantation, not because of the implantation. Thus, at this time the author is unaware of any complications that can be proven to be due to this phenomenon. No fatal episodes of hemorrhage from these implants resulting from repeated trauma are known, nor is the author aware of any cases of hypersplenism attributed to splenosis.

Creation of splenosis in the human has been suggested as one means of avoiding total splenectomy in patients with trauma in whom portions of the spleen cannot be salvaged in the normal position.

GASTRIC FISTULA

When performing splenectomy, care must be exercised in dividing the short gastric vessels along the greater curvature of the stomach. These vessels are quite short and friable, and thus may be easily torn.

The vascularity of this portion of the stomach varies, depending upon the age of the patient. It is usually quite good, but in the elderly patient with advanced atherosclerosis it may be less than optimal, with the result that ligation of the vessels along this portion of the stomach may decrease the resistance of this portion of the stomach to trauma or to digestion by enzymes, such as may occur when a pancreatic fistula is present (Fig. 22–14). The most common cause of gastric fistula after splenectomy, however, is a technical error in which a small portion of the wall of the stomach is inadvertently included in a tie placed on the short gastric vessels. The surgical tie may cause necrosis of the portion of the stomach included in it, and thus a fistula appears, with drainage of gastric juice becoming apparent on the fourth, fifth, or sixth postoperative day (Fig. 22–15A).

Treatment of this lesion depends upon the location of the gastric injury and its size. If the fistula results in leakage of gastrointestinal contents into the peritoneal cavity and the development of a frank peritonitis, an immediate operation is indicated to identify the site of the leak, to repair it by proper closure, to irrigate the peritoneal cavity thoroughly, and to drain this area adequately. In the postoperative period, the patient

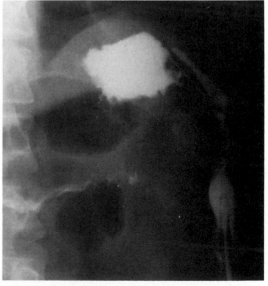

Figure 22–14 Sinogram following drainage of a subphrenic abscess demonstrating the presence of a gastric fistula.

Figure 22–15 *A*, Drawing to demonstrate technical error of including gastric wall in a ligature placed upon a short gastric vessel. This may lead to development of a gastric fistula.

B, Drawing to demonstrate technical error of inadvertently including the tip of the pancreas in the clamp placed upon the splenic vein during splenectomy. This technical error may lead to the development of a pancreatic fistula.

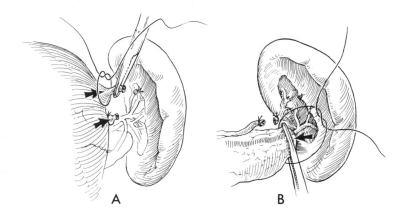

A   B

should be maintained on nasogastric suction and fed intravenously until all evidence of peritoneal irritation has disappeared and normal gastrointestinal function has resumed. Oral ingestion of food should be resumed cautiously, starting with clear liquids and only gradually returning to a full diet. During this period, appropriate antibiotics should be administered, depending upon the result of bacteriologic studies of the contents of the peritoneal cavity. X-ray contrast studies may be useful.

When a drain has been left in the splenic bed, the fistula will appear as drainage of gastric contents along the drain tract without any sign of peritonitis. Under these circumstances, initial conservative therapy is justified. Nasogastric suction should be instituted and the patient should be placed on a regimen including intravenous hyperalimentation to maintain nutrition during this period. The area of drainage should be cultured and appropriate antibiotics should be administered. If the drainage is great in amount, the use of an anticholinergic drug may aid in decreasing its volume. Most fistulas that develop in this manner close spontaneously, and only rarely is operative intervention necessary if there is adequate drainage and infection does not develop.

In the occasional patient in whom closure does not occur spontaneously, operation should consist of complete excision of the area of fistula in the stomach, with removal of all apparently diseased tissue. The stomach may then be closed in layers and the repair covered with omentum to separate it completely from the previous area of the fistulous tract.

PANCREATIC FISTULA

Pancreatic fistula may result from trauma to the tail of the pancreas during splenectomy (Fig. 22–15*B*). Treatment is described earlier in this chapter.

STRESS ULCERATION

Ulceration of the stomach with associated hemorrhage may occur in any patient who has been severely injured. In our experience, stress ulcer occurs in approximately 5 per cent of patients with splenic injury, but it is much more common in patients with multiple organ injuries than in those with a single injury of the spleen. Management of this complication is discussed in detail elsewhere in this volume.

DELAYED RUPTURE OF THE SPLEEN

After external trauma or direct surgical trauma to the spleen, hemorrhage usually occurs and continues until the problem is remedied surgically. In some patients, however, a hematoma develops, either as an intracapsular hematoma or as a perisplenic hematoma. This results in temporary cessation of hemorrhage and a stable state for varying periods of time. Eventually, however, the hematoma may be dislodged by continued oozing, or dissolution of the hematoma may occur before fibrotic healing has resulted, and hemorrhage may recur.

Delayed hemorrhage of the spleen occurs in 10 to 15 per cent of patients sustaining splenic trauma. Some surgeons employ non-operative therapy when the hemorrhage appears to cease spontaneously, especially in children, but this is a dangerous practice. Delayed rupture may occur at any time, from a few hours to several weeks after trauma. In most cases delayed rupture occurs within 2 or 3 weeks after initial trauma, but we have observed episodes of delayed rupture as long as 6 months later.

ATELECTASIS AND PNEUMONIA

These complications may occur after any surgical procedure, particularly when general anesthesia is required. Atelectasis and pneumonia of the left lower lobe is perhaps more common after surgery for splenic trauma than after other operations, because patients with this injury sustain trauma to the left chest in addition to the injury to the spleen. In each patient undergoing splenectomy for trauma, therefore, meticulous tracheal toilet should be done, and care should be taken to ensure that both lungs are well aerated at all times and that support of respiration is provided if fractures of lower ribs on the left prevent adequate excursion of the chest wall.

MORTALITY

The operative mortality rate for splenectomy varies considerably, according to reports in the literature. A good deal of the variance depends upon the spectrum of diseases being treated. Thus, the mortality rate for elective splenectomy is quite low, not exceeding 1 per cent in a number of articles. The mortality rate for splenectomy after trauma to the spleen is considerably higher, however, and is related to the degree of hemorrhage, to the time that elapses between injury and treatment, and to the number of associated organs injured. Hemorrhage represents the most common cause of death; in the report by Shirkey and associates, tabulating 189 consecutive cases of splenic trauma, hemorrhage accounted for 52 per cent of all the deaths.[59] The

hemorrhage, however, is as often from associated injuries as from the spleen itself. In the same study, the second most common cause of death was infection, although it accounted for a mortality rate of only 1 per cent. Other causes of death in this series were primarily related to associated injuries, though there were two patients (1 per cent of patients treated) who died of pulmonary embolus. It is not possible in this group to ascertain whether this was specifically related to splenectomy, however. At the time of the report, the over-all mortality rate for splenectomy following injury was 22 per cent. A more recent unpublished study in our institutions indicates that the over-all mortality rate is 16 per cent and that the mortality rate when the spleen is the only organ injured is 3 per cent.[57]

Bibliography

PANCREAS

1. Arianoff, A. A.: Sphincterotomy: Indications and results in 285 cases. Int. Surg. *46*:363, 1966.
2. Balfour, J. F.: Pancreatic pseudocysts: Complications and their relations to the timing of treatment. Surg. Clin. North Am. *50*:395, 1970.
3. Berne, C. J., Donovan, A. J., and Hagen, W. E.: Combined duodenal pancreatic trauma. Arch. Surg. *96*:712, 1968.
4. Blomstrand, R., Carlberger, G., Forsgren, L., Lundh, G., and Norrbrink, B.: Expiratory pattern of $^{14}CO_2$ after feeding ^{14}C-labelled fats to a patient with total pancreatectomy: Case report. Acta Chir. Scand. *134*:677, 1968.
5. Bolooki, H., Jaffe, B., and Gliedman, M. L.: Pancreatic abscesses and lesser omental sac collections. Surg. Gynecol. Obstet. *126*:1301, 1968.
6. Brawley, R. K., Cameron, J. L., and Zuidema, G. D.: Severe upper abdominal injuries treated by pancreaticoduodenectomy. Surg. Gynecol. Obstet. *126*:890, 1967.
7. Burnett, W. E., Rosemond, G. P., Caswell, H. T., Beauchamp, W., Jr., Tyson, R. R., and Wright, W. C.: Studies in so-called postgastrectomy pancreatitis. Ann. Surg. *149*:737, 1959.
8. Cattell, R. B., and Braasch, J. W.: An evaluation of the long T-tube. Ann. Surg. *154*:252, 1961.
9. Child, C. G., III, Frey, C. F., and Fry, W. J.: A reappraisal of removal of 95 per cent of the distal portion of the pancreas. Surg. Gynecol. Obstet. *129*:49, 1969.
10. Collins, J. J., Craighead, J. S., and Brooks, J. R.: Rationale of total pancreatectomy for carcinoma of the pancreatic head. N. Engl. J. Med. *274*:599, 1966.
11. Dardik, I., and Dardik, H.: Patterns of hemorrhage into pancreatic pseudocysts. Am. J. Surg. *115*:774, 1968.

12. Dunn, D. C.: Diabetes after removal of insulin tumours of pancreas: A long-term follow-up survey of 11 patients. Br. Med. J. 2:84, 1971.

13. Farringer, J. L., Robbins, L. B., II, and Pickens, D. R., Jr.: Abscesses of the pancreas. Surgery. 60:964, 1966.

14. Fish, J. C., Smith, L. B., and Williams, R. D.: Digestive function after radical pancreatico-duodenectomy. Am. J. Surg. 117:40, 1969.

15. Giulian, B. B., Singh, L. M., Mansfield, A. O., Pairent, F. W., and Howard, J. M.: Treatment of pancreatic exocrine insufficiency. Ann. Surg. 165:564, 1967.

16. Hamilton, R. F., Davis, W. C., Stephenson, D. V., and McGee, D. F.: Effects of parenteral hyperalimentation on upper gastrointestinal tract secretions. Arch. Surg. 102:348, 1971.

17. Hori, M., Austen, W. G., and McDermott, W. V., Jr.: Role of hepatic arterial blood flow and hepatic nerves on renal circulation and function. Ann. Surg. 162:849, 1965.

18. Howard, J. M.: Pancreaticoduodenectomy: Forty-one consecutive Whipple resections without operative mortality. Ann. Surg., 168:629, 1968.

19. Howard, J. M., and Jordan, G. L., Jr.: Surgical Diseases of the Pancreas. Philadelphia, J. B. Lippincott Company, 1960.

20. Jordan, G. L., Jr.: Pancreatic fistula. Am. J. Surg. 119:200, 1970.

21. Jordan, G. L., Jr., and Howard, J. M.: Pancreatic pseudocysts. Am. J. Gastroenterol. 45:444, 1966.

22. Jordan, G. L., Jr., and Shelton, E. L., Jr.: Significance of jaundice following pancreatoduodenal resection. J.A.M.A. 162:196, 1956.

23. Kalser, M. H., Leite, C. A., and Warren, W. D.: Fat assimilation after massive distal pancreatectomy. N. Engl. J. Med. 279:570, 1968.

24. LeBauer, E., Smith, K., and Greenberger, N.: Pancreatic insufficiency and vitamin B_{12} malabsorption. Arch. Int. Med. 122:423, 1968.

25. Longmire, W. P., Jr., Jordan, P. H., Jr., and Briggs, J. D.: Experience with the resection of the pancreas in the treatment of chronic relapsing pancreatitis. Ann. Surg. 144:681, 1956.

26. Maki, T., Sato, T., and Kakizaki, G.: Pancreatoduodenectomy for periampullary carcinomas. Ann. Surg. 92:825, 1966.

27. Neville, R. W. J., Stewart, G. A., Sutton, P. M., Taghizadeh, A., and Trethewey, J.: Anti-insulin serum, plasma insulin, and the hypoglycaemia of total pancreatectomy and partial hepatectomy in the rat. Br. J. Exp. Pathol. 52:1, 1971.

28. Partington, P. F.: Sphincterotomy for stenosis of the sphincter of Oddi. Surg. Gynecol. Obstet. 123:282, 1966.

29. Perry, T., Jr.: Postgastrectomy proximal jejunal loop obstruction simulating acute pancreatitis. Ann. Surg. 140:119, 1954.

30. Peterson, L. M., Collins, J. J., and Wilson, R. S.: Acute pancreatitis occurring after operation. Surg. Gynecol. Obstet. 127:23, 1968.

31. ReMine, W. H., Priestley, J. T., Judd, E. S., and King, J. N.: Total pancreatectomy. Ann. Surg., 172:595, 1970.

32. Schumer, W., McDonald, G. O., Nichols, R. I., and Miller, B.: Transgastric cystogastrostomy. Surg. Gynecol. Obstet. 137:48, 1973.

33. Shapiro, H., Ragland, J. B., Sherman, R., and Wruble, L. D.: A study of a patient with an external pancreatic fistula. Am. J. Dig. Dis. 12:1029, 1967.

34. Shires, G. T.: Care of the Trauma Patient. New York, McGraw-Hill Book Company, 1966.

35. Smith, R.: Pancreatic and ampullary carcinoma. Presented at the Postgraduate Course in Diseases of the Liver, Biliary Tract, and Pancreas, 58th Annual Clinical Congress of the American College of Surgeons, San Francisco, 1972.

36. Waddell, W. R., and Loughry, R. W.: Gastric acid secretion after pancreatoduodenectomy. Arch. Surg. 96:574, 1968.

37. Walker, W. M.: Chylous ascites following pancreatoduodenectomy. Arch. Surg. 95:640, 1967.

38. Warren, K. W., Poulantzas, J. K., and Kune, G. A.: Life after total pancreatectomy for chronic pancreatitis: A clinical study of eight cases. Ann. Surg. 164:830, 1966.

39. Warren, K. W., Veidenheimer, M. C., and Pratt, H. S.: Pancreatoduodenectomy for periampullary cancer. Surg. Clin. North Am. 47:639, 1967.

40. Warren, K. W., and Wagner, R. B.: Long-term results of non-penetrating pancreatic trauma. Lahey Clin. Found. Bull. 16:217, 1967.

41. Warren, W. D., Leite, C. A., Baumeister, F., Poucher, R. L., and Kalser, M. H.: Clinical and metabolic response to radical distal pancreatectomy for chronic pancreatitis. Am. J. Surg. 113:77, 1967.

42. Waugh, J. M., and Giberson, R. G.: Radical resection of the head of the pancreas and of the duodenum for malignant lesions: Some factors in operative technique and preoperative and postoperative care, with an analysis of 85 cases. Surg. Clin. North Am. 37:965, 1957.

43. Weitzman, J. J., and Rothschild, P. D.: Surgical management of traumatic rupture of the pancreas due to blunt trauma. Surg. Clin. North Am. 48:1347, 1968.

44. Werschkey, L. R., and Jordan, G. L., Jr.: Surgical management of traumatic injuries to the pancreas. Am. J. Surg. 116:768, 1968.

45. Zeppa, R., Warren, W. D., and Hutson, D. G.: Prevention of postoperative hemorrhage following surgery for pancreatic pseudocyst. Presented at the 84th Annual Seminar of the Southern Surgical Association, Boca Raton, Florida, Dec. 1972.

SPLEEN

46. Applebaum, P. C., Shaikh, B. S., Widome, M. D., et al.: Fatal pneumococcal bacteremia in a vaccinated, splenectomized child. N. Engl. J. Med. 300:203, 1979.

47. Bilski-Pasquier, G., and Bonnet-Gajdos, M.: Risk of infection after splenectomy in children. Ann. Pediatr. 12:110, 1965.

48. Cerise, E. J., Pierce, W. A., and Diamond, D. L.: Abdominal drains: Their role as a source of

infection following splenectomy. Ann. Surg. *171*:764, 1970.

49. Davis, H. H., and Sharpe, J. C.: Splenic vein thrombosis following splenectomy. Surg. Gynecol. Obstet. *67*:678, 1938.

50. Dennehy, T., Lamphier, T. A., Wickman, W., and Goldberg, R.: Traumatic rupture of the normal spleen: Analysis of 83 cases. Am. J. Surg. *102*:58, 1961.

51. Giebink, G. S., Schiffman, G., Drivit, W., *et al.*: Vaccine-type pneumococcal pneumonia: Occurrence after vaccination in an asplenic patient. J.A.M.A. *241*:2736, 1979.

52. Haller, J. A., Jr., and Jones, E. L.: Effect of splenectomy on immunity and resistance to major infections in early childhood: Clinical and experimental study. Ann. Surg. *163*:902, 1966.

53. Lieberman, R. C., and Welch, C. S.: A study of 248 instances of traumatic rupture of the spleen. Surg. Gynecol. Obstet. *127*:961, 1968.

54. Martin, J. C., Jr., and Cooper, M. N.: Complications of splenectomy. South. Surgeon *16*:1047, 1950.

55. Norcross, J. E.: Splenectomy: Its indications and complications. Surg. Clin. North Am. *24*:583, 1944.

56. Olsen, W. R., and Beaudoin, D. E.: Wound drainage after splenectomy: Indications and complications. Am. J. Surg. *117*:615, 1969.

57. Ott, D. A., and Liddicoat, J. E.: Unpublished data.

58. Sherman, R.: Perspectives in management of trauma to the spleen: 1979 Presidential Address, American Association for the Surgery of Trauma. J. Trauma *20*:1, 1980.

59. Shirkey, A. L., Wukasch, D. C., Beall, A. C., Jr., Gordon, W. B., Jr., and DeBakey, M. E.: Surgical management of splenic injuries. Am. J. Surg. *108*:630, 1964.

60. Slate, R. W., Getzen, L. C., and Laning, R. C.: One hundred cases of traumatic rupture of the spleen. Arch. Surg. *99*:498, 1969.

61. Widmann, W. D., and Laubscher, F. A.: Splenosis: A disease or a beneficial condition? Arch. Surg. *102*:152, 1971.

62. Zollinger, R. M., and Williams, R. D.: Surgery of the spleen. Minnesota Med. *42*:881, 1959.

23

COMPLICATIONS OF PORTAL-SYSTEMIC SHUNT SURGERY

Robert B. Smith, III
and Joseph D. Ansley

COMPLICATIONS OF PORTAL-SYSTEMIC SHUNTING

Surgical treatment of portal hypertension may be indicated for one of three major problems: bleeding from gastroesophageal or ectopic varices; massive, medically resistant ascites; and symptomatic hypersplenism. As the medical therapy for cirrhotic ascites has improved over the past decade, and as non-shunting surgical procedures have been introduced for the correction of otherwise intractable ascitic fluid accumulations, the need for portal decompression primarily to relieve ascites has become a thing of the past.[60] Likewise, hypersplenism alone seldom produces sufficient symptoms in the setting of portal hypertension to require surgical intervention. Either of these factors, however, may play a secondary role in the choice of a shunting procedure done for the main indication of bleeding varices. A single, well-documented hemorrhage from varices in an adult with portal hypertension is adequate justification for a portal shunting procedure. However, a more conservative approach may be preferable in the pediatric age group, since younger patients with extrahepatic obstruction generally tolerate rebleeding much better than adult cirrhotics. Prophylactic shunting procedures, performed in the presence of varices that have not yet bled, have been shown in control studies to be of no benefit to the cirrhotic population, as any potential increase in survival resulting from the prevention of variceal hemorrhage is more than offset by an increased rate of late hepatic failure.[6, 12, 28]

Nicolai Eck is credited with reporting the earliest portal-systemic connections in 1877.[14] Whipple and Blakemore reintroduced the concept of portal-systemic shunting in 1945 for relief of bleeding from esophageal varices and ushered in an era of shunting that has continued over the suc-

Robert B. Smith, III graduated from Emory University School of Medicine and took his internship and residency training at Presbyterian Hospital in New York City. He joined the Emory faculty in 1966 as Associate in Surgery and was made Professor of Surgery in 1977. As Chief of Surgery at the Atlanta V.A. Medical Center and Staff Surgeon at Emory University Hospital and Grady Memorial Hospital, he has had a rich experience in the management of portal hypertension and related operations.

Joseph Dickerson Ansley was born in Atlanta and attended Davidson College and Emory University School of Medicine. He took his internship and residency training at Emory and thereafter the Fellowship in Vascular Surgery at that institution. Dr. Ansley is currently Assistant Professor of Surgery at Emory University.

ceeding 35 years.[5, 76] A large number of modifications of their basic portacaval anastomosis have been described during that time, including the use of prosthetic and autogenous interposition grafts. With a single exception, all shunting procedures provide for total (non-selective) decompression of the portal venous system into a lower pressure systemic vein bypassing the liver with most, if not all, of the portal venous flow. Many patients tolerate this portal deprivation poorly, and a relatively large number suffer major morbidity when compared with non-shunted controls. Indeed, the 5-year survival rate is not significantly different between surgical and non-surgical populations; only the mode of death is changed, with shunted patients dying less often from massive hemorrhage.

In 1967, Warren, Fomon, and Zeppa introduced a selective portal decompression procedure, the distal splenorenal shunt, which relieves the elevated pressure within gastroesophageal varices, while it preserves existing hepatopetal blood flow.[72, 74] Experience with this procedure over the past 10 years in a number of centers has demonstrated its superiority over total shunts in terms of preservation of metabolic function of the liver and reduction in the incidence of portal-systemic encephalopathy.[38, 51, 71] However, control studies have yet to show any advantage of this procedure over other shunts in long-term survival following operation.[51] Indeed, life expectancy of the cirrhotic seems to be more related to the underlying disease process in the liver than to the type of surgical procedure used for decompression of the portal system. Pessimism with respect to survival rates is not sufficient reason to withhold operation from patients who would otherwise benefit from protection against recurrent hemorrhage, nor is it reason to perform a total shunt and to subject the patient to a high risk of portal-systemic encephalopathy if a selective distal splenorenal shunt is a feasible alternative.[51]

SELECTION OF SHUNTING PROCEDURE

Deciding which patient should undergo a shunt operation, optimal preoperative preparation, and then the proper choice of shunt for that individual are three vitally important elements in the successful management of portal hypertension. The authors distinctly prefer the selective distal splenorenal shunt (Fig. 23–1*I*) and have found that it can be performed in approximately two-thirds of adult patients who are considered for portal decompression.[73] This operation is admittedly somewhat more difficult technically than a number of the alternatives, especially for the surgeon who only occasionally performs operations for portal hypertension, but the additional effort is justified by the protection that the patient receives against encephalopathy. Individuals are chosen for selective distal splenorenal shunt who have been demonstrated on preoperative angiography to have a patent splenic vein and good to excellent hepatopetal portal flow. Moderate ascites is not a contraindication to this operation, but severe ascites, particularly that which is resistant to diuretic therapy, usually causes us to perform a total decompression. Splenomegaly and hypersplenism are not considered contraindications to the distal shunt, since transsplenic shunting allows for decompression of the congested spleen with gradual improvement in hypersplenic signs in the majority of patients.[18]

Total portal-systemic shunt variations are illustrated in Figure 23–1*A–H*). Except for the end-to-side portacaval shunt, all are hemodynamically and functionally equivalent to the side-to-side portacaval shunt, with the portal vein functioning as an outflow system, if it remains patent.[73] Indications for one of these non-selective decompression procedures include patients with intractable ascites, individuals bleeding from ectopic varices located in other than the gastroesophageal region, patients who have had a splenectomy or those in whom the splenic vein is too small to be used (less than 1 cm.), individuals with demonstrated hepatofugal portal flow or Budd-Chiari syndrome, and persons with a previously performed, but failed, distal splenorenal shunt. Which of the several total shunts is chosen depends to some extent on the personal preference of the surgeon but may also be influenced by technical considerations such as the presence of dense adhesions within the abdomen, whether or not the spleen has been previously removed, the size of the

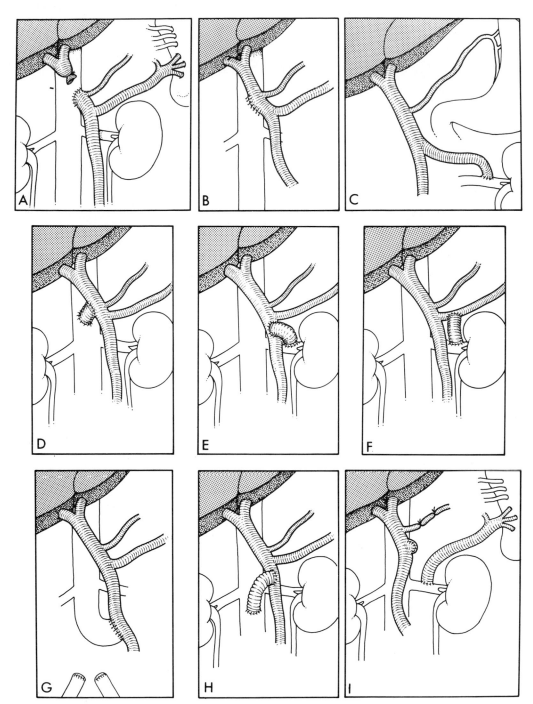

Figure 23–1 Portal-systemic shunts: *A,* End-to-side portacaval shunt; *B,* Side-to-side portacaval shunt; *C,* Proximal splenorenal shunt; *D,* Interposition "H"-graft portacaval shunt; *E,* Interposition "H"-graft mesorenal shunt; *F,* Interposition "H"-graft splenorenal shunt; *G,* Standard mesocaval shunt; *H,* Interposition "H"-graft mesocaval shunt; *I,* Selective distal splenorenal (Warren) shunt.

caudate lobe, and any knowledge of previous shunting attempts. In general, it is preferable to perform a direct vein-to-vein anastomosis whenever possible, as the late patency rates are much better if a prosthetic graft can be avoided. Indeed, we now relegate the prosthetic mesocaval shunt to the infrequent situation in which an emergency decompression is necessary for uncontrollable variceal hemorrhage.[49] Otherwise, the side-to-side portacaval shunt or the autogenous jugular vein H-graft would seem better choices for total shunting. Makeshift shunts done with unnamed collateral tributaries of the portal system are mentioned only to be condemned, as they do not afford adequate protection against recurrent bleeding.[67] Arterialization of the hepatic stump of the portal vein, in association with an end-to-side portacaval shunt, is being studied in several centers but appears to have little promise as a widely used surgical technique.

Nonshunting procedures for portal hypertension are appropriate in highly selected clinical situations. Such non-shunting operations include gastric devascularization (indicated in patients with no patent portal branches), splenectomy (specific therapy for bleeding varices secondary to splenic vein thrombosis), and direct repair of arteriovenous fistulae involving the portal system (shunting procedures here are obviously contraindicated). Because of the high operative mortality rate compared with other non-shunting procedures, esophagogastrectomy with jejunal interposition is rarely performed currently for patients with bleeding varices.[67] Finally, extra-abdominal shunting efforts are sometimes required in patients with Budd-Chiari syndrome who also have significant obstruction of the retrohepatic inferior vena cava and, therefore, no possibility of a successful intra-abdominal decompression. Prosthetic shunts across the diaphragm into the right atrium or the pulmonary artery have been successfully performed in a few such patients to date.[21]

PREOPERATIVE WORK-UP AND PATIENT PREPARATION

When patients with suspected liver disease experience upper gastrointestinal bleeding, it is vital for the surgeon to bear in mind that such bleeding can occur from sources other than varices. Emergency endoscopy should be performed to rule out gastritis, ulcer disease, gastric cancer, or Mallory-Weiss syndrome. After endoscopy has established varices as the most likely bleeding source, all efforts should be made to control the bleeding without operation because of the high mortality that accompanies emergency portal decompression. The patient should be placed in an Intensive Care Unit where minute-to-minute monitoring of vital signs, fluid balance, and gastrointestinal blood loss can be accomplished. A central venous pressure or Swan-Ganz pulmonary artery catheter is placed. Initial treatment consists of blood transfusions and gentle irrigation of the stomach with normal saline. Cimetidine is started, 300 mg. intravenously every 6 hours; if the prothrombin time is significantly prolonged, fresh frozen plasma and vitamin K are administered.[33] When bleeding persists despite these measures, Pitressin is administered, first in a bolus (20 units over 20 minutes in 200 ml. D 5% W), and then as a constant infusion into a peripheral vein (0.3 to 0.5 unit per minute) to provide more sustained lowering of the portal pressure.[33, 46, 58, 62] Some physicians prefer to give the Pitressin via a superior mesenteric artery catheter, but recent evidence fails to show any increased efficacy from that route of administration.[29] Regardless of the route chosen, one must be aware of the risks of Pitressin administration to the patient with atherosclerotic heart disease and be alert to the main side effects of intense hyperperistalsis with cramping and diarrhea and fluid retention.[62] If the bleeding ceases on administration of Pitressin, the infusion is continued for 12 to 24 hours to allow for stabilization. Significant fluid accumulation and weight gain can be expected from the antidiuretic effect of Pitressin; a brisk, spontaneous diuresis usually follows discontinuation of the infusion.

If the bleeding does not respond to Pitressin or the patient rebleeds when the infusion is discontinued, the Sengstaken-Blakemore (S-B) esophageal tamponade tube is inserted.[26, 33] This device is often quite effective in controlling gastroesophageal bleeding, but it is also a potentially harmful weapon and must be used with great care. After the S-B tube has been introduced through the nose into the patient's stomach, 50 ml. of air is injected into the gastric balloon, its position confirmed by an x-ray, and the balloon inflated to a volume of 250 ml. The gastric balloon is then pulled snugly against the diaphragm where it is held in place by attaching the exiting tube to the face mask of a football helmet worn by the patient. Frequently, tamponade by the gastric balloon alone is effective in controlling variceal bleeding. If the bleeding continues, the esophageal balloon is then connected to a mercury manometer and inflated to a pressure of 30 to 40 mm. Hg. This pressure can be maintained for 24 hours and will be effective in controlling the majority of patients in whom it is necessary. After that period of time the esophageal balloon should be deflated and the patient examined for evidence of renewed hemorrhage. If none occurs, tension is released on the gastric balloon after 12 hours and the tube removed at 24 hours. If necessary, the Sengstaken-Blakemore tube and Pitressin infusion can be used simultaneously.

When these techniques are unsuccessful or unsuitable because of inability to insert the S-B tube (nasal obstruction, esophageal stricture, or hiatal hernia) or unwillingness to use Pitressin (known coronary heart disease, angina during its administration, or arrhythmias on EKG monitoring), the patient should be considered for coronary vein embolization.[33, 36] This relatively new technique (pervenous selective catheterization of the coronary vein via the transhepatic or transjugular route to introduce emboli) allows for obliteration of the major feeding collateral to the varices and temporary control of bleeding in patients who might be extremely poor candidates for an emergency shunting procedure (Fig. 23–2). There is a significant risk of rebleeding following coronary embolization and, therefore, it should not be regarded as definitive therapy, but successful embolization should provide a grace period of several weeks during which time the patient can be better prepared for a semi-elective shunt. Sclerotherapy (direct obliteration of varices by endoscopic injection of sodium morrhuate or another sclerosing agent) holds promise as a more definitive treatment for

varices, but in our hands it has not been suitable for the patient with uncontrolled hemorrhage, at least to this time.[30] For the small residual group of patients who continue to bleed despite all efforts or rebleed repeatedly in the hospital, a decision must be made about whether or not an emergency shunt is justified. If the individual is otherwise salvageable and has a reasonable life expectancy, an emergency shunt should be done, usually with the S-B balloon still in place and the Pitressin infusion under way. On the other hand, extremely poor-risk patients are refused operation, as their outlook for survival is essentially hopeless regardless of the therapy used.[16] The latter group generally consists of end-stage cirrhotics who have uncontrolled bleeding in a setting of severe jaundice, massive ascites, nutritional wasting, and coma.

Once active bleeding has been controlled, the patient is subjected to a thorough evaluation of hepatic function, angiographic anatomy, and portal flow characteristics.[51] Standard liver tests are done (bilirubin, albumin, and SGOT), as well as bleeding and clotting studies (prothrombin time and its response to vitamin K, partial thromboplastin time, and platelet count), and, if available, the more refined tests of hepatic metabolic function (maximum rate of urea synthesis, ammonium chloride tolerance, galactose elimination capacity, and antipyrine clearance).[2, 22, 25, 51, 53, 65, 71] A liver biopsy should be done routinely to avoid operating on a patient with extensive necrosis in association with chronic active hepatitis or the cirrhotic with coexistent alcoholic hepatitis, since the mortality of operation is generally felt to be increased in these groups.[42] If the patient has a significant volume of ascites, gradual diuresis should be attempted by sodium restriction and diuretic administration to establish whether or not the ascitic fluid is responsive to the usual medical measures. Standard visceral angiographic studies are obtained to determine the degree of hepatopetal portal flow and to define the venous anatomy available for shunting (hepatic wedge pressure and wedge venogram, superior mesenteric and splenic arteriograms followed through the venous phase, and left renal venogram).[66] Percutaneous splenoportography is rarely done in our center, because of the risk of

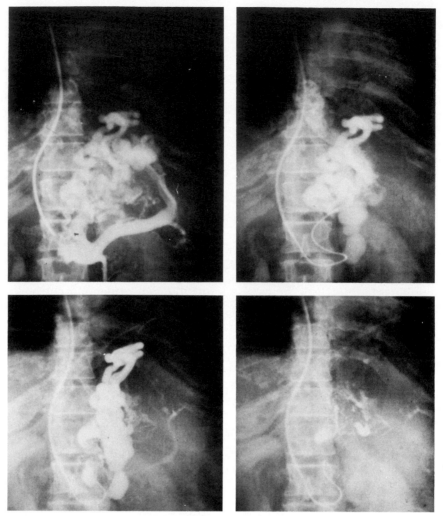

Figure 23–2   Sequential coronary vein embolization via a transhepatic catheter introduced through the jugular vein.

injury to the spleen which might preclude performance of a selective distal splenorenal shunt. We do not hesitate to obtain transhepatic or transjugular portography, however, if further clarification of venous anatomy is needed after the usual indirect angiograms have been done. Throughout this period of preoperative work-up the patient should be observed for evidence of hepatic encephalopathy and treatment instituted as needed. If tolerated, a diet of 1 gm. protein/kg. body weight is given, supplemented by multivitamins.

Having completed all of the abovementioned preoperative assessments, the surgeon is then in a position to decide whether an operation should be done on that hospital admission or postponed to allow for a period of nutritional build-up and recovery from alcoholic hepatitis. Experience has shown that a few weeks of good nutrition and abstinence from alcohol will often allow the cirrhotic to improve a full category in the Child's classification, with resultant reduction in both operative and long-term morbidity rates.[8, 51] Once operation is planned, special attention should be given to preparations for intraoperative bleeding control. If the platelet count is less than 50,000/cu. mm., intraoperative platelet transfusions may be useful. In addition, fresh frozen plasma or fresh whole blood should be available for the patient with vitamin K–resistant elevation of the prothrombin time or other identifiable clotting deficiencies.[33] If the surgeon contemplates entering the gastrointestinal tract during the operative procedure, or if the use of a prosthetic H-graft is anticipated, antibiotic coverage (usually a cephalosporin) is started before the operation.

Elective portal decompression procedures can be done with a hospital mortality of 10 to 12 per cent; emergency shunts, on the other hand, are associated with a mortality rate of 40 to 60 per cent.[7, 15, 16, 27, 35, 38, 46, 61, 63] There seems little doubt that the best single determinant of survival is the patient's hepatic functional status.[69] Other clinical factors that correlate with increased *hospital* morbidity and mortality include advanced Child's classification, marked ascites, preoperative coma, emergency surgical procedure, and intraoperative clotting disturbances. Clinical factors that correlate with increased *late* mortality include advanced Child's classification, preoperative encephalopathy, advanced age at the time of operation, and continued alcohol consumption.[7, 8, 38]

USUAL POSTOPERATIVE CARE

Postoperatively the patient is placed in an intensive care unit for several days to permit continued monitoring of vital signs, fluid balance, body weight, and central venous pressure. Intravenous fluid support consists of $\frac{1}{2}$ normal saline in 5 per cent dextrose, alternating with 5 per cent dextrose in water, plus 50 ml. 25 per cent albumin every 8 hours for the first 2 days. The patient is encouraged to move about actively in bed on the day of operation and is allowed to sit up in a chair on the first postoperative day. Ordinarily, nasogastric intubation is not necessary during the postoperative period. When peristalsis returns, usually by the third postoperative day, a liquid diet is started and advanced progressively. Adequate nutrition in the patient with cirrhosis in the postoperative period is necessary to allow healing of wounds, stabilization of hepatic and visceral function, and maintenance of somatic protein. The patient continues to require sufficient caloric, vita-

min, and mineral intake to maintain homeostasis and to replenish tissues. Sodium content of the diet should be restricted to 2 gm., because of the tendency of cirrhotic patients to retain salt and water; fat content should also be minimized after a distal splenorenal shunt to reduce the possibility of chylous ascites. In the debilitated patient, enteral supplements or an extended intravenous regimen may be necessary. Recent experimental evidence has indicated that, because of the amino acid patterns in the plasma of cirrhotics with encephalopathy, aromatic amines should be restricted in parenteral solutions and branched chain amino acids should be increased.[20] Further documentation of the long-term effects of these mixtures is needed.

If the patient was bleeding immediately prior to the operative procedure, cimetidine is continued intravenously every 8 hours until a regular diet is tolerated. Antibiotics are not given routinely unless a prosthetic graft has been inserted, the G-I tract opened, or the caudate lobe of the liver resected. Because of the combined risk factors of a large upper abdominal incision, postoperative abdominal distention caused by the usual postoperative ileus and ascitic fluid accumulation, and frequent comorbidity from chronic respiratory disease, close attention must be given to pulmonary toilet and respiratory therapy. Skin sutures generally are removed on the eighth to tenth day following operation depending upon the patient's nutritional status and the amount of residual abdominal distention. If no complications occur to delay recovery, the patient is discharged from the hospital on the tenth to twelfth postoperative day. Usually, discharge medications include only a diuretic (spironolactone or furosemide) that may have been restarted in the postoperative period to control ascitic fluid reaccumulation. The occasional patient who has undergone a total shunt may also require moderate dietary protein restriction and lactulose for control of early portal-systemic encephalopathy.

INTRAOPERATIVE COMPLICATIONS

Problems observed during the performance of a portal-systemic shunt can be divided into those common to any shunting procedure and those more specific to a given type of operation. Intraoperative complications will be considered under three categories: general problems, problems specific to the selective distal splenorenal shunt, and problems specific to total shunting procedures.

General Problems

EXCESSIVE INTRAOPERATIVE BLEEDING. Portal shunting procedures can be among the bloodiest operations performed regularly by general or vascular surgeons. This tendency can be attributed to the numerous thin-walled, high-pressure venous collaterals throughout the abdomen and also to the bleeding and clotting deficiencies commonly associated with chronic liver disease and multiple transfusions. To the extent possible, clotting abnormalities should be recognized and treated by vitamin K, whole blood, fresh frozen plasma, or platelet transfusion. If fibrinolysis is definitely diagnosed, epsilon-aminocaproic acid may be administered intraoperatively. Major responsibility for hemostasis in these operative procedures, however, must reside with the surgeon alone, as the volume of blood loss is related chiefly to the degree of attention to meticulous operative technique. Generous use of electrocautery for coagulation of small vessels and the appropriate application of hemostatic clips and suture ligatures assure the maintenance of a dry surgical field.[16] Contrariwise, hasty attempts to clamp a torn vein or to apply metallic clips to an uncontrolled vessel often result in further tears and increased bleeding. It is much better simply to apply fingertip pressure for control of the bleeding vessel, to complete the local dissection exposing the wall of the offending vein or artery, and then, if necessary, to apply a tangential vascular clamp that will allow for precise repair using a fine vascular suture. Careless dissection and coarse tissue handling techniques have no place in successful portal hypertension surgery.

ANATOMIC OBSTACLES. The shunt surgeon must be thoroughly familiar with the usual anatomy of the vessels to be approached and also with the variety of anomalies likely to be encountered. Careful preoperative angiographic studies may alert the surgeon even before the dissection is undertaken to potential problems such as a thrombosed portal trunk or branches, cavernomatous transformation, various left renal vein configurations and anomalies, an unusually high or small splenic vein, hepatic artery originating from the superior mesenteric trunk and ascending lateral to the portal vein, or hepatic vein thrombosis (Budd-Chiari syndrome), with or without caval obstruction. Even the best preoperative angiograms, however, fail to demonstrate a retro-aortic left renal vein, an intrapancreatic splenic vein, or an aberrant left renal artery branch passing anterior to the renal vein.[40] In addition, the shunt surgeon must be prepared for unexpected technical problems, such as those posed by chronic pancreatic fibrosis incorporating the adjacent veins, by marked thickening of the venous wall as a result of thrombophlebitis, or by dense adhesions due to previous operations or infection. Some of these problems can prove to be insurmountable technically and may dictate a change in the type of shunt selected, or, rarely, a switch to a non-shunting procedure such as gastric devascularization. It is well to have mentioned the latter alternative to the patient during the preoperative interview.

TECHNICAL PROBLEMS WITH THE VENOUS ANASTOMOSIS OR THE INTERPOSITION GRAFT. Because of the pliability of the veins involved and the varied anatomical relationships of the structures to be joined, a number of technical problems can develop during creation of a portal-systemic anastomosis.[40] These problems may include tension, kinking, torsion, redundancy, pursestringing of the anastomosis, pleating of the graft, and suture material bridging the anastomosis. Several of these technical obstacles are illustrated in Figure 23–3. Obviously, it is better to avoid these traps by careful planning and execution of the operation, but failing that, the surgeon should be willing to revise or completely redo the anastomosis immediately in order to provide the greatest likelihood of a satisfactory functional result. Certainly, a few additional minutes spent revising the anastomosis at the initial procedure is well justified if it enhances long-term patency.

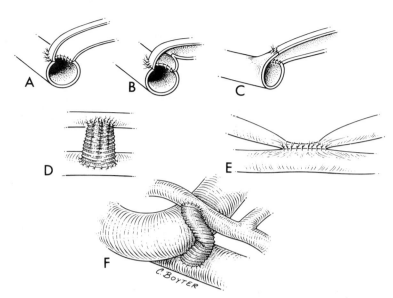

Figure 23–3 Technical problems experienced in the construction of portal shunt anastomoses: *A*, Ideal contour of vein-to-vein connection; *B*, Anastomosis kinked by excessive length of mobilized vein; *C*, Anastomosis narrowed by too much tension on the joined vessels; *D*, Pleating of Dacron "H"-graft as a result of an inadequate size venotomy; *E*, Compromised shunt lumen produced by excessive tension and faulty suture technique; *F*, Torsion and compression of a Dacron mesocaval "H"-graft.

Functional adequacy of the anastomosis can usually be judged intraoperatively by the contour of the sutured vessels, by the thrill produced from a high-volume blood flow, and by the obvious freedom from intraluminal clot when the shunt is compressed between the thumb and index finger. If, after these maneuvers, there still remains a question concerning possible obstruction at the anastomosis, the issue can be resolved easily by measuring the pressure gradient across the shunt or by performing an intraoperative venogram to demonstrate the connection.

ASCITIC FLUID AND LYMPHATIC FLUID LOSSES. The patient operated upon with marked ascites loses not only the volume of fluid in the peritoneal cavity suctioned away at the time of opening the abdomen but also the large volume of transudate that develops during the operative procedure. In order to avoid intraoperative hemoconcentration and hypovolemia, the anesthesiologist must exercise care to replace serum losses concurrently, using both electrolyte solution and colloid. In addition, the surgeon should strive to ligate or to clip the larger lymphatic channels encountered in the retroperitoneum, the hepatoduodenal ligament, or the small bowel mesentery. Mattress sutures are useful for the control of dilated lymphatics, as well as for venous collaterals, located in the edematous tissues surrounding the inferior vena cava and

renal veins. Failure to achieve control of these large lymphatic channels may result in chylous ascites, a particularly troublesome postoperative complication.[39] The surgeon is advised to avoid opening the gastrointestinal tract, if possible, in patients with massive ascites, because of the increased risk of peritonitis in the cirrhotic with impaired defense mechanisms. Adjunctive procedures, such as cholecystectomy, should also be avoided in these individuals, as the use of accustomed abdominal drains (T-tube, Penrose drain, or suction catheter) is totally impractical owing to resultant massive ascitic fluid leakage and the risk of secondary peritonitis.

INTRAOPERATIVE PULMONARY EMBOLISM. Despite the failure to use systemic heparinization during shunt operations, the occurrence of a clinically recognized pulmonary embolus following removal of occluding venous clamps is quite rare. The authors are aware of only two such episodes among the large number of shunts performed at Emory University over the past 10 years. The likelihood of a life-threatening embolus can be minimized by allowing the occluded venous trunks to flush momentarily before completing the anastomosis. If an interposition graft is used, the conduit should be irrigated free of clots using a dilute heparin saline solution just prior to the completion of the anastomosis. In the unlikely event that a small pulmonary embolus should occur, supportive care is all that is indicated; heparin therapy in the perioperative period would be extremely risky in these patients.

Problems Specific to the Distal Splenorenal Shunt

DISSECTION OF THE SPLENIC VEIN. Of the several technical steps necessary in the creation of a distal splenorenal shunt, dissection of the splenic vein is by far the most tedious and potentially the most troublesome. A number of short, small venous tributaries drain from the posterior aspect of the pancreas directly into the anterior and superior aspects of the splenic vein. In addition, one or more coronary branches may arise from the central segment of the splenic vein, and the inferior mesenteric vein frequently converges with the splenic vein along its inferior margin or at the junction with the superior mesenteric vein. Any of these multiple branches can produce serious blood loss if torn during the dissection or if pulled out of the splenic vein by excessive cephalad retraction on the pancreas. Each vessel must be controlled in sequence lest multiple bleeding sites obscure the field. Finger pressure may be used to allow dissection to proceed along the splenic vein to the point that a tangential clamp can be placed across the bleeding site. Occasionally, the splenic vein must be doubly clamped and divided at its portal end before a tear on the posterosuperior aspect can be exposed for precise suture repair. Pertinent hemostatic techniques are illustrated in Figure 23–4.

LOCATION OF THE LEFT RENAL VEIN. Even with the aid of a preoperative venogram to demonstrate the course of the left renal vein, this vein can be quite difficult to locate, because it is frequently concealed by edematous retroperitoneal tissue. Palpation of the contour of the lower pole of the left kidney or detection of the left renal artery pulsation helps to predict the likely location of the renal vein. As the dissection is carried posteriorly through the thickened retroperitoneal tissue, care must be taken to avoid damage to other important structures in the area, especially the duodenum, the left ureter, and the renal artery. In some very obese patients it is useful to initiate this

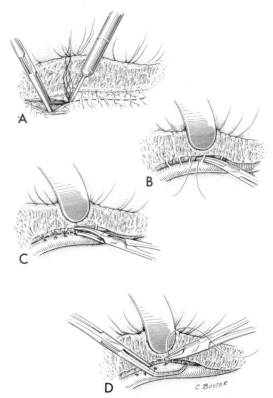

Figure 23–4 Useful techniques to maintain hemostasis during dissection of the splenic vein: *A*, Electrocautery dissection; *B*, Ligation of small venous branches in continuity; *C*, Application of metal hemostatic clips to pancreatic end of veins; *D*, Suture repair of torn vessel under clamp control.

portion of the dissection caudad to the transverse mesocolon and to proceed cephalad along the anterior aspect of the aorta until the renal vein is identified. Once that vessel has been located, attention can be redirected to the previous area of dissection above the mesocolon.

INADEQUATE LENGTH OF SPLENIC VEIN. Most of the time a sufficient length of splenic vein can be mobilized to permit end-to-side anastomosis to the left renal vein without kinking or undue tension. In a few patients, however, especially those with severe inflammatory reaction around the pancreas, or those with an intrapancreatic splenic vein, an adequate segment of vein cannot be developed. Several alternative connections are available to allow safe completion of the distal splenorenal shunt (Fig. 23–5).[73] If the decision is made to disconnect the renal vein, one should preserve as many

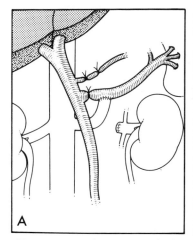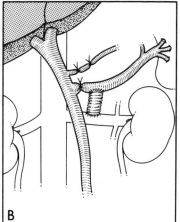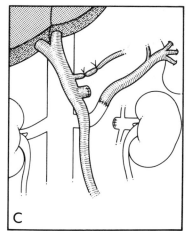

Figure 23–5 Alternative methods for performing a distal splenorenal shunt connection: *A*, Disconnected renal vein anastomosed to the ligated splenic trunk; *B*, Splenorenal "H"-graft interposed with proximal end of the splenic vein ligated; *C*, Both splenic and renal veins disconnected and anastomosed end-to-end.

of its major peripheral branches as possible to allow for adequate venous drainage from the left kidney. Clinically significant renal problems are quite unusual following division of the left renal vein, provided the opposite kidney is normal.

MISCELLANEOUS. In order to avoid intraoperative difficulties, a number of precautions are recommended during performance of the selective distal splenorenal shunt: (a) Do not conduct unnecessary dissection outside of the decompressed left upper quadrant compartment; otherwise, very troublesome bleeding can result from unrelieved portal hypertension. Specifically, one should avoid doing ancillary procedures, such as cholecystectomy, in association with a transsplenic decompression. (b) It is unwise to clamp the left renal artery while the renal vein is occluded to perform the venous anastomosis.[40] Occlusion of the renal artery in a non-heparinized patient may result in arterial thrombosis; moreover, extensive experience has shown that arterial interruption is not necessary to protect the kidney. (c) The temptation to ligate the splenic artery in an effort to reduce portal splanchnic inflow should be resisted, as splenic infarction can result in abscess formation or propagation of clot into the splenic vein. (d) When performing ligation of the coronary vein along its course between the superior border of the pancreas and the gastroesophageal junction, exercise care to avoid passing the ligature also around the hepatic artery.

Problems Specific to Various Total Shunting Procedures

ENLARGED CAUDATE LOBE. A portacaval shunt, either side-to-side or end-to-side variety, can be thwarted by the presence of an enlarged caudate lobe protruding into the foramen of Winslow and separating the portal vein from the inferior vena cava.[40] This mechanical barrier can be overcome in some patients by resection of a part of the caudate lobe using mattress sutures for hemostasis (Fig. 23–6). If needed, additional hemostasis on the cut surface of the liver can be achieved by electrocautery or suture ligatures. Care should be taken to avoid tearing caudate lobe veins that drain directly into the inferior vena cava. If the caudate lobe is removed, the area of resection is not drained, as the tract may allow egress of an excessive volume of ascitic fluid. Some accumulation of subhepatic blood and bile must occur in many of these patients, however, as it is common to observe subcostal tenderness and low-grade fever for several days after caudate lobe resection. Antibiotics should be given to cover the possibility of bacterial seeding of this subhepatic collection.[61]

THROMBOSIS OF THE PORTAL VEIN IN A

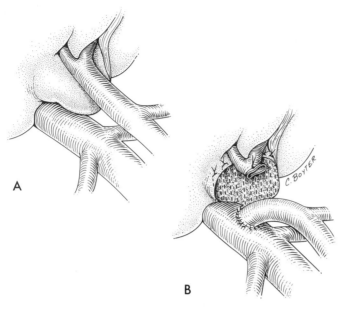

Figure 23–6 Caudate lobe resection to permit an end-to-side portacaval anastomosis.

PLANNED PORTACAVAL SHUNT.   If complete portal angiograms are obtained preoperatively, an occluded portal trunk should be detected in most cases and a shunt selected that avoids that segment of the venous system. In an occasional case, the surgeon is surprised to find recent or old thrombus in a portal vein that has been opened to perform an anastomosis. This is more likely to occur under emergency circumstances when thorough preoperative radiography may not have been feasible, or as a result of spontaneous thrombosis that occurred between the time of the preoperative x-ray studies and actual performance of the operation. If the clot is not densely adherent to the vein wall, it may be successfully extracted by the use of a balloon embolectomy catheter; a brisk gush of liquid blood from the venotomy suggests that an adequate thrombectomy has been achieved. The venous anastomosis may then be completed, but it is desirable to obtain an intraoperative portal venogram subsequently to confirm shunt patency. If the venogram indicates inadequate flow through the anastomosis, or if the thrombus is too extensive or adherent for adequate removal, another shunt site should be selected immediately, using a portal branch shown to be patent on the operative venogram.

TECHNICAL PROBLEMS WITH PROXIMAL SPLENORENAL SHUNT.   The standard, proximal splenorenal shunt has become one of the least commonly performed shunting procedures, and it is also among the most demanding technically.[40] Perisplenitis with dense vascular adhesions between the enlarged, congested spleen and the adjacent diaphragm may be a source of massive bleeding during splenectomy, even if the splenic artery is ligated as a preliminary step. After the spleen has been removed, a second major problem is the mobilization of an adequate length of splenic vein to permit anastomosis to the left renal vein without tension or angulation. This may require resection of a portion of the tail of the pancreas with all the potential risks related to surgical trauma to that organ.[40] Removal of the spleen in the pediatric age group is associated with an increased risk of late sepsis; a problem of similar degree has not been observed in adults undergoing splenectomy.

TECHNICAL PROBLEMS WITH MESOCAVAL SHUNT.   The standard mesocaval shunt, accomplished by disconnecting the inferior vena cava and swinging it up to anastomose end-to-side to the superior mesenteric vein, is essentially reserved for the pediatric age group, as this procedure carries an extremely high risk of disabling leg edema in the adult patient.[7, 9] If a standard mesocaval shunt is performed in the child, one of the most common technical problems is mobilization of a sufficient length of vena cava to permit anastomosis without tension. Extra length can be obtained by dividing the common iliac veins below their confluence and using the opened end of one iliac vein to construct the anastomosis; the second iliac vein stump is simply closed by a continuous vascular suture. Sometimes problems are encountered with the anatomy of the superior mesenteric vein which, after it emerges beneath the inferior margin of the pancreas, may immediately divide into a delta of tributaries. Fortunately, this is an uncommon arrangement, as it makes construction of an adequate shunt almost impossible.

If an interposition mesocaval shunt is planned, the graft should be interposed between the inferior vena cava and the superior mesenteric vein in a gentle curve around the inferior border of the duodenum, care being taken to avoid compression or excessive tension on the graft.[7, 15, 16] Certainly, the H-graft should not be passed through a tunnel between the duodenum and pancreas, as this maneuver is associated with a high risk of post-traumatic pancreatitis and graft failure.[63] If a Dacron graft is selected, a large diameter (18 to 24 mm.) tube has been recommended.[15, 16] The relatively high rate of late graft occlusion observed with Dacron H-grafts in the mesocaval location has led a number of authors to recommend autogenous vein, or, more recently, expanded polytetrafluoroethylene grafts for this purpose.[44, 46, 52, 63]

IN-HOSPITAL POSTOPERATIVE COMPLICATIONS

Recurrent Upper Gastrointestinal Bleeding

Mild gastric bleeding is common in the immediate postoperative period and may require additional blood transfusions. Endoscopy in such patients usually reveals gastritis that may be related to preoperative intubation or to the segmental gastric devascularization performed as a part of a transsplenic decompression procedure. Bleeding of that type is usually brief in duration and small in volume. If more active bleeding occurs, other possible sources, such as peptic ulcer or gastroesophageal varices, must be considered and proven by endoscopy.

Variceal hemorrhage may be simply a continuation of preoperative bleeding or, if the patient was not bleeding at the time of operation, it may be evidence of early shunt failure. When the latter explanation seems more plausible, it is mandatory to establish whether or not the shunt is functional by means of appropriate splanchnic angiography.[66] If the shunt is found to be open but the patient persists in variceal bleeding (a distinctly unusual combination except with ectopic varices in the presence of a distal splenorenal shunt), the radiologist should be asked to look for a patent coronary vein collateral and to attempt coronary embolization for bleeding control.[36] This procedure can be done while the patient is still in the radiology department to save valuable time. If the embolization technique is not available, or when it is unsuccessful, the surgeon should return to the use of intravenous Pitressin and Sengstaken-Blakemore tamponade, hoping that a secure clot will adhere to the varix and allow more permanent control of bleeding.[26] During these maneuvers, clotting deficiencies should be sought and corrected to the fullest extent possible. Generally, non-operative means are successful in controlling recurrent variceal bleeding if the shunt is functional; rarely, it may become necessary to reoperate in order to ligate a bleeding varix in an individual with a widely patent shunt or to revise a stenotic shunt anastomosis.[55] Varix ligation can be performed via either the transgastric or transesophageal route, depending upon the location of the persistent variceal bleeder.

On the other hand, if the shunt is demonstrated to be totally occluded during the early postoperative period, renewed bleeding is presumed to be related to recurrent portal hypertension. Once again, the surgeon is well advised to attempt non-operative control of bleeding by the methods discussed above, in order to permit time for the patient to stabilize and to recover from the recent operative procedure. Thereafter, depending upon the patient's general condition and the ease and completeness of bleeding control, reoperation may be undertaken. Some surgeons have attempted to reopen the previous shunt by thrombectomy, but, in general, we have favored creation of a second shunt, or a switch to gastric devascularization, as more likely to produce long-term success. In the poorer risk categories, sclerotherapy or coronary vein embolization might be a safer alternative than a second major surgical procedure.[30, 36] Obviously, the prognosis for hospital survival is not good for the patient with recurrent bleeding owing to shunt failure in Child's Class C, but some patients can be salvaged by the combined efforts of surgeon, gastroenterologist, and radiologist.[45]

Intraperitoneal Bleeding

Upon completing a shunt anastomosis, the surgeon should make every reasonable effort to secure a dry surgical field before closing the abdomen. Incomplete hemostasis in areas of surgical dissection may result in continued postoperative bleeding with instability of the vital signs and a falling hematocrit. Often these patients respond to transfusion with fresh whole blood and stop bleeding within the first 24 hours, but even if they do cease to bleed, they can be expected to have more prolonged ileus and to face the risks associated with additional units of transfused blood. However, an occasional patient will continue to bleed into the abdomen and require urgent reoperation. At the time of exploratory celiotomy it is usual to find generalized oozing rather than a discrete bleeding site. Clotted and liquid blood should be evacuated and hemostasis accomplished by electrocautery, suture-ligatures, or the use of hemostatic agents such as Gelfoam, Surgicel, or Avitene. Drains are not utilized.

Postoperative Pancreatitis

Considering the amount of dissection necessary to perform certain shunts in the vicinity of the pancreas, especially those involving the splenic vein, it is surprising that there is not more postoperative pancreatitis in these patients.[63] Mild elevation of the amylase in the immediate postoperative period is rather frequent, but clinically recognized pancreatitis is uncommon. If postoperative pancreatitis of any severity does occur, special attention should be given to the patient's blood sugar levels, since hepatogenous diabetes may exist on the basis of

the cirrhosis and can be aggravated by pancreatic disease.[60] If the tail of the pancreas is damaged during the performance of a proximal splenorenal shunt, the full picture of caudal pancreatitis may evolve with ileus, fever, left upper quadrant tenderness, and a left pleural effusion. Conservative treatment is generally effective in these patients, but the occasional individual may develop a traumatic pseudocyst. Operative therapy may be required later if the pseudocyst fails to resolve or if the patient develops evidence of secondary infection.

Peptic Ulcer Disease

The gastric secretory response following various types of portal shunts remains a controversial point, but there is considerable support for the feeling that postshunt cirrhotics have an increased peptic ulcer diathesis. In one large series, Voorhees et al. reported a peptic ulcer complication rate of 12 per cent.[69] Even if the overall incidence in cirrhotics were not higher than in the general population, it is obvious that the severely stressed cirrhotic can ill afford additional complications from a gastric or duodenal ulcer. Peptic ulcer bleeding is a poorly tolerated new problem when superimposed upon the stormy postoperative course often experienced by cirrhotics. Such hemorrhage, which might not otherwise be fatal, can lead to rapid development of hepatic coma and death in the patient with a patent portal-systemic shunt. As a practical matter, in a large shunt experience at Emory University we have diagnosed postoperative peptic ulcer complications quite infrequently over the last few years. Our experience is undoubtedly influenced by the almost routine use of cimetidine in the poor-risk patient or in anyone who develops a major postoperative complication that causes delay in oral alimentation. Prior to the availability of cimetidine, antacids were used generously in the same patient population with a similar degree of protection. Certainly, if the patient has any history of peptic ulcer disease, cimetidine should be given throughout the perioperative period, parenterally at first and then orally when active peristalsis has returned. This drug is continued until the patient is tolerating a full diet and is ready for discharge. Thereafter, antacid therapy is prescribed for a few additional weeks.

Postoperative Ascites

It is common to have a temporary accumulation of ascitic fluid following shunt surgery, even among patients who have had little or no ascites previously. The development of postoperative ascites is fundamentally related to two contributing factors: continued formation of hepatic ascites owing to incompletely relieved hepatic sinusoidal hypertension and the release of lymph and plasma directly into the abdomen from surgically traumatized vessels.[60] The liver, the largest lymph-forming organ in the body, contributes the major volume of lymph that flows through the abdomen. Decompensation of the hepatic lymphatic system is aggravated in the postoperative patient by a reduction in serum albumin production, resulting in diminished oncotic pressure that further enhances the tendency for formation of ascites. Sodium and water retention related to decreased effective plasma volume and secondary aldosteronism also contribute to decompensation, as do alterations in intrarenal blood flow.[17, 23] Reduction of portal pressure by a side-to-side type shunt usually leads to prompt resolution of preexisting ascitic fluid, if there is a satisfactory gradient across the shunt. In instances of elevated inferior vena caval pressure, however, the gradient across the shunt may be less and ascites resolution is retarded.[75] Patients with an end-to-side portacaval shunt seldom have a serious problem with ascites, but an occasional individual will develop truly intractable ascites after that operation (Fig. 23–7).[24, 60] Some ascitic fluid accumulation is almost routinely seen following a selective distal splenorenal shunt, since the intrahepatic venous hypertension is not relieved by that procedure. Leakage of ascitic fluid from the abdominal incision is a serious complication that must be corrected immediately to avoid excessive protein losses and to protect the patient from spreading peritonitis.

In general, the management of postoperative ascites involves restriction of exogenously administered sodium, avoidance of excessive water load, improvement of the colloid osmotic pressure of the plasma, and the use of appropriate diuretic therapy to improve water and sodium excretion.[59] Patients with cirrhosis and ascites have an excess total body sodium, although their plasma sodium concentration may be low owing to the dilutional effect of excess retention of free water. Natriuresis is the goal of therapy, but plasma volume should not

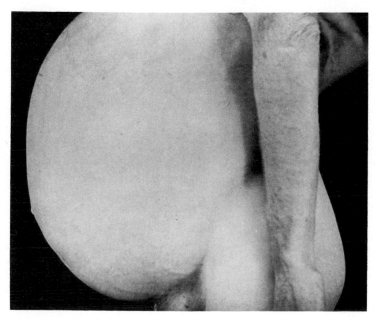

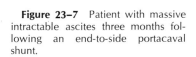
Figure 23–7 Patient with massive intractable ascites three months following an end-to-side portacaval shunt.

be reduced by overzealous fluid restriction and diuresis, as the resultant hypovolemia can be quite detrimental to renal function. Improvement of colloid oncotic pressure of the plasma by infusion of plasma or albumin may be effective in conjunction with diuretic therapy; but unless there is a concomitant improvement in hepatic function, this effect may be only temporary.

In the presence of persistent postoperative ascites a paracentesis is usually done for diagnostic purposes.[27] A small volume of fluid is aspirated for inspection and for laboratory determinations (cell count, protein content, triglyceride content, and bacterial culture). On rare occasions, a patient with tense ascites may require a therapeutic paracentesis to reduce abdominal distention acutely in order to relieve respiratory embarrassment caused by elevation of the diaphragm, or to prevent threatened disruption of the abdominal incision. Removal of the ascitic fluid must be done with care to avoid emptying the abdomen too rapidly or taking off such a large amount as to reduce the circulating intravascular volume. The response of different patients to paracentesis varies greatly and is unpredictable. Some patients become hypotensive with removal of only a small amount of fluid, whereas others tolerate removal of several liters without hemodynamic changes. Since the ascitic fluid collecti n may reaccumulate rapidly, it is necessary to re-expand the plasma volume with exogenous plasma infusions during the paracentesis and for a period after the paracentesis is performed.

Standard diuretic therapy for postoperative hepatic ascites consists primarily of orally administered spironolactone to counteract the aldosterone effect on the renal tubules. In the majority of patients, this drug along with sodium intake restrictions will be sufficient to control ascites. Patients who have more resistant ascites require the addition of a loop diuretic such as furosemide to increase excretion of sodium and water. Spironolactone is generally used in a dosage of 100 to 200 mg. per day and furosemide in a dosage of 40 to 80 mg. per day. Gradual mobilization of ascites is preferred over more aggressive diuresis, because hypovolemia and azotemia can progress to hepatorenal syndrome in the cirrhotic.

A small number of patients have postoperative ascites that proves to be resistant to the standard diuretic and salt restriction regimen described above. In those individuals a diuretic cocktail may be given with salutary effect, provided the circulating blood volume is within normal range. The cocktail consists of rapid intravenous administration of 500 ml. of plasma or 5% albumin followed immediately by 50 gm. of mannitol and 40 to 80 mg. furosemide over a short period of time.[23] Usually a brisk diuresis results. This treatment can be repeated on a daily basis, as needed, but the body weight, hematocrit, creatinine, and blood urea nitrogen must be followed closely to avoid overdiuresis.

Ascitic fluid accumulation is almost routine following a selective distal splenorenal shunt, since sinusoidal hypertension is not relieved by that procedure. In most patients this ascites is relatively mild and can be managed easily by sodium restriction and the use of diuretics. Approximately 5 per cent of distal shunt patients experience a particularly difficult variety of fluid accumulation, chylous ascites, characterized by milky fluid containing high levels of triglycerides.[39] When refractory ascites of this type is encountered a paracentesis will allow for the differential diagnosis. Therapy consists of removal of a major part of the fluid by paracentesis, simultaneous with intravenous administration of plasma. Thereafter, the patient should be maintained on a strict low-fat diet for several weeks to discourage recurrence of the chyle-rich fluid. If all these measures fail, a peritoneovenous shunt may be necessary to relieve intractable chylous ascites.[34]

Patients who are demonstrated to be truly intractable to conservative therapy for ascites, either transudative or chylous in type, are candidates for chronic reinfusion of ascitic fluid by the peritoneovenous shunting procedure described by LeVeen et al.[34, 70] In the postoperative patient the timing of insertion of an ascites drainage device is critically important from three aspects: the stability of liver function, the presence of particulate matter in the peritoneal fluid, and the possibility of bacterial infection of the fluid following operation. Experience at Emory has shown that sufficient clearing of the particulate matter from the fluid and

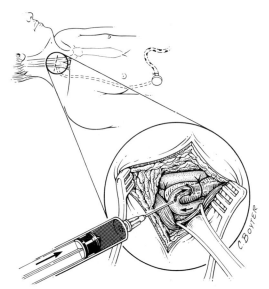

Figure 23–8 Technique of injecting methylene blue into the Silastic tubing of a LeVeen peritoneovenous shunt intraoperatively to demonstrate that the ascites drainage device is functioning properly.

stabilization of liver metabolism requires a minimum of 3 weeks from the time of the initial operation. Patients with unstable hepatic function have an increased risk of complications following peritoneovenous shunting, especially disseminated intravascular coagulopathy.[3, 57] It has been found that a serum bilirubin greater than 4 mg./dl. and a prothrombin time prolonged more than 4 seconds places the patient in a high-risk category for bleeding complications. In addition, the patient's cardiac status and renal function must be evaluated, as successful reinfusion depends upon adequate function of these systems.

The LeVeen peritoneovenous shunting procedure is usually performed under local anesthesia (Fig. 23–8). Following insertion of the reinfusion valve the patient is given furosemide periodically to enhance and sustain the diuresis. Inspiratory exercises are required to improve the transfer of fluid by increasing the pressure gradient from the abdomen to the intrathoracic position of the shunt. In addition, an elastic abdominal binder is applied to increase intra-abdominal pressure. With the resultant movement of large volumes of ascitic fluid into the venous system, the patient has a dilutional fall in hematocrit; transfusion of

packed cells may be necessary to maintain the hematocrit above 26 per cent. In the early postoperative period, excessive potassium losses in the urine may require potassium supplementation. Prophylactic antibiotics are administered for 72 hours to cover insertion of the intravascular foreign body.

Lower Extremity Edema

Pitting edema of the lower extremities is seen in approximately 20 per cent of shunt patients during the immediate postoperative period, regardless of the type of shunt performed. Leg swelling is not due to an increase in inferior vena caval pressure caused by added inflow from the shunt but is thought to be related to the combined factors of reduced colloid osmotic pressure, positive sodium/water balance characteristic of the early postinjury period, and postural effects in the relatively inactive postoperative patient.[60] If the patient has undergone a standard mesocaval shunt with total disconnection of the inferior vena cava, leg edema can be expected in almost every instance. This edema is quite severe and persistent in the adult patient and relatively minimal in the pediatric patient.[7, 60] In addition to leg swelling, individuals who undergo the standard mesocaval operation may also develop signs and symptoms of acute iliac vein thrombophlebitis with lower abdominal tenderness, fever, and leukocytosis. The clinical picture can mimic acute appendicitis or other acute pelvic inflammatory condition. Pelvic phlebitis should be treated expectantly, as the physical findings generally subside within 5 to 7 days, although low-grade fever may persist for 10 to 14 days. Nay and Fitzpatrick reported temporary, unilateral leg swelling in 4 of 22 patients after the external iliac vein was removed to construct a mesocaval H-graft.[44] This complication can be avoided by using the internal jugular vein for the interposition conduit.[63]

Hepatorenal Syndrome

Progressive renal failure following surgery for portal hypertension carries a high morbidity and mortality. Garrett et al. described four patients who developed massive ascites with renal failure following end-to-side portacaval shunt and all four died.[24] Renal failure in the postoperative shunt patient can be traced to preexisting kidney disease or to acute tubular necrosis related to perioperative hypotension in a few individuals, but in most instances it is due to a type of functional renal failure described as hepatorenal syndrome. This rather ill-defined clinical state develops in a setting of severely decompensated liver disease and refractory ascites. When the fragile cirrhotic is subjected to a stress such as hemorrhage, infection, or operation, he may respond with increasing ascites and reduced effective renal plasma flow, resulting in progressive renal failure.[23] The condition is characterized by dilutional hyponatremia, azotemia, and oliguria, with a low urinary sodium excretion and unimpressive urinary sediment. Renal histology is generally non-revealing in this syndrome, and the intrinsic reversibility of the pathophysiology is confirmed by the fact that a kidney from such an individual is capable of normal function if transplanted into another subject. Unfortunately for the cirrhotic, the hepatorenal syndrome, once established, is usually progressive and frequently fatal. Pharmacologic agents are generally ineffective. Spontaneous recovery from severe hapatorenal syndrome has been rare, but survivors have been reported following side-to-side portal-systemic shunts and, more recently, by the reinfusion of ascitic fluid using the peritoneovenous shunt of LeVeen.[4, 57]

In the postoperative period following a portal shunt, renal failure can be precipitated by excessive diuretic therapy, by therapeutic paracentesis, or by insufficient volume replacement. Functional renal insufficiency in its mild form is evidenced by elevation of the blood urea nitrogen and inability to excrete free water. This is accompanied by a decrease in urinary sodium to as low as 5 mEq./l. and usually by hyponatremia. In more advanced azotemia there is an elevation of the serum creatinine. The urine sodium level is a useful differentiating test in evaluation of the cirrhotic with oliguria, but it should be recognized that sodium excretion can be altered by previous administration of diuretics.

All patients with cirrhosis undergoing an operation must be considered potential candidates for hepatorenal syndrome, and prevention is the major consideration. The patient's intravascular volume must be maintained by appropriate administration of plasma and fluids containing a moderate restriction of sodium. In addition, diuretics must be used judiciously with frequent monitoring of body weight, blood urea nitrogen, and serum creatinine. Overzealous attempts to maintain a dry patient can result in progressive renal dysfunction. Patients who have had a distal splenorenal shunt will tend to collect ascites in the early postoperative period, and control of their ascites must be done in such a way that circulating plasma volume is not contracted excessively. If progressive renal failure becomes evident from a rising blood urea nitrogen and decreasing urinary sodium concentration, the first reaction should be to restore intravascular volume. This may result in an initial increase in ascitic fluid collection, but, if the patient maintains adequate renal function, in most cases the ascites will become stabilized over a period of time and respond eventually to gradual diuresis. If the ascites cannot be controlled medically, a peritoneovenous shunting procedure can be done after an appropriate period of time has passed following the initial operation. Internal reinfusion of ascitic fluid restores circulating blood volume and effective renal plasma flow.[70] Schwartz and Vogel reported limited success with this procedure in 5 patients.[57]

Portal-Systemic Encephalopathy

McDermott and Adams first called attention to the syndrome of organic encephalopathy in shunt patients characterized by detectable mental aberrations and an elevated blood ammonia level.[41] The precise mechanism of this non-specific organic encephalopathy is not fully understood, but the following four factors contribute to some degree in all patients: impaired hepatocellular function, portal-systemic shunt, either natural or surgical, protein substrate and bacteria in the intestinal tract, and sensitivity of the central nervous system to certain toxic elements.[56, 60, 69] Ammonia absorbed from the colon is ordinarily carried to the liver via the portal venous system and

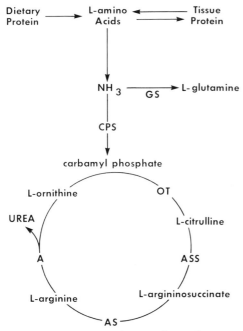

Figure 23–9 Krebs-Henseleit cycle.

converted to urea by reactions of the Krebs-Henseleit cycle (Fig. 23–9).[71] Ordinarily the liver metabolizes more than 80 per cent of ammonia entering via the portal vein on the first passage.[10] To the extent that this mechanism is impaired by whatever cause, or the portal blood diverted from the liver, the blood ammonia is elevated, ammonium intolerance can be demonstrated, and portal-systemic encephalopathy frequently develops. That ammonia toxicity is not necessarily the whole story is evident in the fact that some patients with typical hepatic encephalopathy have normal blood ammonia values at a time when an altered mental state and asterixis are obvious. A number of other changes have been observed in association with this clinical syndrome, including diminished cerebral oxygen utilization, impaired cerebral glucose metabolism, deviations in blood amino acid patterns and short chain fatty acid levels, and elevated ketoglutarate and mercaptans in the blood.[23, 37, 77]

A number of factors common to the postoperative period may contribute, either in combination or any one alone, to the development of encephalopathy in the cirrhotic. These factors include blood in the gastrointestinal tract from continued active bleeding or residual from a previous bleeding epi-

sode; dietary protein; temporarily worsened hepatic cellular function as a result of operative stress and anesthetic agents; postoperative ileus and constipation; electrolyte and acid base abnormalities, especially hypokalemia and alkalosis; certain drugs, particularly sedatives, analgesics, and tranquilizers; azotemia; and infection.[10, 11, 23] The incidence of early postoperative encephalopathy is increased in patients who had coma preoperatively, in those subjected to an emergency shunt procedure, and in persons classified in the most advanced Child's group (Class C).[71] In addition, the type of shunt performed greatly influences the likelihood that the patient may show signs of encephalopathy following operation. The selective distal splenorenal shunt patient is much less likely to have coma than patients with a total shunt, in whom the degree of portal diversion is far greater.

Clinical findings of portal-systemic encephalopathy in the early postoperative patient can be quite variable and, at times, difficult to appreciate. In its milder form the neurologic examination is normal and the syndrome can be elicited only by detecting errors in mental calculation, memory function, or spatial relationships (as may be evident in handwriting).[41] Other individuals may show mental confusion, personality changes, disorders of sleep rhythm, or inappropriate behavior. Later the patient has lethargy progressing to somnolence and then, perhaps, frank coma. A few encephalopaths develop severe agitation or other forms of bizarre behavior; others have fluctuating rigidity of the limbs, reflex grasping, or extensor plantar reflexes.[41] Rarely, one observes an individual with a fixed neurological deficit or seizure activity as a manifestation of hepatic encephalopathy.

The frequency of diagnosis of portal-systemic encephalopathy varies with the diligence with which it is sought. Support for the diagnosis can be derived from electroencephalographic changes, from blood ammonia determinations, and from psychometric testing. It is well known that EEG abnormalities may precede any clinically apparent manifestations of precoma.[11, 48] EEG changes have been graded from A to E according to the Parsons-Smith classification. Typical electrical changes occurring in grades C and D consist of medium-voltage waves, 5 to 6 per second; in grade E slow, high-voltage delta waves are seen.[48] There is an ill-defined correlation of EEG changes with blood ammonia levels, but a fairly consistent reversal of EEG abnormalities does occur following successful treatment of known ammonia elevations. A blood ammonia level of greater than 100 mcg./dl. is considered distinctly elevated in most laboratories.[11, 25] Psychometric testing is another means of identifying subtle deficits before full-blown encephalopathy is evident. In Reitan's trailmaking test the patient connects numbers spatially arranged on a sheet of paper; the test is scored by the time required and the number of errors committed.[48] Such psychometric tests may show definite abnormalities before either of the other two indicators.[77] It must be understood, however, that none of these confirmatory tests is pathognomonic of portal-systemic encephalopathy.

Once the diagnosis of encephalopathy has been made, treatment consists primarily of measures to reduce the load of absorbed ammonia or other biogenic amines from the gastrointestinal tract and to eliminate, insofar as possible, known contributing factors. The urgency and severity of the clinical problem can be quite variable, ranging from slight confusion associated with resumption of a 60 gm. protein diet in one individual to deep coma in another. Obviously, the intensity of therapy required and the ultimate prognosis for survival are much different in these two extremes of the clinical spectrum. The comatose individual requires extremely diligent care in order to avoid problems with aspiration of gastric contents, pulmonary failure, decubitus ulcers, and corneal abrasions; all medications and feedings must be introduced into the alimentary tract via a feeding tube. This contrasts with the patient with milder precoma who is alert and can take both diet and medications orally.

It is important that any active gastrointestinal bleeding be arrested in the encephalopathic patient in order to eliminate that protein substrate from the colon. In addition, the colon should be emptied promptly of any fecal content. A single dose of magnesium sulfate can be given by mouth or via a nasogastric tube and tap water cleansing enemas administered every 12 hours. Soap-suds enemas should not be used, as the soap produces an alkaline pH that enhances ammonia absorption.[11] Dietary protein is reduced to 10 gm. or less, and the content of the diet is altered to avoid foods known to be high in ammonia content, such as gelatin.[23, 54] Caloric intake can be maintained by the use of a high carbohydrate enteral product such as Polycose supplemented by 10% dextrose in water intravenously.[11] Glucose-rich oral feedings are avoided because of their excessive osmotic load; liquids with a high-fat content are also unsuitable, since they tend to produce gastric retention. Concurrently with these dietary changes, the physician should also discontinue any medication suspected of contributing to the encephalopathic state, should correct acid base/electrolyte abnormalities, and should attempt to relieve any contributing element of azotemia or infection. If tube feedings are used, the stomach should be aspirated periodically to prevent regurgitation of retained feedings and possible aspiration.[23] Benadryl is used for sedation in these individuals, in preference to barbiturates or tranquilizers.[11]

Specific drug therapy for portal-systemic encephalopathy consists of two agents with principal action in the colon: neomycin and lactulose. Neomycin sulfate is administered to the patient in acute coma via a nasogastric tube, 1 gm. every hour for 4 doses and then 1 gm. every 4 hours until the syndrome is controlled. In patients with postoperative ileus in whom peristalsis cannot be depended upon to carry the antibiotic into the colon, the drug can be given as a retention enema, 2 gm. every 12 hours. The mechanism of action of this poorly absorbed antibiotic is to reduce the population of colonic organisms capable of generating ammonia. Since neomycin is only minimally absorbed from the intestinal tract, the ototoxic and nephrotoxic side effects observed with its parenteral use are minimized. It is advisable, however, to avoid administration of this agent in patients with known renal impairment.[11, 23]

Lactulose, a more recently approved medication for the management of hepatic encephalopathy, is a minimally absorbed, essentially non-metabolized synthetic disaccharide. Lactulose has two probable mechanisms of action in portal-systemic encephalopathy. It is hydrolyzed by bacteria in the colon to produce acid products that lower the pH of the fecal stream and, therefore, tend to hold ammonia in the stool that would otherwise be transferred across the colonic mucosa into the blood; and it functions as an osmotic cathartic helping to eliminate ammonia-rich feces from the body.[11] The usual dose of liquid lactulose is 30 ml. orally, or via a nasogastric tube every 8 hours, modified according to the number of loose stools per day. Undesirable side effects of lactulose are essentially limited to its tendency to produce flatulence, cramps, and diarrhea. For that reason, it is superior to neomycin for long-term use in patients who require therapy for chronic encephalopathy. Lactulose should be used with caution, however, in diabetic patients as it does contain some digestible sugars. In unusually resistant clinical situations, both neomycin and lactulose can be given simultaneously, although it is seldom necessary to continue such expensive double-drug therapy for more than a few days at a time.

Other medications and mechanical forms of therapy have been subjected to clinical trials over the past two decades but have not been shown to be clearly effective in the treatment of portal-systemic encephalopathy, especially for the cirrhotic with chronically impaired hepatocellular function. These experimental modalities have included corticosteroids, L-dopa, exchange transfusion, cross-circulation, extracorporeal hepatic perfusion, hemodialysis, and liver transplantation.[11, 23]

Hepatic Failure

Following shunt procedures it is common for the patient to show deepening jaundice and to have a brisk rise in the serum bilirubin, alkaline phosphatase, and SGOT. Usually these raised levels return to the preoperative baseline by the tenth to fourteenth postoperative day. If they do not, it may be an indication of more severe hepatocellular dysfunction with a worsened prognosis for extended survival. Indeed, a few shunt patients exhibit a rapid progressive decline in hepatic function in the postoperative period, resulting in early death from fulminant hepatic failure. Still others have a more protracted downhill course over several weeks, leading eventually to death from the same cause. Fortunately, this outcome is quite infrequent among properly selected, well-prepared patients, but it cannot be totally avoided in the current state of the art. Several factors have been shown to contribute to fulminant hepatic failure among shunted patients, including acute deprivation of hepatic portal perfusion in individuals undergoing total shunts or those who develop portal vein thrombosis postoperatively, anesthetic or other drug toxicity, hepatic hypotension or hypoxemia, and hepatocellular necrosis due to alcoholic or viral hepatitis.[64] The clinical picture of postoperative hepatic failure is one of malaise, anorexia, lethargy, and deepening jaundice, usually associated with tense ascites and fetor hepaticus, in a patient with stupor, progressing to Grade IV coma.[64] Generalized bleeding, renal insufficiency, and respiratory depression are frequent elements of the terminal course.

The syndrome of hepatic failure results in an extremely high mortality rate in the cirrhotic, regardless of the type of therapy used.[61] Good general nursing care in an intensive care unit setting is the main element in management of these patients.[77] Careful attention should be given to respiratory support and to nutritional replacement. Initially, the patient is given 25 per cent glucose, multivitamins, and limited albumin as an intravenous infusion; later, enteral alimentation in the form of a high carbohydrate, low protein tube feeding is administered to provide adequate caloric support more safely.[23] Full anticoma measures are required, including neomycin or lactulose via nasogastric tube or by retention enema. Any known septic focus should be treated vigorously and electrolyte abnormalities corrected.[77] Multivitamins, thiamine, folic acid, and vitamin K are given for general support. If a liver biopsy confirms chronic hepatitis as the basic underlying process, moderate doses of corticosteroids may be indicated as well.[23] By diligent application of these measures, a few patients will show spontaneous improvement in hepatic cellular function and survive; however, 90 per cent do not.[64, 77]

A number of experimental forms of treatment have been introduced over the past decade or so in an effort to achieve some improvement in the universally high mortality associated with acute hepatic failure. At best, these modalities have had only sporadic success and then largely in patients who have acute necrosis of the liver with some capability of recovery. The usual shunt patient with underlying cirrhosis obviously is not in that category, as he or she has little likelihood of showing significant improvement in hepatic function during a brief period of heroic support. For that reason, exchange transfusions, ex vivo liver perfusion, total body washout, plasmapheresis, cross-circulation to human or subhuman primates, and various types of dialysis (peritoneal or hemic) all have little to offer the cirrhotic with acute hepatic failure.[1, 11, 27, 32, 64]

Other Complications

In any review of shunt patients there is evident a relatively high frequency of nonspecific complications that can be attributed to some combination of impaired host defense mechanisms, nutritional failure, and co-morbidity conditions so prevalent in these individuals.[35] Septic problems, postoperative fever of unknown origin, pulmonary complications, and neuropsychiatric difficulties related to chronic alcoholism are all common to this patient population. Delirium tremens carries an extremely high mortality in the postoperative shunt patient and is best avoided by delaying the operative procedure, if at all possible, until the patient is safely beyond the likelihood of manifesting DT's.[45] If emergency shunting cannot be avoided and the individual develops DT's in the early postoperative period, aggressive treatment with Librium or other similar agent may allow for survival.

LATE POSTOPERATIVE COMPLICATIONS

Shunt Occlusion with Recurrent Bleeding

In a recent review of 79 patients with Dacron interposition shunts performed at Emory University over an 8-year period, there was a 24 per cent incidence of spontaneous shunt thrombosis. Orloff, in 1977, reported a 32 per cent closure rate of meso-systemic interposition grafts from a worldwide review.[46] Other authors have described a lower incidence of late occlusion with interposition shunts, but there seems to be a significantly increased risk of late failure with prosthetic grafts when compared with direct, vein-to-vein anastomoses.[52, 63] The standard (proximal) splenorenal anastomosis is an exception to this rule, but the higher thrombosis rate with this procedure is probably related to kinking or compression of the splenic vein as it is turned down to join the left renal vein.

Late closure of any type of shunt may occur without detectable clinical sequelae in some cases and will be diagnosed only if late angiograms are done on a routine basis. More often, the patient will have an indication of probable shunt occlusion in the form of recurrent variceal bleeding. Shunt failure may also be signaled in some individuals by the sudden reaccumulation of ascitic fluid, by worsening of hypersplenism, or by spontaneous resolution of chronic portal-systemic encephalopathy. Ordinarily, we do not recommend a second shunt procedure for the patient with an occluded anastomosis unless variceal bleeding recurs and forces the issue. Voorhees et al. described recurrent bleeding as responsible for 11 per cent of the deaths among 748 shunted patients, and Linton et al. reported rebleeding as a complication in 19 per cent of survivors.[35, 69] If late occlusion is not associated with bleeding, the patient may simply be followed for evidence of new complications of portal hypertension. If bleeding does occur, the individual should be considered for another shunt or for a non-shunting procedure. Efforts to approach and reopen an occluded shunt years after the original operation are almost certain to fail and probably would pose a prohibitive surgical risk in many patients. A second shunt is much easier to perform in a different area of the portal system.[15]

Interposition Graft Infection

Delayed infections of the shunt site are extremely rare in direct vein-to-vein anastomoses wherein the endothelium heals promptly with a smooth internal surface. Even in prosthetic graft shunts reports of infection have been quite infrequent and almost always associated with known contamination by gastrointestinal tract organisms at the time of the initial procedure or with late erosion of an adjacent viscus by the graft.[13, 16, 31] H-graft infections have been associated with occlusion of the conduit in most instances but may occur in the presence of a patent graft and can be particularly difficult to diagnose in that setting, since portal angiograms may appear normal.[31] As prophylaxis against prosthetic graft infection, it is advisable to use systemic antibiotics perioperatively and to avoid opening the gastrointestinal tract at the initial procedure, if at all possible.[15]

Successful management of the infected portal interposition graft after it is diagnosed demands removal of the prosthesis and appropriate antibiotic therapy. Whether a second shunt is created at that time or delayed until a subsequent procedure must be decided on an individual basis according to the patient's condition, especially the extent of intra-abdominal sepsis.

Persistent Hypersplenism

Hypersplenism on the basis of portal hypertension is defined as a white blood cell count of less than 4,000 per cu. mm. or a platelet count of less than 100,000 per cu. mm. If hypersplenism is present prior to the portal shunting procedure, the blood count returns gradually to normal over a period of months in approximately one-half of patients. Since chronic congestive splenomegaly is not relieved totally by shunting and some degree of splenic enlargement persists despite a patent shunt, the signs of hypersplenism may not remit completely.[23] Ferrara et al. reported that gradual resolution of hypersplenism can be expected following the majority of selective distal splenorenal shunts.[18] Splenectomy in association with a proximal splenorenal shunt is capable of producing the most dramatic reversal of hypersplenic signs, but this operation is seldom indicated on the basis of hypersplenism alone, since that condition rarely contributes to patient morbidity. If splenectomy is done in the portal hypertensive patient, it is quite uncommon to have rebound thrombocytosis of a sufficient degree to produce hypercoagulability.

Redevelopment of hypersplenism at a time remote from the shunt operation raises the possibility of late shunt occlusion. It is entirely possible that silent thrombosis of a shunt could occur with no clinical signs other than increasing splenomegaly or evidence on routine hemogram of decreasing cell counts. If observed, these changes should prompt a splanchnic angiogram to assess shunt patency. However, reoperation would not be considered for laboratory or x-ray findings alone; rather, a second shunt should be undertaken only if significant new symptoms, such as variceal bleeding, develop.

Late Portal-Systemic Encephalopathy

Portal-systemic encephalopathy may develop months to years following the shunt procedure, either as isolated episodes of mental confusion or as a chronic neuropsychiatric disturbance. Varying clinical manifestations occur from subtle personality changes and errors in judgment to frank hepatic coma. The incidence of late encephalopathy is related to the type of shunt performed, and it is much more common in patients with total shunts than in those who have had a selective splenorenal shunt.[22, 71] The reported incidence of portal-systemic encephalopathy following total shunts varies from as low as 9 per cent to as high as 68 per cent.[7, 16, 35, 43, 45, 46, 61, 63] Undoubtedly, the true incidence relates directly to the vigor with which this complication is sought. In an Emory University randomized controlled study the encephalopathy rate was 52 per cent among patients with total shunt, but only 12 per cent among selective shunt patients followed for a similar period of time.[51] No patient with preservation of portal inflow had encephalopathy in that study. Other investigators have also confirmed the superiority of the selective shunt in terms of metabolic function.[11, 49]

Portal-systemic encephalopathy has generally been thought to be rare among patients undergoing shunts in the pediatric age group for extrahepatic portal venous obstruction. Careful long-term follow-up in a large series of these individuals by Voorhees et al. has shown an unexpectedly high incidence of late neuropsychiatric aberrations and behavior disorders in these patients.[67] In a comprehensive review of adult patients Voorhees et al. observed a direct relationship between the rate of encephalopathy and the duration of follow-up after the operation procedure.[69] They noted a 27 per cent incidence in patients observed for less than 5 years, but a 56 per cent incidence in those followed more than 5 years after the surgical procedure. Additional factors have been shown to correlate with the frequency of encephalopathy among survivors, including more severely impaired hepatic function at the time of operation, older age at the time of operation, emergency status of the procedure, and resumption of alcohol ingestion postoperatively.[45, 68, 69] Preoperative encephalopathy does not necessarily portend postoperative difficulty with this problem.[43]

Late onset of encephalopathy in an individual who has not had previous difficulty with hepatic coma raises the question of deteriorating hepatic function versus possible precipitating factors (occult GI bleeding, azotemia, acid base/electrolyte imbalance, or drug toxicity). All of these possibilities should be investigated and corrected, if possible, in an effort to keep the patient mentally functional. A few individuals require prolonged restriction of dietary protein intake to 40 gm. or less and the daily use of lactulose for extended periods of time. The lactulose dose is titrated according to stool frequency, aiming at two to three semi-formed bowel movements daily.[23] If lactulose is not effective in controlling precoma symptoms, as it may not be in 25 per cent of cases, neomycin sulfate is substituted in a dose of 1 gm. three times a day, provided the patient does not have chronic renal insufficiency.[11]

It has been estimated that only approximately 50 per cent of shunt survivors are able to function normally in society, and it is generally conceded that hepatic coma is the main deterrent to social and economic rehabilitation of this group.[46, 61, 69] Approximately 80 per cent of patients with chronic portal-systemic encephalopathy can be kept functional with standard medical therapy. The remaining 20 per cent have more severe or even intractable encephalopathy and constitute an extremely difficult management problem.[43] These unfortunate persons are totally incapable of providing financial support for their families or carrying out the duties necessary to run a household. Many have been placed in mental institutions or nursing homes as custodial problems. We have observed a few miraculous reversals of incapacitating encephalopathy when the shunt has become spontaneously occluded, especially in patients with Dacron mesocaval shunts. Prompted by that experience, our group has electively closed H-graft shunts in 3 patients surgically, all of whom had improvement in their mental status. Unfortunately, all three died eventually as a result of the surgical procedure. Other investigators have reported a different surgical approach to intractable encephalopathy, namely resection or exclusion of a portion of the colon in order to reduce the ammonia-absorbing surface. A few clinical successes have been reported with colonic procedures, but the operative mortality exceeds 25 per cent in these patinets; consequently, this form of therapy has not been widely accepted to date.[10, 23, 68]

A number of innovative pharmacological approaches have been introduced over the past 20 years to treat hepatic encephalopathy, but none, other than antibiotics and lactulose, has been shown to be effective under rigorous clinical trial. Steroids have been recommended, but no rational basis for their use has been given and the clinical results are nil.[23] Arginine and glutamic acid have been suggested as potentially effective in clearing ammonia from the blood by priming the Krebs-Henseleit cycle or by combining with ammonia to produce glutamine. Likewise, these agents have failed to live up to expectations and are no longer recommended for clinical use in portal-systemic encephalopathy. Similarly, the administration of various branched chain amino acid mixtures has failed to influence the outcome of precoma favorably.[77] More recently, a different approach has been suggested in the pharmacological treatment of hepatic coma, an approach based on the theory that cerebral dysfunction is due to false neurotransmitter amines, such as octopamine, that impair brain function by displacing normal neurotransmitters.[10, 37] L-dopa administered orally has been recommended as a competitor for the false neurotransmitters. L-dopa is known to cross the blood-brain barrier and to enter brain cells in which, it was postulated, it might be capable of restoring central nervous system homeostasis.[19, 47] After initial optimism, this therapy is now being severely questioned because more recent studies have failed to show clinical efficacy.[10, 11, 23, 37, 77] A related drug, bromocriptine, has also failed to reproduce its initial clinical success.[11]

Hepatic Failure

Late hepatic failure in the shunted patient is a frequent mode of death, but it is not so much a complication of the shunt procedure as it is an event in the natural history of chronic liver disease. Experiences reported from a wide variety of centers have shown a remarkably consistent mortality rate among shunted cirrhotics of 50 to 60 per cent at 5 years, regardless of the type of shunt constructed.[7, 35, 38, 45] In a series of 748 shunted patients over a 26-year period, Voorhees et al. observed that liver failure was the most common cause of late death, accounting for 44 per cent of their fatalities.[69] When evidence of progressively deteriorating liver function occurs, the patient should be rehospitalized and supported with nutritional supplements, anticoma measures, and an ascites control regimen. A few patients with late hepatic failure will respond temporarily, especially if they can be effectively withdrawn from hepatotoxic exposure such as alcohol. However, most patients continue a relentless downhill course and die of coma, renal failure, respiratory insufficiency, or a generalized bleeding disorder.

Late Ascites

Development of ascites months to years following portal shunt surgery or sudden worsening of a chronic ascitic condition may be indicative of shunt occlusion, progressive hepatic dysfunction, resumption of alcohol intake, or failure to adhere to a previously prescribed regimen for ascites control. Initial management should consist of a thorough reevaluation of hepatic function and repeat visceral angiography, if shunt occlusion is suspected. A diagnostic paracentesis with appropriate laboratory and cytologic studies will serve to exclude other causes for ascites. After the etiology of the fluid accumulation has been established, intensification of medical therapy should allow for successful control of hepatic ascites in most patients. Sodium restriction and diuretic agents, first spironolactone and then, if necessary, furosemide, will usually be sufficient. If the ascites is chylous, as indicated by elevated triglyceride content, a low-fat diet should be prescribed as well.

A small fraction of patients with ascites become resistant to medical management or develop progressive renal dysfunction on a diuretic regimen. If no contraindications exist, this subgroup should be considered for surgical treatment by the insertion of a peritoneovenous ascites drain as described by LeVeen.[34] Contraindications to this procedure include intraperitoneal infection, variceal bleeding, deteriorating hepatocellular function, cardiac disease with elevation of the central venous pressure, and irreversible renal dysfunction. If inserted, the LeVeen ascites valve has a high rate of success in the control of chronic hepatic ascites.

Bibliography

1. Abouna, G. M., Cook, J. S., Fisher, L. M., Still, W. J., Costa, G., and Hume, D. M.: Treatment of acute hepatic coma by ex vivo baboon and human liver perfusions. Surgery 71:537, 1972.
2. Andreasen, P. B., Ranek, L., Statland, B. E., and Tygstrup, N.: Clearance of antipyrine-dependence of quantitative liver function. Eur. J. Clin. Invest. 4:129, 1974.
3. Ansley, J. D., Bethel, R. A., Bowen, P. A., II, and Warren, W. D.: Effect of peritoneovenous shunting with the LeVeen valve on ascites, renal function, and coagulation in six patients with intractable ascites. Surgery 83:181, 1978.
4. Berkowitz, H. D., Mullen, J. L., Miller, L. D., and Rosato, E. F.: Improved renal function and inhibition of renin and aldosterone secretion following peritoneovenous (LeVeen) shunt. Surgery 84:120, 1978.
5. Blakemore, A. H.: Portacaval anastomosis: A report on 14 cases. Bull. N.Y. Acad. Med. 22:254, 1946.
6. Callow, A. D., Resnick, R. H., Chalmers, T. C., Ishihara, A. M., Garcean, A. J., and O'Hara, E. T.: Conclusions from a controlled trial of the prophylactic portacaval shunt. Surgery 67:97, 1970.
7. Cameron, J. L., Zuidema, G. D., Smith, G. W., Harrington, D. P., and Maddrey, W. C.: Mesocaval shunts for the control of bleeding esophageal varices. Surgery 85:257, 1979.

8. Child, C. G., III: The Liver and Portal Hypertension. Philadelphia, W. B. Saunders Company, 1964.

9. Clatworthy, H. W., Jr., Wall, T., and Watmann, R. N.: A new type of portal-to-systemic venous shunt for portal hypertension. Arch. Surg. 71:588, 1955.

10. Conn, H. O.: Current diagnosis and treatment of hepatic coma. Hosp. Pract. 8:65, 1973.

11. Conn, H. O., and Lieberthal, M. M.: The Hepatic Coma Syndromes and Lactulose. Baltimore, Williams and Wilkins Company, 1979.

12. Conn, H. O., and Lindenmuth, W. W.: Prophylactic portacaval anastomosis in cirrhotic patients with esophageal varices. N. Engl. J. Med. 279:725, 1968.

13. Dennis, M. A., Jr., Monson, R. C., and O'Leary, J. P.: Interposition mesocaval shunt: A less than ideal procedure. Am. Surg. 44:734, 1978.

14. Donovan, A. J., and Covey, P. C.: Early history of the portacaval shunt in humans. Surg. Gynecol. Obstet. 147:423, 1978.

15. Dowling, J. B.: Ten years' experience with mesocaval grafts. Surg. Gynecol. Obstet. 149:518, 1979.

16. Drapanas, T., LoCicero, J., III, and Dowling, J. B.: Hemodynamics of the interposition mesocaval shunt. Ann. Surg. 181:523, 1975.

17. Epstein, M., Schneider, N., and Befeler, B.: Relationship of systemic and intrarenal hemodynamics in cirrhosis. J. Lab. Clin. Med. 89:1175, 1977.

18. Ferrara, J., Ellison, E. C., Martin, E. W., Jr., and Cooperman, M.: Correction of hypersplenism following distal splenorenal shunt. Surgery 86:570, 1979.

19. Fischer, J. E., Funovics, F. J., and Falcao, H. A.: L-Dopa in hepatic coma. Ann. Surg. 183:386, 1976.

20. Fischer, J. E., Rosen, H. M., Ebeid, A. M., James, H. J., Keane, J. M., and Soetens, P. B.: The effect of normalization of plasma amino acids on hepatic encephalopathy in man. Surgery 80:77, 1976.

21. Fonkalsrud, E. W., Linde, L. M., and Longmire, W. P., Jr.: Portal hypertension from idiopathic superior vena caval obstruction. J.A.M.A., 196:129, 1966.

22. Fulenwider, J. T., Nordlinger, B. M., Millikan, W. J., Sones, P. J., and Warren, W. D.: Portal pseudoperfusion: An angiographic illusion. Ann. Surg. 189:257, 1979.

23. Galambos, J. T.: Cirrhosis. Vol. XVII, Major Problems in Internal Medicine. Philadelphia, W. B. Saunders Company, 1979.

24. Garrett, J. C., Voorhees, A. B., Jr., and Sommers, S. C.: Renal failure following portasystemic shunt in patients with cirrhosis of the liver. Ann. Surg. 172:218, 1970.

25. Gerron, G. G., Ansley, J. D., Isaacs, J. W., Kutner, M. H., and Rudman, D.: Technical pitfalls in measurement of venous plasma NH$_3$ concentration. Clin. Chem. 22:663, 1976.

26. Hermann, R. E., and Traul, D.: Experience with the Sengstaken-Blakemore tube for bleeding esophageal varices. Surg. Gynecol. Obstet. 130:879, 1970.

27. Jackson, F. C., Christophersen, E. B., Peternel, W. W., and Kirimli, B.: Preoperative management of patients with liver disease. Surg. Clin. North Am. 48:907, 1965.

28. Jackson, F. C., Perrin, E. B., Smith, A. G., Dagradi, A. E., and Nadal, H. M.: A clinical investigation of the portacaval shunt. II Survival analysis of the prophylactic operation. Am. J. Surg. 115:22, 1968.

29. Johnson, W. C., Widrich, W. C., Ansell, J. E., Robbins, A. H., and Nabseth, D. C.: Control of bleeding varices by vasopressin: A prospective, randomized study. Ann. Surg. 186:369, 1977.

30. Johnston, G. W., and Rodgers, H. W.: A review of 15 years' experience in the use of sclerotherapy in the control of acute haemorrhage from oesophageal varices. Br. J. Surg. 60:797, 1974.

31. Kaminski, D. L., and Warren, W. D.: Infected Dacron mesorenal portasystemic shunt. Arch. Surg. 115:81, 1980.

32. Klebanoff, G., Hollander, D., Cosimi, A. B., Stanford, W., and Kemmerer, W. T.: Asanguineous hypothermic total body perfusion (TBW) in the treatment of stage IV hepatic coma. J. Surg. Res. 12:1, 1972.

33. Koransky, J. R., Galambos, J. T., Hersh, T., and Warren, W. D.: The mortality of bleeding esophageal varices in a private university hospital. Am. J. Surg. 136:339, 1978.

34. LeVeen, H. H., Wapnick, S., Grosberg, S., and Kinney, M. J.: Further experience with peritoneovenous shunt for ascites. Ann. Surg. 184:574, 1976.

35. Linton, R. R., Ellis, D. S., and Geary, J. E.: Critical comparative analysis of early and late results of splenorenal and direct portacaval shunts performed in 169 patients with portal cirrhosis. Ann. Surg. 154:446, 1961.

36. Lunderquist, A., and Vang, J.: Transhepatic catheterization and obliteration of the coronary vein in patients with portal hypertension and esophageal varices. N. Engl. J. Med. 291:646, 1974.

37. Maddrey, W. C., and Weber, F. L., Jr.: Chronic hepatic encephalopathy. Med. Clin. North Am. 59:937, 1975.

38. Malt, R. B., and Malt, R. A.: Tests and management affecting survival after portacaval and splenorenal shunts. Surg. Gynecol. Obstet. 149:220, 1979.

39. Maywood, B. T., Goldstein, L., and Busuttil, R. W.: Chylous ascites after a Warren shunt. Am. J. Surg. 135:700, 1978.

40. McDermott, W. V., Jr.: The techniques of portal-systemic shunt surgery. Surgery 57:778, 1965.

41. McDermott, W. V., Jr., and Adams, R. D.: Episodic stupor associated with an Eck fistula in the human with particular reference to metabolism of ammonia. J. Clin. Invest. 33:1, 1954.

42. Mikkelsen, W. P.: Therapeutic portacaval shunt. Preliminary data on controlled trial and morbid effects of acute hyaline necrosis. Arch. Surg. 108:302, 1974.

43. Mutchnick, M. G., Lerner, E., and Conn, H. O.: Portal-systemic encephalopathy and portacaval anastomosis: A prospective, controlled investigation. Gastroenterology 66:1005, 1974.

44. Nay, H. R., and Fitzpatrick, H. F.: Mesocaval "H"

graft using autogenous vein graft. Ann. Surg. *183*:114, 1976.

45. Orloff, M. J.: Emergency portacaval shunt: A comparative study of shunt, varix ligation and nonsurgical treatment of bleeding esophageal varices in unselected patients with cirrhosis. Ann. Surg. *166*:456, 1967.

46. Orloff, M. J., Duguay, L. R., and Kosta, L. D.: Criteria for selection of patients for emergency portacaval shunt. Am. J. Surg. *134*:146, 1977.

47. Parkes, J. D., Sharpstone, P., and Williams, R.: Levodopa in hepatic coma. Lancet *2*:1341, 1970.

48. Parsons-Smith, B. G., Summerskill, W. H. J., Dawson, A. M., and Sherlock, S.: The electroencephalograph in liver disease. Lancet *2*:867, 1957.

49. Reichle, F. A., Fahmy, W. F., and Golsorkhi, M.: Prospective comparative clinical trial with distal splenorenal and mesocaval shunts. Am. J. Surg. *137*:13, 1979.

50. Reitan, R. M.: Validity of the trailmaking test as an indicator of organic brain damage. Percept. Mot. Skills. *8*:271, 1958.

51. Rikkers, L. F., Rudman, D., Galambos, J. T., Fulenwider, J. T., Millikan, W. J., Kutner, M., Smith, R. B. III, Salam, A. A., Sones, P. J., Jr., and Warren, W. D.: A randomized controlled trial of the selective distal splenorenal shunt. Ann. Surg. *188*:271, 1978.

52. Rosenthal, D., Deterling, R. A., Jr., O'Donnell, T. F., Jr., and Callow, A. D.: Interposition grafting with expanded polytetrafluoroethylene for portal hypertension. Surg. Gynecol. Obstet. *148*:387, 1979.

53. Rudman, D., DiFulco, T. J., Galambos, J. T., Smith, R. B., III, Salam, A. A., and Warren, W. D.: Maximal rates of excretion and synthesis of urea in normal and cirrhotic subjects. J. Clin. Invest. *52*:2241, 1973.

54. Rudman, D., Smith, R. B., III, Salam, A. A., Warren, W. D., Galambos, J. T., and Wenger, J.: Ammonia content of food. Am. J. Clin. Nutr. *26*:487, 1973.

55. Satiani, B., Liapis, C., and Evans, W. E.: Kinking of a Warren shunt as a cause of recurrent variceal hemorrhage. Am. J. Surg. *139*:428, 1980.

56. Schenker, S., Breen, K. J., and Hoyumpa, A. M., Jr.: Hepatic encephalopathy: Current status. Gastroenterology *66*:121, 1974.

57. Schwartz, M. L., and Vogel, S. B.: Treatment of hepatorenal syndrome. Am. J. Surg. *139*:370, 1980.

58. Schwartz, S. I., Boles, H. W., Emerson, G. I., and Mahoney, E. B.: The use of intravenous Pituitrin in treatment of bleeding esophageal varices. Surgery *45*:72, 1959.

59. Sherlock, S.: Diseases of the Liver and Biliary Tract. 5th Ed. Oxford, Blackwell Scientific Publications, 1975.

60. Sherlock, S., Hourigan, K., and George, P.: Medical complications of shunt surgery for portal hypertension. Ann. N.Y. Acad. Sci. *170*:392, 1970.

61. Smith, R. B., III, and Perdue, G. D., Jr.: Early and late morbidity of portasystemic shunts including experience with seven H-grafts. Am. J. Gastroenterol. *58*:396, 1972.

62. Thomford, N. R., and Sirinek, K. R.: Intravenous vasopressin in patients with portal hypertension: Advantages of continuous infusion. J. Surg. Res. *18*:113, 1975.

63. Thompson, B. W., Casali, R. E., Read, R. C., and Campbell, G. S.: Results of interposition "H" grafts for portal hypertension. Ann. Surg. *187*:515, 1978.

64. Trey, C., and Davidson, C. S.: The management of fulminant hepatic failure. Prog. Liver Dis. *3*:282, 1970.

65. Tygstrup, N.: Determination of the hepatic elimination capacity (LM) of galactose by single injection. Scand. J. Clin. Lab. Invest. (Suppl.) *92*:118, 1966.

66. Viamonte, M., Jr., Warren, W. D., Fomon, J. J., and Martinez, L. O.: Angiographic investigations in portal hypertension. Surg. Gynecol. Obstet. *130*:37, 1970.

67. Voorhees, A. B., Jr., and Price, J. B., Jr.: Extrahepatic portal hypertension: A retrospective analysis of 127 cases and associated clinical implications. Arch. Surg. *108*:338, 1974.

68. Voorhees, A. B., Jr., and Price, J. B., Jr.: Surgical treatment of hepatic encephalopathy. Ann. N.Y. Acad. Sci. *170*:259, 1970.

69. Voorhees, A. B., Jr., Price, J. B., Jr., and Britton, R. C.: Portasystemic shunting procedures for portal hypertension: Twenty-six year experience in adults with cirrhosis of the liver. Am. J. Surg. *119*:501, 1970.

70. Wapnick, S., Grosberg, S., Kinney, M., Azzara, V., and LeVeen, H. H.: Renal failure in ascites secondary to hepatic, renal, and pancreatic disease. Arch. Surg. *113*:581, 1978.

71. Warren, W. D., Rudman, D., Millikan, W., Galambos, J. T., Salam, A. A., and Smith, R. B., III: The metabolic basis of portasystemic encephalopathy and the effect of selective vs. nonselective shunts. Ann. Surg. *180*:573, 1974.

72. Warren, W. D., Salam, A. A., Hutson, D., and Zeppa, R.: Selective distal splenorenal shunt. Technique and results of operation. Arch. Surg. *108*:306, 1974.

73. Warren, W. D., Salam, A. A., and Smith, R. B., III: The meso-spleno-renal shunt procedure: A comprehensive approach to portasystemic decompression. Ann. Surg. *179*:791, 1974.

74. Warren, W. D., Zeppa, R., and Fomon, J. J.: Selective transplenic decompression of gastroesophageal varices by distal splenorenal shunt. Ann. Surg. *166*:437, 1967.

75. Welling, R. E., and McDermott, W. V., Jr.: Combined caval and portal hypertension with cirrhosis of the liver. A problem in management. Ann. Surg. *177*:164, 1973.

76. Whipple, A. O.: The rationale of portacaval anastomosis. Bull. N.Y. Acad. Med. *22*:251, 1946.

77. Zieve, L.: Hepatic encephalopathy: Summary of present knowledge with an elaboration on recent developments. Prog. Liver Dis. *6*:327, 1979.

24

COMPLICATIONS OF APPENDECTOMY

W. A. Altemeier
and W. R. Culbertson

The complications of appendectomy are essentially those of acute appendicitis except for those conditions that complicate the operative procedure of appendectomy, anesthesia, or the general postoperative and convalescent states. Furthermore, there are few complications of acute appendicitis as long as the infection is contained within the appendix, but once the infecting bacteria have penetrated the peritoneal appendicular surface or have invaded the regional circulation, any one or more of a series of serious complications may develop. Thus emphasis has been rightly placed on early removal of the inflamed appendix, before perforation has occurred, as the best method of preventing complications.

As with any disease requiring operative treatment, however, complications may result from causes other than the disease itself. Even though appendectomy is not a complex operative procedure, a number of complications may follow it. Most of these are from anesthesia, poor hemostasis, breaks in aseptic technique, atelectasis, pneumonia, phlebothrombosis, pulmonary embolism, associated diseases, and foreign bodies such as sponges accidentally left in the operative wound.

EARLY REGIONAL COMPLICATIONS

PERITONITIS

This complication, which often follows a neglected, undiagnosed, or mistreated case of appendicitis, usually becomes manifest within 48 to 72 hours after the beginning of the attack of acute appendicitis, although it may be evident in less than 10 hours. Its

William Arthur Altemeier, a Cincinnatian by birth, is a product of his home city's elementary, high school, and university educational institutions. He received his graduate training in surgery at the Henry Ford Hospital and the University of Michigan. He progressed through the ranks of the Department of Surgery at the University of Cincinnati College of Medicine to become the Christian R. Holmes Professor and Chairman of the Department of Surgery. He is now the Christian R. Holmes Professor Emeritus of Surgery. Dr. Altemeier is a world leader in the field of surgical infections and has been President of both the American Surgical Association and the American College of Surgeons.

William Richard Culbertson went to Vanderbilt University Medical School by way of Transylvania College. He was trained in surgery at the Cincinnati General Hospital and currently is Professor in the Department of Surgery at the University of Cincinnati. Along with his works in surgical bacteriology, he has maintained a special interest in hemorrhagic and septic shock.

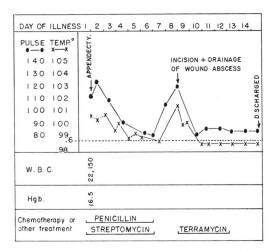

Figure 24–1 Graph of the course of a 5-year-old boy admitted 1 day after onset of symptoms with findings of generalized abdominal tenderness, right lower quadrant spasm, rebound tenderness, and hypoactive peristalsis. Operation revealed acute suppurative appendicitis and localized peritonitis. On the seventh postoperative day fever occurred, and examination showed wound abscess. Drainage was followed by recovery.

onset usually follows appendiceal perforation, and its extent varies greatly. If operation is performed shortly after perforation, the peritonitis usually is still localized to the right lower quadrant or the pelvis (Fig. 24–1). In most instances, however, this proc-

ess exists before appendectomy. Appendectomy may aid in the resolution of this localized peritonitis, or occasionally it may adversely influence it with postoperative continuation and progression of the infection to abscess formation, and spreading peritonitis that may become diffuse and generalized to involve the entire abdominal cavity (Fig. 24–2). Diffuse peritonitis may also result from inadvertent rupture of an acutely inflamed or gangrenous appendix during the course of appendectomy.

Clinically, peritonitis is manifested by diffuse abdominal tenderness, fever, recurrent vomiting, constipation, rigidity of the abdominal wall, hippocratic facies, tachycardia, and leukocytosis. Progression of this process leads to paralytic ileus and abdominal distention with evidence of severe systemic attrition (Fig. 24–3). Development of inflammatory exudation may result in hemoconcentration, reduction in the circulating blood volume, oliguria, and even signs of circulatory collapse or septic shock. The development of paralytic ileus also promotes the stagnation and accumulation of fluids and electrolytes within the lumen of the intestine with resultant greater changes in these parameters of metabolism.

Peritonitis secondary to acute perforated

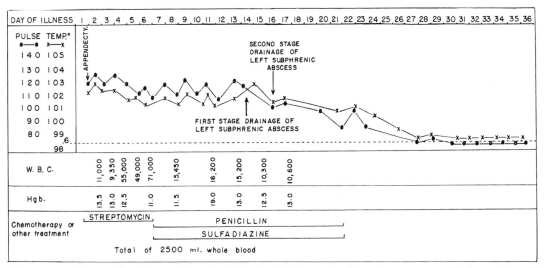

Figure 24–2 Course of a 17-year-old youth admitted with history of 2 days of symptoms and findings of boardlike rigidity of the entire abdomen, generalized abdominal tenderness, and absent peristaltic sounds. Initial x-ray film of the abdomen showed paralytic ileus. Operation revealed suppurative appendicitis with gangrene and generalized peritonitis. A hectic postoperative course was complicated by a left subphrenic abscess which was drained in two stages on the fourteenth and sixteenth days after the onset of initial symptoms.

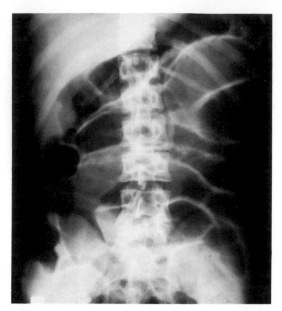

Figure 24–3 Roentgenogram of abdomen of patient whose course is shown in Figure 24–2, showing paralytic ileus. Note diffuse gaseous distention of stomach, small intestine, and colon and the increased space between the contiguous loops of intestine caused by edema and peritoneal exudate.

appendicitis is rarely caused by a single type of bacterium. On the contrary, the bacterial flora of the peritoneal exudate is mixed and varied, and any of the intestinal bacteria may be found in the peritoneal exudate in such cases. In a previous study at the Henry Ford Hospital in 1938, 16 species of aerobic microorganisms and at least 18 species of anaerobes were described by Altemeier in the purulent exudates taken from the immediate vicinity of the perforated appendix of 100 cases. Three or more species of bacteria were recovered from 96 of the 100 cases, and as many as 7 types were occasionally isolated, similar to the findings of Weinberg, Prevot, Davesne, and Renard in 1928. The average number of anaerobic species in a case often exceeds that of the aerobic, agreeing with the previous reports of Veillon and Zuber, and Runeberg and Heyde. Among the aerobes recovered were *E. coli*, streptococci, *B. pseudodiphtheriae*, staphylococci. *S. lactis*, *E. aerogenes*, *B. proteus*, *B. alcaligenes*, *B. subtilis* and *B. mesentericus;* and among the anaerobes were *B. melaninogenicus*, peptostreptococci, peptococci, streptococci, gram-negative diplococci, *B. fragilis*, other Bacteroides species, and members of the Clostridium group.

The pathogenicity of the bacteria most frequently isolated from the peritoneal exudates of 100 cases of acute perforated appendicitis was also studied in experimental animals by Altemeier in 1942. Most of these bacteria, including *E. coli*, did not produce a fatal peritonitis when injected in pure culture. For this and other reasons the ascription of the peritonitis of acute perforated appendicitis to the unaided activity of *E. coli* or other single strains of bacteria seemed to be without sufficient justification in the average case. Many avirulent strains of bacteria, paticularly *E. coli*, became highly virulent, however, in the presence of dead tissue or blood within the peritoneal cavity. In addition, these bacteria showed a synergistic action in mixed culture, producing a high degree of pathogenicity.

On the basis of these findings it was concluded that peritonitis following acute perforated appendicitis is an infection often resulting from the synergistic activities of the various bacterial symbionts present in a given case.

Treatment

There is still no specific treatment for acute septic peritonitis, and successful management is dependent primarily on good surgical intervention, aided by early and correct diagnosis, antimicrobial therapy, and adequate preoperative and postoperative care. The earlier the diagnosis is made, the more effective is prompt treatment. Because of the physiologic effects caused by septic peritonitis, preoperative preparation of these patients is important. This includes the following:

1. Continuous nasogastric suction to overcome the gastrointestinal distention and diaphragmatic elevation, eliminate vomiting, and put the distended inflamed loops of bowel at rest.

2. Correction of dehydration, azotemia, hypochloremia, and toxemia by intravenous infusion of solutions of physiologic saline and glucose in water.

3. Administration of adequate doses of antibiotic agents. The authors prefer the intravenous infusion of aqueous penicillin G in doses of 1,000,000 units and intravenous forms of chloramphenicol or one of the tetracyclines in doses of 500 mg., preopera-

tively and during the operation, to provide an antibacterial concentration in the peritoneal exudate as soon as possible. Alternatives include an aminoglycoside and a cephalothin.

4. Transfusion of adequate quantities of blood or plasma may be useful in some cases.

5. If the condition of the patient is satisfactory, appendectomy is recommended. If the patient is desperately ill or moribund, operation is usually best postponed and conservative but vigorous medical treatment instituted. The operation preferred by the authors consists of the McBurney incision, removal of the appendix, ligation of the appendiceal stump with 0 plain catgut and inversion of it with a purse-string suture of medium silk reinforced with two or three Lembert sutures of the same material.

In making abdominal incisions for peritonitis, it is recommended that one not dissect back the various layers any more than is absolutely necessary, since doing so exposes greater areas of areolar tissue having little resistance to contamination and infection by the mixture of bacteria in the peritoneal exudate.

In established peritonitis the question of drainage is decided on the merits of the individual case. Careful removal of excessive exudate by suction is recommended as part of the operation, but extended efforts to cleanse the peritoneal surfaces with extensive lavage are not recommended by the authors, since they disturb natural protective mechanisms of the peritoneum. There is evidence to indicate that it is unnecessary and useless to attempt to drain the peritoneal cavity in the presence of diffuse peritonitis. Only the presence of foreign bodies, necrotic tissue, and localized collections of pus has been considered an indication for drainage.

Postoperatively, the patient with peritonitis requires vigilant care and adequate supportive therapy. In most cases this consists of the following:

1. Continuation of nasogastric suction.

2. Parenteral infusion of water, electrolytes, and vitamins.

3. No oral intake until peristalsis has returned.

4. Continuation of antibiotic therapy. During the first 4 to 6 days of the disease intravenous administration of 1,000,000 or more units of aqueous penicillin G is recommended along with 500 mg. of tetracycline or chloramphenicol every 6 to 8 hours. Alternatives include an aminoglycoside and a cephalothin. If secondary abscesses or other infections occur, the choice of agents and the dosage are modified as indicated. Review of in vitro studies of sensitivities of the infecting microorganisms may indicate changes in the types of bacteria.

5. Continuous Fowler's position.

6. Oxygen therapy.

7. Blood transfusion may be useful occasionally.

8. Thoughtful dressing care.

9. If septic shock is present even more vigilance and support are needed. Resuscitative measures include respiratory support and the monitoring of adequacy of blood oxygenation, hemodynamic perfusion of brain, kidney, heart, and liver, and renal output. Ventilatory support may be indicated to improve respiratory effectiveness. Fluid replacement is the major need in maintenance of hemodynamic perfusion with use of added vasodilators in instances of refractory septic shock (see Chapter 3). Cortisone or hydrocortisone may be useful in those cases in which it is impossible to restore or maintain the blood pressure by the administration of fluids. An indwelling catheter is recommended to measure the hourly urinary output, which should be maintained between 25 and 75 ml. per hour.

In peritonitis secondary to appendicitis the general mortality rate was reduced at the Cincinnati General Hospital from 14.5 per cent in 338 cases treated without chemotherapy between 1934 and 1938 to 4.9 per cent in 244 cases treated with chemotherapy between 1942 and 1948. The average duration of the infection in the later group was 3.8 days. The results were definitely superior in those cases treated with chemotherapy, not only with respect to mortality, but also in regard to the morbidity and incidence of secondary intraabdominal or wound abscesses.

Originally it was thought that penicillin would be of little or no value in the prevention or treatment of secondary peritonitis because a large proportion of the infecting bacteria were of the gram-negative variety, which were either naturally resistant to the action of penicillin or were producers of enzymes that inhibited or destroyed the action of penicillin. A review of our previous experimental work in peritonitis suggests the explanations for the clinical effectiveness of penicillin.

Many of the gram-positive cocci and bacilli which are associated with peritonitis are susceptible to the action of penicillin. By giving large doses of penicillin one produces a concentration sufficient to inhibit the growth of virulent gram-positive bacteria, particularly the anaerobes, thereby reducing the number of organisms growing actively in the peritoneal exudate and lessening the synergistic effect ordinarily produced. The infection is then more controllable by the normal defensive mechanisms of the peritoneum. This observation supports our previous findings that *E. coli* is not the truly pathogenic organism in the majority of instances.

A review of our previous experimental work suggests that the effectiveness of large doses of aqueous penicillin in acute septic peritonitis is the result of a conversion of a severe synergistic and mixed infection into a simpler one produced predominantly by gram-negative bacteria, usually of lower virulence.

INTRA-ABDOMINAL ABSCESS

Intra-abdominal *appendiceal abscess* is a frequent complication of acute appendicitis and usually occurs 7 to 14 days after the onset of the infection. It may occasionally develop in 5 days and is formed by isolation of the infection to one of several areas by the successful adherence of adjacent structures, particularly loops of bowel and the omentum.

The most frequent location of intra-abdominal abscess after acute appendicitis is the periappendicular area in the right lower quadrant of the abdomen. Should abscess be present before appendectomy or develop subsequent to it, the clinical manifestations are similar: persistent fever, localized abdominal tenderness, the presence of a tender mass in the right lower quadrant, and leukocytosis. The presence of generalized abdominal tenderness and adynamic ileus is unlikely if the abscess is confined to the appendiceal area, though there may be considerable abdominal distention in cases

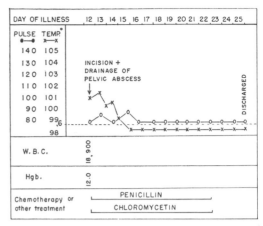

Figure 24–4 Graph of the course of a 16-year-old youth admitted 11 days after appendectomy performed at another hospital for gangrenous appendicitis. Complaints were suprapubic abdominal swelling, nausea, and vomiting. Examination revealed a tender mass filling the lower portion of the abdomen and bulging of the cul-de-sac on rectal examination. Transrectal drainage of the pelvic abscess resulted in rapid recovery.

of abscess that has been incompletely walled-off.

The pelvis is the next most frequent location for the development of postappendectomy abscess. A *pelvic abscess* usually be-

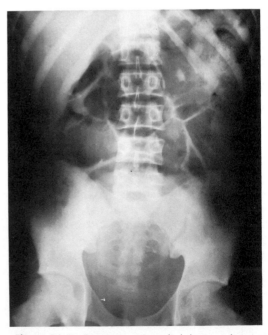

Figure 24–5 Roentgenogram of abdomen of patient whose course is shown in Figure 24–4, showing pelvic abscess. Note displacement of distended loops of bowel from pelvis by symmetrical mass arising in pelvis.

comes manifest within 4 to 5 days after operation, but may be overlooked for 2 or more weeks (Fig. 24–4). Its onset is insidious, and its presence may be relatively obscure. The localizing signs of lower abdominal pain. tenderness, rebound tenderness, muscle spasm, and palpation of an underlying mass may be and frequently are absent unless the mass becomes large enough to emerge from the pelvis. The presence of a pelvic abscess may be suspected in a patient who has increased fever and leukocytosis on the fourth or fifth day after appendectomy in association with the passage of several or more loose stools.

The diagnosis can be made by rectal examination and demonstration of the mass anterior to the rectum in the cul-de-sac. Large abscesses may be detected also by abdominal palpation in the suprapubic or lateral hypogastric area by x-ray examination (Fig. 24–5), and by echogram, gallium scan, or CAT scan.

The treatment of pelvic abscess is early drainage, which may be done through the anterior wall of the rectum in the male, by culpotomy in the female, or through an abdominal incision in the case of the larger or higher abscesses.

In some patients the infection may spread from the pelvis into and along the left paracolic gutter to produce a *left lower quadrant abscess*. When this occurs, it is usually in association with a coexisting or preexisting pelvic abscess. Its presence may be detected by demonstration of a palpable tender mass in this region in a patient who has an increase in fever and leukocytosis. There may also be evidence of colon irritation as expressed by diarrhea with passage of four or more watery stools a day. X-ray examination, echograms, gallium scans, or CAT scans may be of further diagnostic help as in the case of pelvic abscesses.

One of the two most common causes of *subphrenic abscess* is gangrenous appendicitis with perforation (Figs. 24–2 and 24–6). During the postoperative period for perforated appendicitis, extension of infection may progress along the right paracolic gutter and into the right kidney pouch, subhepatic space, and lateral subphrenic spaces. Infection of the bare area of the liver in the subphrenic region may also develop, presumably by extension of the infection along the retroperitoneal lymphatics. The left subphrenic area is involved less frequently in abscess formation, and the route of infec-

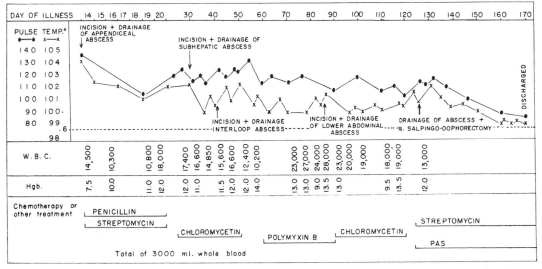

Figure 24–6 Course of an 11-year-old girl admitted with symptoms of 2 weeks' duration, including tender, firm mass filling the entire right lower quadrant and a fluctuant mass filling the cul-de-sac. Incision and drainage of the periappendiceal abscess was the first of a series of operative drainage of abscesses, including a subhepatic abscess on the thirtieth day of illness, an interloop abscess on the thirty-sixth day, and another lower quadrant and pelvic abscess on the one hundred and twenty-fifth day, at which time a right salpingo-oophorectomy was also done. Histologic study of the specimen revealed the process to be tuberculosis. Specific chemotherapy resulted in rapid improvement and recovery by the one hundred and seventieth day.

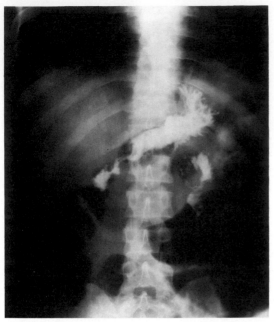

Figure 24–7 Roentgenogram of 27-year-old man showing left subphrenic abscess which was detected on the fiftieth day after appendectomy and drainage of periappendiceal abscess with peritonitis. Note displacement of the fundus of the stomach inferiorly and to the right by the abscess and the increased space between the diaphragm and the most superior portion of the stomach.

tion presumably is along the left paracolic gutter (Fig. 24–7).

The onset and development of subphrenic suppuration usually are insidious and obscure. There are few local signs of inflammation in the majority of patients. The possibility of a subphrenic abscess should be considered in any patient who is not doing well after appendectomy for ruptured appendicitis and who maintains or exhibits an increase in the general signs of infection between the seventh and fourteenth days. Elevation of a sustained type of fever is usually followed by a septic spiking fever associated in some instances with chills and sweats. The white blood cell count characteristically is elevated, and the respiratory rate is increased. Occasionally tenderness of the tip of the twelfth rib posteriorly, intercostal space tenderness or lateral subcostal tenderness, and muscle spasm may be found on careful physical examination. It has been estimated that only 30 per cent of

the patients with subphrenic cellulitis ultimately progress to actual abscess formation.

The diagnosis of subphrenic suppuration may be aided by x-ray examinations showing elevation and impairment of motion of the diaphragm, fixation of the diaphragm, and occasionally an air or fluid level within the abscess cavity itself. Other non-invasive radiographic studies may be helpful in diagnosis of subphrenic abscess. Computerized tomography may reveal occult or small abscesses with accuracy and is of assistance in localizing the position of the abscess for most effective approach for drainage. Echography is also frequently useful, although the usual presence of an ileus with gas present in the lumen of the bowel may interfere with the accuracy. Gallium scan may be used but is often of limited value. Change in position of the patient during x-ray examination may yield useful information about the relative position and size of the abscess containing gas and fluid. In abscesses located in the left subphrenic space the diagnosis may be particularly difficult. Examination of the stomach after ingestion of barium may show displacement of the fundus to the right and inferiorly, with a mass interposed between the elevated diaphragm and the fundus (Fig. 24–7). During this examination it may be helpful to place the patient in the Trendelenburg position, since this gives better delineation of the subphrenic mass. The development of clear fluid in the pleural sac on the involved side is a relatively late sign. As in other intra-abdominal abscesses, echograms, gallium scans, or CAT scans may be of additional diagnostic value.

The treatment of subphrenic abscesses is drainage by one of several approaches placed over the area of the abscess (Fig. 24–8). Operation should be performed as early as possible and not delayed until the x-ray findings have developed. Approaches to abscesses in the subphrenic and subhepatic area may be through subcostal incisions, transverse flank incisions, posterolateral thoracic two-stage procedures through the bed of the eighth rib, and the retroperitoneal approach of Ochsner and DeBakey through the bed of the tenth rib posteriorly. The location and type of incision used

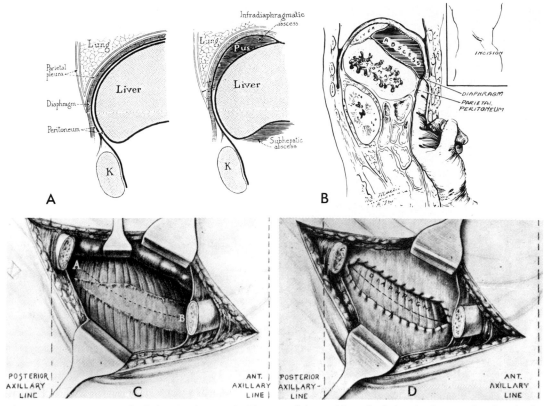

Figure 24–8   Drainage of subphrenic abscess. *A*, Diagram of the position of subphrenic abscess, showing the liver inferiorly and the peritoneum and diaphragm superiorly. *B*, Posterolateral subcostal extraperitoneal approach to left subphrenic abscess. *C*, First stage of lateral transpleural drainage of subphrenic abscess approached through the bed of the tenth rib. *D*, Second stage of lateral transpleural drainage of subphrenic abscess through bed of tenth rib.

should depend upon the location and size of the abscess.

Interloop abscesses may also occur anywhere in the abdominal cavity between loops of small and large intestine. These usually become manifest during the third or later weeks of the disease in the most serious cases. Their presence and location are particularly difficult to ascertain. X-ray examination may be of little or no help. Computerized tomography and echography may be of substantial value in localizing and outlining interloop abscesses.

Occasionally an intra-abdominal abscess may *rupture* as a result of rapid expansion, trauma, or bacterial necrosis of its wall. If this dread complication occurs, an overwhelming generalized peritonitis may develop, characterized by vascular collapse, anuria, and other signs of septic shock. Death may be imminent.

The diagnosis necessarily is made on the basis of the clinical picture, since the grave condition of the patient usually precludes any additional diagnostic procedure. The recommended plan of treatment in this grave situation is essentially the same as that recommended earlier for septic shock in generalized peritonitis.

The prognosis of patients suffering from perforation of intra-abdominal abscess is poor. Under the best forms of available treatment the mortality rate is still 60 to 75 per cent.

SPECIAL COMPLICATING INFECTIONS OR TUMORS

Occasionally a periappendiceal abscess may develop in association with other diseases such as actinomycosis, tuberculosis,

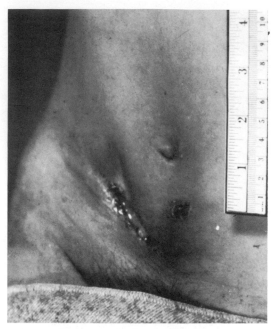

Figure 24–9 Photograph of wound showing actino-mycotic infection complicating McBurney wound for drainage of appendiceal abscess.

carcinoma, malignant mucocele, and lymphoma. Although 45 to 60 per cent of all carcinoid tumors of the alimentary tract have been reported in the appendix, metastasis has been demonstrated in only 2.5 per cent or less. Adenocarcinoma of the colonic type of the mucocele (malignant) is a grade I mucous papillary adenocarcinoma. When ruptured, it may be followed by the distressing development of pseudomyxoma peritonei. Recognition of such complicating or associated lesions is largely dependent upon unusual clinical or operative findings, microscopic examination of biopsied material, or culture.

Upon recognition of these lesions specific chemotherapy or antibiotic therapy for the infection should be instituted. The association of malignant diseases with intra-abdominal abscesses presents problems that can be settled only on the basis of a consideration of the individual case.

amebic infection, or regional enteritis (Figs. 24–6 and 24–9). Neoplasms of the appendix may rarely be associated with perforation of the appendix and abscess formation. The malignant tumors include carcinoid, adeno-

WOUND INFECTION

Infections developing in appendectomy wounds usually become manifest by the fourth to eighth day in the postoperative period (Figs. 24–1 and 24–10). They are usually polymicrobic and complicated by a mixture of gram-negative and gram-

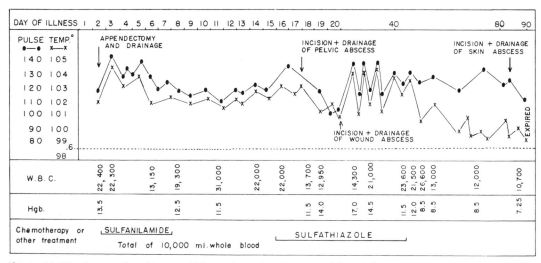

Figure 24–10 Course of an 11-year-old boy admitted on the second day of illness. Operation revealed gangrenous appendicitis with generalized peritonitis. A pelvic abscess developed which was drained on the seventeenth day of illness. On the twentieth day of illness a wound infection was found and was drained. Subsequently he had a staphylococcal septicemia with dissemination to cause multiple subcutaneous abscesses, osteomyelitis, lung abscesses, and death on the ninetieth day of illness.

positive bacteria. On rare occasions, resection of an acutely inflamed appendix incarcerated in an inguinal hernia may become necessary. Wound infection of the hernial wound may follow. The first manifestation of infection is usually *cellulitis. Abscess* may develop, but granulomatous changes in the subcutaneous and areolar tissues are not uncommon. A *crepitant cellulitis* may develop beneath Scarpa's fascia and may extend rapidly into the flank and axilla or into the scrotum, labia, or perineum. It is a necrotizing infection that is rapidly progressive and may be fatal.

The treatment of crepitant cellulitis is early and radical incision and drainage through and beyond the involved areas to provide adequate decompression. In the instance of wound abscesses early drainage by removal of sutures and separation of wound edges is recommended. Supportive and antibiotic therapy should be continued and modified on the basis of the existing bacterial flora and antibiotic sensitivity tests whenever possible.

Chronic progressive cutaneous gangrene fortunately is not seen often in clinical practice. It usually develops around retention sutures in the operative wound as a painful purple pustule on the fifth to ninth day. Ulceration and progressive extension of the ulcer follow. The margin of the ulcer becomes exquisitely tender, painful, undermined, and purplish or purplish black. Surrounding this margin is a zone of red or pinkish erythema. The microaerophilic nonhemolytic streptococcus may be recovered from the area of cellulitis, and the hemolytic *Staphylococcus aureus* from the area of ulceration. The zone of their interaction presumably produces the edge of extending gangrene.

Recommended treatment of this condition consists of radical excision of the ulcerated area and adjunctive antibiotic therapy with large doses of penicillin. Meleney recommended the use of bacitracin in this condition. (See also Chapter 1.)

PYLEPHLEBITIS WITH MULTIPLE LIVER ABSCESSES AND SEPTICEMIA

Pylephlebitis represents a suppurative thrombosis of the portal vein associated with multiple abscesses of the liver and usually septicemia (Fig. 24–10). Its clinical picture is characterized by the development of recurrent chills followed by high fever and drenching sweats. These symptoms usually become manifest 6 to 10 days after appendectomy and are obviously severe. The chills are usually bed-shaking, lasting as long as 30 to 45 or more minutes, and accompanied by cyanosis. Prostration is severe, and jaundice usually follows. The chills are irregularly intermittent and may occur once or more during a 24-hour period or at longer intervals. On physical examination the patient appears to be severely and desperately ill in the advanced cases. The liver becomes enlarged and tender to palpation. Muscle spasm or rigidity of the abdominal muscles in the right upper quadrant is usually present. The cyanosis and rapid respiration in the presence of high fever often lead to a mistaken diagnosis of pneumonia. Patients frequently complain of epigastric or right upper quadrant pain made worse by respiration. Cutaneous petechiae may develop. In patients suspected of having liver abscess, computerized tomography may be of great value in demonstrating the presence and location of the abscesses. In instances of diagnostic difficulty hepatic angiography may be used to show areas with blood flow changes compatible with abscess. Radioisotopic scan may indicate areas of absent liver cellular function.

The prognosis of patients with this complication is grave. Treatment should be directed toward supportive therapy with the intravenous infusion of fluids and blood, and intensive antimicrobial therapy. The responsible agents are often gram-negative aerobic or anaerobic bacilli or anaerobic streptococci. *Escherichia coli, Aerobacter aerogenes* or anaerobic gram-negative bacteroides have been found in association with this condition.

Aqueous penicillin, tetracycline or chloramphenicol should be administered in maximum treatment doses, depending upon the infecting organism. Anticoagulant therapy with heparin or sodium warfarin should be considered to prevent the progression of septic clots into the liver or into the superior mesenteric vessels. Operative ligation of the portal vein has been advocat-

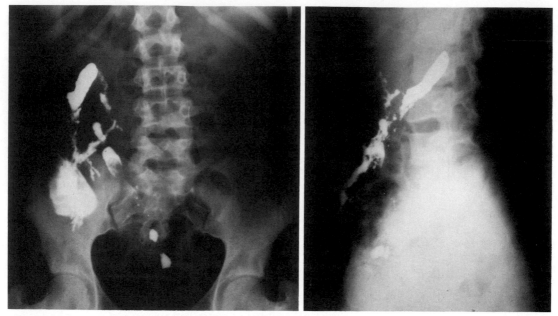

Figure 24–11   Roentgenograms of 17-year-old girl admitted after 5 days of symptoms of abdominal pain, nausea, and vomiting. Findings included fever of 103.8°F., abdominal distention, tenderness, and right lower quadrant rigidity with rebound tenderness. Operative incision with drainage of an appendiceal abscess was done. Her wound continued to drain intermittently and 3 months later showed evidence of having become a fecal fistula. Injection of barium into the sinus tract revealed an abscess cavity with communication with small intestine causing a fecal fistula.

ed, but the majority of present surgical opinion is against the procedure in the presence of pylephlebitis. The desperate condition of the patient and the dissemination of the infection make this procedure impracticable in the opinion of the authors.

Drainage of the liver abscesses is usually not feasible because of their multiplicity and dispersion. If they become confluent to produce one or more large abscesses, surgical incision and drainage is indicated. Again, scanning techniques and hepatic artery angiography may be of value in the diagnosis and localization of such abscesses.

FECAL FISTULA

Development of a fecal fistulous tract from the stump of the appendix into the area of the wound is an infrequent complication (Fig. 24–11). Failure to properly ligate the amputated stump of the appendix and invert it carefully with a silk or other non-absorbable purse-string suture may result in this complication. Other causes include operative injury to the cecum or ter-

minal ileum, coexistent diseases of the ileocecal segment, and appendectomy performed in the presence of active regional enteritis or cystic fibrosis and meconium ileus. Theoretically, there is a possibility of a fecal fistulous tract resulting from erosion of the ileocecal segment by a contiguous periappendiceal abscess. This circumstance, however, has been rare in the experience of the authors, as has been internal fecal fistula between loops of adjacent bowel. Colorectal fistula has been reported following transrectal drainage of a pelvic abscess as a rare complication. The fistula communicates with the cecum at the appendiceal stump area. Its treatment is transabdominal excision.

Conservative treatment in conjunction with active treatment of the postappendectomy state usually permits spontaneous healing of the fistulous tract unless there is distal obstruction of the intestinal tract or specific infection such as actinomycosis. Persistent fistulas may require secondary operative procedures consisting in excision of the tract and closure of the internal opening into the bowel by a double row of interrupted silk sutures.

EARLY DISTANT OR REMOTE INFECTIONS

PULMONARY COMPLICATIONS

Pulmonary abscess may complicate the post-appendectomy state. It may be produced by septic embolization in the course of a septicemia or by direct extension of the infection from the subphrenic areas penetrating the adjacent diaphragm and lung. The former type of pulmonary complication occurs relatively early, whereas the latter is more apt to occur during the third or fourth week of the disease, or later. Communication with the bronchial tree may develop.

The bacterial flora of this type of pulmonary abscess is mixed and similar to that of the peritonitis. Management of these cases with antibiotic therapy alone may be inadequate, and surgical intervention with drainage may be necessary.

Thoracic empyema may occur as an extension of the subphrenic space or as a metastatic lesion. Since the purulent exudate is thick and fetid, treatment requires closed drainage by early insertion of a thoracotomy tube. Antibiotic therapy and supportive therapy are adjunctive measures.

PERICARDITIS

Pericarditis is another rare complication that may be seen during the course of septicemia. Its treatment is essentially that directed toward the septicemia and drainage of the pericardium by aspiration followed by instillation of a solution of the appropriate antibiotic. Occasionally open drainage may be required.

BRAIN ABSCESS

Another rare complication during the postappendectomy period is putrid brain abscess. This complication is prone to develop 4 to 8 weeks or longer after the acute attack of appendicitis, and its presence is obscure unless its position may be deduced from localizing symptoms. The Bacteroides, Peptostreptococcus, and "L" forms may be important etiologic agents. Drainage of the abscess in conjunction with intensive antibiotic therapy is the recommended treatment.

NOSOCOMIAL INFECTIONS

Hospital acquired infections that may occur as complications of appendectomy include bacteremia from infected indwelling intravenous infusion lines or indwelling urinary catheters and respiratory tract infections related to postoperative atelectasis or aspiration.

LATER COMPLICATIONS

SINUS TRACT FORMATION

As a result of recurrent active chronic infection or a retained foreign body in the right lower quadrant of the abdomen, the retroperitoneal space, or the abdominal wall, a sinus tract may develop and persist.

Roentgenographic examination after injection with radiopaque solutions usually yields valuable information as to the nature and extent of the tract. If the tract enters the intestinal lumen, it is correctly designated as a fistulous tract. Important information concerning the delineation and exten-sion of the tract may be documented by injection of Hypaque solution through a Foley catheter inserted and inflated in the fistulous tract.

If conservative treatment is unsuccessful in producing healing of the tract, operative intervention may be necessary, consisting in adequate incision and drainage of underlying abscesses, removal of foreign bodies, or even excision of the tract. It is important that healing progress from the base outward to prevent loculation and recurrent abscesses with recurrence or persistence of the tract.

INTESTINAL OBSTRUCTION

During the postoperative period occlusion of the intestinal tract by contracting adhesions resulting from the inflammatory process or the operative procedure may occur and result in acute mechanical obstruction. This complication may develop after the first week of the postoperative period or may occur as long as many years later. The diagnosis and treatment of this form of mechanical obstruction will not be discussed here other than by emphasis of the importance of early diagnosis, preoperative and postoperative intubation, early operation and supportive treatment. (See Chapter 22.)

HERNIATION

There is an increased probability of postoperative herniation of appendectomy wounds in which there has been active infection with delay in wound healing and septic necrosis of tissue. Prolonged drainage may result in scarring and fixation of the layers of the abdominal wall, leaving a defect through which herniation may later develop. Such scarring of the underlying tissue may be excessive and result in decreased tensile strength.

The diagnosis of this condition is usually obvious on careful examination. Treatment consists in operative repair, which should be delayed until all evidence of infection has disappeared. The authors prefer to postpone operative repairs of this type of herniation that develops in association with infection until at least 6 months after healing has occurred.

"POSTAPPENDECTOMY" APPENDICITIS

Rarely a patient may have appendicitis after apparent appendectomy. This deceiving complication may have as its origin the erroneous assumption by the surgeon that appendectomy has been performed because a right lower quadrant scar exists in a patient who presents himself with symptoms and signs of appendicitis, but gives a history of previous operation for appendicitis. The occurrence of such a complication of operation for appendicitis can be the result of the fact that the preceding operation was done for drainage of an appendiceal abscess without accompanying appendectomy or of incomplete amputation of the appendix in a fashion that failed to include the entire organ and failure to invert the stump. Management of this complication resembles in all aspects the management of original acute appendictis.

OTHER COMPLICATIONS INCIDENT TO APPENDECTOMY

As indicated above, most complications of appendectomy and appendicitis are infectious. As with any surgical procedure, however, certain complications may occur as a result of the operation itself.

Hemorrhage may occur in the abdominal wall, into the peritoneal cavity, or, rarely, into the lumen of the intestine. Hemorrhage into the abdominal wound usually results from failure of the surgeon to ligate one of the vessels of the abdominal wall, and since such vessels are not large in this area, the blood loss is usually not enough to endanger the patient's life. Exploration of the wound and control of the bleeding point may be indicated if the hemorrhage is large or if conservative, less specific measures are unsuccessful.

Intraperitoneal hemorrhage is a much more serious circumstance and usually represents bleeding from the mesentery of the appendix because of either insecure ligation or septic erosion of the vessel. Bleeding from this source may be massive, and if the wound has been closed without drainage, no external evidence can be noted. Symptoms related to sudden severe anemia, abdominal distention with or without pain, tachycardia, and hypotension may be all the patient will show.

Intraluminal colonic hemorrhage following appendectomy is a rare complication resulting from bleeding at the site of amputation of the appendix after the ligature of the inverted stump has sloughed away. This bleeding may be severe and may arouse justifiable suspicions as to other causes for gastroenteric bleeding before relating it to the appendectomy. Bleeding of this sort can most often be controlled by non-operative measures and blood transfusions for replacement.

Wound dehiscence may follow appendectomy, particularly in the case of vertical incisions associated with wound infection, although it may occur in the absence of gross infection. The development of wound dehiscence in a McBurney type of appendectomy wound is much less likely to occur and carries less serious implication than when the same complication occurs in a rectus or midline incision. The latter almost invariably requires reoperation and closure with through-and-through wire sutures to control the underlying evisceration, whereas protrusion of viscera is less likely to occur in a McBurney wound. This is one of the many reasons for our preference for the McBurney incision. Obviously, consideration of the possibility of evisceration should be made when either type of wound dehiscence occurs and emergency operative treatment given should it be present. In the absence of evisceration, wound dehiscence may be treated as a wound infection.

Complications resulting from operative technical difficulties during appendectomy are rarely encountered and are usually the result of accident or unskillful techniques. *Division of cutaneous or motor nerve* of the abdominal wall may result from misplacement of the incision or during enlargement of such incision. If the nerve is a sensory one, minimal discomfort or disability will occur. Division of a motor nerve to the lower abdominal wall may possibly be related to the development of inguinal hernia in subsequent years.

Traumatic perforation of the cecum may occur during operation as a result of manipulation of the structure or because the adjacent inflammation has caused the wall to be extremely friable. It is obviously important that such perforation be recognized and repaired immediately and that drainage of the area be instituted.

Rarely, because of lack of skill or obliteration of normal anatomy, the *right ureter or right iliac vessels* may be damaged. Such catastrophes must be quickly recognized and repaired at the initial operation in order that subsequent fatal effects may be avoided.

Intussusception of the appendiceal stump has been reported as a complication following appendectomy. This very rare lesion occurred in four cases reported by Fraser and in one case reported by Little as early as 12 days and as late as 4½ years after appendectomy. In these instances the lead point of the intussusception was the inverted stump of the amputated appendix.

25

COMPLICATIONS IN SURGERY OF THE COLON AND RECTUM

Stephen E. Hedberg
and Claude E. Welch

Operations on the colon and rectum are attended by numerous complications, many of which are serious or even fatal. A variety of circumstances exist that render large bowel surgery particularly susceptible to complications. For the most part it is not strictly elective, and patients are not as a rule in ideal physical condition. With carcinoma and diverticulitis, patients are apt to be of advanced age and therefore run an increased risk of complications peculiar to geriatrics. Younger patients, on the other hand, usually are suffering from such debilitating diseases as ulcerative colitis, in which malnutrition and previous steroid therapy predispose to complications of wound healing and infection. Obstruction and bleeding, which comprise the most common indications for operations on the colon, cause electrolyte imbalance, anemia, hypovolemia, and hypoproteinemia, and these factors likewise increase the risk of operation.

The peculiar anatomy and physiology of the colon conspire to produce a situation that is much less conducive to a successful surgical outcome than exists, for example, with the stomach. In the colon, collateral circulation is present only between major arterial vessels, and damage to or interruption of major channels is quickly followed by gangrene and anastomotic failure. The colon is the only intraperitoneal organ whose contents consist largely of bacteria, so that infection with indigenous organisms or virulent strains selected by antibiotic treatment is to be expected unless special precautions are taken. Furthermore, a small local infection which might otherwise be controlled by body defenses often produces anastomotic leakage with continued soiling by contaminated material. Wide resections of colon and colonic mesentery for cancer produce large areas that are denuded of peritoneum and are oozing blood, so that intraperitoneal abscesses are likely to develop. Operations on the colon are frequently of long duration; the opportunity for injurious drying of tissues and the possibility of contamination by droplets and airborne bacteria are thereby increased.

Stephen E. Hedberg is a Bostonian, educated at Harvard College and Harvard Medical School. He received his surgical training under Edward Churchill at the Massachusetts General Hospital, where he serves on the staff. His research interests have centered on the field of gastrointestinal surgery and fiberoptic endoscopy.

Claude E. Welch was educated at Doane College, the University of Missouri, and Harvard Medical School. He received his postgraduate training in surgery at the Massachusetts General Hospital. His interests in the field of gastrointestinal surgery and malignant disease were developed at the MGH, where he served for many years as Chief of the Tumor Clinic. This renowned surgeon has served many surgical organizations in positions of leadership, including the presidencies of the American Surgical Association and the American College of Surgeons.

Errors in diagnosis or lack of appreciation of the extent of the disease is much less common than formerly, but these mistakes and the technical or strategic errors that accompany them also cause complications. Singly or in combination, the aforementioned factors may tend to produce bleeding, poor healing, infection, or slow return of normal function, and certain complications common to all colonic operations are apt to result. Sepsis, ileus, hemorrhage, and fistula formation can follow operation on any part of the colon as a direct effect of surgery. There are, in addition, special risks of phlebitis, pulmonary embolism, wound dehiscence, and genitourinary infection, as well as the complications that follow diagnostic maneuvers done in the study of colonic disease.

PROPHYLAXIS OF COMPLICATIONS

Complications rarely occur singly, because the various mishaps of sepsis, ileus, fistula, and hemorrhage tend to have common causes, and the presence of one frequently leads to one or more of the others.

On review of 500 consecutive colectomies and resections of the rectum done at the Massachusetts General Hospital, it was evident that complications tend to be multiple, particularly in the patients who die (Table 25–1).[36] Furthermore, the over-all incidence of complications was much higher than expected, and it was clear that many of them were possibly preventable through more careful attention to the various details of preparation, procedure, and postoperative care. It is appropriate, therefore, in the discussion of complications after colon surgery, perhaps more than in any other field, to devote first consideration to the *prevention* of complications, after which the specific complications and their management will be discussed.

MEASURES USED PREOPERATIVELY IN PREVENTION OF COMPLICATIONS

Accurate diagnosis and thorough preoperative study often uncover or forewarn of diseases which, if unsuspected and untreated, could lead to postoperative trouble. A careful history may elicit symptoms of diabetes, prostatism, pulmonary insufficiency, cardiac failure, or angina pectoris. Any of these conditions, if uncorrected, can be of crucial importance in the postoperative phase. Physical examination likewise may be expected to disclose many potential complicating factors such as abscess, perforation, signs of obstruction, hepatic metastases, malnutrition, dehydration, and pulmonary impairment. Sigmoidoscopy, which is an integral part of the physical examination in all these patients, is essential to assess the state of the lower bowel. Colonoscopy is indicated in many cases in order to evaluate the entire colon. Colonoscopic biopsy or polypectomy

TABLE 25–1 COMPLICATIONS FOLLOWING SURGERY OF THE COLON*

	Right Colectomy (Cancer)	Left Colectomy (Cancer)	Sigmoid Resection (Cancer)	Miles Resection (Cancer)	Sigmoid Resection (Diverticulitis)
Total patients..................................	100	100	100	100	100
Patients with fatal complications†.........	8	9	9	7	2
Patients with nonfatal complications.....	30	26	30	43	21
Total complications...........................	56	46	65	69	21
Complications per patient with fatal complications..............................	1.8	2.0	2.5	1.7	1.0
Complications per patient with nonfatal complications..............................	1.4	1.1	1.4	1.3	1.8

*From Hedberg, S. E., and Welch, C. E.: Complications following surgery of the colon. Surg. Clin. North Am. *43*:775, 1963.

†Includes palliative resections.

may furnish positive indications for surgery or may obviate the need for surgery. Avoidance of surgery via colonoscopy has already proven to be one of the chief contributions of this enormous technical advance. Clearly, there is no more effective way to avoid the complications of surgery than to avoid the surgery. Laboratory work should lead to an evaluation of possible anemia, glycosuria and hyperglycemia, electrolyte imbalance, uremia, hepatic obstruction or dysfunction, leukocytosis, urinary tract infection, and bleeding abnormalities. A preoperative electrocardiogram is of value as a baseline against which postoperative changes may be compared. Roentgenograms of the chest may reveal atelectasis, pneumonia, tuberculosis, or cardiomegaly, which should be treated preoperatively as adequately as possible. A plain film of the abdomen and barium enema may disclose intestinal obstruction, the presence of other colonic lesions (especially diverticula), the location of flexures, and congenital abnormalities. An intravenous pyelogram should be done if there is any question of sacrifice of one kidney or of ureteral involvement, and is also valuable to determine the position of the ureters if sigmoid resection or operations on the pelvic colon are planned. A series of bone films, a bone scan, or a liver scan to detect metastases may be indicated in some cases. However, physical signs of metastatic disease such as hepatomegaly, cervical adenopathy, or a rectal shelf are usually present before osseous lesions are visible radiographically. On the other hand, bone pain in any area should obviously be studied by means of roentgenograms preoperatively. Selective arteriography is very helpful in patients with severe hemorrhage or suspected vascular impairment.

Restoration of homeostatic mechanisms and correction of deficits should be done before operation as far as feasible because the basic disturbance, if uncorrected, will be compounded by the weakening effects of anesthesia and surgery. Losses of fat and lean body mass due to malnutrition usually cannot be restored until the pathologic process leading to starvation has been corrected. Two exceptions, however, can occur. The first exception occurs when a diversionary operation such as defunctioning colostomy or ileostomy improves matters suffi-

ciently to allow alimentation and the restoration of a positive nitrogen balance. In such cases considerable delay before definitive surgery may be indicated if the patient's condition is substantially improved thereby. Second, in patients with debilitating fistulas or chronic inflammatory bowel disease, total parenteral nutrition with complete bowel rest can restore the patient to optimum preoperative condition, sometimes with healing of the fistula or remission of the inflammatory process. Total parenteral nutrition does not obviate surgery as often as had been hoped, so that once a reasonable preoperative condition is attained one should not delay unduly, considering the expense of hospitalization for hyperalimentation and the not inconsiderable risk of the procedure.[1, 23] Indeed, in a recent study made at the Massachusetts General Hospital, total parenteral nutrition decreased the amount of drainage in only a third of the patients in which it was used.

Anemia and electrolyte deficits can and should be corrected before operation; usually 2 or 3 days will be required to relieve hypoproteinemia, hypokalemia, or hyponatremia with safety, because rapid correction with concentrated solutions can lead to serious cardiac or neurologic derangement. An exception to this general rule occurs in the case of electrolyte abnormalities secondary to obstruction and peritonitis, when it may be possible only to correct anemia and hypovolemia before proceeding with emergency resection or diversionary procedure. Even then, however, such fluids as are given for the purpose of restoring blood pressure and urinary output should contain liberal amounts of sodium, potassium, or chloride, depending on the patient's serum electrolyte concentrations and urinary output. Because many of these patients have lost large quantities of protein, both intraluminally and intraperitoneally, large amounts of plasma may be necessary.

Of considerable importance in the avoidance of postoperative septic complications is the preoperative treatment of infectious processes such as pneumonia, abscess, and urinary tract infection. Peritonitis may require early operation, but in most cases intensive preoperative preparation is indicated. The most serious condition apt to be encountered is septic shock due to gram-negative bacteremia. Even when the focus of infection is known with certainty, surgical treatment must await improvement of the patient's general condition, or a fatal outcome is likely. Specimens of blood, sputum, and all excreta are planted in media for culture and determination of antibiotic sensitivities, but vigorous treatment with high doses of broad-spectrum antibiotics is begun immediately, before the nature of the offending organism or its antibiotic spectrum is known. In life-threatening cases the most frequently used combinations are penicillin and chloramphenicol or clindamycin and gentamicin. Cephalosporins such as cefazolin or cefoxitin may be used preoperatively but are more frequently used against a known sensitive organism, or as part of a routine preoperative prophylaxis that also includes kanamycin or neomycin. The massive doses of penicillin we use — up to 60,000,000 units a day — are effective even against some gram-negative organisms. Except for the hazard of allergic reactions, the only toxic reaction to be considered is the possibility of hyperkalemia if the potassium salt of penicillin is used in patients who are oliguric or anuric. When hypotension is resistant to volume replacement, and when replacement has been adequate as measured by return of central venous pressure to normal or levels above normal, then the use of pressor agents must be considered despite their disadvantages in terms of renal and intestinal ischemia. In general, we have preferred to try the effect of intravenous dexamethasone or hydrocortisone before resorting to agents such as dopamine, isoproterenol, epinephrine, or norepinephrine. Needless to say, patients in whom hypotension and oliguria require such vigorous therapy should be operated upon at the earliest possible moment after blood pressure and urinary output have been restored, assuming the focus of infection or contamination is surgically correctable. One should not be encouraged to wait for further improvement, because the "golden moment" is usually transitory, and efforts to bring the patient out of a second hypotensive episode generally fail.

In semielective cases with pulmonary infections such as bronchopneumonia, lobar pneumonia, or chronic emphysematous bronchitis, severe postoperative complications usually can be avoided by vigorous antibiotic and physiotherapeutic measures. Discontinuance of smoking for up to 6 weeks is most important. In chronic or acute pulmonary disease with borderline compensation, preoperative tracheostomy has been recommended on the basis that patients may have an opportunity thereby to adjust to the inevitable superinfection that follows the procedure. In our hands, however, this approach has not proven beneficial, and we prefer to manage such patients postoperatively in the setting of a respiratory intensive care unit, maintaining sedation and retaining the endotracheal tube until ventilatory dynamics and respiratory function are sufficient. Often a brief period of mechanical ventilation is necessary; but only occasionally, after 7 to 10 days of nasotracheal intubation, is it necessary to perform tracheostomy. Urinary tract infections resulting from prostatic obstruction, colovesical fistula, or neoplastic ureteral obstruction are treated by bladder catheter drainage, hydration, and antibiotics according to indications in the particular case. With intraperitoneal abscesses and peritonitis, vigorous treatment with broad-spectrum antibiotics is the general rule, the rationale being avoidance of wound infection, septic emboli, bacteremia, and extension of the local process following operation.

Preparation of the colon itself for surgery consists of mechanical measures to clean the bowel of its contents and also measures to eliminate the resident bacterial flora. It is impossible to sterilize the bowel completely, and prolonged use of antibiotic agents permits the emergence of resistant strains; therefore, some compromise is necessary. In general, the more extensive the preoperative preparation, the greater the danger of postoperative staphylococcal enteritis. The rates of decrease of bacterial concentration and emergence of resistant strains have been the subject of much study, and various regimens have been worked out to take advantage of the several factors involved. An excellent review by Cohn[15] includes much original work supporting the conclusion that kanamycin, 1 gm. hourly for 4 hours, then every 6 hours for 72 hours, is an effective and safe regimen. Pseudomembranous enterocolitis was encountered only once in Cohn's series of 815 patients. Poth[48] also has contributed many studies on various antibiotics. Our own recent preference is for a 24-hour course of erythromycin base and neomycin given orally, supplemented by parenteral cefazolin or clindamycin and gentamicin just before and during the operation.

Despite our respect for the principle addressed by the late Leland McKittrick in his editorial, "The Surgeon's Bib,"[45] we must now agree with Altemeier,[3] that the effectiveness of preoperative and perioperative antibiotic preparation in avoiding postoperative morbidity and mortality is now so well established the use of a placebo group as a control in prospective studies is no longer justifiable. Ethical practice now requires that evaluation of a new regimen be done by comparing it with an established one. Altemeier's contention was subsequently proven scientifically — although with catastrophic results for the experimental subjects — in a study by Clarke et al. that conclusively demonstrated preoperative preparation with erythromycin base was much better than nothing.[13] The results were so bad in half the subjects that the protocol was terminated prematurely, since six patients who died from sepsis in one group were indeed the unfortunate recipients of placebo. Condon stated that a placebo control group was used because it was felt that the "results would be cleaner" than if erythromycin base had been compared against a standard regimen.[16] A more recent study reported in Lancet by Eykyn et al.[22] again used a placebo group in evaluating the effect of metronidazole as prophylaxis. In this instance justification for this approach was that many of the local surgeons used no preparation at all. Finally, in both studies the results in the placebo group were so bad, when compared with historical controls, as to force sad realization that the admonition of McKittrick's Bib is not so outdated as it might seem. The current generally accepted intraluminal bowel preparation is that of erythromycin base and neomycin; in a 1979 report by Condon[17] there was no beneficial effect of cefalothin when given systemically either instead of or in addition to the oral combination of erythromycin base and neomycin.

We feel that effective mechanical cleansing of the bowel is the single most important step in preparation for colonic surgery. Not only does a poorly prepared bowel present a danger from the point of view of an increased risk of contamination, but also the effects of anastomotic leakage are bound to be much more severe if abundant fecal matter remains in the bowel above the point of anastomosis. Measures used to empty the bowel before elective and semi-elective surgery when there is no obstruction include two days of a no-residue diet followed by castor oil or Dulcolax and cleansing enemas the afternoon before. Castor oil in doses of 2 to 4 ounces leaves the bowel completely clean and dry, but it is rejected by many patients for whom Dulcolax is acceptable. A 10 per cent solution of mannitol has been used by some surgeons. Laxatives and enemas must be used with caution in patients with obstructive symptoms of colitis.

In frank obstruction, cleansing of the bowel is impossible. Intestinal intubation and suction may reduce distention and prevent further accumulation of colonic contents, but intubation is ineffective for cleansing of the large bowel. It is dangerous to rely on tubes for decompression in the presence of a competent ileocecal valve, because perforation of the colon can occur in a few hours. Transverse colostomy or cecostomy allows obstructive edema to subside after decompression, so that distal irrigations and gradual removal of fecal matter are possible.

Other measures used more or less routinely include the insertion of a Foley catheter for bladder drainage and a Levin tube, which, in addition to providing postoperative decompression, also prevents annoying distention of the bowel with anesthetic gases that may accidentally be insufflated through the esophagus by the anesthesiologist. Elastic stockings are best applied preoperatively so that patients receive whatever protection they afford during the period of immobility on the operating table. In patients with atheromatous, cerebrovascular, or cardiovascular disease, or active phlebitis, preoperative anticoagulation can be considered, although we have generally avoided it because of the dangers of intraoperative and postoperative bleeding. For patients with phlebitis or a history of pulmonary emboli, plication of the inferior vena cava by application of a DeWeese clip is quick, safe, and effective. The clip application should be done before opening the bowel and walled off with pads before continuing with the colonic procedure. If postoperative anticoagulation is indicated, low doses of heparin are effective in preventing thrombosis and embolism but carry an undetermined risk of bleeding complications that must be considered.[55] Sigmoid resection and operations on the pelvic colon may be facilitated in certain obese patients and patients with retroperitoneal inflammation or neoplasm by the preoperative introduction of ureteral catheters. Though we have not used them, some surgeons rely on them to avoid injury to the ureters.

MEASURES USED AT OPERATION IN PREVENTION OF COMPLICATIONS

Selection of the best incision for colonic operations is a subject that can always be counted upon to excite discussion and differences of opinion among surgeons. Since operations on the colon often require wide mobilization of at least two flexures, an incision capable of easy extension is essential. For this reason in recent years we have preferred the midline incision. The additional advantage of this incision is that the decussating fibers comprising the linea alba constitute a stronger band of tissue than the combined anterior and posterior sheaths used in repairing a paramedian incision. Exceptions are transverse colostomy or resection of the transverse colon, in which transverse incisions are more convenient, and sigmoid resection in the obese patient, in whom an oblique incision may provide considerably better exposure. If possible, old scars should be excised to avoid necrosis between incisions. Colonic or ileal stomas are preferably brought out through auxiliary incisions. Safe conduct of the operation through an adequate incision must be the first concern in colonic surgery. Incisional infection is discouraged by the application of an adherent plastic drape after skin preparation and the insertion of a plastic wound protector as soon as the belly is opened.

After the incision has been made, the peritoneal cavity is explored carefully, and the lesion itself is examined at the last. The liver is palpated with great care. Node-bearing areas along the aorta and elsewhere are likewise examined thoroughly, because the presence of proved metastatic disease in unresectable areas may indicate the performance of a simpler procedure with fewer potential complications. Similarly, the finding of duodenal ulcer, gallstones, hiatus hernia, or other intraperitoneal pathologic changes may provide the surgeon with reason to limit his operation in some way or other. He must weigh the risks and advantages of cholecystectomy or cholecystostomy for removal of gallstones, particularly when a right colectomy is done, or when transverse colostomy is to be performed or is considered a possibility in the postoperative phase. The presence of both kidneys should be verified. The spleen is palpated with great circumspection; numerous diaphragmatic adhesions or a short lienocolic ligament will warn the surgeon that he must be particularly cautious in dissection of the splenic flexure. Finally, the lesion itself is evaluated as thoroughly as possible before undue trauma is inflicted by the opening of tissue planes, which would be undesirable if the surgeon were to decide ultimately that a two- or three-stage operation with preliminary colostomy seemed the safest approach. The strategy of the operation is planned and estimates are made of the length of bowel available for anastomosis and the likely extent of resection necessary. If the operation is for potentially curable malignant disease, the first consideration is a wide excision; on the other hand, one must avoid inadvertent sacrifice of major arterial vessels, as, for example, the superior mesenteric artery, with wide dissection. Hence, blood supply must always be kept in mind.

The procedure itself is conducted with avoidance of contamination or bleeding, and whenever the bowel is opened or appears to be in danger of accidental opening, gauze pads should be used liberally to protect surrounding areas. In the construction of open anastomoses, the surgeon should develop techniques whereby contamination is restricted as much as possible to the tips of his instruments; the first assistant must be aware that suture material is contaminated and that in the process of tying knots or holding the standing end of a running suture his fingertips are also grossly contaminated. Some surgeons always use closed methods of anastomosis; others use them where indicated by poor preparation of the colon. Our preference is for the open method when suturing is used, but in recent years we find that stapling machines offer some advantages in precision, ease, and cleanliness of anastomosing. In low pelvic anastomoses, Goligher has shown, and we agree, that the end-to-end anastomosing stapler can save much time and contamination, with excellent postoperative results.[31] Imperfect anastomoses should be revised completely whenever possible, or at least protected by defunctioning colostomy. Adequacy of colonic blood supply must be verified not only by inspection, but also by observation of arterial bleeding or pulsation at the cut ends of the bowel.

Postoperative hemorrhagic and septic complications will be minimized by accurate dissection in avascular planes with meticulous control of all bleeding points. General lavage of the peritoneum with saline or antibiotic solutions probably distributes bacteria as much as it eliminates them, but irrigation of anastomoses or denuded areas with 0.5 per cent neomycin, kanamycin or povidone-iodine may offer some protection.

The pros and cons of peritoneal drainage are still debated because of the feeling that although a drain in the region of an anastomosis may provide egress for fecal matter if fistulization occurs, the presence of the drain undoubtedly encourages the formation of a fistula. As a rule we do not use drains, but feel that in pelvic anastomoses, removal of accumulating blood and serum by means of small rubber or plastic suction catheters for a period of 24 to 48 hours is safe and beneficial. Mesocolic defects and the traps lateral to colostomy or ileostomy should be closed completely to prevent herniation and obstruction of small bowel loops. The repair of raw surfaces left in the paravertebral gutters after hemicolectomy is controversial, there being increasing evidence that suturing to close these defects actually discourages adhesion-free reperitonealization. Similarly, there has been a resurgence of interest in primary closure of the perineal wound after pelvic colectomy, without repair of the pelvic peritoneum. Intestinal decompression by means of Levin tubes, long tubes, or gastrostomy may be of questionable value in upper intestinal operations, but we believe that some such means or other is vital to the prevention of distention during the period of paralytic ileus that inevitably follows colonic operations. In most cases a Levin tube is the best and entirely adequate solution to the problem, but we use gastrostomy in patients with existing or anticipated pulmonary difficulties and long intestinal tubes in patients with peritonitis or numerous small bowel adhesions, and in those in whom multiple intestinal procedures have been necessary. In such cases we attempt to advance the tube through the full length of small intestine and leave it in place for 5 days to a week postoperatively, because the splinting function of the tube may help to prevent sharp angulation of the bowel and obstructive adhesions. Tubes cannot prevent colonic distention proximal to an anastomosis in the presence of a competent ileocecal valve unless the tip of the tube is actually advanced into the colon. A need for prolonged intestinal suction should be anticipated in patients with malnutrition, diarrhea, peritonitis, obstruction, hypoproteinemia, or hypokalemia. The use of tubes is not without complications, the prevention and treatment of which are discussed in Chapter 20.

In closing the wound, the surgeon must consider the high incidence of infection and dehiscence observed after colonic operations. Collections of blood and serum in wound dead space can set the stage for infection, while dehiscence is caused by inadequate suturing technique or materials. In the preantibiotic era, and in wartime surgery, delayed primary closure was valuable. It was used formerly in many cases at the Massachusetts General Hospital. In recent years, however, most incisions have been closed primarily even in grossly contaminated situations. Colostomy closures provide a case in point. In our personal series there has been no instance of wound or anastomotic complication (infection, dehiscence, fistula, or obstruction) in the last 45 consecutive cases. The technical factors that seem important in reducing the complication rate below the 17 to 30 per cent reported in previous series are avoidance of gross contamination by thorough mechanical preparation of the bowel and meticulous walling-off procedures, perioperative systemic antibiotics, soaking of the wound and anastomosis with 0.5 per cent neomycin solution before closure, musculofascial suture with monofilament polypropylene, a suction catheter to eliminate subcutaneous seroma or hematoma in obese patients, and deep subcuticular closure with polyglycolic acid suture to avoid piercing the heavily contaminated pericolostomy skin.

The same techniques have virtually eliminated wound complications in colonic resections during the past 6 years in which they have been used. In a handful of instances when the abdominal wall was weakened by malnutrition, existing infection, or previous dehiscence, the repair has been done with interrupted all-layer sutures of monofilament wire. The wires are twisted rather than tied so that the tension may be easily adjusted postoperatively as tissue edema occurs and then wanes. The application of povidone-iodine ointment to the skin around these wire sutures can reduce the amount of sepsis, irritation, and necrosis associated with their use.

Closure of wounds around colostomies and ileostomies is most critical at the peritoneal level, where a snug but not tight fit should be provided. This should prove no problem when the stoma is constructed during an operation performed through another laparotomy incision. The difficulties are a little greater when transvere colostomy is done as an independent procedure and greatest when a permanent sigmoid colostomy is brought out through the main incision. With the latter method the risks of herniation, sepsis, and dehiscence are much increased, and we use this technique only when the mesosigmoid is so short that the bowel cannot be brought out laterally.

The question of drainage of wounds rarely arises when anterior fascial stays are used, and delayed primary closure is probably the wiser choice if drainage is seriously considered.

The management of anesthesia and resuscitation must necessarily be assumed by others during operation, and the problems encountered are the subject of Chapter 10. Legally and morally, however, the surgeon shares responsibility; he or she must be constantly aware of any problems that arise and be prepared to offer advice, particularly as regards replacement of blood and plasma.

MANAGEMENT OF OPERATIVE COMPLICATIONS

A certain amount of operative contamination no doubt occurs in every operation upon the colon. Classifiable as a complication, however, is gross contamination by spillage of fecal matter during construction of the anastomosis or accidental perforation during colectomy. Rupture of an unsuspected abscess may lead to wide contamination of the peritoneal cavity with pus. Fecal matter or pus is removed by wiping or aspiration and an attempt is made to control the leak or completely empty the source of contamination by a suction apparatus. The soiled area should be lavaged with antibiotic solution, and broad spectrum antibiotics should be given immediately by the intravenous route. When gross spillage of infected material has occurred, it is probably wisest to drain the area, but care should be taken not to allow the tip of the drain to rest near an anastomosis.

Hemorrhage during operation is usually the result of rough handling of tissues, inclusion of too much tissue in a single ligature for hemostasis, excessive obesity of the patient, or anomalies of the vascular anatomy. Safe control of operative hemorrhage requires adequate exposure and illumination, an effective suction apparatus, and sufficient blood available for transfusion so that the surgeon can confidently and deliberately control the exact bleeding point without resorting to use of mass sutures or ligatures. Bleeding from trauma to the spleen often requires splenectomy, and sufficient exposure should be obtained by extending the incision, if necessary, to assess the damage and to avoid trauma to the pancreas. Conservation of the damaged spleen is frequently possible, so that application of microfibrillar collagen (Avitene), pressure, and suture of a minor tear should be considered before splenectomy. Hemorrhage from the middle colic vessels usually occurs as a result of traction, and it is likely to originate from their junction with the superior mesenteric artery and vein. The only reliable and safe method of control is meticulous suture of the tear with fine cardiovascular suture material. Hemorrhage from the pelvic plexus of veins is perhaps the most common serious bleeding complication encountered at operation. Because of their inaccessible location, attempts to control the bleeding points by clamp or suture are usually inadvisable, and further damage with increased bleeding is often the result. It is better to provide tamponade of the area with a pack, and often, after 5 to 10 minutes, bleeding will have ceased. If not, both hypogastric arteries are ligated at their origin.[38] Even then, it may be necessary to pack the pelvis tightly with gauze that is removed several days later through the perineal wound or through a suprapubic opening left for the purpose.

Operative complications may occur during construction of an anastomosis in the form of inadequate blood supply, subserosal hemorrhage, or excessive tension with tearing of the bowel or cutting of the sutures. The general principle for dealing with this sort of situation is based on the fact that there is always more bowel available for anastomosis; if there is any real question about the integrity of an anastomosis, such further resection as is necessary should be carried out without too much debate. In ileocolic anastomoses there should be no hesitancy whatsoever in resecting the anastomosis and starting over again, because unlimited bowel is available, while the incidence of anastomotic failure and fistula formation is significant, even with this comparatively simple anastomosis. With low pelvic anastomoses further resection may be difficult, so that a transverse colostomy should be performed in all instances in which technical features of the anastomosis have been less satisfactory than is desirable.

MEASURES USED POSTOPERATIVELY IN PROPHYLAXIS OF COMPLICATIONS

Much of the postoperative routine following colonic surgery is directed toward the prevention of complications. After any operation, particularly in the older age group and in patients with a history of pulmonary disease, lung complications are unfortunately common. While the patient is still on the operating table Donaldson[19] massages the patient's legs to move stagnant venous blood and discourage postoperative thrombosis. In the recovery room, while the

patient is still under the effects of anesthesia, prophylaxis of pulmonary complications begins with frequent changes of position of the patient to provide postural drainage, encouragement of deep breathing and coughing, and intermittent positive-pressure breathing by face mask. These maneuvers, designed to prevent the development of atelectasis, are continued throughout the first few days after operation. In difficult cases or when patient cooperation is lacking, pulmonary physical therapists who specialize in these problems are often of great help. If secretions accumulate and atelectasis or pneumonia develops in spite of attempts to avoid them, tracheostomy must be considered for the purpose of keeping the airway clear. Antibiotics should be used in high-risk patients, and nasogastric tubes are to be avoided in such patients if the surgeon feels that gastrostomy will suffice.

Urinary tract infection and obstruction are avoided by catheter drainage in pelvic operations, and urinary antiseptics or antibiotics should always be used in patients who have indwelling catheters. Bladder catheters should be irrigated several times a day, but the most effective form of irrigation is an adequate urinary output, which is related directly to adequacy of parenteral fluid intake.

Myocardial infarction remains a significant factor in the over-all mortality rate after colon resection (Fig. 25–1). Although a certain incidence of coronary occlusion is to be expected in this age group, it seems clear that the effect can be minimized by avoidance of hypotension and maintenance of the blood volume and state of hydration. Measurements of urinary output, hematocrit value, and central venous pressure provide valuable indices for the adequate replacement of volume losses, and central venous pressure measurements in particular help in avoiding overreplacement and resultant congestive failure.

The prevention of intestinal distention is an important part of postoperative prophylaxis. The use of intestinal tubes for decompression has been mentioned already. Tube decompression should be continued until intestinal function has resumed, and we feel that it is better to leave a tube in a day too long rather than to remove it a day too soon.

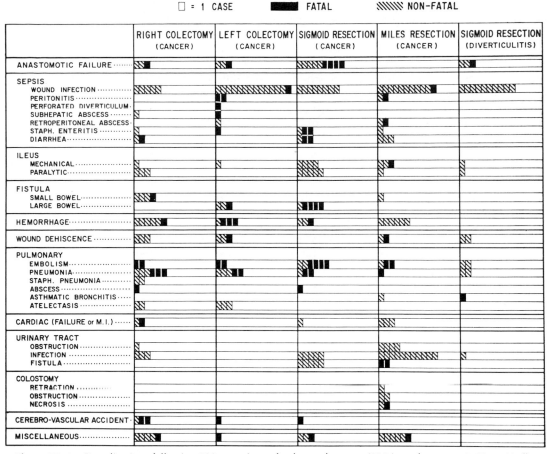

Figure 25–1 Complications following 500 resections of colon and rectum (100 in each category). (From Hedberg, S. E., and Welch, C. E.: Complications following surgery of the colon. Surg. Clin. North Am. *43*:775, 1963.)

Often when there is any question, the tube can be left in place while suction is discontinued. Gravity drainage and siphonage prevent gastric retention but allow passage of intestinal juices if function is adequate for this to occur. Once the tube is finally removed, caution is still in order, and advancement of diet must be done gradually over a space of several days to a week. Patients are kept on a low-roughage diet for about 2 months.

Thromboembolic disease is another serious and common complication following surgery of the colon. Causal factors are not well understood, but postoperative hypercoagulability of blood and muscular inactivity with pooling of blood and sludging in the deep veins of the lower extremities seem to be important. Prevention of phlebothrombosis in every case is, of course, im-

possible, but various measures are used to improve venous circulation and discourage hypercoagulability. Early ambulation, leg exercises, the use of elastic stockings, and avoidance of abdominal binders and of tight bed covers are routine measures. The value of prophylactic anticoagulation with warfarin (Coumadin) or heparin has been proved by Salzman et al.[50] in our hospital in controlled clinical studies, but, because of the potential dangers, we have preferred not to use anticoagulation except in high-risk patients. Formerly, ligation of the superficial femoral veins was done frequently as prophylaxis, but now we would interrupt veins only in very high-risk patients, or patients who have shown signs of deep thrombophlebitis. When embolization has occurred, femoral veins are tied if signs of phlebitis are present. If not, or if the iliac vein is involved, we prefer to treat with ligation or plication of the inferior vena cava, or percutaneous insertion of a caval umbrella.

We use antibiotics prophylactically whenever it is anticipated that the intestine will be opened at surgery. Antibiotics are most effective in preventing postoperative sepsis if they are begun preoperatively. We usually give 1 gm. of cefazolin or cephaloridine intramuscularly before operation, followed by cephazolin intravenously for 2 to 5 days. Alternatively, cefoxitin or combinations of clindamycin and gentamicin, or penicillin with chloramphenicol may be used perioperatively. The known hazards of staphylococcal enteritis, emergence of resistant strains of bacteria in the wound and elsewhere, and overgrowth of monilia and other yeasts must be watched for when antibiotics are used prophylactically.

Pseudomembranous enterocolitis is an important complication that may follow the administration of broad spectrum antibiotics. Ampicillin, Bactrim, and clindamycin, as well as other aminoglycosides, are the most common offenders; since they are used frequently for colonic diseases, or in combination with operative procedures on the colon, careful attention must be paid to all patients who receive these drugs.

The cause of the enterocolitis is believed to be toxin produced by the anaerobe, *Clostridium difficile*. Clostridial growth in the colon is promoted by the elimination of aerobic organisms by antibiotics. Symptoms vary from mild diarrhea to widespread ulceration, shock, and toxic megacolon. Fortunately severe involvement has usually been in the colon rather than the small intestine, so that in severe cases emergency colectomy has been a lifesaving procedure.

The accepted treatment at this time for all cases is the omission of broad spectrum antibiotics that have little or no influence on clostridia, and the administration of specific antibiotics. Vancomycin by mouth is not absorbed from the gastrointestinal tract; Schapira and Dyson advise a 5-day course of 125 mg. of vancomycin every 6 hours, although the manufacturer advises a daily dose of 2 gm. for 5 days.[51] Metronidazole is also effective against *Clostridium difficile* but is absorbed readily through the small intestine and does not reach the colon in sufficient concentration.

MANAGEMENT OF POSTOPERATIVE COMPLICATIONS COMMON TO ALL COLONIC OPERATIONS

A logical discussion of postoperative complications requires a dissection of factors often present in combination, but four main types of complications are apparent without artificial division. They are sepsis, ileus, hemorrhage and fistula. The diagnosis and operative, non-operative, and postoperative treatment of each will be described in turn.

SEPSIS

Sepsis may be manifest as peritonitis, either local or generalized, staphylococcal enterocolitis, septicemia, abscesses in the wound or internally, phlegmons, or other enteric infections such as salmonellosis. Diagnosis may be difficult but is of prime importance in distinguishing surgical from non-surgical infections. Conservative treatment deserves great emphasis, but, depending on the cause and nature of the infection, may have to be supplemented by surgical drainage, bypass, or other procedure.

DIAGNOSIS

In diagnosing postoperative infections, the operative notes and recollections upon unusual features of the operation may be valuable clues. Anatomic anomalies, excessive bleeding in certain locations, raw areas uncovered by peritoneum, anastomotic difficulties, and poorly prepared or distended bowel may help direct the surgeon's suspicions when signs suggestive of sepsis appear. Historic features of poor resistance to infection such as malnutrition or diabetes may make the surgeon particularly wary.

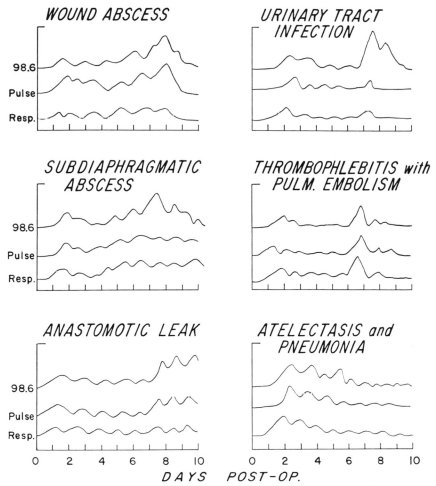

Figure 25–2 Diagrammatic representations of clinical charts. Differential elevations of temperature, pulse, and respiration typically occur at certain stages in the postoperative course. Pulse and temperature build up gradually in wound infection until drainage occurs. In urinary tract infection temperature elevation is out of proportion to rise in pulse and respiratory rate. Subdiaphragmatic abscess resembles wound infection, but with greater increase in respiratory rate. "Allen's sign" is typical of thrombophlebitis. Anastomotic leak often occurs on the seventh or eighth postoperative day after a benign course. Atelectasis and pneumonia, with elevations of all parameters, begin soon after operation and gradually respond to antibiotics and physical therapy.

Chief among the symptoms of infection is pain, but the pain of peritonitis, abscess, or phlegmon is difficult to distinguish from incisional pain in many cases. Incisional pain, however, should decrease daily except in patients with wound infection, in which unusually severe pain may begin within the first few hours after operation. Localized pain may develop in an abscess or near the site of anastomotic leakage, but little if any pain is characteristic of subdiaphragmatic abscess. An exception, of course, is the classic referral of diaphragmatic pain to the shoulder. Nausea and hiccuping may be present as signs of paralytic ileus secondary to sepsis anywhere within or near the peritoneal cavity, but especially in subdiaphragmatic abscesses. Chills are most likely with the spiking fever characteristic of urinary tract infection, or in the periodic bacteremias that accompany abscess formation (Fig. 25–2). Malaise, depression, and a querulous reaction are important neurologic symptoms, and, in the advanced age groups, confusion and even toxic psychosis are common. Because of the great differences that exist in the reactions of patients to operation, more important than absolute subjective sensations is a change for the worse. Particularly difficult are neurotic or overreactive patients, who must be carefully watched because of the unconscious defenses stimulated in the surgeon by the ungrateful reaction of the patient to operation.

Though it is natural for the surgeon to think first of possible technical errors and complications when pain and other symptoms appear, he or she should not overlook the fact that the pain of cardiac and pulmonary disease can often be referred to the abdomen and may mimic peritonitis or other intraperitoneal lesions. Lower lobar pneumonia is notorious for causing abdominal pain and paralytic ileus, and the authors have seen myocardial infarction produce signs and symptoms almost indistinguishable from those of appendicitis.

The signs of sepsis are often marked first by tachycardia with a vague appearance of agitation or distress. The degree of fever and the nature of the fever chart are unreliable in the very young and very old, but are still of especial interest because certain patterns are characteristic or almost diagnostic (Fig. 25–2). Gram-negative septicemia may produce hypothermia, bradycardia, and hypotension. Tachypnea is prominent in pulmonary sepsis, subdiaphragmatic abscess, and, of course, pulmonary embolism, either septic or bland. Abdominal distention without tympany in the presence of a functioning decompressive tube suggests fluid accumulation in bowel (enteritis) or peritoneum (leak or abscess). Tenderness may be difficult to evaluate because of incisional pain, but routine examination, daily or twice daily, renders changes more obvious. Some guarding is to be expected, but it should be minimal within 48 to 72 hours. Peristaltic sounds are usually rare for 2 to 4 days after operation, and the time of their resumption can demand no great attention because it is so variable. Disappearance of bowel sounds after postoperative resumption of peristalsis, however, is extremely important.

The surgical wound must be considered the most likely source of sepsis. A wound infection, however, may occasionally be the first presentation of intraperitoneal abscess and may be the sign of a favorable outcome if drainage is adequate. Another very common source that must be excluded immediately in sepsis is an intravenous catheter. With the occurrence of septicemia all such inlying tubes must be removed and cultured, and replaced if necessary in a different location.

Laboratory signs suggesting sepsis should be investigated thoroughly. A white blood cell count in the first few days after operation can be valuable for later comparison, and a stained smear of the peripheral blood may show a further shift toward immature polymorphonuclear forms. Drainage from the abdominal wound, posterior wound, or drain tracts should be cultured and antibiotic sensitivity tests done. One should not overlook anaerobic cultures; clostridia and bacteroides produce deadly infections and can be diagnosed only by growing the organisms anaerobically. Stained smears and cultures of stool and gastric aspirate can lead to an early diagnosis of staphylococcal enteritis. Bilirubinemia and anemia often accompany the hemolysis of sepsis, but hemoconcentration is more usual. With loss of plasma into the area of infection, the hematocrit level rises and urinary output falls with a coincident rise in specific gravity. Radiographs of the chest and abdomen should be obtained. There is a tendency to use portable equipment so that sick patients will not have to be moved excessively; more useful films, however, are obtained with the larger equipment in the radiology department, and the difference is usually worth the inconvenience and discomfort to the patient. Chest films may show pneumonia or atelectasis and interstitial edema above the diaphragm over an abscess. There may be a slight pleural effusion on the side of a subdiaphragmatic abscess. Upright films of the abdomen almost always show free peritoneal air, which is apt to persist for a week or two after operation, so that this finding is not diagnostic of perforation unless the quantity of air is excessive (Fig. 25–3). Fluid levels seen in gas-containing loops of bowel usually indicate the presence of ileus, which may be either paralytic or mechanical when secondary to abscess or peritonitis. A hazy ground-glass appearance indicates the presence of large amounts of peritoneal fluid. A mass may be detectable on the abdominal film, and the presence of an air-fluid level within the mass strongly suggests an abscess. Often, abnormalities not noticed on a single

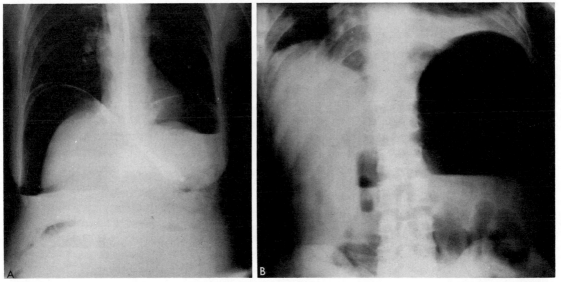

Figure 25–3 *A,* Massive intraperitoneal accumulation of fluid and air may occur rapidly after anastomotic failure or, as in this case, perforation of an obstructing carcinoma. Displacement of the liver away from the right diaphragm and the air-fluid level are clearly seen. *B,* This accumulation of air and fluid beneath a thickened left diaphragm 1 week after sigmoid resection was at first interpreted as gastric dilatation. A nasogastric tube, however, showed the stomach to be collapsed, and this large subdiaphragmatic abscess was then successfully drained. Fluid in the pleural space obscuring the left costophrenic angle remains sterile until diaphragmatic perforation becomes imminent.

radiologic examination will be apparent on comparison with earlier or subsequent films, so that films should be obtained every day or two in difficult cases.

The aphorism, "Pus somewhere; pus nowhere; pus under the diaphragm," does not always hold. It is exceedingly difficult at times to find the abscess that clinical signs indicate must be there. The patient appears too sick to withstand further septicemia, yet too weak to withstand general exploration, lysis of adhesions, and blood loss in the search for a collection of pus whose position is not known. It may be reasoned that if the abscess could be found and drained, the patient would rally and could survive; but if no pus were found then matters would be made worse by the fruitless surgery. This line of thinking is further supported by the fact that the surgical approach to a known abscess is usually direct, may not open free peritoneal or pleural spaces, and represents minimal trauma compared to drainage of the same abscess found during exploratory laparotomy. For these reasons preoperative localization of a septic focus has come to occupy much surgical attention now that radiographic capability extends well beyond

the traditional plain x-ray films. Unless the location of an abscess is known on the basis of clinical signs, it is usually worth the time and expense to use every available means to find it preoperatively. These methods presently include ultrasonography, computed body tomography, and radionuclide scans of liver, lung, spleen, and bone. Radioactive gallium can sometimes be persuaded to concentrate in an abscess wall, although our experience with gallium scans to date has been disappointing. Barium or Gastrografin swallowed or injected into the intestine or into sinus tracts may help visualize a space-occupying lesion, a communication with a collection, or a leaky anastomosis. In a few cases angiography can localize the hyperemic vascular pattern surrounding a localized infection not found by less invasive methods. Recurrent bacteremia of unknown source always raises the question of cardiac valvular origin; even in the absence of a new murmur this unusual cause can now be excluded non-invasively with cardiac ultrasonography. Spectacular as may be the results of some of these newer diagnostic methods, they are not infallible, and a negative result cannot be accepted as meaning no focus. A second examination with the same technique a few days later may show that what was a borderline finding has now become diagnostic.

The thread running through the entire discussion on diagnosis of complications is that absolute observations are much less valuable than changes from hour to hour or day to day. Frequent postoperative examination of patients is therefore indispensable if complications such as sepsis are to be discovered early and treated promptly. The need for surgery is determined by the nature of the septic process and its cause, but exact differential diagnosis of these factors is often impossible.

NON-OPERATIVE TREATMENT

In enterocolitis, gram-negative septicemia, certain forms of peritonitis, occasional abscesses, and phlegmon, and frequently in infections of unknown origin, nonoperative treatment is all that is needed or possible. Every effort should be made to determine the source of infection, since this diagnosis is one of the bases on which the timing of surgery is decided. Non-operative measures are used in the treatment of almost every case, not only in preparation for operation, but also because the differential diagnosis of the infection may become apparent during the time allotted for preoperative treatment. Furthermore, the response to treatment may suggest the diagnosis as well as indicating the need for operation.

Of first importance is maintenance or restoration of blood volume, red cell mass, and blood electrolyte composition that may be deranged by the fluid losses and hemolysis of infection. Staphylococcal enteritis is probably the most difficult to handle in this regard because losses of fluid may reach as high as 16 liters a day, as recorded in one of the cases reported by Speare.[54] Peritonitis and other infections, however, can produce large losses that should be replaced primarily by albumin or plasma. Arterial and venous blood pressures, changes in urinary output, and serial determinations of the hematocrit value are the guidelines for therapy with plasma, blood, and electrolyte solutions.

Paralytic ileus and intestinal distention secondary to infection must be avoided or corrected lest mechanical obstruction by kinking of the bowel be superimposed. At the first sign of ileus, oral intake is discontinued and nasogastric suction begun. Suction should then be carried on until the intestinal tract is functioning normally, even though the septic process may appear to have become localized or otherwise brought under control.

The use of specific antibiotic drugs is discussed in Chapter 1, but in general, broad spectrum drugs or combinations should be used in treating the infections that follow colonic surgery. Penicillin and chloramphenicol are a useful combination, as are clindamycin and gentamicin or tobramycin. These drugs or a cephalosporin alone is used in prophylaxis by surgeons who routinely use antibiotics after operation; they should also be given if pulmonary infection is suspected or if it is not known whether the infection is gram-positive or gram-negative, at least until specific sensitivities of the offending organism are available. Most infections after colonic surgery, including the common urinary complications, are caused by gram-negative bacteria, and treatment should anticipate this finding on culture, except in the case of enteritis, in which antibiotics primarily active against the staphylococci should be given. The combination usually used in these cases is erythromycin and chloramphenicol, which are effective against most staphylococci, and also for salmonellosis and other enteritides. Penicillinase-resistant penicillins are also useful in staphylococcal infections, especially when chloramphenicol may have been etiologic in the infection. If tetanus or other clostridial infections are considered possible, massive doses of penicillin should be given; in very high doses, this antibiotic also is effective against gram-negative organisms, although gentamicin is now frequently the drug of choice. Bacteroides infections, which seem to be increasingly common as anaerobic cultures are done more often, are usually sensitive to tetracycline, and clindamycin is almost always effective against bacteroides of bowel origin. Cefoxitin is effective against a broad variety of gram-negative and gram-positive organisms and has good activity against many anaerobes as well.

The antibiotic to be used should be given

intravenously for most rapid effect, and, of course, the intravenous route is the only reliable one in hypotensive patients. In gram-negative septicemia with shock, cephalosporin and gentamicin are a potent combination; if bacteroides is also suspect, chloramphenicol is added as a third drug, and may be continued if cultures show pseudomonas or proteus. Antibiotics, unfortunately, can seldom be given orally to these patients, though bacitracin, kanamycin, and nystatin are the best drugs to use orally in staphylococcal enteritis and monilial infections. Antibiotics given intravenously should be well diluted to avoid chemical phlebitis and excessive destruction of veins; subclavian vein catheterization allows prolonged antibiotic administration but must be used with caution to avoid the complications of central venous cannulation. Material from pulmonary or enteric staphylococcal infections should be recultured every 5 to 7 days to detect changes in flora and antibiotic sensitivity, which are apt to occur in patients under antibiotic treatment.

In spite of 30 years' experience, the place of steroids is still not established even in the treatment of bacteremic shock, in which these compounds do have at least temporary benefits. The over-all effect of these drugs is understood even less in other infections such as generalized peritonitis, in which steroid treatment has the theoretic advantage of decreasing the rate of adhesion and perhaps thereby discouraging loculation and abscess formation. The lack of information on this subject is due to the great difficulty of setting up controlled studies in desperate clinical situations. We have tended to use steroids in massive doses for bacteremic shock in patients whose condition seems otherwise hopeless because of overwhelming peritonitis or peritoneal contamination. A short course of massive therapy seems most effective and is not supposed to produce adrenal suppression. Most surgeons nowadays doubt the value of steroids in septic shock, but sometimes it appears that the glucocorticoid exerts a permissive effect upon the action of pressor amines. Dexamethasone is a glucocorticoid approximately 35 times as potent as cortisone, and it has been used in doses up to 80 mg. a day for short periods in life-threatening peritonitis or gram-negative septicemia.

When hypotension is persistent in spite of the treatment suggested here, the use of pressor amines must be considered. The indications for their use are few because the effects on intestinal and renal circulation may be disastrous. We have seen several cases of intestinal perforation due to focal areas of gangrene that resulted from the intense vasoconstriction caused by pressor amines. Nevertheless, in certain situations, dopamine, norepinephrine, isoproterenol, or metaraminol may be lifesaving when they maintain circulation in an emergency until more specific treatments have had a chance to have their effect.

The effect of hyperbaric oxygen in gas gangrene is well known. Exploration of the use of high-pressure oxygen in bacteremic shock has been encouraging and suggests that oxygen may be valuable treatment not only in anaerobic and microaerophilic infections, but also with aerobic bacteria.

The non-operative treatment of sepsis is generally administered in graduated doses, according to the severity of the disease. The use of these measures does not preclude surgery and may actually make operation safer.

OPERATIVE TREATMENT

The indications for operation in the treatment of postoperative sepsis are generally determined by the cause of the infection. If an early diagnosis can be made, free anastomotic leak, rupture of an abscess or diverticulum, strangulation obstruction, or ischemic necrosis demands operation as soon as the condition of the patient permits. Any source of continuing intraperitoneal contamination must be controlled. Obviously the diagnosis often cannot be made preoperatively, and laparotomy for diagnosis must frequently be considered. In the absence of a diagnosis as to causation, the indication for surgery may be stated simply as inadequate response to non-operative treatment. A pitfall, however, lies in the seemingly adequate response in surgical sepsis, when failure to recognize that improvement is only temporary may result in loss of the best opportunity for intervention. If the diagnosis is made early, then treatment can be almost immediate and conduct of the operation is little different from the handling of intraoperative contamination. If sepsis is well advanced and the condition of the patient has deteriorated, however, the risks of surgery are great unless the patient is prepared adequately by intensive non-operative treatment already outlined.

If infection is mild or remains localized, the need for operation is not pressing, and one can afford to wait in the hope that non-operative treatment will be sufficient or that localized sepsis will drain through the abdominal incision or back into the bowel. Most intraperitoneal abscesses, except those in the pelvis or subdiaphragmatic space, will eventually drain through the laparotomy incision. Drainage into the bowel is usually a vain hope except when proximal decompression has been provided. In less severe cases in which infection is localized and continuing contamination slow or doubtful, the need for operation may be uncertain, and preparation for operation consists really of a trial of non-operative therapy. Under these conditions the patient remains in generally good or improving condition, and preparation may be considered complete when it is decided that the local situation has not responded or will not respond further.

Recent interest in needle or catheter aspiration of relatively stable abscesses has followed the improved ability to locate and follow these lesions by means of ultrasonography or computed body tomography. In some cases needle aspiration for positive diagnosis and culture has resulted in complete evacuation and cure of the abscess; in other cases, repeated aspirations by needle or implanted catheter have not resulted in resolution of the abscess, and surgery has been delayed at considerable expense. Our present perception is that the procedure may have merit in certain cases, but until the indications are defined more precisely this method should be used only on patients who are under direct surgical control. The decision of when to aspirate or when to operate should be made by the surgeon, not the radiologist or internist.

In severe cases with massive contamination, widespread infection, or overwhelming systemic effects, the need for operation may be clear, but the condition of the patient too parlous to risk it. Here vigorous treatment with nasogastric suction, blood, plasma, water, salt, oxygen, antibiotics, and

hypothermia may improve matters sufficiently so that proximal decompression may be considered. Stable vital signs, defervescence, and satisfactory production of urine are important before such an operation is undertaken. Improvement in these patients may last only a few hours, and the patient must be observed closely lest the only chance for operation escape. Almost always, homeostasis can be artificially restored in this manner *once*, but a second deterioration usually means that the basic process and attendant shock have progressed to irreversibility.

Postoperative sepsis usually originates at the site of the primary operation, but operative treatment may require maneuvers in various parts of the abdomen. Even when simple drainage only is required, the advantages of a good exploration may be considerable or even lifesaving, as when unsuspected leak and obstruction may coexist. Adequate incision is therefore essential with drainage or colostomy planned through separate incisions after exploration.

The earlier the reoperation, the less extensive it need be, perhaps involving only closure of a perforation, local débridement, and proximal colostomy. Later cases may be jeopardized by too extensive dissection with lysis of established, protective fibrinous barriers. In advanced disease, however, it may be necessary to carry out complete refunctionalization of the intestine from the ligament of Treitz to the pelvic floor, with lysis of all adhesions, drainage of abscesses, decompression by enterotomy and suction, splinting of small gut by advancement of a long tube, resection of badly damaged gut, and/or proximal colostomy.[62]

Few universal rules can be formulated, but, in general, operation for sepsis secondary to a low anastomotic failure should always include proximal colostomy. Exteriorization of the anastomosis is a method that may be used higher in the colon, as after ileocolostomy. Irrigation with antibiotics may be of value in early cases, but when fibrin has begun to organize, irrigation will be of little use. Irrigation should be done to remove fecal material, barium, food, or other debris. Solutions of saline, 0.5 per cent neomycin or kanamycin, or povidone-iodine may be used. If the peritoneum is acutely inflamed, iodine may be absorbed in concentrations toxic to the kidneys, while the antibiotics may produce respiratory depression. Saline is undoubtedly safer for the copious part of the irrigation, perhaps finishing with a measured quantity of one of the antibacterial solutions. The temperature of the irrigant should be physiologic or cold, depending upon whether it is desired to lower the febrile patient's body temperature.

In closure of the infected wound, delayed primary closure should be considered, and buried non-absorbable suture material avoided. Single-layer closure with closely spaced sutures of No. 24 stainless steel wire is practically failure proof, and very quick. These heavy wires should be twisted rather than tied so that they can be loosened by untwisting if necessary. Closure of the wound that has been contaminated by pus found within the belly can usually be done successfully using continuous No. 0 polypropylene to fascia after soaking the wound with neomycin solution. We prefer subcutaneous and subcuticular closure with polyglycolic acid over delayed primary closure in this situation. If drains are to be used they should not be brought through a wound closed in this manner, although drainage through a wound closed with all-layer wire is acceptable. Drains are used in areas from which pus has been removed, but drainage of "peritonitis" may be extremely hazardous because of the chance of causing small intestinal adhesions, angulation, and stricture. Drainage of the free peritoneal cavity is rarely beneficial because the drain becomes quickly walled off by intestinal and omental agglutination, and the material drained is usually only that stimulated by the presence of the drain itself.[9]

In addition to colostomy and cecostomy for decompression, the other ancillary operation to be considered in peritonitis is that of tracheostomy, which should be done in patients who have required ventilatory support via endotracheal tube preoperatively. Patients with generalized peritonitis have a restricted vital capacity and tidal volume because of pain, diaphragmatic paralysis, and abdominal distention. As a result the accessory muscles of breathing and the intercostal muscles are exploited to a greater degree than the diaphragm, and this change involves a decrease in breathing

efficiency with an increase in work done per unit volume of oxygen inspired. At the same time the effects of infection and fever increase the oxygen requirement still further, so that despite adequate exchange at the alveolar-capillary level, these patients, if left to their own respiratory devices, may be unable to absorb an amount of oxygen equal to their needs. When this occurs, arterial oxygen saturation falls, respiratory rate rises, the work of breathing increases, effective dead space increases, and a vicious cycle is instituted that has been termed high-output respiratory failure.[12]

The term is a useful one, calling attention as it does to the parallel situation in high-output cardiac failure, in which the myocardium fails in spite or because of increased cardiac output. The respiratory problem has been studied extensively in the respiratory unit at the Massachusetts General Hospital, where many patients who would otherwise have died of "peritonitis" have been saved by the use of intermittent positive-pressure ventilation via an endotracheal tube, which is almost always left in place for at least several hours or days after operation (Fig. 25–4). If there is doubt as to the need for assisted ventilation, serial studies of arterial oxygen tension and oxygen saturation may be used as guides. An increase in respiratory rate accompanied by a decrease in oxygen values constitutes our indication for assistance. The care of patients on respirators is a specialized subject in itself and is attended by numerous complications, which are beyond the scope of this chapter. From the point of view of conduct of the operation in postoperative sepsis, however, the principal complication seems to be the increased strain placed on the abdominal wound by the mechanical respirator, with an increased incidence of wound dehiscence unless the strongest techniques of closure have been used.

Wound abscess may, in many cases, represent the spontaneous resolution of anastomotic leak and intraperitoneal abscess. Traditional treatment involves the wide opening of skin and subcutaneous tissues with gauze packing and secondary closure. We find, however, that in most cases limited drainage between one or two pairs of retention sutures is adequate. This method has the advantages of preserving wound

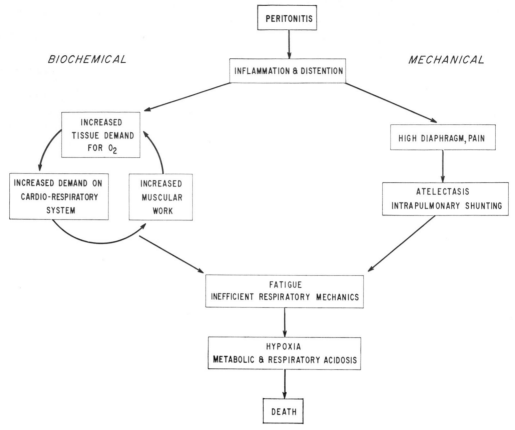

Figure 25–4 This figure depicts the causal relations that Burke[12] has termed "high-output failure." For mechanical and biochemical reasons peritonitis may lead to death through respiratory insufficiency. Both mechanisms are often correctable by means of artificial ventilation with a mechanical respirator.

strength, shortening convalescence, and lessening the psychologic trauma to the patient. The necessity for wider drainage is manifest by failure to respond to conservative drainage. Prolonged drainage may indicate the presence of a fistula.

POSTOPERATIVE MANAGEMENT

In the postoperative phase following exploration for sepsis, complications tend to be multiple. These patients may run the entire gamut of cardiac, respiratory, neurologic, renal, and circulatory problems. With frequent observation and recording of vital data by special nurses and frequent visits of physicians, each setback may be met as it appears, and a large percentage of these patients can be saved. In a very large series the mortality rate after resection of the colon for carcinoma was around 6 per cent and for diverticulitis, about 2 per cent.[64] These relatively high figures, however, seem low when compared with the much higher incidence of serious postoperative complications, most of which obviously have been detected early and treated successfully.

ILEUS

A universal sequel of colonic surgery, paralytic ileus usually lasts 3 to 4 days, if the passage of flatus is accepted as a valid indicator of the termination of this phase. This 3- to 4-day figure is an average, however, and ileus without definable pathologic implication rarely may last for as much as 2 weeks. Although the differential diagnosis between paralytic and mechanical ileus may be easy, at times it is nearly impossible. Treatment for either type can be operative or non-operative, although mechanical ileus usually requires operative correction. The origin of postoperative ileus, like sepsis, may involve several factors, and prevention is at least as important as treatment from the over-all point of view of lowering mortality rate.

DIAGNOSIS

Differentiation between paralytic and mechanical ileus is important in the rare instance in which distention is minimal or controlled by tubal decompression, because persistent mechanical factors demand operative correction. Clues to differential diagnosis may be found in history, physical examination, laboratory data, and radiographic findings. The final diagnostic tool, however, and the only infallible one is exploratory laparotomy.

In many patients there will be particular details of the past history or of the colonic operation that suggest an increased risk of paralytic ileus, such as malnutrition, peritonitis, wide areas of retroperitoneal dissection, the necessity for prolonged retraction on small intestine, and so forth. In others the presence of numerous adhesions, a weak peritoneal floor, or inability to close a paracolostomy or para-ileostomy trap may forewarn the surgeon of an increased danger of postoperative mechanical obstruction. The signs and symptoms of ileus are those of fullness, nausea, vomiting, obstipation, abdominal pain, and distention. Frequently the patient's course appears to run normally, with passage of flatus at the expected time, only to have obstructive symptoms appear after removal of a decompressive tube or resumption of oral intake. The surgeon must be unusually wary in colonic operations because large amounts of fluid and air can collect in the small bowel before symptoms or much distention appears. Discontinuance of suction and advancement of diet in stages are again emphasized. In a relaxed abdomen the first sign of trouble may be the appearance of a visible or palpable loop of distended, nontender small bowel. Percussion of tympanitic areas and flank dullness may be of little use except when shifting dullness can indicate the presence of intraperitoneal as opposed to intraluminal fluid. Auscultation of bowel sounds is most important. According to careful study, sounds of activity never disappear completely after operation, but for 1 or 2 days frequency is so decreased that sounds are seldom heard during the space of several minutes. Continued diminished activity may indicate paralytic ileus on a metabolic or traumatic basis, while loss of activity previously present suggests a septic or vascular complication. Active peristalsis in the presence of obstipation or cramps, a classic sign of mechanical ileus, also occurs regularly with return of function after operation. The rapid appearance of dehydration or distention is a general sign often found in mechanical ileus. Postoperative pain and fever are unreliable signs, but the vague, mild tenderness of distended gut in their absence may be characteristic.

Increased returns from gastric suction and decreased urinary output are signs that accompany obstruction and loss of fluid into the gut. Rapid change of mental status, depression, and a vague (but well communicated) sense of uneasiness may be due to coincident electrolyte shifts.

Leukocytosis may be due simply to hemoconcentration or may indicate accompanying or etiologic sepsis. Differentiation by changes in hematocrit level is sometimes possible; the hematocrit value may fall in sepsis, but will rise in dehydration. Blood smears may show a shift to the left if leukocytosis is real, as in sepsis, whereas the shift is usually absent in the leukocytosis of hemoconcentration. Serum amylase values above normal are found in intestinal obstruction, while ileus, of course, may be due to postoperative pancreatitis. Serum electrolyte concentrations are helpful in suggesting possible metabolic causes of paralytic ileus, whereas a large serum protein deficiency as seen in malnutrition or loss of plasma-rich fluid into the peritoneal cavity is strongly suggestive of paralytic ileus.

When ileus is first suspected, the stomach should be emptied by a nasogastric tube and roentgenograms obtained. Distended loops of small bowel with fluid levels of differing height on plain and upright films suggest mechanical ileus, especially if only a few loops are visible. Numerous loops of moder-

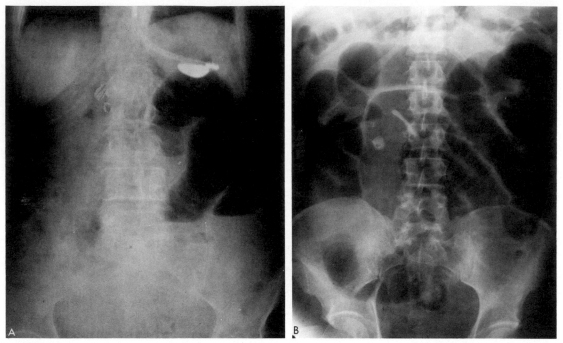

Figure 25–5 *A,* Mechanical small bowel obstruction following colonic operations is too frequently discovered much later than in this case, in which only two distended jejunal loops attest to the need for early exploration. The relative absence of gas elsewhere in the bowel makes interpretation of this plate simpler than usual, because the scattered loops seen in postoperative paralytic ileus often confuse the picture. *B,* This plate is fairly typical of paralytic ileus with numerous loops of small intestine more or less uniformly distended with gas. There is gas present in nondistended colon. This patient's bowel finally resumed function about 2 weeks later, having responded gradually to intubation with a Harris tube.

ately distended small and large bowel containing fluid at the same level are more suggestive of paralytic ileus (Fig. 25–5). Prolapse of a single loop through a trap, mesenteric defect, or peritoneal floor usually causes closed-loop obstruction, and diagnosis by roentgenography is infrequent, because gas in the loop is often absent. The diagnosis of ileus, although not always easy, is easier than the differentiation between mechanical and paralytic ileus. Observation of the clinical course may be the only practical method of differentiation.

NON-OPERATIVE TREATMENT

Because it is impossible in the majority of cases to differentiate between mechanical and paralytic ileus immediately, and because even mechanical obstruction occasionally yields to non-operative treatment, conservative therapy is almost always given a trial first.

Decompression is the first step in treat-

ment and precedes even diagnostic tests. A nasogastric tube usually suffices in early cases when distention is not great, and prevention of further accumulation may be all that is necessary. If the diagnosis is made late, however, long intestinal tube suction should be used. Long intestinal tubes require constant attention, beginning with careful positioning under fluoroscopic guidance. Plain abdominal films are required daily or more frequently to record the progress of the tube and evaluate resolution of distention. The tube must be irrigated frequently to assure its patency, and once it has started into the duodenum it should be advanced a small distance at frequent intervals. Often Harris or Miller-Abbott tubes progress no farther than the ligament of Treitz, and holdup at this level can cause obstruction of the bowel with the air- or mercury-containing bag. In this case, if the tube is functioning, large amounts of drainage will be returned, but no distal decompression will occur. If the tube becomes plugged, however, the rapid onset of vomiting is likely. Occasionally it may be necessary to decompress the stomach with a Levin tube during passage of a long intestinal tube. Sometimes long intestinal tubes are of value in paralytic ileus, but the passage of the tube through the intestine signifies that paralysis is by no means complete.

If gas is visible by x-ray in the colon, and especially if there is colonic distention, passage of a colonoscope can be diagnostic as well as therapeutic. In one instance a transverse colostomy planned for later in the day was avoided by evacuating the colon endoscopically in a case of stubborn postoperative distention. In several other cases anastomotic edema or synechia has been corrected by colonoscopic manipulation or dilatation. These maneuvers should be attempted only by a very experienced colonoscopist because the danger of complication is considerable, although complication has not yet occurred in our experience.

Fluid that is lost into the gut, whether returned by suction or as vomitus, must be replaced by normal saline as accurately as can be estimated. Potassium ion is also lost in variable amounts, and the serum potassium concentration should be maintained at normal by intravenous replacement. Determination of the potassium content of intestinal drainage may be helpful if the quantity of drainage is large or if suction is to be prolonged for a few days. Hypoproteinemia should be corrected by infusion of plasma or albumin. If the patient is already depleted or if resolution does not occur within a day or so, preparation should be made for total parenteral nutrition with installation of a subclavian vein catheter. Vitamin deficiency is of questionable importance in paralytic ileus, but replacement of pantothenic acid and other vitamins should do no harm.

The stimulation of peristalsis in paralytic ileus is a subject of great interest and importance, but little is known about it and few practices are consistently reliable. Warm packs applied to the abdomen provide a comfort, but peristalsis is better stimulated by the application of cold compresses. Urethane, bethanechol (Urecholine), metoclopramide and vasopression have been used to induce peristalsis, but their effectiveness is questionable. Furthermore, it may be unwise to increase bowel activity if mechanical obstruction is suspected.

OPERATIVE TREATMENT

Mechanical obstruction may be caused by distention and angulation secondary to paralytic ileus, adhesions, abscess, internal herniation through traps or the peritoneal floor, volvulus around a colostomy or ileostomy, anastomotic stricture, edema, and so forth. Except in closed-loop or strangulation obstruction, there is a chance of resolution through non-operative treatment. On the other hand, the earlier operation is done, the better is the chance to cure the patient. After 7 to 10 days of obstruction the bowel becomes edematous and difficult to handle. Seven to 10 days might be an average duration for a trial of conservative treatment in a very favorable case. It would be less if strong suspicion of mechanical obstruction existed or if the patient were already depleted of nutrition and available veins by prior events. It would also be less if, after 2 or 3 days of continued ileus, no progress was made in passing a long tube, or distention of gut was unrelieved.

The preparation of these patients for operation is largely anticipated by the measures taken in non-operative treatment of ileus. Coverage by antibiotics given preoperatively should be considered because gross contamination is always a possibility, and is particularly serious in these depleted patients. Insertion of a catheter for measurement of central venous pressure is of great value in managing fluid replacement. The hematocrit value should be measured on the day before operation, and transfusions of whole blood or packed red cells should be given if the red cell volume is under 30 per cent. Several units of blood should be made available for operation if exploration is to take place more than 7 days postoperatively, when adhesions may have become rather vascular.

In anastomotic obstruction of the left colon, signs of sepsis added to those of obstruction indicate thorough exploratory laparotomy and usually transverse colostomy. In the absence of sepsis, cecostomy is indicated and is usually best done under general anesthesia. After right colectomy or when there is ileus of the small bowel only, general exploration should be carried out. A collapsed loop may be located first with a minimal lysis of adhesions, and is followed back to the most distal obstruction, which is relieved. The entire small bowel should then be run back to the ligament of Treitz to exclude other points of obstruction. Sometimes internal herniations, such as through mesenteric defects, may be unnoticed until all the small gut has been eviscerated.

Decompression is the next most important point of procedure, permitting bowel to resume function as soon as motor activity returns, allowing replacement of bowel in gentle curves, and facilitating closure. We prefer to milk the intestinal contents back to the stomach without opening the bowel whenever possible. If this is not possible, then enterotomy and aspiration with a Hodge sump apparatus is efficacious, and we have had good results on the several occasions when we have used the long enterostomy tube recommended by Baker.[6, 7] After decompression in this manner, advancement of long tubes is easier and perhaps even more worthwhile if the tube is left in place as a splint during the healing phase.

Abscesses encountered should be evacuated and often drained externally, but the peritoneal cavity need not be drained simply because of operative or preoperative contamination. In the culture of the organisms contained in these abscesses, one should not omit anaerobic techniques.

Whether or not to break down adhesions in order to inspect anastomoses suspected of being defective is always a dilemma; if the original procedure was sufficiently satisfactory to warrant closure without protective colostomy, and if no gross abscess is found near the anastomosis, it is usually better to leave well enough alone. It is unlikely that any effective repair can be done under these conditions anyway.

Closure in these patients should follow the principles previously discussed in relation to sepsis. except that single-layer sutures of wire are seldom necessary. The incidence of wound infection may be higher after secondary operations so that the use of braided or twisted non-absorbable suture material is to be avoided.

Prolonged ileus after secondary exploration is surprisingly infrequent, probably because of the effect of thorough decompression at the operating table, but these patients, on the other hand, often acquire a variety of pulmonary, urinary, vascular, cardiac, and renal complications before recovery. Perhaps the single most important factor in recovery is the frequency with which the patient is examined, for certain complications can be detected and treated successfully only in the early stages.

HEMORRHAGE

The ability to control hemorrhage is the great advantage of the modern surgeon over his predecessors. It ranges from improved techniques of blood replacement to maneuvers for control of operative hemorrhage, and requires the understanding of various mechanisms and correctable deficits that lead to abnormal bleeding. Nevertheless every surgeon sooner or later will encounter patients who present problems in preoperative, operative, or postoperative hemorrhage.

DIAGNOSIS

Diagnosis in general is obvious, in contrast to the diagnosis of ileus or sepsis. Tachycardia, hypotension, and falling hematocrit level are classic signs even in the absence of gross blood appearing from either end of the intestine or through operative defects in the intestine. Intraperitoneal bleeding may be diagnosed late unless the index of suspicion is high, because generalized distention or a localized swelling is difficult to detect in the postoperative belly.

Preoperative bleeding in polyps, ulcerative colitis, or diverticulitis cannot be classified as a complication of surgery, but failure to investigate thoroughly possible bleeding and clotting defects can lead to major complications. Bleeding time, partial thromboplastin time, and prothrombin time are worthwhile screening tests, and in patients with ulcerative colitis liver function tests may prove diagnostic of dangerous abnormalities. Most abnormalities thus detected can be corrected before major surgery is undertaken. In massive hemorrhage it must be remembered that bank blood lacks labile clotting factors, and so we make it a practice in patients in whom massive replacement is necessary to give one unit of fresh blood for every four units of bank blood. The citrate anticoagulant in bank blood is not a significant factor, and intravenous administration of calcium is therefore rarely indicated. An exception is the situation in which myocardial function may be depressed as a result of large infusions of serum albumin that lower the ionized fraction of calcium. This abnormality may be corrected by administration of calcium chloride, 1 gm. intravenously, or by giving digitalis, which renders the heart more able to use the calcium available. Depression of the prothrombin level as a result of antibiotic preparation is to be kept in mind and counteracted with preoperative use of vitamin K.

MANAGEMENT OF INTRAOPERATIVE HEMORRHAGE

Operative hemorrhage is infrequent with modern techniques, but the problem can present itself in several ways. Generalized oozing is least common and is often the result of some hemostatic abnormality which may have been undetected preoperatively. A prothrombin determination should be done while the patient is on the operating table, and, of course, the anesthesiologist must be sure that poor oxygenation and carbon dioxide elimination are not contributing factors; a mismatched blood transfusion must be considered. Vitamin K is given intravenously, and fresh blood or fresh-frozen plasma may be given empirically. In extreme cases the intravenous use of steroids can be considered. Frequently ligation of several major bleeding points controls what seems at first glance to be a discouragingly general ooze.

Accidental tearing or laceration of a major vessel is not common in colonic surgery, but sometimes may occur when cleavage planes are obscured or when the surgeon is attempting extensive multiorgan or wide en-bloc resections. Blind clamping and deep mass sutures are to be avoided, and the techniques of the vascular surgeon are most helpful in such situations. Usually the bleeding point can be controlled with a fingertip, and deliberate repair of the vein or artery can then be undertaken with precisely placed continuous sutures of 5-0 silk or Mersilene, swaged on a small curved needle. With venous hemorrhage, it is often effective simply to pack the area temporarily with a sponge while dissection continues elsewhere; when the sponge is later removed, the bleeding will have stopped. Strenuous attempts to identify and suture the exact site of venous bleeding may lead to further damage.

Pelvic hemorrhage is still a danger even in the best of hands, sometimes because of aberrant veins or abnormally large arteries and sometimes because the wrong plane is entered in presacral dissection. Ligation of the hypogastric arteries is without complication and may be entirely effective, although it is necessary at times to pack the pelvis with gauze in difficult cases. Splenic tears are relatively common in left colectomy, and the surgeon should be prepared to remove the spleen if bleeding is not readily controlled by pressure or fibrin-foam mats. Microfibrillar collagen (Avitene) has proven very useful in splenic conservation after closed trauma, and our early experience with it in bleeding from intraoperative injury has been encouraging. If the spleen has to be removed, however, platelet determinations must be followed postoperatively and anticoagulants instituted if the count rises above 1 million per cu. mm. Platelet stickiness and thrombotic complications of thrombocytosis are diminished by the administration of as little as 300 mg. of aspirin a day.

MANAGEMENT OF POSTOPERATIVE HEMORRHAGE

Postoperative hemorrhage may be manifested by external bleeding, generalized abdominal distention, or the appearance of an abdominal mass with or without deterioration of vital signs. Once the diagnosis of postoperative hemorrhage is made, the source is usually deducible from the nature of the operation. The treatment of persistent perineal bleeding following a Miles resection will be discussed later under the appropriate heading. Intra-abdominal bleeding must, of course, occur to a certain extent after every colectomy, so that the fact of its detection is not of itself necessarily an indication for operation, although if the diagnosis of more than a minimal amount of bleeding can be made early, immediate exploration is indicated. The peritoneum can clear enormous quantities of blood without complication, provided infection is not present. The therapy of intraperitoneal bleeding then logically comes down to control of continuing hemorrhage and removal of infected hematoma, so that the diagnosis of these conditions is the main question.

Presuming that bleeding is detected first by a change in vital signs, followed perhaps by observation of abdominal distention and anemia, one can reasonably give a transfusion rapidly until blood pressure and pulse return to normal and then more slowly until the hematocrit value reaches a satisfactory level (over 30 per cent). Subsequent deterioration of vital signs or significant fall in hematocrit level is an indication for exploration. If abdominal distention is considerable, exploration is indicated to remove potentially infected blood and probably to control continuing bleeding.

If the first sign of bleeding is an abdominal mass, then the problem is handled somewhat differently because changes in the size of the mass serve as an indication of further bleeding. Usually, if the bleeding point is well enough enclosed so that a mass is formed, cessation of bleeding occurs spontaneously with increasing tissue pressure. One is then left with the decision whether to operate simply to remove a hematoma. In patients who are young and in good condition, removal is justified as prophylaxis. In older, sicker patients, one may decide to wait until signs of infection actually appear, recalling that some tenderness and a degree or so of fever are expected from hematoma even without infection. Changes for the worse are an indication for operation.

Operative treatment of postoperative bleeding does not differ in principle from the methods already discussed that are used in the control of intraoperative bleeding. Insertion of drains is indicated only if infection is found. Exploration for and control of postoperative hemorrhage usually need not foreshadow a complicated course. Indeed, the reverse is often true.

Postoperative bleeding into the lumen of the gut is handled in essentially the same way as bleeding from the same source preoperatively; i.e., diagnosis as to source is the first and often most difficult problem, with surgical intervention determined largely by the response to conservative therapy. Probably one tries to be more conservative because of the recency of major surgery, but there cannot be much leeway in determining the need for operation in uncontrolled gastrointestinal bleeding. The most severe limitation is in the use of diagnostic measures such as gastroscopy and colonoscopy in a patient with postoperative ileus and perhaps a colonic anastomosis. If endoscopy is done, the insufflating gas should be carbon dioxide, which is quickly absorbed from the gut, not air, which can cause persistent distention. The use of barium contrast x-rays is to be discouraged especially in the nonoperated patient, because these x-rays never show an actual bleeding point and always interfere with subsequent endoscopic or angiographic studies that may become necessary. Inspissation of barium sulfate suspension in the postoperative colon can cause severe complications. We now rely heavily on arteriography not only to localize the point of bleeding but also to permit infusion of vasopressin (Pitressin), which often controls this type of bleeding by localized vasoconstriction.

One point that should be mentioned here falls into the area of prophylaxis as much as the area of management of postoperative hemorrhage, and that concerns the patient with ulcerative colitis whose indication for operation is that of severe hemorrhage. It has been our experience that attempts to conserve the rectum in such patients have too often been followed by continuing severe bleeding that then requires proctectomy under desperate circumstances.

Postoperative bleeding resulting from the use of anticoagulants as prophylaxis against recurrent cerebral, coronary, or peripheral thrombosis is always reversible with the appropriate antidote. Such bleeding is sufficiently uncommon that one should not be deterred from maintaining patients in the range of 1 to 1½ times normal prothrombin time if the need exists. If bleeding does occur, once the clotting time has returned to normal, the problem is identical with that of postoperative bleeding in any patient.

FISTULA

DIAGNOSIS

The diagnosis of a fistula is complicated by difficulties of definition. As Moore[47] pointed out, some "fistulas" are really abscesses with drainage to the skin in one direction and into the bowel in another. Determining the cause of a fistula is even more difficult when one attempts to decide whether the abscess caused the anastomotic leak or vice versa. Fistulas used to be more common when drains were left near anastomoses, but whether the drains caused the fistulas or were truly justified because of the high incidence of fistulas secondary to poor preparation and technique is unanswered. At least it is certain that a freely draining colocutaneous fistula is better for the patient than an intraperitoneal abscess or generalized peritonitis, which are the other common sequelae of anastomotic failure. If there is any doubt as to diagnosis, injection of a radiopaque medium such as Hypaque into the sinus or feeding of charcoal powder should quickly and safely settle the question.[26]

Fistulas remain a common complication of colonic resection and anastomosis, having occurred in 3 per cent of 400 cases studied at the Massachusetts General Hospital (see Fig 25–1). Surprising was the fact that anastomotic failure in fistula formation was almost as common after right colectomy as after the traditionally more hazardous left colectomy and sigmoid resection. In the 56 colonic or low ileac fistulas collected from the Massachusetts General Hospital records by Edmunds and others,[20] twenty were due to anastomotic failure and five to surgical injury. In 500 colectomies there were 5 small bowel fistulas, 3 resulting from failure of ileotransverse colostomies and two from surgical injury (see Fig. 25–1). Eight colonic fistulas all resulted from anastomotic failure after left colectomy or sigmoid resection for carcinoma. In Edmund's report it was stated that inflammatory disease was significant in anastomotic failure, and 5 of 20 colonic anastomoses failed because of the presence of diverticulitis at the suture line.

Colonic fistulas practically never present the problems of electrolyte imbalance, fluid loss, and skin digestion that are seen with jejunal and ileal fistulas. A more recent review of the Massachusetts General Hospital series of fistulas by Aguirre and others[1] emphasizes the importance of nutrition via intravenous hyperalimentation and the greater freedom in timing of the surgical intervention that is enjoyed when nutrition

is not a consideration for urgent surgery. The chief complication of colonic fistula is sepsis — phlegmon, wound abscess, intraperitoneal abscess, and generalized peritonitis. Twenty-five per cent of patients in Edmunds's series had generalized peritonitis, while almost half had intraperitoneal abscess.

Because colonic fistulas do not produce debilitating loss of body fluids, and because slightly more than half of them will close spontaneously, the serious consideration in their management is the control of infection.

NON-OPERATIVE MANAGEMENT

After the formation and diagnosis of a fistula, the situation must be studied closely to determine the severity of the accompanying infection and the probable size of the fistula. Local and systemic reaction and the presence of a mass suggesting abscess may well respond to antibiotic treatment and a few days' waiting. If infection is thus controlled, one should wait at least 4 weeks before considering operative intervention of any kind, bearing in mind that many colonic fistulas have closed spontaneously even after that time. Inlying drains and sump suction apparatus are rarely of value in improving drainage or avoiding skin irritation, and their presence may actually inhibit closure. The Goldsmith cup has proven a useful contribution in this area,[28] but usually the fistulous drainage can be managed with the special technique and materials available to the enterostomal therapist.

OPERATIVE TREATMENT

If signs of generalized peritonitis accompany the appearance of a fistula, then all the indications for surgical intervention in sepsis are fulfilled as previously discussed. Until the source of continuing contamination is controlled by closure (unlikely to be successful), diversion, or exteriorization, there can be no hope for recovery. Simple closure is doomed to failure unless accompanied by proximal decompression and drainage, because the factors leading to leak are unchanged except for the *addition* of infection.

In less serious degrees of infection such as phlegmon and abscess, after trial and failure of conservative treatment, the usual management will be twofold: improvement of drainage and defunctioning of the bowel proximally. Resection is rarely indicated, and in general it can be said that the minimal procedure that produces results is best.

When infection has subsided and a productive fistula remains, efforts should be made to determine (1) the size of the colonic defect, (2) the presence of distal obstruction, and (3) the presence of etiologic agents such as carcinoma, diverticulitis, or retained foreign material (suture, needle, sponge). Barium by rectum, colostomy, or the fistula usually produces the answers to these questions.

If there is no obstruction or inciting agent and the opening in the colon measures 1 cm. or less, spontaneous closure may be anticipated; otherwise, operative repair will probably be necessary. In favorable cases it is reasonable to defer defunctioning colostomy for 4 to 8 weeks; but, by that time, defunctioning should be carried out in all cases, not only to improve chances of spontaneous closure, but also to prepare for definitive operation. The best chance for cure exists when defunctioned and noninflamed bowel and fistula are resected en bloc and a fresh anastomosis is performed, although turn-in of the fistula gives surprisingly good results when conditions are ideal.

OTHER COMPLICATIONS

From inspection of Figure 25–1 it is apparent that *pulmonary embolism* remains an extremely important cause of death following colonic surgery, and it actually outranks hemorrhage in that regard. We have not used anticoagulants prophylactically in poor-risk patients, but evidence is accumulating that this may be a worthwhile practice. The danger of hemorrhage appears slight if the prothrombin time is kept between 1 and 1½ times normal. Data derived from a controlled study from the Massachusetts General Hospital indicate that anticoagulants do prevent thromboembolism in high-risk patients.[50] Heparin is more manageable than aspirin or Coumadin because

of heparin's short duration of action. Five thousand international units may be given intramuscularly every 4 hours. There is usually no need for monitoring the effect of low-dose heparin in patients with normal coagulation parameters. Other routine measures for prophylaxis include early ambulation, adequate hydration, elastic stockings, and the avoidance of abdominal binders and behind-the-knee supports. The treatment of thrombophlebitis has been discussed briefly above, and extensively in Chapter 9.

Wound dehiscence occurred in 2 per cent of 500 patients and was associated in most cases with ileus and distention, fistula, or wound infection.[36] In our own experience, dehiscence never occurred when anterior fascial or all-layer retention sutures were used, provided they were placed not more than 2 cm. apart and were not removed too early. We used to use retention sutures after every colonic operation, but our recent experience with monofilament polypropylene and subcuticular Dexon has been equally perfect in avoiding dehiscence, and much better in terms of wound sepsis (one in 287 open-bowel cases), lesser postoperative discomfort, greater convenience (no sutures to remove), and better appearance of the wound.

Urinary tract obstruction and *sepsis* are frequently observed after colonic surgery; to a certain extent they may not be preventable in this elderly group, in whom catheterization is frequently necessary. Urinary fistula, however, constitutes a technical error that should be either avoided or recognized and corrected. In the Massachusetts General Hospital series, 5 patients, who survived, had urinary fistula after sigmoid resections for carcinoma, whereas 2 patients who were found to have fistulas after Miles resections both died. The diagnosis, when suspected, is usually quickly confirmed by intravenous pyelogram; retrograde studies must then be considered. Ureteral fistula is more serious than vesical fistula, which often heals spontaneously with simple bladder catheter drainage. The damaged ureter presents a bigger problem; adequate diversion may be achieved by cystoscopic placement of a splinting catheter, but frequently the catheter will not pass, and repair or open drainage in the operative area can lead to failure, often with stricture and persistent leak. Sometimes the most radical treatment — nephrectomy — in actuality is the simplest and least complicated way out of a life-threatening situation.

Cardiovascular and *cerebral vascular acci-* dents were fairly common causes of death in this group of patients, but there is little that can be done to prevent these complications except that, whenever possible, operation should be delayed for 3 months after a myocardial infarction.

MANAGEMENT OF COMPLICATIONS RELATED TO SPECIAL PROCEDURES

Because different operations upon the colon are so varied in their nature and effects and because the different segments of the colon are in intimate relation to practically every intra-abdominal organ, it is not surprising that each operation carries certain hazards peculiar to it. Much of the pertinent material, of course, has been covered in the previous section, so that only brief mention need be made here in many cases.

COMPLICATIONS OF DIAGNOSTIC PROCEDURES

Except for the all-important rectal examination, the main diagnostic procedures utilized are sigmoidoscopy, colonoscopy, and barium enema. In experienced hands these procedures are extremely safe, although they may be rather uncomfortable for the patient. Under certain circumstances, however, the risk is increased, and they must be performed with extreme care.

In diverticulitis, ulcerative colitis, and carcinoma spontaneous *perforation* may occur. When the colon is hovering near such a state, it is understandable that the addition of a barium enema or endoscopy may be all that is required to convert a weak spot into a perforation. Although, in general, sigmoidoscopy should precede a barium enema, in these cases it is particularly important, because the finding of an obstructive carcinoma that can be biopsied not only establishes diagnosis, but also contraindicates barium enema. Barium enema here is not omitted because of a fear of perforation necessarily, but because with obstructing lesions there is danger that barium may be forced beyond the lesion where it will remain and become inspissated. Occasionally surgical removal of the obstructing and ulcerating plugs is the only effective therapy. Nevertheless, in certain cases in which the diagnosis is seriously in doubt, barium study by an experienced radiologist may be valuable. If the radiologist is forewarned of the problem, he is often able to delineate the obstructing lesion with passage of only minimal amounts of barium beyond it.

Perforation during sigmoidoscopy may be the result of bursting by excessive insufflation of air, tearing by actual pressure of the instrument, or explosion when colonic gases are detonated by a fulgurating device. The treatment is immediate operation, and for maximal safety a decompressive colostomy may be performed in addition to definitive surgery for the perforation and for the original lesion.

Perforation during diagnostic colonoscopy has, in most centers, occurred with an appreciably higher incidence than sigmoidoscopic perforation — approximately 0.2 per cent as compared with 0.01 per cent. Colonoscopic perforation should be diagnosable immediately. Management is the same as for sigmoidoscopic perforation and, as a matter of fact, most colonoscopic perforations do occur in the sigmoid.[40] Colonoscopy is to be avoided in the poorly prepared bowel, in acute diverticulitis, especially when perforation or abscess is suspected, and in severe colitis because of the risk of post-colonoscopic toxic dilatation. Because it is generally impossible to prepare the bowel adequately proximal to an annular lesion, it is risky and usually unproductive to pass the colonoscope beyond such a lesion. However, endoscopy up to that point is useful to exclude distal lesions, which are frequently missed by barium enema.

Perforation during barium study usually involves heavy contamination of the peritoneal cavity with variable amounts of the

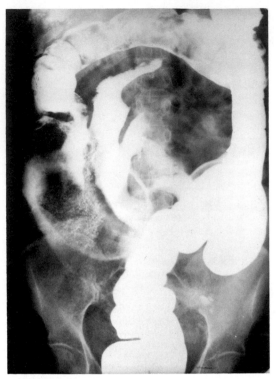

Figure 25–6 A 68-year-old woman with a 6-weeks' history of constipation finally entered after 4 days of severe abdominal pain and total obstipation. Barium by rectum showed normal bowel around to the hepatic flexure, where the combination of obstruction and perforation resulted in extensive extravasation of barium into the peritoneal cavity. The patient died of sepsis several weeks after resection of an unusual napkin-ring lesion of the right colon.

barium-feces mixture (Fig. 25–6). At exploration, which should not be delayed, every effort should be made to remove the last vestiges of barium, because recurrent infection and pernicious adhesive peritonitis result. Irrigation with massive quantities of salt solution and scrubbing with sponges may be necessary to dislodge the adherent substance. Needless to say, many of these unfortunate patients die of infection postoperatively, while those that survive are subject to recurrent bouts of obstruction from adhesions.

COMPLICATIONS OF COLONOSCOPIC POLYPECTOMY

Transcolonoscopic polypectomy has proven to have a lower incidence of fatal and non-fatal complications than polypec-

tomy via laparotomy and colotomy or colectomy. At the Massachusetts General Hospital we have performed over 4000 colonoscopic polypectomies with only one death, which was due to an undiagnosed postoperative perforation. Splenectomy was necessitated in one patient in whom excessive traction was used in rounding the splenic flexure. Pedicle hemorrhage severe enough to require re-snaring, transfusion, or angiography for vasoconstrictive infusion occurred in 2.5 per cent of cases; in no case did postpolypectomy bleeding require laparotomy for its control. In some cases, however, laparotomy was done because immediate histological sections on the excised specimen showed invasive carcinoma, constituting an indication for resection and precluding any dalliance with other methods of bleeding control. It is a fact, perhaps not surprisingly, that hemorrhage, as well as perforation, occurs more frequently from a malignant polyp, so that frozen sections on the excised lesion should be obtained whenever cancer, perforation, or bleeding is suspected or anticipated. The incidence of perforation following polypectomy has been 1 per cent overall, slightly higher with sessile lesions and a little lower with pedunculated ones. When the totally resected lesion is proven histologically benign, the perforation, which is usually walled-off, may be managed conservatively like diverticulitis as long as signs are localized and improving. When the lesion is malignant or has not been totally resectable, or when the progression of local signs and symptoms indicates that the process is not contained, then resection should be done. The need for a staged procedure, as with perforative diverticulitis or cancer, depends upon the patient's general condition and the findings at operation. Contamination is always minimal and primary resection is the usual choice.[40]

COMPLICATIONS OF COLOSTOMY

Colostomy is followed by an extraordinary variety of complications, most of which are not common or serious.

The prevention of complications following colostomy requires attention to the details of operation and consideration of the purposes of operation: namely, decompression and defunctioning of the bowel proximal to an anastomosis or obstruction. Failure to achieve these objectives is a mishap so serious that its classification simply as a complication is open to question. It must be remembered, however, that cecostomy does not defunction the bowel and may fail to decompress it adequately, particularly if there is a great deal of solid material above a left-sided obstruction. Loop colostomy, through spillover, may not defunction the bowel completely and, unless the proximal limb is emptied promptly, may not decompress the right colon soon enough to prevent perforation. Most early complications of colostomy are related to poor fit of bowel exteriorized to the aperture in the abdominal wall. As a general rule there should be room for a fingertip to be placed through the peritoneal opening beside ·the colon. This is true, however, only if the colon is of relatively normal size. Distended or edematous gut will shrink soon after successful decompression, leaving a peritoneal defect that may be many times too large. Evisceration commonly results. In such situations the colon should be emptied in the most sanitary manner possible (depending on the consistency of its contents), and then the serosa carefully attached to the peritoneal ring with interposition of peritoneal, fascial, and skin bridges as the best means of preventing prolapse or evisceration.

TRANSVERSE COLOSTOMY

In a review of 80 consecutive personal transverse colostomies the complications

TABLE 25–2 COMPLICATIONS OF COLOSTOMY

	Sigmoid	Transverse
Number of cases......	104	80
Hernia....................	18	12
Stricture.................	19	0
Bleeding.................	15	8
Retraction..............	4	1
Prolapse.................	4	7
Obstruction	6	2
Abscess..................	2	12
Perforation.............	3	0
Gangrene	1	1
Constipation...........	2	1
Diarrhea.................	14	4
Evisceration	1	1
Fistula...................	0	1
Miscellaneous..........	4	3

listed in Table 25–2 were found. Wound abscess and hernia were by far the most common complications and tended to be associated with each other and with closure of the transverse colostomy. Most of the wound infections required no treatment other than the application of wet dressings, and only one of the hernias required operative treatment. Hemorrhage from the colostomy is generally minor and easy to control with a suture. Obstruction usually responds to finger dilatation, but it may be necessary to remove a stitch or two at the peritoneal level. Prolapse of the colostomy is a spectacular complication in its extreme form, but it usually requires no treatment, since this complication is easily handled by bowel resection at the time of closure of the colostomy. Retraction of the colostomy may require operative correction if early, and dehiscence must be corrected immediately.

In a more recent personal series at our institution a number of changes in technique were made in an effort to reduce the incidence of complications. A larger-diameter plastic rod elevated by a folded gauze sponge was used to minimize spillover. With this modification the colostomy opening could be made longitudinally rather than transversely, and it was therefore not necessary to divide the bowel. Repair of the longitudinal incision was done transversely in Heineke-Mikulicz fashion, with resultant widening of the closure site and much less operative trauma than is involved in resection. Thorough bowel preparation, perioperative systemic antibiotics, meticulous walling-off procedures, wound soaking with 0.5 per cent neomycin solution, primary closure with running polypropylene, polyglycolic acid, and skin tapes completed the routine. With this technique the last 45 consecutive colostomy closures have proceeded without local complication or distal anastomotic complication. Compared with our historical controls and with previous reported incidences of 15 to 37 per cent local complications (abscess, fistula, obstruction, or dehiscence), the present results encourage us to be more liberal in our use of colostomy.[68] In contrast, in recent years there has been a tendency to discourage protective colostomy on the basis that its own complications exceeded the frequency of those it purported to avoid.[66] With the newer techniques we now feel we can take full advantage of the admitted protection offered by transverse colostomy in avoiding the serious and sometimes fatal complications of deep pelvic anastomosis.

SIGMOID COLOSTOMY

In the former study permanent sigmoid colostomies were also reviewed, and the accompanying list of complications was compiled in a personal series of 104 patients (see Table 25–2). Hemorrhage and hernia of the colostomy remain fairly frequent, but the most common complication in sigmoid colostomy is evidently stricture or narrowing at the skin level. Almost all these colostomies were performed by drawing the end of the bowel through a stab wound in the flank and fixing it there with an Allen-Kocher clamp for several days while healing occurred. This method can produce a perfectly adequate stoma, but it is necessary for the patient to insert a finger deeply into the stoma every other day for 6 months or more to prevent the complication of stomal stricture. Late stricture usually responds to dilatation, but if constipation results and dilatation of the stricture is painful, then a simple plastic procedure under local anesthesia should be done. It is possible that some strictures could be avoided by mucocutaneous suture at the time of colostomy, which has the additional advantages of immediate and secure fixation of the colon at the desired level, as well as early maturation that facilitates the patient's adjustment to his stoma and its appurtenances.

In four cases retraction of the sigmoid colostomy occurred, retraction being a complication of colonic surgery in patients with a very thick abdominal wall. Because these are usually permanent colostomies and must function effectively for a long time, operative correction is usually necessary to produce an adequate stoma. Sometimes sufficient length of bowel to reach the skin level comfortably can be obtained only by stepping down the splenic flexure, and occasionally the mesosigmoid is so short that the bowel cannot be drawn laterally through the flank but must be delivered straight up through the incision. When this is necessary the additional complications of wound infection, retraction, and dehiscence are naturally more frequent.

Prolapse was just as common as retraction. Surgery for this condition, of course, is simple, but need not be done unless the patient is having bothersome symptoms.

One of the most interesting complications of sigmoid colostomy is perforation by means of an irrigating catheter, which occurred in 3 of 104 patients. History provides the diagnosis when the patient reports the sudden onset of excruciating abdominal pain during an irrigation after which very little of the solution is returned. On examination, signs of peritonitis exist. The condition is serious, and unless these patients are operated upon soon after perforation, a fatal outcome is a distinct possibility. Closure of the perforation is less desirable than freeing enough bowel within the peritoneal cavity so that the perforation can be exteriorized or resected along with all bowel distal to it.[33]

The one case of gangrene of the stoma in this group was handled by ascertaining in this very obese patient that viable bowel mucosa was present up to the level of the anterior fascia, which was at least 4 inches deep to the skin level. It was necessary later to reoperate upon the patient and bring a new stoma out at a higher level.

Obstruction of the sigmoid colostomy occurred in 6 patients to the extent that obstipation and dilatation of the bowel were noted in the postoperative phase. In only one patient, however, was the obstruction so severe that it did not respond to finger dilatation. The anterior fascial ring was so tight that the patient had to be reanesthetized and the opening enlarged. The postoperative course was subsequently uncomplicated.

The early complications of transverse and sigmoid colostomy discussed here are generally less distressing to the patient than the later abnormalities of function that occur in a few cases. For example, constipation was a problem in 2 patients with sigmoid colostomy and one with transverse colostomy. Diarrhea, on the other hand, occurred with annoying frequency in 14 patients with sigmoid colostomy and was practically continuous in 4 patients with transverse colostomy. These difficulties are only of minor importance in patients with transverse colostomies, since, for the most part, these patients are looking forward to closure of their temporary stoma. In patients with permanent sigmoid colostomies, however, the need for a solution to the problem is more pressing.

Most abnormalities of function, we find, can be successfully controlled by the use of tap-water irrigations every other day, and our patients are routinely begun on such a program as soon as the stoma is sufficiently adherent to the surrounding tissues post-operatively. This occurs between the fifth and seventh days after operation. This system is in contrast with that advocated widely in Great Britain, where the colostomy is allowed to discover its own rhythm, usually functioning about the same time every day. The disadvantage to the patient of this method, however, is the fact that in times of unusual stress such as imposed by social or business events, the colostomy is apt to discharge profusely when least expected or desired. Preferable to this type of accident may be the expenditure of time necessary to perform a thorough irrigation of the bowel every other day. In active patients who are on a diet reasonably free of sugar, legumes, and other gas-forming foods, the stoma frequently needs no more attention than the application of a small gauze pad to absorb mucus. Patients whose movements tend to be abnormally dehydrated benefit from the addition of psyllium muciloid or a detergent such as dioctyl sodium sulfosuccinate to the diet. Mineral oil is less satisfactory because it tends to leak through the stoma even between irrigations.

Colostomy diarrhea may be intermittent when caused by infection or dietary indiscretion, or practically continuous in patients whose residual colonic mucosa never seems to acquire the dehydrating capability of the resected rectosigmoid. No matter how perfect or well regulated the bowel function, we always advise patients to have a standard colostomy appliance on hand for use when the movements are unusually loose or frequent. Patients with chronic or frequently recurring diarrhea sometimes respond to belladonna or diphenoxylate (Lomotil), but in most cases control is achieved only through the use of opiates. The use of adhesive disposable bags (Hollister) is of great comfort to many patients, especially soon after operation.

Small bowel obstruction due to prolapse of bowel along the lumbar gutter lateral to the colon is a potential and serious complication not seen in our series of sigmoid colostomies. This complication has evidently been prevented by careful suturing of the sigmoid mesocolon to the parietal peritoneum, thus closing the trap. Sometimes it is not possible to close this defect satisfactorily with sutures, in which case it is better to leave the trap completely open. Another interesting complication not seen in this series is gangrene of the distal colon secondary to incarceration of a paracolostomy hernia. In one recent case the incarcerated small intestine was found to be completely viable, although the colon was gangrenous from the level of the fascia to the skin because of stretching and compression of its blood supply by the contents of the hernia sac. Most herniations require no treatment; Thorlakson[57] has described the technique of repair when operation is necessary.

Evisceration of small intestine alongside the colostomy in the early postoperative phase is a possibility if the peritoneal opening is made too large or if subsidence of edema in obstructed bowel leaves more room between colon and peritoneum than was anticipated. This complication was not seen in our series and should be avoidable if the peritoneal opening is carefully adjusted in the manner already described. If the colon is swollen, however, it will be necessary to approximate serosa to peritoneum with carefully placed interrupted sutures of catgut so that a paracolostomy defect will not be left when the bowel returns to normal size.

COMPLICATIONS OF CECOSTOMY

Tube cecostomy by the Gibson technique is used less now than formerly, but still has an important place in the management of obstructing lesions of the transverse colon and splenic flexure. Cecostomy, however, never defunctions the bowel and may not decompress it, so that these patients have to be watched postoperatively with great care. The tube used must be of adequate size and should project well into the lumen of the bowel. Irrigations of the right colon with saline and magnesium citrate solutions can also aid in the decompression of the bowel.

Retention of the cecostomy tube for too long a time can cause perforation of the cecum by erosion. Ten days after insertion, adequate healing should have taken place and the sinus will remain open as long as distal obstruction persists. In most cases definitive resection will already have been carried out by this time.

Occasionally the cecostomy wound fails to close spontaneously because of excessive sepsis in the abdominal wall, anastomotic obstruction or edema, epithelization of the tract, or eversion of the cecal mucosa. This occurred in 6 per cent of 240 cases reviewed by Allen and Welch.[2] If the sinus remains patent for more than 6 to 8 weeks, closure can be effected by simple local procedure in the majority of cases, but in some, recurrent drainage necessitates cecectomy and ileocolostomy.

Incisional hernia nearly always follows cecostomy, but it is rarely large enough to require repair.

COMPLICATIONS OF OPERATIONS ON THE RECTUM

Because of its confinement within the pelvis, its retroperitoneal position, and the fact that it terminates at the anal sphincter, the rectum presents the surgeon with unique technical challenges and a correspondingly impressive array of complications. Working space, particularly in the male, may be almost non-existent. Healing of bowel anastomoses depends usually on serosal adhesion first, but in the extraperitoneal rectum the absence of serosa delays healing in every case. Blood supply to the bowel is variable, and minor hematomas assume importance when peritoneum is not nearby to absorb them. Raw surfaces invite the formation of adhesions and obstruction. When resection is carried to a very low level, anastomosis at or near the anus is apt to be attended by incontinence of stool, bladder dysfunction, or sexual impotence.

ANTERIOR RESECTION

Prevention of complications in anterior resection of the rectum is obviously impossible in every case, but meticulous technique is essential if the surgeon is to have even a reasonable chance of avoiding trouble. Sometimes bleeding ooze from raw pelvic surfaces is not completely controllable, and the necessity for a method to remove the accumulated blood is obvious. In other cases gross hemorrhage may not be present at the completion of the procedure, but it must be assumed that some bleeding will occur subsequently, and provision must be made to remove it. Tight closure of the peritoneum over an undrained space is therefore not permissible, and if no drain is used, a defect lateral to the proximal bowel should be provided so that blood may work up into the peritoneal cavity where it will be absorbed. If herniation of small bowel is feared and the space accordingly closed, we feel that drainage with commercially available suction catheters or sumps is preferable to drainage with Penrose wicks, and these tubes may be brought to the skin surface entirely retroperitoneally. Our current favorite is the Jackson-Pratt suction drain, which is more flexible than the Hemovac drain; both have an advantage over sumps in that air-drying of secretions with resultant plugging is avoided. Paracoccygeal drainage is effective, but invites infection ascending from the always contaminated perineum. Furthermore, perineal fistulization from the anastomosis through the paracoccygeal drainage tract is common when this technique is used, and reconstruction or repair when this occurs is very difficult.

Adequate blood supply to both ends of the colon should be verified by the presence of spurting or pulsating vessels prior to anastomosis. Bowel ends must be sutured without tension, and the anastomosis must be watertight. As is often the case when no infallible technique is available, there are many conflicting recommendations for pelvic anastomosis including those advocating both one and two layers of sutures, and proponents of inverting, everting, or end-on anastomoses.[29, 49] Goligher's reports of his experience with the end-to-end anastomosing stapler are most interesting, and our own experience with stapling has been satisfactory, although technical difficulties have occasionally prevented the production of a complete anastomotic ring.[30, 31] The stapled anastomosis, therefore, like any other must be inspected carefully after construction to detect a weak spot in need of a reinforcing suture. An ordinary blunt probe poked along the suture line can be of great value in this way, and the injection of neomycin solution under pressure via an inlying rectal tube can expose a leak.

The beneficial effects of antibiotic irrigation of the pelvis after anastomosis may never be proved, but a 0.5 per cent neomycin wash is so simple, so desirable on theoretical grounds, so free of ill efects, and so satisfying emotionally that we cannot argue strongly against it.[52]

If there is any question about any phase of the operative preparation, performance, or patient, we feel that proximal decompression by means of a transverse colostomy is the single most important aspect of preventive medicine in anterior resection.

As implied earlier, hematoma formation in the pelvis is thought to be the precursor of many complications of anterior resection. The diagnosis of hematoma formation, if not massive, is usually impossible, and preventive measures must be completely reliable if fistulization is to be prevented. Disruption of the anastomosis may be manifested by systemic signs of sepsis, paralytic ileus, peritonitis, anastomotic obstruction, small bowel obstruction, wound infection, or colocutaneous fistula.

Treatment of hemorrhage may require simple evacuation of hematoma and transverse colostomy, but if pelvic packing is required, the anastomosis will usually have to be taken down and a colostomy formed with the proximal limb. Anastomotic leakage and resulting sepsis may be treated with non-operative measures at times, but drainage and diversion are needed in major sepsis. Drainage through the anus or paracoccygeally is seldom sufficient, but there are exceptions. If the proximal colon is clean and well decompressed, anastomotic obstruction is rarely permanent, and anastomosis with only a small sector intact may heal perfectly in time. It is important to begin saline irrigations of the defunctioned bowel distal to the transverse colostomy early and have the patient continue irrigating during the many months of healing that may follow. Regular dilatation of the anastomosis by finger or sigmoidoscope may be crucial, and occasional barium enema radiographs are helpful in estimating progress

and determining the time for colostomy closure.

Later complications of anterior resection are rectal tenesmus with frequency, diarrhea, and even incontinence. These difficulties almost always disappear in time, but opiates or belladonna alkaloids may tide the patient over a trying experience. Late stricture of a functioning anastomosis is rare, and the most likely explanation for obstructive symptoms after resection for cancer is suture line recurrence. Anastomotic recurrence is debatably classified as a complication of surgery; measures used in prevention are thoroughly discussed in articles by Wheelock et al.,[67] Floyd et al.,[24] and Localio.[43-44]

MILES RESECTION

Despite the absence of anastomoses, complications of combined abdominoperineal resection of the rectum are surprisingly frequent. The complications of sigmoid colostomy, an integral part of the Miles resection, have already been discussed. Other complications have to do with the peritoneal floor, the exposed and denervated lower urinary tract, and problems of the eviscerated pelvic dead space.

Hemorrhage in the pelvis during or after a Miles resection has already been mentioned, and the efficacy of ligating the hypogastric arteries should be reemphasized. In contrast to anterior resection, the disadvantages of tamponade of the pelvis with a pack are minor, and it is easily removed later through the perineal wound. Hemorrhage immediately after operation is not common and occurs usually when blood pressure is restored to normal in a patient who may have been hypotensive during operation. If bleeding from the posterior wound is unusually heavy and does not diminish, then reoperation under general anesthesia should be undertaken, although this is a rare occurrence.

Prolapse of small intestine through pelvic peritoneal dehiscence is frequently fatal because the obstructed and later strangulated loop may easily pass undetected for several days. Peritoneum for closure should be carefully preserved and widely dissected. Closure must be meticulous, preferably with two layers of chromic catgut. In the female the uterus can be retroverted to provide an effective buffer to support the suture line. If the peritoneal floor cannot be closed securely, it is better to leave it completely open, with support provided by a gauze pack covered with gutta percha or Silastic. Disadvantages of the pack technique are small bowel adhesions, later herniation, prolapse lateral to the pack, and poor drainage around the pack leading to sepsis, a most dangerous complication in proximity to pelvic venous plexuses. There has been increasing interest in primary closure of the perineal wound as a means of avoiding some of the severe complications associated with leaving it open, or packing. Our method involves suture of pelvic peritoneum as well as perineal subcutaneous tissue and skin, with suction drainage of the closed presacral space. Warshaw has reported good results leaving the peritoneum unsutured, with no instance of perineal herniation or small bowel obstruction.[60] It seems important to use a subcuticular suture for final approximation in order to avoid penetrating the naturally heavily contaminated perianal skin. Altemeier has reported good results with primary closure of the perineum.[4]

Urinary tract sepsis and obstruction following a Miles resection are common in males, owing to the advanced age of these patients, the necessity for catheterization, and the unavoidable partial denervation of the lower urinary tract. Usually these complications respond to adequate hydration, specific antibiotic treatment, and catheter decompression. Occasionally prostatectomy will subsequently be necessary, and this should be done by the transurethral route whenever possible, because of the minimal systemic trauma imposed by this operation. If it can be determined that prostatectomy will almost certainly be required, the perineal phase of the Miles operation provides unexcelled exposure, and prostatectomy at the same sitting adds only a few minutes to the operation. It must, however, be done with great care by an experienced urologist, for a postoperative urinary fistula through the perineum can be troublesome. Most urologists will have more confidence with transurethral resection.

Urinary fistula following a Miles resection is caused by injury to the ureter, bladder, or urethra, all of which are exposed and subject to hazard. Diagnosis is provided by appearance of a blue stain in pelvic drainage after intravenous administration of 5 ml. of indigo carmine solution.

The perineal wound is the source of many complications, although it is surprising how often this enormous space heals rapidly and without untoward event. Leaving the wound open with wide drainage of the space is always safe, although primary closure is recommended by some, particularly after second-stage resection following subtotal colectomy for colitis. The tissues of patients with ulcerative colitis are apt to heal so slowly if the wound is left open that primary closure has considerable appeal, although undrained sepsis may be correspondingly more serious in these patients.

Persistent drainage and failure to heal in cancer patients usually mean recurrent disease in the pelvis, and a painful posterior wound almost always implies the same. Further resection is rarely possible and never curative. The best treatment is supervoltage radiotherapy in high doses; surprisingly, some excellent results have been obtained even with colloid carcinomas. Persistent sinus and pain may sometimes result from simple failure to heal, but recurrence again is more likely. Pain is occasionally relieved by excision of the sinus.

After proctocolectomy for ulcerative colitis non-healing or delayed healing of the perineal wound is common unless primary closure has been successful.[5, 34] Unfortunately, the perianal sepsis preceding operation in many cases is so severe as to preclude primary closure. In achieving healing it is important to recognize the adverse consequence of a bottle-shaped sinus with a narrow opening at the outside. There is a tendency for the skin and immediate subcutaneous tissue to close more rapidly than the deeper defect, producing an infected cavity with poor drainage and a resulting tendency to enlarge rather than heal. Enlarging the opening to eliminate the bottleneck and produce a cone-shaped cavity with the base of the cone to the outside can encourage drainage and promote healing. It may be necessary to repeat this procedure several times, so pernicious is the tendency for the outside to heal prematurely. Creation of an adequate opening may require incision posteriorly lateral to the coccyx. Eventually excision of the coccyx may be necessary,[53] and a few cases finally come to a complex tissue transfer procedure involving the rotation of a buttock flap or a composite vascularized pedicle from the leg to close the defect.[14]

One of the most spectacular late complications is the indolent although widespread sepsis in the perineal wound of patients with ulcerative colitis or Crohn's disease. The process acts like hidradenitis suppurativa, with extension of the infection by sinus tract formation through all the tissue planes and spaces of the perineum and pelvis. The only solution is to follow each sinus to its end, laying the entire network open to heal by secondary intention. Povidone-iodine ointment is a much cleaner and less irritating dressing than the saline or hypochlorite solution pads formerly used.

The most unusual late complication we have seen is evisceration of small bowel through a perineum previously healed except for small sinus. Peritonitis did not result, and healing followed packing with dressings soaked in Dakin's solution. Late herniations with rupture have been reported.

PULL-THROUGH OPERATIONS

We have had little experience with pull-through operations for cancer because we believe that malignant tumors below the peritoneal floor should usually be removed by a Miles resection. Pull-through operations are applicable, however, to certain large villous adenomas, and certain low-grade carcinomas, and to congenital megacolon. Pull-through operations are subject to most of the complications of anterior resection and Miles resection plus a few more. Suture techniques are less apt to produce stricture, but retraction, slough, and anastomotic failure are more likely.[61] Fortunately, direct observation of the suture line is often possible, and strictures can be handled by retrograde dilatation. If slough extends back to the suture line, reoperation and colostomy are usually necessary. The treatment of hemorrhage and septic complications is similar to that in anterior resection. Intestinal obstruction is more frequent than with a Miles resection because of the insecurity of the pelvic floor, and reexploration for this cause is not unusual.

Late complications of pull-through operations are suture line recurrence after resection for cancer, and anal incontinence, the reported incidences of which vary widely. Waugh[61] reported an incidence of 10 per cent perfect results, 30 per cent fair, and the rest more or less incontinent. Sloughing of the bowel occurred in 13 per cent. Black's[10] results are considerably better, "endorectal resection" incontinence occurring in only 7 per cent. Again, Black's most serious complications were slough and pelvic abscess. He states that since the advent of suction catheters for drainage, the incidence of pelvic abscess has been reduced from 20 per cent to less than 1 per cent. After pull-through operations mild incontinence can be controlled with perineal pads, and most patients benefit from daily cleansing enemas as with sigmoid colostomy. Some patients are happier if provided with an abdominal rather than a perineal colostomy, because the former is better positioned for convenience in care.

Swenson's operation for megacolon is followed by incontinence in only about 1 per cent of cases in his experience.[56] A more serious complication is enterocolitis, which seems to have a predisposition in similar episodes that occur during the obstructive phase prior to operation. Colitis may be resistant to all forms of therapy and is the leading cause of late postoperative death in Hirschsprung's disease. Impotence following Swenson's operation is reported to be rare, owing to meticulous care in carrying dissection exactly on the surface of the rectum to avoid the nearby nervi erigentes. The procedure advocated by Soave, in which the outermost layer of the rectum is left in situ, may have the advantage that the pelvic nerves are left completely undisturbed. Both end-to-end and Soave type pull-through operations can be performed with the end-to-end or lateral anastomosing staplers. The staggered double row of tiny B-shaped staples is applied with perfect precision and quickly, so that the surgeon's attention may be directed entirely to the important details of blood supply and freedom from tension. Goligher has reported a number of stapled anastomoses done within a few centimeters of the dentate line,[30] and he now prefers the circular stapler over any type of pull-through procedure. At some level, of course, low anastomosis loses practicality, as there is so little rectum remaining that rectal sensation becomes deficient.

D'ALLAINES PROCEDURE

The d'Allaines operation, which consists of an anterior resection and posterior anastomosis, has achieved some popularity because of the excellent exposure for supra-anal anastomosis that is achieved when the area is visualized through a paracoccygeal or coccyx-resecting incision.[18] In a review by Donaldson, Rodkey, and Behringer[19] of 20 operations performed at the Massachusetts General Hospital, only 4 patients escaped without some sort of complication, either early or late (Table 25–3). Although this figure would appear at first discouraging, comparison of Table 25–3 with other tables of complications in this chapter shows that the complication rate is not strikingly higher and that the complications themselves have not been particularly serious. Except for 2 patients who finally did require permanent colostomy after the d'Allaines procedure, all patients have tolerably good bowel function. Localio reported upon 427 cases of low rectal carcinoma managed by low anterior

TABLE 25–3 COMPLICATIONS OF D'ALLAINES PROCEDURE (20 CASES)

Early

Urinary infection	2
Rectovaginal fistula requiring closure	1
Inability to void	1
Requiring TUR	1
Draining sinus—spontaneous closure	3
Wound infection	1
	9

Late

Tenesmus	2
Occasional incontinence	4
Constipation requiring medication	5
Requiring frequent enemas	1
Requiring regular enemas	1
Anal stenosis requiring dilatation	2
Permanent colostomy	2
	17
Patients without significant complication	4

resection, Miles resection, or abdominosacral resection and anastomosis (d'Allaines).[44] There were 100 of the latter procedures done, with a mortality rate of only 2 per cent, which was intermediate between that of the other two procedures. There was no significant difference in recurrence rate between the abdominosacral resections and the Miles resections for comparable lesions, and Localio believes that ASR permitted permanent preservation of anal continence in over 50 per cent of patients who would otherwise have required a colostomy.[43] From this point of view the final results are comparable with those of pull-through or other operations that have been devised for low anastomosis.

OPERATIONS FOR RECTAL PROLAPSE

The various operations devised for correction of rectal prolapse are directed at the three structural abnormalities characteristic of this disease: the dilated lax perianal musculature, the excessively long pelvic colon, and the poor fixation of the pelvic colon. Simple rectosigmoid resection with deep presacral dissection usually produces enough shortening and fixation to alleviate the prolapse; the complications are identical to those attendant on any rectal resection. Failure to correct the prolapse is a complication that may require additional surgery to narrow the aperture through the perianal musculature. The installation of a Thiersch wire may result in infection or slough, both of which require removal of the wire. Perineorrhaphy carries a high failure rate due to sepsis, although meticulous technique and appropriate use of topical and systemic antibiotics can reduce that rate to an acceptable level. Probably the most popular operation for prolapse today is the Ripstein procedure, in which a band of Teflon felt is used to suspend the rectosigmoid at the pelvic brim.[21, 46] Like the older Moskowitz and similar suspensory procedures, the sutures are not supposed to enter the bowel lumen, and septic complication can result if they do. In addition, sepsis in the Ripstein procedure leads to infection of the Teflon, requiring its removal. If the sling is placed too tightly the bowel may become obstructed, or the sling may cause pressure necrosis with sloughing into the lumen of the bowel. Sometimes redundant sigmoid will angulate across a sling that appears correctly placed, again causing obstruction of the bowel, which may rapidly necrose at the angle where it is stretched over the sling. Late stricture at this level occurs in about 6 per cent of cases.[32] Most of these complications will require removal of the mesh and opening of a defunctioning colostomy at a minimum.[42] Removal of the redundant sigmoid at the same time has a good chance of preventing recurrent prolapse, as mentioned above. Local conditions will determine whether end sigmoid colostomy with anastomosis or sigmoid anastomosis with or without transverse colostomy should be done.

COMPLICATIONS OF SEGMENTAL RESECTIONS OF THE COLON

Resections of the sigmoid for carcinoma in the series reviewed by us carried a surprisingly high incidence of complications, as seen in Figure 25–1. Diagnosis and treatment have been discussed earlier, but the high rate of postoperative difficulty requires explanation, especially in relation to left colectomy, complications of which were unexpectedly somewhat less frequent. We have theorized that several important factors may be operative here: (1) poor-risk patients are apt to have less extensive resection; (2) incurable patients also are apt to have the lesser procedure; (3) diverticula at the anastomosis are more likely with limited resection; (4) tension may be greater when the surgeon hopes to avoid stepping down the splenic flexure; (5) blood supply to the left transverse colon is often better than that to the upper sigmoid; (6) resection of rectum down to spurting blood vessels may be practiced more faithfully if the surgeon is unconcerned about having sufficient bowel to reach; and (7) the lesser resection is perhaps performed more frequently by surgeons of lesser experience. The apparent paradox in the increased incidence of complications in sigmoid resection or left colectomy may be most important, however, because it emphasizes the numerous details of good technique so necessary to successful colonic surgery.

Left colectomy carries the additional hazards of injury to the spleen, left ureteral injury, and bleeding from the colonic bed in the left gutter. These complications are more likely in resections for diverticulitis in which cleavage planes are obscured by inflammatory edema, or the mesosigmoid may be shortened by postinflammatory fibrosis. Frequently, the damage to the ureter is inflicted at a point distant from the place where it is first observed. Certain identification of the ureter before each pair of clamps is applied should avoid injury to the ureter. When the ureter is divided cleanly it may be repaired with interrupted sutures of 6-0 catgut over a 5 or 6 French ureteral catheter splint, the lower end of which is passed down into the bladder for later retrieval. A lateral laceration of the ureter may be repaired without splinting, but the tip of a drain should be placed near the repair. When a segment of ureter is lost, repair will involve retroperitoneal transfer to the right ureter or creation of a bladder tube, and these rather complex urological procedures should be carried out immediately.

In right colectomy there is risk of injury to the duodenum and superior mesenteric vessels. In addition, small bowel fistulization occurs with surprising frequency as a result of anastomotic failure. One can only assume a somewhat overconfident attitude on the part of the surgeon in some of these cases, because anastomotic failure should be practically unknown after this easy anastomosis. In extended right colectomy, when the middle colic vessel is taken at its origin, some difficulty may be encountered with anastomosis between the ileum and the left side of the transverse colon. The necessary mesenteric closure may result in torsion or compression of the bowel. If this occurs, there should be no hesitancy in resecting more colon so that an ileosigmoid colostomy may be performed in more favorable anatomic circumstances.

Operations for volvulus are generally done on patients of advanced age in whom the bowel is dilated, friable, and edematous as a result of obstruction. Recurrent volvulus is common, however, unless cecostomy, right colectomy, or sigmoid resection can be carried out. Often the safest course is exteriorization of the affected sigmoid loop, which is easy in the presence of the usual redundancy. In our experience primary resection and anastomosis have proven safe, provided the serosal sutures are tied with the greatest care. Otherwise anastomotic breakdown is a hazard in these debilitated patients. The Mikulicz resection, which is occasionally elected in this situation, carries certain special risks, most of which can be avoided by careful approximation of the two limbs by interrupted sutures. The area of approximation should be deep enough so that small bowel has no chance of being pinched by the tip of the spur-crushing clamp, and the area should be broad enough so that free perforation does not occur when the clamp cuts through. With proper attention to detail the operation is usually more difficult than primary anastomosis, and it is seldom used.

COMPLICATIONS OF TOTAL AND SUBTOTAL COLECTOMY

Total and subtotal colectomy for ulcerative colitis are hazardous operations because of the poor condition of these patients, not only because of the effects of their disease, but also because of steroid treatment. Ulcerative colitis produces changes in liver, skin, and other organs that can adversely affect recuperative ability. In addition, there seems to be an almost specific defect in the ability to heal wounds, as observed most obviously in the delayed healing of the perineal wounds in these patients as compared with patients who have had rectal resection for carcinoma, for example. Furthermore, many of the sickest patients have been treated vigorously with steroids in a desperate attempt to avoid colectomy. Controlled studies are practically impossible because they would involve a decision to withhold steroids from some patients, randomly selected. It is the clinical impression of many surgeons, however, that patients treated with steroids tend to have more postoperative complications than would be expected. Shock after operation is attributed to adrenal insufficiency and responds to intravenous administration of glucocorticoids. Hayes[35] recommends that any patient who has ever been treated with steroids or ACTH be prepared for operation with steroids and weaned gradually after opera-

tion. We usually use hydrocortisone, 100 mg., intravenously during operation, and start weaning immediately from a dose of about 200 mg. a day to terminate in about 2 weeks. The fact that adrenal suppression seems to persist to some extent for years after steroid treatment suggests that the delayed wound healing observed may be partially caused by subclinical adrenal insufficiency.

Shock in the early postoperative phase should be presumed first to be due to hypovolemia and should be treated with rapid transfusion of blood. If no response is obtained after one or two units (in the absence of observable bleeding), then hydrocortisone should be given intravenously, 50 to 100 mg. directly and 100 mg. in a slow drip. Of course the equivalent of prednisolone, dexamethasone, or other steroid may be used equally well.

Toxic megacolon presents special problems because of the very poor general condition of these patients, the frequency of undiagnosed perforation, the friable condition of the colon, the impossibility of preparing the bowel, the copious liquid content of the colon, and the high risk of manipulative rupture of the bowel. Massive contamination can be avoided by evacuating the colon through a previously placed large bore rectal tube after the abdomen is opened. By working slowly and carefully, the colonic contents can be milked down to the tube, which should be blunt-tipped with numerous extra holes cut in the side. Such evacuation, by reducing the pressure in the bowel, the quantity in the lumen, and the tension in the wall greatly reduces the risk of the sudden, massive contamination that is a virtual certainty if one attempts to mobilize the full colon. The high mortality rate after resection for toxic megacolon caused Turnbull to develop the blowhole procedure, in which no mobilization of the bowel is done, but it is simply evacuated through openings made in the most prominent loops, with circumferential suturing of each colotomy to its overlying peritoneal opening. Colectomy is done later as a semielective procedure when the patient's general condition has improved.[58]

Hemorrhage from the pelvis is more likely after rectal resection for colitis because of the increased vascularity associated with the disease and because dissection in the male is carried as close as possible to the rectum rather than in the avascular plane of the presacral space. The treatment, however, is the same as discussed under Miles resection, with the exception that ligation of the hypogastric arteries is to be avoided in sexually active males.

When the rectum is relatively uninvolved by disease, subtotal colectomy is sometimes recommended so that later ileorectal anastomosis may be considered. If the rectal stump is turned in, harboring disease within it, dehiscence of the suture line may occur, with disastrous consequences. If the rectum is turned in, the anal sphincter must be widely sectioned for drainage, a maneuver that offers adequate protection against infection. In the young male, subtotal colectomy with preservation of a short rectal stump has other complication-averting advantages: a difficult pelvic dissection is avoided; the pelvic peritoneal closure is better supported and more secure; and the nearby innervation of the sexual apparatus is not endangered. In a personal series of such cases, Hedberg has subsequently excised the rectal mucosa from below, with preservation of the anal sphincter through dissection in a submucosal plane. In 14 consecutive patients there were no complications from this minor procedure, and only 3 or 4 days of hospitalization were required in most cases.

A frequent complication after colectomy for ulcerative colitis is small bowel obstruction from abscess or adhesions. The diagnosis may be fairly obvious because the possibilities are limited, owing to absence of the colon, the omentum, and any anastomosis. Early reoperation is the preferred treatment; lysis of adhesions usually suffices, but all peritoneal closures should be inspected for possible defects in need of repair. Only frank abscesses should be drained because of the danger of causing small bowel adhesions to a drain tract.

Late complications of total or subtotal colectomy are concerned mostly with the ileostomy, but obstructions due to adhesions continue to appear with ever decreasing frequency as the years pass after operation.[63] A retained rectum is subject to late complications, the most significant of which is carcinoma that may pass undetected be-

cause atrophic stenosis prevents inspection by sigmoidoscopy or barium enema. Persistent colitis, with passage of small amounts of mucus and blood, is common, and certainly these symptoms contraindicate ileoproctostomy. If ileoproctostomy cannot be carried out within a year or two, then the rectum should be removed, because the symptoms of continuing low-grade proctitis mimic exactly those of carcinoma. In a significant number of patients colitis recurs after ileoproctostomy; in addition, of course, in these patients the rectum must be inspected frequently for the development of a carcinoma even if colitis does not recur.[65] In our own practice ileoproctostomy is successful so infrequently and the complications of the retained rectum are so common that we almost always perform total colectomy except in special circumstances.

COMPLICATIONS OF ILEOSTOMY

The complications of ileostomy are the legacy of colonic surgery, and the striking reduction in the incidence of complications after ileostomy is the result of increased experience with total and subtotal colectomy. Loop ileostomy, rarely performed now, used to be done frequently to defunction the colon prior to resection. Obstruction, electrolyte imbalance, and progression of disease in the colon followed so often that primary resection increased in popularity. Here too, however, complications of terminal ileostomy were originally very common.

In a review of 210 ileostomies done before 1951, Warren and McKittrick[59] found an incidence of ileostomy dysfunction of 62 per cent. Dysfunction, or stomal obstruction, is characterized by crampy pain, profuse ileac discharge, and later distention with vomiting. When an obstructive picture is not preceded by profuse discharge, proximal obstruction is suspected, and the same is true if stomal intubation fails to produce a gush of thin intestinal juice. Enterocolitis, of course, must also be considered in the differential diagnosis, and excluded by appropriate study.

Several refinements of technique have resulted in diminution in the incidence of dysfunction.[25] The frequency of "backwash ileitis" suggested that resection of 6 to 8

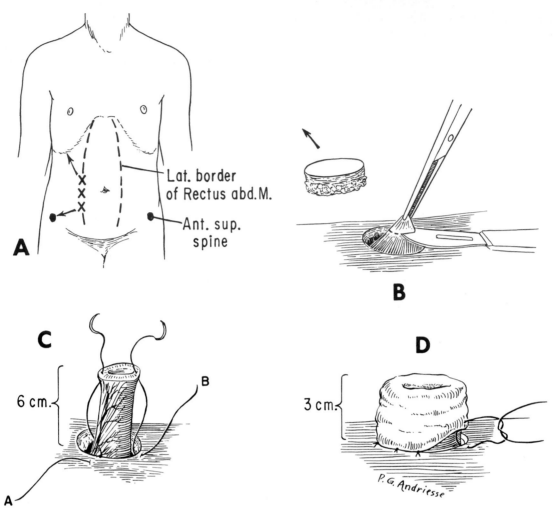

Figure 25–7 *A,* Some patients present considerable latitude in selection of a site for ileostomy (X-X-X), while in others the iliac crest and costal margin are so close to each other and to the lateral border of the rectus muscle that only one spot may be suitable. *B,* A simple stab wound is inadequate for ileostomy. Buttons of skin and fascia must be excised if the incidence of stricture is to be kept at a minimum. *C,* The Brooke mucocutaneous suture does *not* maintain eversion of the ileal bud because the serosa is avoided. Brooke allows placement of a serosal anchoring suture only at the mesenteric border. Primarily, however, eversion depends upon having an adequate length of ileum outside the skin. *D,* The completed ileostomy bud should measure 2.5 to 3.0 cm. in length; whether it will then shorten, lengthen, or remain the same length is unpredictable in an individual case.

inches of terminal ileum should be carried out in continuity with colectomy. Kinking of the prestomal ileum is avoided by careful adjustment of the intraperitoneal segment. Internal herniation lateral to the ileostomy is prevented by careful approximation of ileal mesentery to parietal peritoneum with interrupted sutures. Non-absorbable sutures are used because healing in patients with ulcerative colitis is apt to be slow, and catgut has been observed to dissolve before the mesentery has become sufficiently fixed

to the lateral abdominal wall. Closure of all raw areas is probably unnecessary and may actually promote adhesion formation in some manner.

Perhaps the most important technique developed to discourage dysfunction is the formation of the ileal "bud" by means of the Brooke mucocutaneous eversion stitch[11] (Fig. 25–7). This method, if successfully performed, prevents not only stricture and dysfunction, but also retraction and, to some extent, prolapse and skin irritation.

Among ileostomy patients seen in our Gastrointestinal Followup Unit, it is estimated that 90 per cent of the appliance and skin problems would have been avoided if the patients had at least ½ inch of ileum projecting above the skin level.

Ileostomy stricture at the skin level also occurs when there is insufficient projection of the bud. Excision of a crescentic segment of adjacent skin and mucocutaneous suture in the wider aperture is effective in some cases, but because skin irritation is likely to continue, a new stricture is the common result. It is better, therefore, once it is decided that reoperation is necessary, to free the ileum completely down through the fascia or peritoneal level and refashion an ileal bud by means of the Brooke technique. Stricture at the peritoneal level rarely occurs but is likely to occur at the external oblique fascia unless a button of this structure is excised originally. Further excision of fascia may be necessary if fascial stricture is symptomatic, i.e., produces the dysfunction syndrome.

When dysfunction is established, ileal serositis and edema tend to worsen the condition until complete obstruction occurs. Before the days of the Brooke technique simple incision of the "bishop's collar" that surrounded the maturing ileostomy would relieve nearly all patients and allow proper healing (Fig. 25–8). In other instances the terminal ileum may be put to rest by intubation and drainage, and resolution of the process usually follows. Later stages in which proximal dilatation has occurred must be treated like frank obstruction with nasogastric intubation and all other ancillary measures. Reoperation is rarely necessary, but sometimes terminal ileum must be resected in patients with recurring or unremitting disease. Unrelieved dysfunction may eventuate in perforation of the distended terminal ileum.

Prolapse is sometimes treatable by a fairly simple procedure involving further resection and construction of an everted button. An intraperitoneal procedure may be required ultimately, however, if the difficulty stems from imperfect fixation of the terminal ileum and its mesentery. Retraction almost always requires laparotomy and complete revision.

Other complications of ileostomy include

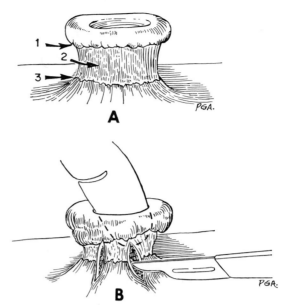

Figure 25–8 *A,* The maturing ileostomy shows advancing mucosa *(1),* granulation tissue overlying serosa *(2),* and advancing skin *(3).* Stricture may result from circumferential contraction of this zone of healing producing a deformity likened to a "bishop's collar." *B,* With a finger palpating the interior of the ileum, the obstructive narrowing is corrected by radial incisions into the constricting collar. The greatest care is necessary in avoiding full-thickness injury to the bowel.

fistula, paraileostomy hernia, and dermatitis. Fistulas occurred in 7 per cent of 139 patients reviewed by Wheelock and Warren.[67] Superficial fistulas may be caused by placement of a serosal bite in construction of the ileostomy bud. Brooke therefore recommends that only one anchoring suture be used, and that that one be placed through the mesentery (see Fig. 25–7).[11] Unification of the two openings by cutting the mucosal bridge is sufficient for cure of superficial fistulas, but the bud effect is thereby lost in this area, and dermatitis may be the result. Fistulas arising below the skin level tend to have more than one opening or tract and generally are not cured by techniques short of resection. They may be caused by placement of fixation sutures from serosa to peritoneum, so that this technique, necessary for some colostomies, is to be avoided in construction of an ileostomy.

Paraileostomy hernia can result from excision of a peritoneal button, which is always unnecessary, since the opening need be large enough only to permit the insertion of a finger tip beside the exteriorized ileum. Repair of a paraileostomy hernia after colectomy is indicated because it contains small intestine that may incarcerate. Recurrence and fistula formation are hazards after repair, which, if performed in a contaminated field, require that absorbable sutures be used. A more secure repair can be done with monofilamentous polypropylene, approaching the hernia from within the belly via a separate incision made at a distance from the stoma.

Digestive dermatitis is the inevitable sequel of contact between ileal content and skin. Many ingenious devices have been invented to prevent leakage, but the most effective means yet discovered depends on the construction of a proper stoma in the correct position. Pitfalls in placement of the stoma include a tendency to use McBurney's point, which, in thin patients, usually puts the stoma uncomfortably close to the iliac crest. In many thin patients the stoma should be opposite the umbilicus or even a little higher and as close to the umbilicus as the proposed bag will permit (but the ileum should always be brought out lateral to the rectus muscle). In fat patients, on the other hand, an even greater problem is encountered because the position of the stoma varies so much from the erect to the recumbent position. It is a good idea to mark the most convenient site on the abdominal wall of a fat patient while he is standing up.

Formerly many patients had a dermatitis in the early days after operation, and the skin problem remained the only complication to delay the patient's discharge from the hospital. This train of events is prevented now by the immediate application of a self-adherent plastic disposable ileostomy bag in which the aperture is custom-tailored to the stoma. Nurse-practitioners involved in enterostomal therapy can contribute a great deal in preoperative teaching and help in selecting the stoma site, and the enterostomal therapist can manage the day-to-day care of the postoperative stoma as well. Following discharge from the hospital almost all of our patients are followed by their therapist in our stoma clinic.

As implied earlier, the perfect ileostomy bud rarely, if ever, gives trouble, but in case of dermatitis several non-operative techniques are useful before resorting to revision of the stoma. First of all, the opening of the disk and its surface should be checked for size and contour. Both stomas and patients are apt to change in size and shape in the first months after ileostomy, and it is routine to have to send for new disks to compensate. Early dermatitis is usually corrected easily by some such simple mechanical adjustment, but in careless patients or patients with massive diarrhea the condition of the skin may be such that the appliance is floated away by serum almost as soon as it is glued in place.

In these difficult cases we have found karaya powder to be indispensable. It may be dusted over the raw, weeping areas until an adherent protective gum is formed, and then the appliance may be glued on as usual. Or, by mixing powder and water, a thick paste can be blended from which one can mold a karaya gum doughnut over which the appliance is pressed. Within the past few years disposable appliances incorporating karaya-gelatin rings have become available. The temporary use of these bags may be followed by prompt healing of the skin.

Sometimes the skin is so sensitive that the slightest contact of ileal content prevents healing, or infection requires the application of ultraviolet light or ointments to the skin. In these cases ileal discharge is kept away from the skin either by a sump suction device or by positioning the patient face down for a few days on a special bed that has a hole in the mattress. Suction catheters should be used with great care not to cause perforation or fistulization of the ileum. Once the skin is healed, the permanent ileostomy bag should again be given a trial, perferably for a few additional days in the hospital.

The construction of a continent ileostomy can avoid many of the problems discussed, albeit with the introduction of some new problems unique to the Kock pouch.[8, 39] The details of operation are still undergoing modification at this time in efforts to avoid some of the more frequent complications such as slippage of the inverted ileal nipple. A collective review of 479 patients by Goldman revealed that 82 to 95 per cent of patients ultimately achieved continence, but reoperation was necessary in 99 patients.[27] Because a few complications of continent ileostomy, such as volvulus or leakage from the pouch, may be fatal, the procedure should not be attempted on patients who are acutely ill or depleted at the time of their colectomy. If the procedure were reserved for the less than 10 per cent of ileostomy patients who are dissatisfied with their Brooke ileostomy to the extent of wishing a continent revision, then the mortality rate for continent ileostomies would immediately be reduced by a factor of 10, not even considering the improved overall status of the patient presenting for elective revision.

Other complications of the continent ileostomy have been dermatitis from leakage, perforation with the catheter and ileitis of the reservoir. Some of these complications can be diagnosed endoscopically with the colonoscope.

Skin problems will continue to plague some patients for as long as they live, but all eventually reach some sort of symbiosis with their stomas; we have never seen a patient permanently crippled by an ileostomy. Before leaving this subject, however, we would be remiss not to mention what for many patients has been the single most important factor in rehabilitation, the Ostomy Clubs. These organizations, all of whose members have ileostomies or colostomies, are distributed widely throughout the United States and abroad. The function of these clubs is to provide information and psychologic support for members, particularly neophytes, and the club is often able to help in a way no physician can.[41] The Ostomy Association of Boston has published a classic manual for the ileostomy patient that has enjoyed worldwide distribution.[37] This booklet should be read by every surgeon, internist, and ileostomy patient.

Bibliography

1. Aguirre, A., Fischer, J. E., and Welch, C. E.: The role of surgery and hyperalimentation in the therapy of gastrointestinal-cutaneous fistulas. Ann. Surg. *189*:393, 1974.
2. Allen, A. W., and Welch, C. E.: Cecostomy. Surg. Gynecol. Obstet. *73*:549, 1941.
3. Altemeier, W. A.: Discussion of paper by Clarke, J. S., et al.: Preoperative oral antibiotics reduce septic complications of colon operations: Results of prospective randomized double-blind clinical study. Ann. Surg. *186*:251, 1977.
4. Altemeier, W. A., et al.: Primary closure and healing of the perineal wound in abdomino-perineal resection of the rectum for carcinoma. Am. J. Surg. *127*:215, 1974.
5. Anderson, R.: The dilemma of Crohn's disease: Management of the posterior wound after colo-proctectomy. Dis. Colon Rectum *20*:393, 1977.
6. Baker, J. W., and Ritter, K. J.: Complete surgical decompression for late obstruction of small intestine, with reference to method. Ann. Surg. *157*:759, 1963.
7. Baker, J. W.: Selective usage of the original and modified Baker intestinal tube. Surg. Gynecol. Obstet. *149*:577, 1979.
8. Beart, R. W., Beahrs, O. H., Kelly, K. A., Dozois, R. R., and Wolf, S. A.: The continent ileostomy. A viable alternative. Mayo Clin. Proc. *54*:643, 1979.
9. Berliner, S. D., Burson, L. D., and Lear, P. E.: Use and abuse of intraperitoneal drains in colon surgery. Arch. Surg. *89*:686, 1964.
10. Black, B. M.: Combined abdomino-endorectal resection. *In* Turell, R. (Ed.): Diseases of the Colon and Anorectum. 2nd Ed. Philadelphia, W. B. Saunders Company, 1969, pp. 555–559.
11. Brooke, B. N.: The management of an ileostomy, including its complications. Cancer *2*:102, 1952.
12. Burke, J. F., Pontoppidan, H., and Welch, C. E.: High output respiratory failure. Ann. Surg. *158*:581, 1963.
13. Clarke, J. S., Condon, R. E., et al.: Preoperative oral antibiotics reduce septic complications of colon operations: Results of prospective randomized double-blind clinical study. Ann. Surg. *186*:251, 1977.
14. Cohen, B. E., et al.: Gracilis muscle flap for closure of the persistent perineal sinus. Surg. Gynecol. Obstet. *148*:33, 1979.
15. Cohn, I., Jr.: Intestinal antisepsis. Dis. Colon Rectum *8*:11, 1965.
16. Condon, R. E.: Discussion of paper by Clarke. Ann. Surg. *186*:251, 1977.
17. Condon, R. E., et al.: Preoperative prophylactic cephalothin fails to control septic complications of colorectal operations: Results of a controlled clinical trial. Am. J. Surg. *137*:68, 1979.
18. D'Allaines, F.: Traitment chirurgical du cancer du rectum. Paris, Editions Medicales Flammarion, 1946.
19. Donaldson, G. A., Rodkey, G. V., and Behringer, G. E.: Resection of the rectum with anal preservation. Surg. Gynecol Obstet. *123*:571, 1966.
20. Edmunds, L. H., Williams, G. M., and Welch, C. E.: External fistulas arising from the gastrointestinal tract. Ann. Surg. *152*:445, 1960.
21. Eisenstat, T. E., et al: Surgical treatment of complete rectal prolapse. Dis. Colon Rectum *22*:522, 1979.
22. Eykyn, S. J., et al.: Prophylactic perioperative intravenous metronidazole in elective colorectal surgery. Lancet *2*:761, 1979.
23. Fischer, J. E.: Parenteral and enteral nutrition. DM *24*:1, 1978.
24. Floyd, C. E., Corley, R. G., and Cohn, I., Jr.: Local recurrence of carcinoma of the colon and rectum. Am. J. Surg. *109*:153, 1965.
25. Garlock, J. H., and Kirschner, P. A.: Prevention of ileostomy dysfunction. Surgery *40*:678, 1956.
26. Goldfarb, W. B., Monafo, W., and McAlister, W. H.: Clinical value of fistulography. Am. J. Surg. *108*:902, 1964.
27. Goldman, S. E., et al.: The continent ileostomy: A

collective review. Dis. Colon Rectum *21*:594, 1978.

28. Goldsmith, H. S.: Control of viscerocutaneous fistulas by a new suction device. N. Engl. J. Med. *265*:1052, 1961.

29. Goligher, J. C., et al.: A controlled comparison of one- and two-layer techniques of suture for high and low colorectal anastomoses. Br. J. Surg. *64*:609, 1977.

30. Goligher, J. C.: Use of circular stapling gun with perianal insertion of anorectal purse string suture for construction of very low colorectal or colo-anal anastomoses. Br. J. Surg. *66*:501, 1979.

31. Goligher, J. C., et al.: Experience with the Russian model 249 suture gun for anastomosis of the rectum. Surg. Gynecol. Obstet. *148*:516, 1979.

32. Gordon, P. H., et al.: Complications of the Ripstein procedure. Dis. Colon Rectum *21*:277, 1978.

33. Green, W. W., and Blank, W. A.: Colostomy perforations by the irrigating tip. Dis. Colon Rectum *8*:59, 1965.

34. Hartz, R. S., et al.: Healing of the perineal wound. Arch. Surg. *115*:471, 1980.

35. Hayes, M. A.: Surgical treatment as complicated by prior adrenocortical steroid therapy. Surgery *40*:945, 1956.

36. Hedberg, S. E., and Welch, C. E.: Complications following surgery of the colon. Surg. Clin. North Am. *43*:775, 1963.

37. Ileostomy-A Guide. United Ostomy Assoc. Inc. 1974.

38. Khubchandani, I. T., and Bacon, H. E.: Bilateral hypogastric arterial ligation in abdominoperineal rectal excision. Pennsylvania Med. J. *68*:25, 1965.

39. Kock, N. G., et al: Ileostomy. Curr. Probl. Surg. *14*:1, 1977.

40. Lahiry, S., and Hedberg, S. E.: Fiberoptic colonoscopy and polypeptomy complications and their management. Dig. Dis. Week Abstr., 1978.

41. Lenneberg, E.: QT Boston — An ileostomy group. N. Engl. J. Med. *251*:1008, 1954.

42. Lescher, J. J., et al.: Management of late complications of Teflon sling repair for rectal prolapse. Dis. Colon Rectum *22*:445, 1979.

43. Localio, S. A., et al.: Abdominosacral resection for carcinoma of the mid-rectum: Ten years experience. Ann. Surg. *188*:475, 1978.

44. Localio, S. A., et al.: Sphincter-saving operations for cancer of the rectum. N. Engl. J. Med. *300*:1028, 1979.

45. McKittrick, L. S.: The surgeon's bib. Surg. Gynecol. Obstet. *99*:374, 1954.

46. Miller, R. L.: Ripstein procedure for rectal prolapse. Am. Surg. *45*:531, 1979.

47. Moore, F. D.: Discussion of paper by Edmunds et al. Ann. Surg. *152*:470, 1960.

48. Poth, E. J.: The role of intestinal antisepsis in preoperative preparation of the colon. Surgery *47*:1018, 1960.

49. Quill, J. R.: Side-to-side colorectal anastomosis with monofilament stainless steel wire. Arch. Surg. *138*:104, 1979.

50. Salzman, E. W., Harris, W. H., and DeSanctis, R. W.: Reduction in venous thromboembolism by agents affecting platelet function. N. Engl. J. Med. *284*:1287, 1971.

51. Schapira, A. H. V., and Dyson, P. H. P.: Vancomycin dose for pseudomembranous colitis. Lancet *2*:204, 1980.

52. Shear, L., Shinaberger, J. H., and Barry, K. G.: Peritoneal transport of antibiotics in man. N. Engl. J. Med. *272*:666, 1965.

53. Silen, W., and Glotzer, D.: The prevention and treatment of persistent perineal sinus. Surgery *75*:535, 1974.

54. Speare, G. S.: Staphylococcus pseudomembranous enterocolitis, a complication of antibiotic therapy. Am. J. Surg. *88*:523, 1954.

55. Stuart, M., et al.: Prophylactic use of low-dose heparin in colorectal surgery. Dis. Colon Rectum *28*:487, 1978.

56. Swenson, I.: Follow-up on 200 patients treated for Hirschsprung's disease during a ten-year period. Ann. Surg. *146*:706, 1957.

57. Thorlakson, R. H.: Technique of repair of herniations associated with colonic stomas. Surg. Gynecol. Obstet. *120*:347, 1965.

58. Turnbull, R. B., Jr., Hawk, W. A., and Weakley, F. L.: Surgical treatment of toxic megacolon: Ileostomy and colostomy to prepare patients for colectomy. Am. J. Surg. *122*:325, 1971.

59. Warren, R., and McKittrick, L. S.: Ileostomy for ulcerative colitis: Technique, complications and management. Surg. Gynecol Obstet. *93*:555, 1951.

60. Warshaw, A. L., et al.: Primary perineal closure after proctocolectomy for IBD. Am. J. Surg. *133*:414, 1977.

61. Waugh, J. M., and Turner, J. C., Jr.: Abdominoperineal resection, with preservation of the anal sphincter, for carcinoma of the midrectum. *In* Turell, R. (Ed.): Diseases of the Colon and Anorectum. 2nd Ed. Philadelphia, W. B. Saunders Company, 1969, pp. 560–570.

62. Welch, C. E.: Treatment of combined intestinal obstruction and peritonitis by refunctionalization of the intestine. Ann. Surg. *142*:739, 1955.

63. Welch, C. E.: Intestinal Obstruction. Chicago, Year Book Medical Publishers, 1958.

64. Welch, C. E., and Burke, J. F.: Carcinoma of the colon and rectum. N. Engl. J. Med. *266*:211, 1962.

65. Welch, C. E., and Hedberg, S. E.: Colonic cancer in ulcerative colitis and idiopathic colonic cancer. J.A.M.A. *191*:815, 1965.

66. Wheeler, M. H., and Barker, J.: Closure of colostomy — a safe procedure ? Dis. Colon Rectum *20*:29, 1977.

67. Wheelock, F. C., Jr., and Warren, R.: Ulcerative colitis. N. Engl. J. Med. *252*:421, 1955.

68. Yajko, R. D., et al.: Morbidity of colostomy closure. Am. J. Surg. *132*:304, 1976.

GENERAL

Adson, M. A., and Waugh, J. M.: Complications of Surgery of the Large Intestine, Including Ileostomy. In Artz, C. P., and Hardy, J. D., eds: *Complications in Surgery and Their Management*. Philadelphia, W. B. Saunders Company, 1961, pp. 764–99.

26

COMPLICATIONS OF GASTROINTESTINAL SURGERY IN INFANCY

Richard C. Miller

Like all complications, those following gastrointestinal surgery in the newborn are best avoided. The skill of the physician in diagnosis, surgical technique, and patient management is of particular importance in the care of the neonatal infant, where there is little room for error, little time for secondary procedures, and lesser patient reserves to withstand excessive surgical trauma, infection, or inadequate nutrition (Fig. 26–1). Because newborn intestinal surgery may carry an increased risk when compared with similar procedures in the adult, the surgeon may be tempted to delay operation, only to further lessen the patient's chances for survival. One should be aware of the distinction between procrastination (the patient's overall condition cannot be expected to improve with time and may actually worsen) and delay with good reason (the patient may be a better candidate for operation at a later time, and there is not undue risk of deterioration with delay). Beyond the time needed for repair of water and electrolyte deficits, restoration of blood volume, and treatment of sepsis, little benefit is gained by additional delay.

Consideration must always be given before and after operation to other neonatal problems that may be present but that are not directly related to the surgical diagnosis. These problems, although often medical in nature, may be accentuated by the surgical lesion and its attendant sequelae — fluid and electrolyte imbalance, operative trauma, and administration of anesthetic agents. Of concern are those abnormalities relating to prematurity, respiratory distress syndrome, abnormal cardiovascular function, neonatal hyperbilirubinemia, hypoglycemia, hypothermia, and associated congenital anomalies. If the need for surgical intervention is not urgent and if delay will not, as far as can be predicted, produce untoward results, it may be preferable to wait until the medical problem is corrected. For example, hyperbilirubinemia in the premature infant may require early exchange transfusion to prevent kernicterus. Similarly, preoperative treatment of respiratory distress secondary to hyaline membrane disease or to aspiration pneumonitis will improve the patient's chances for survival. Although in such conditions as lower intestinal obstruction, Hirschsprung's disease with enterocolitis, and perforations of the gastrointestinal tract, delay of surgery may be contraindicated, upper gastrointestinal obstruction at the

---

Richard Charles Miller, a native of Connecticut, was graduated from Harvard College and Harvard Medical School. He served his internship and surgical residency at the University Hospitals of Cleveland and later was Fellow in Pediatric Surgery at the Royal Children's Hospital in Melbourne, Victoria, Australia. He is currently Chief of Pediatric Surgery at the University of Mississippi Medical Center and Professor of Pediatric Surgery and Associate Dean of the School of Medicine. His special interests have been in gastrointestinal surgery of the newborn, nutrition, and medical education.

INFANT   CHILD   ADULT

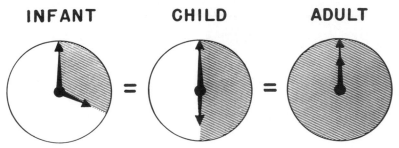

Figure 26–1   Requirements for fluids, electrolytes, and calories per kilogram of body weight demand close attention and frequent reevaluation in all infant patients. Metabolic turnover is such that 4 hours in an infant is equivalent to 6 hours in an older child and to 12 hours in an adult. (From Clatworthy, H. W., Jr.: Complications of gastrointestinal surgery in infancy. *In* Artz, C. P., and Hardy, J. D.: Complications in Surgery and Their Management. 2nd Ed. Philadelphia, W. B. Saunders Company, 1967.)

duodenal or high jejunal levels may be temporarily managed by nasogastric tube decompression for several days. During this interval other entities may be treated so that the patient will be in the best possible condition for operation. In no other age group must the surgeon be so acutely aware of multiple disorders requiring simultaneous treatment and vigilance.

In the over-all management of the neonatal surgical patient, too much emphasis cannot be placed upon the importance of the neonatal intensive care unit. It is these units with their highly trained neonatologists and nursing staffs that have been in large measure responsible for the recent decline in neonatal mortality rates, especially in infants with marked prematurity, respiratory distress, and multiple organ disease. A medical-surgical team approach in the neonatal intensive care unit is to be highly recommended. Although ultimate responsibility for the patient's welfare must reside with one service or the other, an atmosphere of congenial cooperation with frequent consultation is essential to provision of the best care.

The surgeon must be aware that the pathologic processes likely to be seen in the infant are for the most part different from those seen in older children and adults. The large majority of neonatal gastrointestinal problems are congenital and include such entities as atresias, malrotation with or without midgut volvulus, congenital aganglionosis of the colon (Hirschsprung's disease), meconium plug syndrome, meconium ileus, peritoneal bands, and other lesions. Pyloric stenosis is usually encountered in infants a

few weeks of age, whereas idiopathic intussusception has its peak incidence at 5 to 10 months. Except in rare instances, neoplasms do not, as in the adult, involve the gastrointestinal tract. Abdominal neoplasms in the pediatric age group are mainly sarcomatous or teratogenic in nature and are usually retroperitoneal, or, when intraperitoneal, most often involve the liver or ovaries. The gastrointestinal tract may be pushed aside by large bulky abdominal neoplasms, but invasion or obstruction of the intestine does not usually result except as a manifestation of end-stage disease. Perforation of the intestine is not uncommon in infancy and may result from a variety of causes. Complications of neonatal surgery may be expected to be less when the surgeon is prepared, by training and experience, to handle unusual congenital lesions as they are encountered.

SPECIFIC COMPLICATIONS

Distention

When a thoracoabdominal x-ray of an infant with abdominal distention is reviewed, the relatively small thoracic volume compared with that of the abdomen is easily appreciated (Fig. 26–2). Furthermore, when it is realized that the infant relies almost entirely upon diaphragmatic motion for respiration, the deleterious effects of uncontrolled abdominal distention are apparent. Increased intra-abdominal pressure may seriously compromise the tidal volume, which in a small infant may normally be only 15 to 20 cc.

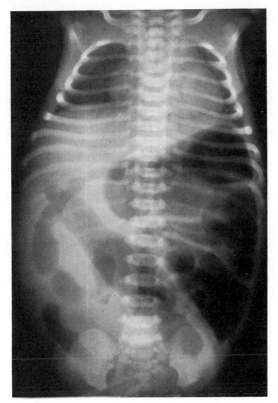

Figure 26–2 Abdominal distention in an infant may produce serious encroachment upon the thoracic volume. The relatively large size of the abdomen is illustrated in this film from an infant with meconium ileus.

NASOGASTRIC DECOMPRESSION. Decompression of the stomach by a nasogastric tube may also effectively evacuate the upper small bowel, particularly when congenital high intestinal obstruction has left the pylorus open and incompetent. A multi-holed plastic catheter (8 or 10 F) may be passed readily via a naris into the stomach of nearly all infants and attached to gentle intermittent or continuous suction. It is a rare infant whose nose is so small that a 5 F catheter will be needed. It has been our experience that pediatric sump catheters work poorly because of the small size of the lumen. Infants are obligate nose breathers and thus one of the nares must always be left clear.

Complications due to malfunction of the suction apparatus may be avoided by frequently disconnecting the tubing and listening to ascertain that there is a vacuum in the line. Long intestinal tubes, such as the Miller-Abbott, have not found general usage in the infant age group.

DECOMPRESSIVE GASTROSTOMY. Because simple nasogastric tubes are well tolerated and may be left in place for several weeks if necessary, elective gastrostomy for decompressive purposes is generally reserved for those patients in whom a prolonged or complicated course may be predicted at the time of initial surgery. In these infants, the gastrostomy is simply accomplished as an adjunct to the primary procedure. Decompressive gastrostomy has also found wide application as a temporizing procedure in patients with esophageal atresia in whom it is desirable to prevent reflux aspiration through a distal-pouch tracheoesophageal fistula. In these infants, the gastrostomy catheter may be used for feeding once the fistula has been divided.

Paralytic Ileus

Paralytic ileus of severe degree is much less common and persistent in the newborn than in the adult patient. Vigorous peristalsis is often noted at the time of laparotomy and may not be diminished appreciably by anesthesia and surgery. Postoperatively, intestinal function may routinely be expected to return within 24 to 48 hours unless other factors such as intraperitoneal infection, generalized sepsis, intestinal obstruction, or wound dehiscence, are present. Persistent intestinal anastomotic dysfunction is not uncommon in infants and may be due to a variety of causes to be discussed in a later section.

Whenever an infant with prolonged postoperative ileus is encountered, a cause and explanation should be actively sought. Sepsis should be treated and electrolyte disturbances corrected. Intestinal and anastomotic function is most easily evaluated by simple abdominal radiographs, using swallowed air as the contrast material. Air visible in the distal small bowel or rectum, for example, usually indicates at least some degree of patency in all proximal areas. Intestinal function may also be evaluated by placing a few milliliters of barium in the stomach, clamping the nasogastric tube temporarily, and obtaining periodic abdominal films to assess progress. Care must be taken, of course, to avoid giving too much barium and risking vomiting and aspiration.

Pulmonary Complications

ASPIRATION PNEUMONITIS. Respiratory complications secondary to the aspiration of vomitus are an important cause of morbidity in a small debilitated infant. Although newborn infants easily vomit and regurgitate gastric contents through the esophagus, they are unable to actively clear the pharynx, an act dependent upon gravity and a turned head. Often unable to move because of restraints, the infant is highly susceptible to aspiration.

Prevention of aspiration depends upon maintenance of a functioning nasogastric tube in proper position. The tube length should be measured before insertion, and its position should be checked by aspiration with a syringe and by blowing in an air bubble while listening with a stethoscope over the epigastrium. Furthermore, the function of the tube and suction device should be checked periodically. A non-functioning suction pump with a closed system is far less desirable than simple dependent drainage. A short, infant-size nasogastric tube or a straight urinary catheter should always be employed in preference to standard adult-length, small-caliber Levin tubes with their attendant and unnecessary resistance to drainage.

Although nasogastric tubes may be irrigated periodically to assure patency, this is seldom necessary unless there is particulate matter in the stomach. Tube dysfunction is most often due to improper positioning or inadequate suction. Usually the tube has been inserted too far and has kinked within the stomach. If irrigation of nasogastric tubes is required, small volumes of fluid should be used.

PULMONARY ATELECTASIS. Atelectasis most often occurs in those patients with aspiration or in those with some measure of preexisting pulmonary disease. Infants should be routinely turned front-to-back and side-to-side at 2-hour intervals so as to avoid dependency of any particular segments of the lung. Even when connected to a respirator, an infant may be periodically turned to all but the face-down position. Pulmonary physiotherapy in the form of chest clapping and vibrating with dependent drainage may be employed, just as in older children and adults.

Hypothermia

The predictable response of the sick and septic newborn infant is lowering of body temperature toward that of the environment. Temperature regulation from exogenous thermal sources is therefore of prime importance. Fever in the neonatal infant is unusual except as a manifestation of an overly warm incubator. Nurseries are generally well equipped to handle temperature-regulation problems, either with heated closed incubators or radiant heaters, but operating rooms rarely are. An infant on the operating table may lose considerable amounts of heat both by convection into the air-conditioned room and by radiation to the cool walls. The resultant low body temperature is one of the most common causes of apnea following general anesthesia. Frequently the infant must be rewarmed before spontaneous respirations resume. It is therefore essential that the infant in the operating room be kept normothermic. All infants should be routinely monitored with indwelling rectal or tympanic membrane temperature probes. Heat loss may be minimized by keeping the patient in the incubator until the last moment, by routinely wrapping all extremities in cotton cast padding, and by exposing as little of the body as possible during induction of anesthesia. Skin preparation solution should be warm and should be used judiciously so that sheets remain dry and further heat loss by evaporation is prevented.

Heat may be routinely supplied by a warming mattress placed just beneath the operating table cover. All towels or rolls used to position the patient should be placed under the mattress so that the heating surface is in close proximity to the patient. Operating room temperature must be increased sometimes to a point at which personnel are uncomfortable (75° to 80° F.) unless there is some other exogenous source of radiant heat for the patient. When operating on small premature infants, we are currently accustomed to working beneath a radiant heater such as are used in many nurseries. Other methods of providing warmth at the operating table have been described.[20] The transport incubator should be kept warm and ready to receive the infant immediately after operation.

Anesthesia

Many abdominal surgical procedures in the newborn infant may be accomplished under local anesthesia, in order to circumvent problems related to general anesthesia. It has been our policy to use local anesthesia for gastrostomy and simple, double-barrel loop colostomy. In addition, laparotomy in most infants weighing less than 2000 gm. may be performed with local anesthesia using 0.2 per cent lidocaine without excessive difficulty. As a general rule, the smaller the infant, the greater the indication for local anesthesia and the greater the ease with which it is accomplished. During all newborn surgery under local anesthesia, an anesthesiologist should be present, and no compromise should be made in regard to monitoring the infant's temperature, electrocardiogram, and blood pressure with the aid of a Doppler flowmeter. Infants in whom respirators are being used preoperatively are simply transferred to the operating room with portable oxygen and then are moved to the operating table for either general or local anesthesia, as indicated.

Infections

Sepsis continues to be a major hazard and complication in infancy. Every effort must be made not only to provide a safe environment to prevent nosocomial infections but also to monitor each patient in order that appropriate cultures may be obtained if infection is suspected. While strict isolation and "clean" techniques are routinely practiced in newborn nurseries, they are too often disregarded when the patient leaves the nursery for the radiology department or the operating room. Surgeons and anesthesiologists, who routinely wash between patients in the nursery, are likely in the operating suite to remove the patient from the incubator and to begin the anesthetic without thought for washing.

Cultures should be obtained at the time of laparotomy if there is any sign of an infectious process or if the bowel has been opened. In the presence of suspected sepsis, blood and other cultures should be obtained and broad spectrum antibiotic coverage initiated. There is not time to await culture data which characteristically become available in 24 to 48 hours. Laboratory antibiotic sensitivity testing should routinely be used to modify the initial therapy when that seems appropriate. The surgeon, with the aid of nursery personnel, should be aware of currently prevailing nursery organisms and their antibiotic sensitivities. He must also be aware of recommended antibiotics along with the dosage and frequency of administration currently being recommended for infants.[11, 12] For some drugs, dosage schedules differ during the first few weeks of extrauterine life until renal function matures.

COMPLICATIONS OF SPECIFIC PROCEDURES

Laparotomy

When a definite operation may be planned in advance (e.g., gastrostomy, colostomy, Ramstedt pyloromyotomy), it is usually possible to use a well placed incision at the site of the disorder and to perform the procedure without regard to other intra-abdominal organs. However, when laparotomy is performed for congenital anomalies, obstructions, or perforations in the newborn, it is essential that the entire small bowel and most of the colon be visualized so that additional unsuspected abnormalities such as defects in intestinal rotation may be visualized. Correctable intra-abdominal lesions should not turn up as needless postoperative complications. The palpating finger should not miss the opportunity to outline the size and consistency of the kidneys, as renal lesions are not uncommon components of multiple anomaly syndromes. Delicate newborn intestine should be handled gently with the fingers rather than with rough forceps so that easily created subserosal and mesenteric hemorrhages are avoided. Similarly, unpadded retractors should be kept away from the fragile liver, which is most difficult to manage once a tear has occurred.

DECOMPRESSIVE ENTEROTOMY. At the time of laparotomy for intestinal obstruction, distention may be so great as to prevent reduction of eviscerated bowel back into the abdominal cavity. Excessive efforts to reduce bowel may quickly produce sub-serosal hemorrhages, seromuscular splits, and areas of denuded mucosa. Closure under these circumstances may be facilitated by enterotomy performed with a No. 18 needle attached to the suction tubing. The needle is placed inside a purse-string suture of 5-0 atraumatic silk that is further tightened as the needle is removed. A few additional inverting Lembert sutures may be used to cover the enterotomy site. If this procedure is properly executed, there should be no spillage onto the peritoneal surfaces, and the danger of fistula formation is essentially nil. We have not encountered complications from enterotomy of this type.

Gastrostomy

Complications of gastrostomy are best avoided by limiting this procedure to those cases in which it is absolutely necessary. Although gastrostomy has been widely used as an adjunct to a variety of intra-abdominal procedures in the newborn, it should be remembered that nasogastric tubes are adequate for the purposes of both aspiration and feeding. Most infants tolerate indwelling nasal tubes for long periods without an undue increase in respiratory complications.

Attention to detail in the construction and management of the catheter gastrostomies is essential if leakage, the principal complication, is to be avoided. The gastrostomy is constructed by placing two concentric purse-string sutures in the anterior wall of the stomach to hold a mushroom or Malecot catheter in place. The ends of the purse string are left long and are subsequently used to anchor the stomach to the anterior abdominal wall by bringing them out along with the catheter and suturing one on each side to the fascia or skin. It is of prime importance that the gastrostomy tube transverse the abdominal wall at right angles and that the emerging tube be held in this position postoperatively. A number of mechanisms may be used to accomplish this, the simplest of which is to wrap a gauze sponge around the catheter and tape it in place. An angled catheter tends to produce, by erosion, a larger than necessary orifice, with resultant leakage of gastric contents and consequent excoriation.

While a mushroom catheter with its unobstructed lumen and short tip is optimal for most gastrostomies, a Foley catheter should be used for replacement if the first tube falls out within the first 10 to 14 days. During this time the seal between the stomach and the anterior peritoneum may not be firm, and the somewhat traumatic insertion of a mushroom catheter may cause leakage. On the other hand, Foley ballooned catheters have a tendency to migrate into the duodenum, where they may cause intraluminal obstruction. Gastrostomy tubes should therefore always be adequately secured with tape after the catheter tip has been pulled back snugly, but it should not be so tightly fixed that there is risk of extrusion.

Small amounts of gastric content commonly leak around the catheter 7 to 10 days after construction, but then, after a tight band of fibrous tissue has formed, tube gastrostomies are usually dry. It is during the early stage that it is particularly essential to maintain the catheter at right angles to the skin to prevent abdominal wall erosion.

Feedings through the gastrostomy may be started within 24 to 48 hours, provided that care is taken not to overdistend the stomach and thereby risk leakage. Adequate gastric decompression may be insured by suspending the end of the open gastrostomy tube above the patient. An open syringe barrel may be attached for convenience. Feedings may thus be added by gravity, and the infant in turn may regurgitate air or fluid into the syringe reservoir. Although this suspension arrangement is not usually necessary beyond the first 2 weeks, it may be used in any patient in whom gastric-emptying difficulties are anticipated and in whom vomiting would be undesirable.

Colostomy

EXCORIATION. Cutaneous excoriation is by far the most common, most often troublesome, and least harmful complication of colostomy. Because of almost continuous fecal soiling, a considerable effort must be expended to keep the abdominal skin clean and dry. Although various appliances and colostomy bags have found wide usage, many parents elect to manage the colostomy by changing diapers, particularly in early infancy. Aside from colostomy bags, two methods of management have evolved: keep the skin dry by fastidious care and exposure, or protect it by various creams. No matter which method is elected, the greatest success always comes to the most diligent nurse or parent.

PROLAPSE. The increased incidence among infants of prolapsing colostomies, particularly of the loop type, has long been recognized. The great majority of prolapses occur in the distal defunctionalized loop. A limited prolapse may be tolerated, particularly when the colostomy is to be temporary, but on occasion the prolapse is of such severity as to defy reduction and require surgical intervention.

Although prolapse may not always be prevented, certain steps may be employed during construction of the colostomy to minimize postoperative difficulties. Fine interrupted sutures are placed circumferentially between the seromuscular coat of the bowel and the abdominal wall muscle and fascia. These sutures serve not only to anchor the bowel but also to prevent pericolostomy herniation of small intestine. The abdominal wall defect should be left just large enough to admit the colon without constriction of its blood supply. Not infrequently, however, the abdominal wall defect ultimately will be too large when the obstructed thick walled colon, for which the colostomy was originally tailored, shrinks to normal caliber. When a prolapse becomes incarcerated, surgical reconstruction of the colostomy stoma becomes necessary. In freeing an incarcerated prolapse it is usually necessary only to free the prolapsing half of the stoma from the surrounding skin and fascia. The stoma is reconstructed by suturing the bowel to all abdominal layers and by closing the fascia to a suitable diameter around the colostomy. Resection is usually not indicated unless infarction has occurred.

STENOSIS AND RETRACTION OF COLOSTOMY STOMA. Once a colostomy is healed and is functioning satisfactorily, there is little tendency toward stenosis. However, if the entire stoma or central limb of a loop colostomy retracts, there may follow cicatricial narrowing of the stoma at the skin level. In the loop colostomy, retraction of the central limb allows spillover into the distal segment, which may be particularly undesirable. Retraction of the central limb is best avoided by leaving the supporting rod in place. A short segment of ¼-inch glass or plastic rod with 1 or 2 cm. of rubber tubing on each end will remain innocuously under a colostomy loop for several weeks or months. It offers little difficulty to the patient. Furthermore, the glass rod usually insures that the two stomas are well separated and that the distal loop is defunctionalized. On occasion a glass rod left in place for several weeks may gradually cut through the loop, producing two stomas separated by scar tissue and pointing in opposite directions. It has been our policy to discharge infants from the hospital with the rod in place, and to remove it at an office visit several weeks later.

If it is important that the distal limb remain defunctionalized once retraction of the central limb has occurred, surgical intervention to reestablish divided stomas with a new rod is the only feasible treatment. Following successful repair of the distal obstructing lesions, spontaneous closure of the loop colostomy has intentionally been allowed to occur when for some reason the central colostomy limb has retracted.

CLOSURE OF COLOSTOMY. Colostomy closure is greatly facilitated if both stomas are in close proximity. When fashioning cutaneous enterostomies, the surgeon should always think ahead toward closure and should avoid widely separated stomas whenever possible. Even when long segments of intestine have been resected, it is usually possible to bring the ends out through adjacent stab wounds. Recently, in premature infants with necrotizing enterocolitis who require bowel resection, we have brought both stomas out through the same wound. This procedure has the advantage that only minimal peristomal dissection is required for early closure.

The two most common and serious complications of colostomy closure are obstruction and leakage at the suture line. A loop colostomy stoma may be closed with very little additional incision other than the circumferential one required to free the bowel from the skin and fascial layers. It makes little difference whether the free peritoneal cavity is entered and the bowel is dropped completely back in, or whether an extraperitoneal closure is effected. It is essential that enough bowel be freed up so that scar tissue may be trimmed away and the bowel anastomosis may be made without angulation.

Although leakage at the colostomy closure site is relatively uncommon, it occurs most frequently if there are problems with the anastomosis or if distal colonic obstruction remains uncorrected. It is therefore axiomatic that a colostomy should not be closed until a radiographic contrast study has shown that the distal segment is clear to the anus. When colostomy closure is of the extraperitoneal type, a subfascial drain may be placed in the pouch surrounding the anastomosis and brought out through the wound. Subcutaneous wound drainage at the site of colostomy closure is almost always indicated, as the infection rate in these contaminated wounds is understandably high.

Intestinal Anastomosis

Intestinal anastomoses in the newborn infant with atresia or other abnormalities often present the surgeon with difficult technical problems. The anastomosis must be constructed so that it will function without obstruction and yet not leak, even though there is a considerable disparity in size between the proximal and distal loops. While it has long been recognized that the dilated, thickened atonic segment proximal

to the atresia should be resected, this is not always entirely possible. In high jejunal atresia, resection is often performed at the level of the third portion of the duodenum, where further dissection is limited by the pancreas. In duodenal obstructions, it is not feasible to resect any of the dilated bowel at all. Thus, in spite of resection, the surgeon is often faced with considerable difference in the diameters of the segments to be anastomosed. Although an end-to-side anastomosis is easily accomplished no matter what the disparity, it should be noted that runoff is determined by lumen size distal to the anastomosis and not by the size of the anastomosis itself (Fig. 26–3). For functional reasons, an end-to-end or "end-to-backside" anastomosis is to be preferred. Thomas[27] has advised tapering jejunoplasty as an alternative. All anastomoses must be accomplished without a significant amount of inversion. To avoid excessive turn-in, the anastomosis may be constructed with a single layer of interrupted 5-0 atraumatic silk sutures with the knots in the lumen. Placing the knots on the inside assures an inverted anastomosis with serosa-to-serosa adaptation. A few additional Lembert sutures may be used on the serosal surface in the last stage of the anastomosis to tidy up any insecure areas. After completion of the anastomosis, saline is injected into the lumen of the proximal bowel with a 25-gauge needle to test for leakage and patency at the suture line.

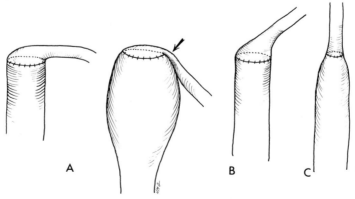

Figure 26–3 Intestinal anastomosis in an infant with atresia, particularly of the high jejunum, may present a technical problem because of disparity in size between the proximal and distal bowel. Although a large end-to-side anastomosis (A) is easily accomplished, runoff is dependent upon the caliber distally. There is a tendency for obstruction to occur postoperatively as the small flaccid distal bowel drapes over a distended proximal pouch. Better function is usually achieved by the end-to-backside oblique anastomosis (B) or by the straight end-to-end anastomosis (C). The last type may be accomplished with a single layer of 5-0 atraumatic silk sutures with the knots in the lumen and strict adherence to proportionate suture placement. Alternatively, the proximal pouch may be tailored as advocated by Thomas.[27]

ANASTOMOTIC DYSFUNCTION. Prolonged postoperative ileus may be due to intestinal anastomotic malfunction. Whereas these functional delays are well recognized entities, there must be constant vigilance for other causes of ileus such as adhesive peritonitis, kinks, abscesses, and suture line infections which require more than a wait and see approach. Reoperation is usually considered only when function has not returned after 14 to 21 days. A mechanically obstructed anastomosis may be found at operation, or the anastomosis may be perfectly intact and anatomically patent. Whether the anastomosis is obstructed or patent and nonfunctioning, the best method of management is resection of a few centimeters of bowel and construction of a fresh suture line.

ANASTOMOTIC LEAKAGE. Anastomotic breakdown and leakage is an ever-present hazard especially when the caliber of the bowel is small and every effort has been made to invert the suture line as little as possible, to avoid obstruction. Unlike the adult patient in whom postoperative intraperitoneal air may persist for several days, evidence of free air in the newborn beyond 24 hours is strongly suggestive of perforation. Repeated abdominal films are always indicated in the presence of increasing postoperative distention, ileus, or sepsis. At times, even in the presence of overt perforation, the infant may seem deceptively well and appear to be without undue distress. However, such a picture is temporary, and marked deterioration of the patient's condition will occur unless the perforation is closed. When anastomotic dehiscence is encountered at laparotomy, the decision must be made either for reanastomosis or for temporary cutaneous enterostomy. In recent years, since the advent of intravenous hyperalimentation, we have increasingly chosen the latter. The anastomosis is simply exteriorized through a single stab wound and opened, much as a loop enterostomy. The enterostomy may be closed subsequently, when peritonitis has subsided and the nutritional balance of the patient has been restored.

Intravenous Nutrition

While intravenous nutrition has accounted for the increased survival of many in-

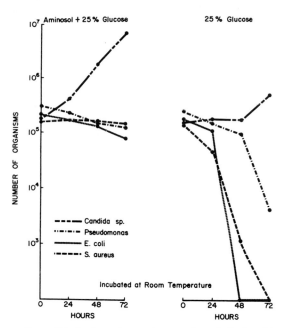

Figure 26–4 Fungal organisms preferentially flourish at room temperature in intravenous nutritional mixtures of glucose and protein hydrolysate.

fants with congenital intestinal anomalies, the procedure is not entirely benign nor without complications. Because of the hazards involved and because of problems related to the placement and maintenance of central venous lines in small infants, we have generally reserved intravenous hyperalimentation for those patients in whom intravenous fluids and nutrition will be needed for more than 7 to 10 days. The principal complications of intravenous nutrition are infection, venous thrombosis, and osmotic diuresis.

INFECTION. Sepsis, particularly that due to fungal organisms, is the most common serious complication of long-term intravenous nutrition. It has been reported in several series of infants to occur at a rate of 15 to 25 per cent when intravenous nutritional catheters have been used for 30 to 60 days. While there is good evidence that intravenous nutritional solutions will support many species of bacteria at room temperature, only fungal organisms seem to proliferate actively under the same circumstances (Fig. 26–4). It is therefore apparent that every effort should be made to avoid contamination during the handling and mixing of all hyperalimentation fluids. In most hospitals, all mixing is performed by special personnel in a bacteriologically safe area and atmosphere.

There is little evidence that patients with sepsis have been infected by way of contaminated infusates, however. In a study of intravenous nutritional infusion systems that employed in-line bacterial filters, Miller and Grogan[14] found very little correlation between organisms recovered from the fluid and filters within the system and those recovered from the patient. These authors suggest that sepsis may also arise from entrance of organisms around the catheter or from sources endogenous within the patient and that the indwelling catheter becomes a secondary nidus for infection.

In any event, septic complications during intravenous infusion may be minimized by adherence to a few simple rules: (1) Fluids should be mixed under aseptic conditions, preferably by a person or team trained for this purpose. (2) In-line bacterial filters should be employed. (3) Fluids should be mixed frequently and old unused stock discarded. (4) The cutaneous entrance site of the catheter should be cleaned and a small amount of antibacterial and antifungal cream applied daily. Although we have routinely left the catheter site on the scalp open to the air, others have advocated sterile dressings and care by a special team. (5) The infusion line should never be entered for the purpose of giving medications or drawing blood. (6) Infusion tubing, except for the indwelling patient catheter, is changed and cultured frequently. (7) If the patient appears septic, blood and urine cultures should be obtained and the indwelling catheter removed. Candida sepsis may be insidious and should be aggressively pursued if the patient "just isn't doing well." Candida is often found in the urinary sediment or in urine cultures several days before the blood culture becomes positive; and if Candida appears in the urine of a patient receiving hyperalimentation, it should be assumed that fungemia is already present.

VENOUS THROMBOSIS. Placement of the catheter tip in a large-bore vessel usually insures adequate flow and mixing so that the hypertonic infusate is immediately diluted and thrombosis is avoided. The superior vena cava is of sufficient size for this purpose in the adult, but its dimension is much smaller in the infant. Accordingly, the catheter tip in infants should be placed in the right atrium, corresponding to the level of the fifth to seventh thoracic vertebra as visualized by chest x-ray.

OSMOTIC DIURESIS. Diuresis due to glucosuria may result during intravenous hyperalimentation if the patient is not able to metabolize the infused glucose. It is therefore a matter of routine in all new patients to increase gradually the concentration of glucose infusate over several days while the patient adapts. The urine should be monitored for glucose with a dipstick every 8 hours as a matter of nursing routine, and the rate of infusion or concentration of the infusate or both should be altered as necessary.

COMPLICATIONS OF SPECIFIC LESIONS

Congenital Hypertrophic Pyloric Stenosis

This lesion, with its characteristic and well known onset at a few weeks of age, is usually a distinct and easily recognizable entity. The diagnostic, olive-size mass may, with patience, be palpated in a high percentage of patients; in only a minority are barium studies necessary. However, when there is any question about the clinical findings, barium contrast films are absolutely essential to rule out pylorospasm or vomiting due to other causes. Unnecessary operations and explorations are to be avoided.

ASPIRATION. Although aspiration is relatively uncommon when the amount of vomiting in pyloric stenosis is considered, it may occur with increased frequency in a hospitalized infant after he is restrained to receive intravenous fluids. When contrast studies have been obtained, most pediatric radiologists routinely empty the stomach of all barium by nasogastric tube prior to returning the patient to the ward. Continuous suction is not usually instituted at the time of admission, but a nasogastric tube should be employed for a few hours immediately before operation to circumvent possible vomiting upon induction of anesthesia.

DEHYDRATION AND ELECTROLYTE IMBALANCE. Severe alkalosis and depletion of water and electrolytes should be corrected before surgery for pyloric stenosis. In severe derangements, adequate correction may take 2 or 3 days. During this period, the infant should receive nothing by mouth, and nasogastric suction should not be used except for initial emptying of the stomach. It is a rare infant with pyloric stenosis who will continue to vomit if he has ingested nothing. Continued suction, on the other hand, will cause unnecessary continued losses of gastric secretions and make correction of alkalosis an even more difficult task. Serum chemistry studies should not be expected to return to normal before operation but should reflect marked improvement in the state of hydration and correction of alkalosis. Postanesthetic apnea is a common sequela to uncorrected alkalosis.

PERFORATION. Detection of a mucosal perforation at the time of Ramstedt pyloromyotomy is essential if this uncommon occurrence is not to have serious sequelae. Because of the configuration of the pyloric hypertrophy, inadvertent perforation almost always occurs at the duodenal end where the tumor ends abruptly (Fig. 26–5). Perforation is prevented by gradual spreading and cracking of the "olive" with a blunt-tipped hemostat or other instrument. It is essential that the tips of the spreading instrument be kept in sight and that they not be allowed to disappear beneath the hypertrophied muscle. At completion of the myotomy, gastric and duodenal contents should be expressed through the pylorus to ascertain that bubbles and bile are not seen. Any perforation should be immediately

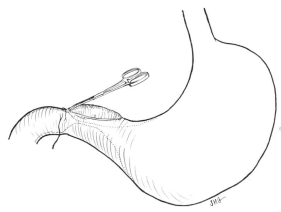

Figure 26–5 Perforation of the mucosa during Ramstedt pyloromyotomy most often occurs at the duodenum where the "tumor" ends abruptly. The tips of the spreading clamp should always be kept in sight. Postoperative obstruction, on the other hand, may occur from incomplete operation at the antral end.

closed with fine 5-0 atraumatic silk sutures, and nasogastric suction should be maintained postoperatively. The incidence of perforation is approximately 2 per cent.[17]

HEMORRHAGE. Operative hemorrhage of significant degree is unusual. In most patients, the Ramstedt procedure is accomplished with only a few ml. of blood loss. We routinely use a small midline incision starting at the xiphoid. Not only is this incision convenient to the pylorus, it also has the advantage of being almost bloodless. Any slight bleeding from the separated muscle edges usually ceases promptly on return of the stomach to the abdominal cavity and venous hypertension, created by the constricting action of the small abdominal incision, is relieved. If hemorrhage continues when the pylorus is again pulled out and inspected a few minutes later, a 5-0 atraumatic silk suture should be passed under the vessel as a suture ligature. Hemostatic clamps will not hold in the friable, cartilaginous, hypertrophied muscle.

Hemorrhagic gastritis, although rarely of severe degree, may occur preoperatively or postoperatively, particularly when there has been long-standing pyloric obstruction of high degree. It is best treated by performance of the pyloromyotomy to relieve obstruction at the earliest possible moment. Periodic administration of antacids through a nasogastric tube may also be useful.

POSTOPERATIVE VOMITING. Continued vomiting following pyloromyotomy is always worrisome, although an incomplete operation is an unusual occurrence. The parents should be warned that the infant who has vomited for a long period preoperatively and who has markedly hypertrophied gastric musculature may be expected to vomit postoperatively. Although pyloromyotomy produces marked improvement, it usually does not produce abrupt relief of all symptoms except when the prodromal period has been short and the diagnosis has been made early. Small amounts of glucose water may be offered 6 hours after operation, but feedings should be stopped if vomiting ensues and then gradually started again the following day. Postoperative intravenous fluid administration is usually necessary for 24 to 48 hours or longer.

Incomplete operations are quite unusual but may occasionally result from failure to extend the pyloric incision proximally to the hypertrophied fibers of the distal antrum.[23] At the time of initial surgery, proximal dissection should be continued until the antral fibers are seen and spread for a short distance. In contrast to the risk at the duodenal end, proximal dissection may be continued without fear of mucosal perforation if reasonable care is exercised. As a general rule, the length of the pyloric split should be approximately one and one-half times the width of the "olive."

Duodenal Obstruction and Anomalies

Partial or complete duodenal obstruction may be associated with a variety of anomalies, including atresia, annular pancreas, malrotation of the colon, and duplications. While the classic "double-bubble" x-ray appearance of complete obstruction will rarely be misinterpreted, incomplete obstructions may be a good deal more insidious and may be manifested by such vague problems as a "poor feeder" or failure to thrive.

Newborn surgery for duodenal atresia or annular pancreas should be designed to relieve obstruction with the shortest possible bypass. In most instances, a duodenoduodenostomy may be performed. If this is not feasible, duodenojejunostomy, but never gastrojejunostomy, is the procedure of choice. When the duodenum is opened, a catheter should be carefully passed in both directions to rule out other unsuspected areas of obstruction. Delayed function of duodenal anastomoses is common. Reoperation for anastomotic failure is therefore generally not indicated for at least 2 weeks, and then only when there is little or no evidence of gas in the small bowel distal to the duodenum. Patience and persistent frequent feedings of small volumes usually will be rewarded by gradually increasing anastomotic function. The proximal duodenal segment may remain dilated for months, as shown by barium studies, even though the patient is entirely asymptomatic.

While waiting for a sluggish anastomosis to begin to function, the surgeon should be constantly vigilant lest dysfunction be secondary to suture line disruption or intraperitoneal infection. Careful attention to

any sign of sepsis and repeated x-ray studies to assess progress and to look for extraluminal air are indicated.

Patients with congenital duodenal obstruction often have other severe anomalies unrelated to the gastrointestinal tract. Of particular importance is the high incidence (20 to 30 per cent) of Down's syndrome, prematurity, and esophageal atresia. It is these other life-threatening anomalies with their own attendant complications that, for the most part, account for the deaths related to duodenal atresia.

Distal Small Bowel Lesions

Lesions of the distal small bowel and mesentery may be manifest by immediate symptomatology in the newborn infant or conversely may remain dormant for years. Almost all lesions attracting attention within the first few days or weeks of life are associated with signs and symptoms of intestinal obstruction or perforation. Those lesions presenting in later infancy and childhood are often manifested by hemorrhage, abdominal pain, or acquired obstruction.

JEJUNAL AND ILEAL ATRESIA. When the Gross textbook of pediatric surgery[5] was published in 1953, the majority of distal small bowel atresias seemed to arise in the ileum. Dr. Gross' experience, based upon children seen at the Boston Children's Hospital, involved 140 cases of intestinal atresia: duodenum, 32; jejunum, 19; ileum, 72; ileocecal valve, 2; colon, 6; and multiple, 9. More recently, our experience at the University of Mississippi Medical Center[13] suggests that far fewer ileal atresias are currently being seen and that there is a marked trend toward complicated, multiple atresias involving the jejunum. Of 45 infants with intestinal atresia, 16 were in the duodenum, 24 in the jejunum, and 5 in the ileum. Only 3 patients of the 24 with jejunal atresia had a single area of obstruction. The remaining atresias have been associated with other severe gastrointestinal anomalies, multiple areas of atresia, or the Christmas tree deformity.[29] While the mortality rate in duodenal atresia relates principally to other anomalies such as Down's syndrome, morbidity and mortality in jejunal atresia patients are much more apt to be associated

TABLE 26–1   SMALL INTESTINE ATRESIAS AT THE UNIVERSITY OF MISSISSIPPI MEDICAL CENTER*

	Patients	Patients Requiring Multiple Operative Procedures	Lived	Died	Per Cent Survival
Duodenum	16	3	11	5	69
Jejunum (all)	24	12	19	5	79
Single	3	0	3	0	100
Multiple	7	5	6	1	86
Other GI anomalies	5	2	4	1	80
Christmas tree deformity	9	5	6	3	67
Ileal	5	0	5	0	100
Total atresias	45	15	35	10	78

*Forty-five patients seen at the University of Mississippi Medical Center over a 12-year period illustrate the current predominance of patients with complicated jejunal atresias. Mortality in the duodenal group has been principally associated with other anomalies such as Down's syndrome and congenital heart disease, while mortality in the jejunal group has been associated with the intestinal anomaly itself. (Adapted from Miller, R. C.: Complicated intestinal atresias. Ann. Surg. *189*:607, 1979.)

with the severity of the intestinal lesions themselves (Table 26–1).

Many of the complications associated with small bowel atresia have previously been discussed in the section dealing with intestinal anastomoses. The surgeon must be aware that multiple areas of atresia are not uncommon and that atretic areas distal to the first one may not be apparent on external inspection of the bowel. Occasionally a clue to other areas of obstruction is provided by segmental collections of small amounts of meconium. In all cases of intestinal atresia, it is mandatory to flush the entire distal small bowel and colon with saline to insure internal patency. This may be conveniently accomplished with a syringe and 25-gauge needle inserted into the lumen just distal to the most proximal atresia. In cases of multiple atresias, a choice must always be made between conserving bowel and an excessive number of suture lines. Multiple adjacent obstructions may be converted by resection into a single anastomosis. Most difficult, however, are those cases in which multiple equidistant atresias exist, in which resection would result in undue loss of intestinal length, and in which multiple anastomoses are required. Obstruction and leakage of multiple distal anastomoses are common and the mortality rate is correspondingly high. Simple per-

forating procedures of distal webs have also been reported.[4]

The unique lesion of high jejunal atresia associated with failure of formation of the mesentery (the "apple-peel" or "barber-pole" deformity) deserves special attention. In this deformity the ends of the jejunal atresia become widely separated, so that the distal jejunum and ileum hang suspended on a short mesentery around the superior mesenteric artery, producing the barber-pole appearance. It is essential that proximal resection be carried back to smaller-caliber bowel although the dissection is limited by the proximity of the pancreas. Secondly, it is advisable to resect a short segment of the distal unused bowel, since the incidence of anastomotic and intestinal dysfunction has been particularly high in these patients. Intravenous nutrition will almost always be required in patients with this deformity.

MECONIUM ILEUS.   Infants with cystic fibrosis and meconium ileus present a difficult challenge in terms of both the technical management of intestinal lesions and pulmonary complications, which may be unusually severe. It is absolutely essential that every effort be made to prevent pulmonary problems and that pediatric personnel experienced in the management of cystic fibrosis be consulted from the start.

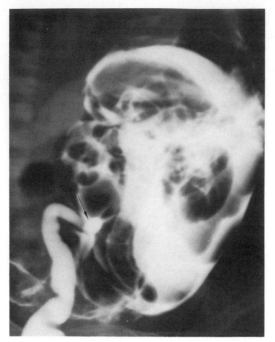

Figure 26–6   Perforation of the colon (*arrow*) occurring during Gastrografin enema for attempted relief of meconium ileus. Fortunately, the infant survived.

Since Noblett's report[16] of successful management of meconium ileus with relief of obstruction by Gastrografin enema, experience with this procedure and its hazards has accumulated slowly.[28] It appears that best success with washouts will be obtained in milder forms of meconium ileus when there is not marked dilation of the ileum and when complications such as prenatal volvulus, perforation, or atresia have not occurred. Perforation of the small bowel or colon is a definite hazard of the Gastrografin procedure (Fig. 26–6).

Following relief of meconium ileus, the most prevalent surgical problem is that of continued intestinal obstruction. For this reason, we favor the construction of a vented ileostomy, as described by Bishop and Koop,[2] which not only allows for resection of markedly dilated or atretic segments but also permits postoperative antegrade irrigations of the unused distal ileum and colon with saline, mineral oil, and N-acetylcysteine mixtures. These ileostomies may subsequently close spontaneously or, if persistent, may be electively turned in and sutured at a later date when the infant is thriving.

MECKEL'S DIVERTICULUM, DUPLICATIONS, AND OTHER LESIONS. This miscellaneous group of problems, usually presenting at some time after the newborn period, most often come to the attention of the parents and physician because of secondary manifestations. Both Meckel's diverticulum and duplications may be associated with asymptomatic lower gastrointestinal hemorrhage or with symptoms related to intussusception or perforation. Operative complications of these lesions therefore become closely associated with those reasons for which surgery is being performed. Particular attention must be directed toward replacement of blood and fluids and toward the treatment of sepsis.

Postoperative complications are generally those related to laparotomy and leaking anastomoses, abscess formation, or peritonitis. In the presence of significant intraperitoneal infection, cutaneous enterostomy rather than anastomosis may be indicated to avoid undue risk of suture line dehiscence.

Malrotation

Malrotation of the intestine may present with several clinical syndromes, any of which may be apparent in the immediate newborn period or in older patients. Most commonly malrotation presents as a problem of partial or complete duodenal obstruction due to extrinsic duodenal bands. These bands, being nothing more than folds of peritoneum passing from the malpositioned colon to the right upper quadrant, produce obstruction by extrinsic pressure on the second and third portions of the duodenum. However, intrinsic webs and stenoses, unrecognizable from the exterior serosal surface, may also be present. It is therefore not sufficient during procedures for malrotation to simply release the extrinsic bands; intrinsic defects must also be ruled out. It is most embarrassing to have overlooked an intrinsic web that continues to cause obstruction postoperatively. Intrinsic defects may be ruled out by a small antral gastrotomy through which a Foley catheter (10 or 12 F) is introduced distally as far as the proximal jejunum. The Foley balloon, having been pretested for size, is blown up to approximately 1 cm. and pulled back through the duodenum. Occasionally in a premature infant, a smaller balloon must be used. If at any point the balloon becomes snagged, an intrinsic obstruction should be suspected and the duodenum opened. Webs may be handled conveniently by longitudinal duodenotomy over the point of obstruction, simple division of the web, and closure of the duodenum in the transverse direction, providing for a wider-than-normal lumen. Since these obstructions are often located in the second portion of the duodenum and may be intimately associated with the ampulla of Vater, division of the web should always be accomplished on the anterolateral margin. It is not uncommon for the bile duct to drain through the very edge of the web.

MIDGUT VOLVULUS. Malrotation may also present as a midgut volvulus due to lack of fixation of the small bowel mesentery to the posterior abdominal wall. With this anatomic arrangement, the midgut may twist upon the axis of the superior mesenteric artery, with resultant infarction of the entire small bowel from the ligament of Treitz to the transverse colon. As this devastating complication may result in the death of the patient, operation should never be delayed if malrotation with volvulus is suspected. However, it is quite unusual to find infarcted small bowel due to malrotation and volvulus unless distended loops are visible by x-ray.

Incomplete surgery for malrotation may result in continued obstruction and risk for midgut volvulus. In the standard Ladd procedure,[7] it is important that the entire ligament of Treitz be taken down so that the duodenum and jejunum hang vertically on the right side of the abdomen with the colon falling where it will. Incidental appendectomy is indicated to avoid the confusion and possible complications of undiagnosed appendicitis in future years. The parents should always be informed that the appendix has been removed, and this information in later years should be passed on to the patient.

When severe compromise of intestinal circulation due to volvulus has occurred prior to surgery, derotation with return of circulation may produce areas of questionable viability. If the entire small bowel is involved and if resection would therefore unduly compromise chances for long-term survival, the entire intestine may be placed back in the abdominal cavity and reexploration carried out the following day. With suitable attention to circulating blood volume, fluids, and antibiotics, it may be possible thus to identify and save any areas of gut that were of questionable viability at initial operation and therefore would have been resected. In general, however, infarction of the entire midgut is a fatal disease or at least one that will require ongoing intravenous nutrition.

Intussusception

Not a problem of the newborn, intussusception of the idiopathic variety has a peak incidence at 5 to 10 months of age and characteristically occurs in large healthy male infants (60 to 70 per cent of cases). Complications associated with intussusception should be minimal if the diagnosis is promptly suspected and treatment is initiated before the patient reaches the stage of advanced strangulated bowel obstruction manifested by marked distention, dehydration, and sepsis. While the basic pathophysiology of intussusception is that of a strangulating obstruction, the patient may seem deceptively well. Peritonitis does not usually result, because the infarcted intussusceptum is sleeved in the outer, viable intussuscipiens. While all surgeons would agree that signs of peritonitis are an absolute indication for a primary operative approach, reduction may be accomplished by hydrostatic barium enema in a considerable number of patients with less advanced disease. Except in markedly ill infants with advanced obstruction, we have attempted enema reduction with a success rate of just over 40 per cent.[8]

Prior to attempted hydrostatic reduction, fluid volume should be restored by intravenous fluid therapy and the patient made ready for laparotomy should that become necessary. Although this slight delay could conceivably result in some loss of intestinal viability, the ability of the patient to withstand any necessary procedure is of far greater importance. The presence of the surgeon during the barium enema procedure will prevent further delay entailed in moving the patient to the operating room if reduction is incomplete or in the rare instance of perforation. Hydrostatic pressure should be limited to 36 inches.[18]

At the time of surgery, reduction is accomplished by pushing the intussusceptum backward in the distal direction, rather than by pulling. When reduction is impossible — usually because infarction has occurred —a maximal amount of viable bowel should be preserved. Usually the resection will involve the terminal ileum and cecum, resulting in an end-to-end ascending ileocolostomy.

During resection of an intussuscepted segment, care must be taken to divide the mesentery as close to the gut margin as possible so as to avoid other mesenteric vessels that may have been attenuated and drawn in with the intussuscipiens. Mobilization of the bowel and resection is always made more difficult by the shortened mesentery, which is also intussuscepted.

Recurrent intussusception occurs in less than 5 per cent of all cases[18] whether reduction has been accomplished by surgery or by hydrostatic enema. At laparotomy, all ileocecal bands and peritoneal folds should be lysed, particularly if the lead point was the ileocecal valve itself. These bands may act to produce chronic prolapse of the ileocecal valve into the cecal lumen. When the lead point was at the tip of the cecum (cecocolic intussusception) or the base of the appendix, appendectomy with inversion of the stump may serve to alter the anatomic configuration and thus discourage recurrence.

In older infancy and childhood, the relative incidence of pathologic lesions as the lead point steadily increases. Thus, laparotomy should be strongly considered in this age group as primary treatment, and certainly if there is recurrence after hydrostatic reduction.

Hirschsprung's Disease (Congenital Aganglionosis of the Colon)

Hirschsprung's disease, like malrotation, may present with a variety of clinical syndromes. On one hand the patient may be referred with complete intestinal obstruction in the newborn period, and on the other, may present with chronic constipation several years later. Although there is often little relationship between symptomatology and the level of aganglionosis, it may generally be stated that the longer the aganglionic segment, the more severe the symptoms and the earlier the age of referral.

In the newborn infant, the clinical presentation may be confused with a variety of problems including distal ileal and colonic obstructions, paralytic ileus, and the meconium plug syndrome. The latter problem, not related to meconium ileus and cystic fibrosis, is permanently relieved once the inspissated meconium plug (actually a cast of the distal colon often extending as far as the splenic flexure) has been evacuated.[3] On the other hand, evacuation of meconium in congenital aganglionosis produces only temporary improvement, followed by recurrent constipation, obstruction, and enterocolitis.

The diagnosis of Hirschsprung's disease is usually easily established by demonstration on barium enema of a change in colonic caliber at the transitional zone; it is confirmed by biopsy of the aganglionic segment. However, changes in bowel caliber may not be readily apparent by x-ray in the newborn infant, nor are they seen when the disease exists in very low segments, below the pelvic levator sling, or when there is complete aganglionosis extending to the small bowel.

COLOSTOMY. A colostomy for symptomatic Hirschsprung's disease in infancy is best placed at the distal end of the normally ganglionic colon. Since the rectosigmoid area is most commonly involved, a small transverse incision may be made in the left lower quadrant just lateral to the rectus muscles. In the newborn, in whom the lower abdominal wall segment is relatively short, the incision usually falls almost at the umbilical level. If the incision is made just large enough to deliver the colon, very little abdominal wall closure will be needed and the colostomy can be constructed as previously described. The colostomy must be placed in dilated bowel just proximal to the narrowed aganglionic segment, and the presence of ganglion cells at the colostomy site must be confirmed. We routinely open and primarily "mature" all colostomies. While the everted bowel is being sutured to the skin, the pathologist examines the frozen section for confirmation of ganglion cells. Although placement of the colostomy in dilated intestine proximal to any narrowed segment provides reasonable assurance, confirmation by frozen section leaves no doubt in the mind of the surgeon that adequate decompression will be achieved.

When the narrowed aganglionic segment is readily available in the surgical field at the time of colostomy, a seromuscular biopsy specimen taken there will document the presence of distal aganglionosis, thereby avoiding the need for subsequent rectal biopsy. Rectal biopsy is generally not indicated as a prerequisite to emergency colostomy in the distended and ill newborn in whom the barium enema appears diagnostic.

ENTEROCOLITIS. One of the most common neonatal complications of Hirschsprung's disease is enterocolitis. While complete intestinal obstruction is readily recognized and surgical consultation is promptly obtained, enterocolitis usually presents as undefined diarrhea, and the patient is likely to be found on the pediatric isolation ward rather than on the surgical division. The diagnosis of enterocolitis associated with Hirschsprung's disease should be actively entertained in any newborn with diarrhea and abdominal distention of unknown cause. Stool cultures usually reveal normal flora. Because of the high risk of bacteremia, emergency colostomy is mandatory.

PULL-THROUGH PROCEDURES. Potential complications during definitive operations for repair of Hirschsprung's disease are related mainly to injury to the urinary tract and to inadequate vascular supply of the ganglionic bowel to be pulled through to the perineum. During dissection and mobilization of the colon, the course and position of both ureters must always be kept in mind; since ureters are not firmly fixed, they may be pulled up into the base of the sigmoid mesentery as the bowel is mobilized. This is especially true on the left side.

When much of the sigmoid colon is involved by aganglionosis, it is often impossible to provide an adequate length of bowel for pull-through without division of the inferior mesenteric artery pedicle. This artery should be divided proximally near its origin so as to avoid interference with the collateral circulation of the marginal vessels. If mobilization of the ganglionic bowel is completed early in the operative procedure,

there will be enough time for assessment of the terminal circulation before the actual pull-through procedure. When there is any question regarding adequate circulation of the bowel as it rests in the abdominal operating field, it is certain that further compromise will occur when the bowel is stretched to enable placement in the confining areas of the pelvis and anal canal. Inadequate circulation is best corrected by mobilization of an additional amount of colon at the time of initial surgery.

The principal serious postoperative pull-through complication is that of fecal contamination following vascular compromise, disruption of the pelvic suture line, or retraction of the ganglionic segment back in the pelvis and abdomen. These complications may occur with any of the currently employed procedures and may result in rapidly overwhelming sepsis and death unless it is recognized and promptly treated by a diverting colostomy. Leakage should be suspected in any child in whom sepsis develops after a pull-through procedure or if there is x-ray evidence of free extraluminal air in the pelvis. In performing the endorectal pull-through procedure, it has been our practice to leave at least several centimeters of bowel protruding through the anus, as originally described by Soave.[24] In this manner, blood supply problems and retraction are readily visible during the postoperative period. The excess bowel may be trimmed and sutured to the anus without difficulty at 5 to 7 days. However, many surgeons perform the Soave procedure, making a primary anastomosis without protruding bowel.

In the Duhamel procedure, in which anterior aganglionic rectum is left in place and ganglionic bowel is brought down posteriorly, incomplete crushing of the septum between the two pouches may result in stenosis, partial obstruction, and fecal impaction. This complication may be avoided by primary anastomosis of the two pouches above and below, with the crushing clamp extending the entire length of the rectal segment,[10] or by primary division of the septum with the use of a double-row stapling device.[26] When division of the septum has been incomplete, reapplication of the crushing clamp or secondary surgical division may be necessary.

Strictures at or just inside the anal orifice

are usually not persistent problems if an adequate pull-through has been performed and if there has not been postoperative leakage and pelvic inflammation. On occasion, however, anorectal dilatations may be required if a firm fibrous band develops. More severe strictures involving longer segments of bowel have developed when there have been problems with inadequate blood supply.

POSTOPERATIVE COLITIS.   Enterocolitis is occasionally encountered following a pull-through procedure, especially if a segment of aganglionic rectum has been retained. In patients so affected, abdominal distention may be marked. On occasion, distention and air-fluid levels may appear in the small bowel with a clinical picture that might be confused with higher intestinal obstruction. While a single-finger rectal examination is usually rewarding, two-finger dilatation of the anus may allow for explosive decompression of the colon between the spread fingers. Suitable draping is advised.

ANAL SPHINCTEROTOMY.   When an excessive length of aganglionic bowel has been left in place or when there is recurrent anal spasm that has not responded to repeated dilatations, internal sphincterotomy or partial sphincterectomy may relieve the symptoms of constipation and recurrent colitis. These procedures are similar to those that have been advocated as primary treatment for low-segment Hirschsprung's disease.[1, 9, 19]

Imperforate Anus

Since the ultimate goal in infants with imperforate anus is to provide the patient with a lifetime of normal bowel control, care and caution must be exercised in the newborn infant to avoid any surgery that will be deleterious to anorectal function. It must be appreciated that the term imperforate anus encompasses a wide variety of anomalies of the rectum, anus, and perineum and that treatment is contingent upon a knowledge of the embryology involved.[25] A basic distinction must be made between those patients who have "low" anal and perineal anomalies and those who have "high" anorectal agenesis. The defect in the former group is almost always amenable to repair by primary anoplasty, usually performed under local anesthesia, whereas patients in the latter groups, including those with fistulas to the urinary tract or vagina, should be treated by temporary colostomy. Although the abdominal-perineal pull-through procedure has been accomplished in newborn infants with high anomalies, it is not to be recommended. The principal concern of such procedures must be the dissection and preservation of the levator (puborectalis) muscle sling as the primary mechanism of fecal continence. This muscle may be irreversibly injured by injudicious dissection in a newborn infant. Colostomy is therefore advised as a temporary procedure until the infant weighs 20 to 25 pounds, at which time definitive repair can be accomplished.

OPERATIVE COMPLICATIONS.   Complications arising during the pull-through procedure for high imperforate anus are primarily those affecting the urinary tract and those related to dissection of the puborectalis muscle sling. In the female infant, vaginal injury may occur but this is of far less immediate importance than a urethral tear or transection in the male. The sacrococcygeal-perineal operation of Stephens has been of signal benefit during the isolation and atraumatic dissection of the puborectalis. This direct posterior approach allows for mobilization of the muscle sling and creation of the tunnel for pull-through under direct vision.[25]

The Stephens procedure also minimizes the chance for urethral injury by allowing dissection inside the sling along the posterior urethral wall with a urethral sound in place. In this manner the position of the urethra may be constantly visualized and palpated. Most urethral injuries occur in the area of the rectourethral fistula at the level of the prostate. It is here that dissection is most difficult, because the blind-ending colon and the urinary tract are closely adherent and the precise point of the fistula is hard to visualize. When this portion of the dissection is carried out through the posterior approach, it is helpful to open the blind rectal pouch and to view the fistula from within. Once the bowel has been completely separated from the urinary tract, the urethral sound is removed and replaced by a Foley catheter, which is guided into the bladder so that it does not push through the posterior urethral suture line. If a urethral tear develops or if the fistula is difficult to close, healing is usually not a problem provided that the urethra is protected by catheter drainage.

We have not employed abdominal-perineal procedures for repair of imperforate anus for several years. Except when the colon ends above the pubococcygeal line and the fistula enters the bladder rather than the urethra, it has been possible to accomplish the repairs entirely through the sacrococcygeal-perineal approach.[15] The colostomy is closed at a later time, when the perineum is healed and the new anus is soft and well dilated.

ANAL STENOSIS. One of the most common problems following surgery for imperforate anus is postoperative stenosis. It may occur regardless of whether repair has been accomplished by primary anoplasty or by a later pull-through procedure. It is essential to calibrate the anus with sounds at the time of surgery and to continue dilatations in the postoperative weeks and months as long as there is any tendency toward recurrent stenosis. When the anal opening easily admits a finger without tightness or induration, dilatations may be discontinued. If there is any real degree of stenosis, it is generally inadequate for the mother to perform dilatations with her finger as she may be hesitant and finger dilatation difficult. It is far better to provide a Hegar uterine dilator of appropriate size and to periodically exchange it for a larger one as daily dilatations proceed. If postoperative calibration of the anus and dilatations are performed as a matter of routine, severe, obstructing anal stenosis should not occur. Should stenosis result from lack of follow-up, operative intervention to divide the stenotic ring and long-term dilatation usually become necessary.

FECAL INCONTINENCE. Problems with fecal control are unusual in patients with low anomalies. However, in high anorectal agenesis, all hope of fecal continence must rest upon a functioning puborectalis sling. In these infants, the internal sphincter, which is embryologically associated with the circular smooth muscle of the bowel, is nonexistent, and the external sphincter may be malformed and of little use. Not only must the surgeon use due care during pelvic dissection but he or she must be sure that the pull-through occurs inside (anterior to) the muscle sling. A posterior tunnel in the presacral space, although easily accomplished, usually results in little more than a perineal colostomy. If by error the pull-through has occurred posterior to the sling mechanism and incontinence results, consideration may be given to complete release of the levator ani sling as described by Kottmeier.[6] However, for the most part, secondary surgical procedures for fecal incontinence have been unrewarding.

The great majority of children with anorectal agenesis achieve continence when the levator muscle sling has been properly utilized during repair. However, as the sling mechanism relates to more gross levels of control, it is not unusual for some seepage and soiling to result if diarrhea develops. A similar problem may exist in regard to control of flatus in the absence of the finer sphincter mechanisms.

URINARY COMPLICATIONS. Urinary tract problems related to imperforate anus include both congenital anomalies and acquired infections.[21, 22] Abnormalities that may involve both the upper and lower urinary tract are more commonly seen in patients with high anorectal deformities. Therefore, in all patients with imperforate anus, intravenous urography should be performed routinely.

Urinary infections usually result from fistulous communications to the rectum. Following colostomy in the newborn, washout of the distal colonic segment is important if continued contamination of the urinary tract is to be avoided. Periodic urinalyses and cultures are indicated.

Finally, when a colostomy has been constructed for a patient with anorectal agenesis and rectourethral fistula, urinary reflux into the colonic segment during micturition may result in hyperchloremic acidosis. Although reflux into the colon is unusual, any watery discharge from the distal colostomy stoma should be noted and the serum electrolytes evaluated. If severe acidosis results, it may be necessary to proceed with definitive repair sooner than originally planned.

Bibliography

1. Alexander, J. L., and Aston, S. J.: A technique for posterior myectomy and internal sphincterotomy in short-segment Hirschsprung's disease. J. Pediatr. Surg. 9:169, 1974.

2. Bishop, H. C., and Koop, C. E.: Management of meconium ileus. Ann. Surg. *145*:410, 1957.
3. Clatworthy, H. W., Jr., Howard, W. H. R., and Lloyd, J. R.: The meconium plug syndrome. Surgery *39*:131, 1956.
4. El Shafie, M., and Rickham, P. P.: Multiple intestinal atresias. J. Pediatr. Surg. *5*:655, 1970.
5. Gross, R. E.: The Surgery of Infancy and Childhood. Philadelphia, W. B. Saunders Company, 1953.
6. Kottmeier, P. K., and Dziadiw, R.: The complete release of the levator ani sling in fecal incontinence. J. Pediatr. Surg. *2*:111, 1967.
7. Ladd, W. E.: Congenital obstructions of the duodenum in children. N. Engl. J. Med. *206*:277, 1932.
8. Larsen, E., and Miller, R. C.: Clinical aspects of intussusception. Am. J. Surg. *124*:69, 1972.
9. Lynn, H. B.: Rectal myomectomy for aganglionic megacolon. Mayo Clin. Proc. *41*:289, 1966.
10. Martin, L. W., and Altemeier, W. A.: Clinical experience with a new operation (modified Duhamel procedure) for Hirschsprung's disease. Ann. Surg. *156*:678, 1962.
11. McCracken, G. H., Jr., Eichenwald, H. F., and Nelson, J. D.: Antimicrobial therapy in theory and practice. I. Clinical pharmacology. J. Pediatr. *75*:742, 1969.
12. McCracken, G. H., Jr., Eichenwald, H. F., and Nelson, J. D.: Antimicrobial therapy in theory and practice. II. Clinical approach to antimicrobial therapy. J. Pediatr. *75*:923, 1969.
13. Miller, R. C.: Complicated intestinal atresias. Ann. Surg. *189*:607, 1979.
14. Miller, R. C., and Grogan, J. B.: Incidence and source of contamination of intravenous nutritional infusion systems. J. Pediatr. Surg. *8*:185, 1973.
15. Miller, R. C., and Izant, R. J., Jr.: Sacrococcygeal perineal approach to imperforate anus. Am. J. Surg. *121*:62, 1971.
16. Noblett, H. R.: Treatment of uncomplicated meconium ileus by Gastrografin enema: A preliminary report. J. Pediatr. Surg. *4*:190, 1969.
17. Ravitch, M., Welch, K. J., Benson, C. D., Aberdeen, E., and Randolph, J. G.: Pediatric Surgery. Chicago, Year Book Medical Publishers, 1979.
18. Ravitch, M. M.: Intussusception in Infants and Children. Springfield, Ill., Charles C Thomas, 1959.
19. Shandling, B., and Desjardins, J. G.: Anal myomectomy for constipation. J. Pediatr. Surg. *4*:115, 1969.
20. Shaw, A., Franzel, I., and Bordiuk, J.: Prevention of neonatal hypothermia by a fiber optic "hot pipe" system: A new concept. J. Pediatr. Surg. *6*:354, 1971.
21. Singh, M. P., Haddadin, A., Zachary, R. B., and Pilling, D. W.: Renal tract disease in imperforate anus. J. Pediatr. Surg. *9*:197, 1974.
22. Smith, E. D.: Urinary anomalies and complications in imperforate anus and rectum. J. Pediatr. Surg. *3*:337, 1968.
23. Smith, E. I., Stone, H. H., and Swishchuk, L. E.: The importance of Torgersen's muscle in the diagnosis and treatment of infantile hypertrophic pyloric stenosis. South. Med. J. *64*:1010, 1971.
24. Soave, F.: Hirschsprung's disease: Technique and results of Soave's operation. Br. J. Surg. *53*:1023, 1966.
25. Stephens, F. D., and Smith, E. D.: Ano-Rectal Malfunctions in Children. Chicago, Year Book Medical Publishers, 1971.
26. Talbert, J. L., Seashore, J. H., and Ravitch, M.: Evaluation of a modified Duhamel operation for correction of Hirschsprung's disease. Ann. Surg. *179*:671, 1974.
27. Thomas, C. G., Jr., and Carter, J. M.: Small intestinal atresia: The critical role of a functioning anastomosis. Ann. Surg. *179*:663, 1974.
28. Wagget, J., Bishop, H. C., and Koop, C. E.: Experience with Gastrografin enema in the treatment of meconium ileus. J. Pediatr. Surg. *5*:649, 1970.
29. Weitzman, J. J.: Jejunal atresia with agenesis of the dorsal mesentery. Am. J. Surg. *111*:443, 1966.

27

COMPLICATIONS OF HERNIAL REPAIR

Lloyd M. Nyhus

The repair of groin hernias is the second most common non-gynecologic operation performed in hospitals of America today, removal of tonsils and adenoids being the most common procedure. More than 550,000 hernial repairs are performed yearly. Fortunately, complications are uncommon, yet an over-all complication rate of only 1 per cent would affect 5500 patients, and of 5 per cent, 27,500 patients; the magnitude of the problem is apparent.

Certain complications are well recognized; others are not. The purpose of this chapter will be to cover many of the common and uncommon complications that relate to groin (indirect and direct inguinal and femoral) hernias. Complications of hernial repair in other anatomic sites, i.e., ventral, lumbar, and pelvic, have many similarities to those seen in the groin, and therefore will not be discussed.

PREOPERATIVE COMPLICATIONS

Correct diagnosis is the key to good therapy.

DIFFERENTIATION OF HERNIAL TYPE

The preoperative differentiation between a direct and an indirect hernia is frequently discussed; however, since similar approaches are used for both, the importance of this diagnostic exercise has diminished. This is fortunate, since current studies have shown that the differentiation by a clinician between indirect and direct inguinal hernias

at the time of physical examination is little better than a chance estimation.[19] Contrariwise, the femoral hernia should be recognized as a distinct entity because of the different operative approach it usually demands. Further, the presence of a femoral hernia should alert the surgeon to the increased hazards of intestinal incarceration and strangulation.

It is usually taught that a femoral hernia passes into the upper thigh beneath the inguinal ligament, appearing at the saphenous opening in the deep fascia. Unfortunately, the thickened fat and fascia layers of

---

Lloyd Milton Nyhus was born in Mount Vernon, Washington, and received his medical education at the Medical College of Alabama. After obtaining his surgical training at King County Hospital, Seattle, Washington, he was appointed to the faculty of the University of Washington School of Medicine. In 1967, he became the Warren H. Cole Professor and Head, Department of Surgery, The University of Illinois College of Medicine, Chicago. His abundant research and clinical contributions to the study of peptic ulcer disease have established him as an authority in that field. He is also deeply interested in hernias and has published a monograph on this subject, now in its second edition.

the hernial sac wall are fixed, and reduction of the lump may be impossible. Further, it may be difficult to determine its relation to the inguinal ligament. Confusion also may occur because an enlarged inguinal lymph node, lipoma, saphenous varix, or psoas abscess may mimic a femoral hernial enlargement in many details. The surgeon, having blundered into a pointing psoas abscess on a morning set aside for a clean femoral hernia repair, would agree that more care should have been taken in making a correct diagnosis.

The late Sir Heneage Ogilvie[16] has given us considerable insight into how we may prevent making these disastrous errors in diagnosis.

The differential diagnosis of a femoral hernia will depend on whether it is reducible or not.

The common femoral hernia is irreducible but symptomless. The sac contains nothing but a tag of adherent omentum and the outer coverings are fat laden and bulky. There is no impulse on coughing. Such a swelling is merely a rounded elastic tumour in the inner half of Scarpa's triangle that must be distinguished from an enlarged lymph gland and a lipoma, the only conditions which it resembles.

The distinctive feature of the hernia is that it has a neck, and the neck passes backwards below Poupart's ligament and medial to the femoral vessels. When the lump is moved about this deep attachment becomes obvious. A lymphatic gland lies in the plane of the superficial fascia, and in that plane it can be moved to an approximately equal extent in all directions. A single enlarged inguinal gland is in any case unusual. A lipoma is in the subcutaneous fat, and can be lifted off the deep fascia. A femoral hernia can be moved in circles within the range allowed by its "stalk," like the joy-stick of an aeroplane: in most cases the "stalk" can be traced to Poupart's ligament.

A reducible femoral hernia may be quite clearly a hernia, that is it is reduced by manipulation, and returns not immediately, but after coughing or straining. Reduction and reappearance are accompanied by the gurgle of intestine, and the swelling is resonant to percussion. The only difficulty in such a case is the distinction between a femoral hernia lying over the external ring and an inguinal hernia.

The distinction between femoral and inguinal hernia rests on two points; on the relation of the swelling to the pubic spine, and whether the swelling after reduction reappears above or below Poupart's ligament. An inguinal hernia that has reached the external ring overlies the pubic spine, but the spine can be felt by putting a finger below and lateral to the swelling and displacing it inwards. In femoral hernia the pubic spine can be felt only by a finger placed above and medial to the swelling. After reduction of a hernia whose nature is in doubt, a finger should be kept on the inner end of Poupart's ligament while the patient coughs. It can then be determined whether the swelling reappears from below the ligament, that is from the crural canal, or above it from the inguinal canal.

Two reducible swellings in Scarpa's triangle, saphenous varix and psoas abscess, may be mistaken for the femoral hernia by the inexperienced or over confident. Both are reducible swellings below Poupart's ligament, but neither has the true characters of a hernia. Both appear in the erect position and disappear on recumbency, and neither has the firm rounded outline of a hernia, gives a gurgle when handled, or is resonant to percussion.

Ultrasonography may be useful in the diagnosis of the femoral hernia that is not palpable.[22] Real-time ultrasonic techniques also will be of use in differentiating vessels and possibly psoas abscess from unusual femoral hernia presentations.

DIAGNOSTIC AID IN INFANTS. The exploration of an asymptomatic groin in an infant or child with negative findings at operation must be considered an error in judgment.[10] Yet it remains accepted practice to explore the contralateral side following the repair of a groin hernia in children. Will the new technique of herniography prevent these unnecessary operations? Thompson et al.[24] believe that many fewer explorations will be performed following use of the diagnostic herniogram. Herniography in their practice gave a diagnostic accuracy of 88 per cent, which compared favorably to the usual clinical diagnostic accuracy of 50 to 60 per cent. They recommend the procedure for all children with unilateral hernia and those with a history of a bulge unconfirmed by physical findings. Major complications (abdominal wall cellulitis with septicemia and hematoma of bowel wall with intestinal obstruction) have occurred following herniography.[3] As with any invasive diagnostic method, indiscriminate use must be avoided.

INCARCERATION AND STRANGULATION

The evolution from simple hernia to one of intestinal incarceration and strangulation

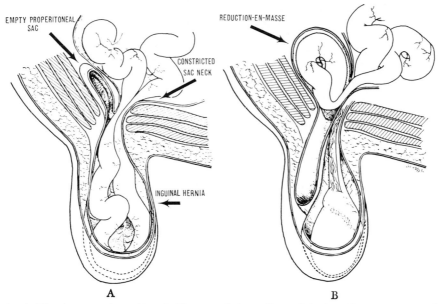

Figure 27–1 *A,* Bilocular properitoneal hernia. The constriction at the neck is above the common opening of the two sacs. Attempted reduction could cause the situation represented in *B. B,* Reduction en masse. The constriction above the common opening has prevented reduction of the inguinal sac contents into the peritoneal cavity. They have entered the properitoneal sac, but the bowel is still strangulated. (From Altman, B.: Interparietal hernia. *In* Nyhus, L. M., and Condon, R. E. (Eds.): Hernia. 2nd Ed. Philadelphia, J. B. Lippincott Company, 1978.)

is the basic problem of all hernias. It is usually easy to make the diagnosis of incarceration; however, one of the most difficult diagnostic skills encountered in medicine is recognition in a fixed hernial mass of the process of strangulation. Because of this deficiency in our diagnostic acumen, the empiricism of early operation for irreducible acute hernial incarceration developed.

In our zeal to prevent prolonged incarceration, excessive attempts made to reduce the hernia may result in "reduction en masse."[1] The contents of the hernial sac would then be displaced into a preformed interparietal sac, while the constriction at the sac neck still remains (Fig. 27–1). The continuation of symptoms of intestinal obstruction following apparent reduction of an incarcerated hernia is suggestive of this phenomenon.

INTESTINAL OBSTRUCTION

One of the easiest pitfalls in the erroneous diagnosis of the cause of intestinal obstruction relates to hernia. The failure to look for "lumps and bumps" in the groin is inexcus-

able. In the absence of external findings, the occult and, fortunately, more uncommon hernial causes of intestinal obstruction must be considered: (1) internal — paraduodenal and hernias of the foramen of Winslow, mesenteric, retroanastomotic, interparietal, and supravesical; (2) pelvic — obturator, sciatic, and perineal; and (3) ventral — umbilical, epigastric, Spigelian, lumbar, and incisional.

The partial enterocele, or Richter's hernia, is treacherous because it does *not* cause intestinal obstruction early. Thus the partial incarceration may surreptitiously progress to necrosis of the bowel, converting a simple problem to one of complexity.

CONCOMITANT DISEASE

It is well known that obstructive uropathy and chronic pulmonary disease must be treated before an elective hernial operation is undertaken. It is not so well recognized that change in intraperitoneal pressure dynamics caused by carcinoma of the pancreas and colon or by cirrhosis with subclinical ascites may transform an otherwise asymptomatic hernia of 20 years' duration into a hernia causing real annoyance. These possibilities must always be considered in the older patient who suddenly, after years of procrastination, desires an operation. Particular attention must be given to the system review of the patient's history as well as to the performance of a careful physical examination. Sigmoidoscopy and barium enema should be performed as a routine portion of a preoperative workup in patients over 50 years of age.

Terezis et al.[23] documented this phenomenon as it relates to the colon. In an analysis of 107 consecutive male patients with clinically proven cancer of the large intestine, 17 per cent first sought medical assistance because of symptoms referable to an inguinal hernia. These symptoms included pain or discomfort at the hernia site, recent increase in size of a preexisting hernia, or sudden recurrence of a previously repaired hernia. The yield of examination for occult colon carcinoma in patients with asymptomatic inguinal hernia[5] will be small, but this does not negate the value of the opportunity to screen a large number of older patients for colorectal lesions.

OPERATIVE COMPLICATIONS

HEMORRHAGE

Hemorrhage may occur during the course of any operative procedure. Significant hemorrhage may occur in hernial repair as a result of trauma to three different vessels: (1) pubic branch of the obturator artery (so-called corona mortis); (2) inferior deep epigastric vessels; and (3) external iliac artery and vein. Damage to the first two is troublesome, but after extension of exposure, these vessels may be ligated with impunity because of rich collateral connections. Injury to the major artery or vein to the thigh and leg is a different matter. Careless deep placement of sutures into the anterior femoral sheath or iliopubic tract will assure a high incidence of this complication. These fascial structures should be "tented up" when the needle is passed. Upon discovery of this complication, there is always the tendency for the surgeon to tie the suture, but the safest practice is to withdraw the suture and apply pressure. If this does not control the hemorrhage immediately, the operative wound must be enlarged and the vessel exposed. Adequate exposure will allow effective local tamponade, or the rent may be sutured with fine vascular suture material. Ligation of these major vascular trunks would be catastrophic and must be done only to save the patient's life.

SEVERANCE OF THE VAS DEFERENS

Because there are two vasa deferentia, this accident in the child or young adult may be considered of minimal importance by some surgeons. This should not be the attitude, however, and the severed vas should be repaired immediately. Urologic surgeons have been exceptionally successful in the secondary repair of this structure. Although it is difficult to evaluate results after an operation of this type, approximately 50 per cent of vasa repaired are considered to be functional.

The cut ends of the vas are approximated with very fine catgut, and an internal splint of catgut is also used (Fig. 27–2). It has been suggested that the defect be bridged with a fine stainless steel wire brought through the wall of the vas deferens on each side of the anastomosis through the fascial layers to the skin and tied over a bolus of gauze. This "pull-out" splint may be removed after 7 to 10 days. Finally, if an operating microscope

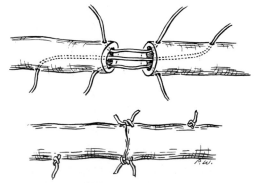

Figure 27–2 Method of repairing severed vas deferens using fine catgut suture material as an internal splint.

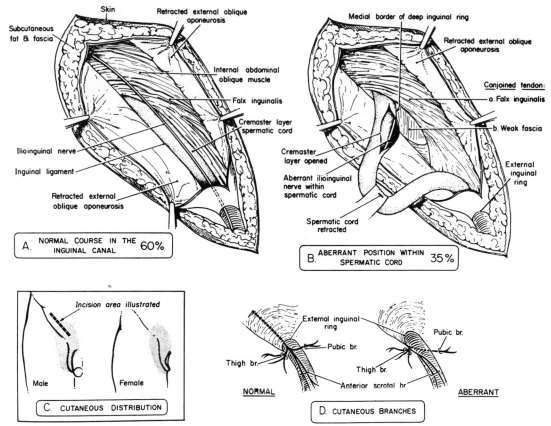

Figure 27–3 Course, distribution, and branches of normal and aberrant ilioinguinal nerves in the inguinal region. (Courtesy of: Moosman, D. A., and Oelrich, T. M.: Prevention of accidental trauma to the ilioinguinal nerve during inguinal herniorrhaphy. Am. J. Surg. *133*:146, 1977.)

is available in the surgical suite, an end-to-end anastomosis with interrupted 6-0 silk to the wall of the vas deferens is recommended. Under these conditions no splint is necessary.

SEVERANCE OF NERVES TO LOWER ABDOMINAL WALL

ANATOMY

The lower abdominal wall is rich in nerve fibers. The fibers important to hernial repair are two branches of the first lumbar nerve, the iliohypogastric and the ilioinguinal. The iliohypogastric nerve penetrates the internal oblique muscle and runs medially beneath the fascia of the external oblique aponeurosis cephalad to the inguinal canal. It supplies the suprapubic area with the sensory fibers.

The ilioinguinal nerve — usually seen during early dissection of the inguinal canal — also perforates the internal oblique muscle approximately 1 to 1.5 cm. from the anterior iliac spine. It then passes beneath the external oblique fascia in or near the inguinal canal to the subcutaneous inguinal ring, where it exits to provide sensory innervation to the base of the penis, part of the scrotum, and comparable areas in the female (Fig. 27–3). It should be noted that there is an interchange of fibers between the twelfth thoracic, first lumbar, and second lumbar nerves, and that there is a segmental overlapping of the area supplied by the nerve immediately above and below. These nerves also give off motor fibers to adjacent muscles.[11]

Although the iliohypogastric and ilioinguinal nerves are given greatest consideration, surgeons should be aware of other nerves in the area that could conceivably give rise to similar complications. The penile skin and the immediate scrotal area are supplied by sensory fibers from the sacral plexus. The genitofemoral nerve, arising from the first, second, and third lumbar nerves, supplies the scrotum and upper part of the thigh with sensory fibers as well as motor fibers to the cremaster muscle by way of the genital branch. The genital branch reaches the inguinal canal at the internal abdominal ring in its medial aspect and continues to the skin of the scrotum. The femoral branch accompanies the femoral artery beneath the inguinal ligament to innervate the femoral triangle with sensory fibers.

OPERATIVE CONSIDERATIONS

Since the ilioinguinal nerve lies just beneath the external oblique fascia near the inguinal canal, it is particularly vulnerable when this fascial layer is incised. The iliohypogastric nerve is endangered when a relaxing incision is made during a Cooper's ligament repair, or during the medial exposure of a preperitoneal approach. If one of these nerves is accidentally cut, it is of no practical value to attempt repair. The nerve end should be freshened and a silver clip carefully applied to the end. This allows the neurilemma to close accurately and keeps the axon elements of the nerve away from the mesodermal cells, the latter being the sine qua non of neuroma production.

Fortunately, the cross-connections and segmental overlap between nerve trunks just mentioned may prevent prolonged anesthesia of the affected skin. The nerve entrapped in a suture may cause prolonged symptoms; thus, each nerve must be protected from both severance and entrapment.

These same observations apply to the branches of the genitofemoral nerve. The genital branch in the spermatic cord probably is more vulnerable. Certainly in those operative procedures in which the cremaster muscle is incised and excised at the level of the internal inguinal ring, it may be cut. Patients rarely complain of loss of sensation or loss of contractile response following section of the genital branch, but on occa-

sion a patient will note that the testis on the side operated on rests in a more dependent position than preoperatively. This latter complaint probably relates to manipulation of the cremaster muscle rather than severance of the genital nerve. Areas of postoperative anesthesia usually resolve after several months because of the aforementioned cross-communication of the nerves.

DAMAGE TO ARTERIAL BLOOD SUPPLY TO TESTIS

Every precaution should be taken to prevent damage to the vascular bundle in the spermatic cord during mobilization of the hernial sac. Despite this care, laceration of the vessels occurs. The vessels are very small, making repair impractical. Ligation is indicated here. Does ligation of the major artery to the testis at the level of the internal inguinal ring or in the inguinal canal preclude subsequent atrophy of the testis?

CIRCULATION OF THE TESTIS

The internal spermatic or testicular artery, arising from the front portion of the abdominal aorta, is the main arterial supply to the testis. This artery joins the cord structures at the level of the internal inguinal ring. The external spermatic artery, a branch of the inferior epigastric artery, joins the spermatic cord and passes through the inguinal canal adjacent to the vas deferens and supplies the cremaster muscle. Loosely incorporated in the sheath of the vas deferens is the artery to this structure, a branch of the superior vesical artery. There is free communication between the deferential artery and the internal spermatic artery.

COLLATERAL CIRCULATION

There is a rich collateral circulation between the major testicular vessels. Distal to the external inguinal ring, there are anastomoses between branches of the vesical and prostatic arteries and the internal spermatic and deferential arteries at the upper end of the testis. Further, scrotal arteries, branches

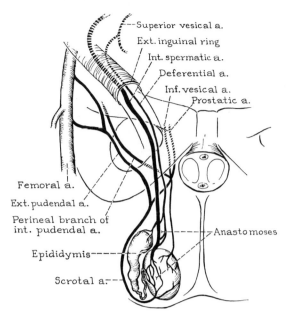

Figure 27–4 Schematic drawing of both primary and collateral circulation to the testis.

of the internal and external pudendal arteries, freely anastomose into this collateral system (Fig. 27–4).

OPERATIVE CONSIDERATIONS

As just indicated, these multiple arterial connections allow a certain margin of error for accidental damage to vessels in the spermatic cord. It must be emphasized that removal of the testis from the scrotum will destroy this collateral circulation distal to the external ring.[6]

These same observations apply to elective removal of the spermatic cord from the inguinal canal. The occasional hernial repair will be enhanced by excision of the spermatic cord at the level of the internal ring or within the inguinal canal. This is particularly true during the repair of recurrent hernias.[8] It may be difficult, however, to know whether dislocation of the testis occurred during the previous repair or repairs; thus, a cautious approach must be taken under these circumstances. Further, a rare patient may not have sufficient collateral circulation to allow for transection of the cord. Whenever the possibility of this maneuver is contemplated preoperatively, all the ramifications should be discussed with

the patient, and a document granting permission should be signed by him.

DAMAGE TO ABDOMINAL VISCERA

HIGH LIGATION OF SAC

Meticulous attention must be given to the placement of each suture during this portion of the operation. Blind suturing here is not acceptable. Fecal fistula, abscess, and intestinal obstruction are a few of the sequelae that may follow accidental suturing of the bowel to the proximally ligated hernial sac. When this is recognized at the time of the operation, removal of the misplaced suture will suffice.

INJURY TO CECUM OR SIGMOID IN SLIDING HERNIA

Two operative complications are recognized from the pulling type of sliding hernia. The bowel may be entered or the bowel wall may be devascularized prior to recognition of the pathologic condition involved. Because the hernial sac is usually placed anteriorly, dissection of all hernial sacs should be started from this aspect. When a rare sacless sliding hernia occurs, or whenever the hernial sac seems excessively thickened, extreme caution is indicated.

Since the blood supply to the bowel enters at the posterior aspect of a sliding hernia, dissection of this posterior portion will result in hemorrhage or necrosis of the bowel from compromise of the vascular supply. If the peritoneum is incised about 1 inch laterally and medially to the sliding component, these complications may be avoided (Fig. 27–5).

If the colon has been entered, a careful two-layer closure (4-0 catgut to mucosa and 4-0 silk to the serosa) must be performed. The closure is followed by massive irrigation of the wound with normal saline solution. Compromise of the vascularity of the bowel wall is more difficult to ascertain. If unquestioned devascularization has occurred, the individual situation will dictate the course of action, which may include (1) lateral wedge resection, closure, and proximal temporary diversion of bowel content; (2) Mikulicz

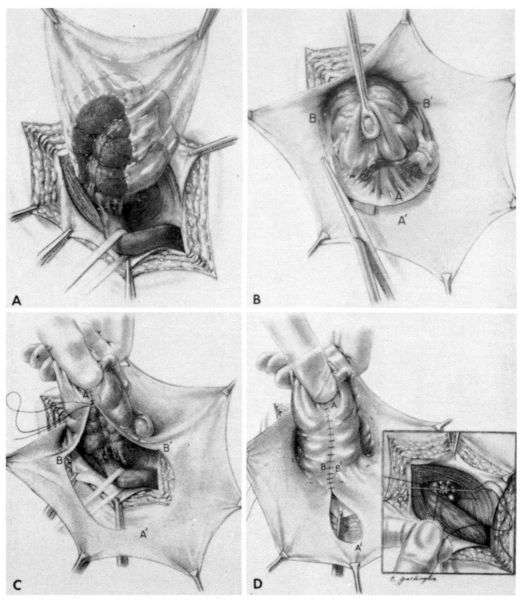

Figure 27–5   *A,* Repair of sliding hernia of cecum—inguinal approach. The hernial sac has been partially dissected and is held upward, exposing the large retroperitoneal portion of the cecum posteriorly, still somewhat attached to the cord structures. *B,* The hernial sac has been opened anteriorly, exposing the peritonealized portion of cecum. The peritoneum is being incised about 2 cm. from the cecal edges. *C,* The posterior surface of the cecum has been dissected away from the cord structures and the floor of the canal well into the abdominal cavity. The cut edges of peritoneum are being sutured together behind the cecum, forming a mesentery covering the small nutrient vessels to the cecum. *D,* The peritoneal closure has been continued on the posterior abdominal wall down to the sac. A purse-string suture is applied under direct vision at a point which will assure a high ligation of the neck. In the inset the purse-string suture has been tied, and the excess sac trimmed away. A transfixing suture is applied through the sac just distal to the pursestring for reinforcement. (From Moretz, W. H.: The special problem of sliding inguinal hernia. *In* Nyhus, L. M., and Harkins, H. N. (Eds.): Hernia. Philadelphia, J. B. Lippincott Company, 1964.)

exteriorization; or (3) colectomy and primary anastomosis with or without proximal venting of bowel content. The seriousness of this complication is obvious.

INJURY TO URINARY BLADDER

The medial side of a direct inguinal hernia often contains bladder wall (a sliding hernia). A hole may be made accidentally in the bladder when the direct sac is opened (since most direct sacs have a broad neck, many surgeons do not open the peritoneum here, thus avoiding this complication). As with many of the complications mentioned in this section, the familiar saying, "It isn't so bad to make the complication, but it is inexcusable not to recognize *and* repair the defect," pertains.

The defect in the bladder wall should be sutured in two layers (watertight) with 00 chromic catgut. An indwelling urethral catheter should be inserted, placed at straight drainage, and left in for 4 days. The hernial repair may proceed as a matter of routine after the bladder closure. After this course of action, most patients will have an uneventful recovery.

VIABILITY OF STRANGULATED BOWEL

The accurate determination of bowel viability is difficult. The large number of tests proposed to aid in this decision is indicative that no one test is superior. Fortunately, most bowel is immediately recognizable as viable — rapid return of good color and contractility — or non viable — failure of return of these same characteristics. Additional techniques include (1) fluorescein injection and examination under ultraviolet light; (2) use of vasodilators and study of temperature changes; and (3) administration of oxygen in high concentrations to accentuate the color changes previously mentioned. Regardless of these techniques, the best method remains careful clinical observation, tempered with experience, of the color and serosal shine, presence or return of peristalsis, pulsation of mesenteric blood vessels, and odor and general nature of the peritoneal fluid. The best treatment

here is to resect the affected bowel whenever there is doubt of viability. If questionable bowel is returned into the peritoneal cavity, the patient must be observed carefully for a number of days for evidence of peritoneal irritation. If symptoms of the latter complication occur, immediate abdominal exploration is necessary.

THE QUESTION OF APPENDECTOMY

A total of 2200 Americans die annually of appendicitis, and anyone living 70 years will have approximately one chance in three of having appendicitis and requiring an appendectomy.[4] These observations indicate why surgeons often wish to combine right inguinal hernial repair with appendectomy.

Several factors have prevented this combination of procedures from becoming routine practice. Increased operating time, infection, and recurrence have been the prime considerations. The increase in time, if not inordinate, should not be a factor in this decision. On the other hand, an increase in infection rate or recurrence rate could not be condoned. Most reports indicate that when the setting is appropriate, appendectomy can be performed without an increase in morbidity. As suggested by Eiseman,[4] concurrent appendectomy is permissible *only* if the following prerequisites are met: (1) There is no complicating disease to contraindicate a slight prolongation of the operative time. (2) The entire appendix from tip to base can be easily delivered into the wound so that the stump can be amputated and secured with good exposure without enlarging the hernial defect or the neck of the sac.

Thus, a moderate course between *never* and *every* is recommended.

MISCELLANEOUS CONSIDERATIONS

LOSS OF "RIGHT OF DOMAIN"

This author viewed a filmstrip on the repair of a massive scrotal hernia. During the operation the colon was resected so that the hernial defect could be closed. In the 1940's, Moreno originated the concept of preoperative progressive pneumoperitoneum in preparation for repair of massive ventral and inguinal hernias.[12] My colleagues and I have used this method for more than 30 years and have never resected bowel to allow wound closure.

THE PROBLEM OF THE MISSED HERNIA

The second hernia on a given side is often missed. Thorough finger exploration of the posterior inguinal wall through the opened indirect hernial sac is mandatory. The region of Hesselbach's triangle and the femoral canal may be easily palpated by this technique. Similar finger and direct visual exploration of the posterior inguinal wall is practiced with the preperitoneal approach.[14]

LOSS OF STRANGULATED BOWEL INTO PERITONEAL CAVITY

Section of the constricting band at the neck of a hernial sac may release the entrapped intestine with great rapidity. Unless the operating team is alert to this possibility, the bowel may suddenly disappear into the peritoneal cavity. The dilemma is apparent. Was the bowel viable or not? If a standard groin approach was used, it may be necessary to make a separate formal laparotomy to answer this question. When there is doubt, the bowel *must* be visualized. As suggested, this complication should not occur in the presence of an alert operating team.

SELECTION OF OPERATION

Surgeons must learn to pattern their operative approach to the individual problem encountered. The simple indirect hernia in the child or young adult may be handled satisfactorily by a classic anterior approach and high ligation of the hernial sac with or without closure of the internal ring. Contrariwise, the massive direct hernia, the sliding hernia, the strangulated hernia, or the recurrent hernia may more appropriately be approached preperitoneally with concomitant iliopubic tract repair. The skillful surgeon should be practiced in both approaches. Furthermore, his or her ability to cope with *potential* operative complications will be greatly enhanced.[15]

POSTOPERATIVE COMPLICATIONS

EARLY COMPLICATIONS

GENERAL

Systemic complications of hernial repair occur at a rate comparable with the complication rate of other operative procedures of the same extent. Rydell[21] reported an incidence of systemic complications following inguinal hernia repair in the adult of 6.9 per cent (Table 27–1). Miscellaneous complications in this series included gout and single occurrences of acute cholecystitis, intestinal obstruction, gastrointestinal hemorrhage, renal calculus, herpes zoster, liver necrosis, and acute psychosis. The mortality in this series was 0.3 per cent. These figures are representative of the incidence of general complications following inguinal hernial repair in the United States today.

RELATION OF ANESTHESIA TO EARLY COMPLICATIONS. Urbach et al.[25] studied the difference between spinal and general anesthesia in relation to the postoperative complications of inguinal hernial repair. Their data indicated that there is an increased risk of vomiting, but not of nausea, after general anesthesia. Spinal anesthesia does not prevent respiratory complications.

TABLE 27–1 SYSTEMIC COMPLICATIONS IN ADULTS FOLLOWING INGUINAL HERNIA REPAIR: 961 OPERATIONS*

	Number	Per Cent
Cardiovascular-pulmonary	39	4.1
Atelectasis, pneumonitis	24	2.5
Thrombophlebitis	13	1.4
Coronary occlusion	2	0.2
Urinary retention (req. T.U.R.)	10	1.0
Urinary infection	5	0.5
Miscellaneous	12	1.3
Totals	66	6.9

*From Rydell, W. B., Jr.: Inguinal and femoral hernias. Arch. Surg. *87*:493, 1963.

The rare major neurologic complication of spinal anesthesia must be balanced against the higher risk of vomiting, with the possibility of aspiration, and greater incidence of cardiac arrest reported during general anesthesia.

Urinary retention occurred with similar frequency in the two groups studied, i.e., in about 30 per cent of patients. To minimize the incidence and sequelae of this complication, Urbach and his colleagues suggested the avoidance of excessive use of pain control medications—atropine and scopolamine, postoperative narcotics for pain, prolonged sensory block by spinal anesthesia, and prolonged recovery from general anesthesia. Finally, prompt catheterization is mandatory if urinary retention persists beyond 12 hours, lest overdistention and permanent damage to the bladder occur.

The place of local anesthesia in hernial repair is well established. These techniques should be studied and practiced frequently.[17] The surgeon adept in the use of local anesthesia will be well rewarded by lower complication rates. Leaverton and Garnjobst[7] found that repair under local anesthesia was followed by a much lower rate of urinary retention necessitating catheterization (6.2 per cent) than repair under spinal anesthesia (16.2 per cent).

LOCAL

Table 27–2 summarizes the experience of local complications in a large series of patients treated for groin hernia at the Mary

TABLE 27–2 LOCAL COMPLICATIONS IN ADULTS FOLLOWING REPAIR OF 1053 HERNIAS*

	Number	Per Cent
Wound	21	2.0
Major infection	14	1.3
Hematoma	7	0.7
Scrotal and cord (924 male hernias)	62	6.7
Marked swelling	24	2.6
Testicular atrophy	16	1.8
Postoperative hydrocele	5	0.5
Ilioinguinal neuritis	14	1.5
Cut vas deferens	3	0.3
Totals	83	8.7

*From Rydell, W. B., Jr.: Inguinal and femoral hernias. Arch. Surg. *87*:493, 1963.

Hitchcock Memorial Hospital in New Hampshire. The author presents his data in a refreshingly candid manner, and again, this study probably represents an accurate reflection of the incidence of these early local complications seen generally today.

WOUND. *Major wound infection* should be infrequent. An occasional severe infection, however, will follow treatment of advanced strangulation of the intestines. Local and systemic measures will usually resolve both superficial and deep infection in this area. An unfortunate sequela of deep fascial infection is a high incidence of hernial recurrence. *Hematoma* of the wound is uncommon; however, after dissection of a scrotal hernia, formation of a hematoma is assured unless meticulous attention is given to immediate hemostasis. Local pressure may abort an early hematoma. If bleeding continues after local measures have been tried, reoperation may be necessary. The chronic hematoma may be aspirated, but special precautions must be taken to prevent infection.

SCROTUM AND TESTIS. *Swelling* of the scrotal skin and testis may occur. The exact cause of this complication is obscure, but probably relates to the closure of the internal ring. Venous obstruction with resultant engorgement and tissue edema is the probable mechanism. All young surgeons are admonished not to close this ring too tightly. The incidence of testicular atrophy subsequent to this complication is high. Thus, meticulous closure (between Scylla and Charybdis—too tight or too loose) of the internal ring about the spermatic cord is extremely important. The swelling and discomfort are alarming, and treatment consists of bed rest, scrotal support, and ice compresses.

FEMORAL VEIN COMPRESSION AND THROMBOPHLEBITIS. A key portion of the Cooper's ligament (McVay) repair for femoral and direct groin hernia is the approximation of transversalis fascia to Cooper's ligament below the level of the femoral vessels. If this row of sutures is carried too far laterally (prior to the transition suture) actual encroachment of the femoral vein may occur when the sutures are tied. Brown and colleagues[2] have studied this specific problem and suggest an incidence of about 1.2 per cent of significant femoral vein compression and subsequent ipsilateral thrombophlebitis after this type of repair. The same anatomic structures are used with the iliopubic tract repair, but visualization of the femoral vein is superior with the preperitoneal approach. It would be of interest to know the incidence of this complication following this latter operative approach.

LATE COMPLICATIONS

HYDROCELE

This scrotal collection of fluid may result from leaving a distal hernial sac in situ after transecting the sac at the hernial neck and high ligation of the proximal stump. Regardless of the cause, most of these will either resolve spontaneously or not recur after several separate needle aspirations.

SINUS TRACTS

With the increasing use of plastic meshes to buttress fascial repairs, chronic infection may become a problem.[20] Fortunately, this has not been the record to date. If evidence of chronic deep infection occurs, it is most likely due to use of silk or other non-absorbable suture material different from that of the mesh itself. If the infected material can be retrieved through the sinus tract with a crochet hook or other device, the wound will heal. We have not found it necessary to remove the mesh buttress because of chronic deep wound infection.

NEUROMA

Ilioinguinal neuritis or the actual formation of neuromas following section of a nerve in this region can occur. Patients complain bitterly when afflicted with this complication. The incidence, at least of the neuritis, is markedly increased in the compensation-prone patient. Most of the twinges will resolve without treatment, and those that persist should be treated by local nerve blocks. In a few patients the wound must be explored. Accurate preoperative localization of the point of pain will help the surgeon to find the elusive neuroma. After the neuroma has been excised, the cut end

of the nerve must be handled with the silver clip as described earlier.

TESTICULAR ATROPHY

This serious complication develops after episodes of postoperative testicular swelling and testicular ischemia as detailed earlier. It is difficult to denude the testis of its arterial supply by trauma to the vessels at the level of the internal ring or inguinal canal without the removal of the testis from the scrotum. Koontz[6] made an important medicolegal observation, i.e., "atrophy of the testicle sometimes follows a simple primary operation for inguinal hernia repair, in which neither the collateral nor primary circulation has been molested as far as the surgeon is aware." It may be important to reassure the patient early that the absence of one testis will not diminish his sexual potency, propagating powers, and internal secretion.

HERNIAL RECURRENCE

The 6-year recurrence rates reported by Rutledge[20] for indirect, direct, and recurrent hernias were 0.6, 2.4, and 2.2 per cent, respectively. Marsden[9] reported a recurrence incidence of 5.2, 7.4 and 19 per cent, respectively. The latter results are representative, whereas those presented by Rutledge[20] are superb, and his methods should be reviewed carefully.

Postlethwaite[18] has summarized causative factors as follows:

I. Age and general condition of patient
II. Type of primary hernia
III. Conduct of the operation
   A. *Indirect hernia*
     1. Sac not found, incomplete dissection, low ligation
     2. Internal ring not snug
     3. Direct or femoral hernia missed
   B. *Direct hernia*
     1. Inherent weakness of tissues
     2. Incorrect suturing
       a. Bites too large
       b. Improper interval
       c. Tied too tight
     3. Excessive tension

4. Indirect or femoral hernia missed

C. *General*
1. Sutures: type, absorption, cutting, breaking, knots insecure
2. Extensive dissection, excessive trauma, incomplete hemostasis, presence of foreign bodies
3. Bilateral simultaneous repair
4. Inadequate anesthesia
5. Surgical skill

IV. Postoperative period
A. *Early*
1. Strain due to cough, vomiting, distention, retention
2. Hematoma
3. Infection
B. *Late*
1. Direct trauma
2. Strain, lifting, etc.
3. Delayed infection
4. Tissue atrophy
5. New hernia

The high recurrence rate reported from good medical centers indicates a need for continued diligence in our approach to this common problem. Memorization of this long list of causative factors will not prevent hernial recurrence entirely, but it will help.

Surgeons are constantly looking for one operation, one suture material, or one reconstructive mesh that will be the panacea. There is no panacea in hernial repair.[15] The practice of good surgical judgment and good surgical technique will be the best prophylaxis against all the complications mentioned in this chapter.

Bibliography

1. Altman, B.: Interparietal hernia. *In* Nyhus, L. M., and Condon, R. E. (Eds.): Hernia. 2nd Ed. Philadelphia, J. B. Lippincott, 1978.
2. Brown, R. E., Kinateder, R. J., and Rosenberg, N.: Ipsilateral thrombophlebitis and pulmonary embolism after Cooper's ligament herniorrhaphy. Surgery 87:230, 1980.
3. Ducharme, J. C., Guttman, F. M., and Poljicak, M.: Hematoma of bowel and cellulitis of the abdominal wall complicating herniography. J. Pediatr. Surg. 15:318, 1980.
4. Eiseman, B.: Simultaneous herniorrhaphy and appendectomy. *In* Nyhus, L. M., and Harkins, H. N. (Eds.): Hernia. Philadelphia, J. B. Lippincott, 1964.
5. Juler, G. L., Stemmer, E. A., and Fullerman, R.

W.: Inguinal hernia and colorectal carcinoma. Arch. Surg. *104*:778, 1972.
6. Koontz, A. R.: Atrophy of the testicle as a surgical risk. Surg. Gynecol. Obstet. *120*:511, 1965.
7. Leaverton, G. H., and Garnjobst, W.: Comparison of morbidity after spinal and local anesthesia in inguinal hernia repair. Am. Surg. *38*:591, 1972.
8. Ljungdahl, I.: Inguinal and femoral hernia: Personal experience with 502 operations. Acta Chir. Scand. (Suppl.) *439*:1, 1973.
9. Marsden, A. J.: Inguinal hernia. A three-year review of two thousand cases. Br. J. Surg. *216*:384, 1962.
10. McGregor, D. B., Halverson, K., and McVay, C. B.: The unilateral pediatric inguinal hernia: Should the contralateral side be explored? J. Pediatr. Surg. *15*:313, 1980.
11. Moosman, D. A., and Oelrich, T. M.: Prevention of accidental trauma to the ilioinguinal nerve during inguinal herniorrhaphy. Am. J. Surg. *133*:146, 1977.
12. Moreno, I. G.: The rational treatment of hernias and voluminous chronic eventration. *In* Nyhus, L. M., and Condon, R. E. (Eds.): Hernia. 2nd Ed. Philadelphia, J. B. Lippincott, 1978.
13. Moretz, W. H.: The special problem of sliding inguinal hernia. *In* Nyhus, L. M., and Harkins, H. N. (Eds.): Hernia. Philadelphia, J. B. Lippincott, 1964.
14. Nyhus, L. M.: The preperitoneal approach and iliopubic tract repair of all groin hernias. *In* Nyhus, L. M., and Condon, R. E. (Eds.): Hernia. 2nd Ed. Philadelphia, J. B. Lippincott, 1978.
15. Nyhus, L. M., and Bombeck, C. T.: Hernias. *In* Sabiston, D. C., Jr. (Ed.): Davis-Christopher Textbook of Surgery. 11th Ed. Philadelphia, W. B. Saunders Company, 1980.
16. Ogilvie, H.: Hernia. London, Edward Arnold Publishers, Ltd., 1959.
17. Ponka, J. L.: Seven steps to local anesthesia for inguinofemoral hernia repair. Surg. Gynecol. Obstet. *117*:115, 1963.
18. Postlethwaite, R. W.: Recurrent inguinal hernia. Am. J. Surg. *107*:739, 1964.
19. Ralphs, D. N. L., Brain, A. J. L., Grundy, D. J., and Hobsley, M.: How accurately can direct and indirect hernias be distinguished? Br. Med. J. *1*:1039, 1980.
20. Rutledge, R. H.: Cooper's ligament repair for adult groin hernias. Surgery *87*:601, 1980.
21. Rydell, W. B., Jr.: Inguinal and femoral hernias. Arch. Surg. *87*:493, 1963.
22. Spangen, L.: Spigelian hernia. Acta Chir. Scand. (Suppl.) *462*:1, 1976.
23. Terezis, N. L., Davis, W. C., and Jackson, F. C.: Carcinoma of the colon associated with inguinal hernia. N. Engl. J. Med. *268*:774, 1963.
24. Thompson, W., Longerbeam, J. V., and Reeves, C.: Herniograms: An aid to the diagnosis and treatment of groin hernias in infants and children. Arch. Surg. *105*:71, 1972.
25. Urbach, K. F., Lee, W. R., Sheely, L. L., Lang, F. L., and Sharp, R. P.: Spinal or general anesthesia for inguinal hernia repair? A comparison of certain complications in a controlled series. J.A.M.A. *190*:25, 1964.

28

COMPLICATIONS FOLLOWING THE SURGICAL TREATMENT OF WOMEN WITH POTENTIALLY CURABLE CARCINOMA OF THE BREAST

Guy F. Robbins*

The mortality associated with the surgical treatment of women with carcinoma of the breast is under 1 per cent. However, physical and psychologic situations that may produce troublesome morbidity do occur. The degree of severity of these complications largely depends upon the preoperative preparation of the patient, the surgeon's expertise, and the patient's response to the combined effort of the health professionals to assist her readaptation to society. Efforts toward prevention of physical complications are important. The psychological impact of

*This chapter is a revision of the chapter written by Charles T. Fitts and Curtis P. Artz for the second edition of this volume.

breast cancer can be kept at a minimum if preventive measures and early postoperative assistance are applied vigorously.

PREPARATION FOR SURGERY

An internist and anesthetist are involved in consultative capacities. The method of treatment should be selected after analysis of the data base and the best possible correction of recognized deficiencies. The data base must include the patient's history and the findings of physical examination, hemogram, blood chemistry studies, urinalysis, chest roentgenography, and electrocardiography. For a patient whose disease is consid-

Guy F. Robbins was born in Indiana and received his college and medical education at Northwestern University. Beginning as Instructor in surgery in 1950, he is now Clinical Associate Professor at Cornell University Medical College. At Memorial Hospital for Cancer and Allied Disease, he has had extensive experience in various fields of oncology. He is currently the senior attending surgeon, Breast Service, in the Department of Surgery at Memorial Hospital. Dr. Robbins is eminently qualified to discuss postoperative problems as related to breast surgery.

ered clinically borderline and potentially curable, or who has bone pain, a bone scan or skeletal survey is a necessity. We do not do bone scans or skeletal surveys routinely. Our data show that only 19 per cent (61 of 321 patients in 1960) of our potentially curable patients with invasive breast cancer incurred bone metastasis during the 10 years after their primary surgery. We do obtain postoperative bone scans as a baseline for follow-up care on patients with postsurgical pathologic stages II and III disease.

The plethora of reports in the lay and medical journals concerning unproven innovative conservative methods of treatment has resulted in an increased need for detailed explanations of the therapeutic options available. Multicentricity of breast carcinoma, inaccuracy of clinical evaluation of the status of axillary nodes, and the importance of long-term survival statistics must be presented in an understandable form to patients and their families. In addition, the advantages and disadvantages of the two-step surgical procedure must be explained.

Women's fears of breast cancer make preoperative psychologic support by health professionals a must. Usually a patient who has been advised properly of the events associated with admission and contemplated hospital procedures will be more sanguine about the entire situation.

The use of the two-step surgical procedure has resulted in many patients seeking second, third, and fourth opinions. Unfortunately, many of these patients leave their original surgeons and are eventually operated upon by a "specialist." Because of the delay between the two procedures, infection can be and has been a problem. Therefore, we recommend that prophylactic antibiotics be utilized prior to and following the definitive surgical procedure.

Whole blood and plasma should be available prior to surgery. Antibiotics prophylactically are indicated if the patient is a diabetic or has some intercurrent infection or an ulcerated breast lesion. We apply elastic stockings or Ace bandages to the legs before surgery in women over 40 years of age and to younger ones if phlebitis is a recognized problem. Although carious teeth are a recognized source of postoperative upper re-

spiratory infections, such deficits are corrected infrequently prior to breast surgery.

Great care should be exercised in positioning the patient on the operating table so that when both arms are outstretched at right angles they are not permitted to fall backward. The brachial plexus can be injured in an unconscious patient if the arm is forced backward to an unreasonable extent.

SELECTION OF SURGICAL PROCEDURE

The medical condition of a patient, the histologic characteristics of the cancer, and its anatomic location should dictate the selection of a specific surgical procedure. Elderly patients, patients with severe cardiac disease, and diabetics are prone to complications including acute cardiac episodes and poor wound healing. For these patients with invasive carcinoma the procedure of choice is modified radical mastectomy or total mastectomy. The former is defined as a total mastectomy plus removal of the pectoral fascia, the axillary nodes and fat, and the nodes and fat between the pectoralis major and minor muscles. At times the pectoralis minor muscle is resected. If the dominant lesion is deep in the breast, it is prudent to remove a segment of the underlying pectoralis major muscle. Those patients whose lesions are in the lateral half of the breast are subjected to a standard radical mastectomy when the tumor is greater than 2 cm. in diameter or when there is gross evidence of involvement of the axillary nodes. Those patients with small (<2cm.) lesions are subjected to modified radical mastectomies, provided the dominant lesion is in the outer half of the breast and the axilla is clinically uninvolved with axillary metastasis. In patients with small central or inner quadrant lesions, the internal mammary nodes are biopsied. If the biopsy results are negative, a modified radical mastectomy is performed. If positive, an extended radical mastectomy is carried out.

Patients with pure intraductal carcinoma, lobular in-situ carcinomas, and non-infiltrating Paget's disease of the nipple are subjected to total mastectomy and low axillary dissection. Patients with invasive carcinoma of the center or inner half of the breast are subjected to extended radical mastectomy — either the Urban procedure, consisting of a classic radical mastectomy plus excision of segments of the ribs, the internal mammary nodes, and the underlying pleura, or the extrapleural extended radical mastectomy, which includes radical mastectomy plus removal of the internal mammary nodes extrapleurally. The contralateral breast biopsy, provided a gener-

ous segment of breast tissue is obtained, alerts one to the preclinical existence of precancerous areas and at times even to non-invasive or invasive carcinomas. The frequent multicentric existence of non-invasive and invasive breast carcinoma renders partial mastectomy useful only in those few patients who are deemed medically unable to withstand the potential dangers of more extensive procedures.

COMMON TECHNICAL ERRORS

INCISION

The Meyer and Halsted incisions are the ones most commonly used. One of the serious errors in technique is to carry the skin incision into the hollow of the axilla. A vertical band of scar tissue will form across the axilla, like a bowstring, and arm motion will be restricted.

An inadequate incision may lead to local recurrences. A margin of at least 2 inches from the outermost edge of the tumor on all sides must be maintained. Halsted believed that it was better to remove too much skin than too little. The important aspect in making the incision is to eliminate the malignant lesion; closure can be effected by means of a skin graft if necessary.

Cosmetically, a transverse incision merits consideration because the normal neck line is preserved. The improved breast reconstructive efforts of plastic surgeons are enhanced when a transverse incision is utilized. A lateral cephalic extension affords excellent exposure of the axillary components. In preparation for a modified radical mastectomy, the arm should be draped free. This added mobility with the aid of upward retraction of the pectoralis major and minor muscles provides additional visualization of the axillary contents.

PREPARATION OF THE FLAPS

Defining of the thin fascial layer just beneath the skin is essential to the development of proper skin flaps. There is a ten-

dency to leave more fat on the edges of the flaps than near their base; this destroys the circulation to edges, with their resulting slough. Short flaps plus a skin graft are indicated in patients with diabetes and associated arteriosclerosis. One will note very little bleeding from the flaps if the subcutaneous fascial plane described is utilized as a landmark and followed.

AXILLARY DISSECTION

Rough handling of tissues and unnecessary traction on the vessels and nerves in this area will tend to produce serious sequelae including lymphedema, vessel thrombosis, and excessive bleeding. Under no circumstances should retractors be applied to or near the brachial plexus. Partial paralysis has been noted when such pressure has been applied for as little as 15 to 30 seconds. A small retractor can be applied carefully for short intervals to the axillary vein without danger.

In dissection of the axilla it is most important to remove all the fat, lymph nodes, and areolar tissue that lie below the axillary vein. In the routine radical mastectomy any dissection carried above the axillary vein to the axillary artery or brachial plexus is usually considered unnecessary and may result in a rare but painful brachial neuralgia.

Occasionally the axillary vein may be torn. Sometimes it can be closed with one fine suture; in other instances in which bleeding cannot be controlled it may be necessary to ligate the vein. It is doubtful whether ligation of the axillary vein increases the incidence of edema of the arm, but every effort should be made to repair the vein if a small tear occurs.

If the axillary artery is injured and profuse bleeding occurs, small bulldog clamps should be applied above and below the site of injury. As soon as hemorrhage has been controlled the laceration in the artery may be sutured with fine silk.

Running vertically outward and downward from behind the axillary vein is the thoracodorsal nerve, which innervates the latissimus dorsi muscle. This nerve lies in close proximity in its course to the subscapular vessels. A decision must be made whether to sacrifice or preserve the nerve. It is unreasonably hazardous to try to dissect the nerve out from along lymph nodes if it is likely that they contain metastases. The nerve should be saved when possible, however. If it is cut, paralysis of the latissmus dorsi muscle results, with a slight weakness of abduction and internal rotation of the arm. This nerve is frequently sacrificed in the standard radical mastectomy procedure, and the weakness in arm motion is scarcely perceptible.

The long thoracic nerve of Bell comes out of the apex of the axilla and courses downward along the lateral aspect of the serratus muscle. This nerve must be preserved. As the axillary vein is dissected free on the medial end near the apex of the axilla it can be lifted with a small vein retractor. The dissection then proceeds laterally. A mass of tissue between the medial portion of the vein and the chest wall is dissected downward and outward off the surface of the subscapular muscle. The long thoracic nerve then comes into view. Great care should be taken to identify this nerve because under no circumstance should it be cut. Cutting the nerve produces wing scapula, an ugly deformity, and patients in whom the nerve has been cut or damaged complain of a great deal of shoulder pain for several months.

PERFORATING ARTERIES

One of the most troublesome technical complications is bleeding from one of the perforating vessels. These vessels come through the intercostal muscles and are encountered when the pectoral muscles are removed. They should be clamped with blunt-nosed hemostats applied parallel to the chest wall. If the perforating artery is not properly grasped it may retract between the intercostal muscles and cause serious bleeding. When this occurs, it is usually wise to separate the intercostal muscles and ligate the internal mammary artery above and below the bleeding point.

Sharp-pointed hemostats applied at right angles to the chest wall may perforate the pleura and produce a pneumothorax.

CLOSURE OF WOUND

Before the wound is closed its entire extent should be irrigated with saline and inspected to make sure that it is dry. Hemostasis must be painstaking. Special precaution should be taken so that no gauze sponges or lap pads are left beneath the flaps or in the axilla. The flaps should be sutured together at the upper and lower ends of the wound with fine interrupted sutures. Great care must be taken in handling the edges of these flaps so that they will not be traumatized and become necrotic. If it is found that the flaps cannot be brought together and held with 3-0 or 4-0 silk, then it is probably wiser to cover the remaining defect with a skin graft. Wound closure is facilitated when several stents are fixed at several levels along the lateral flaps. This maneuver diminishes the probability of tension on the suture line, a precursor of poor wound healing. In addition it aids in causing adherence of the flaps to the underlying chest wall.

WOUND DRAINAGE

The extensive surfaces of the wound flaps, denuded chest wall, and axilla are prone to postoperative oozing, even though proper drainage is instituted and pressure dressings are applied. Fluid may accumulate in three areas: the axilla, the upper arm, and the lower part of the wound. Involvement of the lower area is only a nuisance,

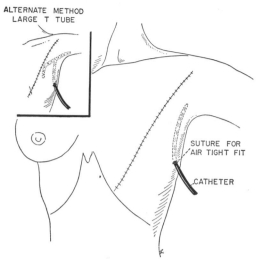

Figure 28–1 Methods for applying negative pressure to flaps after mastectomy to prevent the collection of serum under the flaps and in the axilla. A 16 or 20 French catheter is inserted through a stab wound low in the lateral flap posteriorly. The catheter should have several holes cut in the side. The tip of the catheter is placed in the axilla. It is extremely important that a suture be placed in the skin to make the stab wound tight around the catheter so that negative pressure can be maintained. Sometimes, as shown in the inset, an alternate method is the use of a large T-tube with multiple holes. Suction should be applied to the catheter at the operating table to make sure that the negative pressure pulls the flaps down to the chest wall.

but fluid in the other two areas may increase the tendency toward limited arm motion and lymphedema of the arm. Therefore these areas must be drained adequately (Fig. 28–1). We have drained the upper arm through a stab wound approximately 10 cm. from the shoulder, removing the drain after 24 hours. The other two areas are drained by a Hemovac unit or two Penrose drains beneath the medial and lateral flaps. The lateral drain extends up into the axillary component of the wound. The drains are shortened and removed as indicated. The Hemovac tubes are aspirated daily or the unit is removed when the fluid yield diminishes to a few milliliters (usually in 5 to 7 days).

Following extended radical mastectomy of the Urban type, underwater drainage is established for 1 or 2 days depending on the status of the underlying lung as demonstrated by x-ray findings. The actual drainage of the wound itself is similar to that of the standard radical mastectomy wound.

Patients subjected to modified radical mastectomy do not need arm drainage. The chest wall and axilla are drained by the Hemovac unit or with Penrose drains beneath the flaps as previously described.

POSTOPERATIVE COMPLICATIONS

HEMORRHAGE AND SEROUS DRAINAGE

Postoperative drainage may be hemorrhagic or serous. If pocketing occurs, aspiration or insertion of new drains may be necessary. Gross bulging of the axillary component of the flaps usually indicates bleeding from a major axillary vessel due to the loss of a vessel tie. The situation requires surgical exploration of the wound, preferably under general anesthesia. Hematocrits of 9 to 10 ml. per 100 ml. are common following mastectomy. Iron replacement by mouth usually rectifies the anemia. Transfusion of packed cells is recommended if one finds a hematocrit below 8 or 9 ml. per 100 ml. In most instances minimal postoperative hemorrhage is controlled by pressure dressings.

PNEUMOTHORAX

Occasionally unilateral pneumothorax will occur at the time of the operative procedure. It may be unrecognized and not manifest itself clinically until after operation. This complication arises when a sharp-pointed hemostat perforates the pleura as one attempts to clamp a bleeder in the intercostal muscles.

Pneumothorax is more common after extended radical mastectomy. Continuation of the routine underwater drainage (closed thoracotomy) with x-rays of the chest wall as a surveillance measure is recommended.

INFECTION

Infection is a most serious complication after mastectomy. There are thin flaps on the chest wall and compromised lymphatic drainage around the axilla. Every effort should be made to prevent infection. Many surgeons use prophylactic antibiotic therapy. The fact that the wound is open for a long period and that the flaps are thin with limited blood supply makes for a potential area of infection. Should wound infection occur, it must be treated vigorously with antibiotics. If there is abscess formation, drainage is indicated. Fortunately gross infection is not common.

NECROSIS OF SKIN EDGES

One of the common complications of radical mastectomy is poor wound healing and necrosis of skin edges. If the necrosis is minimal, the area may heal if it is kept clean. When the necrosis is appreciable, it is injudicious to wait a long time and permit constant inflammation and infection. Excision of the dead tissue with skin grafting will prevent low-grade infection and fibrosis of delicate and scarce collateral lymphatic channels.

The area affected by the necrosis of flaps determines the seriousness of this complication. Deviations from normal wound healing of the axillary component of the wound often produce the major factors — fibrosis and infection — in the development of postoperative lymphedema of the arm.

Frequent 1 per cent acetic acid soaks will result in epithelization of defects as large as 4 or 5 cm. in diameter. Pinch or postage-stamp grafts are superior to sheets of split-thickness skin because their "take rate" in an infected base is usually better. Débridement of necrotic tissue is done periodically. Necrosis of the chest wall flaps usually responds satisfactorily to the outlined treatment and with only minor sequelae, provided the flaps are not in the axillary component of the wound. If this complication occurs, one can expect sequelae that include a long-term period of healing and potentially persistent arm edema.

LIMITATION OF MOTION OF THE ARM

Limitation of motion of the arm will occur unless proper measures are taken to prevent it. Early in convalescence the patient

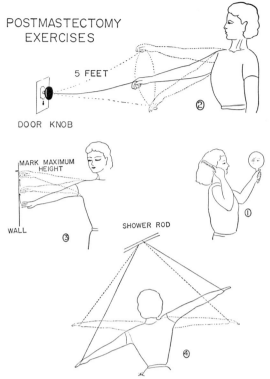

Figure 20–2 Exercises for the patient after breast surgery to prevent limitation of motion of the arm. *1,* Brushing and combing the hair. *2,* Swinging a rope tied to a door handle increases motion at the shoulder girdle. *3,* Walking the wall: the patient raises the arm to as high a level as possible and walks the fingers up the wall. She then puts a mark on the wall and at the next exercise period attempts to achieve a higher position. *4,* Pulley exercise increases abduction. The rope is put over a shower rod, and a pulley motion is used in which the good arm tends to pull on the affected arm.

should be encouraged to use but not abuse her arm. Under the supervision of trained physiatrists, trained nurses, volunteers from the American Cancer Society's Reach to Recovery Program (with patient's and surgeon's approval), exercises are instituted during the second or third day post mastectomy. There are two exceptions to this dictum — patients who were subjected to extended radical mastectomy and those in whom skin grafts were used as part of the wound closure are usually started on an exercise regimen 3 to 4 days after operation.

There are four types of exercises that will help the patient to regain a freely movable arm and axilla (Fig. 28–2).

HAIRDRESSING EXERCISE. Combing and brushing the hair allows the patient to improve her appearance while elevating her upper arm and making use of her hand and forearm.

WALL-CLIMBING EXERCISE. The patient is instructed to stand facing the wall, placing her fingers against it at shoulder level. The fingers are used to walk the arm slowly well up over the head. The arm is elevated as high as possible, and the level is marked on the wall. This is repeated several times a day. The object is to increase the height at each exercise period.

ROPE-TURNING EXERCISE. The patient is told to tie a piece of clothesline approximately 5 feet long to the knob of a door. Taking the loose end of the rope in the hand on the treated side, and keeping the arm rigidly extended, she turns the rope with a rotating shoulder motion. The speed and size of the circle in this exercise are gradually increased.

PULLEY-MOTION EXERCISE. The patient places a rope over a shower curtain rod and holds an end of the rope in each hand with the arms fully extended sideways. She then slides the rope up and down over the rod in pulley fashion.

AXILLARY CONTRACTURE

Sometimes with infection and poor wound healing there may be contracture of the skin in the axilla. Occasionally this occurs because the incision has been carried across the anterior axillary fold. Some contractures of the axilla may be corrected by the use of a Z-plasty. In other instances it may be necessary to remove the scar tissue, release the contracture, and cover the defect with a thick split-thickness skin graft.

EDEMA OF THE ARM

The major postoperative complication of radical mastectomy is edema of the arm. Many patients have a slight transitory increase in the diameter of the arm after radical mastectomy. Such edema usually disappears with restoration of arm function. Occasionally there is a baggy enlargement of the ventral aspect of the upper arm. This is seen in obese patients with relaxed tissues and results from severance of the axillary fascia. In obese women this can hardly be avoided. Patients who have local recurrence of carcinoma in the axillary or supraclavicular region may have edema of the arm, but this is not a true complication of radical mastectomy.

Edema of the arm as a complication of modified or radical mastectomy may be of two types: (1) immediate postoperative edema, which may be regarded as transitory and frequently is the result of some fault in technique, and which is usually corrected by compression with Ace bandages and exercise of the arm; and (2) secondary or persistent edema developing and remaining for months or years after operation.

INCIDENCE OF PERSISTENT EDEMA. Percentage figures on incidence of edema vary greatly, owing to three factors: (1) precise definition of edema, (2) different techniques of radical mastectomy, and (3) the kind of patient upon whom the operation is performed. Obviously if the surgeon is operating upon patients with extensive axillary metastases and routinely uses radiation therapy, the incidence of edema may be high. Conversely, if careful surgical technique is used in selected cases without radiation therapy, the incidence is lower. It appears that persistent edema occurs in 8 to 50 per cent of patients.

Fitts and co-workers reported that half of the 130 patients in their series had appreciable swelling of the arm after radical mastectomy. Veal and co-workers performed examinations from 6 months to 11 years after operation on 100 patients who had been subjected to radical mastectomy. An analysis of these cases indicated that some degree of lymphedema of the arm was present in 70 per cent. Twenty-six per cent had swelling with an increase in circumference of 3 cm. or less, 33 per cent had swelling with an increase of 3 to 6 cm., and only 11 per cent had swelling of more than 6 cm. increase in circumference. In his personal series of 356 patients, Haagensen noted edema in the immediate postoperative period in 4.8 per cent of the patients. None of these had severe edema. The incidence of late persistent edema was 7.6 per cent. In almost all those who had late edema it was possible to identify the portal of entry of infection.

CAUSES. There are apparently many causes of edema. Different authorities have different opinions as to the most predominant cause. Basing their belief primarily on clinical appraisal, both Evans and Smedal have stated that postmastectomy lymphedema usually results from thrombophlebitis and recommend prophylactic anticoagulation beginning 3 days after operation. Veal states that he observed an increase in venous pressure and confirmed the presence of venous obstruction by venography in patients with postmastectomy edema. He feels that edema resulting from obstruction of the axillary vein is by far the most common cause of swelling of the arm following operation. His thesis is that lymphatic obstruction is usually a secondary result of venous obstruction which, if prolonged, leads to permanent blockage of the lymphatic flow. Since his study, however, ample evidence has accumulated to demonstrate that venous obstruction is not the primary cause. Many times the axillary vein is sacrificed without development of postoperative edema. Several workers, including Neuhof and MacDonald, have independently noted no significant increase in the incidence of edema when ligation of a portion of the axillary vein was performed as a part of radical mastectomy.

From the best evidence that has accumulated it would appear that the cause of lymphedema after mastectomy is insufficiency of the lymphatics due to either obstruction or destruction. Anything that tends to obstruct the lymphatics after their channels have been interfered with by axillary dissection may lead to moderate or severe edema of the arm. This includes wound infection, collections of serum in the axilla, unusual trauma to the axilla with malignant nodes, radiation therapy, recurrence of metastasis, and, finally, infection in the arm as a separate entity after mastectomy. When infection develops from an injury to the arm or a paronychia, the compromised lymphatics may become inflamed and fibrosed with subsequent blockage and edema of the arm. If this edema persists, it may become difficult to manage. On the other hand, if it can be eliminated before fibrosis occurs in the lymphatics, there may be no further swelling.

Bower and his associates have shown that there is considerable variation in the number and size of lymphatic channels in normal subjects. Using preoperative and postoperative lymphangiography, they have been able to show that patients who subsequently have edema of the arm had minimal lymphatic drainage pathways prior to operation. These findings tend to explain the apparently capricious development of postmastectomy lymphedema. Some women apparently have abundant lymphatic channels and no tendency to lymphedema. Others have very few and are probably predestined to suffer edema after radical mastectomy. A third group undoubtedly exists with minimal lymphatic channels preoperatively who can tolerate uncomplicated radical mastectomy without edema developing. Any added insult, however, such as infection will destroy enough lymphatic drainage to produce edema.

As pointed out by Bower and associates, it is possible that with unlimited acquisition of data and knowledge in this field postsurgical edema may be predictable on the basis of preoperative lymphatic visualization. Mustard and Murillo reduced the incidence of postmastectomy lymphedema from 51 per cent to 4 per cent by leaving the areolar tissue around the axillary vein in 121 patients. Overall 5-year survival was 58 per cent in this group and 50 per cent in a group of 90 patients subjected to standard axillary vein dissections the previous 5 years. Although it is doubtful whether this compromise procedure will ever be used on all patients, it is possible that it would find a place in patients with documented preoperative lymphatic insufficiency.

PREVENTION. When the swelling of the arm occurs and persists, treatment by either conservative or surgical means is seldom satisfactory. Several factors may be helpful in the prevention of postmastectomy edema. The axilla should be carefully dissected with as little trauma as possible to minimize local injury and prevent local recurrence. Some authors feel that excision of the clavicular head of the pectoralis major muscle is associated with an increase in lymphedema, but this view is not shared by all authorities. Great care should be taken to achieve primary wound healing without skin slough or infection. Fluid accumulation in the axillary dead space must be eliminated. The use of an elastic bandage on the arm in the postoperative period has been recommended and successfully used for both prevention and treatment. When radiation therapy is used, it should be administered carefully to avoid the hazards of radiation dermatitis and infection. Injections of any kind in the affected arm are contraindicated. Early mobilization and graded exercises of the arm may prevent some minor edema. Great emphasis should be placed upon weight reduction in obese women.

Most important of all, care should be taken to avoid even minor infections in the arm and hand. These infections may lead to recurrent episodes of erysipelas. Should this condition develop, prompt and intensive antibiotic therapy is indicated. Rigid hygiene of the hand is essential in prophylaxis. The patient must realize that any trauma to the arm or hand that provides a portal of entry for bacteria may lead to infection and edema. Cuts and minor burns are the most frequent sources of infection. When even a minor infection develops in an arm after mastectomy, immediate antibiotic therapy should be instituted.

A list of do's and don'ts relating to the care of the hand and arm is given to patients upon their discharge.

SUGGESTED HAND CARE FOR POSTMASTEC-TOMY PATIENTS

After a radical mastectomy, an arm may swell because lymph nodes and lymph vessels are necessarily removed and the body is therefore less able to combat infection in this extremity.

Make every effort to avoid all cuts, scratches, pinpricks, hangnails, insect bites, burns, and use of strong detergents, as these can lead to serious infection with increased swelling.

SOME DON'TS

Do not hold a cigarette in this hand.

Do not carry your purse or anything heavy with this arm.

Do not wear a wristwatch or other jewelry on this arm.

Do not cut or pick at cuticles or hangnails on this hand.

Do not work near thorny plants or dig in the garden.

Do not reach into a hot oven with this arm.

Do not permit injections in this arm.

Do not permit blood to be drawn from this arm.

Do not allow your blood pressure to be taken on this arm.

SOME DO'S

Do wear a loose rubber glove on this hand when washing dishes.

Do wear a thimble when sewing.

Do apply a good lanolin hand cream several times daily.

Do contact your doctor if your arm gets red, warm, or unusually hard or swollen.

TREATMENT. Every effort should be made to prevent edema of the arm, but in spite of firm preventive measures this crippling complication of mastectomy does occur. Its treatment is extremely difficult and frequently unsuccessful. The large number of operative procedures designed to achieve reduction of the size of the swollen arm attests the fact that no single surgical measure has been developed to cope successfully with the problem. Various procedures have been proposed to create new lymphatic channels. Stellate ganglion block has been used but is of little value. Extensive resection of the subcutaneous tissue down to muscle with the application of split-thickness grafts has been tried. The success of all surgical procedures has been limited, and benefits have been transient. It is doubtful whether any kind of operation is worth trying. When total disability with excruciating suffering demands drastic treatment, amputation may be a last resort. This heroic treatment is rarely required but may be indicated for the alleviation of agonizing pain and relief of an immensely swollen arm in certain unfortunate patients.

Several conservative measures may be of value. The affected arm should be elevated at every possible opportunity even to the point of resting the arm on several pillows during the hours of sleep. Massage toward the heart each evening for 10 minutes increases the speed of lymph flow. Mechanical massage with a sleeve containing rubber balloons inflated by a mechanical pump is sometimes of great assistance. Three such devices are available. The Vaso-pneumatic machine* has a number of rubber cuffs that are inflated in distal-to-proximal succession. The Jobst intermittent compression unit† is

---

*Manufactured by the Poor and Logan Manufacturing Company, North Hollywood, California.

†Manufactured by the Jobst Institute, Toledo, Ohio.

a single-chambered inflatable sleeve in which periods of inflation and deflation are regulated by a timer. The Circulator* has several chambers that are inflated in distal-to-proximal succession, with pressure maintained in each chamber after it has been inflated. Each of these pumps appears to work equally well. They may be used for an hour or two each day. Foam rubber pads applied lightly to the arm and held in place with an elastic bandage may be of value at night. The arm is then connected by means of rope and pulley to counterweights which balance the weight of the arm comfortably and keep it elevated. This enables the patient to move about in bed without disturbing the degree of elevation of the arm. When the patient is ambulatory, an elastic support in the form of a fitted appliance or a rubberized elastic bandage is essential to prevent loss of tissue elasticity.

At the onset of therapy it may be well to have the patient in the hospital and put her on a dehydration regimen. She should be given a salt-restricted diet and daily mercurial diuretics. If she is overweight, strict weight reduction schedules should be followed.

Constriction around the shoulder should be avoided, because after removal of the lymphatic channels in the axilla the lymphatic flow from the arm passes through new channels located about the shoulder. In so doing it must traverse beneath the strap of a brassiere. The pressure of the strap then becomes of extreme importance as a limiting factor in withdrawal of fluid from the arm. It is always wise to advise the use of a brassiere with no strap at all on the involved side.

Lymphangiosarcoma in the Lymphedematous Arm

One of the more serious but rare complications of lymphedema following mastectomy is the development of lymphangiosarcoma. Since 1948, when Stewart and Treves first described this clinical entity in the postmastectomy lymphedematous arm, approximately 76 cases have been reported. Bowers

---

*Manufactured by Circulator Therapeutics, Inc., Freeport, New York.

discussed 15 reported cases and one of his own. In these patients the interval between radical mastectomy and the appearance of lymphangiosarcoma varied from 2 to 14 years, the average being 9 years. Almost all the patients died or had widespread metastases within 9 months of discovery of the tumor. The tumor starts as a mildly tender cutaneous nodule, purplish and usually on the anterior surface of the upper arm. Satellite nodules may appear and coalesce or become widely disseminated. The tumors are highly malignant.

Various surgical procedures have been advised, from wide excision followed by irradiation to interscapulothoracic amputation. Bowers's patient was treated with interscapulothoracic amputation and survived for more than 2 years. It seems important that the lymphedematous arm be observed frequently and a biopsy performed at the first sign of a lesion. If there is lymphangiosarcoma, a radical procedure would seem indicated, although radiation therapy has occasionally resulted in spectacular short-term results. Occasionally, these patients respond to various combinations of chemotherapeutic agents. Immunotherapy has been recommended, but none of these agents is consistently effective.

COMPLICATIONS FOLLOWING RADIATION THERAPY

Postoperative prophylactic adjunct radiation therapy has resulted in an increased incidence of lymphedema. However, with the discard of the direct axillary port, a marked reduction of this complication has been noted. Investigators at the M. D. Anderson Hospital have reported delayed wound healing when preoperative radiation therapy is used.

COMPLICATIONS FOLLOWING ADJUNCTIVE CHEMOTHERAPY

The majority of chemotherapeutic agents currently prescribed in the management of patients with potentially curable breast cancer are known to produce side effects. It is mandatory to explain these potential complications to each patient. Each patient must be monitored constantly by the physician responsible for the chemotherapy.

PSYCHOLOGICAL SUPPORT AND ADJUSTMENT

The loss of a breast has tremendous impact upon the patient, although at times her husband and family seem to be more affected than she is. Health professionals can be most helpful during this period of readjustment. In addition, we have found that assistance afforded by the volunteers of the American Cancer Society's Reach to Recovery Program has been a major adjunct in assisting the mastectomy patient readapt to society. These volunteers become involved only if requested by the patient's surgeon. They do not usurp the surgeon's role; on the contrary, they add a dimension to the surgeon's efforts — assistance from one who has actually experienced the problems facing the patient.

Another area of concern is whether the cancer will recur. In fact, this may be the prime concern of the postoperative patient. It is important to her to know that this fear is shared with many others. Nothing of what patients are thinking is "foolish," "silly," or "stupid," and their fears should be sought out and listened to with sympathy and reassurance based on the fact that approximately 85 per cent of those whose breast cancer is treated before it spreads to the lymphatic system survive five years or longer. In addition, between 65 and 80 per cent of those who undergo biopsy for a breast lump are found to have a benign condition.

The wife of a United States Senator who underwent a mastectomy gave great credit to the "perfect stranger" who came to visit her in the hospital to talk to her about her own breast surgery. That perfect stranger was a member of the Reach to Recovery Program of the American Cancer Society.

Bibliography

1. Bower, R., Danese, C., Debbas, J., and Howard, J.: Advances in diagnosis of diseases of the lymphatics. J.A.M.A. *181*:687, 1962.

2. Bowers, W. F., Schear, E. W., and LeGolvan, P. C.: Lymphangiosarcoma in postmastectomy lymphedematous arm. Am. J. Surg. *90*:682, 1955.

3. Coller, F. A., Crook, C. E., and Iob, V.: Blood loss in surgical operations. J.A.M.A. *126*:1, 1944.

4. Economou, S. G., Southwick, H. W., and Slaughter, D. P.: Chest repair following mammary lymphadenectomy. Arch. Surg. *83*:231, 1961.

5. Evans, J. A.: Treatment of acute thrombophlebitis of the arm after radical mastectomy. Angiology *12*:155, 1961.

6. Fitts, W. T., Jr., Keuhnelian, J. G., Ravdin, I. S., and Schor, S.: Swelling of arm after radical mastectomy; Clinical study of its causes. Surgery *35*:460, 1954.

7. Haagensen, C. D.: Symposium on cancer of breast; Technique for radical mastectomy. Surgery *19*:100, 1946.

8. Haagensen, C. D.: Diseases of the Breast. 2nd Ed. Philadelphia, W. B. Saunders Company, 1971.

9. Haberlin, J. P., Milone, F. P., and Copeland, M. M.: A further evaluation of lymphedema of the arm following radical mastectomy and postoperative x-ray therapy. Am. Surg. *25*:285, 1959.

10. Halsted, W. S.: Swelling of arm after operation for cancer of breast: Elephantiasis chirurgica — Its cause and prevention. Bull. Johns Hopkins Hosp. *32*:309, 1921.

11. Lasser, T.: Reach to Recovery. New York, Simon & Schuster, 1972.

12. Lewison, E. F.: Breast Cancer and Its Diagnosis and Treatment. Baltimore, Williams & Wilkins Company, 1955.

13. MacDonald, I.: Resection of axillary vein in radical mastectomy; Its relation to mechanism of lymphedema. Cancer *1*:618, 1948.

14. Moloney, G. E.: Apposition and drainage of large skin flaps by suction. Aust. N. Z. J. Surg. *26*:173, 1957.

15. Mustard, R. L., and Murillo, C.: Prevention of arm lymphedema following mastectomy. Ann. Surg. *154* (Suppl.):282, 1961.

16. Neuhof, H.: Excision of axillary vein in radical operation for carcinoma of breast. Ann. Surg. *108*:15, 1938.

17. Smedal, M. I.: The cause and treatment of edema of the arm following radical mastectomy. Surg. Gynecol. Obstet. *111*:29, 1960.

18. Stewart, F. W., and Treves, N.: Lymphangiosarcoma in postmastectomy lymphedema: Report of 6 cases in elephantiasis chirurgica. Cancer *1*:64, 1948.

19. Tamoney, H. J., Jr., and Stent, P. A.: A dermal graft for chest wall repair. Surg. Gynecol. Obstet. *118*:289, 1964.

20. Treves, N.: An evaluation of the etiologic factors of lymphedema following radical mastectomy: An analysis of 1,007 cases. Cancer *10*:444, 1957.

21. Urban, J. A.: Extended radical mastectomy for breast cancer. Am. J. Surg. *106*:399, 1963.

22. Veal, J. R.: Pathologic basis for swelling of arm following radical amputation of breast. Surg. Gynecol. Obstet. *67*:752, 1938.

29

COMPLICATIONS OF
ADRENAL SURGERY

Charles Eckert

In recent years our knowledge of the pathophysiology and biochemistry of the adrenal cortex and medulla has increased considerably. The role of surgery in the treatment of adrenal diseases has also undergone changes so that for some diseases increased numbers of operations are done, whereas for others non-operative treatment has supplanted surgery. With increased knowledge there has also been a decline in the risk of operations on the adrenal glands, and procedures that were formerly trying experiences for both patient and surgeon are now much less formidable events. It is our purpose in this chapter to discuss the complications that occur in the course of operations on the adrenal glands from the standpoint of their frequency, causation, and prevention. In doing so we will stress those that are more or less specific for adrenal surgery without repeating material that has been well covered in other portions of this book.

The complications that are more or less unique to adrenal surgery are derived from two main sources: first, the protected anatomic location of these structures, which leads to technical difficulties; and second, the complex metabolic effects of the adrenal hormones, which are altered either by the pathologic process or by surgery.

There are four routes of access for removal of the adrenal glands — transabdominal, through the flank, transthoracic, and thoracoabdominal. In the operation through the flank the patient may be positioned either on his side or prone. The same layers are traversed in either position and the exposure is also much the same. Use of the prone position permits bilateral operation either sequentially or simultaneously, in either case without moving the patient. Each surgical approach is associated with complications that are more or less specific and that in some measure determine which approach the surgeon will select.

Despite the voluminous literature on surgery of the adrenal glands there are few reports specifically describing the complications of these operations. Three such reports are those of Franksson and Hellstrom, Pezzulich and Mannix, and Auda, Brennan, and Gill. For the purposes of this chapter we have also reviewed and added the complications occurring in our own series of adrenal operations.

Franksson and Hellstrom described a series of 118 adrenalectomies all done

---

Charles Eckert was born in Denver, Colorado, and received his medical education at Washington University. He has been Professor of Surgery and Chairman of the Department at Albany Medical College. Before his appointment at Albany in 1956 his professional life was spent at Washington University and Barnes Hospital in St. Louis, where, as a member of the Department of Surgery, he was in charge of the tumor clinic. In this capacity his interest in adrenal surgery was stimulated by studies of adrenalectomy for advanced hormonally dependent cancer. He has been Chairman of the American Board of Surgery and First Vice President of the American College of Surgeons.

TABLE 29–1 COMPLICATIONS OF ADRENAL SURGERY

Surgical Approach	Franksson & Hellstrom	Pezzulich & Mannix		Eckert				Auda, Brennan & Gill		
	Flank	Flank	Abdomen	Flank	Abdomen	Thoraco-abdominal	Trans-thoracic	Flank	Abdomen	Thoraco-abdominal
Number of patients	118			61	139	6	1	17	32	1
Number of operations*	236	136	74	135	46	6	1	27	32	1
Operative mortality	4	5		2	2	0	0	0	5	0
Injury to spleen	0	0	6	0	7	0	0	1†	5	0
Injury to pancreas	0	1	5	0	1	0	0	0	1	0
Injury to pleura	32	18	0	13	0			0	0	0
Injury to vena cava	11	3	0	3	1	0	0	0	0	0
Injury to renal vein	3			1	1	0	0	0	0	0
Injury to portal vein	0	0	2	0	0	0	0	0	0	0
Adrenal insufficiency	13	10		3	0	0	0	0	0	0
Miscellaneous (pulmonary, wound, thrombophlebitis, pulmonary embolus, etc.)	14	38		28				7	11	0

*Each bilateral flank operation is counted as two, regardless of whether done in one or two stages.
†Splenic artery injured.

through a flank (posterior) approach. Of these, 98 were one-stage and 20 were two-stage procedures. The major indication for operation was disseminated mammary cancer, although surgery was performed for adrenal hyperplasia, malignant hypertension, and other conditions. There were 4 deaths (3.4 per cent).

Pezzulich and Mannix described 210 operations on the adrenals in 152 patients. Seventy-four operations were done through an abdominal approach and 136 operations through a flank approach. The indications for operation were Cushing's syndrome (77), breast carcinoma (22), pheochromocytoma (19), hyperaldosteronism (13), adrenogenital syndrome (6), and other miscellaneous indications (15). There were 5 deaths (3.3 per cent of patients).

Our own series consists of 107 patients. Of the operations, 39 were done through an abdominal approach, 61 through flank incisions, 6 through a thoracoabdominal approach, and 1 through a transthoracic approach. The indications for operation consisted of breast cancer (62), Cushing's syndrome (19), pheochromocytoma (13), functioning adrenocortical carcinoma (8), hyperaldosteronism (3), and miscellaneous indications (2). There were 4 deaths (3.7 per cent of patients).

Auda, Brennan, and Gill reported on their experience with 50 patients with primary hyperaldosteronism operated upon over a period of 22 years. The in-hospital 30-day mortality was 10 per cent (5 patients). Causes of death included hemorrhage at operation, myocardial infarction, and acute left heart failure. All patients who died were operated upon through an anterior transperitoneal approach. There have been no deaths since 1970.

The complications encountered in these patients are shown in Table 29–1. The relation between the anatomic route of access and the type of associated injury is striking. Injury to the spleen often necessitating splenectomy in the course of left adrenalectomy through an abdominal incision occurred in 6 of 74 patients in the Pezzulich-Mannix series, in 7 of 39 patients in the Eckert series, and of 32 patients in the Auda, Brennan, and Gill series, five sustained inadvertent splenic laceration, but the laceration was repaired in all five, thereby avoiding splenectomy. Pezzulich and Mannix attribute splenic injury to the exposure of the adrenal by means of mobilizing the spleen, tail of the pancreas, and splenic flexure of the colon medially rather than exposure through the gastrocolic ligament in which the pancreas is mobilized anteriorly. In the latter exposure, however, injury to the pancreas was more frequent in their series.

In patients operated on through flank incisions the pleura and the vena cava were the structures most likely to be injured. However, there were no deaths attributable to either exsanguinating blood loss or opening the pleura.

Pulmonary complications, urinary tract complications, thrombophlebitis, pulmonary embolism, wound infection, and so forth, occurred in nearly 12 per cent of patients in the combined series. The type of incision appears to be unrelated to the frequency with which these complications are seen. Thus atelectasis, pneumonia, or empyema appears to be no more likely after operations during which the pleura is injured than after operations done through a flank incision without injury to pleura or operations done through an abdominal incision.

Patients with either primary or secondary hypercorticism (Cushing's "disease" or Cushing's syndrome) usually tolerate surgery poorly. Pezzulich and Mannix found an increase in operating time, a higher incidence of splenic injury, more frequent pulmonary embolization, and more frequent wound infection in these patients as compared with those operated upon for other indications. The difference in frequency of wound infection in this study was not statistically significant.

SURGICAL ANATOMY

The adrenal glands are paired structures located in the retroperitoneum paravertebrally at or about the level of the eleventh thoracic vertebra. A few examples of congenital absence of one adrenal have been reported, but more common than unilateral adrenal absence is atrophy of one gland. Overproduction of hydrocortisone by func-

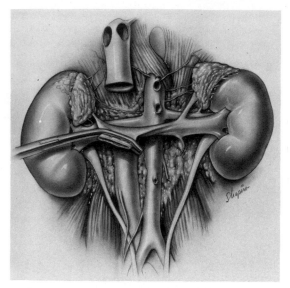

Figure 29–1 Anatomic relations and blood supply of the adrenal glands. The vena cava has been cut and is retracted inferiorly.

tioning cortical tumors (Cushing's syndrome) causes inhibition of pituitary corticotropin (ACTH), which in turn results in atrophy of the opposite adrenal. Since obesity is a prominent manifestation of this syndrome, the atrophic adrenal may be overlooked at the time of surgical exploration. This explains some, but not all, cases of "adrenal absence" reported after operation.

The adrenal glands are closely approximated to the superior and mesial aspect of the kidneys and along with the kidneys lie within the renal fascia. They are more intimately adherent to the fascia than to the kidneys; accordingly, mobilization of the kidneys usually leaves the adrenals above in contact with the diaphragm. Because of the relation between the adrenals and the kidneys, expanding adrenal tumors frequently produce renal displacement that can be visualized roentgenographically and is of diagnostic importance. Inferiorly, the adrenals at times extend to the level of the renal arteries. On the right the gland is in relation to the vena cava, and on the left the adrenal lies close to the aorta. These vascular structures are all vulnerable to injury in the course of operative dissection of the adrenals.

The right adrenal lies above the reflected peritoneum in contact with the bare area of the liver and the diaphragm. On the left the inferior portion of the adrenal is traversed by the splenic vessels and tail of the pancreas. Examination of the adrenals at the time of abdominal exploration through the intact peritoneum is unsatisfactory. To determine the size of the glands or to be certain a small tumor is not present, the peritoneum must be incised and each gland partially mobilized.

The size and weight of the adrenals vary considerably in proportion to body size during different periods of life and different physiologic states. Their average weight is 3 to 5 gm. Their length is 40 to 60 mm. and their width 20 to 30 mm. The right adrenal is pyramidal in shape and is thicker than the left, which is crescentic.

As in other endocrine glands, the blood supply is rich. Three arteries are usually present on each side, arising from and named for the inferior phrenic, aorta, and renal arteries, respectively. The veins exit from a central hilus; on the right the vein is short, emptying directly into the vena cava; the vein on the left is larger and longer, draining into the renal vein.

The principal lymphatics course to nodes in the renal hilus and to periaortic nodes, and communicate directly with nodes above the diaphragm in the posterior mediastinum.

The innervation is mainly by the splanchnic nerves. Small twigs from the vagus and phrenic nerves along with the splanchnic fibers form the adrenal plexuses. These in turn communicate with the renal and celiac plexuses and the celiac ganglia.

Each adrenal consists of an inner medullary portion derived from embryonic ectoderm of the neural crest and an outer cortical portion derived from embryonic mesoderm between the dorsal mesentery and genital ridge. The neural crest cells, from which the medulla is derived, go largely to form the sympathetic ganglia; the smaller portions form the paraganglionic chromaffin system, so designated because of the peculiar staining affinity of the cells with chromium salts. The carotid and aortic bodies are a part of this system, and the paraganglionic cells may be found anywhere from the base of the skull to the coccyx. The primordial cell, the sympathogonia, differentiates along two lines, into neural elements and chromaffin (pheochrome) elements. Tumors arise within either of these, the neuroblastoma or ganglioneuroma from neural elements and the pheochromocytoma from chromaffin elements. In about 80 per cent of cases the tumors arise within the adrenal and in 20 per cent from the extra-adrenal paraganglionic tissues.

Accessory cortical tissue also has been found in divergent areas. It is most common in the region of the adrenal glands but is not infrequent in the testes, ovaries, broad liga-ment, retroperitoneum, pancreas, and mesentery. In some cases larger accessory cortical nodules will also be found to contain medullary tissue, in which case they truly represent accessory adrenal glands. The existence of accessory cortical tissue is important not only because tumors can arise from such tissue, but also because when total adrenalectomy is contemplated, it is necessary to examine the periadrenal areolar tissue to find and remove accessory nodules.

COMPLICATIONS RESULTING FROM TECHNICAL DIFFICULTIES

It is apparent that the adrenal glands, in addition to being remarkably inaccessible, are in relation to important structures that are susceptible to operative injury. The likelihood of inadvertent injury is increased when a malignant tumor is to be removed, for such a tumor tends to infiltrate extensively in the local area. Good exposure and careful dissection in a dry field are general principles that must be followed if injury to adjacent structures is to be avoided. Good exposure requires good anesthesia to provide adequate relaxation with safety. It also requires the selection of the surgical incision that best meets the needs of the individual situation. There has been an unfortunate tendency for surgeons to familiarize themselves with one of the several different avenues of access and then champion this method of exposure to the exclusion of all others, regardless of the lesion, the habitus of the patient, or the comparative risk incurred. We believe that it is best to alter the surgical approach depending upon these criteria.

ABDOMINAL APPROACH

This is particularly useful when need exists to explore the abdominal viscera, to perform other procedures simultaneously with adrenalectomy, or to explore both adrenals before deciding upon the actual procedure to be followed. In thin patients the exposure will be sufficient for all indications with the exception of malignant adrenocortical tumors. Obesity, however, is a serious drawback to this approach.

When normal adrenal glands are to be removed for treatment of disseminated breast or prostatic cancer or for essential hypertension, the exposure obtained transabdominally will almost always suffice. In women with breast cancer, oophorectomy is ordinarily done before adrenalectomy. Although both pairs of glands can be removed through a long vertical incision, removal in one stage is not usually advisable because the advantage of noting the response to the removal of the ovaries is lost, the exposure of the adrenals is not as satisfactory as with a long transverse incision, and, of greatest importance, the tolerance of the patient may be exceeded.

Our present methods of evaluation of adrenal function are sufficiently precise to permit an accurate differential diagnosis between Cushing's "disease" (hyperplasia) and Cushing's syndrome (tumor). Nevertheless, even when a tumor is identified preoperatively, the opposite adrenal should be explored before the tumor is removed. For this reason, a transverse upper abdominal incision is a good approach, for it permits bilateral adrenal exploration and can be converted to a thoracoabdominal incision when necessary.

It is in the surgery of medullary tumors that the advantage of complete exploration is greatest. Multiple pheochromocytomas have been reported in 6 to 15 per cent of cases. Most of them were bilateral medullary tumors, but in some patients, multiple extra-adrenal tumors were present, and in others an intramedullary tumor was found in conjunction with an extramedullary lesion, located within the abdomen (Graham). In Sipple's syndrome (medullary carcinoma of the thyroid, pheochromocytoma, parathyroid hyperplasia or adenoma) bilateral pheochromocytomas have been reported in 65 per cent of cases. They are familial in approximately 35 per cent of instances, and in the kindred bearing pheochromocytomas they appear to be inherited as an autosomal dominant trait. The removal of only one of two functioning medullary tumors is poorly tolerated by the patient, who continues to suffer the effects of oversecretion of pressor amines. When only one of two pheochromocytomas is removed, the continued excessive secretion will necessitate control with alpha-adrenergic blocking agents, and if arrhythmias occur, beta-adrenergic blocking agents may be required as well. At operation arrhythmias may develop which can eventuate in ventricular fibrillation unless control is promptly effected.

An additional advantage of the abdominal approach to these tumors is early access to the blood supply. Manipulation of the tumor before it is isolated from the general circulation leads to the release of epinephrine and norepinephrine; therefore early ligation of the adrenal vein is desirable.

The main complications of the surgical treatment of neuroblastomas are related to their highly anaplastic, locally invasive tendencies. The parietes and adjacent viscera are frequently infiltrated; consequently complete surgical removal is seldom possible. The kidney is almost always involved and must be sacrificed, at least in part. At times removal of the tumor in continuity with infiltrated segments of the liver, spleen, tail of the pancreas, or colon is feasible. Obviously, if this is to be done, an abdominal or thoracoabdominal incision is mandatory. The large size of these lesions often leads to injury to adjacent structures even when they are not directly involved.

Removal of the right adrenal through the abdominal approach can be facilitated by mobilizing the renal fascia from the inferior surface of the diaphragm before opening the fascia, thereby bringing the adrenal closer to the surgical field. The central vein on the right side is short, emptying directly into the vena cava. It is in the dissection of this structure that the vena cava is most likely to be injured. The hepatic flexure of the colon is retracted downward, and in some cases it is necessary to mobilize the second portion of the duodenum by dividing its lateral peritoneal attachments and retracting it toward the midline. Injury to the duodenum is possible in the course of this maneuver, but it should not occur if the peritoneal incision is made under direct vision.

Removal of the left adrenal through the abdominal approach is likely to be more difficult. Access to the gland is obtained either directly through the lesser peritoneal sac or by mobilizing the spleen, tail of the pancreas, and splenic flexure of the colon toward the midline. The direct approach through the lesser sac involves division of the gastrocolic and splenocolic ligaments with downward retraction of the splenic flexure while the stomach and spleen are retracted upward and the pancreas is retracted anteriorly. This approach is most useful in removal of the normal or hyperplastic gland but is not suitable for removal of a neoplasm, for which better exposure is needed. In either case the tail of the pancreas, the splenic vessels, and the spleen must be handled carefully if injury is to be avoided.

The splenic vessels are, of course, large, and if they are torn, profuse hemorrhage will result. Bleeding from this source can be controlled by digital pressure proximal to the bleeding point to allow repair in a dry field.

The result of pancreatic trauma is unpredictable; at times apparently severe damage will heal without difficulty, and lesser injury will lead to traumatic pancreatitis, abscess or pseudocyst formation, or pancreatic fistula. If a portion of the pancreas is devitalized, it should be removed. Injury, with or without devitalization, is an indication for drainage. For this purpose a sump drain is recommended because of the possibility of pancreatic fistula. If drainage is profuse, the sump is left in place for 5 to 7 days. By this time a well defined tract should be present. Prolonged use of sump drains is undesirable because they are constructed of rigid or semirigid materials that are conducive to pressure necrosis if they are long in place.

Laceration of the splenic capsule may

occur in the course of mobilization of the spleen or from forceful retraction. When the spleen is mobilized, blunt dissection should not be used. With proper exposure the lateral splenic attachments can be cut with scissors under direct vision. Bleeding from the spleen will necessitate splenectomy for certain control.

Some degree of adynamic ileus is to be anticipated after operations on the adrenals, regardless of the route of exposure. The degree of ileus is usually greater, however, after transabdominal exposure than when the operation is entirely extraperitoneal. In either case it is best to decompress the gastrointestinal tract through a Levin tube for 24 to 48 hours. In the absence of pancreatitis or peritonitis of other origin, serious ileus is rare. Decompression for 48 hours will usually suffice, but evidence of normal peristaltic activity should be present before the tube is removed and oral feeding allowed.

LUMBAR APPROACH

This is an entirely extraperitoneal exposure that is well tolerated even when bilateral one-stage adrenalectomy is performed. It is most useful for removal of normal or hyperplastic adrenals but is less satisfactory for adrenal tumors, for which better exposure is desirable.

The patient is placed in the prone position after the induction of anesthesia and insertion of an endotracheal tube. Some surgeons continue to use the lateral decubitus and turn the patient if bilateral operations are to be done. To obtain adequate exposure, the twelfth rib is removed, and in obese patients posterior division of the eleventh rib may also be necessary.

The pleura extends to the level of the twelfth rib posteriorly; therefore precaution must be taken to avoid its injury either during the subperiosteal removal of the rib or as the dissection is carried through the underlying muscles. It is usually not difficult to visualize the pleura, but inadvertent injury to this structure is not serious unless it goes unrecognized. The anesthesiologist should be immediately notified of the event so that increased positive pressure can be applied to maintain pulmonary expansion.

Unless this is done, inadequate oxygenation and accumulation of carbon dioxide will ensue. Prolonged pulmonary collapse during operation will also increase the frequency of postoperative atelectasis and pneumonia. Efforts to close the rent in the pleura are unnecessary. When closure of the wound is started, a 16 French soft rubber catheter is placed in the pleural cavity and clamped; the tube is aspirated after completion of the closure and removed when no further air is obtained. Serious sequelae are prevented by this simple expedient, even when the pleura is opened on both sides.

When the adrenal is exposed through the lumbar approach, the blood supply is less accessible than it is when the abdominal approach is used. Therefore the gland must be mobilized before the vessels are clamped. The risk of hemorrhage is greater on the right side, where the adrenal vein is short and easily torn. Tearing this vein will give rise to troublesome hemorrhage, and if the tear extends onto the vena cava, the wound will rapidly fill with a pool of blood. Efforts to clamp the bleeding point under these circumstances are more likely to compound the injury than to accomplish satisfactory control. A large pack should be placed on the bleeding point and pressure applied. If pressure is maintained for an adequate period, bleeding will either be stopped or slowed sufficiently to allow accurate placement of a vascular clamp or suture. Larger tears in the wall of the vena cava are handled by mobilizing the vein sufficiently to allow placement of a partially occlusive vascular clamp; as this is done, bleeding is controlled by digital pressure. The defect is then sutured with 5-0 silk. Tears in the renal vein are handled in the same manner. Troublesome bleeding of arterial origin is infrequent.

TRANSTHORACIC INCISION

This route of exposure has been used for the removal of adrenal tumors and for the hyperplasia of Cushing's disease. Exposure of the left adrenal is excellent with this approach, but the right adrenal is less accessible. We have not used this incision because in cortical hyperplasia we have found either the transabdominal or the lumbar incision

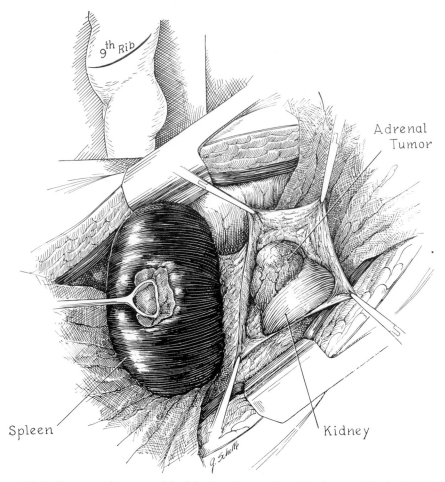

Figure 29–2 Exposure of a tumor of the left adrenal cortex through a thoracoabdominal incision.

entirely satisfactory; for cortical neoplasms we have preferred the thoracoabdominal incision, and for pheochromocytomas the advantages of the abdominal incision have been previously enumerated. Furthermore, the risk of pleural and pulmonary complications is greater with this approach than with the lumbar or abdominal approach and is comparable to that taken with the thoracoabdominal incision. Despite these objections, the fact remains that the transthoracic incision has been used with satisfaction by experienced surgeons.

The patient is placed in the prone position for bilateral operation and in either the lateral or prone position for unilateral procedures. Endotracheal anesthesia is necessary. The incision follows the eighth or ninth rib or the corresponding intercostal space. Upon opening the pleura the lung is retract-

ed upward, but expansion should be maintained by gently assisted respirations. The diaphragm is sectioned posteriorly, with care to avoid the major branches of the phrenic nerve.

The complications most likely to occur when this approach is used are diaphragmatic hernia, particularly on the left, pulmonary atelectasis, pneumothorax, hemothorax, empyema, and bronchopneumonia. None of these should be frequent, provided good surgical technique is used and the details of postoperative care necessary after thoracotomy are carefully followed. (See also Chapter 15.)

Closure of the diaphragm with catgut is conducive to herniation through this structure, but herniation is infrequent when careful two-layer closure with non-absorbable sutures is used. Accurate hemostasis is important and, when obtained, greatly reduces the likelihood of hemothorax. Before closure of the incision, anterior and posterior intercostal tubes are inserted and connected to underwater drainage bottles. The lung should be inspected to ascertain that it is completely expanded and has not been injured by retraction.

In the postoperative period coughing and frequent changes in position are encouraged. If secretions accumulate in the tracheobronchial tree, endotracheal suction with a sterile disposable plastic catheter or bronchoscopy is performed. The use of brochodilator drugs in nebulizers, along with "blow-bottles" or intermittent positive-pressure breathing apparatus, is helpful in eliminating the hazard of atelectasis and assists in maintaining pulmonary expansion. The routine use of antibiotics is not recommended.

THORACOABDOMINAL INCISION

This incision is used only to provide the exposure needed for wide removal of cortical tumors, which are frequently malignant and, when malignant, have been infrequently cured or controlled in the local area. We believe that this danger exceeds the increased risk of postoperative pulmonary complications. For other adrenal lesions use of this incision is not justified.

The patient is placed on his back with the side to be operated upon elevated approximately 45 degrees. The abdominal portion of the incision is made first to confirm the diagnosis and the need for opening the chest. It consists of an oblique incision from the midline, just above the umbilicus, to the costal margin opposite the ninth costal cartilage. In opening the thorax the costal margin is incised and a portion of cartilage removed to prevent friction. Unless this is done, movement of the cut costal margin will give rise to troublesome symptoms postoperatively. The ninth costal cartilage and rib are removed to the angle of the rib. The diaphragm is incised in line with the incision. On the right the liver is retracted upward into the chest, and on the left the spleen, splenic vessels, and tail of the pancreas are separated and retracted toward the midline. If any of these structures are adherent, they are resected en bloc with the tumor. Dissection of the tumor itself begins mesially, to control its blood supply before manipulation of the tumor and by so doing to limit venous spread during removal.

The problems of pulmonary expansion, intercostal tube drainage, and postoperative care are similar to those previously described under the Transthoracic Incision.

OPERATIVE COMPLICATIONS

ACUTE ADRENAL INSUFFICIENCY

A most serious although completely avoidable complication encountered in the course of adrenal surgery is acute adrenocortical insufficiency. It is to be anticipated whenever a total or subtotal adrenalectomy is done, regardless of the surgical approach. As previously mentioned, tumors producing Cushing's syndrome usually suppress function of the uninvolved gland. Tumors resulting primarily in the production of androgens or estrogens, with little disturbance of cortisol production, may or may not be associated with atrophy of the opposite adrenal. Since this is impossible to predict before removal of the tumor, however, the same postoperative care is indicated as for patients with Cushing's syndrome.

We use essentially the same preparation for patients with functioning tumors as for those who are to undergo complete adrenalectomy, despite the presence of an apparent excess of hydrocortisone in Cushing's syndrome. The postoperative management differs in that the totally adrenalectomized patient is fairly rapidly titrated until his basal requirements are determined, while the patient with residual adrenal tissue disturbed by operation or atrophied will go through a careful period of "weaning" to promote gradual return of function of residual adrenal tissue ultimately sufficient to maintain the patient without exogenous supplementation. The atrophic gland can be expected to resume function, but the functional capacity of residual adrenal tissue after subtotal adrenalectomy is unpredictable. If the blood supply is prejudiced, the residual tissue will be unlikely to survive. Many patients in whom partial adrenalectomy has been performed need permanent substitution therapy.

An alternative to continued replacement therapy is the autotransplantation of adrenal cortical tissue into a peripheral muscle, most frequently the sartorius. This was first suggested by Franksson et al. in 1956 and has subsequently been carried out by numerous surgeons. Most recently Hardy reported on 8 patients with Cushing's disease in whom autotransplants were used in an effort to obviate the need for replacement therapy. "All eight exhibited biopsy or functional evidence of some degree of graft survival. One patient stopped steroid replacement permanently and another developed recurrent Cushing's syndrome from the graft."[16] The role of this experimental procedure remains to be defined.

PREPARATION OF THE PATIENT FOR ADRENALECTOMY. Preparation is directed toward supplying an excess of active adrenocortical substance in the tissues and plasma during the period of operation and immediately thereafter. Although many different steroidal compounds having physiologic activity have been isolated from the human adrenal cortex, two principal corticoids are found in adrenal venous blood. These are hydrocortisone (cortisol, compound F) and aldosterone. The activity of cortisone is dependent upon its conversion to hydrocortisone.

We usually perform bilateral adrenalectomy on patients prepared with cortisone or hydrocortisone alone, but for maximal safety the addition of small amounts of a mineralocorticoid such as fludrocortisone acetate (Florinef), 0.1 mg. orally, or desoxycorticosterone acetate (DOCA), 5 mg. intramuscularly, is desirable as the dose of glucocorticoid is reduced toward physiological requirements. Some of the newer adrenal steroid compounds that have been developed for their anti-inflammatory effects are less complete in the spectrum of adrenocortical function than cortisone; therefore they should not be used for substitution therapy in place of cortisone. The dosage schedule given in Table 29–2 has been found to provide a satisfactory margin of safety for adrenalectomy or removal of a functioning cortical tumor.

TABLE 29–2 CORTISONE DOSAGE SCHEDULE FOR ADRENALECTOMY

Day before operation	Cortisone 50 mg. I.M. at 6:00 P.M.
Day of operation	Cortisone 50 mg. I.M. 1 hour before operation. Add 100 mg. cortisone to each liter of intravenous fluids during operation.
Postoperatively	Cortisone 50 mg. I.M. every 6 hours until on oral intake, then start cortisone by mouth 50 mg. every 8 hours and decrease successively until on maintenance dose of 50 mg. per day in four divided doses.

If sodium declines and potassium rises, a mineralocorticoid, fludrocortisone acetate (Florinef), may be added.

The dosage is successively halved until the daily intake is 50 mg. of cortisone. Infrequently patients will feel weak or anorectic with this dosage, but are symptom-free when given 75 mg. each day. Orally administered cortisone is rapidly conjugated in the liver, mainly into inactive glucuronides; therefore it is best to divide the maintenance requirements into four equal doses taken at 6-hour intervals. In our early experience 25 mg. taken twice each day did not uniformly prevent pigmentation of the skin, weakness, and anorexia, the symptoms of chronic adrenal insufficiency. The same dose when distributed in four equal portions effectively prevented these symptoms.

During operation an intravenous infusion of 5 per cent dextrose in 0.85 per cent saline solution to which has been added 100 mg. of cortisol per liter is given.

The signs of acute adrenal insufficiency in the anesthetized patient or the one whose reactions are incomplete are hypotension and tachycardia. The same signs, of course, may result from blood loss and drugs used before and during anesthesia. With the outlined regimen we have not seen adrenal insufficiency during operation.

The hazard of acute adrenal insufficiency is greatest in the first 72 hours after operation. The symptoms are apathy or restlessness, weakness, anorexia, nausea, and vomiting. The temperature and pulse rate rise, and the blood pressure falls. It is of interest that during the early period the serum sodium and potassium levels are normal, a fact that suggests that the regulatory effects on these ions are not the main factor. The blood urea nitrogen level is usually moderately elevated. Unless appropriate treatment is promptly given, a shocklike state and death will follow. Treatment consists in immediate intravenous infusion of saline to which has been added 100 mg. of hydrocortisone per liter.

Chronic adrenal insufficiency also may occur in the adrenalectomized patient who for some time is apparently well maintained. Patients with breast or prostatic cancer for whom this operation is done are usually kept on minimal replacement dosage not for economic reasons, although cortisone is expensive, but because in the process of the metabolism of cortisone, compounds having estrogenic or androgenic activity may be formed. Stressful situations such as prolonged exposure to heat or cold and infection are particularly likely to produce a relative adrenal insufficiency in these patients unless the dose of cortisone is increased during the period of stress.

Special precautions are needed for the diabetic whose adrenals are removed, for it is likely that the insulin requirement will be lessened after adrenalectomy. If infection should occur, however, both the insulin and corticoid requirements will be increased; failure to appreciate this may lead to adrenal insufficiency or diabetic coma.

Because of the hazards the adrenalectomized patient faces, it has been recommended that all such patients be provided with identification cards engraved with the statement, "I am an adrenalectomized patient. In an emergency I will need cortisone."

The period of withdrawal or weaning from corticoids required in the patient with adrenal atrophy or residual fractions of adrenal tissue should be prolonged and gradual. We have seen adrenal insufficiency develop in a 6-year-old boy with Cushing's syndrome 5 weeks after removal of a malignant cortical tumor. The use of ACTH is of little value, for although it stimulates the adrenal, it does not facilitate pituitary secretion of ACTH. Our current practice is to decrease the cortisone dosage by 5 mg. each week until withdrawal is complete or a maintenance level is reached. During this period close contact is kept with the patient or his family, and adjustments to this schedule are made according to the patient's

response. In most instances in which an atrophic adrenal remains, the foregoing regimen will be found to be conservative, but in subtotal adrenalectomy a level will be reached below which adrenal insufficiency will develop. The dose should be continued in quantity sufficient to prevent symptoms.

HYPERFUNCTION OF THE ADRENAL CORTEX

Adrenocortical hyperfunction results in some of the most unusual metabolic and gonadal disturbances found in medical practice. In recent years improved methodology for the analysis of steroid hormones in urine and plasma has led to better understanding of these alterations, and in spite of the many deficiencies in our knowledge of their pathogenesis, the defects that exist can be classified with some degree of accuracy.

The clinical manifestations of adrenocortical hyperfunction depend on the age at onset, nature of the defect, the sex of the patient, the hormone or hormones secreted in increased amount, and the underlying pathologic process. Hyperplasia of the adrenal cortex occurring in utero results in female pseudohermaphroditism. After birth precocious sexual development or heterosexual changes occur either alone or in conjunction with the signs of Cushing's syndrome. Females are involved much more frequently than males, and the frequency of Cushing's syndrome exceeds that of the adrenogenital syndrome or primary aldosteronism. Feminizing changes in men are rare, and the cases thus far reported all result from malignant cortical tumors.

In adrenal hyperplasia due to Cushing's disease the principal changes are metabolic, resembling those seen with excessive glucocorticoid therapy. Facial hirsutism, acne, and amenorrhea commonly accompany these metabolic changes. In Cushing's syndrome due to a functioning tumor the signs may be identical with those of hyperplasia, but at times virilization is more striking or may be the dominant clinical feature. In virilization due to tumor some evidence of increased 17-hydroxycorticosteroid overproduction exists. This is in contrast to the adrenogenital syndrome with hyperplasia in which the primary defect is inadequate synthesis of cortisol. In this situation cortisone is effective in replacing the corticoid deficit and decreasing androgen production.

The metabolic changes that follow the prolonged hypersecretion of hydrocortisone in Cushing's syndrome and disease influence the preoperative and postoperative care of the patient. Carbohydrate intolerance and protein catabolism are seen, and there is a decrease in lean muscle mass. Hyperglycemia and a diabetic glucose tolerance curve may be present. The muscular wasting is manifested not only in decreased diameter of the extremities but also by a decrease in the efficiency of muscular contraction. Fat metabolism is also altered, as seen by the obesity and buffalo hump fat pad. Severe long-standing Cushing's syndrome may be associated with osteoporosis and, rarely, pathologic fractures. Renal tubular absorption of sodium is increased, with a corresponding decrease in potassium absorption. Hypokalemia, hypochloremia, and alkalosis may be present, depending upon the adequacy of the potassium intake. Of great importance is the decreased resistance and tolerance to infection.

There is increasing evidence to support Cushing's concept that the disease that bears his name is caused by basophilic adenomas of the pituitary. By means of increasingly sophisticated roentgenological techniques microadenomas of the anterior pituitary have been demonstrated with increasing frequency. For this reason there is a trend toward the transsphenoidal microsurgical removal of these tumors in the primary treatment of Cushing's disease. It is likely, therefore, that neither adrenalectomy nor heavy particle irradiation of the pituitary will continue to be used except in unusual circumstances.

In preparation of the patient for operation the anabolic effects of androgens have been demonstrated to result in positive nitrogen and calcium balance. Testosterone propionate, 50 mg. intramuscularly 3 times a week for several weeks, is effective in decreasing nitrogen and calcium losses. Correction of the potassium deficit and the concomitant metabolic alkalosis is accomplished by adding 5 mg. of potassium chloride to the daily diet. Anesthesia and surgery are poorly tolerated in the presence of severe uncompensated metabolic alkalosis.

When acne is present, particularly in the region of the surgical incision, efforts are made to promote healing by regular cleansing with hexachlorophene soap and water and the application of bacitracin ointment. Pus, if present, should be cultured to determine sensitivity to the antimicrobial agents. Sepsis has been one of the more common complications of surgery in these patients; therefore every effort must be made to avoid contamination of the wound.

If adrenalectomy for Cushing's disease is considered necessary, the operation of choice today is bilateral total adrenalectomy. This is most easily done through bilateral flank incisions with the patient in the prone position.

An interesting complication of adrenalectomy for adrenal hyperplasia is the development of corticotropin-secreting tumors of the pituitary. First reported by Nelson in 1958, the tumors are manifested clinically by hyperpigmentation of the skin and visual field defects 3 or more years after adrenalectomy. Roentgenograms of the skull show enlargement of the sella turcica. In a report from the Mayo Clinic, 12 of 122 patients with Cushing's disease and adrenal hyperplasia had chromophobe tumors of the anterior pituitary before or after adrenalectomy. Hopwood and Kenny reported on 31 children from 10 months to 16 years of age who were treated with total bilateral adrenalectomy. Postadrenalectomy hyperpigmentation was reported in 18 patients. Sella enlargement was detected in 8 patients after 1 to 5½ years postoperatively. Five of these patients had documented pituitary adenomas. This incidence is higher than that reported in adults (10 to 16 per cent). No pituitary tumors were seen in 34 patients who had Cushing's syndrome associated with adrenocortical tumors, and no pituitary tumors have been reported following bilateral adrenalectomy for other conditions.

Another form of hyperactivity of the adrenal cortex is primary aldosteronism or Conn's syndrome. This usually is caused by a benign adenoma of the adrenal cortex that hypersecretes aldosterone. The tumors are small and occasionally multiple and bilateral. The common symptoms are muscle weakness, intermittent paralysis, polyuria, polydipsia, and headache. There is usually significant hypertension, and laboratory studies show increased excretion of aldosterone, hypokalemia, mild hypernatremia with a normal sodium intake, and alkalosis. Plasma renin levels are low. Sampling adrenal vein blood for calculation of the ratio of aldosterone to cortisol may be useful. In a hyperfunctioning gland this ratio is usually 6 or higher (mean 33) and the ratio for the contralateral gland is 3.6 or less (mean 1.3).

Treatment is surgical removal of the involved adrenal or adrenals. Because of the small size of these tumors, preoperative localization is difficult and requires special techniques in most instances. Pyelography, carbon dioxide injection, body-section reoentgenography, and aortography are seldom helpful. Catheterization of adrenal veins through the vena cava (and renal vein on the left) for the collection of venous blood for aldosterone assay is helpful. At the same time venography will frequently outline the tumor. Rupturing of small venous channels with extravasation of the radiopaque contrast material is frequent. Following venography there has also been reported cessation of function of an aldosterone-secreting adenoma. This has been attributed to necrosis. It is of interest that this technique has been deliberately used for adrenal ablation in patients with disseminated breast cancer. The services of one skilled in venous catheterization is most essential if this technique is to be successful. Isotopic definition of functioning adenomas using ^{131}I-19-iodocholesterol and the computer-assisted Anger camera was reported by Conn to be useful in defining adenomas in a small series of cases.

Primary aldosteronism has also been treated medically by means of an aldosterone antagonist, spironolactone, or other experimental inhibitors of adrenal function such as aminoglutethimide. This drug blocks the biosynthesis of all adrenal steroids. There is compensatory stimulus of cortisol secretion by ACTH, but there is no compensatory increase in aldosterone secretion. For this reason adrenal insufficiency does not occur but the primary aldosteronism is controlled.

ROENTGENOLOGIC DIAGNOSIS OF ADRENAL TUMORS

Roentgenologic diagnosis of enlargement or tumors of the adrenal glands has been revolutionized by the development of computerized tomography. Although costly and associated with somewhat greater radiation exposure than previously used methods, it shows the adrenal glands in over 95 per cent of patients and can define masses less than 2 cm. in diameter. Since it is non-invasive and highly accurate, it has replaced such previously used techniques as excretory urography with nephrotomograms, presacral gas insufflation, and selective arteriography and venography.

CT scanning is particularly useful in demonstrating adrenal cortical tumors and pheochromocytomas; in both instances it is nearly 100 per cent accurate. It is also very accurate in detecting tumors in aldosteronism.

Gray scale ultrasonography has also been used for adrenal imaging but is not as satisfactory as CT scanning.

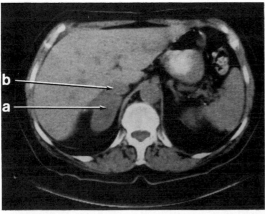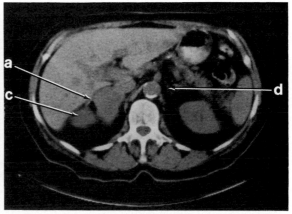

Figure 29–3   CT scans of the abdomen showing adrenal mass: a, adrenal corticocarcinoma; b, inferior vena cava; c, upper pole of the right kidney; d, normal left adrenal gland.

COMPLICATIONS OF ADRENAL STEROID THERAPY

Continued use of adrenal steroid hormones in excess of physiologic requirements is attended by potentially serious consequences that must be considered when these substances are prescribed. The anti-inflammatory properties of the glucocorticoids are those mainly desired in general therapeutic use. Great effort has been expended to develop compounds that have potent anti-inflammatory action but are devoid of other physiologic effects of cortisone. These efforts have been only partially successful, and to our knowledge none of the steroids is entirely free of undesirable activities or complications. Because experience has been greatest with cortisone and corticotropin, the complications described will refer specifically to these substances rather than to the newer steroids.

The administration of cortisone eventually results in atrophy of the adrenal cortex, while the giving of ACTH induces pituitary inactivity. The end result following the withdrawal of either substance is temporary adrenal insufficiency. The patient is frequently without symptoms; at times he may feel somewhat weak and easily fatigued and may have anorexia, nausea, and diarrhea. When he is subjected to stress of sufficient magnitude, such as major surgery, acute adrenal insufficiency will be precipitated. This is particularly likely to happen when an accurate history of previous steroid therapy is not obtained or is overlooked.

Operations can be safely carried out, provided cortisone is given. The dosage schedule outlined for complete adrenalectomy (see Table 29–2) will confer the protection needed. Specific questioning about steroid intake during the previous year should be an integral part of the history. Our present practice is to supply supplementary cortisone when there has been cortisone intake exceeding 2 weeks in duration during the year preceding operation.

Failure to obtain an accurate history will lead in most cases to unexplained hypotension and tachycardia. The intravenous infusion of 0.85 per cent sodium chloride solution to which has been added 100 mg. of hydrocortisone will in most cases suffice to correct the adrenal insufficiency. Cortisone is subsequently supplied intramuscularly and gradually reduced. In many cases other explanations for the hypotension are overlooked and corticoids are needlessly given.

The duration of treatment and the dose influence the development of complications. Short-term treatment seldom produces ill effects, but with continued treatment all the changes of Cushing's syndrome will be produced. These include obesity with the development of an upper dorsal fat pad, moon facies, troublesome mental aberrations, thin red skin, muscle wasting, hypertension, occasionally sodium retention and edema, the accelerated development of arteriosclerosis, osteoporosis, hypokalemia, and metabolic alkalosis. Testosterone propionate will counteract many of the metabolic changes, but in women will produce masculinization if used in dosage sufficient for maximal effects. When 25 mg. is given twice a week, the loss of nitrogen, phosphorus, and calcium will be retarded, and masculinization will occur only after prolonged usage. Moderate sodium restriction is advisable, particularly in the presence of edema. Potassium and calcium should be added to the diet.

The anti-inflammatory properties of the corticoids also reduce resistance to infection. In some overwhelming infections, however, adrenal insufficiency occurs; under these circumstances cortisone should be given along with antimicrobial agents to which the offending organisms are susceptible. Whenever cortisone is used in the presence of infections, bacterial sensitivity should be checked at frequent intervals to be certain that no change has occurred; otherwise the infection will be potentiated.

The same mechanisms whereby cortisone exerts anti-inflammatory action have been demonstrated in animal experiments to retard the healing of wounds. In human beings, however, there is little evidence that, in the usual dosage range of cortisone, wound healing is significantly retarded. In this regard it is important not to confuse wound infection, which does of course delay the healing of wounds, with the process of healing in clean surgical wounds.

During cortisone therapy patients with gastroduodenal ulceration have increased ulcer activity, and the frequency of bleeding and perforation is greater. The perforations are likely to be peculiar in that the signs and symptoms tend to be obscured. We have seen patients with distended abdomen, absent bowel sounds, and free air under the diaphragm, but without complaints. We have also observed massive, uncontrolled arterial hemorrhage in the base of enormous penetrating ulcers requiring subtotal gastrectomy in patients with minimal ulcer complaints preceding the hemorrhage. The development of new ulcers is also increased by the giving of adrenal steroids. Experimental studies of the influence of cortisone on gastric secretion have yielded conflicting results. Although it appears that increased acid-pepsin secretion is not the mechanism of action, patients with a history of ulcer disease who require cortisone therapy, or patients who have symptoms while being so treated, should be placed on a satisfactory ulcer regimen.

When corticoids are used in patients with ulcerative inflammatory disease of the gastrointestinal tract, such as idiopathic ulcerative colitis or Crohn's disease, relatively asymptomatic perforation into the general peritoneal cavity may occur, and under these circumstances the mortality rate is high. Toxic megacolon in ulcerative colitis has also been attributed to the use of steroids, but the evidence that this relationship is a causal one is not strong. Perforation of various portions of the small and large intestine has also been reported in patients without preexistent evidence of ileocolic disease. We have seen one patient with 12 perforations of the terminal ileum apparently confined to the areas of Peyer's patches. There was no previous history of intestinal complaints. Recovery followed resection of the distal 2 feet of small intestine.

PHEOCHROMOCYTOMA

The operative mortality rate from the removal of pheochromocytomas up to 1951 as reported by Graham was 26 per cent (33 deaths in 125 cases). Most of the deaths were due to uncontrolled shock, but cardiac failure, hyperpyrexia, hemorrhage, and uremia also contributed to the mortality. Since 1951 the risk has decreased and at present should be almost non-existent for the removal of benign tumors, provided the patient is properly prepared for operation and the anesthetic management and operation are competently performed.

It is our present practice to prepare all patients with pheochromocytoma with adrenolytic therapy prior to operation for at least 3 days and preferably 2 weeks, regardless of whether they have sustained or paroxysmal hypertension. For this purpose we use the alpha-adrenergic blocking agent phenoxybenzamine (Dibenzyline). Although in the past we were fearful of using this drug lest a refractory state to norepinephrine infusion occur when norepinephrine is needed for control of a hypotensive crisis at operation, increased experience has proven this fear to be unfounded. The dosage of Dibenzyline depends on the response of the blood pressure and associated symptoms.

We have found a reduced plasma volume in most patients with pheochromocytoma and for this reason we give 2 liters of Ringer's lactate solution the night before operation and continuously during operation. With preoperative preparation that includes alpha blocking agents and restoration of plasma volume deficits, the intraoperative course has been much smoother than previously.

The precise anesthetic agent selected is not as important as the facility with which it is used and the expertness with which the blood pressure fluctuations during operation are controlled. Cyclopropane is generally felt to be contraindicated because of the danger of ventricular fibrillation in the presence of increased circulating epinephrine. Perhaps unjustly, use of spinal anesthesia has been avoided because of the hypertension. A quiet induction without excess preoperative medication is desirable and can be achieved with thiopental. An endotracheal tube is inserted after induction and anesthesia is subsequently continued with either nitrous oxide and ether, muscle relaxants with ethylene, halothane, or other agents as preferred by the anesthesiologist. (See also Chapter 10.)

Careful monitoring of the blood pressure,

preferably continuously through an intra-arterial needle or catheter, is essential. Abrupt rises in pressure are controlled by phentolamine (Regitine). The dose of phentolamine is 5 to 10 mg. given slowly with close attention to changes in pressure. A rise in blood pressure is most likely to occur during induction or as the tumor is manipulated by the surgeon. Our objective is to maintain the systolic pressure below 200 mm. Hg and the diastolic pressure below 120 mm.

The other critical point in the operation is at the time of separation of the tumor from the systemic circulation; at this time the blood pressure is likely to fall precipitously to dangerous levels. This event has been infrequent since we have instituted our program of preoperative preparation. Nevertheless, the anesthesiologist should have available a solution of norepinephrine, in concentration of 4 mg. per liter of Ringer's lactate solution, for use in the event that such a hypotensive crisis does occur. This infusion is started at the first sign of a fall in pressure. The rate of infusion is determined by the blood pressure response and is carefully monitored for the remainder of the operation as well as in the postoperative period.

It is at times necessary to continue norepinephrine administration for 24 hours or longer before the blood pressure remains stable without its vasoconstricting action. We have found placing the patient in the Trendelenburg position to be helpful in this weaning process. If absolutely necessary, substitution of intramuscular injections, as needed, will suffice.

Whenever this potent vasoconstrictor is given intravenously, particularly when long continued or in high concentration, there is danger of devitalization of skin. It is therefore important to limit the infusion of norepinephrine solution to the shortest possible period.

Bibliography

1. Auda, S. P., Brennan, M. F., and Gill, J. R., Jr.: Evaluation of the surgical management of primary aldosteronism. Ann. Surg. 191:1, 1980.
2. Bigos, S. T., Somma, M., Rasio, E., et al.: Cushing's disease: Management of transsphenoidal pituitary microsurgery. J. Clin. Endocrinol. Metab. 50:348, 1980.
3. Cahill, G. F., Loeb, R. F., Kurzrok, R., Stout, A. P., and Smith, F. M.: Adrenal cortical tumors. Surg. Gynecol. Obstet. 62:287, 1936.
4. Conn, J. W., and Louis, L. H.: Primary aldosteronism: A new clinical entity. Ann. Intern Med. 44:1, 1956.
5. Conn, J. W., Morita, R., Cohen, E. L., Beierwalters, W. H., McDonald, W. J., and Herwig, K. R.: Primary aldosteronism, photoscanning of tumors after administration of [131]I-19-Iodocholesterol. N. Eng. J. Med. 277:1050, 1967.
6. Cope, O., and Raker, J. W.: Cushing's disease: The surgical care in the management of 46 cases. N. Engl. J. Med. 253:119, 1955.
7. Cowley, D. J., Montgomery, D. A. D., and Welbourn, R. B.: Management of paroxysms of hypertension in patients with pheochromocytomas. Br. J. Surg. 57:832, 1970.
8. Fisher, C. E., Turner, F. A., and Horton, R.: Remission of primary hyperaldosteronism after adrenal venography. N. Engl. J. Med. 285:334, 1971.
9. Fracchia, A. A., et al.: Results of bilateral adrenalectomy in the management of incurable breast cancer: Report of 155 cases. Cancer 12:58, 1959.
10. Franksson, C., and Hellstrom, J.: Bilateral adrenalectomy, with special reference to operative technique and postoperative complications. Acta Chir. Scand. 111:54, 1956.
11. Germuth, F. G., Jr.: Role of adrenocortical steroids in infection, immunity and hypersensitivity. Pharmacol. Rev. 8:1, 1956.
12. Gitlow, S. E., Pertsemlidis, D., and Bertani, L. M.: Management of patients with pheochromocytoma. Am. Heart J. 82:557, 1971.
13. Goldenberg, M.: Adrenal medullary function. Am. J. Med. 10:637, 1951.
14. Goldenberg, M., Snyder, C. H., and Aranow, H., Jr.: New test for hypertension due to circulating epinephrine. J.A.M.A. 135:971, 1947.
15. Graham, J. B.: Pheochromocytoma and hypertension: An analysis of 207 cases. (Int. Abstr. Surg.) Surg. Gynecol. Obstet. 92:105, 1951.
16. Hardy, J. D.: Surgical management of Cushing's syndrome with emphasis on adrenal autotransplantation. Ann. Surg. 188:290, 1978.
17. Hopwood, H. J., and Kenny, F. M.: Incidence of Nelson's syndrome after adrenalectomy for Cushing's disease in children. Am. J. Dis. Child. 131:1353, 1977.
18. Huggins, C., and Bergenstal, D. M.: Inhibition of human mammary cancer and prostatic cancer by adrenalectomy. Cancer Rev. 12:134, 1952.
19. Huggins, C., and Scott, W. W.: Bilateral adrenalectomy in prostatic cancer. Ann. Surg. 122:1031, 1945.
20. Kahn, P. C., and Nichrosz, L. V.: Selective angiography of adrenal glands. Am. J. Roentgenol. 101:739, 1967.
21. Karstaedt, N., Sagel, S. S., Stanley, R. V., et al.: Computed tomography of the adrenal gland. Radiology 129:723, 1979.
22. Lukens, F. D. W., Flippin, H. F., and Thigpen, F. M.: Adrenal cortical adenoma with absence of the opposite adrenal: Report of a case with

operation and autopsy. Am. J. Med. Sci. *193*:812, 1937.

23. Mayo, C. H.: Paroxysmal hypertension with tumor of the retroperitoneal nerve: Report of a case. J.A.M.A. *89*:1047, 1927.

24. Melby, J. C., Spark, R. F., Dale, S. L., Egdahl, R. H., and Kahn, P. C.: Diagnosis and localization of aldosterone-producing adenomas. N. Engl. J. Med. *277*:1050, 1967.

25. Moore, T. C., and Shumacker, H. B., Jr.: Adrenalin producing tumors in children. Ann. Surg. *143*:256, 1956.

26. Nelson, D. H., Meakin, J. W., Dealy, J. R., et al.: ACTH-producing tumor of the adrenal gland. N. Engl. J. Med. *259*:161, 1958.

27. Nelson, D. H., Meakin, J. W., and Thorn, G. W.: ACTH-producing pituitary tumors following adrenalectomy for Cushing's syndrome. Ann. Intern. Med. *52*:560, 1960.

28. Pezzulich, R. A., and Mannix, H., Jr.: Immediate complications of adrenal surgery. Ann. Surg. *172*:125, 1970.

29. Ransom, C. F., Landes, R. R., and McClelland, R.: Air embolism following retroperitoneal pneumography, a nationwide survey. J. Urol. *76*:664, 1956.

30. Rivas, M. R.: Roentgenological diagnosis, generalized subserous emphysema through a single puncture. Am. J. Roentgenol. *64*:723, 1950.

31. Salasna, R. M., Kearns, T. P., Kernohan, J. W., Sprague, R. G., and MacCarty, C. S.: Pituitary tumors in patients with Cushing's syndrome. J. Clin. Endocrinol. *9*:1523, 1959.

32. Sipple, J. H.: The association of pheochromocytoma with carcinoma of the thyroid gland. Am. J. Med. *31*:163, 1966.

33. Souttar, R. D., and Ziffren, S. E.: Adrenocortical steroid therapy resulting in unusual gastrointestinal complications. Arch. Surg. *79*:346, 1959.

34. Wells, S. A., Jr., Santen, R. J., Lipton, A., et al.: Medical adrenalectomy with aminoglutethimide: Clinical studies in postmenopausal patients with metastatic breast carcinoma. Ann. Surg. *187*:475, 1978.

30

COMPLICATIONS OF COMMON FRACTURES AND DISLOCATIONS

Alan E. Freeland

Complications constitute the foremost problems in the management of fractures and dislocations. A fracture or dislocation by itself may cause little temporary or permanent impairment, but a complication may lead to increased morbidity, permanent functional loss, amputation, and even death. The economic deprivation to the patient and the patient's family can be equally devastating.

The best treatment of any complication is prevention. For those complications that cannot be prevented, early recognition and prompt appropriate response are essential. A high index of suspicion and anticipation of potential complications followed by vigilant monitoring of the patient will lead to the early identification of complications.

Complications of common fractures and dislocations may be classified as immediate and delayed. Immediate complications occur at the time of injury or promptly thereafter, as a result either of the trauma producing the fracture or dislocation or of the secondary trauma produced by sharp ends of bone. Immediate complications are not preventable.

Delayed complications occur later at varying times after the fracture or dislocation. Some are preventable, while others are unpreventable. Some occur as a direct result of the trauma producing the fracture or disloca-

tion or are predetermined by the extent and location of the fracture or dislocation. As such, they are largely, if not entirely, unpreventable. Other delayed complications occur, however, as a direct result of improper or faulty treatment or of inadvertent breaks in technique. As such, they are largely, if not entirely, preventable.

IMMEDIATE COMPLICATIONS

Intra-Abdominal Injuries

Fractures of the lower ribs, pelvis, or spine may be associated with life-threatening injuries to such organs as the spleen, liver, kidney, duodenum, or bladder or major blood vessels. Except for some injuries of the kidney, each of these complicating injuries is an indication for prompt operative intervention. Early diagnosis is of prime importance. The diagnosis of an associated intra-abdominal catastrophe is likely to be made if the possibility is considered and diagnostic measures are instituted. Aspiration or, if aspiration is negative, lavage of the peritoneal cavity may give valuable information about intra-abdominal bleeding. The liver or spleen may be damaged in association with fractures of the ribs. The left upper portion of the abdomen may

Alan E. Freeland is an Ohioan by birth and graduated from Johns Hopkins University and from George Washington University, where he was elected Alpha Omega Alpha. He received his postgraduate training in orthopaedics at Johns Hopkins Hospital, Letterman Army Medical Center, and Shriner's Hospital for Crippled Children, Los Angeles. He has had special experience in injuries of the extremities. At present he is Associate Professor of Orthopaedic Surgery at the University of Mississippi Medical Center.

present a triad of injuries, such as fractured ribs, splenic hemorrhage, and rupture of the left kidney. A large, soft tissue mass on transabdominal x-ray may indicate a hematoma; this is often found in the left upper quadrant of the abdomen in the presence of a ruptured spleen. Splenic hemorrhage usually demands splenectomy. Delayed bleeding from the spleen may occur dramatically weeks after initial trauma.

Injury to the right rib cage may be associated with serious injuries to the liver, right kidney, and duodenum. Continuing liver hemorrhage must be controlled by suture, resection of damaged liver, or ligation of bleeding intrahepatic vessels.

Rupture of an intra-abdominal hollow viscus may also result from the same force that produces a fracture of the pelvis or of a vertebral body or, particularly, multiple fractures of the transverse processes. Plain films of the abdomen with the patient in the decubitus or upright views may demonstrate free air, indicating rupture of a hollow viscus. A ruptured hollow viscus must be repaired or the damaged area resected.

The abdomen should be opened if the suspected intra-abdominal injury cannot be ruled out. In doubtful situations, operation is preferable to watchful waiting. An unnecessary laparotomy is preferable by far to an ignored life-threatening injury. Failure of the patient to respond to blood and fluid replacement of the loss reasonably estimated as part of the known injuries indicates continued hemorrhage or massive soiling of the peritoneum. Under these circum-stances, the abdomen should be opened for correction of the intra-abdominal injury as other resuscitative methods are continued. It should be remembered, postoperatively, that laparotomy increases the possibility of ventilatory insufficiency through diaphragmatic splinting and disturbance of the ventilation of basal pulmonary segments.

In an analysis of approximately 4,750 cases of pelvic fractures in the literature, Kane[93] computed that the average rate of major urinary tract complication is 13 per cent. He states that all pelvic fracture patients must be assumed to have urinary tract injuries until proven otherwise and that the presence or absence of hematuria has little or no pathognomonic significance.[93, 104] The inability to void following pelvic trauma may be indicative of serious urologic injury, or it may be simply due to hemorrhage and edema causing bladder displacement and subsequent urethral stretching and sphincter spasm. While patients with fractures or dislocations of the anterior pelvis, such as symphyseal separations, Malgaigne fractures or fracture dislocations, and fractures of both pubic rami, and especially those patients with bilateral fractures of both the superior and inferior pubic rami (butterfly fractures), are more likely to have urinary tract injuries, they can also occur in instances of undisplaced fractures of the pelvis such as in the case of rupture of a distended bladder by sudden compression.[92, 108] Therefore, a cystourethrogram should be performed on all patients with a disrupting pelvic fracture (Fig. 30–1).

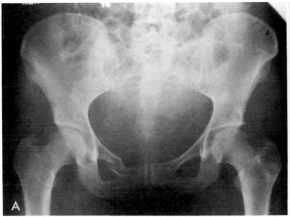 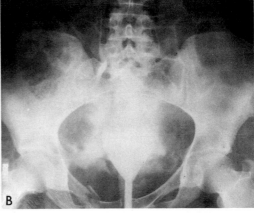

Figure 30–1 Fractures of pelvis, undisplaced, complicated by a ruptured bladder. *A*, Multiple fractures of pelvis with little or no displacement. *B*, Cystogram shows rupture of bladder, which is elevated by hematoma formation.

Rupture of the urethra associated with fractures of the pelvis is virtually limited to the male. Rupture of the anterior urethra may be seen with straddle injuries and is accompanied by contusions and ecchymoses of the perineum and penis as well as signs of extrapelvic extravasation of urine. Rupture of the posterior urethra is usually in the membranous rather than the prostatic portion and is the commonest lower urinary tract injury seen with pelvic fractures in the male. This injury is most commonly seen in pelvic crushes with severe anterior pelvic displacement. The patient is unable to micturate despite a desire to do so. Bleeding at the external urethral meatus is commonly seen but is not pathognomonic. Usually a catheter cannot be passed into the bladder. Rectal examination discloses cephalad retraction of the prostate from its normal position and this retraction is pathognomonic. A urethrogram confirms the diagnosis of urethral tears.

Bladder rupture occurs in 4 per cent of pelvic fractures and may be extraperitoneal or intraperitoneal. The retrograde cystogram is critical in diagnosing a ruptured bladder.[43, 140] A cystogram should be performed by instilling, by gravity flow or gentle injection, 250 ml. of a 30 per cent solution of an excretory urography medium. If the anteroposterior view shows no extravasation, an additional 150 ml. is instilled to overcome the tamponade effect of the perivesical hemorrhage and hematoma and another film is taken. The bladder is then emptied and given a saline washout, and another film is taken to detect extravasations that may have been obliterated by a bladder full of dye.[33] Since both the cystogram and the urethrogram may show extraperitoneal extravasation of dye, the cystogram is done before the urethrogram in males, except in straddle fractures and when it is impossible to pass a catheter into the bladder.

Following evaluation of the lower urinary tract, an intravenous pyelogram should be done in cases of gross hematuria or microscopic hematuria (10 red blood cells per high powered field) to evaluate renal trauma or trauma to the upper urinary tract. The intravenous pyelogram will be unsuccessful if the patient is in shock and may be delayed until systolic blood pressure is restored to at least 100 mm. Hg and, if necessary, may be done intraoperatively.

Some lower urinary tract injuries will require only indwelling catheter drainage, but others will demand open operation. Again, in doubtful situations operation is preferable to watchful waiting. The principal objective is to establish free urinary drainage to avoid extravasation of the urine through fascial planes. Cystostomy should be done in virtually all instances when urinary extravasation is present. Bladder ruptures may be repaired with 2-0 chromic catgut. Urethral tears are repaired over a small inlying urethral splinting catheter via a perineal approach, and cystostomy drainage is maintained for at least 2 weeks. Preventive antibiotics are used. Lower urinary tract injuries occurring in association with pelvic fractures can be a cause of death, particularly if diagnosis is delayed.

ILEUS

Transient ileus due to retroperitoneal hemorrhage is extremely common in patients with thoracolumbar vertebral body fractures, with one or more fractures of the transverse process, or with a pelvic fracture. These patients, therefore, should be admitted to the hospital, placed on a liquid diet, and observed carefully. If ileus develops, all oral intake should be stopped. Nasogastric suction and intravenous fluids with electrolyte replacement should be instituted. Ileus may take 24 hours to develop. It seldom lasts longer than 3 to 5 days.

Intrathoracic Injuries

Fractures of the ribs or sternum may cause serious life-endangering intrathoracic injuries. Hemothorax, pneumothorax, hemopneumothorax, flail chest, and lung contusion are common complications of these bony injuries. Pulmonary insufficiency may occur. This may be life-threatening, especially in association with multiple injuries, particularly when there are fractured long bones requiring treatment in skeletal traction or a fracture or dislocation about the hip. Recent studies strongly indicate that early stabilization of long bone fractures with either cast braces or internal or external fixation within 24 to 48 hours after injury, so that the patient can get into a vertical position on a tilt table or chair, allows much more effective ventilatory therapy and markedly diminishes the mortality from pulmonary failure.[96, 116, 197] It is important to stabilize fractures about the hip and femoral fractures associated with thoracic injuries within the first 24 to 48 hours after injury whenever possible, as these fractures, if unstabilized, cause the most difficulty in getting the patient into a vertical position.

Head Injuries

In spastic, brain-injured patients whose fractures cannot be controlled with traction in bed, internal fixation or external fixators should be used.[71] This also facilitates respiratory and skin care for these patients.

Hemorrhage (External or Internal) and Shock

Open fractures can be complicated by shock caused by external hemorrhage either from a major artery lacerated by a sharp bony fragment or, more commonly, from the bony fragments and torn muscles. Until definitive care can be initiated, hemorrhage from open fractures of the extremities is controlled by a sterile compression dressing, elevation, and splinting. Neither a tourniquet nor clamps should be used. An improperly applied tourniquet can produce a peripheral nerve injury, while a properly applied tourniquet left unattended can result in irreparable ischemia. Clamps directly applied to severed vessels may preclude restoration of continuity, while clamps applied indiscriminately in the wound can damage vital structures.[88]

Shock can also occur in closed fractures, particularly with fractures of the pelvis, spine, and femur and is caused by internal hemorrhage. As much as 1000 to 1500 ml. of whole blood and the same amount of extracellular fluid may be lost into the tissues of the thigh from a closed comminuted fracture of the femoral shaft and the associated soft tissue injury.

Approximately 40 per cent of all patients with pelvic fractures require a transfusion.[83, 93] Unstable fractures with a double break of the pelvic ring require transfusion more frequently than other pelvic fractures and also require more in amount of blood replacement.[83] Mortality in patients with pelvic fractures ranges from 5 to 20 per cent.[39, 67, 83, 104, 138] Hemorrhage is the most serious complication of pelvic fractures and is directly responsible for nearly 50 per cent of the fatalities.[15, 83, 138, 193] In one series, 75 per cent of the fatalities were due to hemorrhagic shock or renal failure.[39] The presence of shock secondary to retroperitoneal hemorrhage from a fractured pelvis can be overlooked, especially in an unconscious or obtunded patient. Contusion and ecchymosis in the soft tissues about the pelvis and pelvic instability in response to compression testing may be evident, but all patients with multiple trauma should have an x-ray of the pelvis because of the frequency and severity of pelvic fractures in the patient with multiple injuries.

A radiolucent litter reduces the number of moves for the trauma patient from the scene of the accident to the time of definitive therapy.[153] Early reduction and immobilization are important in the treatment of hemorrhage from pelvic fractures,[130, 138, 153] but the crucial therapeutic measure for treating the resulting hypovolemic shock is blood replacement by transfusions in quantities sufficient to replace the estimated loss. Estimated losses of extracellular fluid should be compensated by intravenous isotonic sodium-containing fluids. Ordinarily, retroperitoneal tamponade controls the bleeding, but the physician must be prepared to replace 15 or more units of blood in a severe pelvic fracture.[138, 144] External counterpressure suits such as the G suit or Military Anti-Shock Trousers (MAST) have been used successfully in controlling hemorrhage from pelvic fractures.[9] Laparotomy is dangerous and is often unsuccessful and should be reserved as an absolute last resort.[144] A non-enlarging retroperitoneal hematoma should not be disturbed or the tamponade effect will be lost and infection could be introduced. Hypogastric artery ligation is usually ineffective, since the same rich anastomotic blood supply that renders it safe also renders it futile.[123, 134] It also has no effect in instances of venous injury.[70]

Hemorrhage and shock uncontrolled by massive transfusion and external counterpressure suits may indicate major arterial or venous injury. In these instances, arteriography and venography should be done to identify the site of injury. Iliac venography via femoral vein catheter should be done first and followed by transfemoral aortography.[5, 111, 146] Few injuries involve major arteries. These are usually to the internal iliac artery and injury of that artery should be suspected in instances of limb ischemia or whenever pulses distal to the fracture diminish or disappear following reduction of the fracture, whenever a bruit is auscultated, whenever an extremely large or pulsating hematoma is present, and whenever there is severe or recurrent hemorrhage through an open wound.[167] Standard precepts of surgical repair with anastomosis and grafting are used. More often, the injury involves the obturator or internal pudendal arteries or their branches and, if the capability is present, hemorrhage can be controlled safely by embolization of autologous clot or introduction of Gelfoam into the injured artery through the selectively placed angiographic catheter.[149]

Injuries to Major Arteries in the Extremities

Vascular injuries in association with fractures and dislocations tend to occur where vessels pass adjacent to bone or are fixed to bone. The subclavian artery, therefore, is most vulnerable as it traverses the thoracic outlet between the first rib and the clavicle. The brachial artery is vulnerable where it is adjacent to the humerus and particularly at the elbow, where it may be entrapped by dislocation or lacerated by fracture fragments. The entire superficial femoral artery is vulnerable to laceration in association with femur fractures but particularly so where it is tightly fixed adjacent to the femur in the adductor canal. The popliteal artery and vein are especially vulnerable to injury, since they are tethered at the hiatus of the adductor magnus superiorly and at the tendinous soleus origin inferiorly. The collateral circulation about the elbow is more extensive and reliable than that about the knee, so that damage to the brachial artery is less likely to lead to gangrene and amputation

than damage to the femoral or popliteal arteries in instances when recognition or treatment is delayed. In dislocation of the knee, there is injury to the popliteal artery in 20 to 35 per cent of the cases. Many of these result in amputation owing to delay in diagnosis and poor collateral circulation.

Major vascular injuries must be recognized promptly for optimal limb salvage.[65, 118] The diagnosis of "arterial spasm" must be rejected. Clinical signs of vascular injury include extensive swelling, an enlarged or pulsatile hematoma, a bruit, severe or recurrent hemorrhage through an open wound, diminishing or absent pulses, coolness of the extremity, slow capillary filling, mottling, pallor, progressive edema, paresis or paralysis of distal musculature, paresthesias, hypesthesia, and anesthesia. It is equally important to recognize that pulses, pink color, good capillary filling, and a warm extremity may be present initially in cases of intimal tears and in cases of complete occlusion or transection in which adequate collateral blood flow exists. The surgeon must maintain a high degree of suspicion. The Doppler ultrasound device, pulse volume recordings, and other noninvasive techniques may be helpful but often beg the issue and lose time in the case of the limb at risk. If an arterial lesion is suspected, the sine qua non for diagnosis is an arteriogram and this must be done as rapidly as possible (Fig. 30–2). Venography is done when concurrent major venous injury is suspected. In cases in which life or limb is in jeopardy, the patient may be taken directly to the operating room for arterial exploration and arteriogram, if necessary. In cases of major arterial injury, an arteriogram done after arterial repair checks patency and determines if there is a second lesion distal to the first. The major complications of arteriography are allergic sensitivity to the contrast material and local complications and discomfort of arterial puncture. With the advent of computerized intravenous tomography, the complications of arterial puncture will be diminished.[186]

The high amputation rate of extremities in patients with major arterial injuries in World War II, when these injuries were treated by ligation,[47] was improved upon during the Korean War by reparative surgery.[90] Earlier treatment made possible by

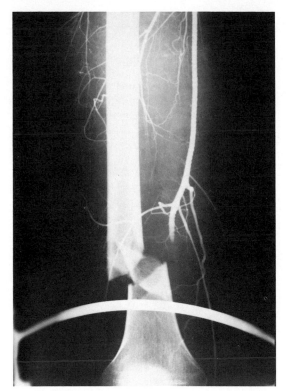

Figure 30-2 Fracture of shaft of femur complicated by laceration of the femoral artery. The arteriogram shows a complete interruption of arterial flow at the level of the fracture. (Courtesy of Dr. James Stokes.)

decreased evacuation time to a definitive treatment center and by continued efforts directed at repair or reconstruction of the arterial injury and major venous injuries, especially those of the popliteal vein, increased the yield of viable extremities even further.[65, 147] Adequate fasciotomies should be done along with arterial and venous repair and reconstruction.

Combat injuries are generally open and contaminated with extensive blast injury and soft tissue destruction. The use of internal fixation for fracture stabilization along with arterial repair was associated with a high incidence of infection, often requiring removal of the fixation. For war wounds and severe or contaminated civilian wounds with open fractures and major arterial injuries, skeletal traction[148] or external fixators provide the best method of fracture stabilization.

Civilian vascular trauma for non-penetrating injury may be due to entrap-

ment, internal traction, torsion, or laceration from bone fragments. For these closed fractures and for selected open civilian fractures in which tissue trauma and contamination are eliminated, skeletal traction or external fixators are satisfactory methods of handling the fracture,[38] but timely internal fixation has worked very well, too.[37, 52, 122, 172] In addition, internal fixation provides the added benefit of definitive fracture treatment that will allow early mobilization of the patient from the bed as well as early joint and muscle rehabilitation.

Fasciotomy should be done in conjunction with major vascular repairs or reconstruction.[38, 133] Four-compartment fasciotomies of the leg may be performed by double incision fasciotomy technique,[47, 50, 126] parafibular release,[113] or fibulectomy.[62, 63, 97] Alternative methods to fibulectomy should be chosen in instances in which there is an associated tibial fracture, because fibulectomy makes the management of a coexisting tibial fracture extremely difficult.

The advent of microsurgery has improved the yield of repairs and reconstructions of peripheral artery injuries distal to the elbow and knee. While arteries distal to the brachial and popliteal arteries may or may not be associated with a limb-threatening situation, their repair provides better extremity perfusion and decreases late complications such as cold intolerance.

Compartment Syndromes and Volkmann's Ischemic Contracture

A compartment syndrome occurs when increased pressure within a closed space compromises the circulation and tissue function within that space. Muscles and nerves are particularly vulnerable. This situation is an imperfect application of Pascal's principle to a biologic system.* Fractures and dislocations about the elbow and distal portion in the upper extremity and about the knee and distal portion in the lower extremity are particularly likely to develop a compartment syndrome. The in-

---

*Pascal's principle states that pressure applied to an enclosed fluid is transmitted undiminished to every portion of the fluid and to the walls of the containing vessel.

creased volume within the non-compliant compartments of the forearm and leg occurs from bleeding from fracture fragments, muscular, venous, or arterial bleeding, and from edema secondary to soft tissue trauma. Later, postischemic edema can add to the volume. Compartment syndromes have also been reported with tight external dressings, including plaster,[13] skin,[69, 133] and epimysium.[55] Volkmann's ischemic contracture was initially described by Richard von Volkmann in 1881. All compartment syndromes can progress to Volkmann's ischemic contracture of the muscles as well as cause fibrosis of the nerves contained within the compartment.

In 1940, Griffiths[76] described the 4 P's associated with Volkmann's ischemic contracture: *pain, *pallor, *pulselessness, and *paralysis. These signs and symptoms are unreliable. Pain, in itself, is expected in any traumatized extremity, varies in degree, and is difficult to quantitate and evaluate. Moreover, anesthesia, a late finding in ischemia, may be misinterpreted and lead to dire consequences. Since most compartment syndromes occur between 30 and 60 mm. Hg and the normal systolic arterial pressure is 120 mm. Hg, pallor and pulselessness usually never occur in compartment syndromes, particularly if the radial artery, which is extracompartmental, is the artery that is monitored. Paralysis is a late finding and may occur after irreversible neuromuscular damage. We should revise Griffiths' 4 P's to a new 8 P's: *Pain on passive stretch of the fingers or toes, decreased two-*point sensory appreciation, increased *pressure in the involved portion of the extremity with swelling and tenseness, flexed *posture of the fingers or toes in the involved extremity, *pulses present, *pink color, *paresthesias, an early finding that may be fleeting, and *paresis.

Clinical signs of compartment syndromes may be confusing, particularly to the novice. There are accurate methods for measuring interstitial tissue pressure to aid in diagnosis and decision making.[112, 125, 195] Neuromuscular deficits are related to both the magnitude and the duration of tissue pressure elevation.[82, 154, 173] Myoglobinuria and acute renal failure can occur in more extreme cases.

The frequency and severity of complications are inversely related to the promptness of decompression. The prime indications for surgical decompression are clinical signs and symptoms of a compartment syndrome or patients with ambiguous or equivocal clinical signs and an interstitial fluid pressure of 30 mm. Hg or above. The technique of fasciotomy is similar to that described for major arterial injuries. Tissue pressures can be used to monitor adequacy of incisions; in addition, tissue pressures are most helpful in distinguishing a neuropraxia from a compartment syndrome when the diagnosis is in doubt, as well as in making objective determinations for operation, particularly in uncooperative or comatose patients. Tissue pressures are also helpful if, later, one wishes to close the wound by delayed primary closure and to be able to check that a compartment syndrome is not being recreated. It is usually safer to close these incisions by skin graft if coverage is necessary. When a compartment syndrome occurs in a patient in traction or with an external fixator, these devices should be released as an initial effort in overcoming the problem. The affected limb should *not* be elevated in patients with suspected or established compartment syndromes, particularly if they are in shock.

Injury to Major Peripheral Nerves

Nerves, like arteries, are more vulnerable to injury from fractures when they are in close proximity to bone and from dislocations in areas where they are tethered to or adjacent to joints. A careful motor and sensory neurologic examination should be carried out and recorded in every injured extremity prior to any treatment. This examination should be repeated after reduction of the fracture or dislocation. The presence of a nerve deficit following reduction that was not present prior to reduction is reason for immediate exploration of the involved nerve. If such an exploration is performed, the fracture should be stabilized with internal or external fixation whether or not the nerve is in continuity or requires repair.

Radial nerve paralysis occurs in about 11 per cent of fractures of the humerus.[7] When these fractures are in the middle one-third of the humerus, the radial nerve is protected by the deep head of the triceps. Spontaneous recovery in 3 or 4 months or less is the rule in this circumstance. When the fracture is at the junction of the middle and distal thirds of the humerus and has a sharp lateral spike on the distal fragment, the radial nerve is particularly susceptible to injury because it is located directly on the "bare spot" of the humerus.[87] These fractures should be fixed and the nerve explored at the time of admission.

Ulnar nerve injury occurs most frequently in cases of elbow dislocation, usually in association with fracture of the medial condyle.[40, 105] Median nerve injury is less frequent.[110] Both median and ulnar nerve injuries about the elbow heal spontaneously and seldom require operative intervention. The posterior interosseous nerve may be injured in a dislocation of the radial head.

The incidence of axillary nerve injury in anterior dislocation of the shoulder is about 30 per cent. The injury is more frequent with increasing age, is frequently overlooked, and almost always resolves spontaneously.[10, 24]

The sciatic nerve or its peroneal component is injured in roughly 10 per cent of posterior hip dislocations or fracture dislocations. Spontaneous functional recovery occurs in 60 to 80 per cent of the cases.[91, 168, 178, 184] Thomas splints should not be used in these injuries nor should the knee be extended on a flexed hip.

Nerve injuries occur in 25 to 35 per cent of knee dislocations, often in association with arterial injuries. Common peroneal nerve palsy should be suspected in any varus injury to the knee when there is damage to the lateral ligaments and capsular structures, in fractures of the proximal fibula, and in dislocation of the proximal tibiofibular joint, particularly posterior dislocations. Unlike arterial injuries, peripheral nerve injuries associated with fractures and dislocations usually do not demand prompt corrective measures. A majority of these nerve injuries are only contusion neuropraxias, and approximately 85 per cent of the nerve injuries associated with fractures of shafts of long bones recover spontaneously within 4 months.[129] Nerve injuries caused by a dislocation or fracture dislocation are often stretch or traction injuries to a nerve tethered across a joint. These stretch or traction injuries are less likely to have a spontaneous return of function than those nerve injuries associated with a shaft fracture. Recovery of function of a contused nerve may be rapid, but it may be slow if the neurons have been killed and have undergone peripheral degeneration. In cases in which the nerve is in continuity and the neurons distal to the injury have undergone peripheral degeneration, regeneration of the nerve occurs from proximal to distal at a rate of about 1 mm./day. An estimate of the approximate time of recovery can thereby be made by measuring the distance from the site of injury to the level of the first muscle innervated distal to the injury. An electromyogram will detect signs of muscle recovery from nerve injury at least 2 weeks before there are any clinical signs.

Early exploration of the nerve is indicated only in unusual situations. Occasionally the presence of a major peripheral nerve injury in association with a fracture may balance the scales in favor of open reduction and internal fixation of the fragments, even though other methods might give adequate reduction. Open reduction of the fracture permits exposure of the injured nerve trunk, its release from the fracture site, and an accurate appraisal of the injury. Radial nerve injuries at the junction of the middle and distal thirds of the humerus with a sharp lateral spike on the distal fragment should be explored early and repaired if severed. If internal fixation is used to treat a fracture, an associated nerve injury can be explored and treated at the same time. Otherwise, if a nerve has been severed (a relatively rare complication of a fracture), end-to-end nerve suture should be performed after healing of the fracture. Intrafascicular nerve grafting[119] may be done, in preference to end-to-end suture under undue tension and in instances of segmental nerve loss. Nerve deficits that have shown no sign of return should be explored within 6 months, since the chances for successful nerve suture or grafting decline after that time. In cases of neuroma in continuity caused by stretch injuries, acceptance of incomplete spontaneous recovery is preferable to attempts at excision of the damaged nerve and repair. But, if at 4 or more

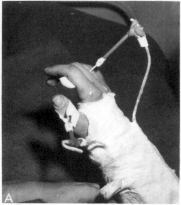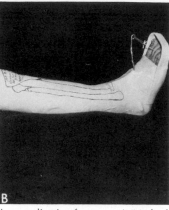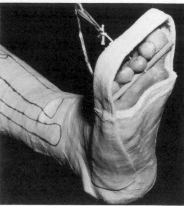

Figure 30–3 Peripheral nerve paralysis complicating fractures. *A,* Method of supporting paralyzed digits in a patient with radial nerve paralysis complicating a fracture of the shaft of the humerus. The elastic supports which hold the thumb and the proximal phalanges of the fingers in extension permit active flexion of all digital joints, thereby minimizing permanent loss of motion. *B,* Method of supporting toes in neutral position in a patient with a peroneal paralysis complicating a fracture of the proximal portion of the fibula. The cast supports the foot at a right angle. This type of support for the toes avoids a fixed plantar contracture and permits active exercise of the digits. (From Hampton, O. P., Jr.: Wounds of Extremities in Military Surgery. St. Louis, C. V. Mosby Company, 1951.)

months after injury there is no sign of spontaneous nerve recovery, the nerve may be explored. If a neuroma in continuity is then found, function will recover in 90 per cent of cases, provided an evoked action potential can be recorded across the neuroma. If no evoked action potential can be recorded across the neuroma in continuity, it should be resected and interfascicular nerve grafting performed.[99]

By appropriate splinting, deformity from unopposed contracture of unparalyzed muscles should be prevented, but the splinting should permit active and passive exercise of the involved joints to avoid permanent restriction of motion (Fig. 30–3). Usually, the splinting is merely supplementary to that of the fracture. Splinting is often omitted if a tendency toward contracture is not present. In complete high median or ulnar nerve injuries or a combination of the two, intrinsic muscle return is infrequent and long delayed in those instances when it does occur. The use of early tendon transfers as internal splints is instrumental in restoring hand function and avoids the complication of a stiff useless hand.[29]

Injuries to the Spinal Cord

Fractures and fracture dislocations of the spine may be complicated by injury to the underlying spinal cord, which multiplies the seriousness of the injury a hundredfold. Fracture dislocations of the cervical and upper dorsal spine are more commonly associated with spinal cord damage.

In the presence of a known or even a possible bone injury to the spine, an immediate careful neurologic examination is mandatory to determine the function of the spinal cord before the patient is moved. All patients with suspected fractures of the spine deserve careful handling; those with evidence of damage to the cord demand it. Motion in all directions in the injured segment of the spine is to be avoided. Patients should have a spine board and straps applied at the scene of the accident and should be transported to and within the hospital on this spine board, until the degree of injury is determined. If an unstable spinal fracture is present, the patient should not be moved from the spine board until an alternative method of stabilization has been established. The spine board may then be slid from beneath the patient with a minimum of motion at the injured spinal segment. The straps used with the spine board permit the entire spine, including the cervical portion, to be immobilized even if the board is turned onto its side, as may be necessary to prevent the patient from aspirating secretions or vomitus. The board is radiolucent and, therefore, adequate roentgenograms can be obtained with the patient strapped to it. If in-hospital transportation on a spine board is not provided, a stretcher used for transportation should have only minimal padding. Several people should aid in lifting or turning the patient so as to avoid all motion of the spine.

Any patient with a head injury or multiple trauma should have cervical spine roentgenograms.[45] The lower cervical spine must be visualized. Many diagnoses are missed for a lack of adequate visualization. If this cannot be done by pulling the shoulders down, a swimmer's view may be helpful. If conventional views or a swimmer's view does not adequately visualize the spine, tomograms must be obtained.

Quadriplegia, when it occurs, causes a generalized sympathectomy of the trunk and lower extremities for up to 24 to 48 hrs. This causes the syndrome of spinal shock, in which the blood pressure may drop to approximately 90 mm. Hg systolic and 50 mm. diastolic. This should not be confused with hemorrhagic shock and is distinguished from it by knowledge of the lesion and a pulse that is within normal limits.

It is extremely important to distinguish a complete from an incomplete lesion of the spinal cord. Careful motor and sensory examinations are mandatory but, again, the rectal examination is critical to verify the impressions gained by the sensory and motor examinations. If the patient cannot feel a pin prick on the anal skin or the gloved finger in the rectum, there is a complete sensory lesion. If there is no reflex or voluntary rectal sphincter contracture about the gloved finger and there is no voluntary motor power below the upper extremities, complete motor paralysis is present. If the bulbocavernosus reflex is not present and does not return after the resolution of spinal shock in 24 to 48 hours after injury, the diagnosis of a complete lesion is confirmed.

A complete spinal cord lesion lasting 48 hours or more carries a hopeless prognosis. On the other hand, a patient with a partial spinal cord lesion who shows early and rapid spontaneous recovery has a good prognosis. In general, laminectomy for decompression is contraindicated unless there is a progressive neurologic deficit, because laminectomy is a relatively ineffective method for decompression and often causes or increases spinal instability. In addition to spinal instability, complications associated with the early care of the quadriplegic include respiratory insufficiency with atelectasis and pneumonia, pressure ulceration of the skin over bony prominences, gastrointestinal bleeding from hemorrhagic gastritis, urinary retention with bladder distention and calculus formation, contractural deformities of joints, skeletal osteoporosis, and psychological withdrawal.

Displaced spinal fracture dislocations with spinal cord injury should be reduced and stabilized no later than 12 hours after injury if at all possible. Early reduction is the best method of decompression of the spinal cord.[11] Stability of the cervical spine in the cord-injured patient should be by means of a halo and jacket or by internal fixation and arthrodesis. This is particularly important in the quadriplegic, who can breathe only with his diaphragm and has a markedly compromised vital capacity, often only 25 per cent of normal. The thoracolumbar spine is best stabilized by open reduction, internal fixation, and arthrodesis. Stabilization of the spine in all cord-injured patients avoids further cord injury and improves pulmonary function, rehabilitation, mental outlook, and skin care. The incidence of thrombophlebitis and pulmonary embolism is decreased, and the possibility of the late complications of pain and deformity due to progressive gibbus is also diminished.

In the spinal cord–injured patient with long bone fracture, early stabilization with internal fixation or external fixators is important for the same reasons as achieving early spinal stability.

High velocity missile wounds to the spinal cord must be debrided, but low velocity gunshot wounds need not be debrided as a matter of routine unless they involve the esophagus or colon.[11]

Burns, Fractures, and Dislocations

When burns and fractures or dislocations co-exist in the same extremity, one complicates the care of the other. Plaster casts do not allow burn care in cases of major burns and should be avoided in these patients. Although internal fixation has been used successfully in burn patients provided operation is performed within the first 24 hours, the incision is made through unburned skin and the wound is left open.[187] All burns are contaminated, and open reduction and internal fixation should generally be avoided because of the risk of infection. While open reduction and internal fixation of fractures in the minimally burned extremity and minimally burned patient may have a place in treatment, the exact role of open reduction and internal fixation in burn patients has not been definitively established. In patients with a seriously burned extremity or with serious generalized burns, bacteremia and septicemia are late complications and put hematomas associated with fractures and fractures treated with metallic implants at grave risk of infection. Therefore, skeletal traction or external fixators, which are indeed a form of portable traction, are preferred for stabilizing fractures associated with burns whenever possible, as these methods of treatment provide fracture stability while allowing access to the burns. In the case of external fixators mobility of the patient for Hubbard tank treatments and accessibility for range of motion exercises to prevent joint contractures are provided, pulmonary function is improved, and morale of the patient is improved.[94, 142] Joints may also be splinted in functional positions between therapy sessions as a measure to prevent contractions. The threaded pins of external fixators and skeletal traction have a very low infection rate, provided there is good daily pin care.[142] It may be prudent to reconstruct a delayed union, a non-union, or a malunion rather than risk infection to the bone by early internal fixation. If internal fixation is used, intravenous antibiotic coverage for both gram-negative and gram-positive organisms should be used along with minimal osteosynthesis.[187]

DELAYED COMPLICATIONS

Fat Embolism Syndrome

The role of post-traumatic fat embolism or lipidemia is not clear but is associated with fat embolism syndrome and may be the major component or a contributing factor to this post-traumatic respiratory distress syndrome. Post-traumatic lipidemia is common after severe or multiple trauma with one or more fractures, multiple fractures, and even isolated fractures, particularly those of the pelvis, hip, and long bones of the lower extremities. About 70 per cent of patients with isolated skeletal injuries will have inapparent hypoxemia, i.e., an arterial oxygen pressure of 70 to 80 mm. Hg but no clinical signs or symptoms of respiratory distress in the first 36 hours after injury.[200] About 25 per cent will develop severe hypoxemia, an arterial oxygen pressure of 60 to 70 mm. Hg, but no clinical signs or symptoms of respiratory distress in the first 36 hours. These patients are at risk for fat embolism syndrome. Two per cent develop respiratory distress, that is, an arterial oxygen pressure of less than 60 mm. Hg, a carbon dioxide retention in the peripheral arteries of 50 mm. Hg or more, and clinical findings of pulmonary distress within the first 36 hours after injury.[200] 85 per cent of patients who develop fat embolism syndrome do so within the first 48 hours after injury.[170] The clinical signs of fat embolism syndrome are fever, tachycardia, tachypnea, and progressive cerebral changes of restlessness, disorientation, confusion, stupor, and coma. Long tract signs may occur with progressive cerebral involvement. There may be an early, so-called "lucid interval." Petechiae clinch the diagnosis and may be fleeting. They are characteristically found on the chest, trunk, root of the neck, axillae, and conjunctivae. Free fat may be found in the blood, urine, and eyegrounds. While these findings may raise the suspicion of fat embolism syndrome, they are not diagnostic and neither are the anemia, thrombocytopenia, hyperbilirubinemia, or electrocardiographic changes often found in association with fat embolism syndrome. The chest x-ray may demonstrate changes of pulmonary edema when this is present but is otherwise non-specific. "Snowstorm cloudiness" of the lung field on x-ray reflects a well-established syndrome and is a sign of a poor prognosis. Serum lipase is demonstrated rather late, 3 to 6 days from onset, and is of little diagnostic significance at that time. The critical laboratory finding that identifies both the syndrome and its severity is the arterial blood oxygen concentration.

Mortality varies and is probably minimized by early recognition and aggressive treatment, since fat embolism syndrome is self-limited and responsive to treatment. Patients in whom diagnosis or treatment is delayed are at risk of death or permanent neurologic deficit from brain injury, including mental retardation. While once thought to be largely a form of adult acute respiratory distress syndrome, this entity definitely occurs in children and is probably underestimated in incidence and less easily recognized than in the adult. This has led to high mortality and morbidity.[194]

The changes in the lung parenchyma are simple mechanical blocking of capillaries by fat droplets and interstitial hemorrhagic pneumonitis. This leads to impaired alveolo-capillary diffusion and decreased lung compliance, respectively. Surfactant activity is decreased, and there is shunting, which may be determined by alveolar arteriolar blood gas comparisons. A self-perpetuating hypoxic spiral is established and can lead to multiple organ system involvement, particularly pulmonary failure, and death can occur unless there is intervention.[72, 127]

The best treatment of fat embolism syndrome is prevention. In lieu of prevention, suspicion of the entity with early identification and treatment will produce a favorable outcome in most if not all instances. Splinting of all fractures should be performed at the scene of the accident for transportation to and within the hospital. Gentle handling should be provided for all patients with skeletal injuries. Blood volume should be replaced early and adequately to prevent the effects of shock synergistic with fat embolism syndrome and to keep the oxygen-carrying capacity of the blood high. Arterial blood gases should be drawn upon arrival in the emergency room for baseline values in all patients at risk for fat embolism syndrome and should be continuously monitored in accordance with the patient's condition. Arterial blood gas determinations every 24 hours for the first 72 hours after injury are appropriate. If there is no trend toward hypoxia and if there are no clinical signs of respiratory distress or cerebral compromise, blood gas monitoring may be discontinued at that point. The most important differential diagnoses are direct intracranial or intrapulmonary trauma. Arterial oxygen concentrations should not be lowered by intracranial trauma alone. It may be important to rule out delirium tremens and a past history of alcoholism may be helpful in this regard. It is important to remember that fat embolism syndrome can co-exist with and compound any of these other conditions.

Peltier[139] has demonstrated that the use of tourniquets during operations on bones decreases the incidence of traumatic lipidemia and fat embolism in the brain, lungs, blood, and kidneys.

Oxygen should be given routinely to trauma patients by nasal cannula or mask, provided the arterial oxygen remains above 70 mm. Hg. Failure of the patient to maintain the arterial oxygen above 70 mm. Hg, progressive hypoxia with clinical manifestations of pulmonary distress or with change in the level of consciousness, or an arterial blood oxygen below 50 mm. Hg for any reason requires sedation, usually with Valium, endotracheal intubation, and mechanical assistance of ventilation with a volume-cycled respirator. A cascade-type humidifier and side-arm nebulizer are preferred to an in-line ultrasonic nebulizer to avoid risk of bacterial contamination.[145] Because oxygen toxicity is both concentration- and time-related, inspired oxygen concentration whenever possible should be maintained at the lowest levels consistent with the delivery of adequate tissue oxygen, 85 to 95 per cent saturation of arterial oxygen. Positive end-expiratory pressure up to 10 cm. H_2O may be used to overcome decreased lung compliance. If continued ventilation is still necessary at 4 days or so, a tracheostomy is often done to prevent tracheal necrosis and permanent vocal cord damage by the endotracheal tube. Diuresis with Lasix (furosemide) or Edecrin (ethacrynic acid) in a dosage of 20 to 25 mg./kg./24 hr. is used along with fluid restriction, to minimize interstitial fluid accumulation in the lungs and pulmonary edema. Sodium is also restricted for the same reasons. In patients at risk for or with established respiratory distress syndrome, the central venous catheter should be replaced with a Swan-Ganz pulmonary artery catheter to monitor both pressure and mixed central venous oxygen tension. An increase in pulmonary artery pressure indicates impending pulmonary insufficiency, while an increase in capillary wedge pressure indicates left-sided heart failure and the need for cardiotonic drugs.

Steroids such as Solu-Medrol (methyl-prednisolone succinate) should be given in divided doses of 30 mg./kg./24 hr. The use of heparin and low molecular weight dextran is controversial and not well established. There is increasing evidence that early fixation of long bone fractures, particularly those of the femur, which allows the patient to assume a vertical posture, may reduce the incidence of fat embolism syndrome or complement its treatment and avoid prolonged cardiopulmonary failure that leads to death.[150]

Thromboembolic Disease

There is an increased incidence of thromboembolic disease in all traumatic fractures of the spine, pelvis, and lower extremities, particularly in hip fractures.[6, 34, 121, 171] Patients with these injuries who are treated with preventive anticoagulants have a significantly decreased incidence of thromboembolic complications.[34] The problem of selecting specific patients for anticoagulation is that both deep vein thrombosis and pulmonary embolism are often silent.[177, 199] In addition, two-thirds of fatal pulmonary embolisms are fatal within 30 minutes. Patients under 20 years of age are at low risk and need no prophylaxis against thromboembolic disease unless they have a malignancy or a prior history of thromboembolic disease. High-risk and very high-risk patients with the above fractures should be considered for preventive anticoagulation therapy after fracture bleeding has been controlled, unless there are specific contraindications. The high-risk profile includes one or more of the following: age over 40 years, increased extent and duration of surgery, increased degree and length of immobilization, increased severity of underlying systemic disease, obesity, multiple injuries, multiple operations, diabetes, cardiovascular or pulmonary disease, prior thromboembolic disease, prior venous surgery in the lower extremities, malignancy, women on contraceptive estrogens, and paraplegics.[175, 185] The very high-risk profile includes one or more of the following: age over 60 years, prior thromboembolic dis-

ease, prior lower extremity venous surgery, or venous insufficiency. The type of preventive anticoagulation is controversial.[6, 36, 68, 79, 107, 155, 171, 188] Preventive anticoagulation does not seem to prevent deep venous thrombosis or pulmonary embolism in patients with fractures, but it does seem to prevent mortality when pulmonary embolism occurs. The concern about thromboembolic problems should be tempered with the problems related to their treatment, specifically, increased incidence of hematoma and subsequent increased infection as well as delayed fracture healing.[86, 179, 180, 182, 198] Important to treatment are early rigid fracture stabilization and early mobilization of the patient, including use of the tilt table, Buerger-Allen exercises, and active and passive leg muscle exercises, along with decreased blood loss at surgery, good hemostasis, good postoperative wound drainage, decreased operative time, compression dressings, anti-embolic stockings, elevation, and monitoring for deep vein thrombosis.[52] Non-invasive methods of evaluating deep vein thrombosis include labeled I[121] fibrinogen uptake test, cuff impedance phlebography, pneumatic plethysmography, and Doppler ultrasound. Venography is an invasive test but is more accurate than non-invasive methods. An intraluminal filling defect is diagnostic. Patients with deep vein thrombosis or pulmonary embolism should be fully anticoagulated unless there are specific contraindications.

Post-Traumatic Reflex Sympathetic Dystrophy

Reflex sympathetic dystrophies encompass a wide spectrum of vasomotor and trophic conditions of uncertain origin that are poorly understood. They may follow trauma, infection, or thrombophlebitis. Fractures and dislocations are among the injuries to the extremities that may be complicated by a reflex sympathetic dystrophy. In spite of the fact that many of these injuries seem quite innocuous, they may be followed by this rather bizarre phenomenon.

Although it is far from entirely clear, the pathophysiology of reflex sympathetic dystrophies seems to include a painful lesion leading to continued irritation of peripheral sensory nerve fibers, a susceptible patient, who may be emotionally unstable and who has a low pain threshold and may overreact to pain, and an abnormal autonomic reflex.[51, 54, 103, 106] It has been postulated but not proven that this reflex occurs through the internuncial cells at the spinal cord level.[106] As early as 1902, Sudek[181] noted that changes did not occur if the reflex arc was broken, as occurs in such diseases as syringomyelia and poliomyelitis.

Reflex sympathetic dystrophies are divided into five clinical forms of increasing severity: minor causalgia, minor traumatic dystrophy, shoulder-hand syndrome, major traumatic dystrophy, and major causalgia.[103] Trauma to a purely sensory nerve causes a minor causalgia. Minor non-nerve trauma causes a minor traumatic dystrophy and includes the majority of cases of reflex sympathetic dystrophies. Shoulder-hand syndrome is a distinct entity that tends to occur in the older age group and often after visceral dysfunction, i.e., cerebral vascular or coronary occlusion, but it can also occur after fractures or dislocations, particularly those about the neck and shoulder.[176] The more severe types of non-nerve trauma that produce a more severe reflex sympathetic dystrophy are called major traumatic dystrophies. Reflex sympathetic dystrophy caused by a major mixed-nerve injury was first described by Mitchell[120] in the Civil War and should be classified as a major causalgia. Major causalgia is usually, if not always, the result of a partial nerve lesion.

Reflex sympathetic dystrophies go through three stages characterized by pain, tenderness, and hyperesthesias. These dystrophies involve the foot and ankle or the hand and wrist and, if the site of the injury is higher in the extremity, they usually extend up to that level. The first or early stage is characterized by a soft puffy edema, redness, heat and constant burning, aching, and cutting or searing pain that is out of proportion to the severity of the injury. One of the earliest signs in the hand is redness over the metacarpophalangeal joints and proximal interphalangeal joints. There is hyperesthesia, and fixed contractures are usually absent. This stage lasts for about 3 months. At the end of 3 to 4 weeks there may be spotty demineralization of the bones on x-ray. At 6 to 8 weeks this may progress to generalized or polar osteopenia. Hyperhydrosis is seen late in this stage. During this stage the pain causes extreme guarding of the involved extremity by the patient and may be intensely aggravated by environmental stimuli including movement, vibration, examination, dependency, heights, touching dry objects, noise, excitement, emotional upset, laughter, peculiar noises, hearing or using certain words, or deep breathing. The patient may be reluctant to move the injured part even in physical or occupational therapy.

In the second or dystrophic stage, the edema becomes fixed, the swelling becomes fusiform in the digits, and the skin becomes brawny and even cyanotic and in some instances, cold, tight, and shiny. Hyperhydrosis persists well into the second stage. There may be hyperemia in the flexor creases later. Flexor and extensor wrinkles are lost. Palmar fasciitis with tender erythematous nodules occurs especially in women. These nodules should never be excised but may respond to steroids. Range of motion decreases and joints may become fixed. Subcutaneous atrophy, especially in the fat pads of the digits, causes tapering of the digits. The x-ray shows generalized osteopenia. This stage lasts 3 to 6 months.

The third stage may last indefinitely. The skin and muscles atrophy. The extremity is pale, cool, and dry, and the skin is thin, tight, and glossy. Swelling decreases but joints stiffen. The neuralgia spreads and may involve the whole limb; and while it may decrease in some instances, in others it becomes intractable. Homogeneous osteopenia persists on x-ray.

Prophylactic measures include early and precise reduction of a fracture; avoiding edema, both dependent and that due to constricting bandages; splints; casts; immobilization of joints in functional positions and early active exercise of all unimmobilized joints and musculature of the extremity. Early functional treatment using plaster,[49] such as walking casts, or early internal or external fixation[85, 124] may be of considerable benefit in preventing post-traumatic reflex sympathetic dystrophy. The key to treating reflex sympathetic dystrophy is early recognition. Reflex sympathetic dystrophy should be suspected when pain, swelling, and stiffness are out of proportion to the severity of the injury and when there are color, temperature, or pseudomotor changes, atrophy, and osteopenia. Although the etiology remains an enigma, it is well-established that the condition is a result of sympathetic overactivity and therapy must be directed at the sympathetic nervous system. One or a series of sympathetic blocks with Marcaine, usually one a day for 3 or 4 days, may be both diagnostic and therapeutic. In about half the cases, this will be curative. If blocks give temporary relief, but this improvement is only transient, sympathectomy should be performed. The sympathectomy must be extensive enough to achieve a warm, flushed, and dry foot or hand, the presence of which should be confirmed before the operation is discontinued. While a Horner's syndrome is helpful in evaluating the adequacy of a chemical sympathetic block, surgical sympathectomy should be performed through a transthoracic approach and should be done sufficiently low enough to prevent the complication of a permanent Horner's syndrome. Surgery should be reserved as a last resort and used only when it is certain that the condition is not going to resolve without it.

Adjunctive therapy in the form of patient support and encouragement; elevation of the involved extremity; heat; gentle, progressive, active range of motion exercises within the patient's pain tolerance; nerve blocks; corticosteroids; vasodilators; intra-arterial reserpine; beta blockers; central acting drugs; psychological or psychiatric guidance, such as is given in a pain clinic; and transcutaneous nerve stimulators have been of some help.

If there is a specific operable lesion causing the reflex sympathetic dystrophy, this should be corrected. Otherwise, elective surgery should not be done until the dystrophy is resolved.

Avascular Necrosis of Bone

Post-traumatic avascular necrosis of bone occurs at the time of fracture, dislocation, or a combination of the two when a region of the bone or one or more fragments become isolated from their blood supply and undergo subsequent osteonecrosis. Those areas of bone predisposed to post-traumatic avascular necrosis have in common a precarious blood supply which, in order for this complication to occur, is either disrupted or blocked. The incidence of post-traumatic avascular necrosis is related to the severity of the injury and consequently to the amount of displacement and disruption of both the hard and soft tissues. Although osteocytes have been observed to remain alive in devascularized femoral heads for as long as 15 days,[35] most observers believe that the destiny of the bone in question is determined in a matter of hours after the injury.[12, 18, 35] It is possible in those instances in which interruption of the blood supply is by blockage rather than disruption that early reduction and stabilization may be of benefit[18] and therefore should be performed.

Post-traumatic avascular necrosis is most frequently observed in the femoral head, scaphoid, lunate, talus, patella, and humeral head (Fig. 30–4). It occurs in the femoral head after epiphyseal fractures in children and after intracapsular fractures in older adults. It also occurs in dislocations and fracture dislocations of the hip, more so in adults than in children. Post-traumatic osteonecrosis of the femoral head is particularly devastating in femoral neck fractures in children, especially over the age of 10,[31] and also in young adults between the ages of 20 and 40.[141]

The more proximal the scaphoid fracture, the more likely that the proximal fragment will undergo avascular necrosis. The lunate, too, may undergo osteonecrosis in cases of dislocation or dissociation in which its blood supply is interrupted. The body of the talus may undergo avascular necrosis in fractures of the neck of the talus, especially if there is displacement of the fracture. If there is dislocation of the body of the talus in addition to a displaced fracture of its neck, the incidence of avascular necrosis approaches 100 per cent. In fractures of the patella, the proximal pole often undergoes avascular necrosis.[165] In four-part fractures of the humeral head, avascular necrosis of the humeral head consistently occurs.[128]

In the femoral head, avascular necrosis may be apparent within a few months of injury or, peculiarly, may not appear for a few years. In fractures of the scaphoid,

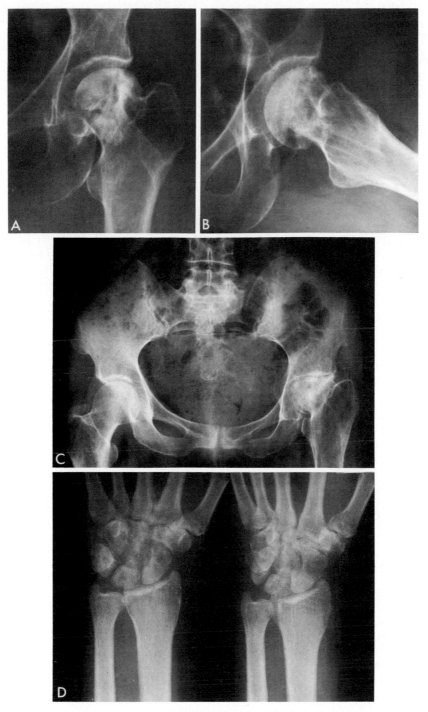

Figure 30–4 Avascular necrosis of bone complicating fractures. *A* and *B,* Anteroposterior and lateral roentgenograms of hip showing avascular necrosis of femoral head, but with union of the fracture. Note relatively increased density of the head of the femur and separation of triangular-shaped fragment of head. *C,* Anteroposterior view of the pelvis showing avascular necrosis of the femoral head with deformity secondary to fracture of the neck of femur which united. *D,* Anteroposterior and oblique views of wrist showing avascular necrosis of proximal fragment of united fracture of carpal navicular.

lunate, talus, patella, and humeral head, avascular necrosis may be diagnosed before union of these fractures and is seldom a very late complication. Avascular necrosis of bone is recognized on roentgenograms by a relative increase in density of the avascular area in comparison with a well-vascularized area of bone (Fig. 30–4). The possibility of avascular necrosis developing in the situation outlined previously should be anticipated. The comparative density of the fragments should be studied on serial roentgenograms in order that the condition may be detected as early as possible. The use of radioactive isotope scanning techniques, venography, arteriography, intra-osseous oximetry, and biopsy may be useful in confirming suspected cases, particularly if the diagnosis is not yet apparent on x-ray in a patient whose symptoms suggest the possibility of avascular necrosis.

Often fractures will unite while the avascular necrosis of one or more fragments is becoming apparent. Avascular necrosis does, however, predispose to delayed union or non-union, since the healing process depends entirely upon the living fragment. Also of concern is subchondral collapse in the region of the adjacent joint leading to post-traumatic arthrosis. A joint in which avascular necrosis has occurred in one of the bones composing the joint must be protected from compressive forces until revascularization reconstitutes the area involved if this is possible and practical. In patients who have no subchondral collapse, decompression with or without bone grafting may facilitate reconstitution.

Delayed Nerve Paralysis

Delayed nerve paralysis is practically always secondary to faulty treatment. Bandages, straps, splints, or plaster casts applied improperly so that they compress peripheral nerves to the point of paralysis may be the cause of this complication. The peroneal nerve is easily compressed against the neck of the fibula by an improperly molded plaster cast or an improperly placed strap of a Thomas splint. The peroneal nerve also may be compressed against the neck of the fibula when the extremity is rotated against a hard bed for several hours. The sciatic or posterior tibial nerve may be compressed by a tight bandage or strap of a Thomas splint. The ulnar nerve at the elbow may become paralyzed because of an abnormal pressure against the medial condyle of the humerus by a bandage or plaster cast. The radial nerve may be compressed against the shaft of the humerus by a crutch or the top of a long-arm plaster cast. The sciatic or radial nerve may be excessively compressed by improperly designed or improperly applied tourniquets about the thigh or arm. Delayed nerve paralyses must be considered preventable complications.

Preventive measures are of paramount importance. In the application of bandages, splints, or plaster casts, pressure at vulnerable points should be avoided or minimized by distributing pressure over broad areas. With these precautions, a pressure paralysis is unlikely.

Circular bandages about vulnerable points should be applied loosely and with care. They should not be applied to remain under plaster casts and seldom under splints. Subsequent swelling of the part can convert a loose circular bandage into a constricting bandage. Pressure points should be well padded before splints are applied. The straps or slings supporting a lower extremity in a Thomas splint should be well-padded and placed so as to avoid pressure on the neck of the fibula and the overlying peroneal nerve. Padding beneath plaster casts should be applied smoothly and lumps of padding at vulnerable points should be avoided. The plaster should be applied smoothly to avoid point pressure, particularly that of the tips of the fingers of an assistant holding the extremity. Actually, as the plaster is setting, it may be molded in a way that minimizes or eliminates pressure at these points. The top of a short-leg plaster cast should terminate either above or below the neck of the fibula. The extremity in a long-arm plaster cast should not hang unsupported but should be kept in a sling or supported by a loop at the wrist to avoid the pressure of the rim of the cast against the back of the arm where the radial nerve passes.

Later the patient should be questioned about points of pain and the presence of referred pain and sensory distributions. In this way, impending paralysis can be detected and the point pressure relieved by removal, lifting, or adjustment of the offending bandage, splint, or cast.

Tourniquets are valuable and indicated appliances in the operative treatment of many fractures, but they must be used properly. A non-elastic tourniquet or rubber strap must not be used on the arm and is undesirable on the thigh. Pneumatic tourniquets with pressure properly regulated are an adequate safeguard against tourniquet paralysis and should be the only tourniquets used in the operative treatment of fractures. The axillary end of crutches should be properly but not excessively padded. Padding can be so bulky as to cause the pressure it is intended to avoid. The patient should be instructed in the proper use of crutches, i.e., to carry weight on the hands and not the axillae. In these ways "crutch paralysis" of the radial nerve may be avoided.

Definitive treatment of delayed nerve paralysis is merely relief of the offending pressure on the nerve trunk and appropriate splinting to avoid contracture deformities. An operative attack at the point of pressure is not indicated. With a paralyzed peroneal nerve, the foot should be supported at 90 degrees to avoid plantar flexion contracture. With a paralyzed radial nerve, the wrist should be supported in slight dorsiflexion and the thumb in some extension and abduction. Such splinting should not go unattended. It should be removed at times to permit some active exercise of the involved joints. Preferably the splinting is dynamic in that paralyzed muscles are supported by the tension of an elastic material that can be stretched by active contracture of the unparalyzed muscles (see Fig. 30–3).

Delayed nerve paralysis seldom if ever occurs from compression of nerve trunks by the healing callus of a fracture. Functioning nerve trunks have been observed to pass through a tunnel in the callus of a fracture. Bony irregularities at points where nerve trunks must glide as joints are moved, however, will produce a traumatic neuritis and loss of function of a nerve. An example is the ulnar nerve rubbing over an irregularity of the medial humeral condyle after a fracture has healed. Preventive treatment is precise reduction of the fracture to avoid the irregularity. Definitive treatment is excision of the bony irregularity or, in the example just cited, anterior transplantation of the ulnar nerve.

Late or Tardy Nerve Paralysis

A true tardy nerve paralysis after a fracture occurs only at the elbow and in only one situation. The ulnar nerve at the elbow, because of a cubitus valgus deformity, may undergo gradual stretching until the nerve fibers distal to the elbow cease to function. The original injury is a fracture of the lateral condyle of the humerus in childhood. Usually, inadequate reduction was obtained. Subsequent growth of the lower portion of the humerus is restricted on the lateral side but proceeds normally on the medial side. As the cubitus valgus deformity develops, the ulnar nerve is stretched around the medial condyle. With strenuous use of the extremity in adult life, the stretching is increased. Gradually the ulnar nerve ceases to function (Fig. 30–5).

The important treatment is preventive. Fractures of the lateral condyle in children must be held in accurate reduction. To achieve this, open reduction of displaced fractures is frequently indicated. If doubt exists as to the quality of reduction, the operative procedure should be carried out.

After union of a fracture of the lateral condyle has taken place, growth of the elbow should be followed by serial roentgenograms until assurance is gained that growth is proceeding symmetrically. If a cubitus valgus is developing, growth of the medial condyle should be stopped at the appropriate time by epiphyseal arrest or the deformity corrected by osteotomy of the lower end of the humerus.

After the tardy ulnar nerve paralysis has developed, the simplest measure that may be of benefit is forward transplantation of the ulnar nerve at the elbow. If this is carried out early, as the process is developing, it is much more likely to be of benefit than if it is done after all nerve function has been lost.

Malunion

Malunion of a fracture denotes union along with a deformity that results in a significant impairment in function, cosmesis, or both. The deformity may result from

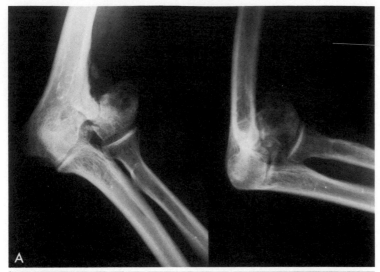

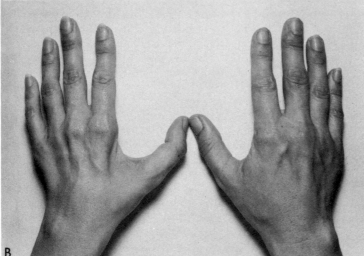

Figure 30–5 Tardy or late ulnar nerve paralysis as a late complication of fracture of lateral condyle of humerus in a child. *A,* Anteroposterior and lateral roentgenograms of ununited fracture of lateral condyle of humerus with valgus at the elbow in a patient 33 years of age. The patient sustained the injury when she was 6 years old. At age 17 she first noticed numbness in the ulnar nerve distribution. Gradually this increased, and she lost power in the intrinsic muscles of the hand supplied by the ulnar nerve. *B,* Photograph of hands of the same patient. Note atrophy of intrinsic muscles of left hand from ulnar nerve paralysis.

displacement, angulation, malrotation, shortening, or lengthening of the bone (Fig. 30–6). Many fractures unite in some degree of deformity without significant effect on function or appearance. Functional treatment of selected fractures in plaster need not have an anatomic reduction to achieve excellent functional and cosmetic results. These are not considered malunions.

In instances of malunion, function may be impaired by alteration of normal joint dynamics. Shifting of the weight-bearing axis of a joint may alter the biomechanics and may lead to uneven weight distribution, uneven wear patterns, joint incongruency, and arthrosis. This may occur in joints adjacent to the site of fracture or even in joints distant from the site of fracture, as in the development of pelvic obliquity, scoliosis, and back pain secondary to leg length inequality due to overriding of fracture fragments and bone shortening or overgrowth of a femoral fracture in a child resulting in bone lengthening.[57, 74, 75, 143]

The degree of actual deformity is not necessarily related to the degree of functional loss. A deformity in the shaft of a long bone has more forgiveness in regard to good function than a deformity near a joint, particularly when the deformity is not in the plane of motion of the joint.[156] Rotation or angulation of a malunited fracture in a lower extremity may interfere with proper balance or gait. A rotational deformity inap-

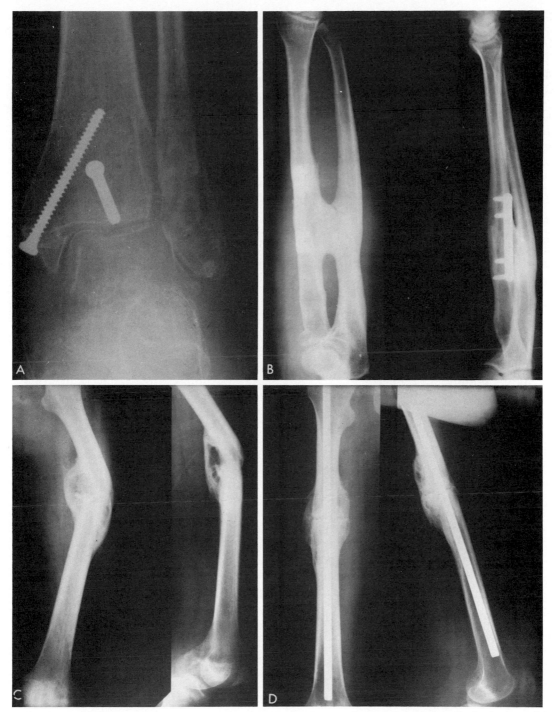

Figure 30–6   Malunion of fractures. *A,* Anteroposterior roentgenogram showing a united bimalleolar fracture of the ankle with fragments and talus displaced laterally in spite of an open reduction. *B,* Synostosis of radius and ulna, a form of malunion, following fracture of both bones of forearm. *C,* Malunion of fracture of femur; note lateral and anterior angulation with resulting functional shortening of nearly 2 inches. *D,* The same femur united in excellent alignment and near-full length after osteotomy, intramedullary nailing, and bone grafting. (Courtesy of Dr. James T. Green.)

parent on roentgenograms may be disabling and even require surgery, for example, a rotational deformity of a metacarpal or phalangeal fracture causing overlapping of the fingers.

Children's fractures are particularly prone to malunion, while deformities of alignment in children under the age of 9 years may be corrected spontaneously with growth, provided the epiphyseal plate is not injured. Those fractures in which the epiphyseal plate is fractured or crushed are particularly predisposed to develop progressive angular deformity, progressive limb length discrepancy, and joint incongruity with resultant post-traumatic arthrosis. Particular care must be taken to achieve anatomic reduction by appropriate closed or open methods with stabilization when necessary in fractures that cross the epiphysis in children. Alterations of growth patterns in fractures and dislocations of children also include avascular necrosis of the epiphysis, crushing or infection of the epiphyseal plate, bony bridge formation at the periphery joining the epiphysis and the metaphysis, non-union, and hyperemia producing local overgrowth.[143] While deformities due to crushing injuries of the epiphyseal plate cannot be prevented, the family of the patient should be advised and the patient carefully monitored so that corrective surgery can be properly timed when it is necessary.

In patients with bony bridge formation between the epiphysis and metaphysis, the bridge may be surgically removed and the defect filled with medical grade Silastic[21] or fat.[102] This should be done as soon as the bridge is discovered and preferably before any deformity has occurred.

Children with proximal tibial metaphyseal fractures tend to develop valgus deformities that may be due to medial overgrowth[42, 131] or inaccurate reduction of the fracture with the knee in a flexed position.[143] These fractures should be treated in long-leg plaster casts with the knee in full extension to avoid malreduction, and they must be carefully monitored. Children with femoral shaft fractures are treated with overlapping of not more than 1 cm., since permanent overgrowth of about 1 cm. due to hyperemia can be anticipated in these fractures, particularly in children under 10 years of age.[57, 74, 75, 143] There must be long-term and short-term monitoring of children's fractures with known potential for malunion because of the fracture configuration.

Malunion may result from treatment failure such as inaccurate reduction or the loss of position due to inadequate immobilization that might have been prevented by more skillful management of the fracture. Often a malunited fracture is a fracture in which displacement or malalignment was not detected or corrected during a critical healing period. A good fracture reduction with adequate stabilization must be achieved and maintained during the critical healing period. Adequate follow-up with serial roentgenograms as well as patient compliance with the treatment plan is essential to achieve this goal.

Malunion can be overcome only by operative intervention. Because such operative procedures carry some risk and the results are not always ideal, the loss of function must be carefully documented and both the patient and the doctor must be certain that the functional impairment is sufficient to justify surgery. Surgery is rarely justified for cosmetic reasons alone. Operations for malunion vary somewhat with the site and type of deformity. Osteotomy is the basic surgical procedure, usually followed by rigid internal fixation of the osteotomized fragments and often accompanied by an autogenous cancellous bone graft. Correction of angulatory and rotational deformities in the shafts of long bones of the lower extremities gives the best results. Attempts to correct malposition of fragments containing portions of articular surfaces are the least likely to lead to satisfactory results. Leg length discrepancy can be corrected by epiphysiodesis in children and by osteotomy and shortening of the uninjured contralateral bone or by leg lengthening following internal fixation by plating and bone grafting.[190] Arthrodesis may be appropriate treatment for painful arthrosis. Surgery should not be performed until an extremity is well rehabilitated and muscle atrophy and disuse osteoporosis are treated.

Delayed Union and Non-Union

Delayed union is prolongation of the healing time of a fracture beyond a theoreti-

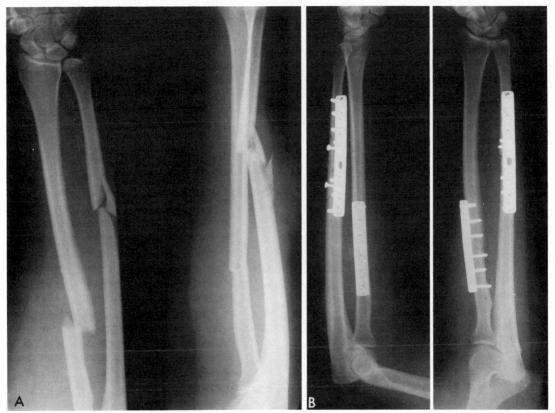

Figure 30–7 Delayed union of fractures. *A,* Delayed union of fracture of both bones of forearm. In this stage only delayed union is present, but non-union is a strong possibility. Prompt operation with bone grafting is indicated not only to increase the chances of union of the fractures but also to improve the apposition and alignment of the fragments. *B,* Apposition and alignment of fragments obtained at operation. Iliac bone grafts about each fracture site are poorly shown.

cal average for the location and configuration of a fracture in a given patient (Fig. 30–7). The term indicates that healing of the fragments is taking place but is progressing more slowly than anticipated. Delayed union is not a distinct clinical or pathologic entity. A diagnosis of delayed union usually indicates only continuation of treatment with the anticipation that bony union will follow. Delayed union may be preliminary to non-union and requires careful clinical and radiographic follow-ups.

Non-union of a fracture is a distinct clinical, pathologic, and radiographic entity (Fig. 30–8). Clinically, there may be tenderness, swelling, erythema, and increased heat at the non-union site. Motion may be present at the fracture site when it is stressed. Pain is often present and is often increased by manual stress testing or by attempts at functional use of the involved extremity. Patients with non-unions of the lower extremities

often walk with an antalgic gait. There may be persistent edema in the involved extremity, with brawny induration and pitting edema of the skin. Often there is muscle atrophy and loss of joint motion or even joint contractures.

Radiographically, the non-union may demonstrate one or more of the following characteristics: a persistent radiolucent fracture line extending from outer cortex to outer cortex, sclerosis of the fracture margins, submarginal cyst formation, linear osteoporosis of disuse, medullary sealing with cortical bone, increased width of the ununited radiolucent fracture line, progressive rounding, molding or mushrooming of the fracture margins, or a complete absence of any bony reaction at one or both of the fracture ends.

A non-union is a failure of progression of fracture healing. This diagnosis should be considered whenever a fracture does not

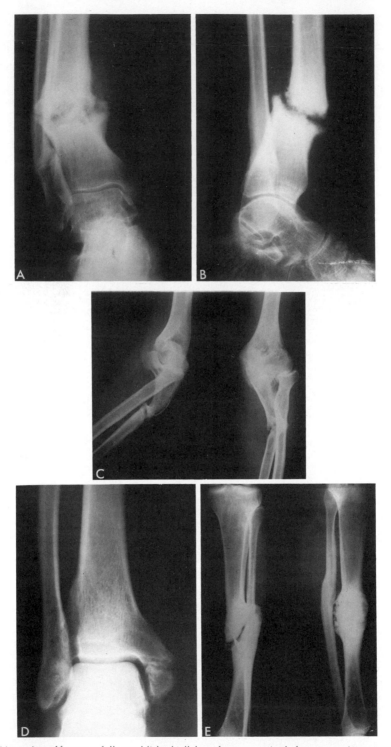

Figure 30–8   Nonunion of fractures fully established (all these fractures united after appropriate surgery, including bone grafting). *A* and *B*, Anteroposterior and lateral roentgenograms of nonunion of fracture of tibia in lower third. The fracture of the fibula united. *C*, Roentgenograms of nonunion of fracture of proximal third of ulna. The radial head is dislocated posteriorly (reverse Monteggia). *D*, Anteroposterior roentgenogram showing nonunion of fracture of medial malleolus of 20 years' duration. *E*, Anteroposterior and lateral roentgenograms showing nonunion of a fracture of the tibia of 22 years' standing. Note exuberant bony callus. The tiny plate represents the height of absurdity in internal fixation.

unite by the clinical criteria previously described according to the anticipated time for the location and configuration of the fracture, and three consecutive monthly x-ray evaluations show one or more signs of non-union and no further evidence of progression of healing. For cases of non-union, four x-rays should always be taken; anteroposterior, lateral, and left and right oblique views. Tomograms and bone scans[169] may be useful both in diagnosing non-union and in determining whether the non-union is hypertrophic, atrophic, or a true pseudarthrosis. A true pseudarthrosis is the end stage of a non-union in which a false joint occurs, with sealing of the medullary cavity and formation of a fluid-filled cavity surrounded by pseudosynovial cells. A true pseudarthrosis rarely occurs and, for all practical purposes, the terms non-union and pseudarthrosis are synonymous.

One or more of the following factors cause or contribute to non-union: an open fracture; infection; a segmental fracture, usually with impaired blood supply to the middle fragment and non-union at the distal fracture site; severe comminution; severe soft tissue and bony loss; soft tissue interposition at the fracture site; persistent separation or distraction at the fracture site; inadequate reduction or fixation; repeated manipulation of the fracture; insufficient length of time of immobilization; and treatment by ill-advised open reduction.[14] Factors of blood supply make certain locations of fractures prone to non-union. These include Type II odontoid fractures, forearm fractures, carpal scaphoid fractures, subcapital fractures of the hip, and fractures of the lower third of the tibia. The more severe the fracture, the displacement, the bone loss, and the soft tissue loss, the greater the chance of non-union. General systemic factors that may adversely influence fracture healing include old age,[23] poor nutrition, a catabolic state, a state of anticoagulation,[86, 179, 180, 182, 198] presence of tumor, diabetes,[41] and hormonal disorders.[115] The use of methyl methacrylate concurrently with internal fixation in pathologic fractures or impending fractures due to metastatic tumors retards fracture healing.[61] Avascular necrosis may lead to delayed union or non-union. The interruption of a precarious blood supply is the common denominator in this problem.

There are four types of pseudarthrosis or non-union: anticipated pseudarthrosis, non-infected pseudarthrosis, previously infected pseudarthrosis, and infected pseudarthrosis. An anticipated pseudarthrosis is one in which bone and soft tissue loss make a pseudarthrosis inevitable. This can be recognized at the time of injury. This must be controlled as soon as possible, preferably with not more than three to four débridements of the fracture done within not longer than a week's time. Early stabilization of the fracture with appropriate internal or external fixation or plaster is appropriate. Delayed primary or early intercalary bone grafting is performed. Simultaneous coverage with a skin graft or pedicle or free flap should be considered, especially if there are unprotected exposed deep structures.

Ninety per cent of non-infected pseudarthroses are hypertrophic, reactive, and vascular. They are often the result of fracture treatment by plaster. They have proliferative callus at the bone ends. They respond to alignment, apposition, fixation, and compression. A bone graft is not required in hypertrophic pseudarthrosis provided rigid fixation and apposition are present and compression is applied.[124, 192] Many surgeons who deal with fractures use a bone graft for assurance of healing or in special situations in which fixation is not used in treating non-unions.

The remaining 10 per cent of non-infected pseudarthroses are atrophic, non-reactive, and frequently avascular. These non-unions require stable fixation with compression when possible and always a bone graft.[124, 192] Some surgeons recommend decortication. This type of pseudarthrosis is more often seen in cases of non-union occurring with the use of internal fixation.

Previously infected pseudarthrosis may be in contact or have a defect. If the fragments are in contact, axial compression achieved with either an external fixator or plate and screws is appropriate. A cancellous bone graft and decortication must be done in those areas that were not previously infected. In previously infected pseudarthrosis with a defect, the bone ends are resected, appropriate plates are applied, and the defect is filled with cancellous bone.[30, 124, 192] Perioperative antibiotics are used.

Infected, draining pseudarthroses present two problems: consolidation of the pseudarthrosis and clearing of the infection. The prime goal in infected, draining pseudarthrosis is union.[66, 124, 192] Once the pseudarthrosis is solid, the infection can be eradicated by sequestrectomy followed by cancellous grafting, if necessary, or in the case of an infected medullary nail by further reaming of the medullary canal by 2 mm. Perioperative antibiotics are used. All infected and necrotic bone and soft tissue are excised and a specimen should be sent for culture. Metal implants may be left in place if they provide stability or may be added for the same purpose. The defect is filled with cancellous bone.[30, 117, 192] Compartmentalization of the leg allows posterior bone grafting of the tibia through the sterile deep posterior compartment while drainage almost always seeks the path of least resistance through the anterior compartment.[66] Once the bone is stable, drainage will stop provided only the soft tissues were infected. If there is chronic osteomyelitis, as evidenced by the presence of its sine qua non — one or more sequestra — further sequestrectomy and bone grafting can be done later. A chronic osteomyelitis can be treated by en bloc resection of all involved bone and soft tissue and plate stabilization with cancellous bone grafting of the defect.[30, 117]

Invasive and non-invasive methods of electrical stimulation have been used successfully in selected cases of hypertrophic non-infected pseudarthrosis with a gap between the bone ends of less than 1 cm.[8, 22]

Excessive Atrophy of Musculature

Some atrophy of musculature is a natural consequence of many fractures. The inactivity imposed by the injury and the immobilization of the part to hold reduction lead to unavoidable restriction of muscle action, and some shrinkage and weakness of muscle masses are likely to follow. Some atrophy of musculature is an unpreventable complication of most fractures.

Excessive atrophy of musculature, on the other hand, is usually a preventable compli-

cation. By early, active exercise of every muscle in the injured extremity that will not disturb reduction of the fracture and of every muscle group in the other extremities, atrophy can be minimized. Rehabilitation of the patient begins on the day of injury.

The only treatment is preventive. Whether the patient is bedridden, ambulatory, or leads a wheelchair existence, every unimmobilized joint should be moved actively with force through a full range of motion many times daily. Such exercises tend to maintain muscle strength and also to avoid subsequent restriction of joint motion. Full active motion of the fingers or toes provides exercise for the muscles of the forearm or the leg.

Exercise of muscles may be beneficial even though the joints they move are immobilized. For example, the quadriceps musculature of the thigh may be contracted over and over again by a patient in a long-leg cast or even a hip spica cast. The repeated contraction maintains in part the strength of the quadriceps and also prevents its gliding mechanism near the knee from adhering to the femur. Strenuous quadriceps drills are an important part of the management of every fracture of the lower extremity. Ambulation, when the patient is treated in functional lower extremity casts or braces, helps prevent muscle atrophy as do functional muscle exercises in functional upper extremity casting and bracing.

Muscle atrophy is part of the cast syndrome which also includes joint stiffness, edema, and osteopenia. When it is appropriate for fracture treatment, open reduction and internal fixation with rigid stabilization of the fracture help to allow early rehabilitation to prevent muscle atrophy.

Loss of Motion in Joints

Some permanent restriction of motion in the joints adjacent to fractures necessarily immobilized as part of treatment is probably second only to muscle atrophy as a complication of fractures. The older the patient is, the more likely that immobilization will result in some permanent restriction of motion. Loss of joint motion also results from injury to the ligamentous tissues about them, with resulting scar formation, from injury to adjacent muscles that limits their subsequent function, and from intra-articular lines of fracture that damage the articular cartilage of the joint and may lead to intra-articular adhesions and post-traumatic arthrosis. In many instances, loss of motion in joints must be considered an unpreventable complication that can be minimized if joints are held in a functional position (Fig. 30–9).

Immobilization of fractures should be avoided when it is not required. For example, an impacted fracture of the surgical neck of the humerus really needs no immobilization, although a few days of immobilization at the side in a sling and a Velpeau bandage may be advisable for relief of severe pain. Early active exercises should be instituted, especially in the pendulum position. A mildly depressed fracture of the lateral condyle of the tibia requires no immobilization, although the knee may be splinted for a few days during the acute stage of the injury. Thereafter, immobilization is a liability, since only protection from weight-bearing is necessary. Active motion of the knee and ankle and active exercises of the musculature of the extremity should be carried out repeatedly.

Open reduction and internal fixation of fractures may offer, among other advantages, early motion of joints and active exercise of musculature. An outstanding advantage of intramedullary nailing of fractures of the femur is the freedom from external immobilization it affords and the active exercise it permits. Internal fixation of condylar fractures of the femur and tibia should provide the best obtainable reduction of the fragments that minimizes the tendency toward traumatic arthritis and at the same time reduces the time of immobilization. When the fixation is rigid and stable, immobilization may be discontinued after the operative wound has healed and exercises may be instituted promptly. In general, fractures about joints require the most precise reduction; therefore, open reduction and internal fixation are indicated frequently. After a technically splendid operation providing rigid stabilization of the fragments and a good fit of the articular surfaces, the additional advantage of early mobilization should not be lost by unnecessary prolonged immobilization.

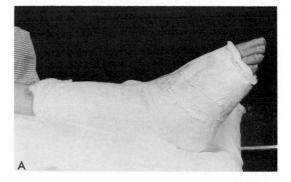

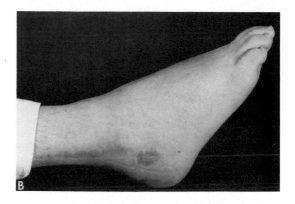

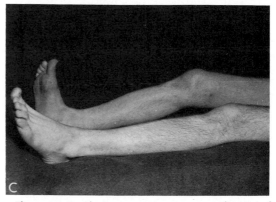

Figure 30–9 Flexion contractures as a complication of fractures. *A,* A poor plaster cast predisposing to fixed plantar flexion of the foot. Moreover, the cast is too short. As a rule, plaster casts applied to the leg and foot should hold the foot at a right angle and extend to a level above the calf of the leg. *B,* A foot in fixed plantar flexion (equinus) because it was immobilized in this position for 3 months in a plaster cast used for treatment of fractures of both bones of the leg. *C,* Photograph of lower extremities of a patient whose right lower extremity was immobilized for several months in skeletal traction as treatment of a comminuted fracture of the femoral shaft. During this period the knee was held flexed to an angle of 45 degrees. Now it cannot be extended past 20 degrees, which is exceedingly disabling. Note atrophy of the right quadriceps musculature. Quadriceps exercises cannot be carried out with the knee flexed past 20 degrees.

Decubitus Ulcers — Pressure Sores and Bedsores

Pressure sores are practically always secondary to faulty medical treatment and bedsores to faulty nursing care, although, in an occasional patient, either of these kinds of decubitus ulcers may occur in spite of every effort to prevent them.

PRESSURE SORES

Pressure sores are the result of excessive long-continued localized pressure to the point of necrosis from ischemia. Pressure over a long period is usually required for the development of delayed nerve paralysis. Plaster casts, coaptation splints, or straps, slings, or other supports attached to splints are the offending agents. Pressure sores practically always occur over bony prominences, but occasionally they develop over prominent tendons poorly protected by the underlying soft tissues. Although they are more likely to occur in senile or poorly nourished patients, they are really the result of faulty technique of application or faulty supervision of casts or splints. Pressure sores, therefore, are preventable complications in most patients (Fig. 30–10).

Plaster casts should be applied snugly but smoothly without reverse turns of the plaster bandages. The problem is not merely the application of padding, as non-padded casts, not so popular in recent years, may be applied without causing a pressure sore. Padding beneath casts must be applied smoothly without wads or lumps, particularly over bony prominences. Joints should be held in the desired position during application of the plaster. For example, a foot should not be allowed to drop into plantar flexion as the plaster turns are taken about the ankle and then pushed up to an angle of 90 degrees (usually the desired position) as the plaster hardens. This procedure tightens plaster about the heel and dorsum of the foot and predisposes to pressure sores. Similarly, to bend the knee a few degrees after plaster has been applied with the knee in full extension may cause a pressure sore over the patella and, in very thin patients, over the hamstring tendons.

Many pressure sores result from faulty holding of the extremity during plaster application. The fingers of the assistant often cause indentations in the plaster; if one of these is over a bony prominence, a pressure sore can follow. Excessive pressure over the heel or the medial condyle of the humerus may easily result, for example, if the holding hand flattens the plaster in either of these regions. The extremity must be held at non-vulnerable points with the entire palm of the hand, without point pressure of the fingertips. If broad indentations result, these may be eliminated by careful molding as the plaster is setting. In addition, the plaster should be molded so that it conforms smoothly about bony prominences.

Plaster should not be applied over circular bandages or traction hitches, even though hitches theoretically can be slipped out after the plaster has hardened. Swelling can cause circular bandages to become excessively tight and produce deep cuts into the flesh, and traction hitches can lead to the same sort of complication.

Pressure sores need not occur when splints are used. Pressure of emergency splints on bony prominences such as the malleoli, the medial condyle of the humerus, or the styloid of the ulna may be kept within safe limits by appropriate padding and care. Vulnerable areas of a lower extremity in a traction splint must be safeguarded. The ring must not jam against the perineum. The heel cord area particularly must not go unprotected at the point at which it rests on the distal sling or support. Actually, a long, broad strip of felt placed between the entire extremity and the slings, from the ring to the heel, is an excellent precaution against excessive pressure of the supports for the leg at all points.

Adequate care soon after application of splints or plaster casts will prevent pressure sores even though excessive pressure is being placed on vulnerable points. As soon as the patient recovers from anesthesia after either closed or open reduction of a fracture, or during the prereduction stage while an emergency splint is in place, the patient should be asked about points of pain. Some pain is to be expected, but it should be localized to the general area of the fracture. All complaints of pain should be investigated as to cause. Sedatives, particularly opiates, should not be given merely because

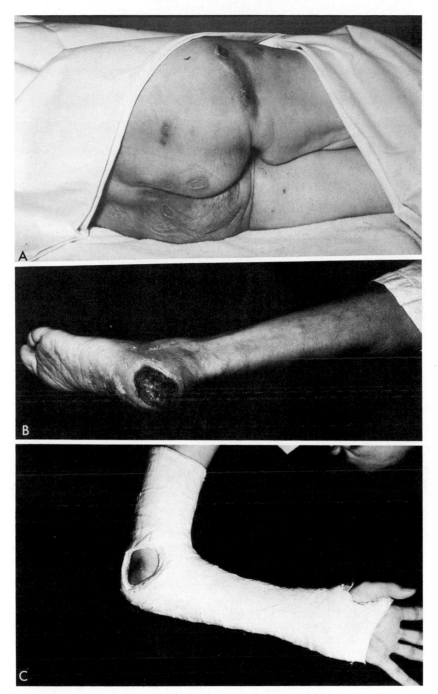

Figure 30–10 Decubitus ulcers. *A,* Necrotic skin over proximal portion of thigh as a result of excessive pressure of the ring of a Thomas splint (a preventable complication) and bedsores over the buttocks and sacrum (usually a preventable complication). *B,* A tremendous pressure sore over the heel which occurred beneath a plaster cast. Proper care in application of the plaster will avoid such a complication. *C,* A pressure sore over the medial epicondyle of the humerus which occurred beneath a plaster cast. Removal of a circular area of plaster is more likely to solve the problem at this pressure point than at others.

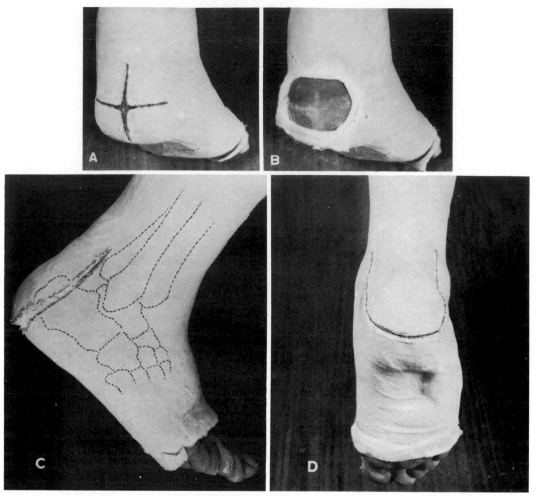

Figure 30–11   Relief of pressure over the heel. *A,* The cruciate incision over the pressure area. Each quadrant of plaster should be elevated slightly so as to relieve the point pressure. *B,* The circular window for relief of pressure. This is not a desirable method, since it creates a circular rim against which the heel must rest so that other pressure areas may develop. The bulging soft tissue may become edematous and increase the pressure on the circular rim. *C* and *D,* The flap or tongue method of cutting a cast to relieve painful pressure over the heel.

the patient complains of severe pain. Close questioning may reveal that the disturbing pain is at a bony prominence remote from the area of the fracture. In these instances the surgeon must "do something, not give something." Nursing staff and house staff must be drilled thoroughly in this philosophy.

When the patient indicates that pain is localized beneath a cast or splint over a bony prominence, the offending pressure must be relieved promptly. The method varies with the type of immobilization. Coaptation splints may be adjusted or reapplied, and the offended bony prominence may be pad-

ded to avoid excessive pressure. The ischial ring or the supports for an extremity in a traction splint must be adjusted to relieve the pressure.

Plaster casts must be cut and the offending portion elevated (Figs. 30–11 and 30–12). This may be achieved in several ways, depending upon the fracture and the necessity for maintaining the same degree of immobilization. At times, the cast may be split on one or both sides over part of or the entire length and the two parts separated to relieve pressure. More often the cast is cut only at the painful point. It must be cut properly. The ideal way is to produce a

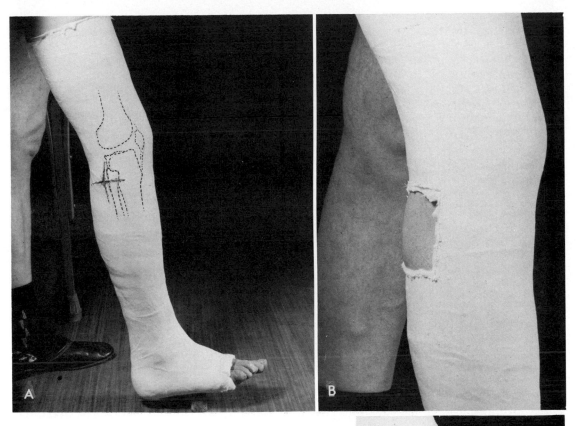

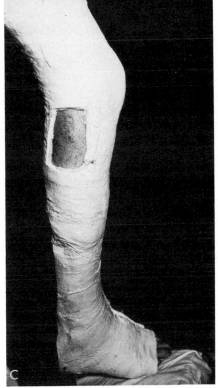

Figure 30–12   Relief of pressure over the peroneal nerve. *A,* The cruciate incision with elevation of the flaps to relieve pressure over the peroneal nerve. The center of these cuts in the cast should be posterolateral rather than directly lateral. *B,* The window method. This is an uncertain way to relieve the pressure. Note that the soft tissue bulges through the window. The peroneal nerve is beneath the most superior edge of the window. Pressure on the nerve may continue. *C,* A lateral window which leaves sufficient plaster posteriorly may relieve the pressure.

cruciate (+) incision over the painful point and to elevate the four small flaps slightly. The point pressure may be relieved by cutting the plaster in order to create a tongue that can be elevated. Occasionally "trap doors" may be created and elevated slightly. In these ways the excessive pressure is relieved, but sufficient pressure is maintained to prevent the formation of "window edema." Usually it is wrong to remove a circular portion of plaster over the painful area. This permits bulging of the soft tissues through the circular window, with resulting edema, and predisposes to necrosis of tissue around the margins of the opening. The edema that follows adversely affects the healing of any preformed skin lesion.

Definitive management of pressure sores varies with the severity of the lesion. Excessive pressure must be relieved promptly by one of the methods just described. In many instances the necrotic soft tissue is allowed to separate spontaneously from underlying and surrounding viable tissue and the resulting ulceration is allowed to heal by granulation and scarification or, if it is not full-thickness, by epithelialization. Occasionally a pressure sore will require surgical excision of the necrotic tissue and, after proper preparation of the bed, covering with a split-thickness or pedicle skin graft.

BEDSORES

Bedsores result from pressure of the patient's body incident to his position in bed. The most common site is over the sacrum, but they occur not uncommonly over the outer side of the heel and occasionally over the prominences of the back of the elbow, shoulder blades, and trochanters. They are most likely to occur in debilitated patients and particularly in paraplegics. Bedsores are preventable complications in many instances, but in others they will occur in spite of every effort to prevent them. In any event, their incidence can be minimized by good nursing care.

Pressure over vulnerable points must be minimized. If treatment of the fracture does not contraindicate, the patient must be turned from side to side and face down frequently and kept off the back as much as possible. When the patient is on the back,

the sacral area should be protected as well as possible by rubber rings. In some instances these must be used to protect the trochanters when the patient is on the side. Pillows should be placed lengthwise under the legs to keep the heels from resting continually on the mattress. Pillows also may be used to protect the points of pressure on the scapulae and elbows. The skin over the vulnerable areas should be kept clean, dry, and powdered and its vitality stimulated by frequent massage.

An alternating-pressure air mattress or a mat of sheep's wool placed on top of the regular mattress is a valuable preventive measure for patients who must remain on their backs for prolonged periods. Mats of sheep's wool are valuable also to protect other parts of the body that are subject to maximal pressure as the patient is placed in varying positions. The alternating-pressure air mattress and the mats of sheep's wool, singly or in combination, are likely to make the patient more comfortable.

A bedsore is more difficult to treat than to prevent. When the first break in the skin appears, efforts to avoid pressure on this point must be redoubled. Local treatment should be drying. The area should be painted two or three times a day with tincture of benzoin and then well powdered. Ointments and dressings are preferably avoided, since they lead to maceration.

When a full-thickness necrosis of the soft tissue over the bony prominence has developed, treatment is much more complex. When the area is small, the eschar may be trimmed away and the area allowed to granulate to healing with scar formation. Larger areas require radical débridement and covering with skin grafts. Pedicle grafts are often necessary.

COMPLICATIONS OF OPEN FRACTURES

An open wound communicating with the fracture site increases the seriousness of the bony injury in proportion to the degree of soft tissue bony injury, including the amount of soft tissue and bony loss when such loss occurs.[59, 124] In the open fracture there are two problems: the wound and the fracture. Both are threatened by infection and impaired healing. The primary goal of treatment of open fractures is to achieve bony union without infection.[30, 66, 124, 192]

Problem of Fracture Healing

Open fractures carry an increased incidence of delayed union and non-union in comparison with similar closed fractures. Open fractures are associated with more trauma to bones and soft parts than are closed fractures. The greater the trauma, the greater the disturbance of blood supply and, therefore, the greater the threat to bone healing. Increased trauma and a disturbed blood supply increase the hazard of infection as well. Infection at the fracture site is the greatest deterrent to union because persistent drainage of any degree interferes with the physiology of fracture healing.

Problem of Wound Infection

By far the most significant and potentially devastating local complication of open fractures is wound infection. In the management of open fractures, every consideration is given to the prevention or eradication of infection. Wound infection may be classified as invasive infection, wound suppuration, and surface infection. Invasive infection is a bacterial invasion and destruction of previously living tissue by bacteria primarily or secondarily implanted in the wound. This is a spreading infection with all the cardinal signs of inflammation. Examples are streptococcal cellulitis and gas gangrene (clostridial myonecrosis). Wound suppuration is a collection of purulent material within a wound (abscess formation) resulting from the septic breakdown of dead and devitalized tissue, including blood clot. The process is augmented by further destruction of tissue as a result of the proteolytic action of enzymes in the pus. Surface infection is a collection of pus on a granulating surface of an open wound such as that presented by a third-degree burn.

Wound infections complicating open fractures practically always fall within the wound suppuration group. For the septic process to develop, dead tissue and bacterial contamination are necessary. All wounds have contamination, the presence of foreign bodies, and tissue injury.[28] The difference is one of degree. The risk of infection in each instance increases with the severity of the open fracture, the degree of injury to the blood supply, and the time interval between the contamination at the time of injury and definitive débridement and irrigation.[124] The bacteria contaminating an open fracture need not have invasive qualities and may be capable only of decomposing retained dead tissue and collections of blood and serum into pus. In some wounds, a suppurative process develops because unprotected fascia, tendon, cartilage, or cortex of bone remain exposed as a result of the loss of soft tissue or merely the presence of a gaping open wound. These tissues cannot survive if they remain exposed in a wound. They desiccate, die, and become a nidus for wound suppuration.[137] The ultimate effect of an open wound that leaves these vulnerable tissues exposed is a wound infection beginning in dead tissue.

Regardless of how and why a suppurative process develops in an open fracture, it is a most serious complication. Union of the fracture is further delayed and may be prevented. A scourge of the septic process, as in all wound infections, is the necrosis of previously living tissue that is certain to follow. Massive sequestration of bone may take place. Sequestration of bone is the sine qua non of chronic osteomyelitis, a very serious complication.[191] Adjacent joints can be invaded and destroyed. An infection can become so extensive that it can warrant amputation as a life-saving measure. At best, wound healing will be slow, with excessive scar formation, and this alone can impair the function of the extremity.

In addition to other bacterial infections, open fractures can be complicated by specific infections leading to gas gangrene and tetanus.

GAS GANGRENE

Gas gangrene results from inadequate treatment of an open wound. There is no active immunization against gas gangrene. Gas gangrene most often occurs with a deep penetrating wound that involves muscle and is sealed off from the surface. Although found in large concentrations in soil and in the intestines of animals, including humans, gas-forming clostridial organisms are ubiquitous. They are obligate anaerobes and cannot multiply in healthy tissues with normal oxygen concentrations. It is not the virulence of the organism that causes infection, but rather the unique local conditions, including necrotic tissue, ischemic tissue, or both. Although gas gangrene has been traditionally thought to occur in war wounds, an alarming increase has been noted among civilian injuries, including some with an initially innocent appearance.[25, 48, 64] Open fractures in which there is gross soiling, difficulty in ascertaining tissue viability at the initial débridement, or both, are particularly susceptible. Such open fractures include those sustained in war; during natural disasters such as hurricanes, tornados, floods, earthquakes, mine cave-ins, plane crashes, and train crashes; soiled wounds, especially those from the farm and from meat, poultry, and fish-packing houses; and those resulting from crush injuries, rotary lawn mower injuries (mini-tornados), high velocity gunshot wounds, and close-range shotgun wounds. Undebrided first-degree open fractures with puncture of the bone through the skin from the inside out[64] and inadequately debrided open fractures,[25] particularly those that are closed primarily, are extremely susceptible to this complication. Tight casts and compartment syndromes that cause ischemia can create the proper environment for clostridial infection. Clostridial organisms in an open fracture, dislocation, or fracture dislocation can be of three types: clostridial contamination, clostridial cellulitis or fasciitis, or clostridial myonecrosis.[1, 2] Clostridial contamination requires only adequate débridement and preventive antibiotics. There is no systemic effect. Clostridial cellulitis or fasciitis usually occurs after several days, with rapidly spreading emphysematous infection with extensive gas formation along fascial planes. Systemic toxicity is mild or absent. Incision, débridement, and open wound care along with antibiotics, preferably high dose intravenous aqueous penicillin, are usually all that is needed. Clostridial myonecrosis is the severe form of infection and, since the incubation period of gas-forming clostridial organisms is 12 to 24 hours, it occurs early

after open fracture. Clostridial organisms multiply and produce toxins that diffuse into the surrounding tissues and devitalize them, allowing progressive clostridial colonization.[48] Disproportionate local pain; a brown, watery, musty, malodorous seropurulent drainage; local edema; and, if gas formation is present, crepitus, occur early. There is an early dissociation of pulse and temperature with an initial tachycardia. As toxemia sets in, the temperature elevates. The progress of the disease is rapid. Gas formation is not always present and therefore is not always seen on radiograph. Jaundice, hemoglobinemia, and hemoglobinuria can occur. Profound shock, coma, and death follow. The mortality rate can be as high as 25 per cent, even with treatment.

Prevention of clostridial myonecrosis is effected by adequate débridement, particularly of all non-viable muscle, wound cleansing, and open wound care. Open wound care must be instituted in any case in which the extent of tissue damage or the thoroughness of débridement is in question. Closing wounds loosely over a drain is of no preventive benefit. Clean wounds can be closed. Preventive antibiotics must be used but are no substitute for adequate débridement or open wound care. High doses of aqueous intravenous penicillin remain the treatment of choice.

The treatment of clostridial myonecrosis is by complete decompression of the infected area and meticulous débridement. Muscle involvement is invariably greater than the skin changes might indicate.[73] The muscle is edematous, gray or dark red, and ischemic. Contractility is absent in involved muscle and gas may bubble from it. Again, high doses of intravenous aqueous penicillin are preferred. Hyperbaric oxygenation is beneficial and also has the specific effect of neutralizing the toxin.[152] The patient should be supported, particularly with appropriate fluid and electrolyte replacement. Polyvalent antitoxin is of no proven benefit. Amputation may be a life-saving measure.

TETANUS

Clostridium tetani is an obligate anaerobe and is non-invasive. Local proliferation causes release of exotoxins that spread rapidly into the muscles. They reach the myoneural junction, where the most potent exotoxin, tetanoplasmin, blocks inhibitory synapses along motor neurons resulting in blockage of spinal inhibition. Muscle hyperirritability, increased deep tendon reflexes, and spasms at the site of injury occur. More areas become involved in muscle spasms as the exotoxins spread from distal to proximal along the peripheral nerve to the central nervous system, where involvement again spreads from distal to proximal. Trismus, risus sardonicus, difficulty in swallowing, and opisthotonos can occur. If the brain becomes involved, the patient can experience headaches and restlessness, and generalized tonic convulsions can result. There are no sensory changes in this disease. Sympathetic involvement is manifested by cardiovascular instability, including tachycardia, an increased metabolic rate, hyperthermia, and intense diaphoresis. Death occurs in 50 per cent of cases and is caused by asphyxia associated with unremitting laryngeal and respiratory spasm.

Tetanus is an inexcusable complication[56] and is prevented by active immunization supplemented by tetanus immune globulin when appropriate.[3] Treatment of established cases of tetanus includes adequate wound débridement and open wound care. Human tetanus immune globulin is used to neutralize the exotoxin. Intravenous aqueous penicillin in high doses is the antibiotic of choice. Tetracycline is the second-line antibiotic used in patients allergic to penicillin. Intravenous diazepam (Valium) is the drug of choice to control spasms or convulsions. Endotracheal intubation and a volume-controlled respirator are necessary with heavy sedation. The disease is self-limiting.

Management of Open Fractures

The management of open fractures is designed to achieve union of the fracture in good position without suppuration of the soft tissues or bone. The most important preventive measure against infection is wound débridement (Fig. 30–13). Necrotic and devitalized tissue and old blood clots, the pabulum of wound infection, must be eliminated. During the so-called contaminated period, the depths and recesses of the wound must be cleaned of dirt, debris, and foreign material, especially all organic matter.

TECHNICAL CONSIDERATIONS

In order that all devitalized tissue may be removed surgically, exposure of the depths of the wound must be ample. As a rule, the open wound must be extended in the direction that will afford adequate access to the depths without injury to important structures such as nerve trunks and without unnecessary exposure of those tissues likely to die if they remain uncovered. Extensions are usually made parallel to the long axis of the extremity from normal tissue proximally to normal tissue distally. Only the devitalized skin of the wound margins should be excised.

A long incision in the fascial layer usually exposes foreign bodies and devitalized muscle, excision of which is the principal objective of débridement of a wound. Débridement removes all devitalized tissue that might act as a culture medium to allow an increase in bacterial concentration. Healthy tissue will resist contamination of up to 100,000 bacteria/cu. cm., while ischemic tissue will almost invariably become infected.[27, 95, 151] Color, consistency, contractility, and capillary bleeding are assessed in determining muscle viability.[166] Contractility, when present, is the most reliable of these parameters and clearly establishes viability. Ischemia occurring with shock may mask the evaluation of capillary flow. Color is the least reliable indicator of muscle viability.

Small devascularized pieces of cortical bone should be removed from the wound. Large fragments of bone with soft tissue connections should be retained, especially if their small vessels bleed onto their exposed surfaces, and even if they require trimming to eliminate contamination. A large fragment with tenuous or no soft tissue connection has a real value in reconstituting a defect but is also a potential sequestrum. There are no absolutely clear criteria about retaining such a fragment. Its potential value as an in situ bone graft is evident. The degree of contamination of the fragment and of the wound and the vascularity of the

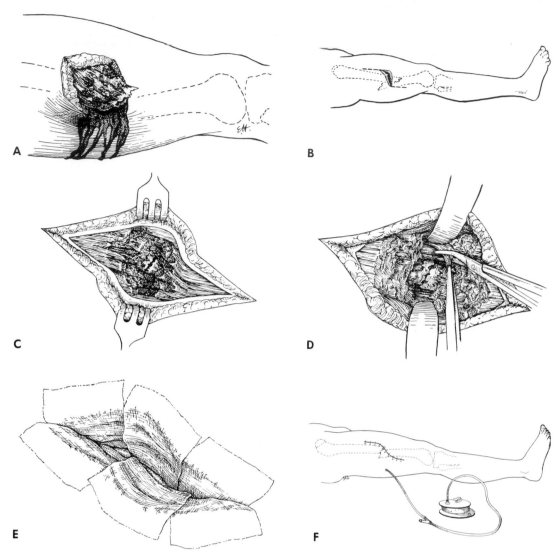

Figure 30–13   Artist's drawings of débridement of an open fracture. *A,* Open fracture of the shaft of the femur with the distal end of the proximal fragment protruding through a jagged open wound on the lateral surface of the thigh. *B,* The first step in débridement is adequate enlargement of the incision. A transverse or near-transverse wound should be enlarged by longitudinal extension proximally and distally at opposite ends of the open wound. These are illustrated by dotted lines. This creates a type of Z incision which facilitates wound closure. Definitely an incision should not be made across the center of the wound which would create a cruciate type of wound. The protruding bone was well cleaned and any obvious tags of dead muscle were excised before the fragment was reduced into the depths of the wound. *C,* The fascia has been split so as to facilitate exposure of the depths of the wound and excision of destroyed muscle tissue. *D,* Devitalized tags of muscle tissue are excised. While skin incisions should be made with a knife, excision of muscle with scissors is highly acceptable. *E,* Proper dressing of the wound if it is to remain open. *F,* If primary suture of the wound is selected, dependent drainage for a few days through the posterolateral fascial plane is a safeguard against deep abscess formation. (Courtesy of Miss Edna Hill.)

adjacent tissue influence the surgeon's judgment. If the fragment is retained it is a calculated risk.

In open fractures presumably opened from within out and first-degree open fractures, wide exposure and débridement are indicated as a safeguard against wound infection, tetanus, and gas gangrene. Clostridial organisms are ubiquitous and can be drawn into the wound. Considerable dirt and foreign material may be introduced into the wound of a fracture that is opened from within out. The degree of bacterial contamination, foreign material, and devitalized tissue cannot be ascertained without débridement. The risk of catastrophic complications such as gas gangrene, wound infection, compartment syndrome, and osteomyelitis is too high not to perform a complete incision and débridement of these initially innocuous appearing first-degree open fractures. These fractures are particularly prone to the complications previously described, if not adequately debrided.

While open fractures caused by high-velocity missile wounds and close-range shotgun wounds[132, 174] must be adequately incised and debrided, the routine débridement of open fractures caused by low-velocity gunshot wounds is controversial[80, 89, 98, 201] unless they enter into joints in which exploration, débridement, and irrigation are mandatory.[4, 46, 81, 135, 183] It is always wise to debride open fractures caused by low velocity missiles if there is any question about tissue viability or foreign body or bacterial contamination, or if there are other specific indications.

In open fractures in which there is difficulty in ascertaining tissue viability at the initial débridement, open wound care should be instituted. Staged wound care should be provided and these patients must be redebrided and re-evaluated every few days until wound control is achieved. Closure at the proper time is highly desirable to minimize scarring, but more so to protect those tissues vulnerable to exposure[137] and to avoid secondary contamination. An immediate successful suture of the wound is most advantageous, but an unsuccessful suture because of abscess formation or necrosis of skin margins due to excessive tension produces worse results than leaving the wound open to heal by granulation. The price of either of these complications is additional necrosis of soft tissue that further retards and may prevent healing of the wound. Closure by suture of a clean, well-debrided wound of a first-degree or mild second-degree open fracture may be permissible except in military circumstances, particularly if the time lag after injury is not too prolonged and provided closure can be carried out without excessive tension both at the time of closure and later after swelling of the tissue margins has occurred. Many wounds may be closed primarily after thorough débridement 12 to 16 hours after injury. On the other hand, if the surgeon has any doubt that the wound has been debrided of devitalized tissue or that closure by suture can be achieved without excessive tension on the wound margins, particularly after swelling has taken place, then an open wound is preferable despite its inherent hazards. At times, a long, full-thickness relaxing incision parallel to but several inches from the proposed suture line may serve to avoid excessive tension. However, every precaution must be taken to insure that the bipedicle flap created has an adequate arterial supply. If the decision is made to leave the wound open, an active effort should be made to achieve wound control and either delayed primary closure or coverage by skin grafting or flap should be performed within 1 week from injury, if possible. This will keep scarring to a minimum. The decision to close or cover a wound is based on clinical appraisal of gross cleanliness. This can be confirmed by bacterial colony count studies provided one has or assumes a homogeneous wound. Dead space must always be obliterated or drained dependently. Hemostasis must be complete and excessive tension on skin and subfascial structures must be avoided (Fig. 30–14).

Management of the wound and management of the fracture go hand in hand. Both the wound and the fracture require stability in order to provide the proper environment for healing or reconstruction and to prevent or control infection. Stability prevents motion, particularly shear motion, which would be disruptive of capillaries and granulation tissue forming between opposing bone ends or skin edges in instances of primary healing, or between bone edges and bone graft and between soft tissues and either skin graft or flap in secondary healing with reconstruction.

As far as the management of the fracture is concerned, the fragments must be placed and held in adequate apposition and alignment. A good reduction not only favors union of the fracture with minimal deformity but also is an additional measure against the development of wound infection. The fragments are held in good position, dead space (that around unreduced fragment ends) in which contaminated blood clot and

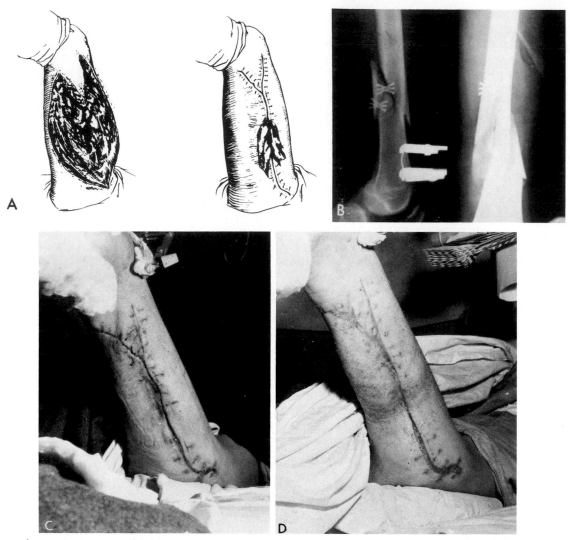

Figure 30–14 Successful delayed primary closure of wound of open fracture of femoral shaft. *A,* Artist's drawing showing the huge wound compounding fracture of the femoral shaft and closure of the wound with drainage 5 days after thorough débridement. *B,* Lateral and anteroposterior roentgenograms showing comminuted fracture of femoral shaft at the junction of the middle and lower thirds. The fragments are in acceptable position. Actually, skeletal traction is being made on a wire through the tibial tubercle, but in addition another wire placed through the distal fragment is being used to elevate it into alignment. *C,* The healing wound 10 days later after removal of the sutures. *D,* The healed wound 4 weeks after débridement and closure. (From Hampton, O. P., Jr.: Wounds of Extremities in Military Surgery. St Louis, C. V. Mosby Company, 1951.)

wound exudate can collect is avoided, pressure of fragments against the under surface of the skin which can cause tissue necrosis does not occur, wound margins are more easily approximated without tension, and repeated, traumatizing efforts at reduction are unnecessary. In these ways, reduction of the fracture inhibits infection in the wound of an open fracture.

In open fractures, the fracture can be reduced and placed at rest either in plaster[26, 157-164, 196] or by means of internal fixation[60, 114] once the wound is controlled. At the same time, functional treatment in plaster that includes ambulatory treatment in plaster of fractures of the lower extremity or active range of motion with joint and muscle rehabilitation may be instituted in those cases in which internal or external fixation is used. The same methods are applicable to open as to closed fractures. In open fractures, however, the question of internal fixation at the time of débridement of the wound is often of paramount importance. When contour of the fracture will permit adequate stabilization, the decision must be made on the basis of whether or not the wound is controlled. Only first-degree and very mild second-degree open fractures that have occurred within the previous 24 hours should even be considered for osteosynthesis at the time of initial débridement. Other fractures should be treated either in plaster or with external fixators until such time as wound control is achieved. Stabilization with internal fixation may then be considered along with closure or coverage. If there is any question about wound control at the time of stabilization, the fracture should be left open. These decisions require expert judgment.

With well-debrided wounds that can be closed by suture or in which heavy masses of muscle tissue will fall over and protect the bone and metal from exposure, internal fixation through the open wound, if really indicated for the fracture, may be carried out. It may also be carried out through a more appropriate separate incision while leaving the wound open for drainage and later closure or coverage. Minimal osteosynthesis requiring little or no periosteal stripping may be preferable (Fig. 30–15).

When factors likely to lead to infection of the wound are present, internal fixation is probably too hazardous. In doubtful instances, another method of management should be selected for the fracture and every effort directed toward obtaining early healing of the wound without infection. Then, if adequate reduction of the fracture has not been maintained, delayed open reduction and internal fixation through a healed skin envelope may be performed. Bone grafting may be performed at this time using autogenous cancellous bone graft or incorporating a corticocancellous bone graft into the rigidly fixed reduction. In this regard, however, it is to be emphasized, as has previously been stated, that an adequately stabilized fracture in good position may actually favor rather than retard healing of the wound. Of some importance is the fact that staged wound care, if indicated, is possible without fear of loss of reduction of the fragments with a fracture stabilized in a reduced position.

Danis,[44] Ehrlich,[58] Hcim,[84] and Küntscher[100] were early advocates of internal fixation for severe open fractures in Europe. Later, in the 1940's and 1950's, Haebler,[78] Brav and Jeffress,[20] Carr and Turnipseed,[32] and Brav[16, 19] advocated internal fixation for severe open fractures in the United States. McNeur[109] expressed similar sentiments about the same time in England. In cases in which other deep structures are to be repaired, the bone must be stabilized. More sophisticated methods of rigid internal and external fixation have been developed by the European Association for the Study of Internal Fixation (ASIF). They have provided reliable guidelines for patient and fracture selection and for the techniques to be used, based upon a degree of contamination and the extent of tissue damage. When internal fixation in open fractures fails, it is usually due to a violation of judgment in selection of the patient or the fracture, a technical error in the application of the implant, or imprudent wound closure. The ASIF method uses the principles of anatomic reduction of the fracture, stable, rigid internal fixation with compression whenever possible, preservation of the blood supply, and early active mobilization of the muscles and joints adjacent to the fracture. Aseptic technique, hemostasis, gentle handling of tissues, and appropriate drainage are important factors in wound healing. Elevation of the injured part and good nutrition of the patient are important in the immediate postoperative period.

After the wound is controlled and the bone is stabilized, an autogenous cancellous iliac bone graft is used for any defect of the cortex opposite a plate, any segmental defect in the bone, and in severely comminuted fractures. This may be done primarily if the destiny of the wound and its cover is certain or may be delayed until such time that this requirement is satisfied. If the bone is stabilized and the autogenous cancellous bone graft will be surrounded by a well-vascularized muscle and fascial structures, the bone graft may be inserted and, in cases of uncertainty of wound control at the conclusion of the procedure, the wound may be left open until its destiny is assured. Then cover may be applied.

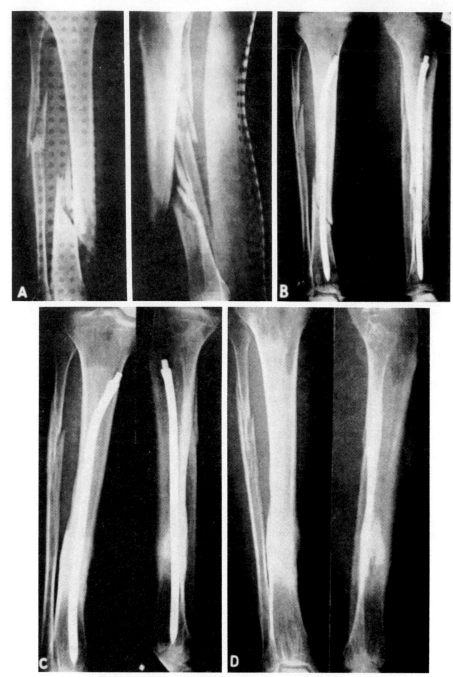

Figure 30–15 Open fracture of both bones of the leg with a fragment of tibia protruding through a long anterior wound. *A,* Anteroposterior and lateral views of open fracture of both bones of the leg. The distal end of the proximal fragment was protruding through the open wound when the patient arrived at the hospital. (From Hampton, O. P., Jr., and Holt, E. P., Jr.: The present status of intramedullary nailing of fractures of the tibia. Am. J. Surg. *93*:597, 1957.) *B,* Anteroposterior and lateral roentgenograms showing excellent reduction of the fragments maintained by an intramedullary nail in the tibia. After thorough débridement of the wound the fragments were stabilized in reduction by insertion of the nail, and the long wound over the fracture site was closed by suture. It healed by first intention. *C,* Anteroposterior and lateral roentgenograms showing the united fractures several months later. *D,* Anteroposterior and lateral roentgenograms showing the splendid end result after removal of the intramedullary nail. (From Hampton, O. P., Jr., and Fitts, W. T., Jr.: Open Reduction of Common Fractures. New York, Grune & Stratton, Inc., 1959.)

ANTIBIOTIC THERAPY

Adjunctive preventive antibiotic coverage is indicated in open fractures and is initiated promptly after the patient has been admitted to the hospital and before the operation on the wound is carried out. Preventive antibiotics are maintained for approximately 48 hours. Cephalosporins[77, 136] are currently thought to be the antibiotics of choice. Cultures of tissues exposed by open fractures taken prior to débridement and just prior to the initiation of antibiotics give the highest yield. If antibiotics are to be continued after 48 hours, these cultures will indicate the antibiotic of choice. Again, antibiotics should not be substituted for adequate débridement and wound care. The condition of the wound is as important, or more important, than its bacterial flora in the development of wound suppuration.

SEPTIC OPEN FRACTURES

The principles for the management of open fractures with established wound suppuration are identical with those for open fractures in the contaminated stage. The depths and recesses of the wound must be explored and cleaned of dirt, debris, and dead and devitalized tissue, including that resulting from the injury and that resulting from the septic process itself. Dead space in which purulent exudate might collect must be drained adequately by dependent drainage. Often a counterincision is necessary for dependent drainage. Although partial closure may be appropriate to cover unprotected deep structures, staged open wound care is the rule. Delayed closure may be performed when the wound becomes clinically clean and controlled. As soon as cultures are taken from the depths of the wound, antibiotic therapy should be instituted. A broad spectrum antibiotic such as a cephalosporin or a combination of oxacillin and an aminoglycoside may be used initially. No more than two antibiotics should be given concurrently. When the results of sensitivity tests made on cultures taken from the wound depths are known, the appropriate antibiotics may be substituted when necessary. Antibiotic therapy is continued until the septic process is controlled and wound healing is in progress, usually for 5 to 10 days.

Fractures must be placed in adequate reduction and held by effective immobilization in plaster, skeletal traction, or external fixators. Precise reduction and immobilization of the fracture help to overcome the wound infection by providing stability and eliminating dead space. In certain circumstances, some form of internal fixation of the fracture, usually with minimal osteosynthesis, may be justified.[30]

COMPLICATIONS OF OPEN REDUCTION OF FRACTURES

Patients with fractures treated by open reduction and internal fixation are subject to about the same complications as those with fractures treated by other methods. The operative method may reduce the incidence of some complications but also may increase the risk of others, particularly wound infection.

Shock

Shock from operative blood loss may be a serious complication of open reduction. In fact, if anesthesia is of high quality and the patient is not suffering from adrenocortical insufficiency, shock developing during open reduction is almost always the result of excessive loss of blood without adequate blood replacement.

Before operation for open reduction of a fracture, blood transfusions should be given in an amount calculated to compensate adequately for blood loss through open wounds or into the tissues. Failure to do this invites shock on the operating table. In the aged, blood replacement must be adequate, but there is a high incidence of pulmonary edema and myocardial failure and a high death rate in elderly patients who are given massive transfusions in an effort to overcome a chronic anemia theoretically associated with a contracted blood volume. Although blood replacement should be adequate to compensate for blood loss and to avoid hemorrhagic shock, considerable caution is indicated in the use of preoperative blood transfusions except to compensate for acute blood loss.

During the operation, sufficient blood should be given to balance the blood lost during the operation, a loss that must not be underestimated. Patients undergoing operation for internal fixation of intertrochanteric hip fractures may lose as much as 1,000 ml. of blood during the operation. Even more blood may be lost during open reduction of fractures of the femoral shaft.

The loss of blood during operation may be minimized by good operative technique. Fracture sites should be approached through fascial planes; actively bleeding vessels must be ligated; portions of the operative wound not needed should be packed while the actual operation is going on at a different part of the wound; and fragments should be reduced promptly after the fracture site has been exposed in order to minimize blood loss from the medullary canals.

The use of compression tourniquets will minimize blood loss in many instances. They are indicated whenever they are practical. A tourniquet may be left safely in place without release for approximately 1½ hours. If the operation is not complete when 1½ hours have elapsed, the wound should be packed and the tourniquet released for 15 minutes. Then, after elevation and exsanguination of the extremity, it may be reapplied. The tourniquet may then be left in place for an additional 1½ hours without danger to the extremity. This period should be ample for the completion of any operation of open reduction and internal fixation of a fracture.

An increasing number of patients are being treated with adrenal steroids. The surgeon operating on a patient previously under treatment with steroids should plan for the administration of steroids before, during, and after operation. In this way, the shock of adrenocortical insufficiency may be avoided.

Fat Embolism Syndrome

The incidence of fat embolism syndrome theoretically should be increased by intramedullary nailing of fractures. This has not been the case. There is no proof that open reduction of a fracture increases the risk of fat embolism syndrome.

Thromboembolic Disease

Patients with fractures of the lower extremities, particularly those in the older age groups, are susceptible to the complications of thromboembolic disease. Many necessarily must remain recumbent in bed for extended periods with some degree of immobilization of the injured lower extremity. Exercise of the muscles and joints of the injured extremity is often minimal, and the prophylactic value of muscle activity is lost.

Open reduction of fractures may increase the danger of thromboembolism. A period of hypotension during the operative procedure creates some venous stasis. The trauma of retractor pull and manipulation of the fragments within the wound may mechanically retard blood flow through the veins caudad to the operative field. The pain produced by the incision itself acts as a deterrent to active exercise of the extremity during the early postoperative period.

On the other hand, open reduction may reduce the incidence of thromboembolism. With the fragments stabilized in reduction, the patient may be turned in bed frequently and be promptly placed in a chair. Early active exercises of the joints and muscles of the lower extremities may often be instituted. The injured extremity may be adequately elevated to promote venous return. Especially in fractures about the hip in the aged, these advantages of open reduction and internal fixation tend to reduce the incidence of thromboembolism in comparison with closed methods of treatment.

With open reduction, a number of prophylactic measures against thromboembolism must be taken. Adequate oxygenation, adequate blood replacement, and minimal operative trauma will avoid periods of hypotension during operation. Compression bandages should be applied from the base of the toes to well above the operative wound at the completion of the operation. The compression bandage should extend in spica fashion about the hip after operations near the hip. Wrapping of the opposite extremity with an elastic bandage is an added precaution. To promote venous return, the extremity operated on should be elevated so that the ankle is slightly higher than the knee, and this in turn slightly higher than the hip. Particularly, a pillow should not be placed so as to flex the knee and thereby place the ankle lower than the knee. Early active exercises of all the muscles of both lower extremities should be instituted. As rapidly as possible, the patient should be turned frequently in bed and mobilized at least to the sitting position. When the patient is sitting, the knees should not be flexed with the legs and feet hanging unless active exercise of the knees and ankles is being carried out almost continuously.

Wound Infection

By far the most significant and potentially catastrophic local complication of open reduction is wound infection (Figs. 30–16 through 30–19). No precaution against it should be omitted.

Wound infections complicating open reduction and internal fixation of fractures fall within the wound suppuration group. Because bacterial contamination is a prerequisite for wound suppuration, every precaution must be taken against errors of omis-

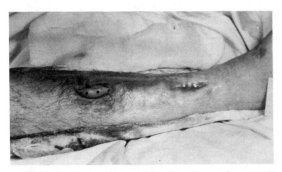

Figure 30–16 Failure of wound healing with necrosis of exposed bone. Photograph of leg showing unhealed operative wound with exposed sequestrum of bone. A fracture of both bones of the leg was treated by open reduction and internal fixation of the fracture of the tibia with a bone plate. The operative wound was closed under considerable tension. Necrosis of a portion of the wound margin followed. When the dead skin had separated and sloughed off, cortical bone and a portion of the plate and several screws were exposed. Of course the cortical bone underwent necrosis and became a sequestrum. The screws became loose, and they and the plate were removed through the open wound. This case illustrates the hazard of wound closure under excessive tension.

sion and commission violating sterile technique. Probably of greater importance, every precaution is necessary to hold to the minimum residual dead tissue and collections of blood and exudate remaining within the wound. These are the media for bacterial action to produce wound suppuration. Even with excellent technique, small particles of devitalized tissue remain in the wound (e.g., ligated vessel ends), and some postoperative oozing of blood and serum into the depths of wounds will occur; hence the importance of a rigid aseptic technique in preventing wound infection.

Precautions designed to avoid wound infection may be classified as preoperative, operative, and postoperative.

PREOPERATIVE PRECAUTIONS

Preoperative precautions against wound infection are comparable to those for all operations. The general condition of the patient must be equal to the anesthesia and the contemplated procedure. Red cell and plasma values must be at adequate levels for the particular patient and operation. Diabetes, if present, must be under control. Cardiac decompensation should have been overcome by appropriate medical therapy.

The skin at the site of the proposed incision should be healthy and have both adequate arterial supply and venous drainage. Above all, furuncles and other skin lesions that could harbor infection must not be present. The postoperative edema at this site must not be so great as to jeopardize closure of the operative wound because of excessive tension.

OPERATIVE PRECAUTIONS

Strict attention to the many details of good operative technique is an excellent precaution against wound infection. Preparation of the skin should be thorough over a large field. Draping of the operative field must be carried out with great care. Aseptic technique must be continually guarded. Devitalization of tisssue by the trauma of the operation must be minimized. Large fragments of tissue must not be clamped and ligated. The trauma of retractor pull must

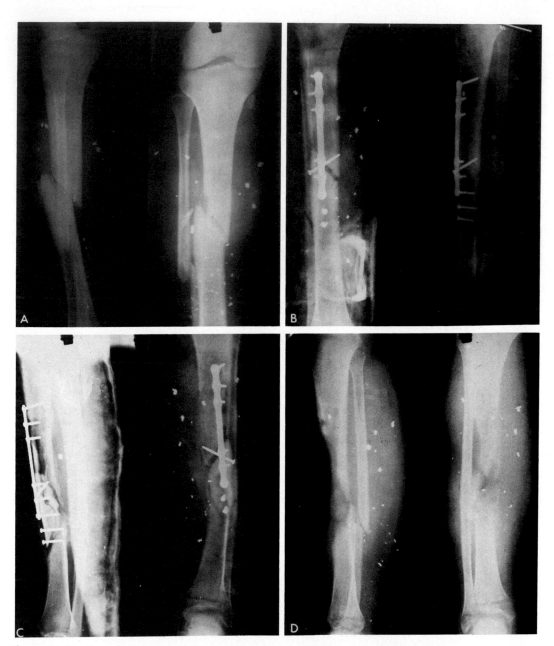

Figure 30–17   Open fracture of both bones of the leg treated by open reduction and internal fixation followed by infection and massive sequestration. *A,* Anteroposterior and lateral roentgenograms before operation. *B,* Anteroposterior and lateral roentgenograms after internal fixation of the fracture with a long plate and screws supplemented by additional screws. Actually the fracture was plated in some distraction despite all the metal. *C,* Anteroposterior and lateral roentgenograms after sepsis had developed. Note the massive sequestration and the loosening of the screws. *D,* Lateral and anteroposterior roentgenograms after removal of the metal and the sequestra. Note the extensive loss of bone from sequestration. The extensive periosteal stripping that was necessary for this internal fixation subjected the patient to the hazard of massive sequestration. The scourge of infection is the necrosis of tissue that may follow.

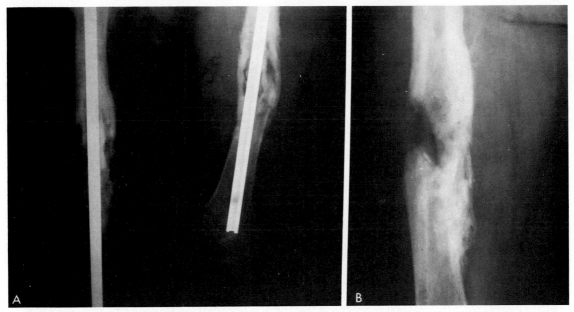

Figure 30–18   Fracture of the femoral shaft treatment by intramedullary nailing followed by infection. *A,* Anteroposterior and lateral roentgenograms showing the united fracture, but with considerable sequestration, particularly surrounding the intramedullary nail. The wound had been draining constantly for 6 months when these roentgenograms were made. *B,* Anteroposterior roentgenogram after removal of the nail and the sequestra. Note the massive defect when the dead loose bone had been removed. Although the fracture has united, union is precarious, and refracture is a possible complication.

be held to a minimum. Arterial supply of muscles should be safeguarded. Hemostasis must be adequate to prevent a postoperative hematoma in the depths of the wound. Tags of devitalized or badly traumatized soft tissue should be trimmed and discarded after internal fixation of the fracture has been completed. At the conclusion of the procedure, thorough irrigation of the wound depths and crevices is indicated to flush out small blood clots and loose bits of soft tissue. The operative wound should be closed in a manner that obliterates dead space but is loose enough to allow for egress of unavoidable serum and blood exudates from the depths of the wound, especially during the first few hours after the operation. Continuous closed suction of large deep wounds for 24 to 48 hours offers distinct advantages.

POSTOPERATIVE PRECAUTIONS

The precautions outlined earlier for preventing thromboembolism are also valuable precautions against a postoperative wound infection. The compression dressing helps to obliterate dead space and to minimize edema about the wound and thereby tends to prevent excessive tension on the sutured wound margins. Excessive tension can lead to ischemia and necrosis of wound margins and subsequent wound infection. Compression bandages should be considered part of the dressing following every open reduction and internal fixation. A plaster cast applied over the operative wound serves as the compression bandage.

Postoperative elevation of the extremity is indicated to aid venous return through the extremity. The degree of elevation must not be sufficient to retard the arterial flow to the extremity.

Prophylactic Antibiotics

Antibiotics in adequate dosage given systemically tend to prevent invasive infection of living tissue by organisms sensitive to them. Antibiotics will not sterilize dead and devitalized tissue, including massive blood clot, that remains in a wound and will not neutralize the proteolytic enzymes in un-

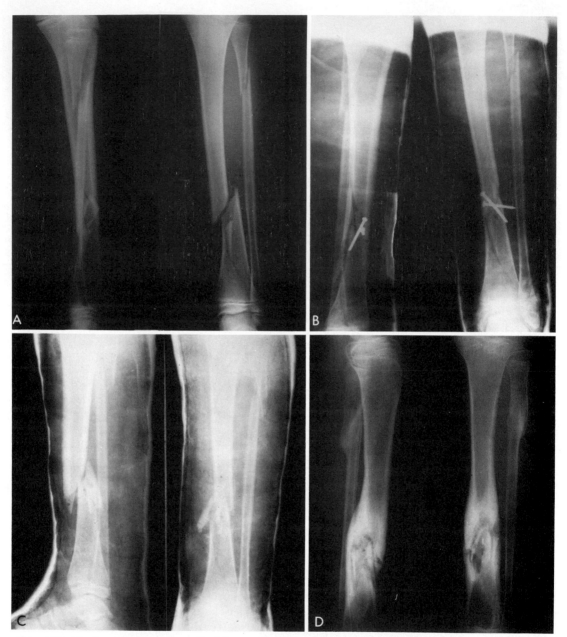

Figure 30–19   Comminuted fracture of both bones of the leg in a 12-year-old boy treated by open reduction and internal fixation followed by infection. *A,* Anteroposterior and lateral roentgenograms showing fracture of both bones of the leg on admission to the hospital. The decision to operate upon this fracture and attempt to fix it internally seems most unwise. In the first place, fracture of the shafts of long bones in growing children seldom if ever present an indication for open reduction and internal fixation. Moreover, in this instance the degree of comminution precluded a stable internal fixation. *B,* Anteroposterior and lateral roentgenograms made after the operative procedure. The direction of the screws is undesirable. The best technique places multiple screws parallel with each other and at 90 degrees to the long axis of the bone. *C,* Anteroposterior and lateral roentgenograms made after sepsis had intervened. The wound had been opened widely and the screws removed because they were loose. *D,* Anteroposterior and lateral roentgenograms showing that the fracture is united in considerable overriding, but with considerable loss of bone from sequestration and with other sequestra remaining.

drained pus. They therefore can never serve as the sole preventive measure against wound suppuration.

Although prophylactic antibiotic therapy, in association with clean elective surgery, is somewhat controversial, many reported clinical and research experiences support its use in patients undergoing extensive, prolonged open reduction and internal fixation of fractures. Moreover, prophylactic antibiotics may prevent urinary and pulmonary complications, particularly in patients in the older age groups.

When used prophylactically, antibiotics in doses adequate to insure an effective blood level should be given perioperatively, i.e., preoperatively, during operation, and postoperatively, for a few days. Provided the patient has no history of sensitivity to the agent, cephalosporins are probably the antibiotics of choice.

When antibiotics have not been given preoperatively and a definite break in sterile technique is discovered during the operation, antibiotic therapy initiated immediately by the intravenous route is appropriate.

MANAGEMENT OF POSTOPERATIVE WOUND SUPPURATION FOLLOWING OPEN REDUCTION AND INTERNAL FIXATION OF FRACTURES

The treatment of postoperative wound infection after internal fixation of a fracture is primarily surgical (Fig. 30–20). In the operating room, usually under anesthesia, the wound should be opened widely by removal in most instances of all the superficial and deep sutures. The objective is to unroof completely the abscess cavity. Material for culture and sensitivity tests should be taken from the depths of the wound. Appropriate antibiotics should be given.

The wound should be explored, with adequate retraction of wound margins, and

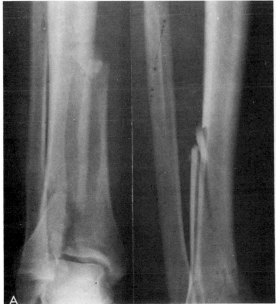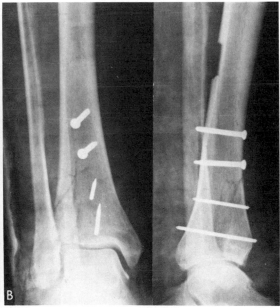

Figure 30–20 Management of wound infection after open reduction of fracture of lower portion of tibia. A, Anteroposterior and lateral roentgenograms of comminuted fracture of the distal portion of the tibia with gross distortion of the distal articular surface. B, Anteroposterior and lateral roentgenograms showing excellent restoration of normal anatomy of the lower portion of tibia, including the articular surface obtained at open reduction with internal fixation.

Unfortunately on the fifth postoperative day a rather severe postoperative wound infection was discovered. In the operating room, under anesthesia, all sutures were removed, all crevices of the wound and the ankle joint were thoroughly irrigated, and tags of devitalized tissue were excised. Enough suture of capsular and ligamentous structures was carried out to close off the ankle joint, but the remainder of the wound was left open. Five days later in the operating room the wound was uncovered and found to be clinically clean in every way. Delayed closure of the wound was then carried out followed by prompt healing. The fracture went on to union in excellent position, and a splendid functional end result was obtained.

thoroughly debrided of debris and tags of devitalized tissue. Thorough irrigation serves as a valuable cleansing method and should be carried out repeatedly during the operative procedure. The wound should be left open as a rule to obtain the best possible drainage, and frequently, in addition, dependent drainage to the wound depths should be established through a separate stab wound.

This recommended program is in contrast with the all-too-often used regimen of removal of two or three sutures, separation of the margins of this portion of the wound to permit the egress of pus, and "sticking in a drain," an inadequate approach to the problem. With an opening in the wound, pus is liberated and is no longer dammed back under pressure, fever may subside, and pain may be alleviated, but the septic process is likely to continue. The small opening in the wound is merely a safety valve. Purulent exudate containing proteolytic enzymes capable of destroying collagenous tissues bathes all parts of the wound. Devitalized tissue incident to the trauma of the operation or to the action of the pus itself remains deep in the wound. The substrate of sepsis persists. If this is to be eliminated and the wound prepared for a possible delayed closure, the program recommended in the foregoing paragraph must be instituted.

In many instances, the opened operative wound may be closed by delayed suture within a few days after it has been opened, provided it is free of dead tissue and is clinically clean. If the wound margins fall together with a good compression dressing, closure by suture is really of no significance, since the wound can heal promptly if the suppurative process has been eliminated. On the other hand, if the open wound tends to leave bony cortex, tendon, cartilage, or metallic internal fixation exposed, enough closure of the wound by suture to cover these structures is indicated and should be carried out if it appears surgically feasible.

As a rule, internal fixation devices should not be removed. The metal may prove to be a deterrent to wound healing, but at this particular time the stability it provides is most advantageous not only in maintaining reduction of the fracture but also in combating the septic process by providing thorough immobilization of the fragments. If wound healing is not obtained within a reasonable time, the matter of removal of metal may be considered. Provided continuing wound suppuration is controlled, it should remain in place until enough bony union has occurred to stabilize the fracture. Loose metal, however, is a deterrent to wound healing and is ineffective for immobilization of the fragments. Loose metal usually should be removed promptly.

NERVE OR VASCULAR INJURY

Injury to a major peripheral nerve trunk or artery during open reduction and internal fixation of a fracture is an avoidable complication. It may be obviated by proper operative technique. Occasionally minor sensory nerves or arteries must be sacrificed for better exposure, but they should be safeguarded as much as possible. Knowledge of the best operative approaches to bones and of the anatomic relations of nerves and arteries is a fundamental prerequisite to selection of the method of open reduction and internal fixation.

For indicated treatment of injured nerves or blood vessels, reference should be made to standard texts and current literature.

DELAYED UNION AND NON-UNION

Despite careful selection of cases for open reduction and internal fixation and despite precise operative techniques, delayed union or non-union of some fractures will follow. Their incidence can be minimized, however, by adherence to established principles, techniques, and precautions. Violation of these is likely to lead to delayed union and non-union that would have been preventable.

When the anticipated time for union of a fracture after open reduction and internal fixation has been reached or exceeded without roentgenographic evidence of union, some additional surgery may be advisable. A state of non-union should not be allowed to go on and on because the complication is either not recognized or accepted, as may occur when the internal fixation is providing so much stability that signs of non-union on physical examination are masked. The non-union must be recognized and an ap-

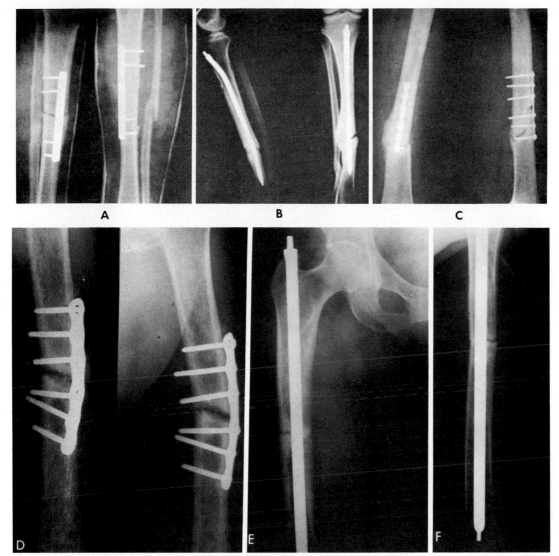

Figure 30–21   Errors in technique that predispose to delayed union and nonunion. *A,* Lateral and anteroposterior roentgenograms showing fracture of tibia plated in some distraction with a rather short plate which was placed on the anteromedial surface of the tibia. Such technique predisposes to non-union. *B,* Lateral and anteroposterior roentgenograms showing non-union of fracture of tibia that had been treated by intramedullary nailing. The nail is entirely too short and provides only minimal fixation of fragments. Note that the fibula united. The impending non-union might have been recognized early. Appropriate operative treatment would have included fibula osteotomy to permit some impaction of the tibial fragments, replacement of the short nail with one of adequate length, and bone grafting of the fracture site. *C,* Anteroposterior and lateral roentgenograms showing non-union of oblique fracture of shaft of femur that was fixed internally with a plate and screws. The plate was too short; no real fixation distal to the fracture site was provided. The distal screw merely encroached on the fracture site and contributed nothing. Actually, this fracture might have been better stabilized and a more desirable end result obtained by intramedullary nailing, perhaps with some supplemental fixation. (Courtesy of Dr. E. C. Holscher.) *D,* Anteroposterior and lateral roentgenograms showing non-union of fracture of the humerus which was fixed in distraction by a plate and screws that were too long. Plating in distraction practically ensures non-union. Screws of such excessive length predispose to injury to major peripheral nerves and blood vessels. *E* and *F,* Anteroposterior and lateral roentgenograms showing delayed union of transverse fracture of femoral shaft 4½ months after internal fixation with an intramedullary nail. Actually, the nail did not fill the canal so as to provide splendid immobilization of the fragments. This delayed union was recognized and appropriate treatment instituted. A larger nail was inserted, and iliac bone grafts were placed about the fracture site. Prompt union was obtained.

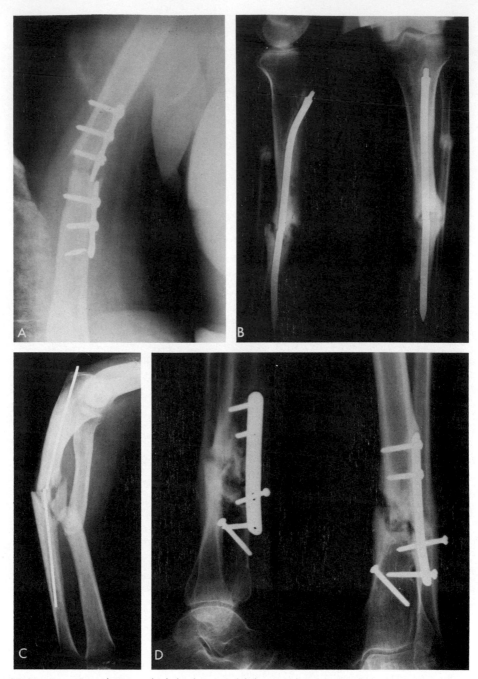

Figure 30–22   Errors in technique which lead to metal failures and non-union. *A,* Anteroposterior roentgenogram showing broken plate and non-union of fracture of shaft of humerus. The fracture was plated in some distraction; a screw was inserted practically into the fracture site; a drill bit was snapped off to remain embedded in the bone. *B,* Lateral and anteroposterior roentgenograms showing broken intramedullary nail at site of nonunion of tibia. The nail was inserted with the takeoff point too low, the fragments of the tibia angulated laterally and with the fragments of the fibula end to end. With this method for treatment of fractures of the tibia the takeoff point should be high, the fragments in good alignment (after the nail has been inserted it may be bent forcibly to correct malalignment such as that shown in this illustration), and fibula fragments should be offset to permit them to override and permit impaction of the tibial fragments. *C,* Roentgenogram of forearm showing broken pin at fracture site of ulna. The pin is entirely too small to be effective, especially for a comminuted fracture. The fragments of both the radius and the ulna should have been stabilized in excellent apposition and alignment. A frank non-union is impending. *D,* Lateral and anteroposterior roentgenograms showing non-union of fracture of tibia. Both plate and screws were too short. The fibula fragments should have been offset to permit them to override slightly, and a slotted plate should have been used on the tibia. (Courtesy of Dr. Fred C. Reynolds.)

propriate operation performed, usually bone grafting. This procedure may be indicated in the stage of delayed union as a safeguard against non-union. At operation for either delayed union or non-union, replacement of the internal fixation may be advantageous. To delay reoperation excessively risks breaking of the internal fixation device from long-continuing strain on the metal.

The outstanding symptoms of non-union are persistent low-grade pain at the fracture site and restricted function of the extremity. The important signs are tenderness and pain on rotatory and angulatory strain at the fracture site. The diagnosis is really made by careful study of the roentgenograms. Exuberant callus about fragment ends, but not actually bridging them, must not be interpreted as healing in progress. Slightly overexposed roentgenograms are preferable when assessing the status of union of a fracture.

ERRORS IN TECHNIQUE AND METAL FAILURES. Errors in technique and metal failures may singly or in combination result in delayed union or non-union (Figs. 30–21 through 30–23). Although either may independently lead to such complications, these two factors are not unrelated in their effect on the healing process. Failure to properly insert or apply metallic devices diminishes their immobilizing effect, which in turn predisposes to failure of union. Both improper technique of application and an impaired healing process place undue and continuing strain on the metal, which is likely to bend or even break under the stress. Failure to provide adequate external immobilization such as a plaster cast for fractures fixed internally also may lead to fatigue fracture of the metal. The majority of internally fixed fractures require additional external immobilization. Fractures of the femur stabilized with large Küntscher intramedullary nails are glaring exceptions. Once the metal has broken, non-union is almost certain.

A metallic internal fixation device must meet two basic requirements: it must have sufficient strength and rigidity, and it must not corrode within the tissues. Either Vitallium or 317 S.M.O. stainless steel when properly annealed and passivated meets these requirements.

The internal fixation device must be con-structed of sufficient mass of material and be designed and fashioned properly so that it will withstand the postoperative strain of normal muscle pull that continues even in a plaster cast. Stainless steel must not have been age-hardened or excessively work-hardened; otherwise, the internal fixation device may not have sufficient strength. All stainless steel for internal fixation of fractures should be of a uniform Rockwell hardness of C35, which provides enough stability and still enough ductility to permit precise designing. Occasionally an item for internal fixation must be molded slightly at the operating table so that it will conform to the contour of the bone in the region of the fracture, as in the plating of a fracture 4 inches below the knee. The metallic device, however, should not be bent back and forth in repeated efforts to achieve the desired degree of molding, since bending weakens the metal considerably and predisposes to subsequent breaking. As will be pointed out, even a single molding carries the hazard of initiating corrosion.

Every precaution must be taken against electrolytic reaction within the tissues that would lead to corrosion of metal, resorption of bone, and loosening of the implanted metal. Metals of different composition should not be used in the same internal fixation. This means that Vitallium and stainless steel should not be used together; moreover, different items of S.M.O. stainless steel of varying composition and properties (such as different degrees of Rockwell hardness) should not be used together.

The metal should not show imperfections or be scratched, dented, or otherwise marred. Such blemishes break the polished protective coat of chromic oxide and set the stage for electrolysis and corrosion. Efforts to bend or mold metallic devices at the operating table create the same defects and series of events. A common site for a break in the protective seal is the hole in a plate where it is scored by a screw. Re-use of internal fixation devices is to be condemned for obvious reasons. Fatigue stress and corrosion potentiate each other. Fatigue stress cracks the protective seal over the surface of the metal and corrosion begins; or corrosion begins at a defect in the metal that is weakened and may break at this point under fatigue stress.

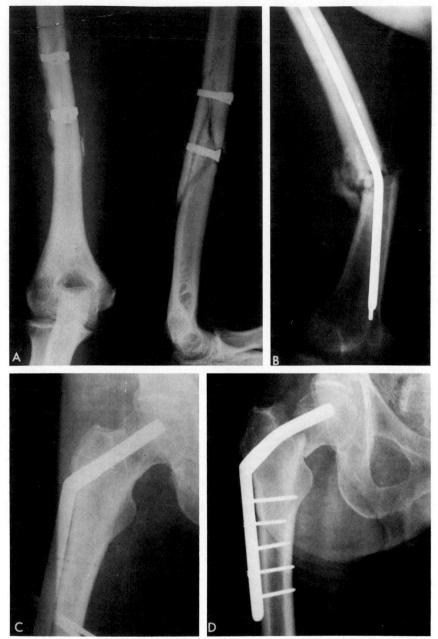

Figure 30–23   Metal failures that predispose to non-union. *A*, Anteroposterior and lateral roentgenograms showing non-union of fracture of humerus that was fixed internally with Parham-Martin bands. These were applied too tightly. Apparently blood supply to the butterfly fragment was strangulated. The bands have caused necrosis and cut into the cortex. (Courtesy of Dr. E. C. Holscher.) *B*, Anteroposterior roentgenogram showing bent intramedullary nail and impending non-union of fracture of femoral shaft. Apparently this nail was fashioned from a soft stainless steel that bends too easily for fractures of the femoral shaft. When this complication is encountered, the nail should be straightened forcibly to permit removal and replaced with a nail of adequate size and strength. Bone grafting of the fracture site is usually desirable. *C*, Anteroposterior roentgenogram showing fracture of neck of femur stabilized by one-piece nail plate. This roentgenogram was obtained in the operating room just before placement of the screws through the holes in the plate. The lateral roentgenogram also showed excellent reduction of the fracture and placement of the nail. *D*, Anteroposterior roentgenogram 2 weeks later shows the metal failure. The nail bent at the fracture site, allowing displacement of the fracture. The only explanation is that the nail was made of too soft a metal.

The ASIF compression plating material meets all desired criteria and when used according to the recommended technique, on proper indications and with proper precautions should hold delayed union and non-union to the minimum. Internal fixation of fractures is a precise surgical procedure to be performed with full appreciation of the physiology of healing of fractures, the advantages and disadvantages of the operative method and the limitations and requirements of the metallic devices to be used. Adherence to the ASIF principles will pay dividends in the form of a low incidence of metal failures, non-union of fractures, and infections.

Bibliography

1. Altemeier, W. A.: Diagnosis, classification and general management of gas producing infections, particularly those produced by *Clostridium perfringens*. *In* Brown, J., and Cox, B. (Eds.): Proceedings of the Third International Conference on Hyperbaric Medicine, Washington, D.C., National Academy of Sciences, National Research Council, 1966.

2. Altemeier, W. A., and Culbertson, W. R.: Acute nonclostridial crepitant cellulitis. Surg. Gynecol. Obstet. *87*:206, 1948.

3. American College of Surgeons Committee on Trauma. A Guide to Prophylaxis Against Tetanus in Wound Management. Bull. Amer. Coll. Surgeons, *57*:32, 1972.

4. Ashby, M. E.: Low-velocity gunshot wounds involving the knee joint: Surgical management. J. Bone Joint Surg. *56A*:1047, 1974.

5. Athanasoulis, C. A.: Angiography to assess pelvic vascular injury. N. Engl. J. Med. *284*:1329, 1971.

6. Atik, M.: Platelet adhesiveness and thromboembolism. 5th European Conference on Microcirculation, Gothenburg, 1968. Bibl. Anat. *10*:494, 1969.

7. Barton, N. J.: Radial nerve lesions. Hand *5*:200, 1973.

8. Bassett, C. A. L., Pilla, A. A., and Pawluk, R. J.: A non-operative salvage of surgically-resistant pseudoarthrosis and non-unions by pulsing electromagnetic fields: A preliminary report. Clin. Orthop. *124*:128, 1977.

9. Batalden, D. J., Wickstrom, P. H., Ruiz, E., and Gustilo, R. B.: Value of the G-suit in patients with severe pelvic fracture. Arch. Surg. *109*:326, 1974.

10. Blom, S., and Dahlback, L. O.: Nerve injuries in dislocations of the shoulder joint and fractures of the neck of the humerus. Acta Chir. Scand. *136*:461, 1970.

11. Bohlman, H.: The pathology and current treatment concepts of cervical-spine injuries: A critical review of 300 cases. J. Bone Joint Surg. *54A*:1353, 1972.

12. Bonfiglio, M.: Aseptic necrosis of the femoral head in dogs: Effect of drilling and bone grafting. Surg. Gynecol. Obstet. *98*:591, 1954.

13. Bowden, R. E. M., and Gutmann, E.: The fate of voluntary muscles after vascular injury in man. J. Bone Joint Surg. *32B*:354, 1949.

14. Boyd, H. B., Lipinski, S. W., and Wiley, J. H.: Observations on non-union of the shafts of the long bones, with a statistical analysis of 842 patients. J. Bone Joint Surg. *43A*:159, 1961.

15. Braunstein, P. W., Skudder, P. A., McCarroll, J. R., Musolino, A., and Wade, P. A.: Concealed hemorrhage due to pelvic fracture. J. Trauma *4*:832, 1964.

16. Brav, E. A.: The management of open fractures of the extremities. *In* American Association of Orthopedic Surgeons, Instructional Course Lectures. Vol. XIII, Ann Arbor, J. W. Edwards, 1956, p. 227.

17. Brav, E. A.: Further evaluation of the use of intramedullary nailing in the treatment of gunshot fractures of the extremities. J. Bone Joint Surg. *39A*:513, 1957.

18. Brav, E. A.: Traumatic dislocation of the hip joint. J. Bone Joint Surg. *44A*:1115, 1962.

19. Brav, E. A.: Open fractures: Fundamentals of management. Postgrad. Med. *39*:11, 1966.

20. Brav, E. A., and Jeffress, V. H.: Modified intramedullary nailing in recent gunshot fractures of the femoral shaft. J. Bone Joint Surg. *35A*:141, 1953.

21. Bright, R. W.: Operative correction of partial epiphyseal plate closure by osseous-bridge resection and silicon-rubber implant. J. Bone Joint Surg., *56A*:655, 1974.

22. Brighton, C. T., Friedenberg, Z. B., Mitchell, E. I., and Booth, R. E.: Treatment of non-union with constant direct current. Clin. Orthop., *124*:106, 1977.

23. Brooks, M.: The Blood Supply of Bone. New York, Appleton-Century-Crofts, 1971.

24. Brown, J. T.: Nerve injuries complicating dislocation of the shoulder. J. Bone Joint Surg. *34B*:526, 1952.

25. Brown, P. W., and Kinman, P. B.: Gas gangrene in a metropolitan community. J. Bone Joint Surg. *56A*:1445, 1974.

26. Brown, P. W., and Urban, J. G.: Early weight bearing treatment of open fractures of the tibia. An end-result study of sixty-three cases. J. Bone Joint Surg. *51A*:59, 1969.

27. Burke, J. F.: The effective period of preventive antibiotic action in experimental incisions and dermal lesions. Surgery *50*:161, 1961.

28. Burkhalter, W. E.: Open injuries of the lower extremity. Surg. Clin. North Am. *53*:1439, 1973.

29. Burkhalter, W. E.: Early tendon transfer in upper extremity peripheral nerve injury. Clin. Orthop. *104*:68, 1974.

30. Burri, C.: Post-Traumatic Osteomyelitis. Bern, Hans Huber Publishers, 1975.

31. Canale, S. T., and Bourland, W. L.: Fracture of the neck and intertrochanteric region of the femur in children. J. Bone Joint Surg. *59A*:431, 1974.

32. Carr, C. R., and Turnipseed, D.: Experiences with intramedullary fixation of compound fe-

moral fractures in war wounds. J. Bone Joint Surg. *35A*:153, 1953.

33. Cass, A. S.: Urinary tract trauma. Minn. Mcd. *57*:15, 1974.

34. Castle, M. E., and Orinion, E. A.: Prophylactic anticoagulation in fractures. J. Bone Joint Surg. *52A*:521, 1970.

35. Catto, M.: Histological study of avascular necrosis of femoral head after transcervical fracture. J. Bone Joint Surg. *47B*:749, 1965.

36. Checketts, R. G., and Bradley, J. G.: Low-dose heparin in femoral neck fractures. Injury *6*:42, 1974.

37. Cole, W. G.: Fractures and dislocation compounded by distal ischemia. Med. J. Aust. *1*:98, 1975.

38. Connolly, J. F., Whittaker, D., and Williams, E.: Femoral and tibial fractures combined with injuries to the femoral or popliteal artery. J. Bone Joint Surg. *53A*:56, 1971.

39. Conolly, W. B., and Hedberg, E. A.: Observations on fractures of the pelvis. J. Trauma *9*:104, 1969.

40. Cotton, F. J.: Elbow dislocation and ulnar injury. J. Bone Joint Surg. *11*:348, 1929.

41. Cozen, L.: Does diabetes delay fracture healing? Clin. Orthop. *82*:134, 1972.

42. Crawford, A.: Fractures about the knee in children. Orthop. Clin. North Am. *7*:638, 1976.

43. Culp, O. S.: Treatment of ruptured bladder and urethra: Analysis of eighty-six cases of urinary extravasation. J. Urol. *48*:266, 1942.

44. Danis, R.: Theorie et Pratique de l'Ostiosynthèse. Paris, Masson, 1947.

45. Davis, D. D., Bohlman, H. H., Walker, A. E., Fisher, R., and Robinson, R. A.: The pathologic findings in fatal craniospinal injuries. J. Neurosurg. *34*:603, 1971.

46. Davis, G. L.: Management of open wounds of joints — Experience during the Vietnam War. A preliminary study. J. Bone Joint Surg. *51A*:1032, 1969.

47. DeBakey, M. E., and Simeone, F. A.: Battle injuries of the arteries in World War II. An analysis of 2,471 cases. Ann. Surg. *123*:534, 1946.

48. DeHaven, K. E. and Evarts, C. M.: The continuing problem of gas gangrene: A review and report of illustrative cases. J. Trauma *11*:983, 1971.

49. Dehne, E.: Ambulatory treatment of the fractured tibia. Clin. Orthop. *105*:192, 1974.

50. Dennis, C.: Disaster following femoral vein ligation for thrombophlebitis: Relief by fasciotomy: Clinical case of renal impairment following crush injury. Surgery *17*:164, 1945.

51. deTakats, G.: Sympathetic reflex dystrophy. Med. Clin. North Am. *49*:117, 1965.

52. Doran, F. S. A., White, M., and Drury, M.: A clinical trial designed to test the relative value of two simple methods of reducing the risk of venous stasis in the lower limbs during surgical operations, the danger of thrombosis, and a subsequent pulmonary embolus, with a survey of the problem. Br. J. Surg. *57*:20, 1970.

53. Doty, D. B., Treiman, R. L., Rothschild, P. D., and Gaspar, M. R.: Prevention of gangrene due to fractures. Surg. Gynecol. Obstet. *125*:284, 1967.

54. Druken, W. R., Hubay, C. A., Holden, W. D., and Bukornic, J. A.: Pathogenesis of posttraumatic sympathetic dystrophy. Am. J. Surg. *97*:454, 1959.

55. Eaton, R. G., and Green, W. T.: Epimysiotomy and fasciotomy in the treatment of Volkmann's ischemic contracture. Orthop. Clin. N. Am. *3*:175, 1972.

56. Edsall, G.: The inexcusable disease. J.A.M.A. *235*:62, 1976.

57. Edvardsen, P., and Syversen, S.: Overgrowth of the femur after fracture of the shaft in childhood. J. Bone Joint Surg. *57B*:338, 1976.

58. Ehrlich, W.: Bisherige Ergebnisse unserer operative Knochenbruchbehandlung, unter besonderer Berucksichtigung des Küntscher-Nagels. Arch. f. Orthop. u. Unfall-Chir. *42*:377, 1943.

59. Ellis, H.: The speed of healing after fracture of the tibial shaft. J. Bone Joint Surg. *40B*:42, 1958.

60. Elstrom, J. A., Pankovich, A. M., and Egwele, R.: Extra-articular low velocity gunshot fractures of the radius and ulna. J. Bone Joint Surg. *60A*:335, 1978.

61. Ennis, J. E.: Effect of methylmethacrylate in osteosynthesis. Clin. Orthop. *105*:283, 1974.

62. Ernst, C. B., and Kaufer, H.: Fibulectomy-fasciotomy. An important adjunct in the management of lower extremity arterial trauma. J. Trauma *11*:365, 1971.

63. Feagin, J. A., and White, A. A., III: Volkmann's ischemia treated by transfibular fasciotomy. Milit. Med. *138*:497, 1973.

64. Fee, N. F., Dobranski, A., and Bisla, R. S.: Gas gangrene complicating open forearm fractures. J. Bone Joint Surg. *59A*:135, 1977.

65. Fisher, G. W.: Acute arterial injuries treated by the United States Army Medical Service in Vietnam 1965–1966. J. Trauma *7*:844, 1967.

66. Freeland, A. E., and Mutz, S. B.: Posterior bone-grafting for infected ununited fractures of the tibia. J. Bone Joint Surg. *58A*:653, 1976.

67. Froman, C., and Stein, A.: Complicated crushing injuries of the pelvis. J. Bone Joint Surg. *49B*:24, 1967.

68. Gallus, A. S., Hirsh, J., O'Brien, S. E., McBride, J. A., Tuttle, R. J., and Gent, M.: Prevention of venous thrombosis with small, subcutaneous doses of heparin. J.A.M.A. *235*:1980, 1976.

69. Gaspard, D. J., Cohen, J. L., and Gaspar, M. R.: Decompression dermotomy, a limb salvage adjunct. J.A.M.A. *220*:831, 1972.

70. Ger, R., Condrea, H., and Steichen, F. M.: Traumatic intrapelvic retroperitoneal hemorrhage: An experimental study. J. Surg. Res. *9*:31, 1969.

71. Glenn, J. N., Miner, M. E., and Peltier, L. F.: The treatment of fractures of the femur in patients with head injuries. J. Trauma *13*:958, 1973.

72. Gossling, H. R., Ellison, L. H., and DeGraff, A. C.: Fat embolism. J. Bone Joint Surg. *56A*:1327, 1974.

73. Govan, A. D. T.: Account of pathology in some cases of *Clostridium welchii* infection. J. Pathol. Bacteriol. *58*:423, 1946.

74. Griffin, P.: Fractures of the shaft of the femur in children. Orthop. Clin. North Am. *3*:213, 1972.

75. Griffin, P.: Fractures of the femoral diaphysis in

children. Orthop. Clin. North Am. 7:633, 1975.

76. Griffiths, D. L.: Volkmann's ischemic contracture. Br. J. Surg. 28:239, 1940.

77. Gustilo, R. B., and Anderson, J. T.: Prevention of infection in the treatment of one thousand and twenty-five open fractures of long bones. J. Bone Joint Surg. 58A:453, 1976.

78. Haebler, C.: Experiences with the marrow nail operation according to the principles of Küntscher. Gunshot fractures of the femur. U.S. Armed Forces Med. J. 1:65, 1950.

79. Hamilton, H. W., Crawford, J. S., Gardinier, J. H., and Wiley, A. M.: Venous thrombosis in patients with fracture of the upper end of the femur. J. Bone Joint Surg. 52B:265, 1970.

80. Hampton, O. P., Jr.: The indications for debridement of gunshot (bullet) wounds of the extremities in civilian practice. J. Trauma 8:475, 1968.

81. Hampton, O. P., Jr.: Editorial. Management of open fractures and open wounds of joints. J. Trauma 8:475, 1968.

82. Hargens, A. R., Romine, J. R., Sipe, J. C., Evans, K. L., Mubarak, S. J., and Akeson, W. H.: Peripheral nerve conduction block by high muscle-compartment pressure. J. Bone Joint Surg. 61A:192, 1979.

83. Hauser, C. W., and Perry, J. F., Jr.: Massive hemorrhage from pelvic fractures. Minn. Med. 49:285, 1966.

84. Heim, H.: Marknagelung von Oberschenkelschussfrakturen. Chirurg 15:387, 1943.

85. Heim, V., and Pfeiffer, K. M.: Small Fragment Set Manual. New York, Springer-Verlag, 1974.

86. Heiple, K. G.: The pathologic physiology of nonunion. Clin. Orthop. 43:11, 1965.

87. Holstein, A., and Lewis, G. B.: Fractures of humerus with radial nerve paralysis. J. Bone Joint Surg. 44A:1382, 1962.

88. Hoopes, J. E., and Jabaley, M. E.: Soft tissue injuries of the extremities. In Ballinger, W. F., II, Rutherford, R. B., and Zuidema, G. D. (Eds.): The Management of Trauma. Philadelphia, W. B. Saunders Company, 1973.

89. Howland, W. S., and Ritchey, S. J.: Gunshot fractures in civilian practice. An evaluation of the results of limited surgical treatment. J. Bone Joint Surg. 53A:47, 1971.

90. Hughes, C. W.: Arterial repair during the Korean War. Ann. Surg. 147:555, 1958.

91. Hunter, G. A.: Posterior dislocation and fracture dislocation of the hip. J. Bone Joint Surg. 51B:38, 1969.

92. Kaiser, T. F., and Farrow, F. C.: Injury of the bladder and prostatomembranous urethra associated with fracture of the bony pelvis. Surg. Gynecol. Obstet. 120:99, 1965.

93. Kane, W. J.: Fractures of the pelvis. In Rockwood, C. A., Jr., and Green, D. P. (Eds.): Fractures. Philadelphia, J. B. Lippincott, 1975.

94. Kaplan, J. Z., and Pruitt, B. A.: Burns and fractures. In Heppinstall, R. B. (Ed.): Fracture Treatment and Healing. Philadelphia, W. B. Saunders Co., 1980.

95. Kass. E. H.: Asymptomatic infection of the urinary tract. Assoc. Am. Physicians, 69:56, 1956.

96. Keever, J. E., Rockwood, C. A., and Heckman, J. D.: Flail chest and fractures aided by cast brace and mobility. J.A.M.A. 239:1839, 1978.

97. Kelly, R. P., and Whitesides, T. E., Jr.: Transfibular route for fasciotomy of the leg. In Proceedings of the American Association of Orthopedic Surgeons. J. Bone Joint Surg. 49A:1022, 1967.

98. Kinman, P. B., Catanzaro, R., and Brown, P. B.: Gunshot wounds of extremities. J. Bone Joint Surg. 57A:1029, 1975.

99. Kline, D. G., and Hackett, E. R.: Reappraisal of timing for exploration of civilian peripheral nerve injuries. Surgery 78:54, 1975.

100. Küntscher, G.: Die Marknagelung von Knochenbrüchen. Arch. f. Klin. Chir., 200:443, 1940.

101. Küntscher, G., and Maata, R.: Technik der Marknagelung. Leipzig, Georg Thieme, 1945.

102. Langenskjöld, A.: An operation for partial closure of an epiphyseal plate in children and its experimental basis. J. Bone Joint Surg. 57B:325, 1975.

103. Lankford, L. L., and Thompson, J. E.: Reflex sympathetic dystrophy, upper and lower extremity: Diagnosis and management. American Association of Orthopedic Surgeons Instructional Course Lectures. Vol. XXVI, St. Louis, Mosby, 1977, p. 163.

104. Levine, J. I., and Crampton, R. S.: Major abdominal injuries associated with pelvic fractures. Surg. Gynecol. Obstet. 116:223, 1963.

105. Linscheid, R. L., and Wheeler, D. K.: Elbow dislocations. J.A.M.A. 194:1171, 1965.

106. Livingston, W. R.: Pain Mechanisms. A Physiologic Interpretation of Causalgia and Its Related States. New York, Macmillan, 1943.

107. MacIntyre, I. M. C., Vasilescu, C., Jones, D. R. B., et al.: Heparin versus dextran in the prevention of deep venous thrombosis. Multi-unit controlled trial. Lancet 2:118, 1974.

108. MacKinnon, K. J., and Susset, J. H.: Urinary complications of fractures of the pelvis. In Moseley, H. F. (Ed.): Accident Surgery. Vol. 2. New York, Appleton-Century-Crofts, 1964.

109. McNeur, J. C.: The management of open skeletal trauma with particular reference to internal fixation. J. Bone Joint Surg., 52B:54, 1970.

110. Mannerfelt, L.: Median nerve entrapment after dislocation of the elbow. J. Bone Joint Surg. 50B:152, 1968.

111. Margolies, M. N., Ring, E. J., Waltman, A. C., Kerr, W. S., Jr., and Braum, S.: Arteriography in the management of hemorrhage from pelvic fractures. N. Engl. J. Med. 287:317, 1972.

112. Matsen, F. A., III, Mayo, K. A., Sheridan, G. W., and Krugmire, R.B., Jr.: Monitoring of intramuscular pressure. Surgery 79:702, 1976.

113. Matsen, F. A., III, Winquist, R. S., and Krugmire, R. B.: Diagnosis and management of compartment syndromes. J. Bone Joint Surg. 62A:286, 1980.

114. Matter, P., and Rittman, W. W.: The Open Fracture. Bern, Hans Huber Publishers, 1977.

115. Mayer, P. J., and Evarts, C..: Nonunion, delayed union, malunion and avascular necrosis. In Epps, C. H., Jr. (Ed.): Complications in Orthopedic Surgery. Philadelphia, J. B. Lippincott Co., 1978, p. 159.

116. Meek, R. N.: Personal communication. 1980.

117. Meyer, S., Weiland, A. J., and Willeneggar, H.: The treatment of infected nonunion of fractures of long bones. Study of sixty-four cases with a five to twenty-one year follow-up. J. Bone Joint Surg. 57A:836, 1975.

118. Miller, H. H., and Welch, C. S; Quantitative studies on the time factor in arterial injuries. Ann. Surg. 130:428, 1949.

119. Millesi, H., Meissl, G., and Berger, A.: The interfascicular nerve-grafting of the median and ulnar nerves. J. Bone Joint Surg. 54A:727, 1972.

120. Mitchell, S. W., Morehouse, G. R., and Keen, W. W.: Gunshot Wounds and Other Injuries of Nerves. Philadelphia, J. B. Lippincott, 1864.

121. Morrell, M. T.: The incidence of pulmonary embolism in the elderly. Geriatrics 25:138, 1970.

122. Morton, J. H., Southgate, W. A., and DeWeese, J. A.: Arterial injuries of the extremities. Surg. Gynecol. Obstet. 123:611, 1966.

123. Motsay, G. J., Manlove, C., and Perry, J. F., Jr.: Major venous injuries with pelvic fracture. J. Trauma 9:343, 1969.

124. Müller, M. E., Allgöwer, M., Schneider, R., and Willenegger, H.: Manual of Internal Fixation. New York, Springer-Verlag, 1979.

125. Murbarak, S. J., Hargens, A. R., Owen, C. A., Garetto, Z. P., and Akeson, W. H.: The Wick catheter technique for measurement of intramuscular pressure. A new research and clinical tool. J. Bone Joint Surg. 58A:1016, 1976.

126. Murbarak, S. J., and Owen, C. A.: Double-incision fasciotomy of the leg for decompression in compartment syndromes. J. Bone Joint Surg. 59A:184, 1977.

127. Murray, D. G., and Raca, G. B.: Fat embolism syndrome. J. Bone Joint Surg. 56A:1338, 1974.

128. Neer, C.: Fractures and dislocations of the shoulder. In Rockwood, C., Jr., and Green, G. (Eds.): Fractures. Philadelphia, J. B. Lippincott, 1975.

129. Omer, G. E., Jr.: Injuries to nerves of the upper extremities. J. Bone Joint Surg. 56A:1615, 1974.

130. Orr, H. W.: Osteomyelitis and compound fractures of the pelvis. Surg. Gynecol. Obstet. 54:673, 1932.

131. Pappas, A.: Fractures of the leg and ankle. Orthop. Clin. North Am. 7:657, 1976.

132. Paradies, L. H., and Gregory, C. F.: Early treatment of close-range shotgun wounds. J. Bone Joint Surg. 48A:425, 1966.

133. Patman, R. D., and Thompson, J. E.: Fasciotomy in peripheral vascular surgery. Arch. Surg. 101:663, 1970.

134. Patterson, F. P., and Morton, K. S.: Neurologic complications of fractures and dislocations of the pelvis. Surg. Gynecol. Obstet. 112:702, 1961.

135. Patzakis, M. J., Dorr, L. D., Ivler, D., Moore, T. M., and Harvey, J. P.: The early management of open joint injuries. A prospective study of one hundred forty patients. J. Bone Joint Surg. 57A:1065, 1975.

136. Patzakis, M. J., Harvey, J. P., and Ivler, D.: The role of antibiotics in the management of open fractures. J. Bone Joint Surg. 56A:532, 1974.

137. Peacock, E. E., and VanWinkle, W., Jr.: Surgery and Biology of Wound Repair. Philadelphia, W. B. Saunders Company, 1970.

138. Peltier, L. F.: Complications associated with fractures of the pelvis. J. Bone Joint Surg. 47A:1060, 1965.

139. Peltier, L. F.: Fat embolism. Orthop. Clin. North Am. 1:13, 1970.

140. Prather, G. C., and Kaiser, T. C.: Bladder in fracture of bony pelvis: Significance of "tear drop bladder" as shown by cystoscopy. J. Urol. 63:1019, 1950.

141. Protzman, R. R., and Burkhalter, W. E.: Femoral-neck fractures in young adults. J. Bone Joint Surg. 58A:689, 1976.

142. Pruitt, B. A.: Other complications of burn injury. In Artz, C. P., Moncrief, J. A., and Pruitt, B. A. (Eds.): Burns, A Team Approach. Philadelphia, W. B. Saunders Company, 1979, p. 533.

143. Rang, M.: Children's Fractures. Philadelphia, J. B. Lippincott, 1974.

144. Ravitch, M. M.: Hypogastric artery ligation in acute pelvic trauma. Surgery 56:601, 1964.

145. Reinarz, J. A., Pierce, A. K., Mays, B. B., and Sanford, J. P.: The potential role of inhalation therapy equipment in nosocomial pulmonary infection. J. Clin. Invest. 44:831, 1965.

146. Reynolds, B. M., and Balsano, N.A.: Venography in pelvic fractures. A clinical evaluation. Am. Surg. 173:104, 1971.

147. Rich, N. M., Baugh, J. H., and Hughes, C. W.: Acute arterial injuries in Vietnam: One thousand cases. J. Trauma 10:359, 1970.

148. Rich, N. M., Metz, C. W., Hutton, J. E., Baugh, J. H., and Hughes, C. W.: Internal versus external fixation of fractures with concomitant vascular injuries in Vietnam. J. Trauma 11:463, 1971.

149. Ring, E. J., Athanasoulis, C., Waltman, A. C., et al.: Arteriographic management of hemorrhage following pelvic trauma. Radiology 109:65, 1973.

150. Riska, E. B., vonBonsdorff, H., Hakkinen, S., Jaroma, H., Kiviluoto, O., and Paavilainen, T.: Prevention of fat embolism by early internal fixation of fractures in patients with multiple injuries. Injury 8:110, 1975.

151. Robson, M. C., Lea, C. E., Dalton, J. B., and Heggers, J. P.: Quantitative bacteriology and delayed wound closure. Surg. Forum 19:501, 1968.

152. Roding, B., Groeneveld, P. H. A., and Boerema, I.: Ten years of experience in the treatment of gas gangrene with hyperbaric oxygen. Surg. Gynecol. Obstet. 134:579, 1972.

153. Root, H. D., and Van Tyn, R. A.: A device and method for the atraumatic transportation of the injured patient. Surgery 58:327, 1965.

154. Rorabeek, C. H., and Clarke, K. M.: The pathophysiology of the anterior tibial compartment syndrome: An experimental investigation. J. Trauma 18:299, 1978.

155. Sagar, S., Massey, J., and Sanderson, J. M.: Low-dose heparin prophylaxis against fatal pulmonary embolism. Br. Med. J. 4:257, 1975.

156. Salter, R., and Harris, W.: Injuries involving the

epiphyseal plate. J. Bone Joint Surg. *45A*:587, 1963.

157. Sarmiento, A.: A functional below-the-knee cast for tibial fractures. J. Bone Joint Surg. *49A*:855, 1967.

158. Sarmiento, A.: A functional below-the-knee brace for tibial fractures. A report on its use in one hundred thirty-five cases. J. Bone Joint Surg. *52A*:295, 1970.

159. Sarmiento, A.: Functional bracing of tibial and femoral shaft fractures. Clin. Orthop. *82*:2, 1972.

160. Sarmiento, A.: Functional bracing of tibial fractures. Clin. Orthop. *105*:202, 1974.

161. Sarmiento, A., Cooper, J. S., and Sinclair, W. F.: Forearm fractures. Early functional bracing — A preliminary report. J. Bone Joint Surg. *57A*:297, 1975.

162. Sarmiento, A., Kinman, P. B., Galvin, E. G., Schmidt, R. H., and Phillips, J. G.: Functional bracing of fractures of the shaft of the humerus. J. Bone Joint Surg. *59A*:596, 1977.

163. Sarmiento, A., Kinman, P. B., Murphy, R. B., et al.: Treatment of ulnar fractures by functional bracing. J. Bone Joint Surg. *58A*:1104, 1976.

164. Sarmiento, A., Latta, L., Zilioli, A., et al.: The role of soft tissue in the stabilization of tibial fractures. Clin. Orthop. *105*:116, 1974.

165. Scapinelli, R.: Blood supply of the human patella. Its relation to ischemic necrosis after fracture. J. Bone Joint Surg. *49B*:563, 1967.

166. Scully, R. E., Artz, C. P., and Saco, Y.: An evaluation of the surgeon's criteria for determining muscle viability during debridement. Arch. Surg. *73*:1031, 1956.

167. Seavers, R., Lynch, J., Ballard, R., Jernigan, S., and Johnson, J.: Hypogastric artery ligation for uncontrollable hemorrhage in acute pelvic trauma. Surgery *55*:516, 1964.

168. Seddon, H. J.: Surgical Disorders of the Peripheral Nerves. 2nd Ed. Edinburgh, Churchill, Livingstone, 1975.

169. Segmüller, G., Cech, O., and Bekier, A.: Diagnostic use of eighty-five strontium in the preoperative evaluation of nonunion. Acta Orthop. Scand. *41*:150, 1970.

170. Sevitt, S.: Fat embolism. London, Butterworth, 1962.

171. Sevitt, S., and Gallagher, N. G.: Prevention of venous thrombosis and pulmonary embolism in injured patients. Lancet *2*:981, 1959.

172. Sher, M. H.: Principles in the management of arterial injuries associated with fractures/dislocations. Ann. Surg. *182*:630, 1975.

173. Sheridan, G. W., Matsen, F. A., III, and Krugmire, R. B., Jr.: Further investigations on the pathophysiology of the compartment syndrome. Clin. Orthop. *123*:266, 1977.

174. Sherman, R. T., and Parrish, R. A.: Management of shotgun injuries: A review of one hundred fifty-two cases. J. Trauma *3*:76, 1963.

175. Silver, R., and Moulton, A.: Prophylactic anticoagulant therapy against pulmonary emboli in acute paraplegia. Br. Med J. *2*:338, 1970.

176. Steinbrocker, O., and Argyros, T. G.: The shoulder-hand syndrome: Present status as a diagnostic and therapeutic entity. Med. Clin. North Am. *42*:1533, 1958.

177. Sternlieb, C. M.: Incidence of silent postoperative pulmonary emboli in geriatric patient. J. Am. Geriatr. Soc. *18*:242, 1970.

178. Stewart, M. J., and Milford, L. W.: Fracture-dislocation of the hip. J. Bone Joint Surg. *36A*:315, 1954.

179. Stinchfield, F., et al.: The effect of anticoagulant therapy on bone repair. J. Bone Joint Surg. *38A*:270, 1956.

180. String, S. T., and Barcia, P. J.: Complications of small dose prophylactic heparinization. Am. J. Surg. *130*:570, 1975.

181. Sudek, P.: Ueber Die akute (trophoneurotische) Knockenatrophie nach Entzundungen und Traumen der Extremitaten. Dtsch. Med. Wochenschr. *28*:336, 1902.

182. Teal, P. V.: The effect of anticoagulation on fracture healing. J. Bone Joint Surg. *55A*:425, 1973.

183. Thompson, J.E., and Berry, F. B.: Penetrating wounds of major joints. Ann. Surg. *126*:947, 1947.

184. Thompson, V. P., and Epstein, H. C.: Traumatic dislocation of the hip. J. Bone Joint Surg. *33A*:746, 1951.

185. Tubiana, R., and Duparc, J.: Prevention of thrombo-embolic complications in orthopaedic and accident surgery. J. Bone Joint Surg. *43B*:7, 1961.

186. Turnipseed, W. D., and Crummy, A. B.: Computerized intravenous arteriography. J.A.M.A. *244*:537, 1980.

187. Vandenbussche, F., Butrville, V, Courtin, V., Vandevord, J., and Decoulx, P.: Fractures in burns. Abstracts of the 5th International Congress on Burn Injuries, Stockholm, Sweden, 1978, p. 93.

188. vanVroonhoven, T.J.M.V., vanZiji, J., and Muller, H.: Low-dose subcutaneous heparin versus oral anticoagulants in the prevention of postoperative deep-venous thrombosis. A controlled clinical trial. Lancet *1*:375, 1974.

189. Volkmann, R.: Die Ischaemischen Muskellamungen and Kontrakturen. Cbl. Chir. *51*:801, 1881.

190. Wagner, H.: Surgical lengthening or shortening of femur and tibia. Technique and indications. Prog. Orthop. Surg. *1*:71, 1977.

191. Waldvogel, F. A., and Vasey, H.: Osteomyelitis: The past decade. New Engl. J. Med. *303*:360, 1980.

192. Weber, B. G., and Čech, O.: Pseudoarthrosis, Pathology, Biomechanics, Therapy, Results. Bern, Hans Huber Medical Publishers, 1976.

193. Weil, G. C., Price, E. M., and Rusbridge, H. W.: The diagnosis and treatment of fractures of the pelvis and their complications. Am. J. Surg. *44*:108, 1939.

194. Weisz, G. M., Rang, M., and Salter, R. B.: Post traumatic fat embolism in children: Review of the literature and experience in the Hospital for Sick Children, Toronto. J. Trauma *13*:529, 1973.

195. Whitesides, T. E., Jr., Haney, T. C., Mosimoto, K., and Hirada, H.: Tissue pressure measurements as a determinant for the need of fasciotomy. Clin. Orthop. *113*:43, 1975.

196. Witschi, T. H., and Omer, G. E., Jr.: The treatment of open tibial shaft fractures from the Vietnam War. J. Trauma *10*:105, 1970.

197. Wolff, G., Dillman, M., Rüedi, T. H., Buchmann,

B., and Allgöwer, M.: Koordination von Kurgie und Intensive-Medizin zur Vermeidung der posttraumischen respiratorischen Insuffizienz. Unfallheilkunde *81*:425, 1978.

198. Wray, J. B.: Treatment of ununited fractures of the long bones: Factors in the pathogenesis of nonunion. J. Bone Joint Surg. *47A*:168, 1965.

199. Wright, I. S.: Pulmonary embolism: A most un-derdiagnosed and untreated disorder. J. Am. Geriatr. Soc. *22*:433, 1974.

200. Wrobel, L. J., Virgilio, R. W., and Trimble, C.: Inapparent hypoxemia associated with skeletal injuries. J. Bone Joint Surg. *56A*:346, 1974.

201. Ziperman, H. H.: The management of soft tissue missile wounds in war and peace. J. Trauma *1*:361, 1961.

31

COMPLICATIONS OF TRANSPLANTATION

Charles W. Putnam
and Thomas E. Starzl

During the last decade whole-organ transplantation, particularly of the kidney, has become increasingly established as a sophisticated kind of patient service. As a consequence, transplantation centers have been started in almost every part of the world. In the United States there are few major medical schools that do not have the capability of carrying out transplantation of at least the kidney. Medical students, house officers, and faculty members are being called upon increasingly to participate directly or indirectly in the management of the resulting complications and problems.

It is the purpose of this chapter to discuss the many things that can go wrong after whole-organ transplantation and to indicate what may be done of a corrective nature. As will become evident, the complications stem from one or more of the following etiologic factors: (1) preexisting organ failure; (2) technical imperfections in the performance of transplantation; (3) inability to control rejection of the new organ; (4) side effects of immunosuppressive agents given to prevent rejection; and (5) other coincidental disease not related either to organ failure or to immunosuppression.

SPECIAL ANESTHETIC CONSIDERATIONS

With transplantation of either the kidney or liver, the patient enters the operation with a well defined loss of certain metabolic pathways by which anesthetic agents are detoxified or excreted or both.

Renal Transplantation

The anesthetic complications facing renal homograft recipients during their transplantations are the consequence of uremia.

Charles W. Putnam was born in Massachusetts and was elected to Alpha Omega Alpha at Northwestern University Medical School. He served his internship and residency at the University of Colorado Medical Center, and was awarded a USPHS Post Doctorate Surgical Traineeship. His experience in transplantation is reflected in his extensive publications in this field of research and practice. He is now Associate Professor of Surgery, University of Arizona College of Medicine, and Chief of Surgery, Tucson VA Medical Center.

Thomas E. Starzl was born in Iowa and attended Westminster College. He received both the M.D. and Ph.D. degrees from Northwestern University, where he was elected to Alpha Omega Alpha. Following internship and residency training at the Johns Hopkins Hospital and the University of Miami, he was named a Markle Scholar in Medical Science. An early worker in the newly applied clinical science of tissue transplantation, he is universally recognized as a world leader in organ transplantation in man. He established the University of Colorado as a mecca for those interested in the art and science of organ transfer. Dr. Starzl is now Professor of Surgery at the University of Pittsburgh.

If homograft function is prompt and adequate, many of the potential problems such as fluid overload or hyperkalemia will be speedily relieved. However, not all homografts achieve a remedial level of function intraoperatively, and the safest approach to the anesthetic management of these patients is to assume that prompt urine excretion will not occur.

There are no specific contraindications to any of the common inhalant anesthetic agents. Considerable care must be exercised in the choice and administration of muscle relaxants, however. In 1964, Virtue cautioned against the use of the depolarizing agent succinylcholine in recently dialyzed patients, in whom hepatic pseudocholinesterase, upon which succinylcholine inactivation depends, may sometimes be nearly absent. Although Sarmina et al.[101] have utilized succinylcholine in their recipients without incident, our anesthesiologists generally prefer to limit its use to induction, particularly if the patient has any evidence of hepatic insufficiency or hyperkalemia.

Prolonged muscle paralysis following successful transplant procedures was observed by Aldrete et al. in 10 (4.8 per cent) of 206 patients who received the non-depolarizing agents gallamine or d-tubocurarine (Table 31–1) for muscle relaxation.[1] In addition to decreased muscle strength, respiratory function was inadequate in these patients and prolonged ventilatory support was required. The complication occurred significantly more frequently with gallamine than with d-tubocurarine. With either agent, the paralysis was not uniformly prevented by the administration of appropriate doses of anticholinesterase-type drugs.[1] It is hardly surprising that this problem does occur, since gallamine in normal animals and man

is excreted almost entirely by the kidney and d-tubocurarine is removed by a renal pathway at about a 90 per cent level.

In renal recipients, continuous electrocardiographic surveillance intraoperatively is essential to detect and treat cardiac arrhythmias before potentially lethal conduction defects supervene. Most such arrhythmias are directly related to disordered potassium balance. Of particular concern are preoperative serum potassium concentrations above 6 mEq./l. or below 2.5 mEq./l. Attention should be directed to the serum potassium concentration before the final pretransplantation dialysis. If this value exceeds 6 mEq./l., it may be lowered temporarily by a single hemodialysis but a rebound hyperkalemia will frequently occur intraoperatively, as has been emphasized by Aldrete.[2]

A fall of 25 per cent or more of the systolic blood pressure is common during renal transplantation.[1] Since most recipients enter the operating room hypertensive, such a decline is rarely of clinical importance. In actuality, it frequently signifies a restoration toward normal physiology by virtue of removal of the diseased kidneys and the provision of adequate renal function.

Chronic anemia also is a nearly universal preoperative finding and need not cause concern. Patients with uremia tolerate this condition well and preparatory transfusion is usually not indicated. In fact, transfusions in the immediate preoperative period may precipitate cardiac failure, since a compensatory increase in plasma volume has usually already occurred.[40] Instead, blood loss is replaced volumetrically during the transplantation with packed red cells.

Aldrete has described intraoperative hyperpyrexia in a few cases of renal homo-

TABLE 31–1   INCIDENCE OF PROLONGED MUSCLE PARALYSIS*

Muscle Relaxant Drug	Number of Patients	Number with Prolonged Weakness	Percent	Significance
Gallamine	15	3	20	p = <0.01
d-Tubocurarine	191	7	3.6	
Total	206	10	4.8	(of all cases)

*From Aldrete, J. A., Daniel, W., O'Higgins, J. W., Homatas, J., and Starzl, T. E.: Analysis of anesthetic-related morbidity in human recipients of renal homografts. Anesth. Analg. *50*:321, 1971.

transplantation. The explanation for this complication has not been defined, although it may have been related to the prior administration of heterologous antilymphocyte globulin (ALG). In any case, it is important to monitor the intraoperative body temperature.

Hepatic Transplantation

With transplantation of the kidney, pharmacologic considerations must take into account the loss of a renal excretory pathway. With hepatic replacement the problem is infinitely more complex, since so many anesthetic drugs commonly used are either processed by the liver or else have the capability of injuring the liver.

In addition, the liver operations tend to be long and bloody. Finally, with liver replacement (orthotopic transplantation) a major hemodynamic insult is incurred intraoperatively when the inferior vena cava and portal vein are temporarily occluded during the anhepatic phase while the new organ is being sutured in place. Pappas et al.[80] have shown that the cardiac output during this critical time may be reduced to one-half or less of the prior state.

The complex anesthetic management problems of liver transplantation were worked out and described in detail by Aldrete. The essentials for success include extensive monitoring of such diverse measurements as arterial and central venous pressures, electrocardiogram, urine output, blood pH, electrolytes, glucose, and blood gases. There must be provision for multiple intravenous inlets. When possible, Aldrete has preferred inhalation anesthesia with enflurane added to a nitrous oxide–oxygen mixture and combined with muscle relaxants as needed.

Other Organs

For heart, pancreatic, and lung transplantation, there have not been such specific problems of drug detoxification.

TECHNICAL COMPLICATIONS

Errors in technique during the performance of renal or hepatic transplantation

have made substantial contributions to the post-transplantation morbidity and mortality. Because of the obviously greater technical complexity of hepatic transplantation, technical complications have been and continue to be more frequent after this procedure than after renal transplantation. Moreover, with either procedure a technical error that in the ordinary surgical setting might be of little or no consequence may, in the face of immunosuppression, prove to be a clinically devastating or fatal one. For this reason, every effort must be made to achieve an anatomically and physiologically acceptable result at the time of surgery.

Renal Transplantation

The techniques used in the construction of the vascular anastomoses in renal transplantation have been well standardized,[112] and it is extremely unusual to encounter vascular problems postoperatively. For example, in our first 64 cases of renal transplantation, there was only one case of arterial thrombosis and none of venous occlusion. Since that time, there have been reports of complications related to both vascular anastomoses, including renal artery stenosis[102] or renal artery occlusion requiring thrombectomy,[59] arteriovenous fistula of the transplant vessels,[9] rupture of the homograft caused by renal vein thrombosis originating from iliofemoral thrombophlebitis,[34] and major arterial hemorrhage postoperatively, almost invariably related to an infected arterial suture line.[78]

From time to time, in the course of revascularization, the arterial supply of the donated kidney has been such that it has been impossible to completely revascularize it. Most frequently, a small polar arterial branch must be sacrificed in the course of donor nephrectomy or else it proves to be too tiny for successful reanastomosis. The consequence of accepting incomplete revascularization is the production of a regional infarct which, in certain instances, may be as large as one-third of the kidney mass. In our experience the only adverse effects of even a large infarct have been transient hypertension and early postoperative hematuria.

In contrast to vascular problems, urinary tract complications have been encountered frequently. Several of the leading centers in renal transplantation have extensively reviewed their experiences with this kind of complication.[62, 63, 79, 95, 116] However, for the purposes of this discussion, we have chosen as illustrative material a review of 216 consecutive patients from our series.[116]

In these 216 recipients, 234 kidneys were transplanted. In 178 instances, urinary drainage was reconstituted with ureteroneo-

cystostomy as depicted in Figure 31–1. The urinary tracts of the other 56 kidneys were reconstructed with ureteroureterostomies (Fig. 31–2). In most instances, this latter procedure was performed even though ureteroneocystostomy was technically feasible. However, in a minority, ureteroureterostomy was performed either because the homograft ureter was too short to reach the

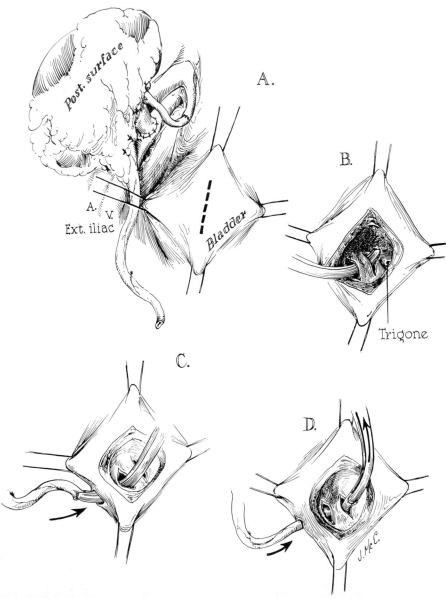

Figure 31–1   Ureteroneocystostomy. *A*, The incision in the dome of the bladder is usually no more than 1.5 cm. *B*, Development of the submucosal tunnel. Often the more lateral counterincision is not necessary. *C* and *D*, Placement of the ureter within the tunnel. The passage through the muscular layers should be widely dilated.

Illustration continued on opposite page

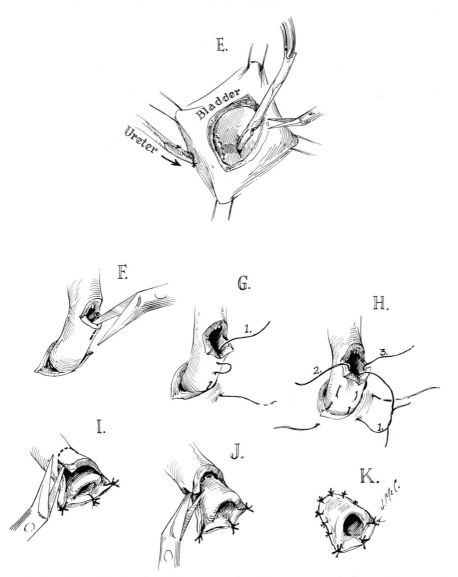

Figure 31–1 *Continued. E* and *F,* Trimming of the ureter. *G* through *J,* Formation of a flat nipple. *K,* Completed ureterovesical anastomosis. The sutures are placed with 5-0 or 6-0 plain catgut on a swaged needle. (From Starzl, T. E., et al.: Urological complications in 216 human recipients of renal transplants. Ann. Surg. *172:*1, 1970.)

bladder, or because of other anatomic considerations such as scarring of the bladder from previous surgery.

With both kinds of ureteral reconstruction, there is approximately a 10 per cent incidence of serious urologic complications. However, the two procedures differ in both the timing of the complication and its character. With ureteroneocytostomy the most frequent complication (3 per cent) was late stricture that usually required reconstruction. Early complications such as urinary

fistula were less common and were usually caused by necrosis of either the distal ureter or the renal pelvis. In contrast, with ureteroureterostomy there was a relatively high incidence of early complications; urinary fistula occurred in 6 (10.9 per cent) of the 56 primary ureteroureterostomies. Late stricture was not seen with this kind of reconstruction.

With the development of a urinary tract complication, prompt reoperation is indicated, particularly if the difficulty occurs in the

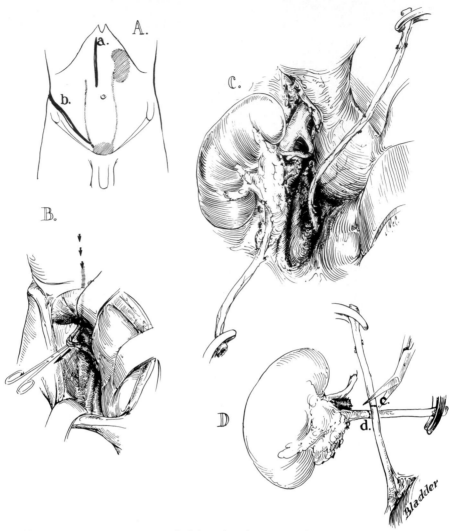

Figure 31–2   Ureteroureterostomy. *A*, Incision for bilateral nephrectomy and splenectomy: The ureter is tied just below the ureteropelvic junction (a). The lower incision (b) is for kidney transplantation. *B*, Recipient site for transplantation, showing the recipient ureter being delivered into the iliac fossa by gentle traction. *C* and *D*, The vascular anastomoses have been completed. The donor and recipient ureters are positioned to be adjacent to each other and are tailored.

Illustration continued on opposite page

early postoperative period. This urgency for reestablishing a watertight urinary system has no parallel in standard urologic practice. In a patient who has the normal capability to heal and resist infection, most urinary fistulas would be expected to eventually close spontaneously. The same cannot be said for the recipient of a renal homograft, who must be treated with potent immunosuppressive agents that predispose to infection in the transplant wound and retard the healing process that would ordinarily close the fistula. Because of these special

considerations, our policy has been to attempt to close urinary fistulas surgically before the supervention of wound sepsis.

Since potentially life-threatening complications have been observed with approximately equal frequency after each kind of reconstruction, a categoric recommendation for one method in preference to the other may not be warranted on statistical grounds. Nevertheless, it is our recommendation that ureteroneocystostomy usually be the first choice, since it requires less technical finesse, is associated with a lower incidence of urinary fistula, and ensures the preservation of long segments of both the donor and recipient ureters for later anastomosis should that become necessary.

Lymphoceles have been diagnosed by ultrasonography[111] or detected at intravenous pyelography by external compression of the patient's bladder or homograft ureter (Fig. 31–3). In several instances, hydronephrosis had developed with concomitant diminution of renal homograft function. Drainage of the lymphocele through the transplant incision, intraperitoneally[13, 76] or by means of closed drainage systems, such as Jackson-Pratt drains, results in relief of the hydrone-

phrosis and improvement in renal function.

Other reported urologic complications include calyceal-cutaneous fistulae[33] and renal calculi, which are, however, exceedingly rare.[73]

Hepatic Transplantation

After renal transplantation, the life-threatening vascular or urinary tract complication may be averted when necessary by removal of the homograft. With hepatic transplantation, however, this ultimate re-

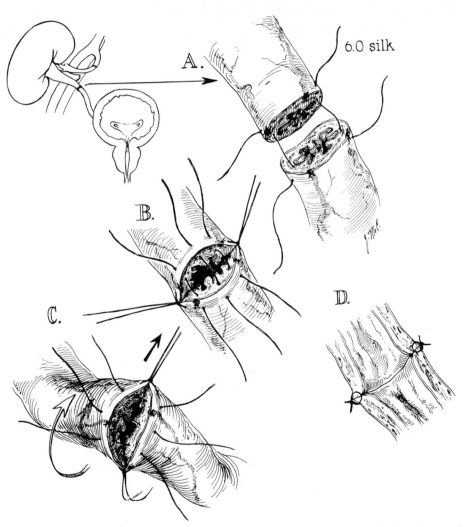

Figure 31–2 *Continued.* Single layer anastomosis performed with 6-0 or 7-0 silk swaged on fine cardiovascular needles. In *D* is shown a longitudinal section with correct placement of the silk sutures. Note the intact mucosa, with no sutures extending into the lumen. (From Starzl, T. E., et al.: Urological complications in 216 human recipients of renal transplants. Ann. Surg. *172*:1, 1970.)

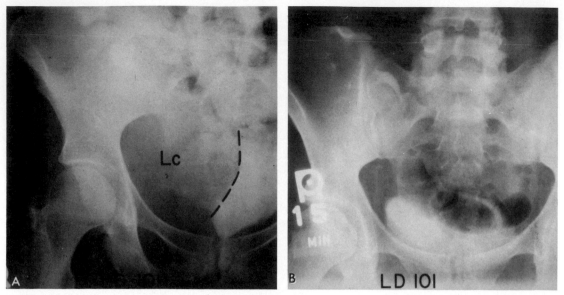

Figure 31–3 *A,* Ureteral obstruction 3 months postoperatively, caused by a large lymphocele (Lc) in the transplant wound. The bladder deformity is evident. *B,* After drainage of the lymphocele the hydronephrosis was completely relieved. The patient is alive 3½ years after operation. (From Starzl, T. E., et al.: Urological complications in 216 human recipients of renal transplants. Ann. Surg. *172*:1, 1970.)

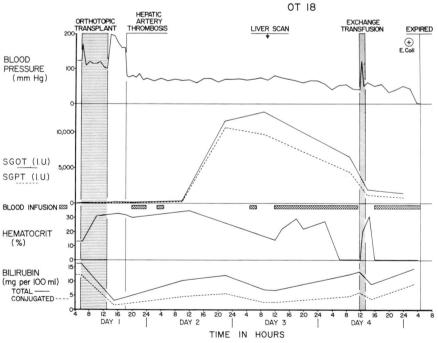

Figure 31–4 The course of a 1-year-old child with extrahepatic biliary atresia who was treated with orthotopic liver transplantation. The hepatic artery of the homograft apparently underwent thrombosis within a few hours after operation, but this fact was not reflected in transaminase level rises until almost a day later. The eventual drop of the hematocrit to almost zero was due to massive hemolysis. (From Starzl, T. E., Brettschneider, L., Penn, I., Bell, P., Groth, C. G., Blanchard, H., Kashiwagi, N., and Putnam, C. W.: Orthotopic liver transplantation in man. Transplant. Proc. *1*:216, 1969. By permission of Grune & Stratton, Inc.)

medial step cannot be taken, and preservation of the patient's life depends upon successful treatment of the complication without homograft hepatectomy. Thus, it is not surprising that technical misadventures have made a major contribution to both the mortality and the morbidity following liver transplantation.[113]

In the two major series of liver transplantations, those compiled at the University of Colorado by Starzl[113, 117, 120, 127] and at Cambridge-King's College by Calne and Williams,[17, 19, 20, 143] the early experience was characterized by a high mortality rate, the main causes of which were technical or mechanical problems. These included instances of excessive ischemic damage to the homografts by the events of donor death or during organ preservation, of thrombosis or kinking of the blood supply to the transplanted liver, of intraoperative cerebral air embolism originating from the homograft, and of biliary duct obstruction.

VASCULAR COMPLICATIONS. If hepatic arterial occlusion occurs early after transplantation, the complication is uniformly lethal. Death may occur almost immediately from massive hepatic necrosis (Fig. 31–4). Alternatively, delayed death from regional hepatic infarction with concomitant sepsis may follow this kind of complication.

Venous thrombosis following liver transplantation is rare. In the Denver series there has been one such complication; in this instance, anatomic anomalies of the recipient portal vein and hepatic artery probably played an important role.

The frequent use of microsurgical techniques, particularly in pediatric recipients, has made a major contribution to the prevention of vascular complications.[117, 127]

BILIARY RECONSTRUCTION. The major technical pitfall of liver transplantation has been the biliary tract. Changing strategies in biliary reconstruction are evident in both the Colorado and the British experience. Until 1976, we routinely performed cholecystoduodenostomy. Its simplicity, however, was negated by a 30 per cent incidence of obstruction or bile fistula, both frequently fatal.[64, 126] Moreover, bacterial contamination of the homografts via the cholecystoduodenal anastomosis often resulted in cholangitis and systemic infection. Unfortunately, many of these biliary complications were not diagnosed until autopsy.

The Colorado group now believes that biliary reconstruction is best achieved with choledochocholedochostomy (Fig. 31–5A), employing a T-tube stent that is left in place for 1 to 2 years.[117] Alternatively, when a common duct anastomosis is not feasible, as in the case of children with biliary atresia, a cholecystojejunostomy (Fig. 31–5B) is performed. With this reconstruction, however, obstruction of the cystic duct has necessitated conversion to choledochojejunostomy (Fig. 31–5C) in nearly one-third of the cases.

It should be emphasized that the frequent

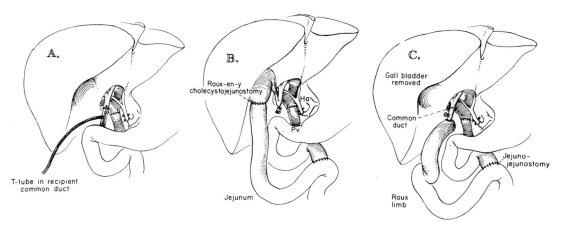

Figure 31–5 Techniques of biliary duct reconstruction used for most of the transplantation recipients in the Colorado series. A, Choledochocholedochostomy. Note that the T-tube is placed, if possible, in recipient common duct. B, Cholecystojejunostomy. C, Choledochojejunostomy after removal of gallbladder. (By permission of Med. Clin. North Am. 63:507, 1979.)

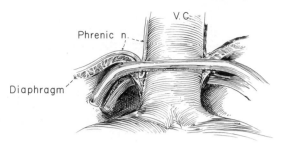

Figure 31–6 Probable mechanism of operative injury of the right phrenic nerve in four pediatric recipients of orthotopic liver homografts. Note the inclusion of the nerve in the bite of the vascular clamp, which has been placed across the suprahepatic vena cava and which has also included a piece of diaphragm. (From Starzl, T. E.: Experience in Hepatic Transplantation. Philadelphia, W. B. Saunders Company, 1969.)

use of T-tube, transhepatic,[127] or endoscopic retrograde cholangiography[117] (the choice being dictated by the method of reconstruction) is mandatory in the rapid identification of biliary difficulties.

Calne's group[16] has advocated an alternative approach in which the common duct and gallbladder are interconnected to form a common chamber; the fundus of the gallbladder is then anastomosed to the recipient common duct or to a Roux-en-Y limb of jejunum. A T-tube stent of the anastomosis enables frequent irrigation and cholangiography. With this technique they have reduced their incidence of biliary complications.

CEREBRAL AIR EMBOLISM. Focal cerebral infarctions occurred in nearly 10 per cent of the first 48 patients in the Colorado series. Air emboli from the homografts were identified as the cause.[130] Apparently, air released into the pulmonary circulation gained access to the systemic arterial system, including the cerebral vessels, by passage through right to left veno-arterial shunts, which are common in liver disease. Prevention is simple: during revascularization of the homograft, a portal venous cannula is infused with electrolyte solution; air bubbles escape through the vena caval cuff as that anastomosis is completed.

OTHER TECHNICAL PROBLEMS. Other complications directly or indirectly attributable to technical errors at the time of hepatic transplantation include hemorrhage caused by a generalized bleeding diathesis,[37] right diaphragmatic palsy apparently caused by the vascular clamp placed too far superior on the suprahepatic inferior vena cava (Fig. 31–6), and infarction of the right adrenal gland in the course of recipient hepatectomy. This last complication is an important one for the surgeon to understand, since it may be the cause of uncontrollable hemorrhage. The basis for the complication is the need to sacrifice the right adrenal vein which drains into the excised retrohepatic vena cava (Fig. 31–7). In about 20 per cent of our cases of orthotopic transplantation, the adrenal gland then has undergone venous infarction and has become the site of hemorrhage that can be controlled only by removal of the gland.

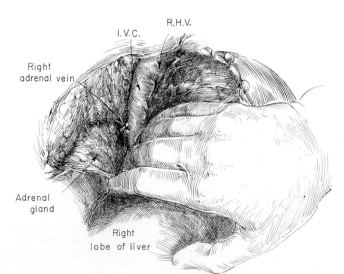

Figure 31–7 Ligation of the right adrenal vein in the course of recipient hepatectomy. Opening of the bare area of the right hepatic lobe has exposed the adrenal gland. The right adrenal vein, which is usually the only posterior tributary to the retrohepatic vena cava, is then ligated and divided. In about 20 per cent of cases, the adrenal gland will undergo infarction and become the site of hemorrhage that can be controlled only by right adrenalectomy. (From Starzl, T. E.: Experience in Hepatic Transplantation. Philadelphia, W. B. Saunders Company, 1969.)

In one case, this kind of regional venous hypertension with hemorrhage necessitated reoperation and probably contributed to the death of the patient.

REJECTION

The central issue in transplantation of any organ is control of the immunologic process by which tissue that is not genetically identical is normally repudiated. Thus rejection — its diagnosis and its prevention — dominates and influences all other events of the postoperative period.

Hyperacute Rejection

This is the most convulsive and ruinous immunologic complication that may be visited upon homografts. The explanation for hyperacute rejection was well worked out a decade ago.[54, 110, 114, 118, 135, 142] As far as can be determined, the initiating event is exposure of the transplant to host blood containing preformed antibodies possessing anti graft specificity. Most commonly, these antibodies are of the cytotoxic variety and are the result of presensitization by exposure to histocompatibility or other antigens by blood transfusions, during pregnancy, or in the course of an earlier transplantation. Cross-reacting antibodies to streptococcal antigens have also been implicated by First et al.[29] In some patients whose homografts undergo hyperacute rejection, no preformed antibodies can be identified but the assumption that they are present is usually made.

The possibility that cytotoxic IgM in the homologous plasma used in ex vivo perfusion will cause immune injury and precipitate an accelerated rejection has also been raised in two cases reported by Light et al.[60]

The events of hyperacute rejection occur with great rapidity. After an organ is revascularized it fails to assume a normal pink hue or it initially has this color but loses it within a few seconds to hours and becomes cyanotic. Not only are antibodies absorbed by the transplant, but essentially simultaneously there is sequestration within the organ of white cells, platelets, and red cells. Finally, there is clearance by the graft of clotting

factors. In this way, the blood supply of the graft becomes plugged with complex thrombi, and this leads to its almost instant devascularization.

Once hyperacute rejection has occurred, there are no known remedial steps that can be taken. The best course is to recognize that the homograft has been lost and in the case of the kidney to remove it promptly since it will predictably undergo ischemic necrosis. If a patient undergoes one hyperacute rejection, the chances of this accident occurring again are greatly increased, and special efforts should be made to identify preformed antigraft antibodies before proceeding with a secondary transplantation.

Delayed Rejection

If homograft rejection occurs despite treatment with immunosuppressive agents, the process usually begins relatively early, within a few days or weeks after operation, when the onset might have been expected had no therapy been given. In Figure 31–8 are illustrated some of the findings of renal homograft rejection in a patient whose initial treatment was with azathioprine. Typically, there is an initial period of satisfactory homograft function followed by deterioration of this function. In the case shown, the kidney performed perfectly at first, but after about 16 days the BUN began to rise, the creatinine clearance fell, proteinuria increased, there was a tendency to hypertension (controlled by medication), and relative oliguria occurred. At the same time, the patient became febrile and had a leukocytosis. In short, there were the findings of secondary failure of the homograft in a patient who exhibited a systemic febrile illness.

It is now well known that the onset of rejection is no cause for despair since this process is so readily reversible. In the case shown (Fig. 31–8), the primary treatment with azathioprine was reinforced with heavy doses of prednisone with a resulting prompt reversal of all the adverse findings. Later, it became possible to reduce drastically the doses of prednisone required to prevent a recurrence of rejection, and after 5 months the steroid therapy was stopped altogether. For 9½ of the 10 years since transplantation, this patient has been treated with

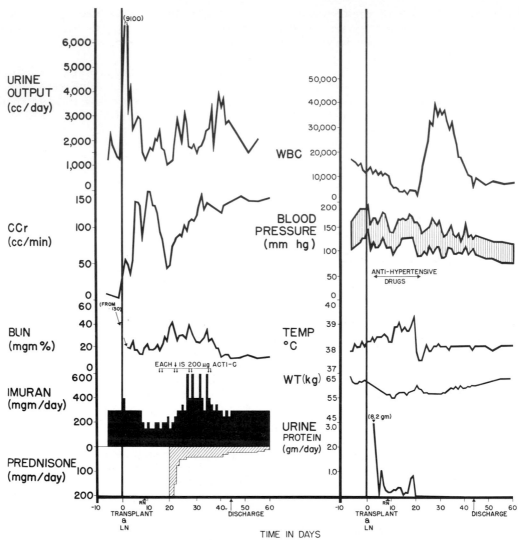

Figure 31–8 Classic rejection crisis in a patient being treated with the double-drug combination of azathioprine (Imuran) and prednisone. Deterioration of renal function began 17 days after transplantation. All stigmata of rejection are present except for acute hypertension and weight gain, which were successfully prevented by medical treatment. The homograft, transplanted on April 17, 1963, still functioned normally 10 years post transplantation. Its appearance at biopsy after 2 years was normal. Acti-C, actinomycin C; LN, left nephrectomy at the time of transplantation; RN, right nephrectomy. (From Starzl, T. E., et al. The reversal of rejection in human renal homografts with subsequent development of homograft tolerance. Surg. Gynecol. Obstet. *117*:385, 1963. By permission of Surgery, Gynecology & Obstetrics.)

smaller doses of the drug azathioprine than those that failed at the beginning of treatment to prevent the onset of a moderately severe rejection crisis.

It would be superfluous to devote more time to a description of the findings of rejection in organs other than the kidney since the changes can be so easily deduced from the natural functions of the organ in question. Suffice it to say that the cardinal features of delayed rejection are those of

deterioration of homograft function plus the same systemic manifestations as just described in kidney recipients. As with the kidney, the reversal of the rejection process has been well documented with every organ so far tested. The specific manifestations in all the various organs, including the kidney,[112] liver,[113] heart,[134] lung[146] and pancreas,[47, 107] have been the subject of books, monographs, or articles.

No matter which organ has been transplanted, the magnitude of immunosuppression required to prevent rejection becomes the dominant factor in determining the incidence and severity of the complications the discussion of which will constitute much of the remainder of this chapter. If the immunologic barrier encountered is a low one, the amount of prednisone and other drugs required to prevent the onset of rejection will be small and the complications of immunosuppression will be accordingly reduced. In contrast, if major problems are encountered with rejection, high doses of the various agents must be used with predictably adverse effects upon the recipient. In difficult cases, steroid therapy invariably plays a dual role of savior and villain. Since steroids are the only really dose-maneuverable component of any of the immunosuppressive regimens now in common use, rejection is usually dealt with by an increase in the daily quantities of prednisone. The graft may well be salvaged but the price may prove to be the sometimes devastating side effects that will be described later in this chapter.

At this point, it should be emphasized that the application of immunosuppressive therapy in the renal recipient should be tempered by the realization that sacrifice of the graft and a return to dialysis or retransplantation may well be the more prudent course.

Chronic Rejection

The kind of rejection that was just described is thought to be a manifestation of cell-mediated immunity. Many months or years after transplantation, a different kind of insult may come to affect a chronically functioning transplant. With this latter process, there is involvement of the blood supply of the homograft, with intimal and subintimal thickening and eventual occlusion of the arteries to the transplanted organ.[36, 93, 112, 113] Thus, a transplanted kidney, liver, heart, or other vascularized organ may, in the long run, have its blood supply squeezed off by an attack on the vascular tree (Fig. 31–9). There has been much speculation that this complication represents an indolent humoral antibody attack upon a transplant by a host that has never completely forgotten its presence.

Renal Transplantation, Rejection, and Hypertension

Arterial hypertension occurs in almost 100 per cent of renal homograft recipients at some time after operation. The greatest incidence is during the first 6 months. With rejection, the factors contributing to a rise in blood pressure include fluid overload due to failure of normal urine excretion, the hypertensive effect of high-dose steroid administration, and the presence of a renin-angiotensin response that is apparently caused by the ischemia associated with rejection. Later in the course, this early hypertension very often recedes in successful cases but with chronic rejection it may return. The hypertension in renal homograft recipients has been thoroughly discussed in the literature.[10, 35, 112, 139]

Recurrent Glomerulonephritis

It may be that the glomerulonephritis commonly seen in renal homografts months or years after transplantation is also a manifestation of a humoral antibody phase of rejection.[5, 62, 124] Two kinds of glomerulonephritis have been seen in transplanted kidneys. In one variety, anti-glomerular basement membrane (anti-GBM) antibody has been found by immunofluorescence techniques, giving the typical appearance of the single glomerulus depicted in Figure 31–10. This glomerulonephritis is the human analogue of the experimental pathologic process known as Masugi nephritis in which the antibody directly attacks glomerular basement membrane.[26]

The other kind of glomerulonephritis observed in transplanted kidneys is comparable to experimental serum sickness nephritis in which antigen-antibody complexes are formed outside the kidney but eventually trapped there because of the peculiarly effective filtration of the renal microcirculation. When such complexes are trapped within the kidney, their immunofluorescent appearance is like that shown in Figure 31–10. The kidney slowly undergoes damage over the ensuing months or years by the attraction of host inflammatory responses including the deposition of immunoglobulin and complement.[26] By light microscopy, the histopathologic manifestations of these

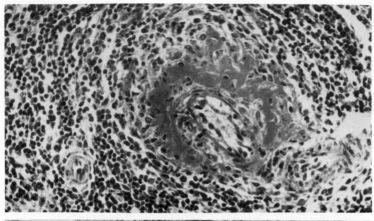

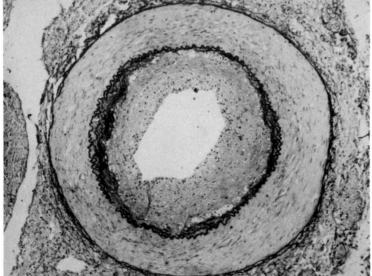

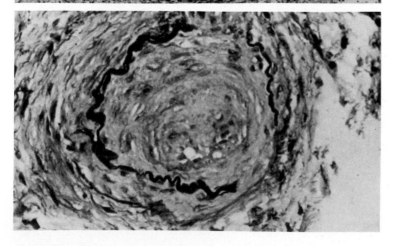

Figure 31–9 Vascular changes in canine renal homografts. *Top,* Renal homotransplant at 19 days from a dog treated with azathioprine and actinomycin C. There is fibrinoid necrosis of the whole wall of an interlobular artery, and the surrounding tissues are heavily infiltrated by cells. H and E (× 180). *Middle,* Renal homotransplant at 739 days from a dog treated with 6-methyl mercaptopurine. An interlobular artery shows diffuse intimal thickening by fibrous tissue. Elastic counterstained with hematoxylin and van Gieson (× 30). *Bottom,* Renal homotransplant at 330 days from a dog treated with azathioprine and actinomycin C. An interlobular artery shows marked fibrous intimal thickening which has almost obliterated the lumen of the vessel. The internal elastic lamina has been ruptured. Elastic counterstained with hematoxylin and van Gieson (× 160). (From Starzl, T. E.: Experience in Renal Transplantation. Philadelphia, W. B. Saunders Company, 1964.)

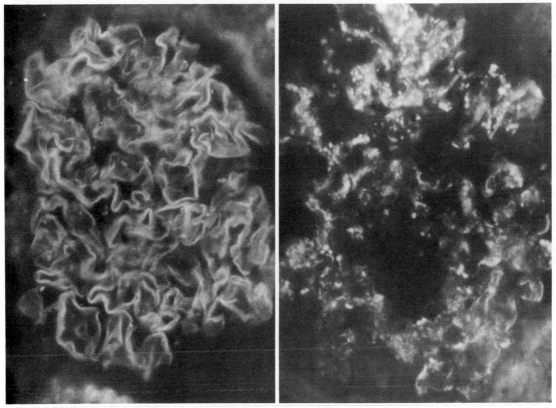

Figure 31–10 Immunofluorescent photomicrographs of typical glomerular lesions in renal homograft biopsies. *Left,* Typical linear fixation of IgG on glomerular walls of a biopsy specimen obtained 23 months post transplantation. The patient had normal renal function at the time of biopsy. *Right,* Typical discontinuous granular deposits of IgG 30 months post transplantation.

events or those with anti-GBM nephritis may be proliferative, lobular, or other kinds of glomerulonephritis, that have distinction by their morphologic characteristics (Fig. 31–11).

The development of glomerulonephritis in transplanted kidneys has been well documented by reports from a number of institutions.[38, 39, 57, 67, 68, 75, 91, 124] At one time, the major emphasis was placed on the "recurrence" of the original disease. It is true that the chance of glomerulonephritis developing in a renal homograft is greater if this was the original diagnosis, and in a number of such cases the appearance of the recurrent disease has been precisely the same as that of the original disease in the native kidneys. However, it has also been well documented that glomerulonephritis may occur in kidneys transplanted to recipients whose original kidneys had been destroyed by other than autoimmune processes.[124] Thus, glo-

merulonephritis has been seen in renal homografts transplanted to patients with polycystic disease, cystinosis, and pyelonephritis, to mention only three examples.

Once glomerulonephritis has developed in a renal homograft, there is no specific therapy. These kidneys almost always leak protein, and the proteinuria may become so extreme as to necessitate transplant nephrectomy. More commonly, the proteinuria is only one manifestation of deteriorating function in a course that leads to retransplantation or a return to dialysis. In a few of our patients with otherwise good renal function, stable severe proteinuria with albumin losses of 5 to 10 gm. per day has developed. When efforts have been made late after transplantation to reverse proteinuria with increased doses of steroids, the results have usually been disappointing in that the objective of reversing the late changes is not realized and at the same time

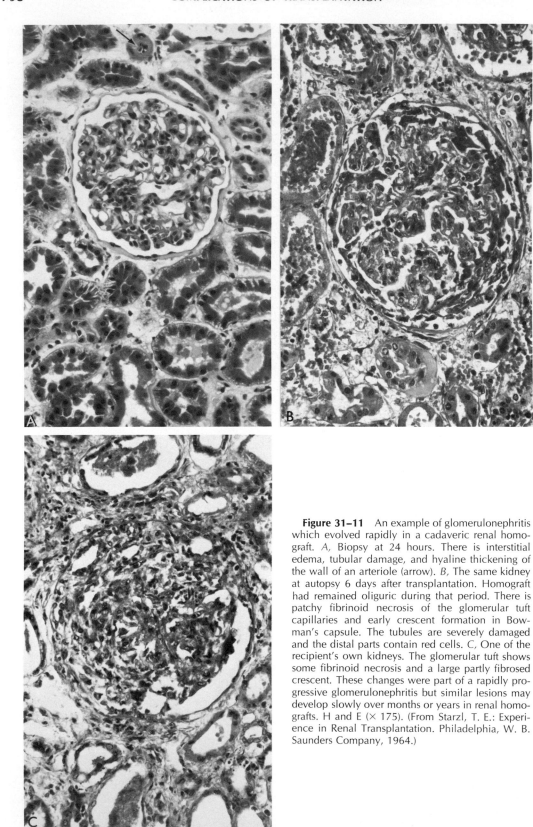

Figure 31–11   An example of glomerulonephritis which evolved rapidly in a cadaveric renal homograft. *A,* Biopsy at 24 hours. There is interstitial edema, tubular damage, and hyaline thickening of the wall of an arteriole (arrow). *B,* The same kidney at autopsy 6 days after transplantation. Homograft had remained oliguric during that period. There is patchy fibrinoid necrosis of the glomerular tuft capillaries and early crescent formation in Bowman's capsule. The tubules are severely damaged and the distal parts contain red cells. *C,* One of the recipient's own kidneys. The glomerular tuft shows some fibrinoid necrosis and a large partly fibrosed crescent. These changes were part of a rapidly progressive glomerulonephritis but similar lesions may develop slowly over months or years in renal homografts. H and E ($\times$ 175). (From Starzl, T. E.: Experience in Renal Transplantation. Philadelphia, W. B. Saunders Company, 1964.)

the penalties of increased immunosuppression must be paid. Thus, in most cases, we accept the residual function these homografts can provide and then remove them when the clinical result is no longer acceptable.

IMMUNOSUPPRESSION AND ITS CONSEQUENCES

As already stated, the condition that makes organ transplantation different from other surgical undertakings and that endows it with special hazards is immunosuppression. In essence, it is necessary to systematically weaken the immune system of the recipient so that a vigorous reaction against the alien tissue does not occur. The means by which this objective is achieved are variable.

The Different Therapeutic Regimens

The "modern" era of whole-organ transplantation was ushered in in 1962 by the use together of the two agents azathioprine and prednisone, as described earlier (see Fig. 31–8). In our center, and in virtually every other one that was active in that era, these two agents provided the essence of treatment.[45, 70, 121, 145] As already noted, the heaviest immunosuppression was required early after transplantation, but subsequently it often became possible to reduce the dosage required to maintain chronic function of the homograft. If minimal doses sufficed to prevent rejection long after operation, the prognosis of the patient proved to be good, whereas if protracted heavy immunosuppression, particularly with steroids, was required, the outlook was far less favorable. The use of azathioprine and prednisone together has often been referred to as "double-drug" therapy.

In 1966, heterologous antilymphocyte globulin (ALG) was introduced at the University of Colorado as an addition to azathioprine and prednisone in a multiple-agent regimen that has been known as a "triple-drug" program.[119] With this triple-drug regimen, ALG is used for the first few weeks or months after transplantation, during that time when the need for aggressive immuno-

suppression is the greatest. After its discontinuance, long-term therapy with azathioprine and prednisone is continued (Fig. 31–12).

In early 1971 at our institution, a systematic trial was undertaken to evaluate cyclophosphamide, an alkylating agent, as a substitute for azathioprine.[128, 129] In all new cases of renal as well as hepatic transplantation, initial therapy with cyclophosphamide, prednisone, and heterologous ALG was given.

Later in the postoperative course, after some weeks or months, azathioprine was usually substituted for cyclophosphamide, mainly because there is far more information about the long-term use of azathioprine in human beings than is available for cyclophosphamide (Fig. 31–13). It is interesting that cyclophosphamide as the primary cytotoxic agent produced comparable results to azathioprine but the latter agent has proven to be more easily manipulated.

Recently, Starzl, Weil, and their co-workers[132, 133] have reported an extensive trial of thoracic duct drainage, a procedure that had been tried and largely abandoned years earlier.[30, 31, 71] TDD was used in combination with azathioprine, prednisone, and, in most instances, antithymocyte globulin. Recipients of renal homografts had thoracic duct drainage established either at the time of transplantation or 17 to 58 days preoperatively; it was continued for up to 115 days post-transplantation. Thoracic duct drainage was found to be of particular value when pretreatment for four or more weeks was accomplished in recipients of cadaveric[132] homografts and in recipients with positive cytotoxic antidonor crossmatches.[133]

In addition to these major treatment programs, a number of adjuvant measures have been described, although none is sufficiently potent to prevent the onset of early homograft rejection. These measures include splenectomy,[112] thymectomy,[123] local homograft irradiation,[44] and intravenous actinomycin C.

A most promising new immunosuppressive agent currently undergoing clinical trials is cyclosporin A, a fungal extract. Calne et al.[18] have treated patients receiving renal, pancreatic, and hepatic transplants without adjuvant steroid therapy; Starzl et al.[131] have combined cyclosporin A with

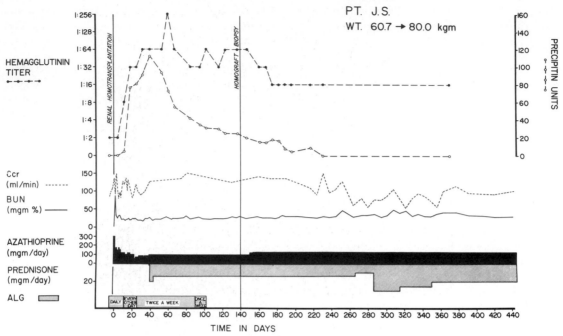

Figure 31–12　The course of a patient who received antilymphocyte globulin (ALG) before and for the first 4 months after renal homotransplantation. The donor was an older brother. There was no early rejection. Prednisone therapy was started 40 days postoperatively because of the high rises in the serologic titers that indicated a host response against the injected foreign protein and that warned against a possible anaphylactic reaction. Note the insidious onset of late rejection after cessation of globulin therapy. This was treated by increasing the maintenance dose of steroids. (From Starzl, T. E., et al.: Heterologous antilymphocyte globulin, histoincompatibility, matching, and human renal homotransplantation. Surg. Gynecol. Obstet. *126*:1023, 1968. By permission of Surgery, Gynecology & Obstetrics.)

prednisone. The ultimate role in organ transplantation of cyclosporin A as well as its toxicity remains to be defined by these and other trials.

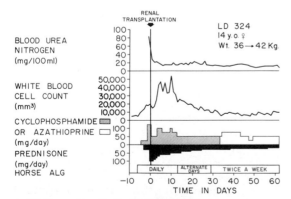

Figure 31–13　Typical triple-drug immunosuppressive therapy with cyclophosphamide (Cytoxan) after renal transplantation. Cyclophosphamide was begun the day before transplantation and continued postoperatively until there was a tendency toward leukopenia. At that time, therapy with cyclophosphamide was interrupted, and azathioprine was begun. Chronic immunosuppressive therapy has been continued with azathioprine.

Problems of Intrinsic Toxicity

The side reactions of immunosuppressive agents may be mediated by a straightforward mechanism of drug toxicity.

AZATHIOPRINE. In dogs, this agent has easily demonstrable hepatotoxicity. Doses comparable to those used in humans produce increases in SGOT and SGPT in essentially every animal (Fig. 31–14). The animals depicted in Figure 31–14 also lost weight and became anemic. Although jaundice was not noted in these 18 dogs, icterus has also been observed in this kind of canine experiment.

An extreme degree of hepatotoxicity of azathioprine is apparently a relatively species-specific finding in the dog. Fortunately, it is not a consistent problem in the human being. Even so, we believe that liver injury from this agent has been seen in patients, as will be demonstrated later.

It goes without saying that the most striking and specific toxic effect of azathioprine is bone marrow depression if the drug is given in excessively large doses.

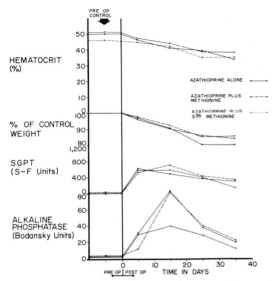

Figure 31–14 The toxicity of azathioprine when used alone or in combination with ^{35}S-methionine. Six dogs were in each of the three test groups. There were easily detectable abnormalities of liver function but jaundice did not develop. The azathioprine doses were 1 to 4 mg. per kilogram per day. Note that the animals tended to lose weight and become anemic. (From Starzl, T. E., et al.: Factors determining short- and long-term survival after orthotopic liver homotransplantation in the dog. Surgery 58.131, 1965.)

PREDNISONE. The other immunosuppressive agent that has extremely important direct toxic effects, particularly on the gastrointestinal tract, is prednisone. The adrenal corticosteroids, when administered over long periods of time, can (1) cause fatty infiltration or even cirrhosis of the liver, (2) induce pancreatitis and diabetes mellitus, and (3) cause ulceration of the duodenum and other parts of the bowel with gastrointestinal hemorrhage or perforation, to mention only a few of their effects.

Among younger patients, the life-threatening complications of prednisone may be of less immediacy than the cosmetic effects. To a sensitive teenager, the most dreaded changes may be the development of severe acne, other unacceptable facial disfigurations, a buffalo hump, and striae of the abdominal wall or elsewhere. More will be said later about the role of prednisone in causing skeletal changes.

CYCLOPHOSPHAMIDE. As is the case with azathioprine, cyclophosphamide administration must be monitored scrupulously because of its ability to cause profound bone marrow depression. In addition, cyclophos-phamide may have important effects upon the gastrointestinal tract. When used alone in large doses, it has caused diffuse or discrete gastrointestinal ulceration or massive hepatic necrosis.[6] Hemorrhagic cystitis has come to be recognized as a classic complication of administration of the same doses.[99]

Until recently, cyclophosphamide has been used for its immunosuppressive qualities most extensively by those interested in bone marrow transplantation.[100] The agent was given for a few days at doses as high as 100 mg./kg./day in an effort to induce tolerance. In whole-organ recipients, cyclophosphamide has been used quite differently, usually in doses that are little greater than 1 mg./kg./day but on a chronic basis. Under these circumstances, cyclophosphamide has seemed neither more nor less dangerous than azathioprine.[128, 129]

HETEROLOGOUS ALG. Some of the most important side effects of ALG afflict the kidney. Renal damage may result if the ALG contains specific anti-GBM antibody that attaches to and injures the glomerular basement membrane. More commonly, antibodies may be generated extrarenally in response to the injected antigen. Then, circulating soluble antigen-antibody complexes are formed that may lodge in the kidney and cause a lesion analogous to serum sickness nephritis. Fortunately, these kinds of nephritis have been seen very rarely.[56, 125, 138]

The most dreaded complication of heterologous ALG is the development of anaphylactic reactions, which have been analyzed by Kashiwagi.[52] In our center, these reactions have caused the deaths of two patients. An anaphylactic reaction is thought to result from an antigen-antibody union that secondarily triggers the release of humoral substances (from mast cells and other cells) which in turn may pass to widely distributed targers, especially those containing smooth muscle. The humoral agents that have been implicated in anaphylaxis of experimental animals or man have included histamine, slow-reacting substance (SRS), bradykinin, and serotonin.[77] Since the initiating event in an anaphylactic reaction is an antigen-antibody reaction, it goes without saying that the risk of this complication increases with repetitive exposure to foreign protein, and so the patient receiving ALG chronically should be watched carefully for any suspicious signs.

When an anaphylactic reaction occurs, in retrospect there have usually been plenty of warning signs. A feeling of chest constriction has been a common, seemingly minor complaint. If this is ignored, a later reaction may lead to profound cyanosis. Arterial blood gases were determined in some of our patients and the Po_2 was recorded as low as 20 mm. Hg. In the fatal cases, massive pulmonary edema ensued that was uncontrollable by any means.

In some instances patients may complain of a foreboding of impending death. In fact the two patients who died in our center from anaphylactic reactions both bitterly resisted the last injections of ALG they were given on the grounds of a premonition of death.

Once an anaphylactic reaction has occurred, it must be treated with great decisiveness and vigor. Usually the intravenous injection of 1 gm. of hydrocortisone (Solu-Cortef) will interdict the potentially lethal manifestations. It may also be desirable to give intravenous diphenhydramine (Benadryl) and eventually even intravenous or intracardiac epinephrine may become necessary.

If the ALG has any significant amount of antiplatelet activity it is entirely possible for it to cause profound thrombocytopenia despite the presence of good bone marrow function.

Immunologic Invalidism

The kind of direct pharmacologic toxicity just described must be borne in mind by anyone treating patients chronically with any of the drugs used in the several immunosuppressive regimens that have now been widely accepted. However, far greater in importance than this kind of direct toxicity is the immunologic invalidism that is deliberately produced, and efficiently so, by the agents in question. From this weakening of the immune system derive the most serious and dreaded complications seen in the population of transplant recipients. To the extent that the immune system must be suppressed in order to retain function of the graft, the recipient loses the capacity to react forcibly to other inimical environmental antigens, including those of bacteria.

Thus, an increased susceptibility to infection is the price for survival. If an invading microorganism causing an infection is a common bacterium against which effective antibiotics are available, the resulting problem can usually be dealt with. But if the invading microorganism is an opportunistic one of normally low pathogenicity and for which no effective antibiotic therapy is available, the outcome is commonly tragic.

What has just been described is a loss of the surveillance of the host to bacteria. It has become recognized that the loss of immunologic surveillance may have more wide-reaching effects, including an increased incidence of de novo malignancies, as will be documented, along with a further account of the infectious complications, in the subsequent sections.

COMPLICATIONS AFFECTING THE ESOPHAGUS, STOMACH, AND DUODENUM

ESOPHAGUS. The most frequent disorder of the esophagus post-transplantation has been esophagitis. Invariably, this is associated with stomatitis. If a recipient complains of substernal pain while eating and if ulcerations of the oral mucosa or lips are found, a presumptive diagnosis can be made. The painful lesions of the mouth and lips have been shown to be caused by the herpes simplex virus, but this infection is frequently associated with Candida albicans infestation. Treatment with nystatin (Mycostatin) oral suspension and tablets is instituted to control the Candida infection, but if this does not control the moniliasis, a course of systemic therapy with amphotericin B may be required.

The dangers of monilial esophagitis, particularly when the esophageal mucosa has already been damaged by herpetic ulceration, are perforation and dissemination. A month after transplantation one of our patients incurred diffuse ulcerations and sloughing of the esophagus (Fig. 31–15), as well as of most of the rest of the gastrointestinal tract (Fig. 31–15), leading to death from esophageal perforation within a few

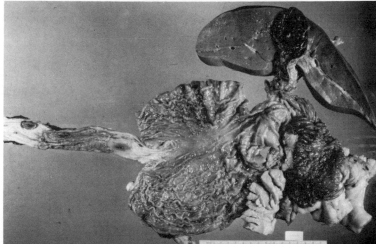

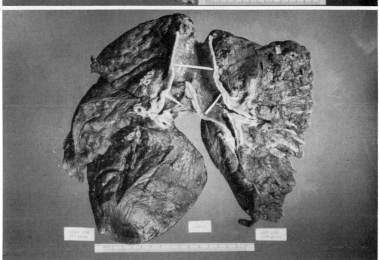

Figure 31–15 An example of monilial esophagitis with diffuse ulcerations and sloughing of mucosa. *Top,* The esophagus and stomach at autopsy. The remainder of the gastrointestinal tract showed similar areas of involvement. *Bottom,* The tracheobronchial mucosa was also the site of ulcerations and sloughing.

days. Several other patients have died of disseminated *Candida albicans* infection with multiple abscesses in several organs.

STOMACH AND DUODENUM. In caring for patients treated with renal homotransplantation, the need often arises to treat surgically a variety of non-urologic intra-abdominal complications. The single most common cause of difficulty has been gastric or duodenal ulceration with perforation or hemorrhage. Some of these complications developed during pretransplantation dialysis. Under these circumstances, vagotomy plus pyloroplasty or gastric resection should be performed before transplantation is done, since after the institution of immunosuppressive therapy the steroid component of treatment may make medical management even more difficult.

In a book published in 1964 based upon fewer than 70 cases of renal homotransplantation, it was pointed out that gastrointestinal hemorrhage occurred during the early postoperative period in 35 of the first 42 cases (83 per cent).[112] During that era, meticulous prophylactic postoperative antacid therapy was not being given. Subsequently, the magnitude of the problems has been reduced by providing all patients on immunosuppressive regimens with a preventive program of either antacids or, more recently, cimetidine. Nevertheless, by 1968, Penn et al.[87] recorded 8 patients from a total of 184 consecutive renal recipients who had required gastric procedures because of gastroduodenal complications — 6 with hemorrhage and 2 with duodenal or gastric perforation.

The problems encountered with the stomach and duodenum under these potentially dangerous circumstances posttransplantation will not be exhaustively discussed, since they are no different from those that have been described in discussions of steroid therapy in patients who have not undergone transplantation. However, a comment is in order about the appropriate gastric procedure, at least if the complication is hemorrhage. A conservative operative procedure has almost always been performed, consisting of vagotomy and pyloroplasty. In the vast majority of cases, the source of hemorrhage has been superficial ulceration of the gastric mucosa or gastritis, whereas in the remainder, relatively superficial duodenal ulcers have usually been responsible. With vagotomy and pyloroplasty, reoperation and resection for continuing or recurrent hemorrhage has been necessary in only one instance.

In the early days of transplantation, it was assumed that perforation of a hollow viscus was almost tantamount to death. However, it has been learned that simple closure of such a perforation, provided this is carried out early, has a good prospect of success. Even under immunosuppression, the peritoneal cavity can withstand a single insult if it is not of great duration and if it is effectively treated.

COMPLICATIONS AFFECTING THE INTESTINES

THE SMALL BOWEL. By far the most common complication affecting the small bowel in transplant recipients is intestinal obstruction from adhesions. There are several obvious reasons. First, abdominal operations have usually been performed, most frequently to remove the diseased native kidneys or to perform splenectomy. Second, many such recipients have had peritoneal dialysis. Finally, the transplantation itself is sometimes performed intraperitoneally, particularly if the recipient is a child[112] whose extraperitoneal space cannot easily accommodate an adult organ. Two of our first 10 pediatric patients who had intraperitoneal homograft placement required reoperation at a later time for lysis of adhesions at the transplantation site.

Occasionally, there may be intrinsic small intestinal lesions. For example, in one of our first recipients of an auxiliary liver homograft, diffuse monilial enteritis developed and caused him to bleed to death.[113] In another patient, a kidney recipient, discrete ulcers, apparently also caused by *Candida albicans,* developed. The conditions first led to small bowel perforation, necessitating resection, and within a few weeks massive hemorrhage from a residual ulcer occurred, requiring a second enterectomy. The patient survived both procedures.

THE COLON. Of all the gastrointestinal complications after organ transplantation, those affecting the colon have been the most uniformly lethal. The first formal report on this subject in the literature was by Penn et al.[83] By 1969 they had collected from the University of Colorado case material eight cases of perforated sigmoid diverticulitis, pseudomembranous enterocolitis, granulomatous colitis, ulcerative colitis, or perforation due to an unrecognized iatrogenic injury. All of these patients died. Since that time, patients with perforated diverticulitis have been successfully treated in two stages, first exteriorization of a perforated sigmoid diverticulum and then closure of the colostomy weeks later. A few other examples of effective treatment of perforating colonic lesions have been reported.[24]

If more survivals are to be obtained when serious inflammatory colonic lesions occur, a high degree of suspicion and early operation will be necessary. In the last few years, a half dozen renal patients have been discovered at autopsy to have large ulcers of the cecum. These renal recipients usually had diarrhea, frequently accompanied by gramnegative septicemia or intermittent bright red rectal bleeding. Barium enema examinations were normal. For such a syndrome we now believe that exploration and consideration of a right colectomy should be entertained.

In addition to the lethal colonic complications, fecal impaction has been common, so severe in one case that operative relief was eventually necessary. There are reasons for this. Disturbances of bowel activity are common in both renal and hepatic homograft recipients. Before the transplant operation the patient may have a hypomotility syndrome, or even frank ileus, because of uremia.[112] After transplantation there may be a period of poor graft function, which may perpetuate a preexisting hypomotility state. As soon as the patient can take liquids by mouth he is given large doses of antacids, as described in the preceding section. At times, the non-absorbable antacid gels may cause constipation or fecal impaction. In order to avoid these problems in organ recipients, the colon is kept empty by preoperative and postoperative enemas, and liberal use is made of stool softeners.

Major colonic complications occur in about 5 per cent of hepatic recipients and include hemorrhage caused by infectious ulcerations or by pneumatosis cystoides intestinalis and perforation from diverticula or from operative trauma. Koep and his associates have reported eight such cases in detail.[55]

PANCREATIC COMPLICATIONS

PANCREATITIS AND HYPERAMYLASEMIA. Elevation of the serum amylase is not an unusual finding after either renal or hepatic transplantation. If the patient is asymptomatic and potential etiologic factors can be excluded, the laboratory finding is probably of little significance. However, when clinical signs and symptoms of pancreatitis accompany the biochemical abnormality, the findings become of grave prognostic significance.

The first report of pancreatitis after renal transplantation revealed that this complication developed in 3 of the first 42 consecutive patients (7.1 per cent) at the University of Colorado.[112] Subsequently, most major transplant centers, when polled by Johnson and Nabseth, reported one or more cases of acute pancreatitis among their renal recipients.[50] The incidence in their collected series was 19 cases among 1074 recipients, or slightly less than 2 per cent. However, the true incidence of this complication can easily be demonstrated to be higher, if clinical and biochemical evidence for the diagnosis is systematically sought.

Penn et al.[86] reviewed 301 consecutive renal homograft recipients; 17 patients (5.6 per cent) were diagnosed as having proven (12 cases) or almost certain (5 cases) pancreatitis (Table 31–2). Eleven of the 12 pa-

TABLE 31–2 INCIDENCE OF PANCREATITIS IN 301 CONSECUTIVE RECIPIENTS OF RENAL HOMOGRAFTS*

Diagnosis	Patients	
Preexisting pancreatitis	5	(1.7%)
Acute pancreatitis	17	(5.6%)
Definite	12	
Suspected	5	
Mortality	11/17	(64.7%)
Hyperamylasemia	43	(14.7%)

*Data from Penn, I., Durst, A. L., Machado, M., Halgrimson, C. G., Booth, A. S., Jr., Putnam, C. W., Groth, C. G., and Starzl, T. E.: Acute pancreatitis and hyperamylasemia in renal homograft recipients. Arch. Surg. *105*:167, 1972.

tients with proven pancreatitis died, and this complication was the major cause of or a factor contributory to death in all 11. The twelfth patient with proven pancreatitis survived, but only after a stormy convalescence (Fig. 31–16). The 5 patients with highly probable pancreatitis survived after protracted illnesses.

In addition to the symptomatic cases of pancreatitis, Penn et al.[86] reported an additional 43 patients (14.3 per cent) who had asymptomatic hyperamylasemia post-transplantation (Table 31–2). Many of these patients, who frequently had had elevations of the serum amylase even before transplantation, probably experienced clinically undetected episodes of pancreatitis at some time in their convalescence but were apparently not thereby harmed.

The etiology of pancreatitis in transplantation patients is probably complex. Inflammatory changes in the pancreas are common in uremia[7] and abnormalities of the gland are frequently noted at the time of bilateral nephrectomy and splenectomy. Operative trauma to the pancreas in the course of the upper abdominal dissection may occasionally aggravate preexisting inflammation or possibly trigger an acute episode of pancreatitis.

Hyperparathyroidism and hypercalcemia, which frequently complicate uremia (see later), may in themselves predispose to pancreatitis. Three of the patients with pancreatitis reported by Penn were found to have parathyroid hyperplasia and five of the

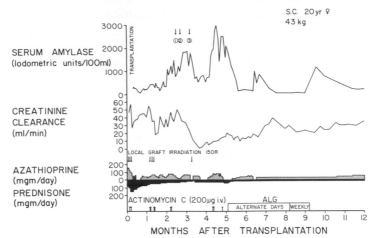

Figure 31–16   Proven pancreatitis in a renal homograft recipient. The pancreatitis was complicated by abscess formation necessitating several surgical procedures. An abscess in the left labium majus was drained 75 days after transplantation ①. Subsequently, a sinogram (Fig. 31–17) demonstrated an extensive proximal extension of the abscess that was then drained through an incision in the left flank ②. Sixteen days later, a large retroperitoneal abscess communicating with the first two abscesses and arising from the pancreas was drained ③. The serum amylase level remained elevated for a prolonged period. Graft function deteriorated during the treatment of the abscesses but partially recovered. (From Penn, I., et al.: Acute pancreatitis and hyperamylasemia in renal homograft recipients. Arch. Surg. *105*:167, 1972.)

patients with asymptomatic hyperamylasemia had concomitant elevations of the serum calcium. One of the latter recipients required emergency parathyroidectomy for hyperplasia 46 months post-transplantation.

Cholelithiasis, hepatitis, and local or systemic infections with bacteria, fungi, or viruses[42] may also cause or predispose to pancreatitis and must be carefully excluded. Less easily documented, but probably more commonly of etiologic significance, are drugs administered post-transplantation. Those implicated include azathioprine,[43] corticosteroids,[21] and the diuretic chlorothiazide.[27]

Finally, renal insufficiency may in itself produce hyperamylasemia by virtue of decreased enzyme clearance.[53] This last consideration may partially explain the large number of patients noted to have asymptomatic hyperamylasemia while on dialysis or during episodes of poor renal function post-transplantation.

Although preexisting pancreatitis is not of itself a contraindication to renal transplantation, every effort should be made to diagnose and correct predisposing factors, including biliary tract disease and hyperparathyroidism. When the diagnosis is made

for the first time after transplantation, efforts are directed toward the correction of inciting factors, vigorous supportive care including antibiotic therapy, and the aggressive treatment of complications, such as abscess formation (Fig. 31–17). Serious consideration should also be given to curtailment of immunosuppression, particularly of the corticosteroid dosage.

HYPERGLYCEMIA AND DIABETES MELLITUS. About one-third of non-diabetic patients awaiting renal transplantation manifest hyperglycemia, usually without glycosuria. The elevated blood sugars are usually a manifestation of the glucose intolerance of uremia and are of little clinical significance.

During the first 24 hours post transplantation, Buckingham et al.[12] documented increases in plasma glucose and insulin which they ascribed to surgical stress and to the administration of corticosteroids intraoperatively. These effects are short-lived, having largely resolved by the second day. Rarely, the hyperglycemic, hyperosmolar non-ketotic syndrome with lactic acidosis may occur.[12]

Later after transplantation, more than half of all recipients will have hyperglycemia of varying severity.[112] In some patients, the biochemical abnormality simply reflects periods of poor renal function from whatever cause and is probably of no greater significance than in the uremic patient who has not undergone transplantation. More commonly, however, the blood sugar elevations parallel the administration of large doses of corticosteroids. The phenomenon is dose-related, usually having its onset when the dose exceeds 2.5 mg./kg./day and usually resolving when the dose falls below 0.7 mg./kg./day.[85] In about 15 per cent of patients (Table 31–3), the hyperglycemia is severe enough to require treatment, and in a few instances prodigious doses of insulin may be required to achieve even mediocre control of the fasting blood glucose level. More frequently, the hyperglycemia is less severe, transient, or inter-

TABLE 31–3 POSTTRANSPLANTATION HYPERGLYCEMIA*

	Patients	Mortality
Severe hyperglycemia, requiring pharmacologic therapy	44 (14.6%)	55%
Hyperglycemia > 30 days, but not requiring treatment	16 (5.3%)	
Intermittent hyperglycemia	52 (17.3%)	
Occasional hyperglycemic episodes	53 (17.6%)	36.5%
Euglycemia	136 (45.2%)	
	301	

*From Penn, I., Durst, A. L., and Machado, M.: Diabetes and hyperglycemia in renal homograft recipients. In preparation.

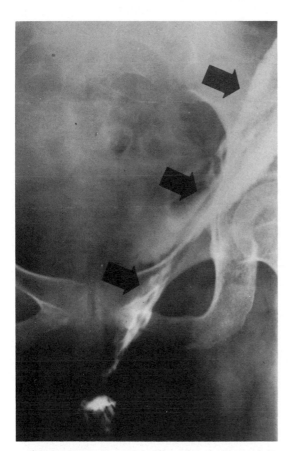

Figure 31–17 Sinogram taken after drainage of the first abscess in the patient whose course is shown in Figure 31–16. A tract (arrows) extends from the left labium majus retroperitoneally into the left flank. (From Penn, I., et al.: Acute pancreatitis and hyperamylasemia in renal homograft recipients. Arch. Surg. *105*:167, 1972.)

mittent and requires no specific therapy other than attention to diet. In these milder cases of diabetes, resolution occurs with reduction in steroid therapy, as mentioned previously.

Not surprisingly, the mortality among patients manifesting hyperglycemia is greater than that among those recipients maintaining euglycemia (Table 31–3). Although an occasional patient may die as a direct result of a diabetic complication such as ketoacidosis, the vast majority of these deaths cannot be attributed directly to hyperglycemia or frank diabetes. Instead, the most frequent cause of death is found to be sepsis, again reflecting the necessity for large-dose steroid administration to combat poor renal function.

Nonetheless, the development of hyperglycemia in a previously euglycemic recipient or of ketoacidosis in the previously well controlled diabetic recipient calls for a vigorous diagnostic evaluation. This should include frequent assessments of renal function and a careful search for infectious complications that might initially otherwise pass unnoticed. Concomitantly, vigorous treatment with dietary control, oral hypoglycemic agents, or insulin should be undertaken to re-establish euglycemia, since ketoacidosis may rapidly become life-threatening.

In recent years, Najarian at the University

of Minnesota and others have recommended a more aggressive attitude toward renal transplantation in diabetic patients. Although the results remain distinctly inferior to those in comparable recipients treated for other renal diseases, the prognosis is nonetheless considerably better than that for diabetics on chronic dialysis. It would therefore seem that diabetes mellitus could, and should, be removed from the list of contraindications to renal transplantation and the prospective diabetic recipient evaluated in light of this more recent experience. Our own experience supports that of Najarian.

HEPATIC COMPLICATIONS

At some time postoperatively, the majority of renal homograft recipients manifest abnormalities of one or more of the standard liver function tests. The immunosuppressive program is presumably responsible for the high incidence of the liver dysfunction, either because of drug hepatotoxicity or because the consequent weakening of the host immune system permits the frequent development of viral hepatitis. The differential diagnosis of hepatotoxicity from hepatitis after transplantation is usually difficult and frequently impossible. Penn's[88] studies have demonstrated the extreme frequency with which such a perplexing distinction should be made, and Torisu et al.[137] have shown how often this may not be possible with any diagnostic tool currently available.

Penn et al.[88] examined the preoperative and postoperative liver function tests in 146 renal recipients. At some time post-transplantation, abnormalities in the serum bilirubin, alkaline phosphatase, SGOT, SGPT, prothrombin time, serum protein concentrations, or sulfobromophthalein (BSP) clearance developed in 88 (60 per cent) of the patients. The hepatic dysfunction usually appeared within the first 6 postoperative months (Fig. 31–18). In most instances the changes were transient and mild. These were accompanied by clinical complaints in only a small minority. In 20 patients, however, the derangements of liver function were severe and persistent; four of the recipients died of hepatic failure 5 to 18 months after transplantation.

It is of some interest that in the series reported by Penn et al.[88] the 66 patients treated with the triple-drug regimen of azathioprine, prednisone, and heterologous antilymphocyte globulin had a somewhat lower incidence (54 per cent) of hepatic dysfunction than the 80 patients who received only azathioprine and prednisone (65 per cent). Moreover, all four of the fatalities were in the group receiving double-drug therapy. It was concluded that the magnitude of the problem had been less since the addition of ALG to the immunosuppressive regimen, (and prior to the widespread routine application of hepatitis virus screening in blood banking and dialysis facilities), probably because of concomitant reductions in steroid and azathioprine dosage.

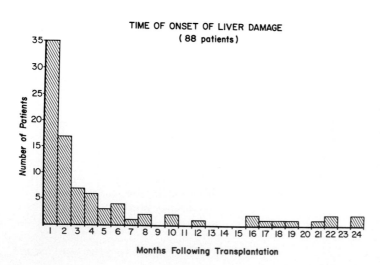

TIME OF ONSET OF LIVER DAMAGE
(88 patients)

Number of Patients

Months Following Transplantation

Figure 31–18 Time of onset in human renal transplant recipients of abnormalities of one or more liver function tests. One hundred forty-six patients were studied. Of these, 88 (60 per cent) had some evidence of hepatic damage, usually during the first 6 postoperative months. This was usually mild, but in 20 patients (14 per cent) it was severe. (From Penn, I., et al.: Hepatic disorders in renal homograft recipients. Curr. Top. Surg. Res. 1:67, 1969.)

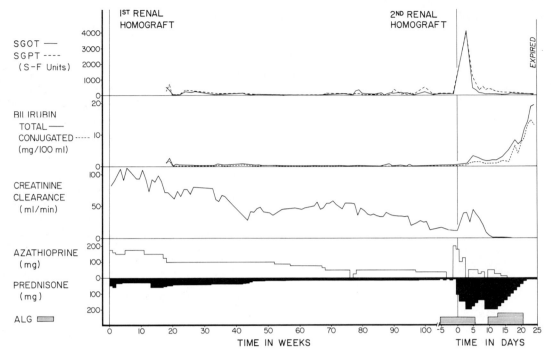

Figure 31–19 The course of a kidney transplant recipient who appeared to have suffered liver damage from azathioprine toxicity. About 5 months after his first renal homotransplantation, low-grade jaundice developed and increases in transaminase levels were seen. The azathioprine dose was cut immediately and further reductions were made at subsequent intervals. The homograft eventually failed and was removed after about 2 years. When retransplantation was performed, four large doses of azathioprine were given just before and after operation. Immediately, the transaminases rose to more than 4000 units. The patient became intensely jaundiced and died of hepatic and renal failure. (From Starzl, T. E.: Experience in Hepatic Transplantation. Philadelphia, W. B. Saunders Company, 1969.)

THE QUESTION OF DRUG HEPATOTOX-ICITY. The two drugs azathioprine and prednisone, commonly employed in modern immunosuppressive programs, are known to be potentially toxic to the liver, as discussed previously. The main attention has been paid to the hepatotoxicity of azathioprine. However, the diagnosis of azathioprine hepatotoxicity in patients has been made with certainty in only a few dramatic cases in which the events of hepatic dysfunction correlated temporally with the duration of or increases in azathioprine dosage. One such case is depicted in Figure 31–19. Nevertheless, when biochemical or clinical evidence of hepatic injury develops in the renal recipient receiving azathioprine, hepatotoxicity should be suspected and consideration given to modification of the immunosuppressive program, as will be discussed later.

HEPATITIS. With the development of serologic tests for the detection of hepatitis-associated antigen (HAA) — also termed

the Australia (Au) or the hepatitis B surface antigen — it became possible to test with greater precision the hypothesis that at least some of these cases of liver damage occurring during treatment with dialysis or after renal transplantation were due to serum hepatitis.

In 1964 Blumberg and his associates reported the discovery of a foreign substance in the serum of Australian aborigines (hence the term Australia antigen). The particle was subsequently identified in the blood of patients with leukemia, Down's syndrome, leprosy, and serum hepatitis.[8] Prince[94] of New York reported in 1968 a similar antigen in the blood of patients with serum hepatitis (hepatitis B). The two substances were soon shown to be serologically identical and have been termed the hepatitis B surface antigen (Hb_sAg).

In the Colorado series of renal recipients, the appearance of the Australia antigen in the bloodstream of a transplant recipient, either preoperatively or in the post-trans-

TABLE 31–4 LACK OF CORRELATION OF AUSTRALIA ANTIGENEMIA AND HEPATIC DYSFUNCTION IN 45 PATIENTS WHO HAD FREQUENT DETERMINATIONS OF LIVER FUNCTION AND IN WHOM SEROLOGIC EVIDENCE FOR AUSTRALIA ANTIGEN OR ANTIBODY WAS SOUGHT*

	Number of Patients Studied	None	Minor†	Major‡	Deaths Attributable to Liver Disease
Au + by all tests	12	5	6	1	0
Au + by complement fixation only	7	4	2	1	0
Au negative	24	10	9	5	3
Anti-Au antibody	2	1	0	1	1

*Data from Torisu, M., Yokoyama, T., Amemiya, H., Kohler, P. F., Schroter, G., Martineau, G., Penn, I., Palmer, W., Halgrimson, C. G., Putnam, C. W., and Starzl, T. E.: Immunosuppression, liver injury, and hepatitis in renal, hepatic, and cardiac homograft recipients: With particular reference to the Australia antigen. Ann. Surg. *174*:620, 1971.

†Minor elevations in the serum transaminases (50–250 I.U.).

‡Elevations of the transaminases > 250 I.U. and/or bilirubin > 2 mg./dl.

plantation period, did not necessarily have an unfavorable prognostic significance in individual cases (Table 31–4).[137]

Two more recent studies also merit comment. Mozes, Najarian, and their co-workers[69] reported in 1978 a retrospective review of 567 patients who had received renal grafts at the University of Minnesota during an 8-year period, 1967–1975. Twenty-two patients developed clinical jaundice. Nine of these recipients died during the initial episode of hepatitis, six died within 3 months of hepatic failure, and four developed chronic liver insufficiency. Only three recovered fully. Of the 22 patients, five had HB_sAg-positive hepatitis, four were proven to have and two were suspected of having cytomegalovirus hepatitis, two had herpes hominis hepatitis, one had varicella zoster hepatitis, and in three, hepatic failure was related to bacterial and/or fungal sepsis. In the remaining five, the etiologic agent was unclear. Drug toxicity was not clearly implicated in any.

A prospective study of 64 recipients was reported recently from the Hôpital Necker, Paris, by Degos et al.[23] Serial liver biopsies were performed at the time of transplantation and 1 and 3 years post-transplantation. At the time of operation, fully 40 per cent of the recipients had chronic hepatitis; 84 per cent of those with hepatitis were HB_sAg-positive. Three years after transplantation, the incidence of hepatitis had increased by only 15 per cent. However, there was an unusually high frequency of evolution from the chronic persistent to the chronic active form of hepatitis post transplantation. The authors concluded that most of the liver disease seen in renal recipients had its origin in events prior to operation, relating to dialysis.

Based on these observations, it would not seem reasonable to forbid renal transplantation to a potential recipient merely because of a positive hepatitis serology. Nonetheless, screening for HB_sAg should be a part of the transplant recipient (and donor) workup, since documentation of positivity has certain practical implications.

First, the finding should prompt a careful evaluation of hepatic function, which, if abnormal, should probably include liver biopsy. If chronic aggressive hepatitis proves to be the diagnosis, the propriety of transplantation should be reconsidered.

Secondly, the patient found to have hepatitis antigen must be regarded as a hepatitis carrier and should be managed as such. Precautions entail proper techniques of isolation, including stool and needle precautions, and education of paramedical personnel. Several transplantation centers have already reported deaths from hepatitis among their nurses, technicians, and other personnel.[137] In this regard, the healthy physician, nurse, technician, or relative is probably at greater risk of developing immediately fatal liver disease than the chronically ill or immunosuppressed dialysis or transplant patient, whereas the prospects of having chronic liver disease have seemed to us much greater in the population under immunosuppression.

Finally, efforts should be made to protect the transplant recipient from unnecessary exposure to hepatitis, such as by Hb$_s$Ag-positive blood products. Hepatitis antigen tests should also be performed on all prospective organ donors.[144] Several cadaveric donors who have been pronounced dead in our hospitals on the basis of irreversible neurologic injury have been discovered to have high titer Hb$_s$Ag antigenemia. If this had not been detected in time, several organs would have been transplanted from each donor with the virtual certainty of transfer of the hepatitis virus to the recipients.

MODIFICATION OF THE IMMUNOSUPPRESSIVE REGIMEN IN THE PRESENCE OF HEPATIC COMPLICATIONS. In the patient with moderate or severe hepatic dysfunction post transplantation or in whom azathioprine hepatotoxicity is suspected — usually on the basis of progressive hepatic disease in the face of a negative result in the search for Australia antigen — consideration should be given to drastic modifications of the immunosuppressive program. Zarday et al.[147] have recommended that in these circumstances azathioprine be discontinued entirely and that the patient be maintained only with steroids.

Alternatively, substitution of cyclophosphamide (Cytoxan) for azathioprine in the immunosuppressive regimen has been carried out.[69, 101] As mentioned previously, cyclophosphamide when used in low doses has little if any hepatotoxicity. The course of a patient in whom such a switch in therapy was made is shown in Figure 31–20. This girl developed fever and extremely severe hepatic dysfunction, including jaundice, while under treatment with azathioprine (Imuran) and prednisone. It was feared at the time that she was dying of liver disease, and cyclophosphamide was substituted for the suspected guilty agent, azathioprine. She completely recovered after the change in therapy and remained well for about 1 year. At that time, azathioprine was restored to the regimen and there was recurrence of high fever, jaundice, and many of the same symptoms that had been present during the previous course of azathioprine. These were all promptly relieved by switching once more to cyclophosphamide.

Among our outpatients being followed for more than a decade after renal transplantation, there are about two dozen recipients who have chronic Australia antigenemia (Table 31–5). Once this serologic finding develops in the immunosuppressed recipient, it does not usually disappear. We have concluded that the treatment with immunosuppression has modified the natural course of the serum hepatitis, that no specific treatment is feasible, and that the best

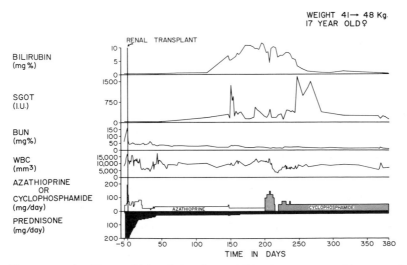

Figure 31–20 The course of a 17-year-old female in whom azathioprine was stopped because of the suspicion of hepatotoxicity. Multiple Australia-antigen tests for serum hepatitis were negative. Note the recession of jaundice after the substitution of cyclophosphamide for azathioprine. (From Starzl, T. E., et al.: Cyclophosphamide and whole organ transplantation in humans. Surg. Gynecol. Obstet. *133*:981, 1971. By permission of Surgery, Gynecology & Obstetrics.)

TABLE 31–5 INCIDENCE* OF Au ANTIGEN BY RANDOM SINGLE SAMPLING IN HOMOGRAFT RECIPIENTS FROM ONE MONTH TO 8 YEARS AFTER OPERATION, USING IMMUNODIFFUSION OR ELECTRO-IMMUNODIFFUSION TESTS FOR SCREENING†

Number of Patients	Au Antigen Positive	Anti-Au Antibody	Negative for Au Antigen and Antibody
89	15 (16.9%)	2 (2.2%)	72 (80.9%)

*The incidence was actually higher than shown, since several additional cases were detected within the negative group by the more sensitive method of complement fixation.

†From Torisu, M., Yokoyama, T., Amemiya, H., Kohler, P. F., Schroter, G., Martineau, G., Penn, I., Palmer, W., Halgrimson, C. G., Putnam, C. W., and Starzl, T. E.: Immunosuppression, liver injury, and hepatitis in renal, hepatic, and cardiac homograft recipients: With particular reference to the Australia antigen. Ann. Surg. *174*:620, 1971.

thing to do is to try to prevent these patients from transmitting the disease to their family members or others.

HYPERPARATHYROIDISM AND BONE DISEASE

The complication of hyperparathyroidism after transplantation is an example of a disorder to the etiology of which preexisting renal failure, as well as the side effects of immunosuppressive agents, are presumed to make important contributions. To begin with, secondary hyperparathyroidism is present in most patients with chronic renal failure. From autopsy studies, it has been known for nearly half a century that parathyroid hyperplasia is a common finding under these circumstances. The pathogenesis of the parathyroid lesion has been relatively well defined.[11, 97] With advanced renal disease and failure of phosphate excretion, hyperphosphatemia develops, with consequent depression of serum calcium. In turn, the hypocalcemia is an effective stimulus for parathyroid hyperplasia and presumably for heightened parathyroid hormone production and release.

It is into this environment that many renal homografts are placed. Since the early days of renal homotransplantation, it has

been thoroughly appreciated that the secondary hyperparathyroidism persists into the immediate postoperative period.[65, 92, 105] Unfortunately, it was originally thought by most of these investigators that resolution of this hyperparathyroidism occurred promptly and almost universally,[3, 48, 49] especially if high serum calcium values are treated with phosphate-containing antacids such as Phosphaljel. With conservative management, severe hypercalcemia post-transplantation became uncommon, and the dogma seemed well established that parathyroidectomy was very seldom required.

The information generated from this center in 1973[32] caused us to alter this conservative position. Although the exact incidence of hyperparathyroidism after transplantation could not be accurately ascertained from our case material, it appeared to be at least 20 per cent. The insidious feature of the complication has been its occult and subtle nature, which in some instances, particularly in children, had permitted progressive bone changes to create a pariah without the features of biochemically florid hyperparathyroidism ever having been demonstrated.

Some of the characteristics of this kind of hyperparathyroidism in 18 patients treated at the University of Colorado are shown in Table 31–6.[32] Before transplantation, all of these recipients had suffered from renal failure for at least several years and all but one had required hemodialysis. There was radiographic evidence of bone disease in 17 of the 18 patients, invariably including osteoporosis. However, 10 also had radiographic or biopsy evidence of osteitis fibrosa cystica or extraskeletal calcification of the arteries or soft tissues or both.

The very serious bone complications[46, 74] in such patients may lead to the kind of tragic disabilities shown in Figure 31–21, with bilateral aseptic necrosis of the femoral neck. The presence of such femoral lesions does not ipso facto make the diagnosis of persistent hyperparathyroidism, although it should arouse suspicion and call for a workup to rule out this diagnosis.

Unfortunately, the determination of total serum calcium and phosphorus concentrations in the renal transplant patient may not provide adequate screening for the diagnosis. In the 18 cases shown in Table 31–6, if

TABLE 31–6 CLINICAL DATA ON EIGHTEEN RENAL TRANSPLANT RECIPIENTS AFTER PARATHYROIDECTOMY*

			Radiographic Findings before Parathyroidectomy		
		Interval between	Bone Disease		
Age (yrs.)	Creatinine Clearance after Transplantation (ml./min.)	Transplantation and Parathyroidectomy (mos.)	Osteoporosis	Osteitis Fibrosa	Calcification
41	95	2	+	−	vascular
22	70	7	−	−	−
21	81	14	+	−	vascular
10	55	18	+	−	vascular
39	49	20	+	−	−
43	90	32	+	+	soft tissue
27	54	47	+	−†	vascular, skin
30	90	54	+	−	−
17	50	63	++	−	vascular, soft tissue
13	51	53	+	−	−
30	53	6	+	+	−
48	89	6	−	+	vascular
32	64	18	+‡	−	−
11	46	19	+	+	soft tissue
39	74	39	+	−	−
24	87	44	+	−	−
40	75	2	+	−†	vascular
39	71	12	+‡	−	−

*From Geis, W. P., Popovtzer, M. M., Corman, J. L., Halgrimson, C. G., Groth, C. G., and Starzl, T. E.: The diagnosis and treatment of hyperparathyroidism after renal homotransplantation. Surg. Gynecol. Obstet. *137*: 997, 1973. By permission of Surgery, Gynecology & Obstetrics.
†Osteitis fibrosa cystica histologically.
‡Aseptic necrosis of femoral head.
+Presence of radiographic bone disease.
−Absence of radiographic bone disease.

an elevation in total serum calcium were a prerequisite for the diagnosis, 8 of the 18 cases of hyperparathyroidism would never have been identified. In our clinics, heavy reliance has been placed upon determina- tion of the ionized calcium. This measure- ment has provided the decisive clue in every case in which it has been performed.[32] More recently, the availability of radioimmunoas- says for parathormone has added an impor-

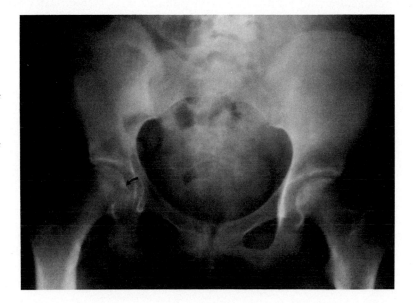

Figure 31–21 Appearance of aseptic necrosis of the femoral head (*arrow*) in a young woman after transplantation. She was on prednisone therapy at the time of this delayed complication. (From Starzl, T. E., et al.: Renal homo- transplantation: Late function and complications. Ann. Int. Med. *61*:470, 1964.)

tant diagnostic dimension and has resulted in a much greater awareness of this complication.

In much of the older literature, the high incidence of osteoporosis and other bone abnormalities in the renal transplant recipient was attributed to chronic therapy with prednisone. This concept undoubtedly has validity. Steroids have the intrinsic capability of causing osteoporosis. In addition, the steroids may contribute to the perpetuation of preexisting hyperparathyroidism. When steroids are administered, they have a depressant effect upon serum calcium concentration[51, 58] and probably a consequent stimulatory effect upon parathyroid hormone induction.[141] Thus, paradoxically, the steroids may help control hypercalcemia at the price of setting up a vicious cycle aggravating hyperparathyroidism.

In the past, the indications for parathyroidectomy after renal transplantation have undoubtedly been too restrictive. It is also clear that efforts to avoid this operation by chronic phosphate administration (as with the use of the antacid Phosphaljel) were self-defeating. If used for long periods of time, the phosphate therapy may itself recreate the parathyroid stimulus by driving down the serum calcium concentration, or it could even, theoretically, aggravate soft tissue calcification.[58, 141] Consequently, parathyroidectomy should be carefully considered after a 3-month period of conservative treatment if there is recurrence of the hyperparathyroid state after phosphate is stopped. The impetus to proceed should be increased if there are bone complications in the background or if there is unexplained deterioration of renal homograft function.

It is of interest that almost two-thirds of the patients reviewed in Table 31–6 had deteriorating renal function prior to parathyroidectomy for hyperparathyroidism. After operation, this decline was either halted or, in almost half the cases, reversed.

In ordinary clinical practice, hyperparathyroidism is usually due to the presence of an adenoma. In contrast, the diagnosis in the renal transplantation patient is almost always diffuse hyperplasia. At operation, before proceeding with resection, it is necessary to identify all the parathyroid glands. After this has been done, a gland with an easily identifiable discrete arterial supply is subtotally amputated with a razor or scalpel, with a small remnant left intact on the vascular stalk. Bleeding from the raw surface is controlled with vascular suture or cautery. Only after the viability of this remnant is established visually are the other glands completely excised. If an accident occurs to the remnant of the original gland, additional opportunities would thereby remain available until the last possible moment.

An alternative method of treatment is to excise all the parathyroid tissue and then carry out free autotransplantation of one fragment into the sternocleidomastoid or a convenient muscle in the forearm. This technique, which has been extensively reviewed by Alveryd,[4] has a major advantage in that it permits precise determination, by simple metabolic studies carried out within the first few postoperative days, of whether all the glands have been identified. If all glands were found and removed, the tubular phosphate reabsorption (TRP) will become 100 per cent within a few days. Failure to demonstrate this finding signifies that the procedure was incomplete and that at least one gland was left behind. After 4 or 5 days, TRP begins to be restored and, in our experience, satisfactory parathyroid function returns.

In this chapter, disproportionate attention has been given to the complication of hyperparathyroidism for a simple reason. The metabolic consequences of this complication have proven to be truly devastating to some of our patients who have been followed for almost as long as a decade. By the time it was realized that this process was going on, irreparable damage had been done to their skeletons, particularly in patients in the pediatric age group, and it is suspected that permanent harm was also done to the renal homograft itself in some cases.

PROBLEMS OF GROWTH

In children with chronic uremia, there is usually a failure of growth. After successful transplantation, the growth retardation associated with the original disease is replaced by whatever inhibition is caused by the administration of large doses of steroids.

Thus, a growth spurt does not ordinarily occur early after renal homotransplantation, and Najarian and his associates[72] concluded that catch-up growth in pediatric patients was not to be expected. However, their observations were based on follow-ups that were, for the most part, no greater than 2 years.

In contrast, our own experience with pediatric patients has been that catch-up growth may be seen an extraordinarily long time after transplantation, even after a delay of as long as 2 to 5 years.[61]

PULMONARY DISEASES

After transplantation of any of the major organs, including the kidney, liver, heart, and pancreas, a major source of subsequent morbidity has been the lung. Pulmonary complications have ranked as either the leading or the second most important cause of death with different reported series of these various kinds of organ transplantation. A very complete analysis of the role of the lung in the deaths of 60 of our early renal transplants has been published by Hill et al.[41] The complications to which the lung is subject in the immunosuppressed organ recipient include infection, thromboembolization, and neoplasia.

PNEUMONITIS. As emphasized earlier, the price for success after organ transplantation under immunosuppression is a partial loss of immunologic surveillance. The most dramatic consequence may be infec-

tion. In concept, until about a decade ago, many people conceived the problem to be insoluble, as depicted in Figure 31–22. The suggestion was that measures to prevent the rejection of grafts would inevitably permit the overgrowth of the contemporaneously present bacteria. The pessimism of this view has been thoroughly disproven. Nevertheless, the margin of safety between therapeutically desirable and lethal immunosuppression may not be great, and in some cases it may not exist at all. As far as the lung is concerned, the margin may be broadened by the clever management of pulmonary infectious complications.

Bacterial Pneumonitis. A variety of gram-positive and gram-negative bacteria may cause pulmonary infections in immunosuppressed organ recipients. The organisms presumably gain entry to the lungs by inhalation or by descent from an upper respiratory tract infection. Because effective antibiotics are available for almost all of the common pyogenic organisms, accurate identification of the organism and determination of antibiotic sensitivities are essential for the successful treatment of bacterial pneumonitides. Because bacteremia frequently accompanies these infections, blood cultures may be useful for isolation of the causative microorganisms, but cultures of tracheal aspirates are usually sufficient for this purpose.

Despite the availability of specific antibiotics for these infections, bacterial pneumonitis has contributed significantly to the mortality following transplantation. In the early

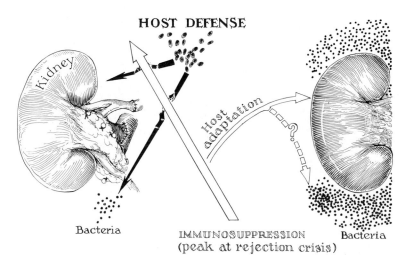

Figure 31–22 Graphic depiction of how immunosuppression, while permitting acceptance of the homograft, may allow the development of infection through a partial loss of immunologic surveillance. (From Starzl, T. E., et al.: Factors in successful renal transplantation. Surgery 56:296, 1964.)

HOST DEFENSE

Kidney

Host adaptation

Bacteria

IMMUNOSUPPRESSION
(peak at rejection crisis)

Bacteria

days of transplantation, there was a tendency to give too much azathioprine, and if bone marrow depression followed, bacterial pneumonitides were frequently fatal.[41] In more recent years, the doses of azathioprine have been smaller, and granulocytopenia has been correspondingly rare. However, bacterial pneumonitis may still cause occasional deaths, particularly if it is complicated by abscess formation, empyema, coexisting devitalization of lung tissue, such as by pulmonary emboli, or the necrotizing vasculitis sometimes seen with *Pseudomonas aeruginosa* pneumonitis.

Fungal Pneumonitis. The avoidance of bone marrow depression has by no means eliminated infections by microorganisms of normally low pathogenicity for which truly effective and safe antibiotic therapy is not available. Fungal pneumonitides have been a common cause of late morbidity and mortality,[41, 108, 112, 113] the most frequently noted microorganisms in our series being *Candida albicans* and *Aspergillus fumigatus*, although in geographic areas in which Coccidioides and Histoplasma[22] are endemic, infections with these fungi might be anticipated with greater frequency. Fungal infestation of the lungs may present as a diffuse pneumonitis or more commonly as a nodular lesion, which subsequently cavitates (Fig. 31–23). The diagnosis should be entertained in any

recipient with a pulmonary infection in whom a bacterial etiology cannot be convincingly established or in whom the lesions are exacerbated by appropriate antibacterial therapy. A definitive diagnosis may sometimes be made from examination and cultures of tracheobronchial aspirates or of material obtained by the endobronchial brush technique of Fennessey.[28] Neither method, however, has proven to be consistently reliable in establishing the etiology of such infections and an open lung biopsy, as recommended by Simmons,[108] may be required, although the risk of this procedure in most acute cases is high.

Amphotericin B is a potent systemic antifungal agent, but the effectiveness of therapy with this drug is severely limited by its toxicity, particularly its nephrotoxicity, which is dose-related. Miconazole is useful in the therapy of certain yeast infections, particularly *Candida albicans*. 5-Fluorocytosine may be administered orally, is usually employed in combination with intravenous amphotericin B, and is much less toxic than the latter drug.

Even with early detection, the results of treatment of pulmonary fungal infections have been disappointing, particularly when the causative organism is Aspergillus. Dissemination, commonly to the brain, may occur before the pneumonitis becomes clini-

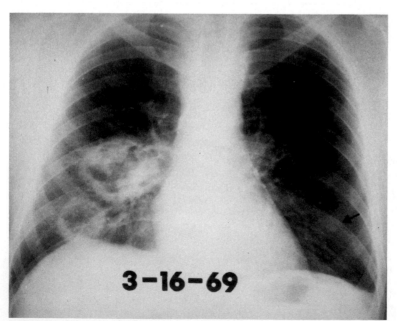

Figure 31–23 Chest x-ray of a patient with fatal *Aspergillus fumigatus* pneumonia. Note the cavitary lesions in the right lung field and the nodular lesions in the opposite lung (arrows). (From Pappas, G., et al.: Pulmonary surgery in immunosuppressed patients. J. Thorac. Cardiovasc. Surg. 59:882, 1970.)

cally evident or even after the institution of vigorous systemic therapy. In recipients of renal homografts, discontinuance of immunosuppression with sacrifice of the transplanted organ and return to hemodialysis may aid in controlling the infection.

In the event a fungus cavity becomes established and increases in size despite therapy with amphotericin B, the possibility of rupture into the pleural cavity becomes a pressing consideration. Under these circumstances, Pappas et al.[81] have recommended early pulmonary resection. We have salvaged several patients by this aggressive approach.

Other Opportunistic Organisms. In a very high percentage of recipients studied at autopsy[41] infection of the lungs with cytomegalovirus (CMV) can be demonstrated. Many recipients carry this virus in their upper respiratory tracts or excrete it in the urine. However, the extent to which CMV causes significant pneumonitis is not known, since it is so commonly found in asymptomatic recipients with normal chest x-rays and since at autopsy the presence of the virus frequently is not associated with any morphologic damage to the lungs.

Until recently, the most common microorganism implicated in lethal pneumonitis had been *Pneumocystis carinii*,[41] an incompletely classified parasite considered to be a protozoan. It is truly an opportunistic organism, since it is pathogenic only in patients with congenital or acquired immune deficiency states or under immunosuppression.

In recipients of organ homografts, this infection usually occurs during the first post-transplantation months. It may present as an acute pneumonitis with cough, a high fever, and rapidly progressive respiratory failure, even when promptly diagnosed and treated. Alternatively, it may have an insidious onset with subtle symptoms and gradual deterioration of respiratory function. In the latter cases, arterial oxygen desaturation without retention of carbon dioxide is one of the most significant laboratory findings. The chest x-ray usually demonstrates bilateral infiltrates, which tend to be most dense in the parahilar areas and lower lobes (Fig. 31–24), and which contrast with the lack of auscultatory findings.

The definitive diagnosis rests upon the

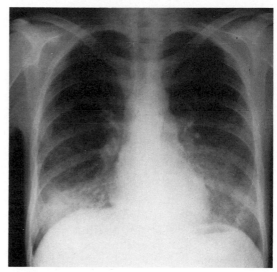

Figure 31–24 Typical appearance of a chest x-ray in *Pneumocystis carinii* pneumonitis, post transplantation. Note the bilateral parahilar infiltrates.

microscopic detection of the pathognomonic cysts in alveolar material stained with methenamine silver. Specimens may be obtained by brush biopsy, which in our experience has proven highly reliable for the diagnosis of this infection, especially in patients having subtle clinical findings.[98]

It was of much greater clinical importance to establish the diagnosis with certainty when the only available therapy was with pentamidine, a drug with considerable nephrotoxicity.[140] More recently, it has been shown that trimethoprim-sulfamethoxazole is highly effective against *Pneumocystis carinii*. Since the latter compound possesses little toxicity, treatment should usually be instituted without delay whenever *Pneumocystis* pneumonitis is suspected, without resorting to potentially dangerous invasive diagnostic procedures.

PULMONARY THROMBOEMBOLIZATION. In the early days of successful renal transplantation, there was an inordinately high incidence of thromboembolic complications. For example, in the first 42 recipients treated by us, there were nine examples of peripheral thrombophlebitis, and in five of these, pulmonary emboli were subsequently proven, either at the time of pulmonary embolectomy or at autopsy.

In 1976, Alexander's group at the University of Cincinnati reported thromboembolic disease in 25 of 100 consecutive renal recipients; nine of these patients died. They estimated the incidence of pulmonary embolism in their series to be 14 per cent.[96]

In more recent years, the incidence has not been so great. In the early cases, the preparation for operation frequently was poor. After transplantation to such "wet" patients, the degree of subsequent fluid loss was so great that as much as 30 kg. of weight was lost in some cases during the first 2 or 3 postoperative days. The resulting major fluid shifts probably predisposed to intravascular clotting.

Although the incidence of thromboembolism has decreased, it is still a significant threat. If thrombophlebitis or pulmonary embolization is suspected, careful heparin therapy is indicated.

OTHER INFECTIOUS COMPLICATIONS

Obviously, infections other than pulmonary ones occur in transplantation recipients but no attempt will be made to tediously document these. Among the most common should be listed pyelonephritis, particularly in kidney recipients, and meningitis. In recipients of renal homografts, and presumably with other organs as well, the combination of infection plus failing

homograft function has been particularly lethal. This fact is indicated in Figure 31–25, in which it is evident that very few infectious deaths occurred in patients who had normal kidney function. The organisms responsible for the deaths in Figure 31–25 are summarized in Table 31–7.

Simmons et al.[109] have emphasized the importance of cytomegalovirus infections in renal transplant recipients. After screening 132 patients, they identified 89 with laboratory evidence of CMV infection. In 83 of the 89, the infection was associated with evidence of rejection, a prompt antibody response to the virus, and recovery. Six more severely immunosuppressed patients, however, showed no antibody response, did not have evidence of rejection, and proved to be susceptible to other opportunistic infections, leading to death.

Descamps et al.,[25] noting the high frequency of antibody rise against a variety of viral antigens in 26 recipients, have suggested that the increases in titer may reflect immunologic dysfunction rather than viral infection. Supporting evidence for this viewpoint included (1) failure to isolate viruses other than those of the herpes group, (2) the occurrence of simultaneous antibody rises against several viruses, and (3) failure to observe the expected clinical signs of viral infection.

In an earlier section, the complication of

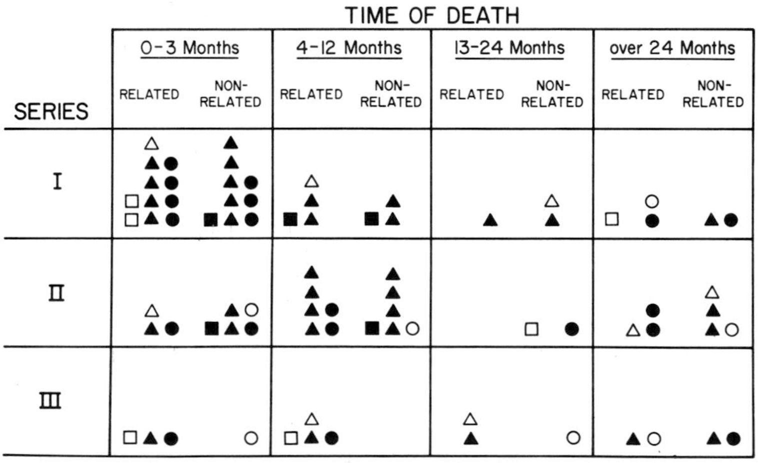

Figure 31–25　The contribution of imperfect or failed renal function and of infections to the deaths of 79 patients. The shading of symbols indicates that infection either caused or was a major contributor to death. The squares indicate excellent premortem renal function. The triangles indicate subnormal but life-supporting premortem renal function. The circles indicate that the homografts had failed. (From Starzl, T. E., et al.: Long term survival after renal transplantation in humans: With special reference to histocompatibility matching, thymectomy, homograft glomerulonephritis, heterologous ALG, and recipient malignancy. Ann. Surg. *182*:437, 1970.)

TABLE 31–7 PATHOGENIC ORGANISMS INVOLVED IN THE DEATHS* OF 79 PATIENTS†

	Number of Deaths with Infection at:		
	0–3 Mo.	4–12 Mo.	Over 12 Mo.
Bacterial			
Staphylococcus aureus	3	4	2
Hemolytic streptococcus	4	0	0
Listeria monocytogenes	0	1	0
Diplococcus pneumoniae	1	0	0
Escherichia coli	8	1	2
Pseudomonas aeruginosa	12	8	5
Klebsiella aerobacter	4	1	2
Proteus mirabilis	3	0	0
Paracolon species	1	0	0
Viral			
Hepatitis	0	1	2
Cytomegalic inclusion dis.	3	1	2
Varicella	0	0	1
Protozoan			
Pneumocystis carinii	1	8	1
Fungal			
Aspergillus fumigatus	2	3	2
Candida albicans and *stelloidea*	4	2	1
Nocardia	0	2	0
Histoplasmosis	0	1	0
Cryptococcus	0	0	1

*Some patients died with two or three types of microorganisms. For each patient the full spectrum of clinically significant microbiologic data has been entered into the table.

†From Starzl, T. E., Porter, K. A., Andres, G., Halgrimson, C. G., Hurwitz, R., Giles, G., Terasaki, P. I., Penn, I., Schroter, G. T., Lilly, J., Starkie, S. J., and Putnam, C. W.: Long-term survival after renal transplantation in humans: With special reference to histocompatibility matching, thymectomy, homograft glomerulonephritis, heterologous ALG, and recipient malignancy. Ann. Surg. *172*:437, 1970.

cholangitis in liver homografts and the role of partial biliary obstruction in this complication were described. An exhaustive review of infections complicating liver transplantation was published in 1976.[104]

DE NOVO MALIGNANT DISEASE

The surveillance hypothesis of malignant disease as proposed by Burnet[14, 15] and Thomas[136] suggested that malignant disease was the result of a failure of immunologic control of abnormal mutant cells. From the premises of Burnet and Thomas, it could have been predicted, and was shown,[106, 112] that an increased incidence of de novo tumors would be found in patients whose immune reactivity was deliberately depressed in order to permit their acceptance of organ homografts. A convincing association between immunosuppression and new malignant neoplasms did not become evident until 1968.[115] Since then there has been an outpouring of reports that have been summarized on several occasions.[82, 89, 90, 122] In addition to carefully studying our own case material, Penn has kept an informal registry of the world experience of this complication. By 1978 he had collected accounts of 529 malignant neoplasms in 506 transplant recipients. The incidence of malignancy was estimated to be 6 per cent, 100 times greater than in the same age group of the general population.[82] Moreover, the incidence appeared to increase with the length of time following transplantation.

The most common malignant growths have been of epithelial origin (213 patients). Squamous cell carcinomas, rather than the usually more common basal cell lesions, predominated. Multiple neoplasms were found in 39 per cent, twice the usual incidence. Ten of the 213 patients died of metastatic disease.

Transplant recipients should be cautioned to avoid excessive or prolonged exposure to the sun. Any skin lesions, particularly of the lip, for which the diagnosis is not certain should be biopsied.

One hundred and nine of the 506 patients had lymphomas, of which the majority (75 cases) were reticulum cell sarcomas, for an incidence 300 times that of the general population.[82] Hodgkin's disease was relatively rare (3 cases). Forty-four per cent of the patients with lymphoma had central nervous system involvement, versus two per cent in the general population. For this reason, neurologic symptoms in a transplant recipient should prompt a thorough neurologic evaluation, including computerized cerebral tomography in many instances.[82]

The frequency of cervical dysplasia in postadolescent female recipients is such that regular pelvic examination with cervical smears is mandatory. The majority of lesions are fortunately in situ and respond favorably to conventional therapy.[82]

It may be that in the highly malignant lymphoreticular tumors, and in the abdominal and thoracic carcinomas, which also carry a grave prognosis in transplant patients, immunosuppression should be stopped to permit reconstitution of immunologic competence and, it is hoped, a renaissance of tumor surveillance. With other tumors such as carcinomas of the skin (except melanoma), lip, and cervix, there is little justification for such a drastic measure since conventional therapy is almost always successful.

From more than a decade of observation, it now seems clear that the threat of malignant disease in organ recipients under immunosuppression is not going to be great enough to cancel the value of organ transplantation. Nevertheless, attention must constantly be focused upon this possibility and the appropriate cancer detection procedures should be mobilized in these patients.

NEUROLOGIC AND PSYCHIATRIC COMPLICATIONS

The brain has proven to be one of the innocent-bystander organs at considerable risk after organ transplantation under immunosuppression. Earlier in this chapter, meningitis was mentioned. In addition, many examples of brain abscess, most commonly of fungal etiology, have been encountered. The de novo lymphoreticular malignant neoplasms mentioned in the preceding section have a predilection for the brain.[103] Cytomegalovirus (CMV) has been found at autopsy in a number of brains. Finally, we have had several patients die, mostly liver recipients, in whom the brains were essentially normal at autopsy in spite of the fact that protracted unconsciousness and grave neurologic impairment had been present for days or weeks before death.

Psychiatric problems also have been extremely common. Among our renal recipients there have been three suicides, one by leaping from an eighth floor window, and two others by refusal to be reentered on effective hemodialysis after failure of their renal homografts. The subject of psychiatric disorders in renal transplant recipients has been discussed by Penn et al.[84]

SUMMARY

In this chapter, an incomplete list has been given of some of the complications of organ transplantation. The need for immunosuppression is by far the most important factor in generating these problems, along with failure of such therapy completely to control rejection. In addition, contributory factors include disabilities from the original disease and technical and anesthetic complications during the operation.

Bibliography

1. Aldrete, J. A., Daniel, W., O'Higgins, J. W., Homatas, J., and Starzl, T. E.: Analysis of anesthetic-related morbidity in human recipients of renal homografts. Anesth. Analg. 50:321, 1971.
2. Aldrete, J. A., O'Higgins, J. W., and Starzl, T. E.: Changes of serum potassium during renal homotransplantation. Arch. Surg. 101:82, 1970.
3. Alfrey, A. C., Jenkins, D., Groth, C. G., Schorr, W. S., Gecelter, L., and Ogden, D. A.: Resolution of hyperparathyroidism after renal homotransplantation. N. Engl. J. Med. 279:1349, 1968.
4. Alveryd, A.: Parathyroid glands in thyroid surgery. Acta Chir. Scand. (Suppl.) 389:1, 1968.
5. Andres, G. A., Accinni, L., Hsu, K. C., Penn, I., Porter, K. A., Rendall, J. M., Seegal, B. C., and

Starzl, T. E.: Human renal transplants. III. Immunopathologic studies. Lab. Invest. 22:588, 1970.

6. Aubrey, D. A.: Massive hepatic necrosis after cyclophosphamide. Br. Med. J. 3:588, 1970.

7. Baggenstoss, A. H.: The pancreas in uremia: A histopathologic study. Am. J. Pathol. 24:1003, 1948.

8. Bayer, M. F., Blumberg, B. S., and Werner, B.: Particles associated with Australia antigen in the sera of patients with leukemia, Down's syndrome, and hepatitis. Nature (Lond.) 218:1057, 1968.

9. Bennett, W. M., Strong, D., and Rosch, J.: Arteriovenous fistula complicating renal transplantation. Urology 8:254, 1976.

10. Blaufox, M. D., Lewis, E. J., Jagger, P., Lauler, D., Hickler, R., and Merrill, J. P.: Physiologic responses of the transplanted human kidney: Sodium regulation and renin secretion. N. Engl. J. Med. 280:62, 1969.

11. Bricker, N. S., Slatopolsky, E., and Reiss, E.: Calcium, phosphorus and bone in renal disease and transplantation. Arch. Intern. Med. 123:543, 1969.

12. Buckingham, J. M., Palumbo, P. J., Woods, J. E., Service, F. J., Aguilo, J. J., and Zincke, H.: Plasma insulin and glucose levels after renal transplantation. Urology 8:210, 1976.

13. Buckingham, J. M., Roses, J., and Zincke, H.: Internal marsupialization of lymphoceles after renal transplantation. Urology 7:486, 1976.

14. Burnet, F. M.: Cancer: A biological approach. Br. Med. J. 1:779, 1957.

15. Burnet, F. M.: The evolution of bodily defence. Med. J. Australia 2:817, 1963.

16. Calne, R. Y.: A new technique for biliary drainage in orthotopic liver transplantation utilizing the gallbladder as a pedicle graft conduit between the donor and recipient common bile ducts. Ann. Surg. 184:605, 1976.

17. Calne, R. Y., McMaster, P., Portmann, B., Wall, W. J., and Williams, R.: Observations on preservation, bile drainage and rejection. Ann. Surg. 186:282, 1977.

18. Calne, R. Y., Rolles, K., White, D. J. G., et al.: Cyclosporin A initially as the only immunosuppressant in 34 recipients of cadaveric organs: 32 kidneys, 2 pancreas and 2 livers. Lancet 2:1033, 1979.

19. Calne, R. Y., and Williams, R.: Liver transplantation in man. I. Observations on technique and organization in 5 cases. Br. Med. J. 4:535, 1968.

20. Calne, R. Y., Williams, R., Dawson, J. L., Ansell, I. D., Evans, D. B., Flute, P. T., Herbertson, P. M., Joysey, V., Keates, G. H. W., Knill-Jones, R. P., Mason, S. A., Millard, P. R., Pena, J. R., Pentlow, B. D., Salaman, J. R., Sells, R. A. and Cullum, P. A.: Liver transplantation in man. II. A report of two orthotopic liver transplants in adult recipients. Br. Med. J. 4:541, 1968.

21. Carone, F. A., and Lieburne, A. A.: Acute pancreatitis lesions in patients treated with ACTH and adrenal corticoids. N. Engl. J. Med. 257:690, 1957.

22. Davies, S. F., Sarosi, G. A., Peterson, P. K., Khan,

M., Howard, R. J., Simmons, R. L., and Najarian, J. S.: Disseminated histoplasmosis in renal transplant recipients. Am. J. Surg. 137:686, 1979.

23. Degos, F., Degott, C., Bedrossian, J., Camilieri, J. P., Barbanel, C., Duboust, A., Rueff, B., Benhamou, J. P., and Kreis, H.: Is renal transplantation involved in post-transplantation liver disease? A prospective study. Transplantation 29:100, 1980.

24. DeLorimer, A. A., Belzer, F. O., Kountz, S. L., and Kushner, J. L.: Simultaneous bilateral nephrectomy and renal allotransplantation for bilateral Wilms' tumors. Surgery 64:850, 1968.

25. Descamps, P., Bedrossian, J., Nochy, D., Duboust, A., Idatte, J. M., Lagranse, P., Acar, J., Leroux, R. C., Sraer, J. D., Kourilksy, O., Meyrier, A., Dupuy, C. A., Huraux, J. M., Nicolas, J. C., and Bricout, F.: II. Renal transplantation and viral infections. III. Clinical and virological correlations. Biomed. 28:113, 1978.

26. Dixon, F. J.: Glomerulonephritis and immunopathology. In Good, R. A., and Fisher, D. W. (Eds.): Immunobiology. Stamford, Conn., Sinauer Associates, Inc., 1971, pp. 167–173.

27. Dreiling, D. A., Janowitz, H. D., and Perrier, C. S.: Pancreatic Inflammatory Disease: A Physiologic Approach. New York, Paul B. Hoeber, Inc., 1964, pp. 37–67.

28. Fennessey, J. J.: A technique for the selective catheterization of segmental bronchi using arterial catheters. Am. J. Roentgenol. 96:936, 1966.

29. First, M. R., Linnemann, C. C., Munda, R., McConnell, C. M., Ramundo, M., and Alexander, J. W.: Transmitted streptococcal infection and hyperacute rejection. Possible cross-reaction of streptococcal antigens and antibodies with mammalian tissues. Transplantation 24:400, 1977.

30. Fish, J. C., Sarles, H. E., Reemers, A. R., Tyson, K. R T., Canales, C. O., Beathard, G. A., Fukushima, M., Ritzmann, S. E., and Levin, W. C.: Circulating lymphocyte depletion in preparation for renal allotransplantation. Surg. Gynecol. Obstet. 129:777, 1969.

31. Franksson, C.: Letter to the Editor. Lancet 1:1331, 1964.

32. Geis, W. P., Popovtzer, M. M., Corman, J. L., Halgrimson, C. G., Groth, C. G., and Starzl, T. E.: The diagnosis and treatment of hyperparathyroidism after renal homotransplantation. Surg. Gynecol. Obstet. 137:997, 1973.

33. Goldman, M. H., Burleson, R. L., Tilney, N. L., Vineyard, G. C., and Wilson, R. E.: Calcyceal-cutaneous fistulae in renal transplant patients. Ann. Surg. 184:679, 1976.

34. Goldman, M. H., Leapman, S. B., Handy, R. D., and Best, D. W.: Renal allograft rupture with iliofemoral thrombophlebitis. Arch. Surg. 113:204, 1978.

35. Greene, J. A., Jr., Vander, A. J., and Kowalczyk, R S.: Plasma renin activity and aldosterone excretion after renal homotransplantation. J. Lab. Clin. Med. 71:586, 1968.

36. Griepp, R. B., Stinson, E. B., and Shumway, N.

E.: Heart. *In* Najarian, J. S., and Simmons, R. L. (Eds.): Transplantation. Philadelphia, Lea & Febiger, 1972, pp. 531–559.

37. Groth, C. G., Pechet, L., and Starzl, T. E.: Coagulation during and after orthotopic transplantation of the human liver. Arch. Surg. *98*:31, 1969.

38. Hallenbeck, G. A., Shorter, R. G., Titus, J. L., Thomford, N. R., Johnson, W. J., and DeWeerd, J. H.: Apparent glomerulonephritis in a homotransplant. Surgery *59*:522, 1966.

39. Hamburger, J., Crosnier, J., and Dormant, J.: Observations in patients with a well tolerated homotransplanted kidney: Possibility of a new secondary disease. Ann. N.Y. Acad. Sci. *120*:558, 1964.

40. Hamper, C. L., Zollinger, R. M., and Skillman, J. J.: Hemodynamic and body composition changes following bilateral nephrectomy in chronic renal failure. Circulation *40*:367, 1969.

41. Hill, R. B., Jr., Dahrling, B. E., Starzl, T. E., and Rifkind, D.: Death after transplantation: An analysis of 60 cases. Am. J. Med. *42*:327, 1967.

42. Hill, R. B., Jr., Rowlands, D. T., Jr., and Rifkind, D.: Infectious pulmonary disease in patients receiving immunosuppressive therapy for organ transplantation. N. Engl. J. Med. *271*:1021, 1964.

43. Hume, D. M.: Progress in clinical renal homotransplantation. *In* Welch, C. E. (Ed.): Advances in Surgery. Vol. 2. Chicago, Year Book Medical Publishers, Inc., 1966, pp. 419–498.

44. Hume, D. M., Lee, H. M., Williams, G. M., White, J. O., Ferre, J., Wolf, J. S., Prout, G. R., Jr., Slapak, M., O'Brien, J., Kilpatrick, S. J., Kauffman, H. M., Jr., and Cleveland, R. J.: Comparative results of cadaver and related donor renal homografts in man, and immunologic implications of the outcome of second and paired transplants. Ann. Surg. *164*:352, 1966.

45. Hume, D. M., Magee, J. H., Kauffman, H. M., Jr., Rittenbury M. S., and Prout, G. R., Jr.: Renal transplantation in man in modified recipients. Ann. Surg. *158*:608, 1963.

46. Ibels, L. S., Alfrey, A. C., Huffer, W. E., and Weil, R., III.: Aseptic necrosis of bone following renal transplantation: Experience in 194 transplant recipients and review of the literature. Medicine *57*:25, 1978.

47. Idezuki, Y., Feemster, J. A., Dietzman, R. H., and Lillehei, R. C.: Experimental pancreaticoduodenal preservation and transplantation. Surg. Gynecol. Obstet. *126*:1002, 1968.

48. Johnson, J. W., Hattner, R. S., Hampers, C. L., Bernstein, D. S., Merrill, J. P., and Sherwood, L. M.: Secondary hyperparathyroidism in chronic renal failure. Effects of renal homotransplantation. J.A.M.A. *215*:478, 1971.

49. Johnson, J. W., Wachman, A., Katz, A. I., Berstein, D. S., Hampers, C. L., Hattner, R. S., Wilson, R. E., and Merrill, J. P.: The effect of subtotal parathyroidectomy and renal transplantation on mineral balance and secondary hyperparathyroidism in chronic renal failure. Metabolism *20*:487, 1971.

50. Johnson, W. C., and Nabseth, D. C.: Pancreatitis in renal transplantation. Ann. Surg. *171*:309, 1970.

51. Jowsey, J., and Balasubramaniam, P.: Effect of phosphate supplements on soft tissue calcification and bone turnover. Clin. Sci. *42*:289, 1972.

52. Kashiwagi, N., Brantigan, C. O., Brettschneider, L., Groth, C. G., and Starzl, T. E.: Clinical reactions and serologic changes following the administration of heterologous antilymphocyte globulin to human recipients of renal homografts. Ann. Intern. Med. *68*:275, 1968.

53. Kevitt, M. D., Rapaport, M., and Cooper, S. R.: The renal clearance of amylase in renal insufficiency, acute pancreatitis, and macroamylasemia. Ann. Intern. Med. *71*:919, 1969.

54. Kissmeyer-Nielsen, F., Olsen, S., Peterson, V. P., and Fjeldborg, O.: Hyperacute rejection of kidney allografts associated with pre-existing humoral antibodies against donor cells. Lancet *2*:662, 1966.

55. Koep, L. J., Peters, T. G., and Starzl, T. E.: Major colonic complications of liver transplantation. Dis. Colon Rectum *22*:218, 1979.

56. Konomi, K., Deodhar, S. D., Tung, K. S. K., and Nakamoto, S.: Immunosuppression with antilymphocyte globulin in clinical renal transplantation. Surg. Forum *19*:194, 1968.

57. Krieg, A. F., Bolande, R. P., Holden, W. D., Hubay, C. A., and Persky, L.: Membranous glomerulonephritis occurring in a human renal homograft. Am. J. Clin. Pathol. *34*:155, 1960.

58. Laflamme, G. H., and Jowsey, J.: Bone and soft tissue changes with oral phosphate supplements. J. Clin. Invest. *51*:2834, 1972.

59. Lee, H. M., Mendez-Picon, G., Pierce, J. C., and Hume, D. M.: Renal artery occlusion in transplant recipients. Am. Surg. *43*:186, 1977.

60. Light, J. A., Annable, C., Perloff, L. J., Sulkin, M. D., Hill, G. S., Etheredge, E. E., and Spees, E. K., Jr.: Immune injury from organ preservation. A potential cause of hyperacute rejection in human cadaver kidney transplantation. Transplantation *19*:511, 1975.

61. Lilly, J. R., Giles, G., Hurwitz, R., Schroter, G. P. J., Takagi, H., Gray, S., Penn, I., Halgrimson, C. G., and Starzl, T. E.: Renal homotransplantation in pediatric patients. Pediatrics *47*:548, 1971.

62. MacKinnon, K. J., Oliver, J. A., Morehouse, D. D., and Taguchi, Y.: Cadaver renal transplantation: Emphasis on urological aspects. J. Urol. *99*:486, 1968.

63. Martin, D. C., Mims, M. M., Kaufman, J. J., and Goodwin, W. E.: The ureter in renal transplantation. J. Urol. *101*:680, 1969.

64. Martineau, G., Porter, K. A., Corman, J., Launois, B., Schroter, G., Palmer, W., Putnam, C. W., Groth, C. G., Halgrimson, C. G., Penn, I., and Starzl, T. E.: Delayed biliary duct obstruction after orthotopic liver transplantation. Surgery *72*:604, 1972.

65. McIntosh, D. A., Peterson, E. W., and McPhaul, J. J.: Autonomy of parathyroid function after renal homotransplantation. Ann. Intern. Med. *65*:900, 1966.

66. McPhaul, J. J., Jr., Dixon, F. J., Brettschneider, L., and Starzl, T. E.: Immunofluorescent examination of biopsies from long term renal allografts. N. Engl. J. Med. *282*:412, 1970.

67. Merrill, J. P.: Glomerulonephritis in renal transplants. Transplant Proc. *1*:994, 1970.

68. Moore, T. C., and Hume, D. M.: The period and nature of hazard in clinical renal transplantation. I. The hazard to patient survival. II. The hazard to transplant kidney function. Ann. Surg. *170*:1, 1969.

69. Mozes, M. F., Ascher, N. L., Balfour, H. H., Jr., Simmons, R. L., and Najarian, J. S.: Jaundice after renal allotransplantation. Ann. Surg., *188*:783, 1978.

70. Murray, J. E., Merrill, J. P., Harrison, J. H., Wilson, R. E., and Dammin, G. J.: Prolonged survival of human kidney homografts with immunosuppressive drug therapy. N. Engl. J. Med. *268*:1315, 1963.

71. Murray, J. E., Wilson, R. E., Tilney, N. L., Merrill, J. P., Cooper, W. C., Birtch, A. G., Carpenter, C. B., Hager, E. B., Dammin, G. J., and Harrison, J. H.: Five years' experience in renal transplantation with immunosuppressive drugs: Survival, function, complications, and the role of lymphocyte depletion by thoracic duct fistula. Ann. Surg. *168*:416, 1968.

72. Najarian, J. S., Simmons, R. L., Tallent, M. B., Kjellstrand, C. M., Vernier, R. L., and Michael, A. F.: Renal transplantation in infants and children. Ann. Surg. *174*:583, 1971.

73. Narayana, A. S., Loening, S., and Culp, D. A.: Kidney stones and renal transplantation. Urology *12*:61, 1978.

74. Nielsen, H. E., Melsen, F., and Christensen, M. S.: Aseptic necrosis of bone following renal transplantation. Clinical and biochemical aspects of bone morphometry. Acta Med. Scand. *202*:27, 1977.

75. O'Brien, J. P., and Hume, D. M.: Membranous glomerulonephritis in two renal homotransplants. Ann. Intern. Med. *65*:504, 1968.

76. Olsson, C. A., Willscher, M. K., Filoso, A. M., and Cho, S. I.: Treatment of posttransplant lymphoceles: Internal versus external drainage. Transplant. Proc. *8*:501, 1976.

77. Orange, R. P., and Austen, K. F.: Chemical mediators of immediate hypersensitivity. *In* Good, R. A., and Fisher, D. W. (Eds.): Immunobiology. Stamford, Conn., Sinauer Associates, Inc., 1971, pp. 115–121.

78. Owens, M. L., Wilson, S. E., Maxwell, J. G., Bordner, A., Smith, R., and Ehrlich, R.: Major arterial hemorrhage after renal transplantation. Transplantation *27*:285, 1979.

79. Palmer, J. M., Kountz, S. L., Swenson, R. S., Lucas, Z. J., and Cohn, R.: Urinary tract morbidity in renal transplantation. Arch. Surg. *98*:352, 1969.

80. Pappas, G., Palmer, W. M., Martineau, G. L., Penn, I., Halgrimson, C. G., Groth, C. G., and Starzl, T. E.: Hemodynamic alterations caused during orthotopic liver transplantation in humans. Surgery *70*:872, 1971.

81. Pappas, G., Schroter, G., Brettschneider, L., Penn, I., and Starzl, T. E.: Pulmonary surgery in immunosuppressed patients. J. Thorac. Cardiovasc. Surg. *59*:882, 1970.

82. Penn, I.: Malignancies associated with immunosuppressive or cytotoxic therapy. Surgery *83*:492, 1978.

83. Penn, I., Brettschneider, L., Simpson, K., Martin, A. J., and Starzl, T. E.: Major colonic problems in human homotransplant recipients. Arch. Surg. *100*:61, 1970.

84. Penn, I., Bunch, D., Olenik, D., and Abouna, G.: Psychiatric experience with patients receiving renal and hepatic transplants. *In* Castelnuovo-Tedesco, P. (Ed.): Psychiatric Aspects of Organ Transplantation. New York, Grune & Stratton, 1971, pp. 133–144.

85. Penn, I., Durst, A. L., and Machado, M.: Diabetes and hyperglycemia in renal homograft recipients. Unpublished observations.

86. Penn, I., Durst, A. L., Machado, M,. Halgrimson, C. G., Booth, A. S., Jr., Putnam, C. W., Groth, C. G., and Starzl, T. E.: Acute pancreatitis and hyperamylasemia in renal homograft recipients. Arch. Surg. *105*:167, 1972.

87. Penn, I., Groth, C. G., Brettschneider, L., Martin, A. J., Marchioro, T. L., and Starzl, T. E.: Surgically correctable intra-abdominal complications before and after renal homotransplantation. Ann. Surg. *168*:865, 1968.

88. Penn, I., Hammond, W., Bell, P., McGuire, R., Hutt, M., and Starzl, T. E.: Hepatic disorders in renal homograft recipients. Curr. Top. Surg. Res. *1*:67, 1969.

89. Penn, I., Hammond, W., Brettschneider, L., and Starzl, T. E.: Malignant lymphomas in transplantation patients. Transplant. Proc. *1*:106, 1969.

90. Penn, I., and Starzl, T. E.: A summary of the status of *de novo* cancer in transplant recipients. Transplant Proc. *4*:719, 1972.

91. Petersen, V. P., Olsen, S., Kissmeyer-Nielsen, S., and Fjeldborg, O.: Transmission of glomerulonephritis from host to human kidney allotransplant. N. Engl. J. Med. *275*:1269, 1966.

92. Pletka, P., Strom, T., Bernstein, D. S., Wilson, R. E., Sherwood, L. M., Hampers, C. L., and Merrill, J. P.: Secondary hyperparathyroidism in human kidney transplant recipients. Proceedings International Congress of Nephrology. Mexico City, 1972, p. 156 (abstract).

93. Porter, K. A., Thomson, W. B., Owen, K., Kenyon, J. R., Mowbray, J. F., and Peart, W. S.: Obliterative vascular changes in 4 human kidney homotransplants. Br. Med. J. *2*:639, 1963.

94. Prince, A. M.: An antigen detected in the blood during the incubation period of serum hepatitis. Proc. Natl. Acad. Sci. (USA) *60*:814, 1968.

95. Prout, G. R., Jr., Hume, D. M., Lee, H. M., and Williams, G. M.: Some urological aspects of 93 consecutive renal homotransplants in modified recipients. J. Urol. *97*:409, 1967.

96. Rao, K. V., Smith, E. J., Alexander, J. W., Fidler, J. P., Pemmaraju, S. R., and Pollack, V. E.: Thromboembolic disease in renal allograft recipients. What is its clinical significance? Arch. Surg. *111*:1086, 1976.

97. Reiss, E., Canterbury, J. M., and Cater, A.: Cir-

culating parathyroid hormone concentration in chronic renal insufficiency. Arch. Intern. Med. *124*:417, 1969.

98. Repsher, L. H., Schröter, G., and Hammond, W. S.: Diagnosis of *Pneumocystis carinii* pneumonitis by means of endobronchial brush biopsy. N. Engl. J. Med. *287*:340, 1972.

99. Rubin, J. S., and Rubin, R. T.: Cyclophosphamide hemorrhagic cystitis. J. Urol. *96*:313, 1966.

100. Santos, G. W., Burke, P. J., Sensenbrunner, L. L., and Owens, A. H., Jr.: Rationale for the use of cyclophosphamide as an immunosuppressant for marrow transplants in man. *In* Bertelli, H., and Monaco, A. P. (Eds.): Pharmacological Treatment in Organ and Tissue Transplantation. Amsterdam, Excerpta Medica Foundation, 1970, p. 24.

101. Sarmina, M. H., Sanchez, R. M., and Ortiz, F. Q.: Tecnica y Agentes Anestesicos en Transplantes Renales. Fev. Mex. Anest. *17*:381, 1968.

102. Schacht, R. A., Martin, D. G., Karalakulasingam, R., Wheeler, C. S., and Lansing, A. M.: Renal artery stenosis after renal transplantation. Am. J. Surg. *131*:653, 1976.

103. Schneck, S. A., and Penn, I.: *De novo* cerebral neoplasms in renal transplant recipients. Lancet *1*:983, 1971.

104. Schroter, G. P., Hoelscher, M., Putnam, C. W., Porter, K. A., Hansbrough, J. F., and Starzl, T. E.: Infections complicating orthotopic liver transplantation: A study emphasizing graft-related septicemia. Arch. Surg. *111*:1337, 1976.

105. Schwartz, G. H., David, D. S., Riggio, R. R., Saville, P. D., Whitsell, J. C., Stenzel, K. H., and Rubin, A. L.: Hypercalcemia after renal transplantation. Am. J. Med. *49*:42, 1970.

106. Schwartz, R., Schwartz, J. A., Armstrong, M. Y. K., and Beldotti, L.: Neoplastic sequelae of allogenic disease. I. Theoretical considerations and experimental design. Ann. N.Y. Acad. Sci. *129*:804, 1966.

107. Seddon, J. A., and Howard, J. M.: The exocrine behavior of the homotransplanted pancreas. Surgery *59*:226, 1966.

108. Simmons, R. L., Kjellstrand, C. M., and Najarian, J. S.: Sepsis following kidney transplantation. *In* Hardy, J. D. (Ed.): Critical Surgical Illness. Philadelphia, W. B. Saunders Company, 1971, p. 559.

109. Simmons, R. L., Lopez, C., Balfour, H., Kalis, J., Rattazzi, L. C., and Najarian, J. S.: Cytomegalovirus: Clinical virological correlations in renal transplant recipients. Ann. Surg. *180*:623, 1974.

110. Simpson, K., Bunch, D. L., Amemiya, H., Boehmig, H. J., Wilson, C. B., Dixon, F. J., Coburg, A. J., Hathaway, W. E., Giles, G. R., and Starzl, T. E.: Humoral antibodies and coagulation mechanisms in the accelerated or hyperacute rejection of renal homografts in sensitized canine recipients. Surgery *68*:77, 1970.

111. Spigos, D. and Capek, V.: Ultrasonically guided percutaneous aspiration of lymphoceles following renal transplantation: A diagnostic and therapeutic method. J. Clin. Ultrasound *4*:45, 1976.

112. Starzl, T. E.: Experience in Renal Transplantation. Philadelphia, W. B. Saunders Company, 1964.

113. Starzl, T. E. (with the assistance of Putnam, C. W.): Experience in Hepatic Transplantation. Philadelphia, W. B. Saunders Company, 1969.

114. Starzl, T. E., Boehmig, H. J., Amemiya, H., Wilson, C. B., Dixon, F. J., Giles, G. R., Simpson, K. M., and Halgrimson, C. G.: Clotting changes including disseminated intravascular coagulation during rapid renal homograft rejection. N. Engl. J. Med. *283*:383, 1970.

115. Starzl, T. E., Groth, C. G., Brettschneider, L., Smith, G. V., Penn, I., and Kashiwagi, N.: Perspectives in organ transplantation. (Proceedings of the Swiss Society of Immunology.) Antibiot. Chemother. *15*:349, 1969.

116. Starzl, T. E., Groth, C. G., Putnam, C. W., Penn, I., Halgrimson, C. G., Flatmark, A., Gecelter, L., Brettschneider, L., and Stonington, O. G.: Urological complications in 216 human recipients of renal transplants. Ann. Surg. *172*:1, 1970.

117. Starzl, T. E., Koep, L. J., Halgrimson, C. G., Hood, J., Schroter, G. P. J., Porter, K. A., and Weil, R., III: Fifteen years of clinical liver transplantation. Gastroenterology *77*:375, 1979.

118. Starzl, T. E., Lerner, R. L., Dixon, F. J., Groth, C. G., Brettschneider, L., and Terasaki, P. I.: Shwartzman reaction after human renal homotransplantation. N. Engl. J. Med. *278*:642, 1968.

119. Starzl, T. E., Marchioro, T. L., Porter, K. A., Iwasaki, Y., and Cerilli, G. J.: The use of heterologous antilymphoid agents in canine renal and liver homotransplantation, and in human renal homotransplantation. Surg. Gynecol. Obstet. *124*:301, 1967.

120. Starzl, T. E., Marchioro, T. L., von Kaulla, K. N., Hermann, G., Brittain, R. S., and Waddell, W. R.: Homotransplantation of the liver in humans. Surg. Gynecol. Obstet. *117*:659, 1963.

121. Starzl, T. E., Marchioro, T. L., and Waddell, W. R.: The reversal of rejection in human renal homografts with subsequent development of homograft tolerance. Surg. Gynecol. Obstet. *117*:385, 1963.

122. Starzl, T. E., Penn, I., Putnam, C. W., Groth, C. G., and Halgrimson, C. G.: Iatrogenic alterations of immunologic surveillance in man and their influence on malignancy. Transplant. Rev. *7*:112, 1971.

123. Starzl, T. E., Porter, K. A., Andres, G., Groth, C. G., Putnam, C. W., Penn, I., Halgrimson, C. G., Starkie, S. J., and Brettschneider, L.: Thymectomy and renal homotransplantation. Clin. Exp. Immunol. *6*:803, 1970.

124. Starzl, T. E., Porter, K. A., Andres, G., Halgrimson, C. G., Hurwitz, R., Giles, G., Terasaki, P. I., Penn, I., Schroter, G. T., Lilly, J., Starkie, S. J., and Putnam, C. W.: Long-term survival

after renal transplantation in humans: With special reference to histocompatibility matching, thymectomy, homograft glomerulonephritis, heterologous ALG, and recipient malignancy. Ann. Surg. *172*:437, 1970.

125. Starzl, T. E., Porter, K. A., Iwasaki, Y., Marchioro, T. L., and Kashiwagi, N.: The use of antilymphocyte globulin in human renal homotransplantation. *In* Ciba Foundation Study Group, Wolstenholme, G. E. W., and O'Connor, M. (Eds.): Anti-lymphocytic Serum. Baltimore, Williams & Wilkins Company, 1967, pp. 4–34.

126. Starzl, T. E., Porter, K. A., Putnam, C. W., Hansbrough, J. F., and Reid, H. A. S.: Biliary complications after liver transplantation: With special reference to the biliary cast syndrome and techniques of secondary duct repair. Surgery *81*:213, 1976.

127. Starzl, T. E., Porter, K. A., Putnam, C. W., Schroter, G. P. J., Halgrimson, C. G., Weil, R., III, Hoelscher, M., and Reid, H. A. S.: Orthotopic liver transplantation in 93 patients. Surg. Gynecol. Obstet. *142*:487, 1976.

128. Starzl, T. E., Putnam, C. W., Halgrimson, C. G., Groth, C. G., Booth, A. S., Jr., and Penn, I.: Renal transplantation under cyclophosphamide. Transplant. Proc. *4*:461, 1972.

129. Starzl, T. E., Putnam, C. W., Halgrimson, C. G., Schroter, G. P., Martineau, G., Launois, B., Corman, J. L., Penn, I., Booth, A. S., Jr., Porter, K. A., and Groth, C. G.: Cyclophosphamide and whole organ transplantation in humans. Surg. Gynecol. Obstet. *133*:981, 1971.

130. Starzl, T. E., Schneck, S. A., Mazzoni, G., Aldrete, J. A., Porter, K. A., Schroter, G. P. J., Koep, L. J., and Putnam, C. W.: Acute neurological complications after liver transplantation with particular reference to intraoperative cerebral air embolus. Ann. Surg. *187*:236, 1978.

131. Starzl, T. E., Weil, R., III, Iwatsuki, S., Klintmalm, G., Schroter, G. P. J., Koep, L. J., Iwaki, Y., Terasaki, P. I., and Porter, K. A.: The use of cyclosporin A and prednisone in cadaver kidney transplantation. Surg. Gynecol. Obstet. *151*:17, 1980.

132. Starzl, T. E., Weil, R., III, Koep, L. J., Iwaki, Y., Terasaki, P. I., and Schroter, G. P. J: Thoracic duct drainage before and after cadaveric kidney transplantation. Surg. Gynecol. Obstet. *149*:815, 1979.

133. Starzl, T. E., Weil, R., III, Koep, L. J., McCalmon, R. T., Jr., Terasaki, P. I., Iwaki, Y., Schroter, G. P. J., Franks, J. J., Subryan, V., and Halgrimson, C. G.: Thoracic duct fistula and renal transplantation. Ann. Surg. *190*:474, 1979.

134. Stinson, E. B., Dong, E, Jr., Bieber, C. P., Schroeder, J. S., and Shumway, N. E.: Cardiac transplantation in man. I. Early rejection. J.A.M.A. *207*:2233, 1969.

135. Terasaki, P. I., Marchioro, T. L., and Starzl, T. E.: Sero-typing of human lymphocyte antigens: Preliminary trials on long-term kidney homo-graft survivors. *In* Histocompatibility Testing. Washington, D.C., National Academy of Sciences–National Research Council, 1965, pp. 83–96.

136. Thomas, L.: Discussion of paper by P. B. Medawar. Reactions to homologous tissue antigens in relation to hypersensitivity. *In* Lawrence, H. S. (Ed.): Cellular and Humoral Aspects of the Hypersensitive States. New York, Hoeber Medical Division, Harper & Row, 1969, p. 530.

137. Torisu, M., Yokoyama, T., Amemiya, H., Kohler, P. F., Schroter, G., Martineau, G., Penn, I., Palmer, W., Halgrimson, C. G., Putnam, C. W., and Starzl, T. E.: Immunosuppression, liver injury, and hepatitis in renal, hepatic, and cardiac homograft recipients: With particular reference to the Australia antigen. Ann. Surg. *174*:620, 1971.

138. Traeger, J., Carraz, M., Fries, D., Perrin, J., Saubier, E., Bernhardt, J., Bonnet, P., and Archimbaud, J.: Preparation, biological activities and long term clinical studies with ALS made from thoracic duct lymphocytes. Transplant. Proc. *1*:455, 1969.

139. West, T. H., Turcotte, J. G., and Vander, A. J.: Plasma renin activity, sodium balance, and hypertension in a group of renal transplant recipients. J. Lab. Clin. Med. *73*:564, 1969.

140. Western, K. A., Perera, D. R., and Schultz, M. G.: Pentamidine isethionate in the treatment of *Pneumocystis carinii* pneumonia. Ann. Intern. Med. *73*:695, 1970.

141. Williams, G. A., Bowser, E. N., Hargis, G. K., Henderson, W. J., Martinez, N. J., Fucik, R., and Kukreja, S.: Effect of glucocorticoids on function of the parathyroid glands in man. Clin. Res. *20*:780, 1972.

142. Williams, G. M., Hume, D. M., Hudson, R. P., Jr., Morris, P. J., Kano, K., and Milgrom, F.: "Hyperacute" renal homograft rejection in man. N. Engl. J. Med. *279*:611, 1968.

143. Williams, R., Smith, M., Shilkin, K. B., Herbertson, B., Jaysey, B., and Calne, R. Y.: Liver transplantation in man; the frequency of rejection, biliary tract complications, and recurrence of malignancy based on an analysis of 26 cases. Gastroenterology *64*:1026, 1973.

144. Wolf, J. L., Perkins, H. A., Schreeder, M. T., and Vincenti, F.: The transplanted kidney as a source of hepatitis B infection. Ann. Intern. Med. *91*:412, 1979.

145. Woodruff, M. F. A., Robson, J. S., Nolan, B., Lambie, A. T., Wilson, T. I., and Clark, J. G.: Homotransplantation of kidney in patients treated by preoperative local radiation and postoperative administration of an antimetabolite (Imuran). Lancet *2*:675, 1963.

146. Yeh, T. J., Toyohara, H., Ellison, L. T., Parker, J. L., and Ellison, R. G.: Pulmonary function in dogs after lung homotransplantation. Ann. Thorac. Surg. *2*:195, 1966.

147. Zarday, Z., Veith, F. J., Gliedman, M. L., and Soberman, R.: Irreversible liver damage after azathioprine. J.A.M.A. *222*:690, 1972.

32

COMPLICATIONS OF BURNS AND BURN TREATMENT

Alan R. Dimick

A patient with an injury as complex as a thermal burn can be expected to have a number of complications. These complications may affect any organ system and may occur at any time from initial care to late convalescence. These complications are directly related to the extent of the burn and the age of the patient. In addition, the variety of treatment modalities used for extensive burn injury predispose the patient to certain complications. The complications of the burn injury and occasionally of burn treatment are sometimes more severe and life-threatening than is the original injury. Some complications are more common than others. In general, the more extensive and more severe the burn, the greater the number of complications. Also, the more prolonged the hospital course, the greater the number of complications. Often, if complications are anticipated, they can be prevented.

PULMONARY COMPLICATIONS

Complications of the respiratory tract fall into two categories: those seen after any type of severe injury and those associated with inhalation of noxious gases and smoke.

It is not unusual in burns about the neck and lower face to see edema of the glottis about 36 or 48 hours postinjury. This edema can be due to the increased capillary permeability in the area of the posterior pharynx that follows deep burns around the neck and chin. One should anticipate such swelling occurring in the critical area of the posterior pharynx and larynx in patients with burns of the face and neck, and in such situations it is best to place an endotracheal tube before swelling obstructs the airway. The edema usually disappears in 72 hours, and the endotracheal tube can be removed if the respiratory status is satisfactory. Since the patient is more comfortable with an endotracheal tube through the nose, this is the preferred route. One should not wait for arterial blood gas analyses to determine if an endotracheal tube is necessary, because frequently in the initial postburn stages, these analyses are normal. If there is any concern for possible obstruction of the airway secondary to edema, it is best to place the tube prophylactically. The tube can then easily be removed later, if it is not needed. Placement of the endotracheal tube is preferred to a tracheostomy, primarily because the edematous tissues of the neck will make tracheostomy a technically difficult procedure.

Alan Robert Dimick was born in Birmingham. He graduated from Birmingham Southern College and the Medical College of Alabama, where he was elected to Alpha Omega Alpha. Following his internship and residency at the University of Alabama Hospitals, he joined that faculty and developed a deep interest in the metabolism and management of trauma, infections, and burns. Dr. Dimick is currently Associate Professor of Surgery and Director of the Burn Service.

Occasionally, pulmonary edema develops in patients without any evidence of inhalation injury. This is more frequent in infants and elderly persons and is usually the result of fluid overload. In extensively burned patients requiring large quantities of fluid for resuscitation, there must be frequent auscultation of the lungs to make sure pulmonary edema is not developing.

Infection in the lungs is one of the common causes of death in major burns. Its exact mode of development is not known. Obviously, the patient who is weak from a severe burn, immobilized in bed, and unable to handle his pulmonary secretions and who has large numbers of bacteria scattered over much of his body surface is an excellent candidate for the development of pneumonia. Should the temperature or respiratory rate increase suddenly, pneumonia should be suspected. Atelectasis occurs frequently in burn patients, probably because secretions are dry and thick. The burn patient loses fluid, lies quietly upon his back for long periods, and receives narcotics to control pain — all of which impede normal respiratory activity. The surgeon who deals with burn patients must anticipate the lethal complication of pneumonia and do everything possible to prevent it. Should it develop, antibiotics must be administered in accordance with the cultures obtained from the sputum, and vigorous respiratory support must be provided. The use of moist air to prevent thickening of secretions, changes of position of the patient, including active exercise, postural drainage, and minimization of the use of narcotics aid in the prevention of pneumonia.

Occasionally, a pneumothorax will occur as a complication of burn treatment. In many extensively burned patients, a subclavian or jugular catheter offers an ideal method of monitoring the central venous pressure as well as a means of administering fluids. The insertion of a catheter may be followed by a pneumothorax, which should be treated by standard methods. Patients with inhalation injury receiving positive end-expiratory pressure (PEEP) also may develop a pneumothorax as a complication of this therapy.

Sometimes the patient's respiratory rate will increase during therapy with Sulfamylon. This increase is due to an attempt by the lungs to compensate by blowing off carbon dioxide, because the buffering ability of the kidneys has been blocked by the acetazolamidelike effect of Sulfamylon. This phenomenon is strictly dose-related. Sulfamylon is easily absorbed, and since it is a strong carbonic anhydrase inhibitor, it will impair the effectiveness of the renal tubular buffering mechanism in maintaining normal body pH. The result is a metabolic acidosis leading to an increased respiratory rate. If a respiratory rate of 40 to 50/min. is observed in a patient being treated with Sulfamylon, the diagnosis of Sulfamylon toxicity should be made. The situation is easily managed by withholding application of Sulfamylon for 48 hours.

Serious complications can occur with tracheostomy. Years ago tracheostomy was performed prophylactically in patients with burns of the face and neck to avoid upper airway obstruction. However, this resulted in a tendency to infection in these patients, especially severe pulmonary infections. Therefore, the placement of an endotracheal tube is preferred to the performance of a tracheostomy in the initial treatment of burns. If the patient requires ventilatory support or cannot clear his secretions for a prolonged period following his burn injury, tracheostomy may be necessary. If so, it should be done in a controlled environment and not as an emergency procedure. For further discussion of the complications of tracheostomy, see Chapter 11.

Inhalation Injury

Inhalation injury not infrequently accompanies burns, especially if the victim is burned in an enclosed space. It is often difficult to determine the exact extent of the injury. It occurs when the victim inhales noxious gases or smoke. These cause irritation of the respiratory tract with an outpouring of fluids and edema of the bronchial epithelium. If the irritant goes deeper into the respiratory tract, bronchiolar edema and bronchospasm occur. This is sometimes referred to as a pulmonary burn; however, it is not actually a burn but an irritation of the respiratory tract. If the injury is particularly severe, pulmonary edema and even extensive pulmonary necrosis may occur. In the less severe forms of injury, damage is limited to the upper respiratory tract and the larger bronchi. This injury is relatively easy to treat and carries with it little mortality. If the injury extends to the lower respiratory tract, involving the bronchioles and alveolae, damage is severe and may lead to death.

Inhalation injury, whose incidence among burn patients approaches 35 per cent, carries an augmented risk of morbidity and mortality. Inhalation injury is recognized clinically by redness and edema in the posterior pharynx, coughing, and hoarseness. Singeing of the nasal hairs may occur. Sometimes there are mucosal burns in the nose or mouth. Such injuries should be suspected when there are flame burns about the face and neck. A delay of several hours or even days in the appearance of clinical signs is characteristic of this damage. Rales, dyspnea, and increased respiratory rate may appear from a few hours until two days after injury. Bronchospasm with prolonged wheezing may be a prominent finding, and increased bronchial markings may be apparent on roentgenographic examination. Initially, the chest x-ray is usually normal but should not fool the clinician. Clinical evidence of pulmonary involvement usually exists many hours before roentgenographic changes are noted. Profuse secretions and bronchial obstruction may occur. These secretions frequently contain a considerable amount of carbonaceous material. One should always suspect pulmonary injury when there is a brassy cough with soot in the sputum. Whenever one suspects pulmonary injury, careful, repeated examinations should be performed. A xenon scan may be helpful. Undoubtedly the best objective data can be obtained from arterial blood gas studies. Such studies provide a valuable means of confirming the over-all clinical impression of diminution in pulmonary function and serve as a yardstick for measurement of the deterioration. However, for good baseline determinations, the patient should be allowed to equilibrate to room air for 3 minutes before drawing the sample for arterial blood gas studies.

Treatment differs according to the stage of the injury. Initially, the primary aim is to provide the patient with moist air to breathe to prevent the secretions from becoming dry and firm, to encourage coughing, and to make sure suctioning of the posterior pharynx keeps the airway as free as possible. Whenever there is a spasm of the bronchioles and the Po_2 falls below 60, three facets of treatment should be instituted: (1) antibiotics, (2) bronchodilators, and (3) insertion of an endotracheal tube, preferably through the nose. Antibiotics should be given to protect against the development of bacterial pneumonia. When severe bronchospasm occurs, bronchodilators such as aminophylline or isoproterenol should be given. An endotracheal tube is usually essential to maintain a clean tracheobronchial tree, as well as to provide those with pulmonary failure the required ventilatory support with large tidal volumes and, when indicated, PEEP.

In the past, tracheostomy was thought to be indicated in patients with respiratory burns, but the large number of septic complications accompanying tracheostomy in patients with respiratory burns has convinced most surgeons that the best initial action is that of placement of an endotracheal tube. If tracheostomy is needed later, it can be accomplished electively over the endotracheal tube.

Several studies have attempted to resolve the issue of whether or not steroids should be used in the acute management of respiratory burns. The combination of burns and inhalation injury creates a high mortality risk and therefore the situation is difficult to evaluate. However, in a discussion of the problem of smoke inhalation at the NIH Consensus Development Conference Concerning Burn Care, in November, 1978, the general consensus was that steroids are contraindicated in the treatment of smoke inhalation.

FLUID OVERLOAD

In the resuscitation of burn patients, fluid overload is more common than inadequate fluid therapy. In the past decade, the utilization of burn formulas has usually ensured that the patient received adequate amounts of fluid. The most common error during the early management of the burn patient is the administration of excessive amounts of fluids. Fortunately, the use of central venous pressure monitoring has prevented fluid overload in many instances. A rapid rise in central venous pressure or above-normal levels of pressure are a sign that excessive amounts of fluids have been given. Fluid overload is more common in infants, elderly persons, and patients who have suffered pulmonary injury. When it occurs, curtailment of fluid administration and administration of diuretics are helpful.

At 4 to 6 days post burn there is a progressive mobilization of massive quantities of edema fluid into the vascular compartment and the eventual elimination of this fluid by the kidneys. This is commonly known as the diuretic phase. In moderate-sized burns it occurs on the third to fifth day, and in more extensively burned patients, it may last from the fifth to the twelfth day. During this time there is a significant overexpansion of the blood volume, and continued administration of large quantities of fluids intravenously during this period can lead to significant clinical overhydration. Therapy is aimed primarily at prevention, but once such a situation exists, simple discontinuance of fluid therapy will suffice in most instances. If congestive heart failure ensues, it may be necessary to resort to the use of rapid-acting digitalis preparations or reduction in blood volume by the use of diuretics.

DEHYDRATION

Dehydration is a surprisingly frequent complication during the course of treatment of an extensive burn. Its occurrence is secondary to the large evaporative water losses through the burn wound. Subsequent to thermal injury to the skin, the keratin layer is destroyed and the water-vapor barrier of normal skin is totally lost. Under such conditions, the rate of evaporation of water from the burn surface is the same as from the surface of an open pan of water under the same ambient conditions of temperature and humidity. Measurements of this evaporative water loss in burn patients indicate it is proportional to the area of burn and particularly to the total area of full-thickness skin loss. In a large burn this may amount to as much as 6 liters a day.

After the initial resuscitation by intraven-

ous fluids, the patient usually takes food and fluids by mouth. If he is quite ill, he may find it difficult to maintain an adequate intake of water. Possibly his hands are burned and he cannot hold a glass. It is rather frequent that attendants fail to offer the patient an adequate amount of water, not realizing that his insensible or evaporative water loss is so high. One cannot depend upon urinary output as a guide to the state of hydration during this part of the patient's course, because the heavy osmotic load of urea that patients with large burns always have will maintain significant urinary output even in the face of severe dehydration.

Severe dehydration is one of the early signs of stress pseudodiabetes in burns owing to osmotic diuresis characterized by severe polyuria. For a complete description of stress pseudodiabetes in burns, see the section later in this chapter.

One simple measurement to determine the state of hydration of burn patients is the daily measurement of urinary sodium concentration. Because of the aldosterone effect, the body retains sodium as the blood volume contracts. Therefore the daily measurement of urinary sodium concentration will serve as a simple guide to the hydration status of the patient.

ACUTE RENAL FAILURE

Although renal shutdown or acute renal failure does not often occur in a well-treated burn patient, it may be seen in very extensively burned victims or in patients who have had insufficient early treatment. It is manifested by a low urinary output in spite of sufficient fluid therapy, a low urine specific gravity, a high urinary sodium level, and rapidly rising blood urea nitrogen and creatinine levels.

One should suspect acute renal failure in any burn patient whose urinary output after the first day is less than 500 ml. with adequate intake. The first aspect of making a diagnosis is the rapid infusion of additional fluid with careful monitoring of the central venous pressure. If resuscitative fluids are infused and the central venous pressure rises to above normal without a significant increase in urinary output, acute renal shutdown should be highly suspected. If the urinary creatinine is not 10 times as great as the serum creatinine, one can feel that there is significant tubular damage and that acute renal failure has occurred. One can also contrast the serum osmolality with the urine osmolality, since the urine osmolality should be 2 to 3 times greater than that of the serum. For a more thorough discussion of diagnosis and management of acute renal failure, see Chapter 6.

OCULAR COMPLICATIONS

Except in cases of contact or chemical burns, direct damage to the globe of the eye itself or to the cornea is extremely unusual. Ocular complications, although not life-threatening, often produce serious morbidity and may cause the loss of vision. About 8 per cent of burn patients admitted to hospitals have ophthalmologic problems in association with their burns. Whenever ocular damage or an ocular complication is present, an ophthalmologist should be called immediately.

Conjunctival problems present on admission are usually associated with direct trauma or irritation by chemical agents. Therapy consists of frequent eye irrigation, eye drops, and topical antibiotics.

Serious injury to ocular structures can occur when infection originating in the burned skin about the eye spreads first to the conjunctiva and then to the deeper structures. This may result from any type of periocular burn. Bacterial colonization that accompanies any burn is increased by the tears from the eyes, which produce a warm, moist environment conducive to rapid bacterial growth. This infection spreads by direct continuity to the conjunctiva, and if strongly proteolytic organisms such as *Staphylococcus* or *Pseudomonas* are involved, there may be destruction of conjunctiva and cornea. In severe cases, the entire globe may become involved with a resulting panophthalmitis, but more frequently, severe cases are characterized by a purulent infection of the anterior chamber following erosion of the cornea, and in the later stage there may be complete dislocation of the lens. Although infection of the periocular tissues cannot be totally prevented, the severity of the infection can be greatly minimized by the use of frequently changed saline compresses that will debride the infected crust and devitalized tissues. Beginning on the third or fourth postburn day, when edema of the lids and face has subsided sufficiently that the conjunctiva can be adequately exposed, the eye should be irrigated and a suitable antibacterial cream placed in the conjunctival sac during each nursing shift.

In partial-thickness burns of the eyelids, edema closes the eyes for a period of 48 to 72 hours. The important therapy during this period is routine eye care, such as irrigation with saline, and the instillation of an antibiotic ophthalmic ointment to prevent infection.

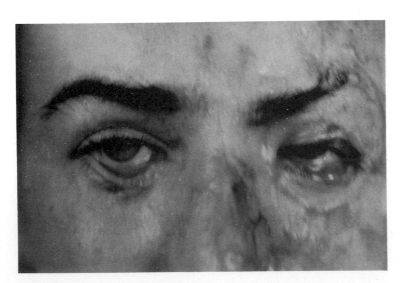

Figure 32–1 Bilateral ectropion. This is a common complication of burns of the eyelid. It can be lessened by tarsorrhaphy and early grafting. Once ectropion develops the contracture should be released with overcorrection of the lid by a split-thickness skin graft.

In full-thickness burns of the eyelids, the chief danger is ectropion formation. The incomplete closure of the lids resulting from the burn causes drying of the cornea and ulcer formation. If infection then supervenes, a panophthalmitis may develop. The primary objective in treatment of burns of the eyelids, therefore, is protection of the cornea. Eversion of the lower lids occurs because of the relative lack of redundant skin in the area and the associated contraction of adjacent burned tissue in the malar area (Fig. 32–1). The large amount of redundant skin in the upper lid and the lesser tendency for contraction of the burned skin of the forehead result in a much lower incidence of upper lid ectropion. Eversion and retraction progress at varying rates, but ordinarily, with proper attention to eye care, they are not of significant concern prior to 3 weeks post burn. By this time, however, retraction of the lids has frequently progressed to such an extent that a portion of the conjunctiva is exposed at all times, with the resultant drying effect and a secondary chronic conjunctivitis.

If the chronic conjunctivitis associated with the ectropion cannot be controlled by local treatment, correction of the ectropion must be accomplished. The lid is freed by a curved incision parallel to the lid margin that is extended to a depth sufficient to loosen the contracted tissues. No tissue is excised, but the widened defect is filled with a split-thickness skin graft. Overcorrection must be accomplished because of the continued retraction of the scar tissue during the subsequent weeks of healing. It is best to avoid correction of ectropion for as long a period as possible, since, in spite of early correction and regardless of the amount of overcorrection, the procedure frequently must be repeated later.

In some instances it is advisable to do a tongue-in-groove tarsorrhaphy to obviate chronic exposure of the globe (Fig. 32–2). This is indicated primarily in those cases in which it is obvious that deep burns of the lids have occurred and a chronic ectropion will undoubtedly form. Simple suturing of the lid margins does not suffice for maintaining long-term approximation, because the sutures usually pull out in a few days. A tongue-in-groove tarsorrhaphy is performed at the time of grafting of the face.

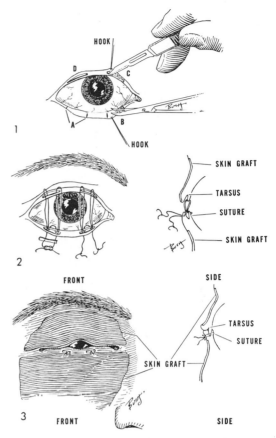

Figure 32–2 *1,* Initial steps in technique of tongue-in-groove type of tarsorrhaphy. Areas are prepared at *A, B, C,* and *D* in order to use the tarsal plate on the upper eyelid as the tongue to be placed in a groove prepared in the lower eyelid. This makes an attachment of the lids on either side of the iris, allowing a peephole in the center. After the sites have been selected the small transverse incisions are made as shown in *A.* Scissors are used to remove a thin strip of epithelium between these incisions as shown in *B.* A knife is used to separate the anterior and posterior layers of the lid as shown in *C.* This separation on the upper lid is carried out anterior to the tarsal plate. Area *D* is then ready for suturing as shown in 2.

2, The lids are sutured together with 5-0 silk. A needle is placed on each end of the suture, and the sutures are started from the posterior aspect of the lower lid. They are carried up through the posterior lip of the upper lid and out through the anterior portion of the lower lid. This brings the posterior portion of the upper (the part containing the tarsus) into the groove of the lower lid. The sutures are tied over a small piece of rubber catheter. Excessive tension must be avoided.

3, Skin grafts are applied after the tarsorrhaphy has been completed. The split-thickness skin should be placed near the margins of the lid and anchored in place with fine interrupted sutures. The sutures in the tarsorrhaphy may be removed between the eighth and tenth postoperative days. (From Moncrief, J. A.: Complications of burns and burn treatment. *In* Artz, C. P., and Hardy, J. D. (Eds.): *Complications in Surgery and Their Management.* 2nd Ed. Philadelphia, W. B. Saunders Company, 1967.)

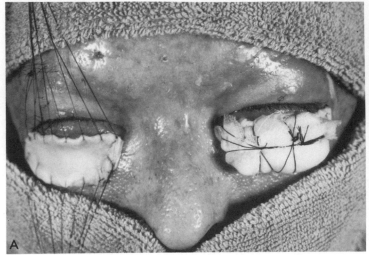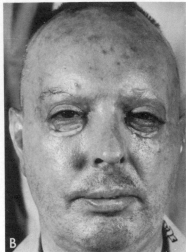

Figure 32–3   *A.* This patient sustained deep burns of the entire face and eyelids 6 weeks before this photograph was taken. There was a contracture of both lower eyelids. After these contractures were released, an overcorrection graft was applied. The graft on the right eye has been sutured in place and is ready to be dressed. A stent-type dressing has been completed over the graft on the left lower eyelid.

B, Both eyelids have healed completely. The thick, split-thickness skin grafts are quite evident. The graft did not contract; hence, a good functional and cosmetic result was obtained.

Grafts may be placed over the lids. A central aperture is left for vision and a medial and lateral one for irrigation and instillation of medication. Such a tarsorrhaphy, even when maintained for several months, does not guarantee the prevention of ectropion. It is not accomplished with such in mind. The purpose of the procedure is to protect the globe, and it should be realized that after release of the tarsorrhaphy, periocular scar tissue contracture may still result in a significant ectropion. This can be corrected later with some type of plastic procedure (Fig. 32–3).

Blindness may be a complication of severe burns, but it is extremely rare. If it occurs early, it is believed to be a manifestation of cerebral damage following hypoxia, edema, and venous sinus engorgement. Most cases of blindness associated with burns occur 2 to 6 weeks after the injury, usually as the manifestation of some type of infection. In some instances it is believed to be an optic neuritis associated with extensive infection in and around the burn wound. Other ophthalmologists feel that it may be the result of a severe encephalopathy associated with overwhelming sepsis. Although there seems to be no cure, the fact that it is a complication emphasizes the importance of calling or

consulting an ophthalmologist whenever ocular symptoms occur in the burn patient.

It should be noted that in patients with high-voltage electrical injury there is a propensity to the early formation of cataracts. Therefore, at the time of discharge from the hospital, patients with electrical injury should be advised to consult an ophthalmologist if they have any difficulty with their vision.

CHONDRITIS OF THE EARS

In deep burns about the head, the thin, delicate ear tissue may be completely destroyed immediately, but more characteristically, the initial damage consists of varying degrees of destruction of the epithelium covering the supporting cartilage. A suppurative chondritis is the most common complication of burns of the ears, but the course of the burn wound subsequent to the initial injury to the ear is completely unpredictable. Patients with obvious full-thickness burns of the ear may never show evidence of gross infection of the cartilage in this area, while others with superficial second degree burns for some reason exhibit a full-blown chondritis, with subsequent loss of most of the supporting cartilaginous substance.

The chondritis characteristically begins in the helix of the ear and is introduced by edema of the area accompanied by aching pain. The pain becomes progressively worse, and the edema causes a stiffening of the rim and base of the ear so that the structure appears to stand out more prominently from the head. In the area of involvement, the ear is exquisitely tender. There may be certain areas of fluctuation. These should be treated by aspiration, warm, wet compresses, and sometimes with a small incision for drainage. If the process continues, it probably means that there is a severe chondritis. The only satisfactory treatment for a fully developed chondritis is an incision along the margin of the helix that allows complete exposure of the involved cartilage. The necrotic cartilage is then removed by sharp and blunt dissection, and the resultant bivalve parts of the ear are kept apart by a thin layer of fine-mesh gauze (Fig. 32–4). Frequent changes of wet compresses are then instituted, and the fine-mesh gauze insert is changed daily. It may

be necessary on occasion to debride the cartilage repeatedly, and in many instances progressive loss of the supporting cartilage results in a totally shriveled and misshapen ear. Auditory impairment is minimal, however.

COSTAL CHONDRITIS

Costal chondritis is a rather unusual complication of thermal injury, but it does occur when the injury is around the costal cartilages. It is most commonly seen as a complication of radical mastectomy, surgery of the biliary tract, or drainage of a subphrenic abscess. In the burn patient, however, it occurs when the injury, whether it be totally thermal or thermal and electrical, damages the skin and deeper tissues over the costal cartilage. Loss or destruction of the perichondrium is followed by necrosis of the underlying cartilage, which then acts as a foreign body, with subsequent sinus tract formation. The most frequently found infecting organism in costal chondritis associated with burn is *Pseudomonas aeruginosa*.

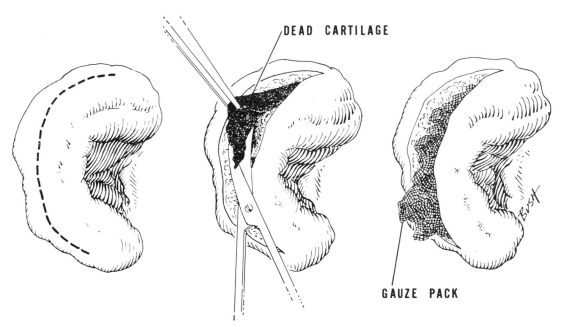

DEAD CARTILAGE

GAUZE PACK

Figure 32–4 In full-thickness burns of the ear the cartilage liquefies and becomes infected. Usually there is considerable edema of the auricle. The preferred method of treatment is a wide, fishmouth type of incision along the helix. The dead cartilage is removed, and the two layers of the ear are held apart with a gauze pack. Warm dressings are applied, and the gauze pack is changed each day. (From Moncrief, J. A.: Complications of burns and burn treatment. *In* Artz, C. P., and Hardy, J. D. (Eds.): Complications in Surgery and Their Management. 2nd Ed. Philadelphia, W. B. Saunders Company, 1967.)

The symptoms are those of draining sinuses of the anterior chest wall in association with fever, a painful, tender area of inflammation, and induration.

Simple local débridement of the involved cartilage is often inadequate. Optimal therapy for costal chondritis of any one of the upper five costal cartilages is complete resection of whichever of these cartilages may be involved. For involvement of any portion of the cartilages composing the costal arch, wide local excision back to an area with intact viable perichondrium is advocated. All operative procedures should be performed after an adequate serum antibiotic level has been obtained.

GENITOURINARY COMPLICATIONS

Cystitis is the most common complication of the genitourinary tract. A certain degree of cystitis always follows the routine use of the indwelling catheter. Rarely is it necessary to leave a catheter in the bladder for a prolonged period of time. A catheter is usually used during the first 3 to 4 days to monitor the urinary output. After that it is too frequently used to prevent soiling of burn dressings. A catheter sets the stage for troublesome infections and should be removed as soon as practicable. Careful attention should be paid to frequent irrigation of the catheter and change of catheters every 5 days.

Occasionally in males a periurethral abscess may form. This follows irritation by the catheter and contamination of the urethra by the bacteria from the burn wound. Frequently the cause of unexplained fever in a burn patient is a periurethral abscess. There is usually drainage of pus through the urethra and tenderness and swelling of the perineum. Periurethral abscesses require appropriate antibiotic therapy and surgical drainage. The formation of periurethral abscesses should be preventable. Currently available plastic collection devices for external application have almost eliminated the need for indwelling catheters over long periods of time in male patients.

Urinary calculi are not an uncommon complication. They may be present in the renal pelvis or in the bladder. Bladder calculi are more frequent than renal calculi. Recumbent posture made necessary by prolonged bed rest causes stasis in the urinary tract and leads to stone formation. Infection in the urinary tract compounds the effects of stasis. Prolonged bed rest is frequently followed by osteoporosis and withdrawal of calcium from the bony skeleton. In addition, dietary imbalances and increased calcium excretion in the urine are factors favoring stone formation. Whenever there are urinary tract symptoms late in the course of the burn, one should suspect stone formation and perform necessary diagnostic roentgenographic studies.

GASTRIC DILATATION

Gastric dilatation is one of the least recognized complications in burns. It is very distressing in the early days after injury to see a burn patient, apparently being well resuscitated, fall victim to an unrecognized acute gastric dilatation, aspirate, and die. Such a series of events is not uncommon and is completely preventable.

Acute dilatation of the stomach may occur at any time during the first 6 weeks postburn. It is seen most often in the first week after injury and is usually due to swallowed air, because the patient has such fear, apprehension, and anxiety. It is a part of the picture of non-specific paralytic ileus that occurs after burning. Sometimes it develops during oxygen therapy, particularly if oxygen is administered by nasal catheter. It accompanies septicemia and is a frequent complication of tube feedings.

The stomach may be enlarged because of simple gaseous distention, or it may be acutely dilated with fluid. Acute dilatation of the stomach is characterized by regurgitation of fluid, upper abdominal distress, dyspnea, dehydration, and, if untreated, circulatory collapse. An early symptom is frequent expectoration of small mouthfuls of fluid. The patient does not vomit but merely spits up the overflow. There may be a persistent hiccup.

Unfortunately, gastric dilatation occurs in the burn patient often with little or no change in the contour of the abdomen, because of a tight eschar over that area. Nurses should be taught the early symptoms of acute gastric dilatation so that it will be recognized before vomiting and aspiration occur. Whenever acute dilatation of the stomach is suspected, a nasogastric tube should be inserted.

PARALYTIC ILEUS

In most burns of more than 15 to 20 per cent of the body surface, peristaltic activity is absent during the first few postburn days. For this reason, extensively burned patients should not receive anything by mouth until there is evidence of good peristaltic activity. In fact, in many patients it is necessary to insert a nasogastric tube during the first 2 or 3 postburn days because of vomiting.

Paralytic ileus after burns appears to be a non-specific manifestation of severe injury. Usually it persists for only a short time and disappears as the patient's condition improves. Persistent paralytic ileus is commonly associated with septicemia. It may also be a prodromal symptom of the development of acute gastrointestinal ulcerations.

PAROTITIS

In severely burned patients parotitis is not uncommon. It usually follows the prolonged use of a nasogastric tube. Because of the fluid problems usually associated with burns, dehydration sometimes occurs, with a diminution in the amount of secretion of the parotid glands. For treatment of parotitis, see Chapter 1.

FECAL IMPACTION

Because the burn patient is immobilized for long periods of time, he is prone to fecal impaction. In fact, this is an extremely common complication unless the attending surgeon is vigorous in efforts to prevent it. Too often the physician is so busy attending to the urgent facets of burn care that routine management of the bowels is neglected. Once or twice a week a rectal examination should be performed to make sure there is

not an impaction. Large doses of a stool softener should be ordered routinely.

Fecal impaction is also a complication of the use of narcotics, especially codeine. The use of active physical therapy and exercise will also help to avoid this complication.

ESOPHAGEAL STRICTURE

Stricture rarely occurs except when indwelling nasogastric tubes are used for prolonged periods of time, such as when a nasogastric feeding tube has been left in place for 3 or 4 weeks. Such strictures are usually benign and respond to esophageal dilatation. They usually manifest themselves several weeks after the patient is completely healed.

ACUTE ACALCULOUS CHOLECYSTITIS

Acute acalculous cholecystitis is a rare complication that appears to be associated with overwhelming bacterial invasion and dehydration. In any patient with jaundice, acalculous cholecystitis should be included in the differential diagnosis. The precise mechanism by which dehydration leads to the development of cholecystitis is a matter of conjecture; however, biliary stasis and sludging with superimposed bacterial seeding seems to be a reasonable sequence of events. Sometimes periduodenal inflammatory changes and edema resulting from Curling's ulcer can lead to cholecystitis because of common duct obstruction. Once the diagnosis is made, cholecystectomy should be performed without undue delay.

SERUM HEPATITIS

Serum hepatitis is a very distressing disease that occurs usually after the patient has been discharged from the hospital. It is usually rather severe in the burn patient. It is directly related to the number of blood transfusions the patient needed during the course of treatment for a burn. Therapy for hepatitis is essentially bed rest and nutritional support. Because most patients exhibit this disease during convalescence, they are in a strong anabolic phase and maintaining a good nutritional intake is easy.

SUPERIOR MESENTERIC ARTERY SYNDROME

This entity occurs occasionally in the burn patient who has lost a very significant amount of weight. When a badly burned patient has lost considerable weight and starts vomiting, one should suspect superior mesenteric artery syndrome. With the loss of fat in the mesentery there is an obstruction of the third portion of the duodenum at the point where the superior mesenteric artery crosses it. An upper gastrointestinal series will confirm the diagnosis. Nonoperative treatments should always be initially employed. During and immediately after meals, the patient should be positioned to promote passage of food beyond the level of the superior mesenteric vessels. Adequate nutrition must be provided, usually by a combination of enteral and parenteral routes to prevent further weight loss and to promote weight gain.

Failure of conservative treatment to relieve the obstruction and inability to resume enteral alimentation within a 10-day period necessitate operative intervention to perform a duodenojejunostomy. The need for operative intervention has been reduced in recent years by the use of improved and more sophisticated alimentation programs.

ACUTE GASTRODUODENAL ULCERATION

The first reported case of gastrointestinal tract ulceration following a burn was by Swan in 1823. In 1842 Curling published a comprehensive report including 10 cases, four of which were his own. Since then acute gastroduodenal ulceration associated with a burn has become known as Curling's ulcer. Originally, all ulcers were thought to be in the duodenum. More recent experience has shown that in about half the patients the ulcers are gastric, in one-third they are duodenal, and in the other patients they are both gastric and duodenal. Occasionally, they may extend into the jejunum but this is rare.

Curling's ulcers are characteristically round, shallow, and sharply demarcated, showing no fibrosis and little inflammatory change. They are frequently multiple. The ulcers associated with massive hemorrhage have eroded into a mural vessel following extension through the muscularis mucosae. About 12 per cent of the ulcers are perforated.

The cause of acute ulceration is unknown. Clinical studies have failed to demonstrate any consistent relation with gastric acid secretion, volume of overnight secretion, or uropepsin secretion. O'Neill found that the absolute quantity of gastric mucus formed is decreased, but the composition is normal.

Burn size is directly related to the occurrence of Curling's ulcer in a dose-response manner, with the incidence of ulceration rising to approximately 40 per cent in patients with burns of 70 per cent of body surface or more. Although there has been considerable debate about the role of sepsis in the development of Curling's ulcer, it appears that a significantly greater incidence of Curling's ulcer is seen in the burn patient with sepsis.

It is extremely difficult to recognize the development of an ulcer in a severely burned patient. There are few prodromal signs. In approximately two-thirds of the patients hemorrhage is the initial sign, and in many instances it may be massive. Usually the surgeon's attention is focused on many facets of care, and what appear to be minor changes in the gastrointestinal tract go unnoticed. Paralytic ileus may be an early sign of the development of an ulcer, but it is not an uncommon complication in many burns and does not necessarily arouse one's suspicion of ulcer formation. Pain as an initial symptom is associated with perforation and occurs in only a very few patients. In about one-fourth of the patients with Curling's ulcer, no symptoms or signs are seen clinically and diagnosis is first made at the autopsy table.

Since Curling's ulcer develops in many extensively burned patients, prophylactic treatment of all patients in this category has been recommended. There is a major difference of opinion throughout the country as to whether or not this is of any value. In some series it has not diminished the incidence of formation of acute ulcers and hemorrhage. The use of an anticholinergic drug can be harmful because it slows the activity of the gastrointestinal tract, leads to constipation, and sometimes diminishes the appetite. Currently the use of cimetidine appears to be beneficial in the prophylaxis of such ulceration.

Fiberoptic gastroduodenoscopy can be helpful in the accurate diagnosis of acute bleeding lesions. The treatment of bleeding Curling's ulcers is the same as the treatment of any other type of ulcer. Initial non-operative treatments should be attempted in all patients unless the hemorrhage is massive. The decision to operate upon the patient with a bleeding Curling's ulcer should be made according to the same criteria as in the patient with a bleeding duodenal ulcer. Too often the surgeon feels that the burn patient is so ill that an operation should not be done. Therefore, the surgeon waits. Procrastination at this time leads to the administration of large quantities of blood and general depletion of the patient. Obviously, patients with perforation must be operated upon immediately.

The choice of operation varies in different types of patients and in different clinics. The most popular operation for bleeding Curling's ulcer is vagotomy and antrectomy. If the ulcer is high in the stomach where it cannot be removed by antrectomy then subtotal gastrectomy is preferred. Subtotal gastrectomy also is preferred in certain instances where it can be accomplished more easily than vagotomy and antrectomy. In adult patients, vagotomy and pyloroplasty is not satisfactory. This operation is followed in a large number of cases with rebleeding. The best evidence, however, is that vagotomy and pyloroplasty is the treatment of choice in children.

DISSEMINATED INTRAVASCULAR COAGULATION

A syndrome of disseminated intravascular coagulation (DIC) is characterized by the sudden onset of diffuse hemorrhage; the consumption of fibrinogen, platelets, and factor VIII activity; intravascular hemolysis; secondary fibrinolysis; and biopsy evidence of microthrombi. It is not a common com-

plication of burns but it does occur. It is frequently associated with septicemia. The disease is suspected because of sudden diffuse hemorrhage that manifests itself as generalized bleeding from the burn wound, from venipuncture sites, and from mucous membranes. The diagnosis can be confirmed by laboratory evidence of consumption of fibrinogen, platelets, and factor VIII activity; intravascular hemolysis; secondary fibrinolysis; and biopsy evidence of microthrombi in unburned skin. Probably the most reliable indicator of DIC is hypofibrinogenemia.

The treatment of disseminated intravascular coagulation must be directed both to correction of the underlying disease and to direct interruption of consumptive coagulopathy. Currently, there is a divided opinion as to the use of intravenous heparin therapy, as well as replacement therapy such as platelet transfusion.

DECUBITUS ULCERS

In some extensively burned patients it is most difficult to prevent the development of decubitus ulcers. These may occur in the sacral regions, over the anterior superior iliac spine, on the posterior aspect of the head, on the back of the heel, and on the lateral aspect of the ankle. In most instances, the decubitus ulcer can be prevented by proper positioning and good nursing care, but in some cases, such as those complicated by multiple open fractures that preclude frequent changes of the patient's position, decubitus ulcers are unavoidable.

Undoubtedly, the best treatment is prevention. Sometimes this can be accomplished by use of a special air mattress or by turning the patient on a CircOlectric bed. The very best preventive means known is use of the air-fluidized bed (Fig. 32–5). Whenever it appears that there is undue pressure on an area, the patient should be transferred to an air bed. It is also excellent for the treatment of decubitus ulcers.

When decubitus ulcers are large, thorough surgical débridement and grafting should be done as soon as possible. In the burn patient, a pedicle flap is rarely indicated as initial coverage; a skin graft for immediate cover is preferred. If it is necessary, a

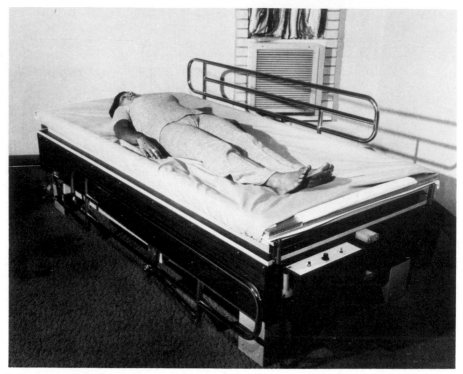

Figure 32–5   Photograph of an air-fluidized bed. This bed prevents undue pressure from being exerted on any point in the body. The patient literally floats in the bed. It is extremely comfortable and prevents the formation of decubitus ulcers. It is also of value in the treatment of small decubitus ulcers. The bed is ideal for burn patients because donor sites on the posterior aspects of the body heal well with the patient lying on his back.

pedicle graft can replace the split-thickness graft after the patient has recovered.

CONSTRICTING ESCHARS

One of the most underestimated complications of thermal injury is the constricting effect of a circumferential eschar of the extremities or of the chest. In the arms and legs, edema forming rapidly beneath the unyielding full-thickness eschar produces pressure sufficient to occlude first the venous circulation and then the arterial, with an ischemic necrosis as the result. The first sign is venous congestion, which may be accompanied by edema of the distal part if it is unburned. It is often difficult to evaluate the circulatory status of a burned extremity. A hand or foot may be pale or cool because of inadequate perfusion or marked edema secondary to the burn. The best indicator of vascular sufficiency seems to be sensation. If there is loss of sensation in an unburned part distal to the constricting eschar, there is

probably a compromise of arterial flow. In edematous extremities it is frequently difficult to palpate the pulse. The use of an ultrasonic flowmeter affords the surgeon the best objective means of measuring arterial flow at the bedside. If flow in the palmar arch or posterior tibial artery is absent, escharotomy is indicated immediately.

Escharotomy is relatively easy because there is no sensation over the full-thickness constricting eschar. Therefore, it can be performed without anesthesia. The preferred sites for escharotomy in the extremities are shown in Figure 32–6. The escharotomy should be of sufficient depth to relieve the pressure, and on occasion this may include incision of the deep fascia overlying the muscle.

The other area in which a constricting eschar is of critical importance is the thorax. This is particularly true in young children and in older people in whom the respiratory reserve is marginal. Since young children have a bony thorax that is more pliable than that of adults, constriction of their chest wall is more severe. The unyielding eschar acts as a tight band restricting expansion of the thoracic cage, and respiratory exchange is limited. Therapy consists of incision of the eschar along the anterior axillary lines bilaterally; then the incisions should be connected transversely across the anterior upper chest from axilla to axilla and over the sternum to provide maximum relaxation of the eschar.

Bleeding from these escharotomies can be brisk when they are done initially, especially in the extremities. This is primarily because of the venous hypertension that is present. One should not attempt to stop the bleeding initially but should apply dressings to the incisions and elevate the extremities above heart level for 3 to 5 minutes to allow the

venous hypertension to subside. Then the extremity can be lowered to its original position, and if bleeders need to be ligated or cauterized, this can be accomplished. Sponges soaked in a solution of epinephrine (10 ml. of 1 to 10,000 in 1000 ml. saline) can be applied to the escharotomy incision to minimize bleeding from small vessels.

FOOT DROP

One of the most common neurologic lesions seen in the burn patient is foot drop due to peroneal palsy. This frequently occurs without a clear cause but on occasion results from pressure on the peroneal nerve at the outer aspect of the leg just below the knee. In burns of the lower extremities, every effort should be made to keep pressure off this area. Once the diagnosis has been established therapy is directed toward maintenance of length of heel cord until regeneration of the peripheral nerve takes place. This is best accomplished by some type of dynamic bracing or, in the bedridden patient, by constant application of a splint or footboard.

SKIN CONTRACTURES

One of the most common complications following burns is contracture of the skin. It can be very disabling and is most likely to occur in the axilla, elbow, neck, fingers, and knee. Flexion contractures of the hip and knee are easily prevented by proper splinting and should not occur. Full-thickness burns of the neck and axilla are almost invariably followed by severe contractures in spite of various measures to prevent them. In general, it is best to prevent these contractures during the treatment of the burn wounds, rather than waiting for full maturation of the scar tissue.

Burns of the face and neck frequently have contractures that become very severe unless aggressive and early treatment is instituted with appropriate splinting and exercise. In patients with burns of the neck, no pillows should be allowed behind the head, with only a small roll being applied behind the neck. Allowing the head to hang over the edge of the mattress while lying on the

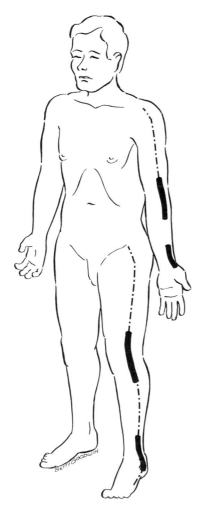

Figure 32–6 Suggested incisions for escharotomy required in circumferential eschars of the extremities.

bed will also assist in prevention of neck contractures.

With the early and aggressive measures for splinting, positioning, and exercise, many of the contractures can be minimized or avoided. With the use of elastic compression garments that are tailor-made for the patient, many contractures can be medically corrected.

However, if contractures have occurred despite these efforts, usually one waits about 6 months after the wound is healed before attempting any reconstruction procedure. In many instances a Z-plasty is very satisfactory, especially if done in older, mature scar tissue. It frequently fails when attempted in young hypertrophic scar areas. For large areas the best means of correction is excision of all the scar along functional lines and replacement with a thick, split-thickness skin graft.

HETEROTOPIC PERIARTICULAR CALCIFICATION

This complication has been observed in the elbow, hip, shoulder, and knee joints in that order of frequency. In about 10 per cent of cases of third-degree burns of the

upper extremity there is periarticular calcification about the elbow (Fig. 32–7). The anatomic distribution of the burn does not dictate the location of the osseous deposits. Although usually heterotopic bone formation occurs about joints underlying areas of burned skin, it has been observed in joints at a distance from the area of burn.

The warning signs of the development of calcification are pain and limitation of motion. Usually it comes on 2 or more months after injury. Symptoms may occur before radiologic evidence of calcium deposition is present.

Early mobilization and active vigorous physical therapy are the best preventive measures. This complication may occur in spite of these measures, however. The presence of heterotopic calcification does not always necessitate surgery. Sometimes there is spontaneous resolution. In adults resorption tends to be very slow, and surgical resection is recommended because it will restore joint motion quickly. In children, resection is usually not required. Surgery is postponed until the surrounding skin is soft and all granulating areas are healed. It is not performed if there is skin infection in any area. Excision should restore a useful or even normal range of motion.

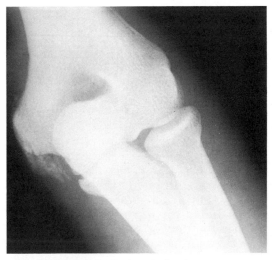

Figure 32–7 Periarticular calcification most commonly occurs about the elbow. Burn over the area is not an absolute necessity for its appearance. Severe limitation of motion may result. (From Moncrief, J. A.: Complications of burns and burn treatment. *In* Artz, C. P., and Hardy, J. D. (Eds.): Complications in Surgery and Their Management. 2nd Ed. Philadelphia, W. B. Saunders Company, 1967.)

DEAD BONE

When bone is exposed but viable periosteum remains, early coverage with skin results in complete protection of the underlying osseous structure. It is not necessary to await the development of granulation tissue, since viable periosteum will support a split-thickness graft without difficulty. If the periosteum is not viable, the outer table of the bone is dead and should be chiseled away (Fig. 32–8). In a few days small granulating buds will grow and provide a good surface upon which a graft may be placed. One should not delay if bone is dead; it should be excised like other dead tissue and the wound closed as soon as possible. One can expect a good take of skin on the granulating buds that grow over recently excised bone.

Decortication of all of the non-viable bone is preferred to the multiple drill-hole technique. More rapid granulation and cover-

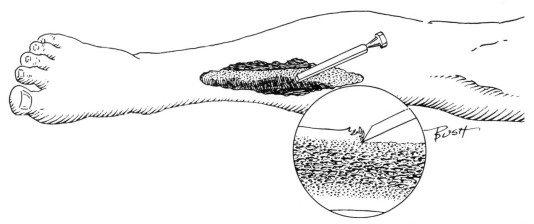

Figure 32–8 Diagrammatic illustration for removal of dead bone after a severe burn. When periosteum is burned, the outer cortex of the bone must be removed. If this is chiseled away, small granulating buds form and provide a surface upon which a graft may be placed. (From Moncrief, J. A.: Complications of burns and burn treatment. *In* Artz, C. P., and Hardy, J. D. (Eds.) Complications in Surgery and Their Management. 2nd Ed. Philadelphia, W. B. Saunders Company, 1967.)

age are provided and infection from foreign bodies of sequestering bone is minimized by the decortication technique. Drilling results in intervening bridges of bone that either sequester or form sinuses and are finally expelled or resorbed. More scarring and poor cosmesis result, as well as impaired graft take and longer hospitalization. The determination of bone viability is sometimes difficult, but bleeding is the best criterion. If there is a large area of decorticated bone it should be covered with a porcine xenograft, which should be changed every 2 days. After about 10 days to 2 weeks, there is usually sufficient granulation tissue to warrant autografting.

MARJOLIN'S ULCER

Marjolin's ulcer is a squamous cell carcinoma that develops in an old burn scar. The celebrated Roman physician Celsus, who lived early in the first century, observed the development of cancer in burn scars. It was Jean-Nicolas Marjolin, however, who gave a complete description of the lesion in 1928. It usually comes on about 25 years after the burn. The age of the scar is more important than the age of the patient. The scar producing Marjolin's ulcer is always of long duration and subject to more or less continuous trauma of tension, friction, or weight-bearing. It is for this reason that most Marjolin's ulcers are found on the extremities.

Usually the ulcer occurs in an old burn scar that has not been grafted. For this reason, Marjolin's ulcers are becoming less frequent in occurrence because in the past 25 years improved methods of burn care have led to early and adequate grafting.

Marjolin's ulcers should be preventable. If there is old scar in an area where there may be continuous trauma, the entire area should be excised and covered with a thick, split-thickness skin graft. Once an ulcer has developed, radical surgical excision of the proven Marjolin's ulcer is the accepted form of therapy. Whenever an ulcer is seen in an old burn scar, it should be biopsied. Tissue from the base as well as from the margins should be taken. In advanced epidermoid carcinoma of the extremities, amputation is preferable.

BURN STRESS PSEUDODIABETES

The syndrome of burn stress pseudodiabetes may complicate the postburn course more often than is realized. It may escape recognition because of a lack of appreciation of the typical features. In most instances, the syndrome develops during periods when there is a high-carbohydrate, high-calorie intake; the first sign may be an intense osmotic diuresis with severe dehydration. The clinical and laboratory manifestations in order of importance are hyperglycemia, glycosuria without acetonuria, high urine specific gravity, and a severe diuresis. These result in marked dehydration, with elevation of the non-protein nitrogen and hematocrit as well as an increase in the serum sodium and chloride. It is more common in patients who have a family history of diabetes. Appropriate therapy consists primarily of vigorous water replacement and sufficient amounts of insulin to control the hyperglycemia.

With the advent of hyperalimentation either by the enteral or parenteral route, frequently a pseudodiabetic state is created requiring the use of insulin to control the hyperglycemia. Also the advent of sepsis will aggravate this pseudodiabetes, and frequently this aggravated state is one of the presenting signs of generalized sepsis.

ADRENOCORTICAL INSUFFICIENCY

Adrenocortical insufficiency is not a common complication of burns, but it does occur occasionally. It should be suspected when very low concentrations of serum sodium and chloride are seen. There is a high concentration of sodium in the urine. Administration of even large quantities of isotonic saline may have little effect on the serum sodium concentration. Treatment consists of the administration of hormones and saline infusions. Usually no medication is required after skin coverage has been achieved.

DISORIENTATION

Undoubtedly one of the most disturbing complications and a frequent one of severe burns is disorientation. Most often it occurs in combination with the type of toxic psychosis that follows severe infection in the burn wound. In other instances it may occur when heavy face dressings close the eyes. It is not uncommon during the first 2 or 3 days after a bilateral tarsorrhaphy. Occasionally, it is seen when the patient is turned face down on a CircOlectric bed. The most disturbing type occurs for no specific reason; some patients who are seriously burned become disoriented, particularly at night, between the second and fifth postburn weeks.

When the patient with obvious sepsis exhibits a toxic psychosis, every effort should be made to eliminate as rapidly as possible infection from the burn wound. At the same time, however, tranquilizers may be of value in minimizing the toxic psychosis.

When dressings occlude the eyes and ears, the patient seems to be isolated from his environment. He may well retain a sense of taste and possibly smell, although the nares are frequently obstructed by dressings. Under such circumstances the previously healthy active person who has now become completely dependent on others for even the most elementary of body functions rapidly becomes disoriented. He characteristically has hallucinations, may be agitated and easily excited, and sometimes reverts to infantile behavior. In such instances, dressings should be removed as soon as possible and possibly another type of local care instituted.

It is important to assure the family that disorientation is not a permanent condition and that the patient's sensorium will be normal after he recovers from the offending condition.

Since a significant number of burn patients have a problem of chronic alcoholism, the disorientation exhibited by burn patients during the first few days post burn should arouse suspicion of the onset of delirium tremens. Vigorous treatment is required in this situation because untreated delirium tremens has a mortality of 25 per cent. Tranquilizers are required as well as maintenance of fluid and electrolyte balance. Remember that tranquilizers, especially Thorazine, are absorbed best when administered orally rather than parenterally. The patient should be kept heavily sedated with tranquilizers until the acute phase of delirium tremens has passed.

INFECTION

Infection is one of the major problems in the treatment of severely burned patients. It is the cause of pain, nutritional disturbances, conversion of second-degree burns to third-degree burns, and failure of skin grafts to take, and it is the most common cause of death. All second-degree burns heal well if kept free of infection. All burns are contaminated. Obviously, the aim in the management of all burns is to treat them in such a fashion that infection is minimized. Considerable progress has been made in this area with the introduction of topical antibacterial agents, such as Sulfamylon and silver sulfadiazine.

LOCAL INFECTION. This type of infection, manifested by cellulitis, lymphangitis, regional lymphadenopathy, fever, and leukocytosis, is usually caused by Group A beta-hemolytic streptococci or staphylococci. Such infection usually complicates partial-thickness burns and donor sites. If the burn is of the deep dermal variety, even a small amount of local infection may destroy the remaining viable epithelium and the injury will be converted to a full-thickness one.

Local infection can be effectively controlled by careful wound hygiene with removal of devitalized tissue when possible and judicious use of topical and systemic antibacterial agents. Penicillin is particularly effective against streptococci, and the semisynthetic penicillins against staphylococci. One can use either wet saline soaks, changed frequently, to keep the wound clean, or the topical antibacterial agents Sulfamylon or silver sulfadiazine to control the bacterial concentration in the wound.

SEPTIC THROMBOPHLEBITIS. This is a complication of burn treatment. It occurs around an intravenous catheter placed percutaneously or by cutdown. The catheter usually has been left in place too long, i.e., longer than 3 days. The organism most frequently encountered is coagulase-positive *Staphylococcus aureus*. Usually when infection develops around a catheter there is a certain amount of redness and the catheter is removed without any serious consequences. When an intravenous catheter is left in for a long period of time, however, the bacterial inoculum originating from the burn wound enters the vein around the catheter, giving rise to a septic thrombus. This thrombus may remain localized as a constant source of bacteremia, or septic emboli may develop and seed various organs of the body. One of the most common causes of staphylococcal bacteremia in burns is infected catheters. Because the saphenous veins so frequently develop thrombophlebitis, it is best to avoid using these veins.

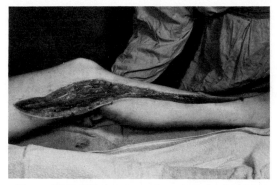

Figure 32–9 Septic or purulent thrombophlebitis is often seen in superficial veins and can be rapidly fatal. It does not usually respond to antibiotic therapy. The only effective treatment is radical excision. The wound is closed secondarily in 5 to 7 days.

Although treatment with the currently available potent antistaphylococcal drugs such as methicillin, oxacillin, and nafcillin ordinarily controls the infection, complete eradication of the sepsis is dependent upon removal of the offending source, namely the indwelling catheter. If the septic thrombus is well established, however, removal of the catheter itself will not result in either control or eradication of the infection. The only effective therapy under such circumstances is removal of the septic thrombus. This must be done surgically by a long incision over the infected vein (Fig. 32–9). After excision of the entire vein, the wound should be left open and wet soaks applied. The wound can be closed a few days later, after all evidence of infection has disappeared.

BURN WOUND SEPSIS. This term describes massive invasive bacterial involvement of burn wound and adjacent tissues. Usually there are 10^7 or 10^9 organisms in each gram of involved tissue. By definition the wound must contain in excess of 10^5 organisms per gram of tissue with invasion of the adjacent area to warrant use of the term burn wound sepsis. It is probably the most serious complication of burns and accounts for more deaths than any other complication. A mixed flora of gram-negative bacteria is the predominant finding on culture.

Blood cultures may or may not be positive. *Pseudomonas*, one of the most common causes of burn wound sepsis, initially involves primarily the lymphatics and may not be found on blood cultures. This complication occurs most frequently in the patients with very extensive full-thickness burns. It is a rare complication of partial-thickness burns that have been treated properly.

The clinical features are those of overwhelming sepsis. The temperature response may vary from 102° to 105°F. to hypothermia of 93° or 95°F., which is not uncommon in severe gram-negative infections. The pulse is rapid, paralytic ileus is common, and disorientation is frequent. Hypotension and oliguria are late preterminal manifestations. Since this is such a lethal complication in burns, every effort in the local treatment of an extensive full-thickness burn should be directed toward minimizing infection in the burn wound and thus preventing burn wound sepsis.

With the onset of generalized sepsis, appropriate cultures should be obtained and coverage with systemic broad spectrum antibiotics should be initiated until the cultures yield bacteria with specific antibiotic sensitivities. Systemic antibiotics are of little value in eliminating or controlling burn wound sepsis because systemic delivery into the avascular area of the infected wound is impossible. Therefore, topical antibacterial therapy is essential both in preventing burn wound sepsis and in active local treatment of it.

Clearing of microorganisms from the bloodstream and eradication of most visceral lesions can be accomplished by appropriate antibiotic therapy. Microorganisms isolated from blood cultures should be tested for sensitivity to several antibiotics. One or more antibiotics to which the invading microorganisms are sensitive should be given in large doses, preferably intravenously. The aim in antibiotic therapy is to diminish the load of bacteria in the bloodstream and to prevent formation of abscesses in internal organs until wound care eliminates the wound as a feeding focus.

In patients with septicemia and bacteremia individualized doses of aminoglycoside antibiotics have yielded improved survival rates.

Wound treatment is extremely difficult. Obviously, every effort should be made to remove the dead eschar. Unfortunately, in a seriously ill patient with eschar over half the body surface, excision is not practical. If the third-degree eschar covers less than 15 per cent of the body surface, excision may be justified. In more extensive burns, appropriate topical antibacterial agents as determined by wound cultures may be used. Dead tissue should be removed with forceps and scissors in such a way that bleeding is minimal. The persistent approach to the elimination of dead tissue permits earlier coverage.

The use of subeschar antibiotics may be of value. The selection of the antibiotic is usually made in accordance with results of sensitivity tests on the bacteria of the wound culture. A daily dose of the antibiotic is diluted in saline, and divided doses are injected at numerous spots beneath the eschar.

Supportive therapy is extremely important. Blood transfusions should be given to maintain the hematocrit above 38. The amount of blood required during sepsis is always more than one expects, primarily due to increased hemolysis.

Insensible water loss in overwhelming sepsis is great. Since paralytic ileus is a common feature and a nasogastric tube usually is in place, large quantities of fluid are lost from the gastrointestinal tract. Adequate fluid and electrolyte infusions are paramount. Nutritional supportive measures are of utmost importance. The patient takes little food by mouth because of gastrointestinal atony. Thus hyperalimentation may be of real value. Corticosteroids, in pharmacologic doses, may be used in the management of shock due to overwhelming sepsis. However, definite proof of their beneficial effect is still lacking.

FUNGAL INFECTIONS. A recent disturbing change in the evolving picture of sepsis in burns is the rising incidence of systemic opportunistic fungus infections. Although many organisms have been cultured, the most predominant one in recent years is *Candida albicans.* Usually sepsis from *Candida* occurs in patients with extensive burns treated by broad spectrum antibiotics and local antibacterial creams. The bacterial growth is minimized and a superinfection with *Candida* occurs. In the burn patient, *Phycomycetes, Aspergillus,* and *Cryptococcus* make up the majority of the remaining secondary fungus invaders.

Unfortunately, there is no characteristic picture of systemic *Candida* infection or septicemia that allows the clinician to differentiate it from gram-positive or gram-negative sepsis. The absence of positive blood cultures in systemic *Candida* sepsis is not unusual and makes the diagnosis doubly difficult. If sepsis persists in a burn patient receiving systemic antibiotics who does not have positive bacterial blood cultures but whose sputum, burn wound, urine, stool, and skin cultures reveal the presence of *Candida*, antifungal therapy should be instituted. Daily urine cultures in such patients will usually reveal *Candida* before it is seen in blood cultures and can be an early sign of *Candida* sepsis.

Consideration should always be given to the prevention of *Candida* infection in extensively burned patients. Fungal infection is more common in patients with impaired glucose metabolism, and *Candida* is seen most often. If such a patient is being given systemic antibiotics, an oral antifungal agent, such as nystatin, 200,000 units six times a day should be administered. Heavy colonization of the burn wound with *Candida* can be treated with amphotericin or nystatin cream. Systemic infection with *Candida*, *Cryptococcus*, *Aspergillus*, or *Phycomycetes* is treated with intravenous amphotericin B given over a 6-hour period. The usual dose is 0.25 mg./kg. on the first day with a gradual increase in the amount given over a period of 3 to 5 days to 1 mg./kg. If the diagnosis of systemic *Candida* infection is correct, clinical improvement is usually seen within 72 hours. Because amphotericin is nephrotoxic, daily determinations of blood urea nitrogen or creatinine and daily urinalyses with careful inspection for casts are imperative.

Bibliography

1. Arney, G. K., Pearson, E., and Sutherland, A. B.: Burn stress pseudodiabetes. Ann. Surg. *152*:77, 1960.
2. Artz, C. P., and Moncrief, J. A.: The Treatment of Burns. 2nd Ed. Philadelphia, W. B. Saunders Company, 1969.
3. Asch, M. J., Curreri, P. W., and Pruitt, B. A., Jr.: Thermal injury involving bone: Report of 32 cases. J. Trauma *12*:135, 1972.
4. Asch, M. J., Moylan, J. A., Jr., Bruck, H. M., and Pruitt, B. A., Jr.: Ocular complications associated with burns: Review of a five year experience including 104 patients. J. Trauma *11*:847, 1971.
5. Bruck, H. M., Nash, G., Stein, J. M., and Lindberg, R. B.: Studies on the occurrence and significance of yeast and fungi in the burn wound. Ann. Surg. *176*:108, 1972.
6. Day, S. B., MacMillan, B. G., and Altemeier, W. A.: Curling's Ulcer: An Experiment in Nature. Springfield, Ill. Charles C Thomas, 1972.
7. McManus, W. F., Eurenius, K., and Pruitt, B. A., Jr.: Disseminated intravascular coagulation in burned patients. J. Trauma *13*:416, 1973.
8. Mandelstam, P., Goldzieher, J. W., Soroff, H. S., and Green, N.: The pituitary-adrenal axis: Acute adrenocortical insufficiency and persistent occult dysfunction following thermal injury. J. Clin. Endocrinol. Metab. *18*:284, 1958.
9. Moncrief, J. A.: Complications of burns. Ann. Surg. *147*:443, 1958.
10. Moylan, J. A., Jr., Inge, W. W., Jr., and Pruitt, B. A., Jr.: Circulatory changes following circumferential burns evaluated by ultrasonic flowmeter: An analysis of 60 thermally injured limbs. J. Trauma *11*:763, 1971.
11. Munster, A. M., Goodwin, M. N., and Pruitt, B. A., Jr.: Acalculous cholecystitis in burned patients. Am. J. Surg. *122*:591, 1971.
12. Polk, H. C., and Stone, H. H.: Contemporary Burn Management. Boston, Little, Brown and Company, 1971.
13. Pruitt, B. A., Jr., Foley, F. D., and Moncrief, J. A.: Curling's ulcer: A clinical-pathology study of 323 cases. Ann. Surg. *172*:523, 1970.
14. Reckler, J. M., Flemma, R. J., and Pruitt, B. A., Jr.: Costal chondritis: An unusual complication in the burned patient. J. Trauma *13*:76, 1973.
15. Salz, J. J., and Donin, J. F.: Blindness after burns. Can. J. Ophthalmol. 7:243, 1972.
16. Schlosser, R. J., Kanar, E. A., and Harkins, H. N.: The surgical significance of Marjolin's ulcer. Surgery *39*:645, 1956.
17. Stone, H. H., and Martin, J. D., Jr.: Pulmonary injury associated with thermal burns. Surg. Gynecol. Obstet. *129*:1242, 1969.
18. Stone, H. H., and Willis, T. V.: Periurethral abscess in patients with major burns. Am. Surg. *38*:318, 1972.
19. The Journal of Trauma *19*:921, 1979 (November supplement).

33

COMPLICATIONS INVOLVING THE NERVOUS SYSTEM

John P. Kapp and Robert R. Smith

Although complications of surgery affecting the nervous system arise infrequently, the results are quite often long-lasting if not permanent and may be sources of ill feelings that at times lead to litigation. Even when all functions seem to be recovering appropriately, bizarre pain syndromes, perhaps associated with personality changes, may appear. In other patients, profound deficits in motor, sensory, or intellectual function require prolonged nursing care from both professional people and family members. Lawsuits may arise from these overwhelming financial burdens.

Some of the complications that involve the nervous system are rare, perhaps being encountered only once in a surgeon's lifetime, and thus no perspective is ever achieved in prevention or treatment, each case being managed primarily on the basis of individual judgment. A "seat of the pants" management plan should never be adopted, however, until a careful search of the literature has been made. Reports of similar cases may be used to help develop a sound management plan. It is also comforting to be backed by the literature when called to the witness stand.

To inform the practicing surgeon that infection, electrolyte imbalance, or arterial hypoxemia may cause confusion, delirium, stupor, or coma seems redundant. However, it is not widely appreciated that these same systemic abnormalities may bring to light previously undiagnosed neurologic disease or cause temporary worsening of an old neurologic lesion, such as a stroke or a head injury.

In a patient with altered sensorium or with other signs of cerebral dysfunction following operation, neurologic evaluation in the following stepwise manner will usually be appropriate and will lead to a correct diagnosis:

John Paul Kapp was born in Virginia and attended both college and medical school at Duke University, where he was elected to Phi Beta Kappa and Alpha Omega Alpha. He also took the degree of Doctor of Philosophy (Anatomy) and his training in neurosurgery at that institution, entering practice in 1972. Dr. Kapp has made numerous contributions to the literature and at present is Associate Professor of Neurosurgery at the University of Mississippi Medical Center.

Robert R. Smith is a Mississippian who graduated from Mississippi State University and from the University of Mississippi Medical School, where he was elected to Alpha Omega Alpha. After receiving his neurosurgical training at his alma mater, he joined the faculty as Instructor in 1967, became Associate Professor in 1970, and was named Professor of Neurosurgery and Chairman of the Department in 1979. Dr. Smith has made numerous contributions to the literature and is widely known for his textbook *Essentials of Neurosurgery*.

1. Careful history of previous neurologic disease or symptoms and history of habitual use of drugs or alcohol

2. Review of operative and perioperative period for events that may be associated with cerebral hypoxia

3. Survey for infection

4. A detailed neurologic examination

5. Serum electrolytes and arterial oxygen analysis

6. Computerized tomographic scan of the brain

7. Electroencephalogram in certain cases

8. Lumbar puncture

Along the way, neurologic consultation will usually be required.

CARDIAC ARREST

The extreme sensitivity of the brain and spinal cord to circulatory arrest is generally known. There is no agreement on the amount of time that the human central nervous system will tolerate total ischemia, although 5 minutes may be considered to be near the upper limit of time tolerated. Several factors affect the tolerance of the nervous system to circulatory arrest, including age of the patient (younger patients have a better prognosis) and preexisting cerebrovascular disease that may predispose to focal infarcts, with brief periods of circulatory arrest or hypotension during resuscitation. More prolonged circulatory arrest may be tolerated if the patient is under general anesthesia because of the metabolic depression of the brain caused by anesthetic drugs and because of hypothermia that may be present. Patients who sustain brief periods of circulatory arrest may have no more sequelae than a transient period of confusion and amnesia followed by complete recovery, or they may have a variable period of coma. The extent of structural damage to the brain can be correlated with the duration of coma. Coronna and Finklestein[11] considered a period of coma lasting 12 hours to be the dividing point, with complete recovery to be anticipated in patients who are in coma less than 12 hours and lasting focal or multifocal motor, sensory, or intellectual deficits likely if the patient is in coma longer than 12 hours.

Focal structural damage in areas of the brain or spinal cord with marginal circulation is often apparent following circulatory arrest. This is most often apparent in elderly patients with preexisting occlusive vascular disease. In patients with normal circulation, infarction may occur selectively in the border zone between the anterior and middle cerebral arteries, resulting in bibrachial paresis sparing the face and legs. Infarction of the occipital lobes may result in cortical blindness or visual agnosia. The arterial supply of the spinal cord is most tenuous in the upper thoracic region, and several cases of cord infarction at this level with paraparesis and without cerebral infarction have been reported.[38] More prolonged circulatory arrest may result in the syndrome of neocortical death, with prolonged coma, unresponsive extremities, and electrocerebral silence, which is characterized pathologically by laminar necrosis of the cerebral cortex[44] or by total cerebral and brainstem destruction (brain death). Ginsberg[16] has recently reviewed the syndrome of delayed neurologic deterioration following hypoxia. This syndrome is usually recognized as a sequela of carbon monoxide intoxication but has been described following cerebral anoxia or ischemia from a variety of causes. Deterioration has been reported to occur 3 days to 3 weeks after the anoxic or ischemic event. Even after other causes of neurologic deterioration, such as electrolyte imbalance, have been excluded, one wonders if this deterioration may not be due to another unrecognized episode of hypotension or hypoxia or simply a separate and spontaneous cerebrovascular accident.

Clarification of the pathogenesis of cerebral damage or death following anoxia was made by Ames in his description of the "no reflow phenomenon." Using India ink as a marker, he showed that spotty areas of the brain are not reperfused following circulatory arrest. Further work demonstrated that the microvascular occlusions were related to reversible cross-linkage of fibrinogen strands and that reperfusion could be accomplished by a period of arterial hypertension following the period of circulatory arrest.[1] On the other hand, severe intermittent hypertension has been reported to have a deleterious effect on neurologic recovery after global brain ischemia in experimental animals.[7]

Treatment otherwise is generally supportive, consisting of measures to assure adequate oxygenation and normal fluid and electrolyte balance and administration of intravenous glucose. Hypothermia and corticosteroid administration is of no proven value. Drugs that dehydrate the brain, such as intravenous urea and mannitol, may be useful if intracranial pressure rises but should probably be used in conjunction with intracranial pressure monitoring.

DURAL VENOUS SINUS THROMBOSIS

Dural venous sinus thrombosis occurs in association with dehydration and cachexia, with malignancy, trauma, and coagulopathy, and as a complication of operative procedures, such as mastoidectomy and radical neck dissection. It may also result from placement of indwelling catheters and transvenous pacemakers in the subclavian vein and superior vena cava. Decreased level of consciousness, with or without focal neurologic abnormality, is a consistent finding. In cases associated with thrombosis of the jugular vein, tenderness and swelling along its course in the neck may be noted. Definitive diagnosis is established by cerebral angiography. A computerized tomographic scan may be useful to exclude hemorrhagic infarction. Heparin anticoagulation is the most widely accepted therapeutic modality, although dexamethasone, mannitol, and even surgical decompression have been advocated.[3, 17]

CEREBRAL AIR EMBOLISM

Cerebral air embolism occurs most frequently as a complication of cardiac catheterization or cardiac surgery. Air trapped in the left heart chambers related to cardiotomy is believed to be the most frequent source, although air may also gain access to the cerebral arterial system during cannulation of the ascending aorta during coronary artery operations without cardiotomy.[6] Air introduced into the venous system on the right side of the heart may pass to the left side and to the arterial system through pulmonary arteriovenous shunts or congenital cardiac defects.

The presentation of cerebral air embolism in a conscious patient is dramatic, with apprehension followed by loss of consciousness or focal neurologic deficits. Usually, however, cerebral air embolism occurs in an anesthetized patient and is suspected because of prolonged unconsciousness following anesthesia or the discovery of focal neurologic deficits as the patient awakens from anesthesia.

Conventional treatment of cerebral air embolism is mainly supportive and includes administration of oxygen and intravenous dexamethasone. Recent reports indicate that mortality can be reduced to approximately 6 per cent with the use of hyperbaric oxygen. Treatment with hyperbaric oxygen is most effective when begun promptly. However, dramatic improvement in neurologic deficit with hyperbaric oxygen treatment has been reported when treatment was initiated as long as 29 hours after the embolization.[29, 32]

FAT EMBOLISM

Fat embolism is covered elsewhere in this volume as a complication of fractures and is mentioned here briefly as a cause of altered sensorium in the postoperative period. The clinical triad of confusion, dyspnea, and petechiae usually begins 2 to 4 days following injury and is usually associated with fractures or intramedullary fixation of long bones. Controversy still exists as to whether the emboli represent displaced marrow fat or arise from hydrolysis of neutral fat droplets by tissue lipase and mobilization of fatty acid stores by catecholamines, glucagon and steroids, or both. It has been suggested that hypoalbuminemia following trauma may decrease serum-binding capacity for free fatty acids and may contribute to the clinical manifestation of fat embolism.

Confusion beginning 2 to 4 days after injury involving a long bone fracture suggests fat embolism, although other causes such as subdural hematoma or electrolyte imbalance should be considered and excluded when appropriate. The presence of arterial hypoxia and a falling hematocrit support the diagnosis, and the finding of petechiae, especially on the lateral aspects of the upper chest and axillae and conjunctiva, is confirmatory. Fever and tachycardia are usually present. The value of examination of urine and sputum for fat globules is questionable, since fat globules are usually present following major trauma whether or not the patient develops other manifestations of the fat embolism syndrome.

Measures that reverse hypoxia form the cornerstone of treatment. This may be accomplished by the use of nasal oxygen or may require endotracheal intubation with a respirator and positive end-expiratory pressure. Frequent arterial gas monitoring is essential, and Po_2 greater than 70 mm. Hg should be maintained. The most effective regimen in treating the fat embolism syndrome has been high doses of systemic corticosteroids. The major basis for action of corticosteroids in reversing the effect of free fatty acids appears to be their anti-inflammatory property. Albumin administered intravenously during the early post-trauma period to reduce the level of free fatty acid has been reported to reduce the incidence of the fat embolism syndrome in patients with multiple injuries. Administration of intravenous ethanol or heparin has been recommended but is of unproven value.[31, 33]

PERIOPERATIVE STROKE

Strokes that occur in the perioperative period, like all strokes, may be classified as ischemic (cerebral infarcts) or hemorrhagic (intracranial hemorrhage). A patient who, for unexplained reasons, fails to awaken from anesthesia or who emerges from anesthesia with a focal neurologic deficit may be considered to have had a stroke of some type. Evaluation will include a detailed neurologic examination, a survey of the history for inciting events, and a computerized tomographic scan to determine the size and location of the lesion and to demonstrate if the lesion is a hemorrhage or an infarct. If these steps are negative or inconclusive, lumbar puncture to rule out subarachnoid hemorrhage should be considered.

Intracranial Hemorrhage

An intracranial aneurysm, arteriovenous malformation, or a small blood vessel in the brain weakened by hypertension and arteriosclerosis may rupture at any time, and the perioperative period is no exception. Periods of hypertension or the use of in-traoperative anticoagulation may precipitate an intracranial hemorrhage. For unknown reasons, perioperative rupture of intracranial aneurysms and arteriovenous malformation has been most frequently associated with obstetric or gynecologic procedures in the authors' experience. Coagulopathy associated with severe trauma or massive transfusion may rarely be connected with intracranial hemorrhage. Intracranial hemorrhage of various types follows cardiac surgery and may be inaugurated by several factors, including anticoagulation and cerebral venous congestion secondary to mechanical retraction of venous channels in the thorax. In addition, reduced intracranial mass owing to reduced arterial perfusion pressure, decreased arterial Pco_2 levels, and hyperosmolality of the perfusate solution may result in stretching and tearing of bridging surface veins or dural stripping and extradural bleeding.[23]

Intracranial hematomas that develop in the perioperative period are potentially treatable lesions and should be managed according to fundamental neurosurgical principles. Factors to be considered include size, location, extent of the associated cerebral damage, and course of the neurologic deficit. Angiography to determine the source of bleeding should be strongly considered in cases in which the cause is not obvious. Whether to use operative or supportive treatment is a decision that should be based on the facts in individual cases.

Cerebral Infarcts

Several intraoperative problems that may culminate in cerebral infarction have been mentioned, including gas, tissue, or cholesterol embolization associated with cardiotomy or aortic perfusion; paradoxical embolization of gas or thrombus through right-to-left shunts within the heart or lungs; and arterial hypoxia or hypotension, which may culminate in focal infarction of areas of the central nervous system with marginal circulation due to preexisting occlusive vascular disease. In addition, dehydration and related increased blood viscosity may predispose the patient to thrombosis of diseased cerebral vessels.

Changes in blood coagulation that accompany surgical operation are variable and are especially influenced by the development of complications.[21, 47] Generally accepted changes in the coagulation mechanism that occur following operations are release of tissue thromboplastin into the circulation; decreased circulating platelets; increased circulating fibrinogen; decreased plasminogen concentration and fibrinolytic activity; increased antifibrinolytic activity; and increased platelet coagulant activity. These changes have been implicated in the pathogenesis of postoperative venous thrombosis. Whether they also increase the possibility of thrombosis of cerebral vessels remains conjectural.

The management of perioperative cerebral infarcts, except in cases of air embolism, is usually supportive. Anticoagulation is not recommended for established infarcts and may be further contraindicated in patients who have had recent surgery. Surgical revascularization of fresh cerebral infarcts is not recommended, although emboli may be surgically removed from cerebral vessels within 4 to 6 hours with occasional gratifying results.

Neurologic response during exposure to hyperbaric oxygen[25] may help to determine whether or not irreversible cerebral infarction has occurred in a patient who develops a perioperative ischemic deficit and in whom surgical revascularization may be contemplated. If the neurologic deficit improves during exposure to hyperbaric oxygen, the patient may be left in the hyperbaric chamber while the operating room is being prepared for the revascularization procedure.

The use of angiography and prophylactic carotid endarterectomy prior to major surgical procedures in patients with asymptomatic carotid bruits has been advocated. However, recent studies have demonstrated no correlation between the presence or absence of carotid bruit and the occurrence of perioperative stroke in patients undergoing cardiac surgery, abdominal aortic operation, or aortoiliac reconstruction.[9, 15, 42] A history of transient episodes of cerebral ischemia should suggest the need for further evaluation of the cerebrovascular system prior to other surgical procedures, however, and non-invasive tests should be used to evaluate the hemodynamic significance of carotid bruits. The symptomatic or hemodynamically significant carotid stenosis may require correction prior to other surgical procedures.[26]

MALIGNANT HYPERTHERMIA

The syndrome of malignant hyperthermia during anesthesia has been recognized for less than 20 years. The typical patient is a previously healthy child or young adult in whom a rapid increase in body temperature occurs during general anesthesia. If body temperature is not being monitored, the first signs to be noted may be hot skin or the development of tachycardia or arrhythmia. By this time body temperature may be 39 to 42°C. In about 75 per cent of patients, there is an associated hypertonus or muscle rigidity. The onset may occur immediately after induction of anesthesia or may be delayed one or more hours.

The etiologic factors responsible for the development of malignant hyperthermia are not completely understood. It is known that this syndrome is based on a hereditary predisposition that is transferred as an autosomal dominant trait and that the syndrome can be triggered by the muscle relaxant succinylcholine or a potent inhalation anesthetic such as cyclopropane, ethyl ether, halothane, methoxyflurane, or enflurane. It has been postulated that at least in rigid forms of malignant hyperthermia, the triggering agent releases calcium from a defective calcium-storing sarcoplasmic reticulum membrane of the muscle cell. The resulting high level of myoplasmic calcium in turn activates phosphorylase kinase, thus accelerating glycolysis; it also activates myosin adenosinetriphosphatase, thus accelerating hydrolysis of adenosine triphosphate to adenosine diphosphate, phosphate, and heat; it inhibits troponin, permitting contraction to occur; and it is taken up into the mitochondria, causing an uncoupling of oxidative phosphorylation.

Therapy should be considered an emergency comparable to a cardiac arrest. The operation is either delayed or concluded within a matter of minutes. Maximum effort is made to cool the patient by surrounding him with ice, administering cold intravenous fluids, instituting ice water enemas and gastric lavage, and washing out any open body cavities with cold saline. Veno-arterial by-pass through an external heat exchanger has been used. The patient is hyperventilated with oxygen; metabolic acidosis is corrected with intravenous sodium bicarbonate; and mannitol or furosemide is given to help maintain urine output and prevent renal shutdown secondary to myoglobinuria. Procaine or procainamide has been suggested to have a specific stabilizing effect on the sarcoplasmic reticulum membrane, and one of these drugs should be administered in doses up to 10 mg./kg. Dantrolene sodium has also been suggested to be of possible benefit.[39]

PERIOPERATIVE CONVULSIONS

The most common cause of convulsions in hospitalized surgical patients in both the preoperative and postoperative periods is omission of anticonvulsant medication. For this reason the admission history should include a careful history of medications, and special attention should be given to continuing anticonvulsants, using the parenteral form if necessary. Abrupt withdrawal of other drugs, especially sedatives or narcotics, or of alcohol may also precipitate seizures in hospitalized surgical patients. The immediate perioperative period is not an appropriate time for planned drug withdrawal. This complication should be anticipated and managed by continuing the necessary medication. In certain instances, prophylactic administration of anticonvulsants may be advisable.

Each individual has a seizure threshold. Numerous factors in the perioperative period may act singly or in combination to produce clinical seizures in individuals who have a low seizure threshold. These include hypoxia; decreased cerebral blood flow secondary to hypotension or decreased cardiac output; electrolyte imbalance, especially hypocalcemia or hyponatremia; water overload; fever; certain drugs, especially local anesthetic or phenothiazines; and deficiency of certain vitamins, especially pyridoxine, in patients receiving prolonged parenteral nutrition. The existence of structural brain lesions such as tumors or brain abscesses should be considered as a cause of lowered seizure threshold. Long-term management

requires a systematic effort to determine the cause of seizures, which generally follows the outline given at the beginning of this chapter.

Acute management of a seizure is generally the same whatever the cause. An adequate airway should be assured, and the patient should be positioned in a lateral or semiprone position so that he will not aspirate gastric contents into the lungs if vomiting occurs. Rapid, if temporary, control of seizures can usually be accomplished by intravenous administration of anticonvulsant medication. Phenytoin or diazepam (Dilantin or Valium) is most commonly used for this purpose. The authors' preference is for phenytoin, since it does not depress respiration, although its rapid intravenous administration may precipitate cardiac arrhythmias. As much as 600 mg. may be given intravenously, but administration should not exceed 50 mg./min. If seizures persist after phenytoin administration, a second drug such as diazepam or an intravenous barbiturate should be added. Cardiac and respiratory function should be carefully monitored when these drugs are used, and facilities for assisted respiration should be at hand. If barbiturates are used, a long-acting barbiturate such as phenobarbital is probably a better choice than a short-acting drug such as pentobarbital. Use of a short-acting barbiturate results in marked fluctuation in drug levels, with poor seizure control and periods of extreme restlessness and hyperactivity.

It is important to achieve complete seizure control as soon as possible. Prolonged convulsions interfere with respiration and may be associated with increased intrathoracic pressure that may be reflected by increased pressure in the venous system and cerebral edema. Prolonged focal seizures may be associated with impairment of consciousness and attendant inactivity, with pneumonia and phlebitis as the ultimate sequelae.

Once seizures have been stopped, the patient should be placed on maintenance doses of anticonvulsants. A combination of Dilantin 100 mg. 4 times/day and phenobarbital 30 mg. 4 times/day is a common starting point in patients who have no history of allergy to these drugs. Dosage may be increased if necessary, usually to a limit of 600 mg./day of Dilantin in an adult. As the surgical stress resolves, dosage may be reduced, and patients should not be routinely discharged from the hospital on large doses of anticonvulsants.

Precautions against seizures should include the use of side rails for the bed or other means of restraint to prevent the patient from injuring himself should he have a convulsion. Under no circumstances, however, should the patient be restrained in the supine position, for example, by securing each arm to the adjacent side rail. If a patient restrained in this manner has a convulsion and vomits, massive aspiration and death will be the likely result.

HYPONATREMIA AND INAPPROPRIATE ANTIDIURETIC HORMONE PRODUCTION

Hyponatremia is probably the most common perioperative electrolyte abnormality. Etiologies of hyponatremia are diverse and include iatrogenic causes such as diuretic administration, excessive parenteral fluids, and a wide variety of pharmacologic agents.[2]

The symptoms of hyponatremia include nausea, emesis, muscular twitching, seizures, and depression of level of consciousness. Preexisting neurologic deficits are exacerbated by hyponatremia. Neurologic manifestations of hyponatremia are usually not obvious until plasma Na^+ has fallen below 125 mEq./l. Severity of symptoms is related to the rapidity of the fall of plasma Na^+.

Increased secretion of antidiuretic hormone is a common cause of hyponatremia in surgical patients that may require specific management. During and after major surgery, antidiuretic hormone release may increase because of medications, hypovolemia, traction on viscera, and pain. Certain tumors, especially bronchogenic carcinoma, may secrete antidiuretic hormone. Pulmonary infections, most notably tuberculosis and pneumococcal pneumonia, are associated with elevated serum levels of antidiuretic hormone and hyponatremia. Patients with acute impairment of brain function from a wide variety of causes may have inappropriate secretion of antidiuretic hormone.

The syndrome of inappropriate anti-diuretic hormone secretion should be suspected in a patient with hyponatremia who has normal renal function and who has not received a water overload or who has no known deficiency in intravascular fluid volume. The diagnosis is confirmed for practical purposes by obtaining simultaneous urine and serum osmolality determinations — the presence of serum hypo-osmolality together with inappropriately high (less than maximally dilute) urine osmolality supports the diagnosis. Actual urine osmolality may range widely but should be above 50 mOsm./kg., with a normal or high urinary sodium concentration. Measurement of plasma vasopressin level is usually not necessary.

Restriction of fluid intake constitutes the first line of therapy and may be the only measure necessary to correct hyponatremia. Daily fluid intake should be limited to less than 1 l./day. Serum sodium levels should be monitored daily and water intake gradually increased as serum sodium rises. Patients with severe hyponatremia (serum Na^+ below 120 mEq./l.) may require more vigorous treatment. Administration of a loop diuretic, such as furosemide, coupled with administration of a fairly large volume of hypertonic NaCl, has been recommended.[20] This form of treatment is not without risk, because of the possibility of rapid extracellular fluid volume expansion in a patient with an already expanded volume. Lithium[46] and demeclocycline[12] (Declomycin) have recently been described as therapeutic agents in patients with a chronic syndrome of inappropriate antidiuretic hormone release. Declomycin appears to be preferable because of both its lack of significant CNS depressant effects and its dose-dependent and predictable effect on water reabsorption.

POSTOPERATIVE PARAPLEGIA

Spinal cord injury during operation on other organs is rare. Injuries to the cervical spinal cord, probably related to position, have been recently reported to be associated with the use of the sitting position for the treatment of acoustic neuromas.[22] Spinal cord compression by epidural hematomas or tight packing within an intervertebral foramen may occur during operations in the posterior mediastinum. In the injured patient, especially those with impairment of consciousness, an undiagnosed spinal fracture may result in spinal cord injury during movement of the patient or positioning on the operating table.

Infarction of the spinal cord has been reported to be associated with periods of hypotension in the absence of interruption of specific vessels supplying the spinal cord.[37] Emboli to the distal aorta may result in spinal cord infarction. Spinal cord injury may occur during aortography, especially if a large amount of contrast medium is injected directly into a radicular artery that is a major source of blood supply for the spinal cord. The incidence of spinal cord damage during aortography is reported to be 0.01 per cent.[40]

Most cases of postoperative paraplegia are associated with surgical interruption of the blood supply to the low thoracic or upper lumbar spinal cord, the radicular artery of Adamkiewicz. The origin of this important artery from the aorta is variable. It commonly arises between the ninth thoracic and second lumbar vertebrae (85 per cent) but occasionally originates as high as T_5 or as low as L_4.[19] In the majority of cases it originates on the left side. Surgical interruption of this artery may occur during resection of aneurysms of the descending aorta with a frequency of occurrence reported to be around 0.2 per cent.[40] In one series, the incidence of paraplegia was 10 times greater in cases of ruptured aneurysms than in cases of unruptured aneurysms. The development of this complication depends on the confluence of several factors in the particular patient, including the anatomic arrangement of the collateral circulation, the presence of occlusive vascular disease, hypotension, and the acuteness of the occlusive process. Measures to prevent cord ischemia during operation on the abdominal aorta include avoiding hypotension intraoperatively and postoperatively and limiting the extent of aortic resection to the diseased aortic segment in order to preserve as many radicular arteries as possible. Re-attachment of the radicular arteries or a portion of the back wall of the aneurysm containing the radicular arteries to the graft may be considered. Preoperative aortography to define precisely the origin of the radicular artery of Adamkiewicz does not appear to be warranted.

Treatment of spinal cord infarction is non-specific. Administration of anticoagulants or steroids, continuous aspiration of cerebrospinal fluid to reduce intradural pressure and thereby increase collateral blood flow to the spinal cord, and surface-induced hypothermia or localized cooling of the involved cord segment with iced Ringer's lactate have been advocated but are of unproven value. Intermittent exposure of the patient to hyperbaric oxygen has been suggested to preserve viability of ischemic neurons,[24] and it might allow time for the development of collateral circulation. This treatment, although rational, remains untested. Therefore, at this time it appears that treatment of the established clinical picture of paraplegia is confined to support, physical therapy, and rehabilitation.

COMPLICATIONS OF SPINAL ANESTHESIA

Immediate complications of spinal anesthesia should be managed by the anesthesiologist and will not be discussed here. Delayed complications are headaches, tinnitus, diplopia, and focal neurologic deficits.[13]

Headache following spinal anesthesia is ascribed to intracranial hypotension secondary to the leakage of cerebrospinal fluid from the subarachnoid space at the lumbar puncture site. The overall incidence is reported to be approximately 11 per cent and can be reduced by the use of very small needles for lumbar puncture. Headache is usually postural, appearing in the head-up position and suggesting that loss of CSF permits traction on pain-sensitive structures. Treatment of headache consists of keeping the patient flat in bed, increasing hydration by the use of forced fluid orally or fluid supplement intravenously, and giving analgesics. Headaches are usually self-limiting. When headache is protracted and severe, epidural injection of 10 to 15 ml. of autogenous blood is recommended. However, back pain and signs of meningeal irritation have been noted after this therapy.

Auditory complaints are reported in 0.4 per cent of patients and consist of buzzing, popping, clogging of the ears, humming, roaring, or loss of hearing altogether, usually associated with postural headache. Visual complaints consisting of double vision, blurred vision, and spots before the eyes also occur in 0.4 per cent of patients. Palsy of the sixth cranial nerve is a well-recognized complication of spinal anesthesia. Auditory and visual complaints are attributed to alterations in fluid pressure in the cochlea and subarachnoid space, respectively.

Permanent neurologic deficit following spinal anesthesia, including paralysis of the lower limbs and urinary and fecal incontinence, may be caused by any one of several mechanisms. Traumatic lumbar puncture may injure nerve roots directly or lead to formation of an intraspinal subdural or epidural hematoma. This problem is more common in patients with coagulation disorders. Epidural abscess may develop if bacteria are introduced at the time of lumbar puncture. Injury to the conus medullaris may occur if the needle is introduced above the L_2 interspace. The complication most feared is chronic progressive adhesive arachnoiditis, which is probably a nonspecific pathologic response to an intrathecal irritant, such as detergent used for cleaning needles and syringes and germicides used for cold sterilization of ampules. Treatment of adhesive arachnoiditis with corticosteroids has been advocated.

COMPLICATIONS OF INTESTINAL BYPASS

Intestinal resection or bypass operation for morbid obesity may affect the absorption of vitamins, electrolytes, or drugs, especially anticonvulsants, which may result in symptoms related to the nervous system. Subacute combined degeneration of the spinal cord as a consequence of vitamin B_{12} deficiency can follow extensive gastric resection or may occur following ileal bypass for morbid obesity.[4] Thiamine deficiency following intestinal bypass may result in peripheral neuropathy.[18] Both syndromes are potentially reversible if appropriate vitamin supplementation is initiated. However, recovery may be slow and incomplete. Hypocalcemia, hypomagnesemia, and hypokale-

mia have been reported following intestinal bypass and may be manifested by paresthesias in the extremities and symmetrical muscular weakness or increased neuromuscular irritability.[28, 38] The symptoms respond to correction of electrolyte imbalance. In most reported cases, symptoms related to both vitamin and electrolyte deficiencies have developed 2 to 4 months following operation.

Operations that reduce intestinal absorption of food may also reduce intestinal absorption of anticonvulsants.[35] If intestinal bypass or extensive small bowel resection is contemplated in a patient with a seizure disorder, adjustment of the dosage of anticonvulsant medication in the postoperative period should be anticipated. High oral doses of anticonvulsant drugs, perhaps double the preoperative dose, may be necessary for seizure control, and obtaining blood levels of these drugs is helpful. Ideally, preoperative blood levels of anticonvulsants should be obtained as a baseline and oral doses increased postoperatively to achieve comparable blood levels.

NEUROLOGIC COMPLICATIONS OF BURNS

Convulsions and a fluctuating level of consciousness that may progress to coma and respiratory arrest occur following thermal burns. These symptoms are most frequently noted in children. When obvious causes of cerebral dysfunction, including hypovolemia, hypotension, hyponatremia, hypoxia, uremia, infection, drug administration, and direct burn injury to the skull and brain have been excluded, a cause remains for which no ready explanation is apparent. This syndrome has been termed thermal burn encephalopathy.[27] The consistent autopsy finding is cerebral edema. Thrombosed vessels and areas of hemorrhagic necrosis have also been reported. Release of a vasoactive substance into the blood from the burned area has been suspected, and increased permeability of brain capillaries has been demonstrated by trypan blue extravasation and electron microscopy[5] following thermal burning of the skin in rats. Treatment is directed at the symptoms. The patient should be observed carefully for signs of respiratory failure, and supportive measures, including tracheal intubation and assisted ventilation, should be taken if necessary. Intravenous administration of a 5 per cent glucose solution has been reported to be beneficial. Whether this is due to its hypertonic effect or to its effect as a substrate for brain metabolism is unknown.[45] Anticonvulsants may be necessary, although anticonvulsants and sedatives that depress respiration should be avoided if possible. The effect of corticosteroid administration has not been evaluated, although this may be contraindicated because of the presence of infection.

PERIPHERAL NERVE INJURIES

The peripheral nerve may actually consist of thousands of axons, each surrounded by a myelin sheath and a sheath of Schwann. Groups of these axons are segmented into bundles by the fibrous perineurium and multiple perineurial bundles by the epineurium, which surrounds the nerve proper. Small nutrient arteries run longitudinally along the epineurium and perforate it at intervals to serve the supporting structures of the nerve. The axon is metabolically dependent upon the cell body.

Based upon anatomic features of the nerve, several levels of injury may be recognized. In *neuropraxia,* both the nerve sheath and the axon are intact, although physiologic interruption has occurred. Complete return of function is the rule and can be expected, although recovery time is variable from a few days to several weeks. In some compression injuries, only the myelin sheath is affected. The injection injuries cause segmental myelin loss due to both toxic and mechanical factors. In this instance, the myelin sheath is replaced by cells of the Schwann layer over a short distance in only a few weeks time. Typically, in Saturday night paralysis, the myelin sheath is affected and recovery usually ensues over the next few days or weeks.

In more severe injuries, both the nerve sheaths and axons are torn, and in this case recovery is extremely slow. Apparently, the smaller axons regenerate at a much faster rate than the larger motor axons, which repair at a rate of about 1 mm. per day or 1

in. per month. Often, however, sweating and pain sensibility mediated by much smaller fibers can be detected long before motor function returns. In *neurotmesis,* total return of function rarely occurs spontaneously, and even after ideal repair, some deficit remains. In these cases, some of the axon sheaths collagenize before the advancing axons can penetrate them and, at other times, motor end-plates degenerate before the advancing axon filament arrives. Aberrant regeneration in which motor and sensory axons become intermingled and penetrate inappropriate sheaths also accounts for the poor results in these severe nerve injuries.

Nerve avulsion occurs in tearing and torsion injuries. The nerve root may be avulsed from continuity or pulled from its insertion into the spinal cord. This injury usually carries a very poor prognosis.

Based on the clinical and laboratory examinations, severity of the nerve injury can usually be approximated and a prognosis established. A number of simple diagnostic maneuvers assist in developing a plan of management. A myelogram, if performed early, is useful in evaluating brachial plexus injuries and may indicate a meningocele at the site of the nerve root that has been avulsed from the spinal cord. Two or more meningoceles along the cervical cord usually indicate a poor prognosis for functional motor recovery. The electromyogram, when it records degeneration or regeneration potentials, is useful. The recording of nerve conduction velocity is helpful in a number of ways. Conduction velocity is determined by stimulating the nerve at two points, one proximal and one distal to the muscle. Actual time is obtained by subtracting the shorter time from the longer time and is expressed in meters per second. Latency studies are performed when a second point of stimulation is not available, but these are particularly useful in evaluating the compression neuropathies. In lesions of the peripheral axon or myelin sheath, conduction velocity is prolonged and the action potential is reduced. In diabetes and other metabolic neuropathies, latency is prolonged and conduction velocity is also decreased. The electromyogram is useful in differentiating atrophy of muscles and in determining whether dysfunction is caused by disease, pain, malingering, hysteria, or true lower motor neuron lesions. The smallest potentials, fibrillations, are usually caused by degeneration of muscle, and regeneration is often characterized by large polyphasic potentials.

Horner's syndrome, which indicates a more central lesion, may be useful in differentiating stretch injuries from nerve root avulsion. The histamine test, which is based on a reflex arc passing from peripheral receptors to cells of the dorsal root ganglion and back, is useful in determining whether the lesion is proximal or distal to the ganglion. If a drop of histamine is placed on the skin and a needle is used to prick the skin through the drop, normally a wheal and flare appear. If the axon is not intact, no flare appears and the lesion is considered to be in the peripheral nerve. If a flare appears, the lesion is central to the dorsal root ganglion and thus is compatible with an avulsion injury.[41]

NERVE INJURIES RELATED TO POSITION ON THE OPERATING TABLE

For the most part, mechanical forces are the most important factors related to nerve injuries that occur during major operative procedures. Patient susceptibility must also play some role, since nerve injuries are more frequently encountered in the diabetic and the cachectic patient and in those patients in whom weight loss has been recorded. Apparently, loss of subcutaneous fat increases the susceptibility of the peripheral nerve to compression. As far as postoperative peripheral neuropathies are concerned, the incidence is about 1 in 1000 operative procedures. Alcoholism and diabetes are predisposing factors, and in patients with cervical ribs, special care must be taken in positioning the upper extremities. In addition to these preexisting conditions, the operation performed, its length, and the body position during the operation are probably equally important. Abduction of the arm is perhaps the most frequent cause of the brachial plexus lesion, which is the most frequent peripheral postoperative neuropathy. The lateral decubitus position, with the leg resting on the operating table, is apparently the leading cause of peroneal neuropathy, the second most frequent postoperative neuropathy. However, metal stirrups, leg stirrups, and inadequate padding have also been implicated. Of the peripheral nerves of the upper extremity, the ulnar nerve seems to be the most susceptible because of its superficial path along the medial elbow joint. These injuries are most frequently caused by contact with the edge of the operating table or the arm board.

The common agent in both stretch and compression injuries of the peripheral nerves may be nerve ischemia. Abduction of the arm greater than 90 degrees results in positional stretch of the plexus, and stretching has been noted to rupture intraneural capillaries. In the brachial plexus lesion, the upper arm is more often involved than the hand and sensory impairment is less significant than motor loss. It also appears that operations lasting 6 hours or longer, muscle relaxants, and hypothermia lead to a greater incidence of postoperative peripheral neuropathy.[34]

Fortunately, recovery in patients with postanesthetic neuropathy can be expected. Less than 10 per cent complain of their deficit after 1 year and over 90 per cent fully recover within 6 months (Table 33–1). In

TABLE 33–1   NERVE FUNCTION RECOVERY TIME IN SIXTY PATIENTS WITH POSTANESTHETIC NEUROPATHIES

Nerve Injury	No. of Patients	No Physical Therapy	Recovery Time	With Physical Therapy	Recovery Time	Residual after One Year
Brachial	25	8	9 days	14	6 mo.	3
Peroneal	13	3	7 days	8	3 mo.	2
Radial	8	2	3 days	6	2 wk.	0
Ulnar	8	3	2 days	5	6 wk.	0
Median	2	2	1 day	0	0	0
Sciatic	2	0	0	2	4 wk.	0
Femoral cutaneous	2	2	6 mo.	0	0	0

Reprinted with permission from: Parks, B. J.: Postoperative peripheral neuropathies. Surgery 74:348, 1973.

those deficits that remain, persistent pain of a causalgia type may be one of the most frequent complaints.

As to avoiding these complications, patients should be placed on the operating table in normal anatomic positions. The arm should not be abducted more than 90 degrees and perhaps even less, especially if the head is laterally rotated. The elbows should be elevated above the table level, and rolled towels should be placed along the upper chest and axilla to prevent plexus injury. The arm board surface should be the same level as the operating table mattress. The pronation of the arm is preferable to supination. Use of gallbladder rests should be discouraged, and a non-slip mattress is essential. Adequate foam rubber padding decreases peroneal nerve susceptibility.[34]

INJURY TO THE ILIOINGUINAL NERVE

Direct accidental trauma to the ilioinguinal nerve during herniorrhaphy is familiar to every surgeon who performs this procedure. This nerve contains both motor and sensory fibers and courses downward and medially through the ilioinguinal canal along the cremaster layer of the spermatic cord or round ligament and passes out of the external inguinal ring. It supplies scrotal branches, crural branches to the upper medial thigh, and a small pubic branch to the base of the penis. Ordinarily, the sensory branch is adherent to the cremaster muscle but in almost one-third of the patients, the sensory trunk may be behind or actually embedded in the spermatic cord. The surgeon, however, must identify this nerve and carefully isolate it to prevent stretching or division during hernia repair.[30] Unusual and unexpected sensory changes or discomfort around the genitalia due to ilioinguinal injury may contribute to the patient's disability, particularly in those cases involved in compensation injury.

INJURY TO THE SPINAL ACCESSORY NERVE

Spinal accessory nerve injury may be both painful and disabling from a motor standpoint. For the most part, these injuries are iatrogenic and because of the subcutaneous position of this nerve, even superficial lymph node biopsy made in the posterior triangle may produce injury. The most frequent complaint is lowering of the shoulder, depression of the scapula, and inability to abduct the shoulder. Most patients complain of pain in and around the shoulder joint, perhaps owing to stretching of the brachial plexus with the shoulder drop. Conservative measures have very little to offer in these postoperative cases, since the nerve has usually been divided. Operative exploration and suture using the operating microscope is the preferred approach, although the shoulder drop may persist for many, many years after successful repair.[43]

INJECTION INJURIES

Irrespective of the care taken by those administering intramuscular injections, injection neuropathies are still encountered. Injury to the sciatic nerve by injections into the buttocks and injury to the radial nerves by injections into the triceps muscle are most common. Both mechanical and chemical factors are probably involved in this injury, although the composition of the injected material is perhaps of greatest importance. Certain compounds, such as penicillin, but also other antibiotics and tranquilizers are most toxic to peripheral nerves. The offending material must be injected into the nerve sheath in order to produce persistent neuropathy. The diagnosis is not always simple. Frank hysteria, malingering, ruptured intervertebral discs, and diabetic neuritis confuse the issue.

If the injected material is known to be caustic, early operative intervention is usually recommended, with neurolysis and irrigation of the toxic material. It has been suggested that in toxic cases, percutaneous irrigation with saline may ameliorate the neuropathy. However, operative irrigation is much more thorough and probably less painful in the long run. Recovery of the function in the first few days after injection indicates that complete restoration is likely to occur. Late and persistent cases require surgical exploration using the microscope. Upon exposure, the nerve may be resected or grafted, or adhesions may be lysed. Resection and primary suture have been suggested when there is complete loss of function, when there is a firm neuroma replacing the nerve, when no evoked potential can be elicited, and when there is adequate length after resection to perform the anastomosis.[10] Cable grafts may also be employed effectively when dense scar tissue has destroyed a section of the nerve. Exploration and neurolysis are recommended when there is incomplete nerve loss.[10] Of course, prevention is the best method of managing the injection neuropathy, and as physicians, we must continue teaching that the upper outer quadrant of the gluteal mass, not the buttock, is the only safe area for injection. The patient should be lying in a prone position, and the needles should be directed perpendicular to the surface of the bed to avoid the sciatic nerve. Needles introduced vertically to the skin surface, particularly in infants, may result in injection of material into the sciatic nerve.[10] Injections in the upper extremity should always be placed in the deltoid muscle rather than the triceps muscle to avoid the radial nerve.[10]

VASCULAR COMPARTMENT SYNDROMES

Vascular compartment syndromes that may result in a peripheral nerve injury are still one of the most neglected areas of neurologic complications. Several theories, including those of arterial spasm, capillary paralysis, and compressive axonal injury, have been offered to explain the devastating effects that result from these injuries. Initially, an arterial lesion with hemorrhage occurs in the confined osseofascial compartment. Edema, swelling, impairment of venous return, and ischemia, both within the compartment and distal to the injury site, are associated with this lesion. The clinical warning signs are pain, pallor, absence of pulses, swelling, paresthesia, and motor weakness. Painful limitation of movement of the extremities is reported by virtually all patients.[14]

In minor cases, the application of ice, elevation of the limb, and observation are recommended. Fasciotomy, using multiple skin incisions, is necessary in progressive cases that threaten to cause distal limb ischemia or profound motor loss due to peripheral nerve compression.[14] Often, the decision of whether or not to operate is a matter

of individual judgment, and there are no clear guidelines as to when conservative measures should terminate and the operative treatment intervene. When sensory or mixed nerves are implicated the result is often a painful, causalgialike syndrome, particularly when the injury occurs in patients of advanced age.

Bibliography

1. Ames, A., III, Wright, R. L., Kowada, M., Thurston, J. M., and Majno, G.: Cerebral ischemia. II. The no-reflow phenomenon. Am. J. Pathol. 52:437, 1968.
2. Arieff, A. I., and Schmidt, R. W.: Fluid and electrolyte disorders and the central nervous system. In Maxwell, M. H., and Kleeman, C. R. (Eds.): Clinical Disorders of Fluid and Electrolyte Metabolism. New York, McGraw-Hill, 1980, pp. 1409–1480.
3. Averback, P.: Primary cerebral venous thrombosis in young adults: The diverse manifestations of an underrecognized disease. Ann. Neurol. 3:81, 1978.
4. Baker, S. M., and Bogoch, A.: Subacute combined degeneration of the spinal cord after ileal resection and folic acid administration in Crohn's disease. Neurology 23:40, 1973.
5. Basch, A., and Fazekas, I. G.: Increased permeability of the blood-brain barrier following experimental thermal injury of the skin. Angiologica 7:357, 1970.
6. Beckman, C. B., Hurley, F., Mammana, R., and Levitsky, S.: Risk factors for air embolization during cannulation of the ascending aorta. J. Thorac. Cardiovasc. Surg. 80:302, 1980.
7. Bleyaert, A. L., Sands, P. A., Safac, P., Nemoto, E., Stezoski, W., Moossy, J., and Ras, G. R.: Augmentation of post ischemic brain damage by severe intermittent hypertension. Crit. Care Med. 8:41, 1980.
8. Brown, B. A.: Sciatic injection neuropathy. Calif. Med. 116:13, 1972.
9. Cavney, W. I., Jr., Stewart, W. B., DePinto, D. J., Mucha, S. J., and Roberts, B.: Carotid bruit as a risk factor in aortoiliac reconstruction. Surgery 81:567, 1977.
10. Clark, W. K.: Surgery for injection injuries of peripheral nerves. Surg. Clin. North Am. 52:1325, 1972.
11. Coronna, J. J., and Finkelstein, S.: Neurological syndromes after cardiac arrest. Current concepts in cerebrovascular disease. Stroke 9:517, 1978.
12. DeTrover, A., and Demanet, J. C.: Correction of antidiuresis by demeclocycline. N. Engl. J. Med. 292:915, 1975.
13. Dripps, R. D., Eckenhoff, J. E., and Vandam, L. D.: Spinal anesthesia. In Dripps, R. D., Eckenhoff, J. E., and Vandam, L. D. (Eds.): Introduction to Anesthesia. Philadelphia, W. B. Saunders Company, 1977, pp. 260–277.
14. Fowler, P. J., and Willis, R. B.: Vascular compartment syndromes. Can. J. Surg. 18:157, 1975.

15. Freiman, R. L., Foran, R. F., Cohen, J. L., Levin, P. M., and Cossman, D. V.: Carotid bruit. A follow-up report on its significance in patients undergoing abdominal aortic operation. Arch. Surg. *114*:1138, 1979.

16. Ginsberg, M. D.: Delayed neurological deterioration following hypoxia. Adv. Neurol. *26*:21, 1979.

17. Girard, D. F., Reuler, J. B., Mayer, B. S., Nardone, D. A., and Jendrzejeuwski, J.: Cerebral venous sinus thrombosis due to indwelling transvenous pacemaker catheter. Arch. Neurol. *37*:113, 1980.

18. Glad, B. W., Hodges, R. E., Michas, C., Moussaviau, S. M., and Righi, S.: Atrophic beriberi: A complication of jejunoileal bypass surgery for morbid obesity. Am. J. Med. *65*:69, 1978.

19. Grace, R. R., and Mattox, K. L.: Anterior spinal artery syndrome following abdominal aortic aneurysmectomy. Arch. Surg. *112*:813, 1977.

20. Hautman, D., Rossier, B., Zohlman, R., and Schrier, R.: Rapid correction of hyponatremia in the syndrome of inappropriate secretion of antidiuretic hormone: An alternative treatment to hypertonic saline. Ann. Intern. Med. *78*:870, 1973.

21. Hirsch, J.: Hypercoagulability. Seminars Hematol. *14*:409, 1977.

22. Hitselberger, W. E., and House, W. F.: A warning regarding the sitting position for acoustic tumor surgery. Arch. Otolaryngol. *106*:69, 1980.

23. Humphreys, R. P., Hoffman, H. J., Mustard, W. T., and Trusler, G. A.: Intracranial hemorrhage complicating surgery of congenital heart disease. Trans. Am. Neurol. Assn. *98*:165, 1973.

24. Kapp, J. P.: Hyperbaric oxygen as an adjunct to acute revascularization of the brain. Surg. Neurol. *12*:457, 1979.

25. Kapp, J. P.: Neurological response to hyperbaric oxygen — A criterion for cerebral revascularization. Surg. Neurol. In press.

26. Kartchener, M.: Stroke prevention. Western J. Med. *130*:254, 1979.

27. Lindsay, W. K., Murphy, E. G., and Birdsell, D. C.: Thermal burn encephalopathy. Canad. J. Surg. *8*:165, 1965.

28. Lipner, A.: Symptomatic magnesium deficiency after small-intestinal bypass for obesity. Br. Med. J. *1*:148, 1977.

29. Mader, J. T., and Hulet, W. H.: Delayed hyperbaric treatment of cerebral air embolism. Arch. Neurol. *36*:504, 1979.

30. Moosman, D. A., and Oelrich, T. M.: Prevention of accidental trauma to the ilioinguinal nerve during inguinal herniorrhaphy. Am. J. Surg. *133*:146, 1977.

31. Moylan, J. A., and Evenson, M. A.: Diagnosis and treatment of fat embolism. Ann. Rev. Med. *28*:85, 1977.

32. Newman, R. P., and Manning, E. J.: Hyperbaric chamber treatment for "locked-in" syndrome. Arch. Neurol. *37*:529, 1980.

33. Oh, W. H., et al.: Fat embolism: Current concepts of pathogenesis, diagnosis and treatment. Orthop. Clin. North Am. *9*:769, 1978.

34. Parks, B. J.: Postoperative peripheral neuropathies. Surgery *74*:348, 1973.

35. Peterson, D. I., and Zweig, R. W.: Absorption of anticonvulsants after jejunoileal bypass. Bull. Los Angeles Neurol. Soc. *39*:51, 1974.

36. Philbin, D. M., and Wang, R. I.: Management of postoperative problems. Wis. Med. J. *70*:165, 1971.

37. Silver, J. R., and Buxton, P. H.: Spinal stroke. Brain *97*:539, 1974.

38. Skausig, O. B., and Iverson, O.: Severe paresis caused by electrolyte disturbances following end-to-side jejunoileostomy for morbid obesity. Danish Med. Bull. *26*:344, 1979.

39. Stephen, C. R.: Malignant hyperpyrexia. Ann. Rev. Med. *28*:153, 1977.

40. Szilagyi, D. E., Hageman, J. H., Smith, R. F., and Elliott, J. P.: Spinal cord damage in surgery of the abdominal aorta. Surgery *83*:38, 1978.

41. Temple, C.: Evaluation of traction injuries to the brachial plexus in adults. South Med. J. *63*:409, 1970.

42. Turnipseed, W. D., Beckoff, H. A., and Belzer, F. O.: Postoperative stroke in cardiac and peripheral vascular disease. Ann. Surg. *192*:365, 1980.

43. Valtonen, E. J., and Lilius, H. G.: Late sequelae of iatrogenic spinal accessory nerve injury. Acta Chir. Scand. *140*:453, 1974.

44. Vogel, F. S.: The morphologic consequences of cerebral hypoxia. Adv. Neurol. *26*:147, 1979.

45. Warlow, C. P., and Hinton, P.: Early neurological disturbances following relatively minor burns in children. Lancet *2*:978, 1969.

46. White, M. G., and Fetner, C. D.: Treatment of the syndrome of inappropriate secretion of antidiuretic hormone with lithium carbonate. N. Engl. J. Med. *292*:390, 1975.

47. Ygge, J.: Changes in blood coagulation and fibrinolysis during the postoperative period. Am. J. Surg. *119*:225, 1970.

34

COMPLICATIONS OF GYNECOLOGIC SURGERY

Michael Newton and John R. Lurain

Gynecologic surgery covers operations on the female genital tract. This may be divided into a lower part, consisting of the perineum, vulva, vagina, and cervix uteri, and an upper part, consisting of the corpus uteri, tubes, ovaries, and surrounding structures and ligaments. The operations performed in these areas, although here included under the general term "gynecology," actually fall into two closely related but separate disciplines, gynecology and obstetrics and the specialties within these disciplines, gynecologic oncology, maternal and fetal medicine, and reproductive endocrinology.

The complications of operations in gynecology and obstetrics differ from those in other surgical fields in several respects. First, many gynecologic patients are young, and preservation of their reproductive function is important. Procedures that either primarily or as a consequence of complications result in the loss of this function mean permanent sterility. In addition to its obvious personal consequences, the termination of the ability to conceive, even for definite medical reasons, poses serious problems for those whose religious beliefs interdict such operations unless they are performed as part of a procedure designed to treat specific disease.

Second, emotional factors are concerned not only with the causes but also with the results and complications of gynecologic

Michael Newton was born in England and received his early education there, including the first two years of medical school at Cambridge University. He came to the University of Pennsylvania School of Medicine on a Rockefeller Medical Studentship and was graduated in 1943. He received his training in surgery and in obstetrics and gynecology at the Hospital of the University of Pennsylvania. From 1955 to 1966, he served as Professor of Obstetrics and Gynecology and Chairman of the Department at the University of Mississippi School of Medicine. He then served as the Director of the American College of Obstetricians and Gynecologists and Professor of Obstetrics and Gynecology, University of Chicago School of Medicine. At present he is Professor of Obstetrics and Gynecology and Head, Section of Graduate Education, Department of Obstetrics and Gynecology, Northwestern University Medical School, and Director of the Division of Gynecologic Oncology, Prentice Women's Hospital and Maternity Center of Northwestern Memorial Hospital.

John Robert Lurain III was born in Illinois and graduated from Oberlin College in 1968 and the University of North Carolina School of Medicine in 1972. He took his residency in Obstetrics and Gynecology at the University of Pittsburgh and had a two-year fellowship in Gynecologic Oncology at the Roswell Park Memorial Institute. He is now Assistant Professor of Obstetrics and Gynecology and Assistant Director of Gynecologic Oncology, Prentice Women's Hospital and Northwestern University Medical School.

operations. These involve such matters as the patient's own concept of herself as a woman, her response to life situations, and her feelings toward her husband or partner and other members of her family.

Third, the interests of persons other than the patient herself are of great importance. Thus, her husband or partner is directly affected either if her ability to have normal sexual intercourse is altered or if she is no longer able to bear children. Moreover, the needs of the fetus are important in obstetric procedures and must be considered at least equally with those of the mother.

Fourth, gynecologic and to a less extent obstetric procedures are more often elective than urgent. Therefore, when a complication occurs, it is usually unexpected and

tends to have the impact of a catastrophe, although this is not necessarily the case.

The complications to be discussed in this chapter will be grouped under three main headings: (1) abdominal gynecologic operations, (2) vaginal gynecologic operations, and (3) obstetric operations. In each main category the complications common to many of the procedures performed will first be covered: these will be divided into those occurring preoperatively, during operation, and postoperatively. Then complications of specific operations will be discussed. In general, only those complications that are related to the gynecologic nature of the operation will be included, and those that might follow general surgical or other procedures will be omitted.

ABDOMINAL OPERATIONS

GENERAL

Preoperative

GENERAL. A patient who is in a good nutritional state is better able to withstand an operative procedure and is less likely to experience postoperative difficulties. Thus, a good preoperative diet, adequate in all essential nutrients, especially protein, is of great value. In certain major operations preoperative enteral or parenteral hyperalimentation may be desirable. Further, simple anemia often accompanies gynecologic disorders. This is best corrected by additional oral administration of iron in the preoperative period.

GASTROINTESTINAL. The stomach and lower bowel should be empty by the time of operation. Special preparation of the intestine by low residue diet, cathartics, enemas, and an intestinal antibiotic is advisable when it is anticipated that the intestine will receive considerable handling or be opened. This is particularly necessary prior to operations for primary and recurrent cancer of the ovary.

LOCAL. Local preparation of the operative area may help to prevent postoperative infection. Thus, the use of a germicidal soap in the preoperative period is helpful. Immediately before operation the bacterial count

of the abdominal skin may be reduced by scrubbing with germicidal solution and painting with povidone-iodine or a similar solution. When the vagina is to be entered, it should be cleansed with an antiseptic solution immediately before the operation.

OTHER. The chance of postoperative complications may be reduced by insuring that serum electrolyte levels (especially potassium because of its possible cardiac effect when low or high), coagulation factors, and respiratory function are within normal limits, as far as is possible. Prophylactic heparin (5000 I.U. given subcutaneously immediately before operation and every 12 hours thereafter until the patient is fully ambulatory) may lessen the chance of thromboembolism. Prophylactic antibiotics (usually a cephalosporin) are advisable when intraoperative bacterial contamination or prolonged urinary tract catheterization is likely.

ANESTHESIA. The choice of anesthesia may affect the patient's response to the operation. When possible, a qualified anesthesiologist should see the patient before operation and discuss with her the anesthesia to be used. When there is serious associated disease, discussion of the situation with the anesthesiologist is of great value. In addition to the possible complications of anesthesia itself, attempts to overpersuade the patient to accept a particular type of anesthesia of which she is afraid may lead to postoperative complications. For example, fear of spinal anesthesia may lead to a postoperative headache.

EMOTIONAL. Because of the emotional aspects of hysterectomy or oophorectomy, women who are to undergo these procedures must be properly prepared for the stress involved. If this is not done, patients may experience postoperative psychological disturbances. Appropriate preparation consists in thorough explanation of the condition present and the necessity of an operation to correct it. It is also important to provide the patient with the opportunity to express her fears about the operation, especially with regard to its effect upon herself and her family. This discussion is best conducted by the patient's physician, whom she trusts, but may be supplemented in certain hospital situations by conferences with nurses, social workers, or others. Available audiovisual aids may be helpful but do not take the place of this discussion. The important thing is to provide a listening ear and help the patient work out a reasonable understanding and solution (albeit temporary) of the problems connected with the operation. This discussion also enables her to give informed consent for the operation.

If attention is to be paid to the patient's emotions as prophylaxis against postoperative emotional disturbance, the patient's husband or partner and the other members of her family require similar attention. This should be on the same lines as for the patient herself and should consist of careful unhurried explanation and listening to and allaying any doubts and anxieties.

Operative Complications

HEMORRHAGE. Excessive bleeding is likely to occur during pelvic operations for several reasons. First, proper exposure may be impeded by the depth of the pelvis and the size of the tumor masses or their adherence to each other, especially when infection, cancer, or endometriosis is present. Second, the normal course of the vessels in the pelvis and the large denuded areas that are left after operation predispose to bleeding from both large and small vessels. Bleeding may be arterial but is more likely

to be venous. It is also likely to be **insidious** in development and to be larger in amount than expected. When considerable blood loss is anticipated, the amount lost should be determined by measuring the quantity of blood suctioned and weighing the sponges before and after use.

The principles of dealing with hemorrhage in the pelvis are similar to those used elsewhere: (1) immediately applying pressure on the bleeding area, (2) obtaining exposure, and (3) attempting to secure individual vessels with hemostatic clips, clamp and ligature, or suture ligature. Right-angled Mixter or similar clamps are useful. If the bleeding is arterial, securing the main vessel, most likely the uterine or ovarian, usually solves the problem. Venous bleeding is more troublesome. Deep in the pelvis it usually comes from a major tributary of the internal iliac vein and may be close to the ligamentous and bony side walls of the pelvis. If serious bleeding continues, whether arterial, venous, or oozing from many small vessels, ligation of both internal iliac (hypogastric) arteries should be considered. Unilateral ligation is usually not successful. Ligation is accomplished by locating the internal iliac artery below the bifurcation of the common iliac artery and passing two 0 silk ligatures around it. These are then tied in continuity. There is no need to divide the artery between the ligatures nor is it necessary to ligate the artery below its superior gluteal branch (Fig. 34–1). At the same time attention should be paid to possible coagulation defects, and blood should be fully replaced.

Hemostatic substances such as Avitene are sometimes helpful in controlling oozing from raw surfaces. As a last resort the bleeding area may be packed with one or more rolls of gauze brought out through the vagina, a lateral lower abdominal stab incision, or the lower part of the main incision. Suction drains reduce postoperative accumulation of blood and other tissue fluids. When possible, they are inserted extraperitoneally and brought out through lower lateral abdominal stab incisions.

INTESTINAL INJURY. This complication may arise during the skin incision when intestine adherent to the abdominal wall is entered. It may also occur during the dissection of small intestine fixed to pelvic

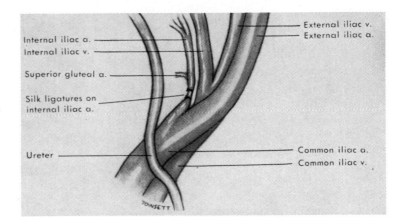

Figure 34–1 Ligation of right internal iliac artery.

Internal iliac a.
Internal iliac v.
Superior gluteal a.
Silk ligatures on internal iliac a.
Ureter
External iliac v.
External iliac a.
Common iliac a.
Common iliac v.

PONSETT

structures or during attempts to detach the bowel from inflammatory or other masses in the pelvis.

Detection of intestinal injury is usually easy because of the sudden appearance of intestinal contents, aided, in the case of the large intestine, by the fecal odor. Small injuries to the serosa alone may not be observed unless one constantly bears this possibility in mind and also carefully inspects all intestine involved in the dissection.

Intestinal repair should be performed promptly. If the small intestine is involved and the lumen has been entered, the bowel should be closed in two layers with an inverting continuous suture of 00 or 000 absorbable sutures through all layers and another layer of inverting interrupted 000 silk sutures through the serosa and muscularis. Closure should be in a transverse direction so as not to narrow the lumen. This should be checked with the finger after the sutures have been tied. When the blood supply has been compromised or the wall so damaged that it cannot be repaired, a wedge resection and an end-to-end anastomosis should be performed, using the same suture material described previously. When the serosa alone has been stripped off, it should be repaired with interrupted 000 silk sutures, again placed transversely so as not to occlude the lumen. Occasionally it may not be possible to complete this closure; then it is better to leave a small raw area rather than to resect the intestine. With injuries to the small bowel the danger of infection is not great. When injuries occur, however, the bowel has often not been prepared.

Therefore, spillage should be minimized and all intestinal fluid removed. A nasogastric tube should be inserted at the end of the operation by the anesthesiologist, and suction should be maintained for 2 to 3 days. The patient should not be given anything by mouth until she has good peristalsis, is not distended, and is passing gas rectally. Broad spectrum antibiotics should be administered for 7 days postoperatively.

Injury to the large intestine is perhaps more common, especially during operations for endometriosis and pelvic inflammatory disease. The same principles of recognition and two-layer transverse closure apply as to the small intestine. Since the danger of infection is greater when large bowel contents are spilled, neomycin (2 gm. in 30 ml. of saline) may be injected into the lumen of the bowel above the site of injury. Proximal colostomy is usually not indicated when there is no evidence of bowel obstruction or when the injury is small. It may be indicated if the bowel is greatly damaged. In this case a loop transverse colostomy over a glass rod should be performed through a separate rectus-splitting incision in the left upper quadrant. After injury to the colon, drainage should be secured by leaving the vagina open or by draining the peritoneal cavity through a right or left lower quadrant stab incision. Use of a T tube, mushroom, or Foley catheter through the vaginal cuff may help to keep it open. After any colon or rectal injury the patient should be placed on broad spectrum antibiotics for at least 7 days.

BLADDER INJURY. Injury to the bladder is most likely to occur either as the abdomen is opened, especially when the bladder is unexpectedly distended, or as the bladder is pushed down off the uterus, cervix, or upper portion of the vagina. Both are more likely to happen when the bladder has been advanced up the uterine wall as in an attempt to cover a cesarean section incision.

A large bladder injury is usually easily recognized by the presence of urine or the sight of the indwelling catheter. A small injury may go unrecognized, unless one is always cognizant of this possibility, since no typical fluid is released and no characteristic odor arises.

The bladder should be repaired as soon as adequate exposure is obtained. Two layers of continuous absorbable 00 sutures should be used. Each should include the muscularis and should be of the inverting type. It may be desirable to avoid penetrating the mucosa with the sutures, but this is not always possible. Non-absorbable sutures should not be used, since they may act as a nidus for stone formation. There is usually no need to perform a suprapubic cystos-

tomy for drainage. An indwelling Foley catheter, left in place for 7 days, is usually sufficient. If damage is extensive, the space of Retzius should be drained.

URETERAL INJURY. The location of the ureter makes it liable to injury in almost every pelvic operation, but especially when there is extensive endometriosis or inflammation, when it is displaced by a large uterine or ovarian tumor, or when radical excision of the pelvic organs is performed for cancer. The most common sites of injury are at the pelvic brim and particularly in its lowest 4 to 5 cm. as it turns to enter the bladder and is closely related to the cervix (Fig. 34–2).

In spite of the greatest care and knowledge of the anatomic relations, the ureter may occasionally be unexpectedly injured. In fact, this may occur more frequently then is usually recognized. Studies of renal function by intravenous pyelography after "simple hysterectomy" have indicated the likelihood of some type of ureteral injury to be as high as 2.5 per cent.[9] It is important to

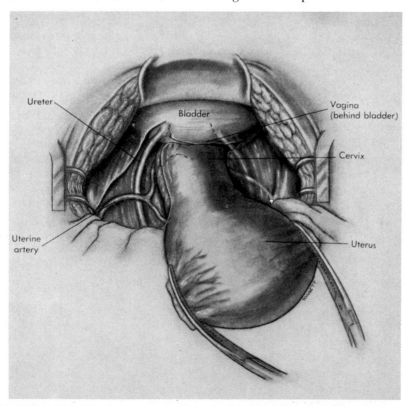

Figure 34–2 Relation of ureter to uterine artery, cervix, and bladder during hysterectomy.

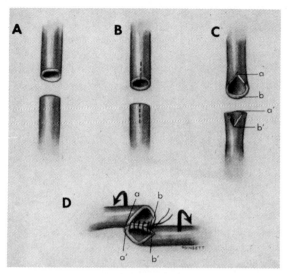

Figure 34–3 End-to-end anastomosis of ureter. *A,* Divided ureter. *B,* Longitudinal incisions. *C,* Opening the ends of the ureter. *D,* Single layer of through-and-through 4-0 chromic catgut sutures.

recognize ureteral injury when it occurs. This can best be done by adhering to the principles that contribute most to avoiding such injuries: palpating or visualizing the ureter at frequent intervals, especially when the dissection is difficult, and avoiding blind attempts to control bleeding.

Partial or Complete Division. If the ureter is incised, it should be repaired, if this can be done with one or two 4-0 interrupted absorbable sutures without narrowing the lumen. If the hole in the ureter is large or the ureter has been completely divided, the site of injury determines the method of repair. At the pelvic brim and down to within about 5 cm. of the ureterovesical junction an end-to-end anastomosis should be performed. The ureter is mobilized above and below the division. A suture in the cut end will facilitate this. Care should be taken to preserve the periureteral tissue as far as possible, since this contains the ureter's blood supply. The ends should then be fish-mouthed (Fig. 34–3) and repair performed with one layer of interrupted through-and-through 4-0 absorbable sutures, reinforced by a few similar sutures through the periureteral tissues if possible. If the ureter has been divided within 5 cm. of the bladder, reimplantation into the bladder is preferable. The distal end is ligated.

The bladder is then opened extraperitoneally and the cut proximal end brought down to it. Mobilization of the bladder will often facilitate this approximation. The bladder can then be fixed by suturing it to the psoas muscle.

There are two effective methods of implanting the ureter. In the first, and most satisfactory, a mucosa-to-mucosa anastomosis is performed with interrupted 4-0 absorbable sutures, and the serosa is then tacked to the muscularis with additional similar sutures. In the second method the ureter is split longitudinally into two halves. One 000 absorbable suture is inserted into one of these halves, passed through the incision in the bladder, and brought out through the bladder wall a short distance from the opening. The other end of the same suture is treated in the same manner, and the suture is then tied on the outside of the bladder. The other half of the cut ureter is sutured in the same manner. The serosa is tacked to the outside of the bladder with interrupted sutures. Occasionally the amount of ureter lost by the operative injury may be so large that end-to-end anastomosis or reimplantation into the bladder is not possible. Then some method of providing a replacement for the lost segment of ureter must be found. This problem is more likely to occur when the injury appears in the later postoperative period and is accompanied by infection. Methods of handling this are described under Postoperative Complications.

After repair or end-to-end anastomosis, the ureter should usually be splinted. This is less necessary when it has been reimplanted into the bladder. Several techniques of splinting are available. First, the bladder may be opened and a No. 5 or No. 6 Silastic catheter passed up to the renal pelvis and down through the urethra. Second, a similar catheter may be inserted upward and downward through the cut ends of the ureter before the anastomosis is made and then extracted from the bladder cystoscopically after operation. Third, a ureteral catheter may be inserted through the cystoscope after operation. Fourth, a T tube may be inserted above the anastomosis and one end passed up to the renal pelvis and the other down the ureter beyond the anastomosis. The authors' preference is for the first or second method. The disadvantage of the third is that it is a blind procedure, while the last involves the creation of an additional hole in the ureter with increased chance for a stricture to develop. After operation the splint is best tied to a Foley catheter and left in place for a minimum of 10 days.

In all cases of ureteral repair extraperitoneal drainage should be established by a Penrose drain, placed close to the site of repair, and brought out through a lower abdominal stab incision. Drainage may be profuse, and the drain should be left in place until after the catheter has been removed.

Follow-up of patients who have had ureteral injuries is essential. Strictures may occur months after repair, and intravenous pyelograms should be obtained at least at 3 and 12 months after operation, as well as before discharge from the hospital.

Clamping or Ligation of the Ureter. It is impossible to determine the amount of injury to the ureter produced by temporary occlusion with a clamp or even by complete ligature. If the ureter regains its normal color and peristaltic waves pass through the area after removal of the constriction, the ureter is probably intact. In this case a Penrose drain should be placed close to the site of injury and brought out extraperitoneally through a lower abdominal stab incision. If the viability of the ureter is in question, a No. 5 or 6 Silastic catheter should be passed up to the renal pelvis, either through the bladder during the operation or afterwards through a cystoscope. The splinting catheter should be handled as previously described. Follow-up intravenous pyelograms are also important.

DENUDATION OF URETER. If the ureter appears to have been stripped bare and to be dusky in color, it is best left alone without splinting. It is impossible to tell the eventual outcome at the time of operation. Healing may occur and further procedures will be unnecessary. An extraperitoneal drain may be used.

Postoperative Complications

HEMORRHAGE. After abdominal operations bleeding may occur early or later. Early hemorrhage may be defined as that which occurs in the first 24 hours after operation. Late hemorrhage may occur at any time within the first 14 days after operation.

Early hemorrhage may occur because a ligature on an artery (or less often on a vein) has slipped or because of continued oozing from a number of small vessels in raw areas. The condition is not usually appreciated until signs of shock appear. Immediate postoperative hypotension due to hemorrhage has to be differentiated from that due to anesthesia, pain, sensitivity to analgesic drugs, or to an acute accident such as a coronary occlusion or a pulmonary embolus. In the early stages differentiation is difficult.

Treatment for early postoperative hemorrhage is empirical, since the cause of the hypotension may not be known. Thus, blood should usually be given immediately. Provided other causes can be excluded, failure of the blood pressure to respond to 1 or 2 units of blood given rapidly supports the belief that intra-abdominal bleeding has occurred. At this point additional signs may appear and other diagnostic measures may be helpful. Thus the abdomen may be distended and a fluid wave elicited. Aspiration of the peritoneal cavity in either lower quadrant with an 18-gauge needle should be performed. Culdocentesis, also performed with an 18-gauge needle, is a valuable but less satisfactory technique because of the difficulty of putting the patient in the lithotomy position at this time. Blood cell counts may not show anemia because hemodilution has not yet occurred.

If the evidence definitely indicates that active bleeding is continuing, the abdomen should be reopened through the same incision and an attempt made to find the bleeding point. The procedures described under operative hemorrhage may then be followed. After reoperation the abdomen is best closed with internal figure-of-eight sutures of the Smead-Jones type.[13]

Occasionally vaginal bleeding may follow abdominal procedures. This should be handled as described later under the general complications of vaginal operations.

Late hemorrhage may be handled in the same way as early hemorrhage. Since the patient will have recovered from the immediate effects of the operation, the symptoms and signs may be more diagnostic. Also, a fall in hemoglobin is likely to occur. It should, however, be remembered that the intraperitoneal bleeding may be caused by some condition remote from the operative area, e.g., from a ruptured spleen.

Hemorrhage may occur without causing the acute picture previously described. In such cases it usually takes place retroperitoneally and is located near the vaginal cuff, either centrally or laterally. The patient usually has no symptoms, and a firm swelling in this area may be felt on pelvic examination. If this is the case, the hematoma will almost always resolve, either without or with vaginal drainage. The patient should be warned of the latter possibility. If the hematoma becomes infected, the patient may have fever and pain in the lower part of the abdomen. Leukocytosis may be present. In the absence of other causes for these findings, a pelvic examination should be performed; rectal examination is particularly helpful in making the diagnosis. Drainage is not usually indicated unless a pointing abscess is found. Often in the course of examination the vaginal cuff sutures are separated, with resulting discharge of bloody purulent material. This should be cultured. Antibiotics may be helpful, and hot baths or heat applied to the lower part of the abdomen may be used.

INFECTIONS. Postoperative infections may occur within the peritoneal cavity, in the retroperitoneal space, or in the incision.

Intraperitoneal infections may occur as a result of spillage of intestinal contents or purulent material from a pelvic cyst or abscess. Symptoms and signs usually appear promptly after operation. The clinical picture is one of abdominal tenderness and rebound tenderness (more pronounced than that usually found after laparotomy), distention, and diminished or absent peristalsis, associated with fever and tachycardia. The condition must be distinguished from paralytic ileus without infection that is simply due to handling of the bowel. The patient's fever may be a guide in this case. Obstruction, especially of the strangulating type, may give a similar picture, but is more likely to occur later. Treatment of intraperitoneal infection is by intestinal suction with a nasogastric or long (Cantor) tube, antibiot-

ics, and rest. The pus may localize in the pelvis, between loops of intestine, or in the subphrenic space. These further complications may be heralded by a persistent swinging type of temperature. Localization of the abscess is often difficult; ultrasonography and gallium scan may be helpful. Treatment is by appropriate drainage.

Retroperitoneal infections follow the course described for retroperitoneal hematoma, except that if infection rather than bleeding is primary, the general symptoms and signs will appear earlier and be more pronounced, e.g., fever, pain, tenderness, and leukocytosis. Again, drainage is indicated when localization occurs.

Wound infections are similar to those encountered after other surgical procedures and are covered in Chapter 2.

INTESTINAL COMPLICATIONS. Intestinal complications of gynecologic abdominal operations include (1) paralytic ileus, (2) intestinal obstruction, (3) pneumoperitoneum, and (4) fistulas. Removal of large tumors or large amounts of ascitic fluid or the presence of pus in the peritoneal cavity, as may occur during removal of a tuboovarian abscess, may predispose to paralytic ileus, in addition to the common causes such as obesity, age, debility, and immobility. Further, large raw areas that may have to be left in the pelvis after the removal of large and adherent tumors or abscesses favor the attachment of loops of bowel and the development of intestinal obstruction.

Pneumoperitoneum occurs to some degree after any laparotomy and may last for as long as 7 days. Persistence of free air may indicate a new leak from the intestinal tract or vagina.

Intestinal fistulas (rectovaginal, enterovaginal, and enterocutaneous) occur rarely after gynecologic operations. They are most likely to follow difficult procedures performed for infection or cancer, especially when the abdomen and pelvis have previously received radiation therapy. The diagnosis of a fistula is usually made by the discovery of discharging intestinal contents. The appearance of ingested charcoal in the discharge is diagnostic. The location of the fistula should be confirmed, if necessary by small or large intestinal x-rays.

Treatment of a rectovaginal or sigmoidvaginal fistula usually requires a preliminary diverting transverse colostomy (in the left upper quadrant of the abdomen). Repair of the fistula should then be deferred for 3 to 6 months to allow the surrounding inflammation to subside. The fistula itself may be closed by the layer technique, the Latzko colpocleisis, or the interposition of a bulbocavernosus fat pad (Martius procedure).[3] Occasionally, an abdominoperineal pullthrough approach may be suitable, or plastic procedures on the colon may be utilized.[4] Rectovaginal fistulas associated with previous radiation treatment are particularly difficult to handle; a bulbocavernosus fat pad procedure is most likely to succeed. With very large fistulas, permanent terminal descending or sigmoid colostomy may be advisable, with the distal end of the colon being turned in.

An enterovaginal or enterocutaneous fistula may be life-threatening because of the great loss of fluids and electrolytes. An additional diagnostic tool is a sinogram — injection of radiopaque material into the fistulous tract. If there has been no previous radiation therapy, gastrointestinal suction with a long tube and parenteral hyperalimentation offer a chance of spontaneous cure, but the intestine must be kept at rest for at least 6 weeks if this method is to have an adequate trial. If this fails or when radiation has been used, operative treatment is usually indicated; a bypass procedure is safer than resection and anastomosis of the bowel because of the poor blood supply.

URINARY COMPLICATIONS

INFECTIONS. The primary factor contributing to urinary tract infections is the use of a catheter. Operative handling of the urinary tract (without direct injury) and other factors are of secondary importance. Insertion of a catheter is routine practice in almost all abdominal gynecologic operations, and rightly so, since it enables the bladder to be identified and injury to be avoided. The precautions taken with an indwelling catheter and the length of time it is left in place greatly influence the development of infection. Strict aseptic technique is essential. Entrance of bacteria is facilitated by attaching and detaching the catheter from a drainage set several times. It should

initially be attached to closed drainage (into a sterile container), and changes of the drainage apparatus should be performed with aseptic precautions, cleaning the ends of the catheter and drainage tube with antiseptics before connecting them.

Catheters should be removed as soon as possible after operation and the number of reinsertions minimized. Urinary acidifying agents or antiseptics (ascorbic acid, cranberry juice, or Mandelamine) or antibiotics (trimethoprim and sulfamethoxazole) should generally be given while a catheter is in place.

Infections may develop in the upper or lower urinary tract. The former is likely to occur earlier and be associated with fever, chills, and flank pain. Examination will usually show some costovertebral angle tenderness, but little else. Urinalysis of a cleancatch specimen will often, but not always, show white cells in larger than normal amounts and possibly in clumps. Treatment should be started promptly, and empirical use of a broad spectrum antibiotic is advisable, together with adequate fluid intake, while awaiting a report on the organism and its sensitivity to the various antibiotics. Failure of infection to respond to the appropriate antibiotic should suggest the possibility of a blocked ureter and indicates further investigation. (See Ureteral Obstruction.)

Of the lower urinary tract infections, cystitis is often difficult to distinguish from the frequency and urgency associated with operations near the bladder and the use of a catheter. When the clinical picture requires clarification, urinalysis and urine culture should be obtained. Treatment is given as previously described. Often sulfonamides are sufficient therapy, since the patient's general response to the infection is not usually great. Urethritis — dysuria or burning on urination — is a common sequela of catheterization. Usually it disappears promptly and gives little difficulty, especially if patients are warned of its occurrence in advance. When it persists, it is often associated with cystitis. Relief of symptoms may be obtained by the administration of adequate fluids and by the use of Pyridium (0.2 gm. 4 times daily) together with antibiotics, if indicated. Persistent urinary tract infection should spur a search for other unsuspected urinary tract disease and is an indication for intravenous pyelography and cystoscopy.

URETERAL OBSTRUCTION. If one ureter has been inadvertently ligated, the patient may have costovertebral pain or may have almost no symptoms. Urinary output may be unchanged or only slightly reduced below normal, and this is difficult to ascertain in the immediate postoperative period. If suspected, the condition can be diagnosed by intravenous pyelography and definitively by ureteral catheterization. Unilateral nephrostomy and later formal reanastomosis of the ureter are preferable to an attempt to remove the ligature and perform an immediate reanastomosis. When both ureters have been ligated, anuria makes the diagnosis clear earlier. Bilateral nephrostomy is the appropriate management.

FISTULAS. Vesicovaginal and ureterovaginal fistulas are both characterized by the discharge of urine from the vagina and may not be easy to distinguish from one another. If they are due to direct injury, unsuspected at operation, leakage may appear promptly. More commonly they are due to necrosis of the wall of the bladder or ureter following unanticipated interruption of the blood supply. In this case, leakage of urine may appear at any time after the fifth postoperative day, although it is commonly noticed between the fifth and tenth days. Many patients have fever prior to this and do not appear to be recovering as well as they should from the operation. Usually there is no sudden gush of fluid. More often a thin fluid will run from the vagina in small amounts for 12 to 24 hours and gradually increase until the quantity and odor make the diagnosis obvious. It is then most important to determine the exact site of the fistula. If this cannot be done on pelvic examination, the simplest test is to insert dilute methylene blue into the bladder while a tampon is kept in the vagina. Blue staining of the upper part of the tampon indicates at least a vesicovaginal fistula. If no dye appears on the tampon, a ureterovaginal fistula is likely. This diagnosis can be confirmed by giving indigo carmine intravenously, with the subsequent appearance of blue dye in the vagina. An intravenous pyelogram is advisable in all cases of urinary fistula to determine the functional state of the upper urinary tract. The side and site of a ureterovaginal fistula can usually be iden-

tified, provided that oblique views are taken. Cystoscopy is also advisable in all cases. The location of a vesicovaginal fistula in relation to the ureters may be determined, and in the case of a ureterovaginal fistula, an attempt (occasionally successful) can be made to pass a ureteral catheter beyond the fistula to serve as a splint for 10 to 14 days around which the ureter can heal.

Repair of a vesicovaginal fistula should generally be delayed until local inflammatory changes have subsided. This usually takes about 90 days. In the meantime, supportive treatment must be given. Some fistulas will heal if an indwelling catheter remains in the bladder. This should certainly be tried. During this time the position of the patient is probably of little importance. If no healing occurs in one week with continuous drainage, the catheter can be removed. While it is in place urinary tract infection should be controlled by appropriate antibiotics.

Formal repair of a vesicovaginal fistula by Marion Sims was one of the earliest operations in gynecology. Although his silver wire sutures are no longer used, some of his principles of repair are still applicable. In general, the first attempt at repair is best made vaginally. If there is doubt about the relation of the fistula to the ureters, ureteral catheters may be inserted preoperatively. There is usually no need to repair the fistula transvesically unless the ureters are directly involved or unless previous failures have indicated the advisability of the suprapubic approach. Two possible techniques may be used vaginally. The first is a partial colpocleisis of the Latzko type. This is most useful if the fistula is small and located at the apex of the vagina. It consists of excluding the fistula, rather than repairing it directly (Fig. 34–4). Its chief disadvantage is that it inevitably results in some shortening of the vagina. The other technique is to dissect out the fistula, freshen the edges, and repair it in three layers if possible with interrupted catgut sutures. For difficult and large fistulas a good technique is that of Moir,[18] in which heavy nylon or prolene sutures are used and are removed in 3 weeks. After any repair of a vesicovaginal fistula an indwelling urethral or suprapubic catheter should be left in place for at least 7 days. Under ordinary circumstances the vaginal approach by either of the two tech-

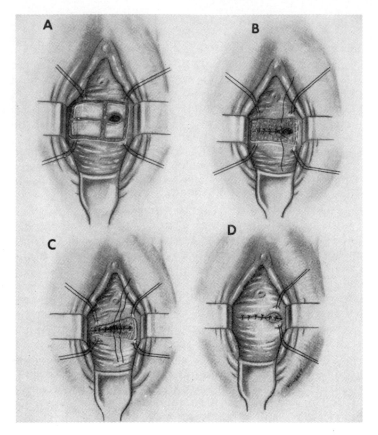

Figure 34–4 Partial colpocleisis for vesicovaginal fistula. *A,* Denudation of vaginal wall. *B,* First layer of sutures, excluding the fistula. *C,* Second layer of sutures. *D,* Closing of the vaginal mucosa.

niques described will result in 80 per cent or more cures at the first attempt. For large or recurrent fistulas, and especially for those that follow radiation therapy, a pedicled bulbocavernosus fat pad can be interposed between the bladder and the vaginal mucosa.[3]

Ureterovaginal fistulas cannot usually be repaired immediately. If a ureteral catheter can be passed initially beyond the fistula, spontaneous healing may occur, but this is rare. Continuous bladder drainage may be of help. It is important to determine renal function in patients with ureterovaginal fistulas. After the initial intravenous pyelogram, others should be obtained at 4-week intervals. Should severe hydronephrosis or decrease in function develop, it may be necessary to perform the repair earlier than planned. Even a diversionary nephrostomy may be indicated. At operation reimplantation of the ureter into the bladder should be attempted as previously described. If the ureter cannot be stretched sufficiently to enable the anastomosis to be made without tension, replacement of the ureter by a tube made from a bladder flap (Boari procedure, Fig. 34–5) or by interposition of a segment of ileum is preferable to performing a nephrectomy. If care is taken to repair the fistula at the right time, success can be achieved in most instances.[27]

Hormonal Changes

Women whose ovaries are removed before the menopause are likely to have vasomotor symptoms (hot flashes) and emotional lability after operation. They are also at greater risk of developing osteoporosis in later years. Unless contraindicated by the fact that the patient had an estrogen-related tumor, such as granulosa cell tumor of the ovary or an adenocarcinoma of the endometrium, it would appear best to forestall the development of these symptoms by the use of estrogens in small doses, starting immediately after operation, at least until the normal age of menopause. The least amount of estrogen that appears to be effective should be given.

Intermittent therapy, i.e., for 3 weeks out of 4 or 5 days out of 7, is advisable to avoid continuous stimulation of other organs such as the breasts. If such prophylaxis has not been used and menopausal symptoms complicate operation, there should be no hesitation in prescribing estrogens. When estrogens are contraindicated, other agents that have occasionally been used with good effect include progestins and vitamins B and E. The patient with menopausal symptoms also needs sympathetic understanding and a listening ear in addition to drug therapy.

Sexual Dysfunction

Occasionally, dyspareunia or lack of libido may follow abdominal hysterectomy or similar procedures. Although local causes should be excluded and estrogen therapy given, it will usually be found that a problem in this area existed before the operation that has been exaggerated by the procedure and by the change in the woman's self-image that it entails. Also important is the possibility that the patient's husband or partner may consider her less desirable because he believes that losing her uterus is synonymous with losing sexual desire. The problem so presented is no different from primary dyspareunia. It requires, in the first instance, reassurance and explanation, but the patient may need prolonged therapy with review of her sexual attitudes in an attempt to get her to change them.

OTHER COMPLICATIONS

SKIN. Special problems in healing are presented by incisions made through previously radiated skin. Closure by internal mattress sutures (Smead-Jones)[31] is advisable

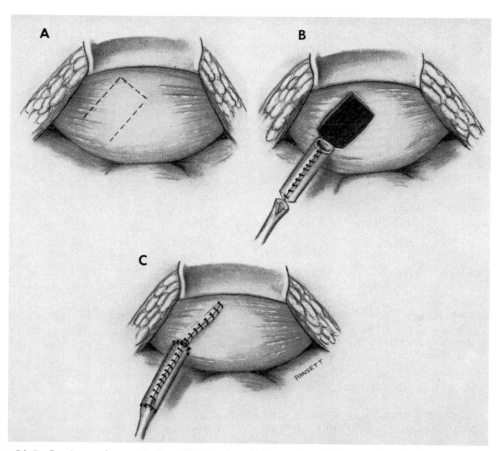

Figure 34–5   Boari procedure. *A,* Outline of bladder flap. *B,* Construction of tube to replace lower ureter. *C,* Completed anastomosis of tube to ureter and closure of bladder.

in these cases. Postoperative problems such as wound infections, dehiscence, or keloid formation are no different from those encountered after other types of surgical procedures and are covered in Chapter 2.

NERVES.   Injury to the femoral nerve is a rare but distressing complication of gynecologic operations. It appears to be related to pressure from a self-retaining retractor and to be more likely to occur with a transverse incision and in thin patients. Careful placement of the retractor with protection of the underlying tissues by a gauze pad may help to prevent this complication.[10]

Femoral nerve injury affects hip flexion (iliopsoas), adduction (pectineus) and rotation (pectineus, sartorius), and knee extension (quadriceps) in varying degrees. Sensory loss is noted on the anteromedial surface of the thigh to the knee and the medial aspect of the leg to the dorsum of the foot. The patient is likely to complain of inability to stand and some numbness of the leg. Treatment is conservative with physical therapy and a knee brace. Eventual return of function can be expected in 3 to 12 months, although occasionally some residual neurologic deficit is noted.

Occasionally, the genitofemoral nerve is injured because of its position on the anterior surface of the psoas. Subsequently, the patient may notice some numbness of the skin over the femoral triangle. This is likely to disappear spontaneously.

SPECIFIC OPERATIONS

Uterus

TOTAL HYSTERECTOMY.   All the complications described earlier for abdominal operations in general may occur after total abdominal hysterectomy. More specific complications may be divided into those that occur abdominally and those that occur vaginally.

Abdominal complications primarily concern the organs left behind — the tubes and ovaries.

The development of cancer in the remaining ovary or ovaries and the high mortality that this disease entails are often cited as reasons for prophylactic oophorectomy at the time of hysterectomy, especially for women over 40. However, the actual risk of ovarian cancer occurring after age 40 is only about 0.8 per cent. Although replacement hormones can easily be given, there may be some advantage to retaining biologic ovarian function. The decision for or against oophorectomy has to be made by surgeon and patient after informed discussion.[22]

The remaining ovary or ovaries may become cystic or may prolapse into the cul-desac. Both these difficulties may be prevented, in part at least, at the time of operation. Thus care should be taken to preserve the blood supply to the ovary both during the removal of the uterus and during the reperitonealization of the pelvis. Also, the ovary should be suspended so that it remains out of the pelvis. This can be done by fixing the ovary laterally under the round ligament with an interrupted absorbable mattress suture (Fig. 34–6). The cystic ovary may not cause any symptoms and may be detected only on pelvic examination. Because of the possibility of cancer, all ovarian enlargements in the woman who has had a total hysterectomy should be regarded with suspicion and the ovaries removed if the mass is 4 cm. or more in diameter or seems to be increasing in size. Prolapse of the ovary may give the patient pain on intercourse or on defecation. If this pain can be reproduced by palpating the ovary during a pelvic examination, removal of the ovary should be considered and weighed against the effect of the resulting castration.

Vaginal complications of total abdominal hysterectomy include (1) incomplete removal of the cervix, (2) granulations and poor healing of the vaginal cuff, (3) dyspareunia, (4) prolapse of a tube through the vaginal cuff, and (5) prolapse of the whole vaginal cuff.

Incomplete removal of the cervix may occur unexpectedly as a result of an operation made difficult by infection, endometriosis, or severe hemorrhage. The remaining portion is usually small and does not cause symptoms. The diagnosis may be difficult, however, when the patient is examined some time after the original procedure. Then a thickened area in the cuff may suggest some type of tumor. Biopsy may be necessary to reveal its true nature. Regular

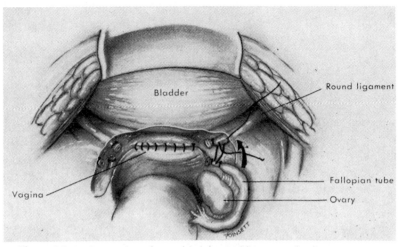

Figure 34–6   Suspension of ovary under round ligament after hysterectomy.

follow-up with cytologic studies is then advisable. The remaining piece of cervix should be removed (see under Subtotal Hysterectomy) if cervical intraepithelial neoplasia develops or if other symptoms occur.

Granulation tissue at the apex of the vaginal cuff is a common complication of abdominal (and also of vaginal) hysterectomy. It may be a little more frequent when the cuff is left open, but closing the cuff is no sure prevention. Usually, at the 6 weeks' check-up, a polypoid piece of red tissue is seen hanging down from the vaginal vault. It should be twisted off and the base cauterized with a silver nitrate stick. This should be repeated as necessary until the granulations have disappeared. Little discomfort is experienced from this procedure, and the patient may expect only a small amount of discharge, perhaps bloody, after it. Occasionally, the granulations do not appear at the 6 weeks' check-up, but only at a later date. Then the patient may complain of vaginal bleeding, especially after intercourse or douches. This is often alarming to her. Examination usually reveals the cause for her symptoms, and the diagnosis is simple, the only confusion perhaps being with a prolapsed fallopian tube. The granulation tissue is removed and sent for pathologic examination. Cauterization is performed as described previously.

Dyspareunia following total abdominal hysterectomy might on theoretical grounds be due to the shortening of the vagina and the reduced distensibility of the vaginal vault, as well as to the absence of the mucus previously secreted by the cervical glands. These are seldom likely to be major factors. In the first place, the vagina is usually not significantly shortened unless the operation is performed for cancer. Second, Masters[15] has shown that sexual lubrication occurs primarily by transudation of fluid across the vaginal wall, and this may occur even in the woman in whom an artificial vagina has been constructed; cervical mucus is not necessary. In these circumstances dyspareunia is probably mainly of emotional origin, and its diagnosis and treatment must be approached on these lines. Frequently a sexual adjustment that was borderline before hysterectomy remains poor or even deteriorates afterwards.

Prolapse of a tube through the vaginal cuff is rare. It may be confused with granulation tissue at the vaginal apex, and only a biopsy may give the correct diagnosis. Treatment is often complicated by not knowing exactly what had been done at the previous operation. When the diagnosis has been made, the tube should be removed, and this should primarily be attempted from the vaginal approach by opening the cuff. If this is impossible, a laparotomy is performed and the tube removed from above.

Prolapse of the whole vaginal vault may follow an abdominal hysterectomy, but it is perhaps more common after vaginal hysterectomy. It is doubtful whether attempts to suspend the vaginal cuff by attaching the round ligaments to it during the abdominal procedure prevent this complication. Utilizing the uterosacral ligaments and the pubocervical fascia in the repair of the pelvic floor may be of some value. Prolapse of the vaginal vault is usually recognized by the patient as a protruding mass. On examination it has to be distinguished from other types of pelvic relaxation. Its treatment will be discussed later under the complications of vaginal operations.

SUBTOTAL (SUPRACERVICAL) HYSTERECTOMY. The complications of subtotal hysterectomy are due primarily to the retained cervical stump. Thus prophylaxis consists in removing all the uterus at the first operation. Forty years ago this was considered difficult; now it should be routine. There are occasions, however, when the prudent surgeon may feel it best not to proceed with total hysterectomy but to leave the cervix in place either because the general condition of the patient is poor or because adhesions or inflammation makes further dissection deep in the pelvis a hazardous undertaking. In this case the patient must be followed at regular intervals with examinations and cytologic studies, just as if the whole uterus were present. If these studies reveal abnormalities, they should be investigated by biopsy, with or without colposcopy, and, if necessary, by conization. Removal of the stump is indicated for cervical intraepithelial neoplasia or if symptoms such as prolapse can be attributed to it. The vaginal route, without entering the peritoneal cavity, is preferable to the abdominal approach.

MYOMECTOMY. Myomectomy is generally performed when the removal of one or more leiomyomas is indicated to improve or preserve fertility. The complications include the recurrence of leiomyomas and the effect of the procedure upon any subsequent pregnancy. Recurrence may be due to the growth of new leiomyomas or to the enlargement of small ones that were not removed at the first operation. This occurs in about 30 per cent of cases, and another operation may be necessary.[8] At the second procedure a total hysterectomy should usually be performed.

The chief obstetric complication of myomectomy lies in the danger of rupture of the uterus at the site of the myomectomy scar. Nothing can be done to mitigate this during pregnancy, when about a third of uterine ruptures occur. Delivery by cesarean section may be indicated in some cases at or near term to prevent rupture during labor. In general, if the myomectomy incision did not penetrate the endometrium and if there is no other obstetric contraindication, vaginal delivery should be permitted. If, however, extensive myomectomy involves entering the endometrial cavity, or if other obstetric indications such as cephalopelvic disproportion exist, then cesarean section is usually indicated.

Tubes

TUBAL LIGATION. Sterilization by tubal ligation may be performed after delivery or as an interval procedure. In the latter case either the abdominal (by laparoscopy or minilaparotomy) or the vaginal route may be used.

The most important complication of this procedure is failure to provide permanent sterilization. Review of all methods of tubal sterilization suggests a failure rate of about 1 to 5 per 1000. Failures of tubal sterilization occur because of recanalization of the tube, formation of a tuboperitoneal fistula, or unsatisfactory initial tubal occlusion. Failure rate is dependent upon the route chosen, the timing with respect to pregnancy, and the type of procedure performed. Generally, with vaginal procedures the failure rate is high and complications, such as bleeding, infection, and rectal injuries, are greater. The failure rate is also higher when tubal sterilization procedures are performed at the time of cesarean section or in the immediate postpartum period. Of the tubal ligations performed abdominally, the Irving and Uchida types seem to be most effective; the Madlener type, the least effective; and the Pomeroy, intermediate. The minilaparotomy technique is cosmetically superior to the longer vertical incision, and it is used widely in developing countries, but it offers no special advantage with regard to success.

Laparoscopic sterilization by coagulation, banding, or clipping has now become the most common method of non-puerperal sterilization. Failure rates are in the range of 2 to 3 per 1000. Complications of laparoscopy are discussed later in this chapter. When pregnancies occur following tubal ligation, an increased percentage are ectopic. Because these pregnancies are unexpected, they can be even more catastrophic than the usual ectopic gestation.

TUBOPLASTY. Tuboplasty is designed to restore patency to the tubes to permit conception. Complications involve failure to restore patency, failure to achieve conception in spite of patent tubes as demonstrated by hysterosalpingogram, and an increased occurrence of ectopic pregnancy if conception does occur. Recent use of microsurgical techniques and better selection of patients for operation have increased the pregnancy rate, but the incidence of ectopic pregnancy remains relatively high.

Ovaries

OOPHORECTOMY. Bilateral oophorectomy involves the general complication of premature menopause but usually does not entail any specific problems. Unilateral oophorectomy may carry the risk of premature menopause, especially if the remaining ovary has a poor blood supply. This possibility should be appreciated when one ovary is conserved, so that appropriate treatment can be initiated if symptoms develop before the expected time of the patient's menopause.

Radical Procedures

RADICAL HYSTERECTOMY. Radical hysterectomy (Type III hysterectomy) involves removal of the uterus and upper one-third of the vagina along with the parametrial and paravaginal tissues out to the pelvic sidewall. It is usually combined with removal of the pelvic lymph nodes from the common iliac artery down to the femoral canal and the obturator nerve. This operation is performed mainly for the cure of early cancer of the cervix (Stage IB).[19] The operative mortality is now less than 1 per cent. Complications peculiar to this procedure involve the bladder, lymphatic system, and vagina.

The ureter is especially liable to injury during radical hysterectomy because it runs directly through the parametrial and para-

cervical tissue on its way to the bladder. Most commonly, the blood supply to the ureter is compromised, leading to necrosis of the wall and development of a ureterovaginal fistula. The incidence of such fistulas has been reduced from 5 to 15 per cent to 1 per cent or less in the last two decades by several techniques: (1) handling the ureter carefully and avoiding stripping of the adventitia through which the blood vessels run; (2) closure of the vaginal cuff and drainage of the retroperitoneal spaces by means of suction catheters; and (3) catheter drainage of the bladder postoperatively for 4 to 6 weeks. The risk of fistula formation is significantly increased after radiation therapy, when the operation is performed for a small central recurrence or persistent disease. The diagnosis and management of a ureteral fistula following radical hysterectomy are similar to those after other abdominal operations.

Injury to the nerve supply of the bladder is inevitable if a radical hysterectomy is properly performed. The result is that the patient is not able to void properly for varying periods after operation. Sensation usually returns before motor power, but the pattern of bladder function may continue to be different for some time. As many as 30 per cent of patients will have some degree of significant bladder dysfunction. The best management is to leave an indwelling catheter in place for 4 to 6 weeks postoperatively. Whenever a catheter is to be left in the bladder for more than 48 hours, the patient should be kept on prophylactic urinary antibiotics, such as a combination of trimethoprim and sulfamethoxazole. After 4 to 6 weeks, the patient can be allowed to void and the catheter left out if the residual urine measures less than 100 ml. The urinary antibiotic should be continued for another 7 days after catheter removal. Rarely does adequate function fail to return. If no progress is made in 6 months after operation, full urologic examination including urodynamic studies, cystoscopy, and intravenous pyelogram is indicated.

Removal of the pelvic lymph nodes may occasionally result in a collection of lymph in the pelvic retroperitoneal spaces (lymphocyst). This can usually be prevented by the use of suction catheters placed in the retroperitoneal space bilaterally at the time of operation and brought out through stab incisions in each lower quadrant of the abdomen. These catheters are kept on continuous suction for a minimum of 3 days, and usually for 5 to 7 days. The length of time is determined by the amount of fluid drained each day; if no fluid is recovered, the catheters are of no value and should be removed. If a lymphocyst develops despite these precautions, it may produce no symptoms and is detected as a mass situated laterally in the pelvis. It may be drained by aspiration on one or several occasions and usually resolves. If infection or ureteral obstruction is associated with a lymphocyst, open drainage through a retroperitoneal groin incision and antibiotics are required.

Decrease in the length of the vagina always occurs as a result of radical hysterectomy. The patient and her husband or partner should be told about this preoperatively. Coitus may be resumed after the apex of the vagina has healed (4 to 6 weeks). This rarely causes problems, as some stretching of the vagina occurs.

PELVIC EXENTERATION. Exenterative procedures in gynecology are usually performed for locally recurrent or persistent cervical cancer after adequate radiation therapy. These procedures are done only with curative intent; if metastatic disease is found outside the pelvis or if the cancer is fixed to bone or the muscles of the lateral pelvic sidewall, it is judged unresectable and the operation is abandoned. Anterior exenteration includes radical hysterectomy, vaginectomy, and total cystectomy with urinary conduit. Posterior exenteration includes radical hysterectomy, vaginectomy, and resection of the rectosigmoid colon with sigmoid colostomy. Total pelvic exenteration involves radical hysterectomy, vaginectomy, total cystectomy, resection of the rectosigmoid colon, and formation of a urinary conduit and colostomy. Total exenteration remains the most commonly performed procedure; posterior exenteration is almost never indicated. With the application of modern radiotherapeutic techniques, there are fewer indications for these procedures. In selected cases, however, they may provide the patient her only chance for survival. Cure rates of approximately 30 to 40 per cent are reported. The operative mortality rate is now about 10 to 15 per cent.[25]

Complications encountered in such radical surgery relate to fluid and electrolyte alterations, blood loss, protracted anesthesia, urinary diversion, sepsis, complications resulting from the denuded evacuated pelvis, and loss of sexual function. Most of these problems have been solved or improvements have been made in the past decade. Fluid and electrolyte problems are well managed by improved monitoring techniques, e.g., Swan-Ganz catheters. Operative mortality is inversely related to operating time and blood loss during operation. Sepsis can now usually be controlled by appropriate antibiotics.

Urinary diversion is usually accomplished by implanting the ureters into an isolated segment of ileum (anterior exenteration) or sigmoid colon (total exenteration). Pyelonephritis and hyperchloremic acidosis are two potential problems with urinary conduits. Using an isolated segment of ileum or colon and keeping the segment of bowel short (12 to 15 cm.) prevent the urine from being stored and thereby chloride absorption is reduced. Also, renal infection is reduced by isolating the conduit from the fecal stream and placing the patient on prophylaxis with trimethoprim-sulfamethoxazole. Strictures at the site of the ureterointestinal anastomosis may occur, leading to obstruction and pyelonephritis. This can be detected by intravenous pyelogram or loopogram. Revision of the anastomosis may become necessary in this case.

Closure of the pelvic cavity continues to be a problem, although recent improvements have been made. There is still an unacceptable long-term incidence of intestinal fistulas and obstruction that result from allowing the small bowel to fall down on the raw pelvic floor. An omental lid to cover the pelvic floor has been devised by freeing the omentum from its attachments along the greater curvature of the stomach except at the superior left border, bringing it down the left paracolic gutter, and sewing it over the pelvic cavity. Improved results have also been reported with use of a peritoneal flap placed over the pelvic floor. Both of these techniques have been significant contributions to the success of the operation and have resulted in the elimination of some complications.

Complications related to the perineal

wound are of concern because of the size of the cavity, the malodorous discharge and chronic infection that result, the time it takes to heal, and the loss of vaginal function. In the woman who was sexually active before operation, creation of a neovagina is an important part of the rehabilitation process.[14] Two satisfactory techniques are the application of a split-thickness skin graft into the perineal defect 3 to 6 weeks postoperatively and vulvovaginoplasty (Williams' procedure). The advantages of the latter procedure are that it can be performed at any time in relation to the exenteration, it does not require skin grafting, and it does not require entering the pelvic cavity and thereby possibly creating a fistula.

Laparoscopy

During the past decade, laparoscopy has become the second most frequent gynecologic surgical procedure. Complications that are unique to laparoscopy include difficulties in establishing the pneumoperitoneum, needle and trocar perforations of abdominal viscera, electrical burns, anesthetic problems, hemorrhage, and sterilization failures. Generally, complications are related to the experience of the laparoscopist and extensions of the indications for the procedure.[13]

An incorrectly placed pneumoperitoneum (Veress) needle may result in insufflation of the abdominal wall, retroperitoneum, mesentery, omentum, or bowel. The most common and least dangerous complication is subcutaneous injection of gas that produces subperitoneal emphysema. Attention to proper technique will usually prevent erroneous placement of gas. The Veress needle must be open and have a sharp point and a functioning spring mechanism. The abdominal wall should be raised upward and the needle should be thrust through it with a rapid motion in a perpendicular direction. During insufflation, no more than 3 liters of CO_2 should be introduced initially into the peritoneal cavity under strict manometric control with the pressure below 20 mm. Hg. Higher pressures may mean subcutaneous or bowel insufflation. The needle should be manipulated or rotated in such a manner that the pressure is kept at its lowest possible level. Percussion of the right upper quadrant of the abdomen during insufflation can determine whether liver dullness disappears. If there is uncertainty about whether the gas is located within the peritoneal cavity, it is best to start again. Aspirating the Veress needle with a syringe, flushing with saline, and then elevating the anterior abdominal wall to see if the saline disappears down the needle may be useful. Severe complications such as mediastinal and neck emphysema, pneumothorax, and cardiac arrest can be avoided by not overinflating, by monitoring the intraperitoneal pressure carefully, and by avoiding vigorous compression of the abdomen.

There are usually no complications following a clean puncture of the colon, small intestine, or stomach with the Veress needle. An attempt should be made to visualize the punctured area, and only if there is a laceration should laparotomy be performed. Perforation of the colon and stomach with the trocar have been reported. This complication may be the result of unrecognized intragastric or intracolonic insufflation of gas, gastric distention during the induction of anesthesia, or defective technique at insertion of the trocar. A site for trocar insertion at least 2 cm. away from previous incisions should be chosen. The patient should be placed in the Trendelenburg position. The trocar should be aimed at the sacral hollow and inserted with a controlled twisting motion. If intestinal perforation occurs with the trocar, immediate laparotomy is indicated. The bladder should be catheterized in order to avoid puncture by one of the trocars.

The most common complication necessitating laparotomy is uncontrolled bleeding, usually from the mesosalpinx during sterilization procedures. This can be the result of insufficient fulguration of the fallopian tube before division or resection, tearing of the mesosalpinx during manipulation, avulsion of the tube, or fulguration too close to the cornual end of the tube. This bleeding can usually be controlled by laparoscopic electrocoagulation. Bleeding from skin incisions is of little consequence, usually ceasing spontaneously when compressed by the trocar and sleeve. Occasionally, bleeding occurs from vessels within the abdominal wall, most significantly from the epigastric vessels, sometimes requiring incision, hematoma evacuation, vessel ligation, and drainage. More serious complications result if the trocar perforates vessels within the mesentery, adhesions, or the retroperitoneal space. Immediate laparotomy is indicated under these conditions. These complications can almost always be avoided by adherence to proper technique, which involves correct trocar insertion, patient positioning, and selection of trocar insertion sites.

Anesthesia for laparoscopy differs from that employed for most other surgical procedures by virtue of the need for pneumoperitoneum, extreme Trendelenburg position, and the use of electrocoagulation. Because of these factors, anesthesia for laparoscopy is attended by various risks and complications. Cardiac arrhythmias, hypotension, hypertension, gas embolization, pneumothorax, hypercarbia, gastric dilatation, and silent gastric regurgitation have all been reported. The anesthesiologist and surgeon must be aware of these possible complications and the factors responsible in order to minimize their occurrence. Excessive pneumoperitoneum and prolonged use of extreme Trendelenburg position should be avoided. Adequate ventilation should be assured. A nasogastric tube should be employed after intubation and before laparoscopy is initiated.

Burns may occur whenever electrosurgical equipment is utilized. The severity of the complication depends on the location of the burn. Abdominal wall burns are upsetting but rarely cause major problems. These can be eliminated by using a system with isolated ground circuitry or bipolar equipment in which the electrical current only passes between the two tongs of the forceps and not the entire body, as it does in unipolar systems. Even if the bipolar forceps is used for tubal sterilization, a unipolar unit should be available for ancillary surgical procedures or control of bleeding. Bowel burns occur by direct application of current to bowel, i.e., by touching the bowel with the hot tip of the coagulation forceps or trocar. Bowel burns are more likely to occur if abdominal distention is allowed to dissipate. If bowel burns are recognized at the time of surgery, a decision must be made between observation of the patient or immediate laparotomy

and repair. If the injury results only in a whitened area on the bowel serosa, the patient may be observed. If the bowel injury results in serosal separation, then laparotomy should be performed and the area repaired by oversewing the defect and inverting it into the bowel lumen. Unrecognized bowel injuries usually follow an uneventful immediate postoperative course. Later, the burned area undergoes necrosis, leading to intestinal perforation several days after operation. The patient develops severe abdominal pain and distention, fever, and chills. This picture needs to be differentiated from an exacerbation of pelvic inflammatory disease. Immediate laparotomy should be performed. In most cases, bowel resection and end-to-end reanastomosis are required, because damage to the bowel may extend several centimeters beyond the area of obvious involvement.

Pregnancies must be considered a complication of laparoscopic tubal sterilization. Many of these pregnancies are luteal phase pregnancies, i.e., operation was performed after ovulation and conception but before the first missed menstrual period. This problem can be avoided by performing laparoscopic sterilization only during the proliferative phase of the menstrual cycle or performing a D and C at the time of operation. Confusing the round or infundibulopelvic ligaments with the fallopian tubes is another reason for laparoscopic sterilization failures. Every effort should be made to identify the fimbriated end of the tube and follow it proximally to the point of coagulation, banding, or clipping.

Urinary Tract

RETROPUBIC URETHROPEXY. Three types of procedures for retropubic urethral suspensions are now generally used for the correction of stress urinary incontinence: sling procedures, the Marshall-Marchetti-Krantz operation, and the Burch modification of the retropubic urethropexy. Each can be used primarily but are more commonly performed after failure of an anterior colporrhaphy. Complications of these procedures include puncture of the bladder while passing the retropubic clamp during sling procedures, creation of a urethrovaginal fistula secondary to pressure necrosis from too tight a sling, osteitis pubis following Marshall-Marchetti-Krantz operations, and placement of permanent sutures into the bladder or urethra.[24] Another problem associated with these procedures is delayed ability to void postoperatively, requiring prolonged catheterization. Bladder infections will inevitably result unless prophylactic antibiotics, such as trimethoprim-sulfamethoxazole, are used. Suprapubic bladder drainage is helpful and avoids repeated catheterizations. Bleeding with hematoma formation in the space of Retzius can sometimes occur; drainage of this space with Penrose drains is recommended by some authors.

VAGINAL OPERATIONS

GENERAL

Comparison with Abdominal Operations

Vaginal procedures are the hallmark of the gynecologist, and there are certain conditions, usually local ones, for which this surgical approach is clearly indicated. When it is utilized for procedures beyond the range of the limited exposure that can be obtained, complications are likely to ensue.

The complications of vaginal operations are somewhat different as a whole from those of abdominal operations. First, vaginal procedures are more likely to be elective rather than urgent, and complications are therefore less acceptable to surgeon and patient alike. Second, sexual problems, as well as being a contributing cause of vaginal operations, are also an important aspect of their complications. Third, vaginal operations do not necessarily involve entering the peritoneal cavity and lack some of the complications due to this. Fourth, vaginal operations are performed near the bladder, urethra, and rectum, and later difficulties are particularly likely to involve these organs. Last, many vaginal procedures are performed for what are simply hernias of the pelvic floor in which the weakness is a result of poor tissues and old age; these factors militate against effective repair and make complications in the form of recurrence more likely.

Preoperative

TIME OF OPERATION. In the woman of reproductive age operative bleeding is likely to be greater in amount at the end of the secretory phase of the menstrual cycle than in the early proliferative phase. Thus, if a choice is possible, the latter time should be selected. This has the added advantage that an unexpected pregnancy will not be encountered.

SEXUAL FUNCTION. In order to avoid postoperative sexual complications, careful inquiry must be made before operation about the patient's desires and feelings in this area. For example, in the repair of relaxation the posterior perineorrhaphy can be performed tightly in the widow of seventy, whereas in the younger woman who is sexually active it may be better to avoid this part of the repair or do a limited procedure because of the dyspareunia that may result from a narrowed introitus or a ridge in the posterior wall of the vagina.

OTHER ORGANS. The amount and type of preparation of neighboring organs vary with the procedure to be done. As far as the rectum is concerned, the problem is to prevent contamination of the operative field. Usually a preoperative enema is all that is necessary. If reconstruction of the bowel is contemplated, as in the repair of a rectovaginal fistula or an old third-degree perineal laceration, additional bowel preparation by means of a low residue diet, cathartics, enemas, and intestinal antibiotics may be advisable. As far as the bladder is concerned, on the other hand, the problem is to prevent infection of the urinary tract. Thus, in minor vaginal procedures the potential danger of introducing infection by way of a catheter can be avoided by having the patient void immediately before the procedure. In major vaginal operations, however, it is a desirable prophylactic measure to empty the bladder immediately before the procedure by means of a catheter.

LOCAL. It is desirable to have the vulvar epithelium and vaginal mucosa as free from bacteria and in as healthy a condition as possible to prevent local infection and promote healing. In the postmenopausal woman whose mucosa is atrophic, the intravaginal application of an estrogenic cream each night for 2 weeks will thicken the mucosa, facilitate dissection, and improve healing. If necessary, estrogens can be given by mouth with the same effect.

The value of preoperative douches and antibiotic suppositories to prevent postoperative infection is ·debatable. Certainly, if a known vaginal infection such as trichomoniasis or candidiasis is present, it should be treated, if possible, before any vaginal operation. Local pHisoHex baths are also of value in cleansing the vulva and perineum of potential contamination from the rectum. In addition, the vagina should be cleansed with an antiseptic such as povidone-iodine just before the procedure is begun.

Operative

There is one general operative problem in vaginal procedures — exposure. Every effort is necessary to improve exposure and avoid dissecting where structures cannot be identified. This means proper positioning of the patient, adequate lighting, competent assistance, and instruments especially adapted for vaginal use. An important corollary is that the vaginal surgeon must not be too proud to conclude a difficult vaginal procedure and perform a laparotomy to complete it so that unidentifiable structures may be seen directly. This can occur, for example, with unexpectedly large leiomyomas or unanticipated pelvic adhesions.

Operative Complications

HEMORRHAGE. This is most likely to be a troublesome, continuous ooze from many small vessels. Large veins may be encountered lateral to the bladder, and also the uterine or ovarian arteries may slip from the grasp of clamps or ligatures. When venous bleeding occurs, local pressure and suture ligature of bleeding points are usually effective. When major arteries slip from a clamp, they usually retract, and finding them again may not be easy. Laparotomy and transperitoneal ligature may be necessary, even to the extent of ligating the hypogastric arteries. Continued oozing at the end of the proce-

dure may be controlled with tight vaginal packing for 24 to 48 hours.

INJURY TO RECTUM, BLADDER, URETHRA OR URETER. As in abdominal procedures, recognition of injury at the time it occurs is important. The rectum is usually entered in the course of a posterior colpoperineorrhaphy. In the repair the mucosa should be inverted by continuous 00 or 000 absorbable sutures and the fascia and vaginal mucosa closed in layers with interrupted sutures of similar material.

No special postoperative therapy is indicated. Similar treatment should be accorded a laceration of the bladder occurring during dissection of the anterior vaginal wall, except that one should be reasonably sure that the ureters are not involved; this may require cystoscopy during the operation. An indwelling catheter should be left in place for 7 days and the patient placed on antibiotics. The urethra may also be entered during repair of the anterior vaginal wall. The mucosa should be closed, transversely if possible, with interrupted 3-0 or 4-0 absorbable sutures and the repair completed in the usual manner. Injury to the ureter during vaginal hysterectomy should be rare if the paracervical tissues are divided close to the uterus. When injury is discovered, it should be handled by the abdominal approach, as described previously, usually by reimplanting the ureter into the bladder (ureteroneo-cystostomy).

Postoperative Complications

HEMORRHAGE. Early hemorrhage (within the first 24 hours) is usually manifested by vaginal bleeding. When this is excessive, the patient must be placed in the lithotomy position, with anesthesia if necessary and the operative area examined, removing the sutures if indicated. The bleeding point, if it can be identified, is ligated. This necessitates good light and appropriate instruments and suture material. Too often it is attempted with inadequate equipment. If no bleeding can be identified, the vagina should be packed firmly with plain or iodoform gauze for 24 to 48 hours.

Occasionally intraperitoneal or retroperitoneal bleeding may follow a vaginal procedure. Intraperitoneal bleeding is recognized and treated as described previously in the section on management of bleeding following abdominal procedures. Retroperitoneal bleeding is more difficult to identify. When it is large in amount, discoloration of the skin of the flanks may occur, but before this there is little to see externally and pelvic examination is often inconclusive. The only sign may be that of the patient's continuing and unresponsive shock.

Later bleeding (after the first 24 hours) may appear as a sudden gush, e.g., from the cervix or vaginal cuff or as a hematoma in the cuff or in the anterior or posterior vaginal walls. The former requires management similar to that used in the early postoperative period, while in the latter case one must wait for the hematoma to be reabsorbed or drain.

INFECTIONS. Good healing is the rule when incisions are made on the vulva or perineum, except in cases in which large amounts of tissue are removed, as in radical vulvectomy with regional node dissection. In the vagina, infection is often associated with a hematoma of the anterior or posterior wall. Pain and fever, confirmed by the finding of induration or a tender mass on pelvic examination, enable one to make the diagnosis. Drainage usually occurs spontaneously but may be hastened, if a fluctuant mass is felt, by breaking down the incision between the sutures or by removing one or more sutures. Cultures should be obtained of any fluid found and the appropriate antibiotics used. Such infections predispose to the recurrence of pelvic relaxation, but little can be done about this except hope for sufficient fibrosis to develop. Immediate reoperation should not be considered.

FISTULAS. Ureterovaginal fistulas are less common after vaginal than after abdominal procedures. On the other hand, rectovaginal, vesicovaginal, and urethrovaginal fistulas are more common. The same necessity of waiting for 3 months before attempting repair applies, and the same principles of reoperation may be used with few exceptions. Small rectovaginal fistulas may close spontaneously or become smaller with only conservative treatment — stool softener, low residue diet, and local cleansing — and colostomy may not be necessary prior to repair. Vesicovaginal fistulas often occur lower down in the vagina than after abdominal procedures and lend themselves more to layer closure than to partial colpocleisis. Urethrovaginal fistulas involve dissecting out the fistula and closing the urethral mucosa if possible. If this cannot be done, available tissues are closed over the urethra in two or three layers. Provided the urethral mucosa is connected at one point or the cut ends are not too far apart, with or without sutures, and catheter splinting is maintained for at least 7 days, closure should be satisfactory.

If the urethra is shortened by loss of its distal end, it can be lengthened by making a tube of vaginal mucosa and closing the fascia and lateral vaginal mucosa below it, using relaxing incisions if necessary.

FUNCTIONAL. The two functions of the lower genital tract that may be affected by the complications of vaginal operations are reproduction and coitus. Delivery after vaginal or perineal repair may break down the sutures and lead to a complication in the form of recurrence of relaxation. Thus, when extensive repairs for incompetent internal os of the cervix, for cystocele or rectocele, or for descensus by parametrial fixation have been performed, cesarean section is usually the method of choice for delivery. After minor perineal repairs, operations on the external genitalia or even closure of a small low rectovaginal fistula or repair of an old third-degree perineal laceration, vaginal delivery may be allowed.

Sexual difficulties may follow any kind of vaginal procedure, whether it produces anatomic changes or not. This complication needs to be specifically investigated, because the patient may not mention it spontaneously. When it is reported, further inquiry should be made of the exact nature of the complaint and thorough examination made for any possible anatomic abnormality. Treatment primarily involves reassurance with consideration of counseling for underlying psychological causes and the operative correction only of definite abnormalities.

RELATED ORGAN SYSTEMS. Major complications in the bladder or rectum include fistula, infection, or prolonged dysfunction. Fistula has been discussed earlier. Infection is primarily a problem in the urinary tract and tends to follow catheterization. This procedure may either exacerbate an existing infection or, by introducing foreign organisms, start a new one. The clinical picture, diagnosis, and management are similar to those described previously in the section on the complications of abdominal operations. Prolonged dysfunction of either organ may follow specific procedures and will be considered later in this chapter.

SPECIFIC OPERATIONS

External Genitalia

REMOVAL OF BENIGN TUMORS. Excision of small cysts and benign tumors such as fibroma, lipoma, or hydroadenoma of the vulva, or of intraepithelial carcinoma, is not usually followed by complications unless the skin fails to heal. In this case warm baths for 15 minutes 2 or 3 times daily together with restriction of activity will normally result in healing. Antibiotics need not be used unless there is a generalized reaction with fever and malaise or lymphadenitis.

Cysts or abscesses of Bartholin's gland present a special problem in complications. Incision of an acutely inflamed abscess is likely to be complicated by recurrence of infection, requiring further incision or marsupialization. Excision, often a difficult task, may also be followed by recurrence if the gland is not completely removed. Marsupialization, probably the most desirable therapy for quiescent cysts or even abscesses, may be complicated by a persistent cavity. This is likely to be of little significance, and the patient who is concerned about it should be reassured, since it may take several months to close completely.

SIMPLE VULVECTOMY. Extensive excision of vulvar tissue or a complete vulvectomy may be performed for widespread carcinoma in situ of the vulva or condylomata acuminata. A similar procedure is extensive cauterization of condylomata. The complications of these operations are similar to those that follow radical vulvectomy in respect to the urinary stream and dyspareunia.

RADICAL VULVECTOMY. Radical vulvectomy with bilateral excision of the inguinal and femoral lymph nodes is the primary operative treatment for cancer of the vulva, whether squamous cell carcinoma, adenocarcinoma, or malignant melanoma. This is a major procedure often performed in older women who are poor operative risks.

Complications are likely to occur and include (1) breakdown and necrosis of the skin incision with hematoma with or without infection, (2) hemorrhage, (3) lymphangitis, (4) edema of the legs, (5) urinary incontinence, and (6) dyspareunia.

1. Failure of the skin incision to heal is common, even if little skin has been removed, because of the undermining edges. It is increased if a hematoma forms under the skin flaps. This can, to a certain extent, be prevented by suction drainage through catheters placed beneath the skin on each side and brought out through separate stab incisions (Fig. 34–7). Suction is continued until drainage is minimal, usually for 4 or 5 days. Early removal may defeat the purpose of the catheters and result in reaccumulation of fluid. It is impossible to predict at operation which incision is likely to break down, although the chances are increased when closure is performed under tension. The most likely place for breakdown to occur is at the center of the crescentic lower abdominal incision over the symphysis pubis, extending outward and downward from this point. The extent of this complication can usually not be determined until at least 7 days after operation and usually after the skin stitches have been removed, although a preliminary idea of the likelihood of breakdowns can be obtained from the color of the skin edges shortly after operation. If they are dusky or black, at least superficial slough of the skin is likely to occur. But if the color of the skin is normal, primary healing cannot necessarily be predicted.

Various methods have been described for preventing skin breakdown. The most important measure is to keep the skin clean and dry. If the edges separate, the incision should be cleaned with hydrogen peroxide 3 or 4 times daily and then dried. Antibiotics appropriate to the organisms cultured from the incision should be given if there is a generalized reaction as indicated, for example, by fever or leukocytosis. Necrotic tissue should also be debrided. Healing by secondary intention takes several weeks unless the area of breakdown is small, but secondary closure or skin grafting is rarely likely to be successful in hastening closure. While healing is taking place, the patient should be encouraged to eat a high protein, high vi-

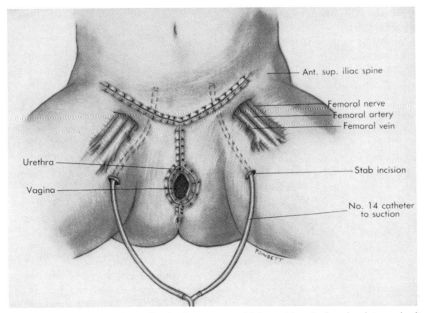

Figure 34–7   Suction drainage after radical vulvectomy and bilateral inguinal and pelvic node dissection.

tamin diet. She need not be confined to bed, since some activity is beneficial. If she has adequate help at home, it is better for her to be there than in the hospital.

2. Hemorrhage from the groin incision is rare, but usually arises from the main vessels — femoral artery or vein — and is associated with wound breakdown and infection. Emergency compression of the bleeding point, transfusion, and, if an artery is involved, replacement by a graft are necessary. When such massive hemorrhage occurs, the outlook for the patient's leg and life is poor.

3. Lymphangitis, involving all the lymph vessels that previously drained into the inguinal nodes, from the leg, buttock, and lower part of the abdomen, is a rare complication. It may occur many months after operation and is apt to be recurrent. It is characterized by high fever, malaise, and pain, and swelling and redness in the affected area. Bed rest and antibiotics are usually successful in treatment. Administration of long-acting penicillin every month for 6 months after operation is advisable as prophylaxis against lymphangitis.

4. Edema of the legs is an almost invariable complication. It does not usually appear until the patient has been on her feet for most of the day, i.e., after she has left the hospital. At first an attempt should be made to control the swelling by having the patient lie down frequently during the day, keeping her feet higher than her abdomen. The use of elastic stockings should be recommended; they should be put on before the patient arises and be worn all day. The swelling usually subsides after 9 to 12 months, as the lymph finds other channels for its return.

5. Urinary incontinence may follow radical vulvectomy if the patient previously had a cystocele with distortion of the urethrovesical angle. Vaginal repair of the cystocele with suspension of the urethrovesical angle may be advisable. Suprapubic vesicourethral suspension is likely to be more difficult than usual after radical vulvectomy and node dissection. It may, however, be necessary to use this should the vaginal approach fail. Usually up to half the urethra can be removed and continence retained. If so much has been removed that control is affected, repair is difficult. Creating a pubic sling vesicourethral suspension by using external oblique or rectus sheath fascia and lengthening the urethra by constructing a tube of vaginal mucosa may be helpful. Such patients are likely to be urologic cripples, however, and urinary diversion may be indicated as a last resort.

6. Dyspareunia following radical vul-

vectomy may be due to the removal of the clitoris and labia which normally supply sexual stimulation, to actual constriction of the introitus by scar tissue, or to the emotional response of the patient or her husband or partner to the operation. Nothing can be done about the first except by explanation and reassurance. The constriction of the introitus may be lessened at operation by dissecting under and everting the posterior vaginal wall at the time the perineum is repaired and by encouraging coitus or manual or instrumental dilatation of the vagina as soon as possible after operation. In persistent stricture a variety of plastic reconstructive procedures may be performed later.[11] When it is apparent that emotional factors are predominant in postoperative dyspareunia, the problem is more complex. Previous sexual difficulties may have become intensified. Resolving these may be hard in the older woman, although reassurance and encouragement can do much.

PLASTIC PROCEDURES. The main purpose of plastic procedures on the external genitalia is to enlarge the introitus. In the pubertal girl this is done because of an imperforate hymen. The complications of this procedure are recurrence of the closure of the introitus and infection, which may extend to the upper genital tract and affect the patient's future reproductive capacity. They may be prevented by adequate initial cruciate incision and the use of antibiotics postoperatively. In the engaged woman a tight introitus may rarely require enlarging by a plastic procedure prior to marriage. An unfortunate complication of this is continued postoperative pain that may interfere with later coitus. This can be prevented by performing such procedures at least 8 weeks before the patient is to be married. Finally, plastic operations may be necessary to release scars resulting from obstetric or gynecologic operations. Here, one must be sure that the difficulty of which the patient complains is due to the scar; otherwise, the operation will be complicated by persistent pain and dyspareunia.

Vagina

MINOR PROCEDURES. Minor procedures on the vagina include removal of small cysts and biopsies of various types of lesions. Complications are usually rare.

PLASTIC PROCEDURES ON THE ANTERIOR VAGINAL WALL. These operations include repair of defects in the musculofascial layers of the anterior vaginal wall such as cystocele and urethrocele. Specific complications involve the function of the urinary tract and include vesicovaginal or urethrovaginal fistulas (see the section on Fistulas), incontinence, and urinary retention.

Urinary incontinence may have been one of the primary reasons for the vaginal repair, or it may occur as the result of operative distortion of the urethrovesical relationships. Whenever the patient complains of incontinence, preoperative urodynamic studies are important.[29] These studies help to differentiate true stress incontinence from urgency incontinence or neurogenic bladder. Operative treatment is usually appropriate for the first but not for the last two conditions. Secondary stress incontinence, occurring after a vaginal repair, is usually best approached by the abdominal route. (See under Radical Vulvectomy.)

In urinary retention the patient cannot void after removal of the catheter or is unable to expel more than a small amount of urine, leaving a large residual volume (more than 100 ml.) in the bladder. Poor bladder function preoperatively may predispose to this complication, as in the case of the neurogenic bladder, and this condition should be excluded when possible by preoperative studies, including a cystometrogram. Otherwise, predisposing factors are not known, and it is usually difficult to predict which patient may have this complication. The tightness of the closure of the bladder wall and of the suspension of the urethrovesical angle may affect voiding ability, as may also the amount of dissection and local trauma occurring during the repair. The length of time the catheter remains in place postoperatively is probably of little importance; the complication occurs with all sorts of regimens.

Management consists in catheterizing the patient as soon as it is realized that she cannot void properly. If she requires catheterization a second time, the catheter is left in place for a further 48 hours and removed again. Removal of the catheter may be accompanied by various measures to aid the patient to void. Since emotional factors may be important, encouragement, mild sedation, and provision of quiet surroundings are of help. Parasympathomimetic drugs such as Urecholine in doses of 5 to 10 mg. every 4 hours, increasing to 20 to 30 mg., may be helpful. Occasionally it may be necessary to have the patient return home with an indwelling catheter in place. She may then remove it several days later and return for a check of the residual urine. Home surroundings may provide the necessary stimulus and relaxation for adequate voiding. Urinary antiseptics or antibiotics should be continued as long as there is need for catheterization and for 48 hours thereafter.

PLASTIC PROCEDURES ON THE POSTERIOR VAGINAL WALL. These procedures are performed to repair a rectocele, rectovaginal fistula, third-degree laceration, or other perineal injuries. Since these conditions usually cause no symptoms except mild difficulty in evacuating the bowel or fecal incontinence, complications are primarily failure of the repair and deserve reoperation if they are severe.

Uterus

DILATATION AND CURETTAGE. This is the most commonly performed gynecologic operation. Complications include perforation of the uterus (by far the most important), intrauterine synechiae, and damage to the internal os of the cervix.

The incidence of perforation of the uterus was found by McElin and Reeves[17] to be 0.63 per cent in 2991 instances of diagnostic curettage. When therapeutic curettages are included, it may be somewhat more frequent. Perforation is usually recognized promptly by the surgeon when the sound or curette goes in farther than seems appropriate. Although certain conditions such as pregnancy, malignancy, and old age predispose to perforation, it may occur at any time. Precautionary measures include (1) careful examination to determine the position of the uterus; perforation at the junction of corpus and cervix is a special hazard when the uterus is retroflexed; (2) the use of great gentleness in instrumentation of the uterus; and (3) caution in dilating the cer-

vix. In the postmenopausal woman especially, the cervix and lower uterine segment are more likely to split as they are dilated.

Once the diagnosis of perforation has been made, two problems present themselves. First, should the diagnostic or therapeutic procedure be continued? If these are important and one is reasonably sure of the site of the perforation, tissue may be removed gently from other parts of the uterus. Generally, however, it is best to desist from further curettage. Second, how should the perforation be managed? Conservative treatment should be considered first. This consists in putting the patient to bed in the semisitting position, keeping her under careful observation, withholding oral intake for at least 24 hours, and giving her antibiotics if infection is present. More active treatment, i.e., laparotomy, may be indicated if hemorrhage occurs, if there is apparent injury to other organs such as bladder or intestine or, in rare instances, if carcinoma of the corpus uteri is present. Hemorrhage may occur from the uterine artery, or its descending branch if the uterus is split laterally, and usually appears promptly. Injury to other organs may not be easy to detect except in the unusual event that a piece of intestine is brought down through the uterus. If the bowel has been damaged, signs of peritonitis may appear and, if persistent, they indicate operation. If the bladder has been injured, urinary output may decrease and the patient's general condition may rapidly deteriorate. Laparotomy should enable the diagnosis to be made. Treatment consists in repair of the perforation. The uterus itself may be closed with absorbable sutures. If the patient's childbearing has been completed, if her condition is good, and if there is an additional indication, such as leiomyomata, hysterectomy may be performed. If the patient becomes pregnant following repair of a uterine perforation, cesarean section should be strongly considered as the method of delivery.

If cancer is present in the uterus when the perforation occurs (the diagnosis having been made preoperatively or by frozen section), immediate hysterectomy may be considered, provided that the tumor is well differentiated and clinically confined to the corpus uteri, because of the danger of disseminating the cancer. In general, however, it is better to wait and carry out definitive treatment in a planned manner.

If no untoward results follow perforation, but a diagnosis of the primary gynecologic problem has not been made, it is wise to wait 6 weeks before attempting to repeat the curettage, and then the utmost caution should be used.

Late complications of dilatation and curettage are rare. They include intrauterine synechiae (Asherman's syndrome) and incompetence of the internal os of the cervix. The former is especially likely to occur when curettage is performed in the postpartum period. It may result in amenorrhea and sterility. Repeat curettage and insertion of an intrauterine device are helpful unless the endometrium has been completely removed. Incompetence of the internal cervical os may lead to second trimester abortion and require a cerclage procedure. Treatment is covered under complications of obstetric operations.

CERVICAL BIOPSY AND CONIZATION. Biopsy and conization of the cervix are primarily performed for the diagnosis of invasive cervical cancer and also for the diagnosis and treatment of cervical intraepithelial neoplasia. Repair of old cervical lacerations may also be an indication.

Complications may be immediate or delayed. Immediate complications include perforation of the uterus and hemorrhage. Perforation may result from overzealous removal of tissue from a short cervix. It is handled in the same way as a perforation occurring during dilatation and curettage. Operative bleeding may be reduced by the injection into the cervix of local anesthetic agents or vasopressors. However, the reactive vasodilation and subsequent bleeding are of concern. Usually bleeding, provided it is not coming from an injured artery higher in the cervical canal, is treated by use of longer-lasting absorbable sutures. The most effective sutures are those placed at the angles of the cervix or those of the Sturmdorf type, inverting the anterior, posterior, or lateral lips (Fig. 34–8).

Late complications of these operations include hemorrhage, stenosis of the cervical canal, obstetric problems, and recurrent cervical intraepithelial neoplasia or invasive cancer. Late hemorrhage may occur at any time up to 14 days postoperatively and its incidence may be as high as 11 per cent.[5] It is usually unexpected as far as the patient is concerned and is not accompanied by pain or other symptoms unless shock supervenes. Immediate examination with the patient in the lithotomy position is indicated, with a good light and adequate instruments at hand. If the bleeding point can be seen, it should be clamped with a right-angled clamp and ligated, although this is usually a difficult maneuver. In any case a vaginal pack of 2-inch plain or iodoform gauze should be inserted tightly against the cervix. The patient should also be treated for shock, if present, with intravenous administration of fluids and blood. The pack should be removed in 24 hours. If bleeding occurs while the pack is in place, the patient should be examined again in the operating room under anesthesia and the cervix sutured as described previously for acute bleeding. Occasionally, persistent profuse bleeding may

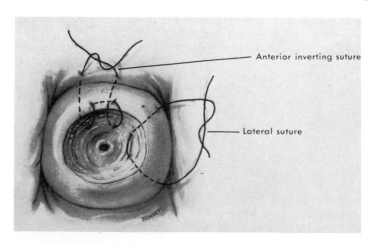

Figure 34–8 Hemostasis and repair after conization of cervix.

necessitate abdominal hysterectomy with or without ligation of the hypogastric arteries.

Cervical stenosis can in part be prevented by testing the patency of the cervical canal postmenstrually on at least two occasions after operation. A uterine sound, thin probe, or the smallest cervical dilator can be used. When this is not done, and sometimes in spite of it, cervical stenosis will occasionally result in the partial or complete retention of menstrual fluid. This causes dysmenorrhea, prolongation of menstrual flow, and occasionally, amenorrhea with hematometra and severe lower abdominal pain. Dilatation must be performed, although it is usually necessary to do this under anesthesia, and it is sometimes difficult to find the external os of the cervix.

The ability to conceive after cervical conization does not seem to be greatly reduced, but obstetric complications may result from damage to the internal os from excessive shortening of the cervix or the formation of scar tissue. The former may result in abortion or premature delivery.[9] The size of the cone may be important.[12] Some type of cerclage operation may be necessary for repeated abortions. Scarring may result in the cervix remaining as a pinpoint opening during labor while effacement takes place in the normal manner. Under these circumstances the tiny os can usually be split open easily with a hemostat or other suitable instrument.

When conization was performed for the treatment of cervical intraepithelial neoplasia, recurrent CIN was found later by Bjerre et al.[2] in 14 per cent, as evidenced by abnormal cytologic studies and pathologic findings. Invasive carcinoma was later found in 9 of 1500 patients (0.06 per cent), and the incidence of later non-invasive and invasive cancer was related to the radicality of the conization, i.e., if the margins were free of disease, recurrence was less likely.

VAGINAL HYSTERECTOMY. Specific complications of vaginal hysterectomy, apart from those related to the hysterectomy itself or to vaginal procedures in general, are chiefly concerned with the support of the vaginal vault. This is more likely to be a problem than with abdominal hysterectomy, since the vaginal operation is often performed because of pelvic relaxation and is associated with weakness of the supports of the anterior and posterior vaginal walls. Loss of support results in the gradual protrusion of the apex of the vagina, leading eventually to complete vaginal prolapse. Symptoms may not be noticed until a mass appears at the introitus, although the patient may be conscious before this of heaviness in the pelvis on standing. Various ways of preventing this complication have been described. They include chiefly different techniques of handling the uterine ligaments at operation. Perhaps of greatest importance is excision of any enterocele that may be present and closure of such uterosacral ligaments as are available.

When vaginal prolapse is found, treatment should be conservative unless it is complete or the patient has symptoms clearly related to the abnormality. Upon examination it is important to distinguish between prolapse of the vaginal vault and enterocele or other types of pelvic relaxation. Treatment may be primarily from below, primarily from above, or by a combined approach. The authors' preference is for the vaginal approach in the first instance, with obliteration of the cul-de-sac, utilizing the type of posterior culdoplasty described by McCall[16]

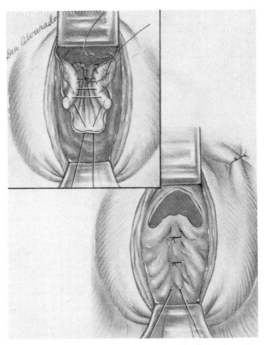

Figure 34–9 Posterior culdoplasty, showing placement of internal and external sutures and external sutures tied.

(Fig. 34–9). If this does not seem practical or does not succeed, abdominal fixation, using strips of fascia from the external oblique muscle, perhaps combined with vaginal repair of associated relaxation, would appear to be useful. A detailed discussion of this problem is given by Symmonds and Pratt.[30] If the patient will not need the vagina for coitus, complete colpocleisis may be advisable.

Salpingo-oophorectomy can usually be added to vaginal hysterectomy with safety.[26] The only additional problem is a slightly increased likelihood of bleeding from the infundibulopelvic ligament or from the surface of the ovary. This should be managed in the same way as any intra-abdominal hemorrhage.

UTERINE REPAIR. Procedures used to repair the uterus, usually for prolapse, include amputation of the cervix and parametrial fixation (Manchester-Fothergill operation). These may lead to obstetric complications, including abortion due to shortening of the cervix and cervical stenosis, which may reduce conception or may alter the pattern of dilation in labor, as previously described.

OTHER VAGINAL PROCEDURES ON THE UTERUS. An additional common procedure performed on the uterus is the application of radioactive substances for carcinoma of the cervix or fundus uteri. Apart from the complications of radiotherapy as a whole, which will not be discussed here, and of vaginal procedures in general, the insertion of radium involves certain specific difficulties. Thus the danger of perforation is greater because of the necessity of pushing the applicator into the uterus. Moreover, the result of perforation can be more serious if the sources come to lie against bowel or other intra-abdominal structures. Thus, postoperative anteroposterior and lateral x-ray studies of the pelvis (with stereoscopic views) are essential after the applicator has been inserted. If perforation is seen, the applicator must be removed. Replacement is probably best delayed for at least 6 weeks, and it is preferable that surgical or other therapy be used. While the applicator is in place, parametrial infection may occur with fever and lower abdominal pain. It is desirable to avoid removing the applicator, since the treatment schedule is compromised thereby, if the patient can be carried through on antibiotics and other conservative measures. Postoperative complications usually relate to the whole course of radiotherapy rather than to the internal therapy alone.

Miscellaneous Vaginal Procedures

CULDOTOMY. Since laparoscopy has become popular, the use of a culdotomy incision for the diagnosis of pelvic conditions and for specific operations on the tubes and ovaries has decreased. Complications usually arise as a result of trying to do too much through a small opening without adequate exposure. Danger of bleeding from an area that cannot easily be reached and inability to perform adequately an operation such as a tubal ligation are two such problems. Culdotomy drainage of an abscess is still a useful technique but should be performed only when the abscess is definitely pointing down the rectovaginal septum. Intraperitoneal rupture of the abscess or creation of a fistula can result from trying to reach too high an abscess. Furthermore, it is important to maintain drainage with a tube or catheter sewn in place to prevent premature closure of the abscess cavity.

CULDOCENTESIS. Insertion of an 18-gauge spinal needle attached to an aspirating syringe into the cul-de-sac provides immediate and useful information for the detection of intraperitoneal bleeding. Complications relate to the size of the needle used and the technique. Very little damage to any organ or blood vessel will be caused by a puncture with this size needle. Inadvertent puncture of the bowel has proven to be of no clinical consequence and requires no treatment. Failure to obtain any fluid (blood or peritoneal fluid) is nondiagnostic and thereby represents a failure or complication of the technique. This is usually due either to inexperience in the proper placement of the needle or poor patient cooperation.

TRANSVAGINAL NEEDLE BIOPSY AND ASPIRATION. These techniques have been used to evaluate pelvic masses and to sample the parametria for persistent or recurrent disease following radiation therapy for cervical or endometrial cancer. Transvaginal needle biopsy of suspicious lesions in the pelvis, employing Vim-Silverman or Tru-Cut needles, yields satisfactory results and the false-negative rate is low, but the procedure requires general anesthesia and complications such as bleeding, infection, and fistula formation have been reported. Thin-needle aspiration using a 22- or 23-gauge needle, on the other hand, is highly accurate, has a low false-negative rate, can be performed without anesthesia, and has caused no complications. The disadvantage of thin-needle aspiration is that only a specimen for cytologic diagnosis is obtained, requiring a well-trained cytologist for accurate interpretation.

COLPOCLEISIS. In addition to the colpocleisis performed for repair of vaginal fistulas, partial colpocleisis (LeFort procedure) may be performed for prolapse in the older woman who does not wish to resume coitus. Theoretically, channels are left lateral to the anterior and posterior apposed walls of the vagina so as to permit the discharge of fluid from above. Obstruction of these channels may occur and result in retention of fluid in the uterus or upper part of the vagina. This may appear in the form of lower abdominal discomfort and must be treated by dividing the adhesions and removing the source of the obstruction.

OBSTETRIC OPERATIONS

GENERAL

The complications of obstetric procedures differ from those of gynecologic operations for several reasons. First, in obstetrics the needs of the fetus equal or surpass those of the mother. As a corollary, the concerns of the baby's father are most important. Second, the pregnant woman is different physiologically in many respects from the non-pregnant woman. Third, many obstetric procedures have to be done in an emergency. Thus, use must be made of the facilities available at the time, and these may not be ideal. Also, necessary preoperative preparations may have to be curtailed. Of these differences, the first is the most important and needs some elaboration.

Concern with the well-being of the fetus implies that during early pregnancy the life of the fetus must not be sacrificed unless the indications are clear and medically, morally, and legally acceptable. Moreover, when there are no indications for the termination of pregnancy, operations that would result in this must be delayed until one is certain that the conceptus is no longer alive. During middle and late pregnancy obstetric operations are conditioned by the necessity of maintaining the fetus in utero until it is viable and of delivering it with the least possible trauma. Finally, obstetric procedures are also concerned with future pregnancies, either that they may occur without **danger** or that they may be prevented.

Preoperative Preparation

FACILITIES. In large part the prevention of the complications of obstetric operations lies in good antepartum care. Since normal delivery is (or should be) an uncomplicated physiologic event and since the majority of deliveries are normal, early identification of the abnormal patient is important. Conditions that put patients at high obstetric risk, likely to require an obstetric operation and to have complications include recurrent abortions, grand multiparity (more than six viable children), hypertension, diabetes, cephalopelvic disproportion, multiple pregnancy, or placental abnormalities. When such a condition has been discovered, preparation should be made for the patient to go to a well-equipped hospital for her delivery (a secondary or tertiary perinatal center, depending upon the complexity of the problem). In this way facilities for anesthesia, blood transfusion, care of the high-risk newborn, and for the management of operative complications are available. Further, since even an apparently normal woman may have a sudden complication such as a prolapsed cord or postpartum hemorrhage, obstetric patients should all be delivered either in or with immediate access to a hospital that has facilities for dealing with these crises.

PREOPERATIVE PREPARATION. Preoperative preparation of the obstetric patient must take into account several factors if fetal and maternal complications are to be avoided.

First, premedication must be such that the fetus is not depressed if it is living. Thus, the use of narcotics such as meperidine is usually contraindicated, although atropine is usually needed when general anesthesia is to be used. Second, because of the urgency of the situation, preparation of bowel, bladder, and skin may have to be abbreviated but must not on that account be neglected. When the patient has recently had a meal and is to receive general anesthesia, the stomach may have to be emptied by nasogastric tube before or during anesthesia to prevent aspiration of vomitus into the bronchial tree. It may not be possible to empty the colon, but the bladder must be emptied, usually by catheterization. Third, scrubbing the skin with germicidal soap is important, although it may not be as complete as in an elective procedure. Fourth, anesthesia must be chosen to give as little fetal depression as possible. Deep general anesthesia for a prolonged period depresses the baby, while spinal anesthesia may lower blood pressure so that the placental blood flow is compromised. Local anesthesia is the safest for the infant, but less desirable from the mother's point of view. Careful evaluation is needed to determine the appropriate anesthesia in the individual case.

Operative Complications

In general, operative complications in obstetrics are little different from those in gynecology.

Postoperative Complications

HEMORRHAGE. Hemorrhage following obstetric operations may be intra-abdominal and similar to that following gynecologic procedures. Vaginal bleeding is more common, however, and may occur after several different obstetric procedures. The majority of these are related to delivery, and hemorrhage following these will be considered here.

Severe vaginal bleeding may complicate both abdominal and vaginal delivery. It is more common in women who have had many children, in those who have had poor health and nutrition during pregnancy, or who have had abnormalities of the placenta or difficult operative deliveries. It is difficult beyond these general considerations to predict which patient is likely to bleed excessively.

Major blood loss usually occurs during and immediately after delivery or in the first 2 hours postpartum. It may occur later, but the incidence and severity usually decrease, the longer the interval after delivery. Since some bleeding is normal, it is important to determine when excessive loss is present. The mean amount lost at delivery was found by Newton et al. to be 625 ml. for primiparas and 314 ml. for multiparas, while the mean loss in the first hour after removal from the delivery table was 20 and 93 ml., respectively.[20] But it is extremely difficult to estimate precisely amounts lost in excess of this. Therefore the patient must be constantly observed, particularly as far as vital signs and size of the uterus are concerned, for at least the first 2 hours after delivery. Also, practice in estimating blood loss is essential, since estimates tend to be low when the loss is large.

When hemorrhage occurs, the possible causes should first be considered. These include uterine atony, retained placental fragments, lacerations of the uterus, cervix, or vagina and, rarely, defects in blood coagulation. Immediate management consists in massage of the uterine fundus (more difficult after an abdominal incision), administration of oxytocin (20 to 40 units in 1000 ml. of 5 per cent dextrose in water or balanced salt solution intravenously), and administration of blood, if necessary. If these measures are ineffective, the whole genital tract must be carefully examined to exclude the other possibilities. This should be done in the delivery room, under aseptic precautions and with an anesthesiologist available to put the patient to sleep if necessary. Retained placental fragments may be removed manually, by sponge forceps, or by a dull curette. Lacerations of the cervix, vagina, or perineum should be sutured. Laceration of the lower uterine segment, which is the most serious problem, usually requires laparotomy and either hysterectomy or repair of the uterus. If no other cause than uterine atony is found, bleeding may be temporarily controlled by compressing the uterus between the vaginal and abdominal hands or by manual occlusion of the abdominal aorta. Rapid administration of blood is necessary and additional intravenous oxytocics in the form of methylergonovine may be useful in the woman who is not hypertensive. As a last resort ligation of the hypogastric arteries may be needed.

INFECTION. The most common infection complicating obstetric operations is intrauterine. In the past this was the principal cause of maternal deaths. Nowadays when aseptic procedures are used for delivery and antibiotics are available when needed, the danger of puerperal uterine infection is small. Nevertheless without these aids it is still a scourge. Infection is usually due to streptococci or *Escherichia coli*, although other organisms may be responsible. It progresses from intrauterine infection (endometritis) to parametritis and thence to pelvic and generalized peritonitis and septicemia. Abscess formation may follow. Endometritis is characterized by the development in the first 3 or 4 days post partum of fever, malaise, and lower abdominal pain. Examination shows the uterus to be larger than expected and slightly tender. Temperature and pulse are elevated. The lochia is not usually foul at first, although foulness soon develops in an untreated case. Leukocytosis is usually present.

In management a cervical smear should first be obtained to identify the responsible organism. Before the report of the culture is obtained the patient should be given antibiotics. A cephalosporin is appropriate, followed by a change to the agent to which the organism is sensitive. The patient also requires oxytocics to cause the uterus to contract, bed rest, and supportive therapy. When the presence of infection has been established, the patient should be isolated and all possible measures taken to prevent its spread to other patients. In most instances prompt treatment on the foregoing lines will result in cure.

Extension of infection may occur, or more widespread involvement may be found initially in the untreated case. Signs of this include a higher pulse and temperature and evidence of peritoneal involvement by reason of abdominal tenderness (lower or generalized), rebound tenderness, and diminished peristalsis. Treatment should be on the same lines as above, but more intensive. For example, this means continued search for the responsible infecting organism and adjustment of the antibiotic coverage to the organism's sensitivities. The development of abscesses is the last stage of puerperal infection. Patients with these complications are often desperately ill. Treatment consists of intensification of the foregoing measures plus intestinal suction and drainage of presenting pockets of pus.

In connection with infections, the term "obstetric morbidity" deserves some discussion. This was a valuable concept 20 or 30 years ago and was used to focus attention on obstetric problems. As generally defined, "obstetric morbidity" consists of a temperature rise to 100.4° F. or greater on any two successive days, excluding the first 24 hours post partum. Although the diagnosis of the exact cause of fever is more important now and, indeed, more practical, the term "obstetric morbidity" still has some value in discussion of generalized problems of infections in hospitals.

SPECIFIC OBSTETRIC OPERATIONS

Vaginal Procedures for Delivery

EPISIOTOMY. Episiotomy is the most commonly performed operation in obstetrics. In fact, it is so common in this country that many have come to regard it as intrinsic to the process of delivery. It still involves a surgical incision, however, and therefore has its complications, which must be remembered in the whole framework of obstetric care. Specific complications include (1) pain, (2) hemorrhage, (3) infection, and (4) functional changes. Similar problems may follow repair of lacerations incurred at delivery.

Pain from an episiotomy is a serious minor problem for the postpartum patient. It is worse if the incision is large, if it is mediolateral or lateral rather than median, if stitches are placed through the skin, or if hemorrhage or infection supervenes. Various immediate prophylactic postpartum measures have been suggested, such as approximating the subcutaneous tissue and skin without sutures but using Allis clamps for 10 to 15 minutes after completing the deep repair or using ice packs or anesthetic sprays on the perineum immediately post partum. The value of these is uncertain. When pain does occur, a heat lamp, anesthetic sprays, or hot baths and analgesics are indicated. Normal discomfort following an episiotomy is worst when edema is at its greatest — 24 to 72 hours post partum — and usually disappears by the seventh to tenth day.

Hemorrhage following episiotomy is peculiar because of the vascularity of the perineal tissues at the end of pregnancy. Thus, it tends to extend upward in the fascial planes of the perineum. The labia become distended and bluish-purple. Blood spreads around the anus and rectum in the ischiorectal fossa and upward beside the vagina, even entering the leaves of the broad ligament. Usually blood does not appear externally. The patient's main complaint is pain, which is sometimes disregarded because it is assumed that pain is normal after operative delivery. Shock may also appear if bleeding is excessive. The diagnosis is easily made by inspection.

In treatment the episiotomy is reopened under aseptic precautions and with the patient under anesthesia, and the clots are evacuated. If the bleeding point can be identified, it is ligated. If it cannot be secured, the incision may be closed again firmly with through-and-through mattress sutures of heavy non-absorbable material, a small drain inserted into the posterior aspect of the incision, and the vagina tightly packed. Packing and drain are removed in 24 hours. Blood transfusion and other supportive treatment are given as indicated. Occasionally, a small hematoma in the episiotomy may simply result in breakdown of the incision without extensive extravasation of blood. If this occurs within the first 48 hours after delivery, the episiotomy should be resutured with through-and-through mattress sutures of non-absorbable material. If breakdown occurs later than this, it is almost invariably accompanied by infection and thus requires special handling.

Infection of an episiotomy is rare if strict aseptic precautions are observed during delivery. In some instances, however, contamination of the perineal area is inevitable. The appearance of an infection is marked by increased pain and fever and redness and tenderness of the episiotomy site. Occasionally a thin purulent discharge may be seen

early. If such is present, a culture is taken. Otherwise, immediate conservative treatment consists of frequent hot baths, compresses of cold witch hazel or other analgesic agents to the perineum, and antibiotics if indicated. Sooner or later in the course of an infected episiotomy, the incision will break down and drainage occur. If the breakdown is extensive and satisfactory cleaning of the wound occurs, secondary layer closure, using interrupted skin sutures, is indicated.

A late complication of episiotomy is pain and scarring. This is likely to be more common after a lateral episiotomy or a mediolateral one incorrectly performed (Fig. 34–10). The patient gives a history of continued perineal pain and dyspareunia. It is important to consider, in addition, psychosexual problems, including the patient's sexual response, her present feelings toward her husband or partner, and her concern about becoming pregnant again. Upon examination the scar is found to be thick and sensitive to touch. Stretching the introitus causes undue discomfort. Occasionally, isolated areas of induration may indicate an unusual reaction to suture material used in the repair. If the mother is breastfeeding her baby, the problem may be compounded by the atrophic vaginal mucosa and lack of lubrication associated with suppression of ovarian function during lactation. Treatment should at first be conservative and consists of local heat in the form of hot baths, anesthetic ointments, reassurance, use of lubricating jelly, and contraceptive advice. Failure of these measures may make plastic procedures necessary. These include secondary hymenotomy to reconstruct the introitus or excision and formal repair of the scar.

OPERATIVE VAGINAL DELIVERY. This term includes the use of forceps, vacuum extractor, rotation of the fetal head, version and extraction, or destructive operations on the fetus. Complications of these operations may involve both the fetus and the mother. In the former, injuries, such as fracture, paralysis, or cranial damage (leading to cerebral palsy or mental retardation) may result in death or long-term disability for which little treatment is available, except continuing care and special education. Prevention, by performing obstetric proce-

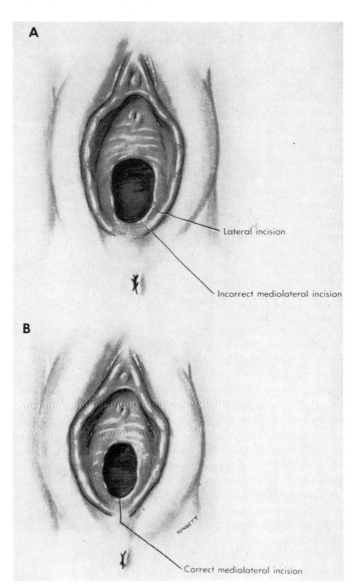

A

Lateral incision

Incorrect mediolateral incision

Figure 34–10 Technique of mediolateral episiotomy. *A,* Incorrect incisions. *B,* Correct incision.

B

Correct mediolateral incision

dures and using obstetric instruments correctly, is most important.

Early recognition of maternal complications, i.e., while the mother is still in the delivery room, is essential. This means appreciation of the amount of blood loss and thorough examination of the birth canal after all operative deliveries. In practice, the perineum and periurethral areas are first inspected. The upper vagina (sulcus) is then visualized, using a vaginal pack and appropriate retractors. The cervix is investigated by palpating its rim between the first two fingers of the examining hand. If this is inconclusive, the cervix is grasped with two ring forceps, and these are then "walked around" its whole perimeter. Exposure is aided by depressing the posterior vaginal wall.

Injuries of the cervix should be repaired if they are over 3 cm. in length. The anterior and posterior vaginal walls are retracted and the cervix grasped with sponge forceps, one in front and one behind the laceration. Interrupted 00 absorbable sutures are then inserted to coapt the anterior and posterior edges of the laceration. To improve exposure the first suture may be inserted in the lowermost part of the cervix and then used for traction to facilitate plac-

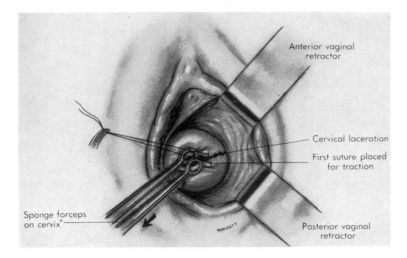

Figure 34–11   Repair of cervical laceration.

ing the higher sutures (Fig. 34–11). Lacerations of the upper part of the vagina (sulcus tears) are repaired with a running locked 00 or 000 absorbable suture, starting above the highest point of the laceration. Perineal repair is performed with similar material, care being taken to reapproximate the muscle layers, including especially the bulbocavernosus, and to conclude with a subcuticular stitch.

Abdominal Procedures for Delivery

CESAREAN SECTION.   The abdominal incision for a cesarean section may be vertical or transverse. The peritoneum over the lower uterine segment is opened transversely and the bladder pushed down. In the most commonly performed operation the uterus is incised transversely. In certain instances, such as with a transverse lie or breech presentation or when there is a complete placenta previa, a vertical incision may be made in the lower uterine segment. Rarely, and usually in an emergency, a vertical incision can be made in the fundus of the uterus (low classic cesarean section). Extraperitoneal cesarean section was formerly performed to minimize potentially untreatable intraperitoneal infection, especially when the uterus was already infected. It is rarely, if ever, indicated nowadays.

The operative complications of cesarean section are similar to those that occur during abdominal hysterectomy, with four exceptions. First, there is greater danger of entering the bladder as the peritoneum in front of the uterus is being opened, since the bladder may be attached higher than expected, particularly if the patient has had a previous cesarean section. The most important thing is to recognize the injury. It should be repaired as described previously as soon as possible after delivery of the infant and immediate control of the bleeding.

Hemorrhage may occur, as the uterus is opened, by lateral extension of the incision to the uterine veins or arteries. This may sometimes be prevented by curving the incision upward at the lateral angles or by adding an upward extension from the middle of the transverse incision, making it into an inverted T. Lateral angle hemorrhage can usually be controlled with figure-of-eight sutures. Occasionally it is so severe as to require hysterectomy. Injury to the fetus can also result from a rapid incision through the uterus and membranes. Finally, in any type of cesarean section, after removal of the baby, especially when abruptio placentae has been the indication, the possibility of uterine atony is likely. This may be prevented or treated by giving oxytocin, usually 20 to 40 units of synthetic oxytocin in 1000 ml. of 5 per cent dextrose in water or balanced salt solution, immediately after the baby has been extracted. Local injection of oxytocin into the uterine muscle may be of help. Continued uterine atony is an indication for hysterectomy.

The early postoperative complications of cesarean section are similar to those that follow any laparotomy. However, infection and anemia are of particular concern. Infection is correlated with the length of labor, the duration of ruptured membranes, and the number of pelvic examinations performed during labor.[23] It is manifested primarily by endometritis, characterized by fever, uterine tenderness, and changes in the lochia, which is often scanty in the early stages but later may become more profuse and foul-smelling. Endometritis may progress to pelvic cellulitis and pelvic thrombophlebitis. Causative organisms (often multiple) include *Escherichia coli*, alpha- and beta-hemolytic streptococci, and various anaerobic bacteria. The initial approach to antibiotic coverage is by using a cephalosporin, to be modified later as indicated by the organism's sensitivities. Anemia is particularly likely to occur after cesarean section because the blood loss may have been higher than estimated. Restoration of the hemoglobin level to at least 10 gm./dl. by transfusion together with administration of iron orally may help to reduce the risk of infection as well as improve the mother's condition after discharge.

The later complications of cesarean section, apart from those common to any abdominal procedure, are concerned with future child-bearing and with uterine function in menstruation. Once a scar has been made in the uterus, the organ may become weaker. The chance of rupture in subsequent pregnancy is difficult to determine. Douglas and Stromme[6] found it to be 1.05 per cent. Vertical (classic) scars are more likely to rupture completely than lower segment transverse scars. But the incidence of incomplete rupture of the latter is likely to be higher than expected, if all incisions are carefully examined. Moreover, the chance of rupture probably increases when the uterus has been opened more than once. However, rupture of a transverse lower segment uterine scar seldom has serious or fatal consequences for fetus or mother. Thus, it is feasible to consider vaginal delivery after cesarean section, provided that the indication for the first cesarean section did not completely contraindicate later vaginal delivery, e.g., major feto-pelvic disproportion.

It seems likely that subsequent menstrual abnormalities are more common if a woman has had a cesarean section than if she has had a vaginal delivery, although it is difficult to be sure of this observation. Studies by Poidevin[21] illustrating deformities in uterine scars after cesarean section, and also the occasional finding of ectopic endometrium in cesarean section scars, suggest that subsequent changes in function are potentially likely. Clinical data obtained by Weed[32] support this. Women who had had cesarean sections were found to have a high incidence of dysfunctional uterine bleeding and subsequent gynecologic operations.

CESAREAN HYSTERECTOMY. Data presented by Barclay et al.[1] suggest that in competent hands cesarean hysterectomy may carry little additional risk beyond that expected for cesarean section alone. This is more likely to be true when the operation is performed electively rather than in an emergency. Even under ideal circumstances, however, the complications may be higher when the operation is performed only occasionally. Then problems occur in the form of excessive bleeding from the vascular structures deep in the pelvis, difficulty of exposure, risk of injuring the bladder or ureter, and identification and complete removal of the cervix.

HYSTEROTOMY. Hysterotomy may rarely be performed for termination of a pregnancy in the second trimester following failure of induction of abortion by intra-amniotic injection of saline or the use of prostaglandin. The complications of hysterotomy are similar to those of laparotomy and cesarean section.

Miscellaneous

ABORTION. The primary operation for abortion is dilatation and suction followed by sharp curettage. The only special complications related to the obstetric aspects of this procedure are the increased ease of perforating the soft uterus, the difficulty of being sure that the uterus is empty, and infection. The risk of perforation can be minimized by giving synthetic oxytocin in doses of 20 to 40 units in 1000 ml. of 5 per cent dextrose in water or balanced salt solution as the procedure is started. The treatment of perforation should follow the lines described above. Failure to remove all the products of conception is most likely to occur if infection has been present, causing the placenta to adhere tightly to the uterine wall, if the uterus is large, or if the procedure is being done for hydatidiform mole. Symptoms include intermittent bleeding that lasts longer than the usual 5 to 7 days and may be accompanied by the passage of clots and lower abdominal cramps. Conservative treatment with ergot derivatives (e.g., methylergonovine maleate, 0.2 mg. every 8 hours for 3 days) is appropriate at first. If this fails, a second curettage should be performed.

Infection primarily involves endometritis and parametritis. Treatment is by the use of appropriate antibiotics after culture of the cervix is obtained. Infection associated with perforation of the uterus and leading to peritonitis may require laparoscopy or even laparotomy for diagnosis. Occasionally hysterectomy may be necessary.

INCOMPETENT CERVICAL OS. Common operations for tightening the internal os of the cervix (cerclage procedures) involve insertion of a synthetic (Mersilene) band in a circular fashion within the substance of the cervix at the level of the internal os (Shirodkar technique) or the use of a purse-string suture of heavy silk inserted relatively superficially at the level of the external os (McDonald technique). These procedures are usually performed in the second trimester of pregnancy. Harger[7] found that both were successful. Shirodkar operations resulted in 87 per cent fetal survival and McDonald operations 78 per cent, compared with rates of 20 and 19 per cent, respectively, for previous pregnancies in the same women. The first and primary complication is fetal loss, usually due to persistent labor (if the procedure was done as an emergency) or to later premature labor. A second complication is the necessity for dividing the band or suture when labor is established at or near term or, alternatively, performing a cesarean section. In the former case the cerclage will have to be repeated in a subsequent pregnancy. Other complications include infection (chorioamnionitis) (0.8 to 3.5 per cent),[8] partial tearing out of the suture and, rarely, annular detachment of the cervix. Infection is managed by appropriate antibiotics. Removal of the band or suture may be indicated in an infection or if it tears out partially. In this case a second cerclage may be performed.

ECTOPIC PREGNANCY. Operation for ectopic (tubal) pregnancy involves removal of the affected tube or in rare instances removal of the pregnancy and reconstruction of the tube. Operative complications include shock due to hemorrhage, requiring rapid removal of the bleeding tube and replacement of blood, and removal of an ovary because its blood supply is compromised by involvement with the affected tube. Postoperative complications include (1) subsequent ectopic pregnancy in the other tube or in the same tube if repair has been attempted; (2) the development of a cornual pregnancy in the medial stump of the tube (note that this can be obviated to some degree by performing a cornual resection) (Fig. 34–12); (3) concurrent intrauterine pregnancy; and (4) the rare abdominal pregnancy usually arising from a ruptured tubal pregnancy with attachment of the placenta to another abdominal organ. This last complication is managed by removal of the fetus through an abdominal incision. At operation catastrophic bleeding can be encountered if an attempt is made to remove a firmly attached placenta from the intra-abdominal organs. It is wiser to leave the placenta behind, although this will result in a persistent mass that may take months or even years to disappear.

OTHER OPERATIONS IN PREGNANCY. Operations for other than obstetric reasons may be necessary during pregnancy and may involve both the extragenital and genital organs. In all cases the complication to be feared is premature termination of the pregnancy. Thus, operations should be performed only in an emergency or when clearly indicated. Procedures that give rise to special concern are those in which the genital tract is involved, such as removal of an ovarian cyst or a pedunculated leiomyoma, or those performed when the patient is in poor general condition, such as with a ruptured appendix.

Prevention of premature labor is most important. When possible, operations should be performed in the second trimester of pregnancy. In the first trimester the danger of abortion is greater, possibly owing to instability of hormone production at this time, while in the third trimester the

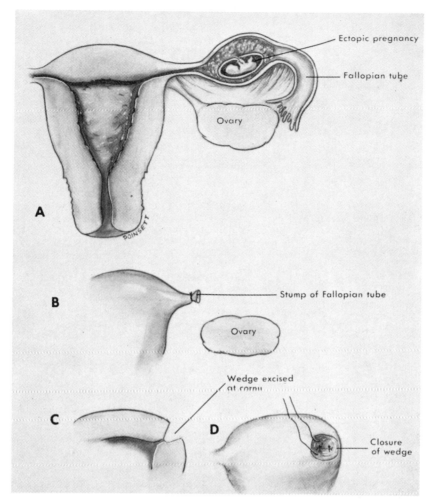

Figure 34–12 Cornual resection after excision of ectopic pregnancy. *A,* Ectopic pregnancy in tube. *B,* After salpingectomy. *C,* Wedge excision of cornu of uterus. *D,* Closure of uterus.

size of the uterus makes abdominal operations difficult. During operation handling of the uterus should be kept at a minimum.

Postoperatively, it may be helpful to try to reduce uterine irritability. Hormonal therapy with a progestin is unlikely to be effective. If uterine contractions begin and persist, uterine relaxants may be used.

Bibliography

1. Barclay, D. L., Hawks, B. L., Frueh, D. M., Power, J. D., and Struble, R. H.: Elective cesarean—hysterectomy—A five year comparison with cesarean section. Am. J. Obstet. Gynecol. *124*:900, 1976.
2. Bjerre, B., Sjöberg, N-O, and Söderberg, H.: Further treatment after conization. J. Reprod. Med. *21*:232, 1978.
3. Boronow, R. C.: Management of radiation-induced vaginal fistulas. Am. J. Obstet. Gynecol. *110*:1, 1971.
4. Bricker, E. M., and Johnston, W. D.: Repair of postirradiation rectovaginal fistula and stricture. Surg. Gynecol. Obstet. *148*:499, 1979.
5. Claman, A. D., and Lee, N.: Factors that relate to complications of cone biopsy. Am. J. Obstet. Gynecol. *120*:124, 1974.
6. Douglas, R. G., and Stromme, W. B.: Operative Obstetrics. 3rd Ed. New York, Appleton-Century-Crofts, 1976, p. 751.
7. Harger, J. H.: Comparison of success and morbidity in cervical cerclage procedures. Obstet. Gynecol. *56*:543, 1980.
8. Hilgers, R. D.: Myomectomy. *In* Sciarra, J. J. (Ed.): Gynecology and Obstetrics. Hagerstown, Md., Harper and Row, 1980.
9. Jones, J. M., Sweetnam, P., and Hibbard, B. M.: The outcome of pregnancy after cone biopsy of

the cervix: A case-control study. Br. J. Obstet. Gynecol. *86*:913, 1979.

10. Klinges, K. G., Wilbanks, G. D., Jr., and Cole, G. R., Jr.: Injury to the femoral nerve during pelvic operation. Obstet. Gynecol. *25*:619, 1965.

11. Körlof, B., Nylén, B., Tillinger, K. G., and Tjernberg, B.: Different methods of reconstruction after vulvectomies for cancer of the vulva. Acta Obstet. Gynecol. Scand. *54*:411, 1975.

12. Leiman, G., Harrison, N. A., and Rubin, A.: Pregnancy following conization of the cervix: Complications related to cone size. Am. J. Obstet. Gynecol. *136*:14, 1980.

13. Levinson, C. J.: Complications. *In* Phillips, J. M. (Ed.): Laparoscopy. Baltimore, Williams & Wilkins Company, 1977.

14. Magrina, J. F., and Masterson, B. J.: Vaginal reconstruction in gynecological oncology: A review of techniques. Obstet. Gynecol. Survey *36*:1, 1981.

15. Masters, W. H.: The sexual response cycle of the human female. I. Gross anatomic considerations. West. J. Surg. *68*:57, 1960.

16. McCall, M. L.: Posterior culdoplasty: Surgical correction of enterocele during vaginal hysterectomy: A preliminary report. Obstet. Gynecol. *10*:595, 1957.

17. McElin, T. W., Bird, C. C., and Reeves, B. D.: Study of uterine perforations occurring during 2991 instances of diagnostic curettage. Int. J. Gynecol. Obstet. *7*:243, 1969.

18. Moir, J. C.: The Vesico-vaginal Fistula. London, Bailliere, Tindall and Cox, 1961.

19. Morley, G. W., and Seski, J. C.: Radical pelvic surgery versus radiation therapy for Stage I carcinoma of the cervix (exclusive of microinvasion). Am. J. Obstet. Gynecol. *176*:785, 1976.

20. Newton, M.: Postpartum hemorrhage. Am. J. Obstet. Gynecol. *94*:711, 1966.

21. Poidevin, L. O. S.: Cesarean section scar safety. Br. Med. J. *2*:1058, 1959.

22. Ranney, B., and Abu-Ghazalek, S.: The future function and fortune of ovarian tissue which is retained in vivo during hysterectomy. Am. J. Obstet. Gynecol. *128*:626, 1977.

23. Rehu, M., and Nilsson, C. G.: Risk factors for febrile mortality associated with cesarean section. Obstet. Gynecol. *56*:269, 1980.

24. Ridley, J. H.: Surgery for stress urinary incontinence. *In* Ridley, J. H. (Ed.): Gynecologic Surgery: Errors, Safeguards, Salvage. Baltimore, Williams & Wilkins Company, 1981.

25. Rutledge, F. N., Smith, J. P., Wharton, J. T., and O'Quinn, A. G.: Pelvic exenteration: Analysis of 296 patients. Am. J. Obstet. Gynecol. *129*:881, 1977.

26. Smale, L. E., Smale, M. L., Wilkening, R. L., Mundy, C. F., and Ewing, T. L.: Salpingo-oophorectomy at the time of vaginal hysterectomy. Am. J. Obstet. Gynecol. *131*:122, 1978.

27. Smith, W. G., and Johnson, G. H.: Vesicovaginal fistula repair — Revisited. Gynecol. Oncol. *9*:303, 1980.

28. Solomons, E., Levin, E. J., Bauman, J., and Baron, J.: A pyelographic study of ureteric injuries sustained during hysterectomy for benign conditions. Surg. Gynecol. Obstet. *111*:41, 1960.

29. Stanton, S. L.: Introduction to the preoperative evaluation of the incontinent patient. *In* Ostergard, D. R. (Ed.): Gynecologic Urology and Urodynamics. Baltimore, Williams & Wilkins Company, 1980.

30. Symmonds, R. E., and Pratt, J. H.: Vaginal prolapse following hysterectomy. Am. J. Obstet. Gynecol. *79*:899, 1960.

31. Wallace, D., Hernandez, W., Schlaerth, J. B., Nalick, R. N., and Morrow, C. P.: Prevention of abdominal wound disruption utilizing the Smead-Jones closure technique. Obstet. Gynecol. *56*:226, 1980.

32. Weed, J. C.: The fate of the postcesarean uterus. Obstet. Gynecol. *14*:780, 1959.

INDEX

Page numbers in *italics* refer to illustrations.
Page numbers followed by (t) refer to tables.

899